CANADIAN MATERNITY, NEWBORN, AND WOMEN'S HEALTH NURSING

Comprehensive Care Across the Life Span

CANADIAN MATERNITY, NEWBORN, AND WOMEN'S HEALTH NURSING

Comprehensive Care
Across the Life Span

SECOND EDITION

Robin J. Evans, RN, PhD, PNC(C)
Associate Professor and Associate Dean
Faculty of Nursing, University of Regina
Regina, Saskatchewan

Marilyn K. Evans, RN, PhD
Associate Professor
Arthur Labatt Family School of Nursing
Western University
London, Ontario

Yvonne M. R. Brown, RN, MCEd
Professor Emeritus, College of Nursing
University of Saskatchewan
Saskatoon, Saskatchewan

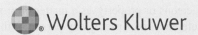

Philadelphia • Baltimore • New York • London
Buenos Aires • Hong Kong • Sydney • Tokyo

Acquisitions Editor: Patrick Barbera
Senior Product Development Editor: Matt Hauber
Marketing Manager: Dean Karampelas
Development Editor: Erika Kors
Senior Designer: Joan Wendt
Manufacturing Coordinator: Karin Duffield
Production Services/Compositor: Aptara, Inc.

ISBN 978-1-4511-9085-4

9 8 7 6 5 4 3 2 1

Printed in China

CIP data available on request from the publisher.

CCS0914

Dedication

This edition is dedicated to the many students and faculty who have told us of their appreciation for an obstetrics textbook that is focused on the Canadian context. We thank them for their support, feedback, and suggestions.

Contributors

Melanie Basso, RN, MSN, PNC(C)
Senior Practice Leader-Perinatal
BC Women's Hospital and Health Centre
Vancouver, British Columbia

Jodie Bigalky, RN, MN, PNC(C)
Lecturer
College of Nursing
University of Saskatchewan (Regina site)
Regina, Saskatchewan

Yvonne M. R. Brown, RN, MCEd
Professor Emeritus, College of Nursing
University of Saskatchewan
Saskatoon, Saskatchewan

Jocelyn Churchill, RN, MN, LCCE, FACCE
Care Manager
Antenatal Community Care Program, Perinatal
    Education and Diversity Liaisons
Alberta Health Services
Calgary, Alberta

Luisa Ciofani, RN, MSc(A), IBCLC, PNC(C)
Associate Director of Nursing - Women's Health
McGill University Health Centre
Faculty Lecturer
McGill University
Montreal, Quebec

Sherrill Conroy, DPhil (Oxford), RN
Associate Professor, Faculty of Nursing, University
    of Alberta
Adjunct Professor, School of Nursing, Dalhousie
    University
Partnerships in Practice Research Team Lead

Robin J. Evans, RN, PhD, PNC(C)
Associate Professor and Associate Dean
Faculty of Nursing, University of Regina
Regina, Saskatchewan

Marilyn K. Evans, RN, PhD
Associate Professor
Arthur Labatt Family School of Nursing
Western University
London, Ontario

Debbie Fraser, MN, RNC-NIC
Associate Professor
Director, Nurse Practitioner Program
Faculty of Health Disciplines
Athabasca University
Athabasca, Alberta

Jean Haase, MSW, RSW
Social Worker, Reproductive Endocrinology and
    Infertility Program
London Health Sciences Centre
London, Ontario

Wendy Hall, RN, PhD
Professor
School of Nursing
University of British Columbia
Vancouver, British Columbia

Kimberley T. Jackson RN, PhD
Assistant Professor
Arthur Labatt Family School of Nursing
Western University
London, Ontario

Lorraine Jarvie, RN, RM, Masters of Midwifery
Clinical Nurse Specialist, Birth Unit
IWK Health Centre
Halifax, Nova Scotia

Janice Kinch, RN, PhD
Assistant Professor
Faculty of Nursing
University of Calgary
Calgary, Alberta

Karen MacKinnon, RN, PhD
Associate Professor and APL Program Coordinator
School of Nursing
University of Victoria
Victoria, British Columbia

Carol McDonald, RN, PhD
Assistant Professor
School of Nursing
University of Victoria
Victoria, British Columbia

Elisha Ogglesby, RN, BScN
Staff Nurse, Reproductive Endocrinology and
    Infertility Program
London Health Sciences Center
London, Ontario

Viola Polomeno, RN, PhD
Associate Professor
School of Nursing
University of Ottawa
Ottawa, Ontario

Deborah Salyzyn, RN, MN
Certified Nurse Specialist, Reproductive Mental
    Health Service
IWK Health Centre
Halifax, Nova Scotia

Erna Snelgrove-Clarke, RN, PhD(c)
Assistant Professor
Dalhousie University School of Nursing
Halifax, Nova Scotia

Taranum Sultana, PhD
Research Associate
Faculty of Nursing
University of Regina
Regina, Saskatchewan

Nancy Watts, RN, MN, PNC(C)
Clinical Nurse Specialist, Maternal/Newborn Care
London Health Sciences Centre
London, Ontario

Reviewers

Esther Aneke, MSN, BSN, RN
Faculty, BSN Program
Douglas College
Coquitlam, British Columbia

Cheryl Besse, BScN, MN, RN
Assistant Professor
College of Nursing
University of Saskatchewan
Saskatoon, Saskatchewan

Shelley L. Cobbett, EdD, MN, BN, RN, GnT
Assistant Professor
School of Nursing
Dalhousie University
Halifax, Nova Scotia

Marianne Cochrane, MHSc(N), RN
Professor, Year Two Coordinator Collaborative BScN
    Program
Faculty of Health Sciences/School of Health &
    Community Services
University of Ontario Institute of Technology/Durham
    College
Oshawa, Ontario

Genevieve Currie, MN, RN
Associate Professor
School of Nursing and Midwifery
Mount Royal University
Calgary, Alberta

Pamela J. Dietrich, MScN, RN
Lecturer, Clinical Instructor
Labatt Family School of Nursing
Western University
London, Ontario

Jodi Found, MN, BScN, RN
Faculty/Undergraduate Adjunct Professor
Saskatchewan Institute of Applied Science and
    Technology (SIAST) School of Nursing/University
    of Regina
Regina, Saskatchewan

Mona Haimour, MSN, RN, MPH(c)
Faculty, Bachelor of Science in Nursing
School of Health and Community Studies
Grant MacEwan University
Edmonton, Alberta

Denise L. Hawthorne, MA, BSN, RN
Faculty, Health Sciences
Douglas College
Coquitlam, British Columbia

Patti Nicks, MSN, RNC
Clinical Nurse Educator
Island Health
Victoria, British Columbia

Margaret Quance, PhD, MN, BN, RN
Associate Professor, Chair of the School of Nursing
    and Midwifery
Mount Royal University
School of Nursing & Midwifery
Calgary, Alberta

Lynn Rollison, MA, BSN, RN, PhD(c)
Nurse Educator
Department of Health and Human Services, BSN
Vancouver Island University
Nanaimo, British Columbia

Candide Sloboda, MEd, BN
Faculty Lecturer
Faculty of Nursing
University of Alberta
Edmonton, Alberta

Wendy M. Wheeler, MN, RN
Instructor
Department of Nursing
Red Deer College
Red Deer, Alberta

Trish Whelan, MHS, BScN, RN, ENC(C)
Assistant Professor
Health and Community Studies
Mount Royal University
Calgary, Alberta

Yvonne Mayne Wilkin, EdD, MSc, BScN, CEFP
Nursing Faculty
Champlain College Lennoxville
Sherbrooke, Quebec

Preface

The majority of textbooks dealing with maternity, newborn, and women's health nursing have been written from an American (United States) context and perspective. The importance of context in this area of nursing cannot be overemphasized. Although there are many similarities between Canada and the United States in relation to basic maternity and women's health care, there are also many differences that need acknowledgement. For example, the ethnic and cultural diversity of Canada differs from that found in the United States. Canada's heritage of the First Nations, Inuit, Métis, Anglophone, and Francophone populations needs to be acknowledged, as does its diverse immigrant population. The significant differences in the makeup of each population result in differences in the health challenges experienced by individuals and the factors that predispose them to those challenges. Differences in the health care systems affect the way that health care is organized and delivered. It is therefore important to address the fundamental ideologies of the Canadian health care system as it pertains to women's health care services.

Many maternity textbooks are limited in their usefulness for faculty and students who are not practicing in the United States. Canadian faculty have had to adapt textbooks that focus on practice in the United States. As a result, students, primarily without prior knowledge of the content area, try to discern information appropriate to the Canadian context and identify gaps. They must then seek appropriate information from many other sources to fill these gaps. Nurse educators and students look for resources that are reflective of Canadian values, beliefs, and culture.

This maternity/women's health textbook is a revision and update of the 2010 adaptation of the US edition and is intended to help address the ongoing need for Canadian content. Canadian society is shaped by historical, political, societal, and cultural influences that are unique and distinctive from other countries. These elements have helped to create a definition of health and a health care delivery system that is characteristic of Canadian way of life. The health and well-being of women and their families are products of these socioecological determinants of health. Nurses who work to help promote the health of women and their families across the lifespan need to remain cognizant of Canadian culture and values.

PURPOSE

This textbook provides a comprehensive resource for nursing students and registered professional nurses that can be used to help plan nursing care for women throughout the life cycle. The text and its supporting products:

- Disseminate up-to-date knowledge within a practical context for use in today's multifaceted health care environment;
- Elucidate the influence of sociocultural beliefs and practices in understanding and identifying health care needs of clients of the same or a different sociocultural group than the nurse;
- Clarify the importance of understanding gender-specific issues, including physical and emotional development.

This product emphasizes sociocultural aspects of client care when working with women and their families at various points throughout the lifespan. In recognizing the importance and uniqueness of the female experience from menarche to postmenopause, the text includes information about every phase from adolescence through older adulthood. It includes content beyond the scope of the average maternity text.

ORGANIZATION

The organization of this text reflects a progressive life-cycle orientation toward the care of women. The book is divided into six units, each emphasizing unique aspects of the client's experience.

Unit 1—Foundations of Maternal, Newborn, and Women's Health Care

Unit 1 introduces foundational content with applications throughout every stage of a woman's life. Chapter 1, "Philosophy and Framework for Women's Reproductive and Sexual Health," introduces women's reproductive and sexual health throughout the life cycle within a broad cultural perspective. It emphasizes the state of women's health care in Canada and explores issues of significant concern to nurses. Chapter 2, "Health Promotion," encompasses areas for preserving and optimizing wellness in women. Chapter 3, "Nutrition for Adolescent and Adult Women," presents nutritional guidelines for different life stages within a multicultural framework. There is a particular focus on women's reproductive years, with emphasis given to nutritional screening, the nurse's role in providing nutritional guidance, and practical applications. Chapter 4, "Medical Alterations in Women During Adolescence and Adulthood," provides comprehensive coverage of physiologic issues that affect quality of life for women. Although it includes significant information about breast disorders, reproductive problems, and sexually transmitted infections, this chapter also addresses diseases with serious implications for women. Examples include autoimmune diseases and cardiovascular diseases. Chapter 5, "Mental Health Concerns for Women in Adolescence and Adulthood," provides an overview of potential changes in women's psychological health. The unit concludes with chapters focusing on two topics relevant to every stage of a woman's life: Chapter 6, "Sexuality and Reproduction," and Chapter 7, "The Family."

Unit 2—Special Reproductive and Health and Concerns

This unit includes issues of special importance to women during their childbearing years, separate from the actual experience of pregnancy, labour, birth, and postpartum care. Chapter 8, "Fertility Control and Contraception," focuses on prevention or timing of pregnancy and related nursing care. Chapter 9, "Voluntary Pregnancy Termination," examines abortion from political, social, cultural, and medical perspectives. Chapter 10, "Fertility Challenges," includes care for families struggling with infertility. Finally, Chapter 11, "Genetics, Embryology, and Preconceptual/Prenatal Assessment and Screening," describes the developmental processes at various stages in utero, threats to embryonic and fetal health, and screening measures prospective parents can take before conception or birth to prevent or manage health challenges in their children.

Unit 3—Pregnancy

Unit 3 covers the unique experience of pregnancy in both normal and high-risk circumstances. Chapter 12, "Process of Pregnancy," lays a foundation for nursing practice that reflects the cultural, psychological, and physiologic influences of pregnancy on a woman and her partner. The focus is on pregnancy without complications. Chapter 13, "High-Risk Pregnancy," assists students to differentiate and apply knowledge regarding expected changes during pregnancy. It also presents detailed information about pre-existing or gestational-onset conditions and associated collaborative management. Chapter 14, "Educational Preparation for Pregnancy, Childbirth, and Parenthood," focuses on the meaning and position of today's methods of childbirth education. It compares various types of preparation and their applications.

Unit 4—Labour and Childbirth

In Unit 4, the reader becomes familiar with normal and high-risk labour and childbirth, as well as pharmacologic methods of managing pain during this time. Chapter 15, "Labour and Childbirth," includes the physiologic and psychological aspects of labour, the mechanisms and stages of normal vaginal childbirth, and collaborative care for each phase of this experience. Chapter 16, "High-Risk Labour and Childbirth," reviews conditions or problems that can interfere with normal labour outcomes and related collaborative management. It also presents detailed information about common obstetrical interventions used to assist labour and childbirth, including labour augmentation and induction, operative obstetrics, and cesarean birth. Chapter 17, "Pharmacologic Pain Management of Labour," presents the etiology of pain during childbirth and the various pharmacologic methods commonly implemented during normal and high-risk labour and birth.

Unit 5—Postpartum Period and Newborn Care

This unit presents postpartum care for the mother, her family/support people, and the newborn. Chapter 18, "Fourth Stage of Labour and Postpartum Period," emphasizes expected maternal physiologic and psychological changes, as well as collaborative care for the new family throughout the first 6 weeks after childbirth. Chapter 19, "The High-Risk Postpartum Woman," explores care for women and families who are experiencing maternal postpartum complications or deviations. The content includes both physiologic problems and psychological maladjustments that may have serious ramifications. Chapter 20, "The Healthy Newborn," enhances students' understanding of the newborn's adjustment to extrauterine life, including assessment findings. It presents comprehensive collaborative care during the neonatal period and concepts of family teaching throughout the newborn's first few months of life. Chapter 21, "Newborn Nutrition," promotes nursing knowledge to facilitate parental decision-making about newborn nutrition. It emphasizes interventions to assist both breast-feeding and bottle-feeding families, describes measures for newborns who need special adjustments, and explores the management of common newborn feeding-related difficulties. Finally, Chapter 22, "The High-Risk Newborn," explores collaborative strategies for newborns experiencing challenges in their transition to extrauterine life. It includes problems related to birth weight, gestational age, acquired conditions, and congenital factors, as well as measures to address them.

Unit 6—Menopause and Beyond

Unit 6 explores the experience of the largest growing segment of today's population—women who are at the end of, or are past, their reproductive years. Chapter 23, "The Menopausal Experience," enhances the reader's understanding of the physiologic, psychological, and cultural factors inherent in the gradual cessation of the menstrual cycle and its effects on women and their significant others. Chapter 24, "The Older Postmenopausal Woman," focuses on health promotion, screening, assessment, common concerns, and common abnormalities for middle-aged and older women. The discussion emphasizes normal female physiology related to aging, along with psychological and sociocultural variations and dimensions for nurses to consider when working with this increasingly influential demographic group.

SPECIAL FEATURES

This book's unique framework reflects emerging views of and attitudes toward women's health. Several key features emphasize the student-oriented focus woven throughout this text and its associated products:

Progressive Case Studies

Each chapter begins with two illustrated scenarios related to the content found within the chapter. Accompanying questions stimulate the student's thought processes about the scenarios and the topics he or she will be exploring. Throughout the chapter, the student will find ongoing questions at relevant points related to the opening case studies. Photographic reminders assist visual learners to recall the scenario and its circumstances when shaping responses. Answers to the questions are provided in the back of the book (Appendix A). In addition, implications for care for the clients in these scenarios are explored in detailed Nursing Care Plans found within the chapters.

Learning Objectives

Objectives at the start of each chapter outline the fundamental goals. They are linked to the summary points at the end of each chapter and provide a framework for instructors to organize their teaching.

Key Terms

Essential vocabulary is presented at the beginning of each chapter. Terms are in bold print, with their explanations in the chapters themselves and reinforced in the book's Glossary.

Collaborative Care

Collaborative Care sections throughout the book are presented in a different text color and review the steps of assessment, diagnosis, planning, implementation, and evaluation relative to the content under consideration. The collaborative care focus emphasizes the nurse's need to work in partnership with the client and her family. It also underscores those areas in which nurses coordinate care with other care team members, emphasizing both independent and cooperative interventions.

Nursing Care Plans

More than 35 care plans related to the progressive case studies are found throughout the chapters. These scenarios and care plans are designed to explore women's health issues and concerns, with appropriate nursing diagnoses, interventions, rationales, and expected outcomes.

Nursing Procedures

Significant skills and techniques are outlined in illustrated procedures throughout the text. Each procedure has a clearly articulated purpose and describes the equipment needed. The steps are organized around the nursing process, providing areas for assessment and planning, relevant interventions and their rationales, and desired outcomes for evaluation. These procedures emphasize variations needed for different life stages or age groups, as well as considerations needed for implementing the skill in community-based settings.

Complementary and Alternative Medicine

Boxes reviewing special issues related to complementary and alternative medicine modalities are found throughout the text.

Teaching Tips

Client and family education are essential for health promotion, disease prevention, and illness management. Appropriate areas for instruction are reviewed in boxes of bulleted points throughout the book.

Pharmacology Boxes

Medications of importance are presented in boxes throughout the book. Such boxes review mechanisms of action, usual dosages, common side effects, and implications for nurses.

Assessment Tools

The book provides tools to assist nurses with health history and physical assessment. These Assessment Tools include well-known instruments, such as the "CAGE Questionnaire," as well as original approaches related to the different topics found across the text.

Research Highlights

Up-to-date, evidence-based research studies are summarized within most chapters to reinforce students' familiarity with the literature and to link results with interventions and best practices as much as possible.

Review Questions

At the end of each chapter, 8 to 10 Review Questions help students to integrate previous learning and test their understanding. Answers with comprehensive rationales are found at the end of the book (Appendix B).

Summary

Bulleted end-of-chapter summaries review pertinent content and help identify the most important considerations. The summaries link to the objectives found at the beginning of the chapter.

Questions to Ponder (Critical Thinking)

These scenarios ask students to apply their knowledge to possible scenarios or developments related to the topics at hand.

References and Resources

Each chapter has been written based on the most current articles, textbooks, websites, and other sources available. Detailed lists of the appropriate citations are found at the end of each chapter. In addition, several chapters contain information on Resources that are helpful for students, nurses, and clients.

Art

One goal of this text was to present a highly visual learning experience for the reader. Beautiful drawings and photos throughout the book underscore important content, highlight complicated issues or care components, and crystallize pertinent information in a way that words alone cannot convey.

TEACHING AND LEARNING RESOURCES

Instructors and students will find valuable resources to accompany the book on at http://thePoint.lww.com.

Resources for Instructors

Comprehensive teaching resources are available to instructors upon adoption of this text and include the following materials.

- A free **E-book** on thePoint provides access to the book's full text and images online.
- A **Test Generator** lets instructors put together exclusive new tests from a bank containing NCLEX-style questions.
- **PowerPoint Presentations** provide an easy way to integrate the textbook with the classroom.
- An **Image Bank** provides the photographs and illustrations from this text for use in course materials.
- **New! Case Studies** with related questions (and suggested answers) give students an opportunity to apply their knowledge to a client case similar to one they might encounter in practice.
- **New! Assignments** (with suggested answers) include group, written, clinical, and web assignments.
- Access to all student resources is also provided.

Resources for Students

Students can activate the code in the front of this book at http://thePoint.lww.com/activate to access the following free resources.

- **Watch & Learn Video Clips** reinforce information in the textbook and appeal to visual and auditory learners.
- **Journal Articles** provided for each chapter offer access to current research available in Lippincott Williams & Wilkins journals.

Acknowledgements

I want to acknowledge and thank my students, nursing colleagues and those who have used the first edition for their feedback, encouragement and support.

Robin J. Evans, RN, PhD, PNC(C)

I extend my gratitude to all my nursing colleagues and students who provided me with continual support, inspiration, and encouragement to work on this second edition.

Marilyn K. Evans, RN, PhD

It has been a privilege and a learning experience to work with my colleagues on this update and revision of a comprehensive Canadian textbook.

Yvonne M. R. Brown, RN, MCEd

We would like to acknowledge:

- Susan Orshan and the contributors of the original textbook. Susan's vision for the textbook and the original work provided a strong foundation for the Canadian edition.
- The Canadian contributors who shared their expertise.
- The editorial staff at Wolters Kluwer who continue to support the development and refinement of books to meet the needs of Canadian nurses, educators and students.

Contents

CHAPTER 5

Mental Health Concerns for Women in Adolescence and Adulthood 175

CHAPTER 6

Sexuality and Reproduction 211

CHAPTER 7

The Family 241

CANADIAN MATERNITY, NEWBORN, AND WOMEN'S HEALTH NURSING

Comprehensive Care Across the Life Span

FOUNDATIONS OF MATERNAL, NEWBORN, AND WOMEN'S HEALTH CARE

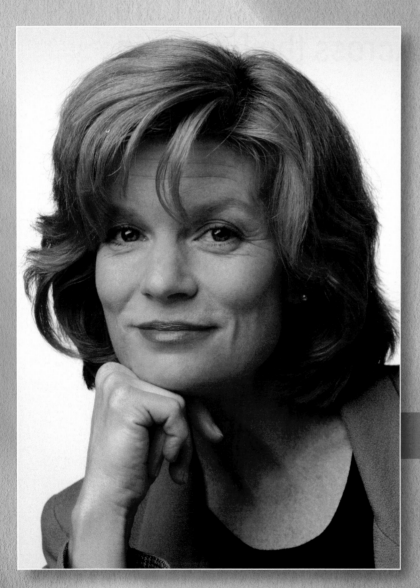

UNIT

1

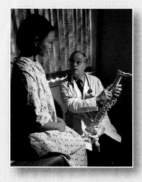 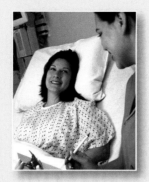 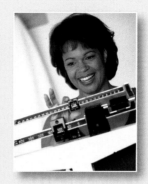 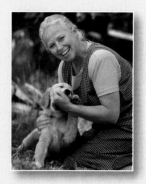

This unit focuses on fundamental components of women's health across the lifespan. The topics are relevant for women of all ages and stages of life. In the 21st century, health care providers need to help women understand how their choices can influence their own and their families' well-being. Nurses need to form partnerships with clients to outline goals and to plan strategies that will maximize wellness, prevent illness, and effectively manage any problems that develop.

Although past paradigms for women's health focused mainly on care during or between pregnancies, this textbook reflects today's philosophy of promoting and optimizing a woman's health from adolescence through the end of life. This unit begins with a framework for current maternal, newborn, and women's health care, providing a context for the rest of the book. Then the focus moves to health promotion and nutrition, including modifications that may be necessary according to life stage, sociocultural variables, and other factors, followed by common medical and mental health alterations, along with relevant collaborative care strategies. Unit 1 ends with chapters on two topics relevant to every stage of a woman's life: (1) sexuality and reproduction and (2) the family.

CHAPTER 1

Philosophy and Framework for Women's Reproductive and Sexual Health

Yvonne M.R. Brown and Susan A. Orshan*

 Taohua, a 22-year-old woman sent by her parents from China to Canada to attend university, was brought to the clinic by her aunt Mei. She has been in Canada for less than a year and is fluent in English, having acted as a translator in a large company in China. Taohua has been experiencing lower abdominal pain and menstrual irregularities for the past few months. Mei says, "I've been urging her to see a doctor, but she says she won't go." Taohua refuses to say anything until her aunt leaves the room.

 Elaine, 45 years old, has three children and works part time as an office assistant. Her blood glucose is elevated and she has developed hypertension. The nurse practitioner discusses the need for lifestyle changes and prescribes medications to help bring her problems under control. Elaine rolls her eyes and says, "I'll try to keep up with the diet and exercise, but I don't know how I will pay for these prescriptions."

These women are two examples of the wide-ranging experiences found in the realm of women's health nursing. Clients and nurses all have stories to draw on and circumstances that shape their attitudes and feelings about wellness, reproduction, motherhood, and aging.

*Contributor to first U.S. edition.

You will learn more about these stories as the chapter progresses. For now, consider the following questions:

- How might age, ethnicity, parenthood, socioeconomic status, fertility, illness, and family relationships shape women's health experiences?
- How will health care costs be covered for Taohua and Elaine?
- What are the implications for her family if Taohua turns out to have a serious health problem?
- What current issues are reflected in these stories?
- How can nurses provide ethically based responses to their clients, while also demonstrating caring and concern?

LEARNING OBJECTIVES

On completion of this chapter, the reader will be able to:
- Discuss demographic and sociopolitical changes during the past decades that have influenced women's health care.
- Examine the Canada Health Act and health care coverage for women in Canada.
- Explore the significance of critical thinking in nursing, particularly related to addressing women's reproductive and sexual concerns.
- Discuss the role of ethics and ethical decision making in women's health nursing.
- Evaluate the significance of informed consent in practice and research.
- Identify procedures and problems for which informed consent is needed when working with women.
- Explore the role of nursing in women's health research.
- Evaluate the significance of evidence-based practice in nursing and women's health care.

KEY TERMS

Aboriginal peoples	fertility rate
best practices	First Nations
birth rate	infant mortality
census family	informed consent
critical thinking	Inuit
determinants of health	maternal morbidity
ethical decision making	maternal mortality
ethical principles	Métis
evidence-based practice	social determinants of health
evidence-informed decision making	

For a better understanding of where women's health, maternal, and newborn nursing are going, it is necessary to recognize where these areas have been and where they are now.

In this chapter we discuss current issues affecting women's health and nursing care. We examine the foundational context within which women's health care is provided, and the important issues currently influencing nursing practice and interactions. The topics discussed in this chapter have implications for and are connected to the content found throughout this book and its supplements. Many of the issues introduced here are described in detail in other sections of this text.

SHIFTING PARADIGMS AND CURRENT CONTEXT

When the 20th century began, most North American families were "nuclear." Men and women in families and communities generally adhered to specific gender roles, and it was normal to have involvement with extended family members, with two or more generations living either together in the same house or in proximity to each other. The dominant perspective in Canada was that of the white Christian male. Women did not have the right to vote, contraceptives were not readily available, abortion was illegal, and laws prohibited some types of non-heterosexual sexual activity.

The world has changed over the past century. Individuals may agree or disagree regarding whether changes are for the better or for the worse, but what all people can generally accept is that understanding the realities of today's women and their families will enable nurses and other health professionals to help clients achieve their health care goals.

Continuity and Change in Canadian Family Structures and Relationships

According to the most recent (2011) census, Canada's population has reached 33.5 million, making Canada the least populous country in the G8 (Statistics Canada, 2012h). Canada has nearly 5 million seniors 65 years and over, accounting for 14.8% of the population (Statistics Canada, 2012g). By 2015, the number of seniors is projected to outnumber the number of children under the age of 15, and by 2031, about one quarter of the population will be 65 and over (Statistics Canada, 2008). However, between 2006 and 2011, there was an 11% increase in the population of children aged 4 and under, the largest growth rate for this age group since the baby boom between 1956 and 1961 (Statistics Canada, 2012g).

Family dynamics have evolved over the past 50 years. In the early 1960s, many people married at a young age and had relatively large families. Later in the 1960s, events such as legalization of the birth control pill, no-fault divorce, and increased participation of women in higher education and in the paid labour force contributed to later marriages, delayed pregnancy, smaller families, and diverse family structures (Statistics Canada, 2012b). The majority of Canadians still live in census families. A **census family** comprises a married or common-law couple, same or opposite sex, with or without children, or a lone parent living with at least one child in the same dwelling (Statistics Canada, 2012f). Married couples were the predominant family structure in 1961, accounting for 91.6% of census families. In 2011, this percentage dropped to 67%, with common-law couples and lone-parent families at 16.7% and 16.3%, respectively (Fig. 1.1) Women head up 80% of lone-parent households (Statistics Canada, 2012f). Canadian families have become smaller over the

past 50 years. The average number of children per family decreased from 2.7 in 1961 to 1.9 in 2011 (Statistics Canada, 2012b). The number of same-sex married couples nearly tripled between 2006 and 2011, reflecting the first full 5-year period for which same-sex marriage has been legal across the country (Statistics Canada, 2012f).

Over a 50-year period, some patterns have remained constant, including higher life expectancy for women than for men. However, the gap is closing. In 1960 the life expectancy at birth was 74 years for women, 68 for men. In 2009, life expectancy for women increased to 83 and men to 79 (Statistics Canada, 2012e). As a result of the narrowing gap in life expectancy between men and women, the proportion of senior women who live alone has declined while the proportion of senior men living alone has remained relatively stable. In 2001, 46.1% of women between 80 and 84 lived alone. In 2011, that number decreased to 40.2% (Statistics Canada, 2012b).

A significant social trend of the past half century is the increasing participation of women in the labour force. In 2012, women comprised 47% of the labour force (Statistics Canada, 2012d). In 2009, 58.3% of women were employed, more than double the number from 1976 (Farrao, 2012). The likelihood of being employed increases with a higher level of education (Farrao, 2012). Since 1976, the number of employed women with children has almost doubled, rising to 72.9%. Women are more likely to work part time than men, with reasons given being child care or other family responsibilities, attendance at school, or inability to find full-time employment (Farrao, 2012).

 The nurse practitioner tries to explore Elaine's situation in more detail. "I've just started this job, now that my youngest is in junior high. Being back to work has increased my stress level, although we need the extra money. We're ordering out more because I don't have the time to plan meals and cook. I know I have to take better care of myself and ask for help, but my husband has never done much around the house." What suggestions might the nurse offer to help Elaine manage her lifestyle dynamics better to improve her health?

Over the 10-year period from 2001 to 2011, couples with children under 14 living at home decreased as a percentage of census families. In 2001, there were more couples with children living at home (43.6%) than there were couples without children (40.3%), whereas in 2011, 39.2% of census families had children living with them and 44.5% did not (Statistics Canada, 2012f). Previous generations of children tended to remain at home with their parents (and possibly their grandparents) until marrying at a relatively young age and starting

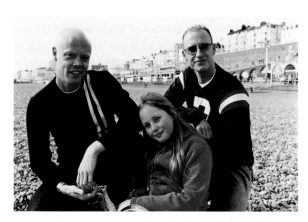
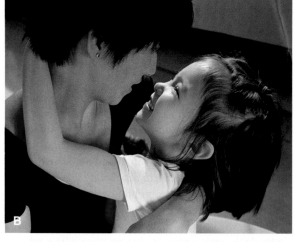
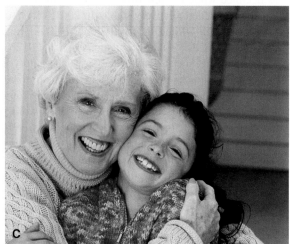
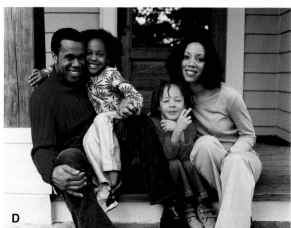

FIGURE 1.1 Notions of what constitutes a family continue to change. Families might be headed by same-sex parents **(A)**, single parents **(B)**, grandparents **(C)**, or heterosexual couples living together who are not married **(D)**.

a family of their own. An increasingly larger number of people in their 20s, however, have either never left home or have returned home after living independently at college or in other circumstances. The proportion of young adults living at home increased from 26.9% in 1981 to 42.3% in 2011 (Statistics Canada, 2012b).

Although multiple-family households are not common in Canada, the proportion has risen slightly since 2001 (Fig. 1.2). These households tend to be more prevalent in areas where there are factors such as housing shortages, high cost of living, and/or cultural preferences. Multiple-family households are also prevalent in areas surrounding the cities of Toronto and Vancouver, possibly reflecting high proportions of immigrant families (Statistics Canada, 2012b). In 2011, 4.8% of all children 14 years and younger lived in households that contained at least one grandparent. In some of these families, there were no parents—the "skip-generation" families. About 20% of people 15 and over did not live with a census family. Some lived alone (13.5%), some with relatives (2.5%) and some with nonrelatives (4.5%) (Statistics Canada, 2012f).

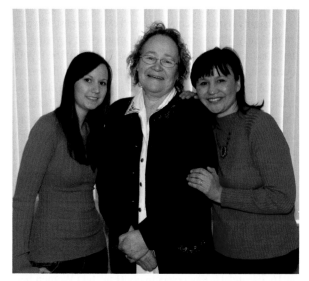

FIGURE 1.2 In multigenerational households, three or more generations are represented as living together under one roof.

Think back to Taohua, the 22-year-old woman who came to the clinic with her aunt. The nurse learned that Taohua recently moved in with her aunt after living in her own apartment for a short time. Taohua's very traditional parents live in China. What influences might these circumstances have on Taohua's state of health and ability to care for herself adequately?

Economic and Sociocultural Influences

Canada's high standard of living and low population replacement rate has led the government to encourage immigration into the country. According to demographic projections, by 2031 the percentage of foreign-born Canadians will be between 9.8 and 12.5 million. Nearly half of the Canadians aged 15 and over will be foreign born or have at least one foreign-born parent (Statistics Canada, 2011a). As well, 29% to 32% of Canadians will belong to a visible minority group, with the largest groups being South Asian, Black, Filipino, Arab, West Asian, and Chinese. Diversity of language and religion is also increasing. In 1981, people whose mother tongue was neither French nor English accounted for less than 10% of the population. By 2006, the proportion had risen to 20% and by 2031 it could be as high as 29% to 32%. Similarly, by 2031, the number of people practicing a non-Christian religion is expected to reach 14%, with half being Muslim (Statistics Canada 2011a).

Canada is multicultural and multilingual, with two official languages. In 1867, Confederation mandated that French and English would be used in parliamentary records and in laws enacted and published. In 1969, the Official Languages Act recognized English and French as the official languages of all federal institutions in Canada. People have the right to receive services in the official language of their choice from federal institutions in certain locations and when appearing before federal courts and tribunals (Government of Canada, 2008). In 1960, the Canadian Bill of Rights, a federal statute, legislated against discrimination on the basis of race, national origin, colour, religion, or sex (Government of Canada, 2012a), and in 1982 the Canadian Charter of Rights and Freedoms formed the first part of the Canadian Constitution (Government of Canada, 2012c).

Following Confederation, Canada's immigration policy was designed to supply a labour pool. Irish and Chinese workers were brought in to build the Canadian Pacific Railway, and American and European farmers were recruited to settle in the west. Attitudes toward immigrants from countries other than Western Europe were not positive, and assimilation was the answer to what was considered to be a "cultural problem." Later, with expansion of the economy after World War II, Canada did not have enough workers, so policies were loosened, and immigrants entered from all parts of Europe and settled mainly in urban areas. In 2010, Canada's economy demanded "a high level of economic immigration to keep our economy strong" and welcomed the highest number of legal immigrants (280,636) in more than 50 years (Citizenship and Immigration Canada, 2011, para. 2). These immigrants were skilled workers who could help fill the gaps in the work force. Increasing numbers of immigrants have come from non-European countries and the developing world. The Canadian Multiculturalism Act of 1985 (Government of Canada, 2012b), recognized cultural pluralism and stated that the blueprint for Canada would be a cultural mosaic, with multiculturalism existing within a bilingual English–French framework.

The "mosaic" has not been without issues. Immigrants are entitled to equal access to jobs, housing, education, and health services, but despite the recent trend to select immigrants for their education, training, and job skills, "it is taking longer for newcomers to achieve income levels similar to those of Canadian-born" (Thomas, 2011, p. 52).

New immigrants initially report better health than do Canadian-born citizens, but in time, the "healthy immigrant effect" appears to diminish, in self-reported health, mental health status, chronic diseases, and birth and death outcomes. The explanation for this phenomenon is complex and includes demographic, socio-economic, and behavioural factors, as well as ability to function in the language of the new country (Ng et al., 2011). The impact of social determinants of health differs according to immigration status, gender, generation, ethnicity, and language (Simich & Jackson, 2010).

Given the projected population of foreign-born Canadians and our increasing diversity, health practitioners are increasingly involved in the care of immigrant populations, including health promotion and health care. Immigrants and their children comprise the majority of physician practices in some areas of the country. "Access to health services and health conditions of some migrant populations differ from patterns among Canadian-born patients, and these disparities have implications for preventive care and provision of health services" (Gushulak et al., 2010 p. 1).

Immigrant women comprise about 20% of the Canadian female population, a proportion that varies according to location. Recently arrived women are more likely to be living in a low income situation than Canadian women (Chui, 2011). Immigrant women's experiences with pregnancy, labour, birth and postnatal outcomes are the subject of ongoing research that focuses on accessibility and acceptability of maternity-related health care (Higginbottom et al., 2012). An international research collaboration is investigating commonalities and differences between countries with respect to maternity and migration, with the aim of developing new approaches to maternity services for immigrant women (Higginbottom, 2013).

Canada's cultural mosaic includes a significant and growing Aboriginal population. Before European settlers arrived in Canada, First Nations and Inuit peoples had the country to themselves. There were six cultural groups: Inuit, Subarctic, Northwest Coast, Plateau Tribes, Plains Tribes, and Eastern Woodlands (EcoKids, n.d). **Aboriginal** was defined in the Canadian Constitution Section 35(2) as including Indian, now referred to as First Nations; Inuit, living mainly in northern Canada; and **Métis**, of mixed Aboriginal and European ancestry (Government of Canada, 2012c). Starting in 1701, in what would eventually become Canada, Britain entered into treaties between First Nations and non-Aboriginal peoples. Treaty rights that predated the year the Constitution Act was passed were recognized in the Constitution (Aboriginal Affairs and Northern Development Canada, 2010b). In 2006, the population reporting Aboriginal identity was just over 1 million (Statistics Canada, 2008) and is projected to increase to between 1.7 and 2.2 million by 2031, about 4% of the total population (Statistics Canada, 2011b).

Canada has not had a stellar track record in its approach to Aboriginal peoples. Colonialism resulted in "diminished self-determination and a lack of influence in policies that directly relate to Aboriginal individuals and communities" (Loppie-Reading & Wien, 2009, pp. 2–3). The loss of land, language, and sociocultural resources has had a significant impact on generations of First Nations, Inuit, and Métis people.

Assimilation policies adopted by the federal government have also had long-lasting effects. In 1879, Prime Minister Sir John A. Macdonald commissioned a study of the US industrial schools for "Indians and Half-Breeds." The author of the study wrote: "If anything is to be done with the Indian, we must catch him very young. The children must be kept constantly within the circle of civilized conditions" (Hanson, 2009). He recommended that Canada follow the United States' example. Macdonald agreed and established a residential school system to be funded by government and administered by churches (Hanson, 2009). The residential school system operated from the 1880s to 1986, when the last school was closed. Children were separated from their families for extended periods of time and forbidden to acknowledge their Aboriginal heritage and culture or speak their own language. Physical, emotional, and sexual abuse was widespread (Hanson, 2009). By the 1950s it became clear that assimilation was not working, and the devastating experiences of the students were acknowledged. Some changes were made to the system, including ending church involvement (Hanson, 2009).

Many Canadians see the residential school system as part of the distant past and thus not important in today's society. However, there are intergenerational effects, including compromised family systems, loss of language, culture, and the teaching of tradition (Hanson, 2009). In 1996 the Royal Commission on Aboriginal Peoples (Parliament of Canada, 2000) brought attention to the residential school system, and in 1998 the Canadian Government publicly apologized and established a $350 million plan to help communities affected by the residential schools. A Truth and Reconciliation Commission (2013) has allowed survivors to share their stories and experiences, and an Indian Residential Schools Settlement began in September 2007, providing monetary compensation to former students of residential schools (Aboriginal Affairs and Northern Development Canada, 2010a).

In addition to the children who lived in residential schools, thousands of Aboriginal children were taken from their homes and adopted into non-Aboriginal homes between 1960 and the mid 1980s. "The 60's scoop" was so named because "children were literally scooped from their homes and communities without the knowledge or consent of families and bands" (Sinclair, 2011, para. 1). Many of these adoptees are now trying to find their birth families and communities, and there are a number of family reunification programs in Canada (Sinclair, 2011).

In the early 1940s, researchers, operating under the auspices of the Canadian government, reported that there might be a connection between the high incidence of malnutrition and health problems such as tuberculosis that existed in northern Cree communities (Mosby, 2013). First Nations representatives proposed that hunger and malnutrition could be ended by more generous relief money during times of extreme hardship, increased rations for the old and destitute, and establishment of fishing reserves so the people could feed themselves. Government response was to commission studies to demonstrate whether addition of food factors that were lacking would result in better health. Over the next decade, in an era when federal policies related to Aboriginal peoples were shifting, the science of nutrition was emerging, and attitudes toward the ethics of experimentation on human subjects were changing, "bureaucrats, doctors, and scientists recognized the problems of hunger and malnutrition, yet increasingly came to view Aboriginal bodies as 'experimental materials' and residential schools and Aboriginal communities as kinds of 'laboratories' that they could use to pursue a number of different political and professional interests" (p. 148). In addition to surveys of the nutrition and health status of northern Cree people and of children in residential schools, researchers conducted double blind studies in which people in the experimental groups received vitamin supplements and those in the control groups did not. Mosby (2013) concludes that these studies had no long-term positive effects on the lives of the people studied or on the quality of the food services in residential schools. He further concludes that the experiments should be "remembered and recognized for what they truly were: one among many examples of a larger institutionalized and, ultimately, dehumanizing colonialist racial ideology that has governed Canada's policies towards and treatment of Aboriginal peoples throughout the twentieth century" (p. 172).

The legacy of assimilation policies, residential schools, racism, and loss of self-determination and cultural identity continues to affect the health and well-being of Canada's Aboriginal population. Health determinants such as unemployment, poverty, crowded living conditions, educational disadvantages, and lack of access to services have an impact on health across the lifespan, and the ensuing health issues create additional determinants that in turn influence health. For example, poverty may lead to substance use, which leads to family disruptions and loss of social support (Loppie-Reading & Wien, 2009).

One of the indicators used as a measure of health is **infant mortality rate,** that is, the number of deaths of infants under 1 year per 1,000 live births. Canada's infant mortality rate in 2011 was 4.92 (Indexmundi, 2011). The infant mortality rate for the Aboriginal population is not available (Health Canada, 2011a). Measuring the rate is complex and challenging because of the inability to link infant birth and death registrations, the lack of First Nations, Inuit, and Métis identifiers in vital statistics databases, and infant deaths that are not reported. According to two recent studies, however, although the First Nations infant mortality rate is declining, it remains considerably higher than non-Aboriginal rates (Health Canada, 2011a).

There are many programs and projects aimed at improving Aboriginal maternal and child health. One of these projects, developed by the Health Council of Canada, is a "Compendium of Promising Practices," part of a multiyear project on Aboriginal health status. Seven consultation sessions were held across Canada and involved front line workers, program managers and coordinators, Aboriginal leaders, academics, health authorities, and government representatives (Health Council of Canada, 2011).

Canada's demographic shift, with an expanding Aboriginal population and increasing immigration, has had an impact on health indicators and overall national wellness. There are many factors that negatively affect the health of Aboriginal peoples and immigrants, including poverty, but the health care system itself also bears responsibility. Many Aboriginal peoples and immigrants do not trust or do not use health services because they feel threatened by racism and stereotyping and because the health system seems intimidating.

The 1982 Charter of Rights and Freedoms includes nondiscrimination legislation in relation to age and disability as well as to race and ethnic origin. In 2009, 12% of Canadian women over the age of 15 (about 1.7 million) reported long-term health conditions that interfered with normal daily life; nearly half of these women were over the age of 60 (Crompton, 2011). The Health

utility index (HUI) used eight components to measure functional health: ability to see, hear, walk, talk, handle objects, remember and think; it also assessed emotional well-being and amount of pain. Of the eight components of the HUI, pain was the major contributor to poor functional health. The most common chronic conditions among women with activity limitations were, in order of frequency, arthritis, back problems, high blood pressure, migraines, mood disorders, anxiety disorders, asthma, bowel disorders, urinary incontinence, heart disease, diabetes, chronic obstructive pulmonary disease, ulcers, effects of a stroke, cancer, dementia. Just over half of the women with activity limitations needed some help with at least one major activity of daily living. Compared with women with no limitations, they were not as well educated, participated less in the workforce, reported a 25% lower personal income, visited the doctor more, exercised less, and were more likely to be overweight (31%) or obese (28%) (Crompton, 2011).

Changes in Political Viewpoints

Politically, sexual and reproductive issues have seen various shifts. Unlike in 1900, contraceptives are available now to people who desire them, although not all types of contraception are accessible to those who want them (see Chapter 8). At present, there are no statutory prohibitions against abortion in Canada. However, access to service providers is uneven across the country, and those who provide abortion services are sometimes threatened by those who do not support abortion. Abortion services continue to be an uncomfortable, value-laden issue for governments. See Chapter 9 for a fuller discussion. Although homosexuality is not universally accepted, Canada legalized same-sex marriages in July 2005 with the passing of Bill C-38, the Civil Marriage Act (Parliament of Canada, 2005).

NORTH AMERICAN HEALTH CARE SYSTEMS

Perspectives on the provision of health care vary greatly around the world. In most industrialized countries, these perspectives fall mainly into two categories: (1) government-sponsored care that is accessible to all citizens independent of their ability to pay for it and (2) health care provided based on each health care consumer's ability to pay for services individually.

This dichotomous approach is represented through the two diverse systems found in North America. The Canadian health care system is government funded and based on the belief that all Canadians should have access to necessary health care according to need rather than the ability to pay (Health Canada, 2012a). However, Canada has moved toward adding some aspects of privatization of health care to its publicly funded system. In the United States, health care is provided mainly by private for-profit organizations. About 60% of American people have employer-provided health care insurance. Others buy private health insurance, and about 2% are uninsured. Two thirds of health care comes from government-sponsored programs for people with low income (Medicaid), the elderly (Medicare), or those on active military status (Gill, 2012). High-quality health care is accessible to people with the ability to pay. There continues to be active debate about health care reform, a politically charged issue.

Canadian Health Care System

Canada has a publicly funded dynamic health care system established in accordance with the 1984 Canada Health Act. Reforms have taken place since its inception, but the basic principle remains the same: "universal coverage for medically necessary health care services provided on the basis of need, rather than the ability to pay" (Health Canada, 2012a, para. 2). Provincial and territorial governments have most of the responsibility for health and social services, while the federal government is responsible for First Nations and Inuit people. Health care is financed largely through taxation. Public health, including sanitation and infectious diseases, is also shared among the federal, provincial/territorial, and municipal governments (Health Canada, 2012a). Health Canada describes its approach to service as primary health care, that is, provision of first-contact services and coordination of services to ensure continuity of care and ease of movement across the health care system (Health Canada, 2012b). The services may vary from community to community, and may include prevention and treatment of common diseases and injuries, basic emergency services, referrals to other levels of care, primary mental health care, palliative and end-of-life care, health promotion, healthy child development, primary maternity care, and rehabilitation services (Health Canada, 2012b). In accordance with the Canada Health Act of 1985, each province and territory in Canada must meet specific national criteria to receive federal money and is subsequently responsible for the health care administration and delivery (Health Canada, 2012a) (Box 1.1). Many Canadians also access additional health coverage through private health plans, either purchased or provided by employers.

Canadians gain access to the health care system through a health care professional or through telephone- or computer-based services (Health Canada, 2012a). Despite the apparently open access to health care in Canada, primary health care services in rural and remote areas are not as available as in urban areas. The definition of "rural" includes factors such as: distance between a site and advanced care, distance between a site and basic care, population number and density. One in five women lives in a rural area, and rural women face "unique health challenges, such as lower than aver-

● BOX 1.1 Principles of the Canada Health Act

The five Canada Health Act principles provide for:

Public Administration

The provincial and territorial plans must be administered and operated on a nonprofit basis by a public authority accountable to the provincial or territorial government.

Comprehensiveness

The provincial and territorial plans must insure all medically necessary services provided by hospitals, medical practitioners, and dentists working within a hospital setting.

Universality

The provincial and territorial plans must entitle all insured persons to health insurance coverage on uniform terms and conditions.

Accessibility

The provincial and territorial plans must provide all insured persons reasonable access to medically necessary hospital and physician services without financial or other barriers.

Portability

The provincial and territorial plans must cover all insured persons when they move to another province or territory within Canada and when they travel abroad. The provinces and territories have some limits on coverage for services provided outside Canada, and may require prior approval for nonemergency services delivered outside their jurisdiction.

Source: Health Canada. (2012). *Health Care System. Canada Health Act: Overview.* Retrieved from http://www.hc-sc.gc.ca/hcs-sss/pubs/system-regime/2011-hcs-sss/index-eng.php.

age life expectancy, and higher rates of disability, infant mortality, and deaths from cancer and circulatory diseases compared with their urban counterparts" (Leipert et al., 2011, p. 37). Nurse Practitioners can play an important role in increasing access to primary health care services, but their inclusion on the health care team has not been widely implemented (Leipert et al., 2011).

Many rural women have limited access to maternity care services. In a joint position paper by the Canadian Association of Midwives, Canadian Association of Perinatal and Women's Health Nurses (CAPWHN) (2011), the College of Family Physicians of Canada, and the Society of Obstetricians and Gynaecologists of Canada (SOGC) (Miller et al., 2012), the authors expressed concerns that maternity programs in rural areas have been cut due to cost reductions, regionalization of care, lack of skilled personnel, and diminished services such as laboratory testing, diagnostic imaging, appropriate equipment, and transport systems (Miller et al., 2012). The first of the 14 recommendations made by the joint task group was: "Women who reside in rural and remote communities in Canada should receive high-quality maternity care as close to home as possible" (Miller et al., 2012, p. 2). Other recommendations addressed issues such as collaborative care, cultural sensitivity, social and emotional needs, innovative remunerative and training models, and ongoing interprofessional continuing education.

Throughout most of the 20th century Canada was the "only western industrialized country with no legal provisions for the practice and profession of midwifery" (Tyson, 2001, para. 1). Early in the century, lay midwives attended births. In subsequent decades, the medical profession provided all primary maternity care, except for remote areas of the country where internationally educated nurse-midwives were employed. In the rest of Canada, midwives were not recognized or licensed. In the 1970s and 1980s there was public dissatisfaction with women's lack of choices in maternity care and a desire for access to midwifery services. In the 1990s Ontario was the first province to integrate midwifery into the health care system (Tyson, 2001). By 2012, midwifery had become legalized and regulated in all provinces and territories, except Prince Edward Island and the Yukon, where the matter is still under consideration (Canadian Midwifery Regulators Consortium, 2012). Not all provinces provide funding for care received from a midwife. The practice of midwifery in Canada is growing, but has not reached the level of acceptance and contribution to maternity services that is seen in other industrialized countries (Malott et al., 2009).

In Canada, nursing and midwifery are regulated separately and it is possible to be licensed as both a nurse and a midwife. Registered midwives provide primary health services within their scope of practice and make referrals to other care providers as necessary. They attend births in hospitals, birth centres, and at home. (Canadian Midwifery Regulators Consortium, 2013). Nurses and midwives work together, "complement and learn from each other, and understand and value each other's roles and experiences . . . [to] foster safe and effective maternity care that responds to the needs of women, families and communities" (CAPWHN, 2013, para. 2).

In 2003, to address concerns about availability of high-quality health care, an agreement was reached among the provincial and territorial health ministers and the federal government to strengthen and renew Canada's publicly funded health system. They agreed to address access to care, health promotion and wellness, primary health care, home care and community care, pharmaceuticals management, health information and communications technologies, health equipment and infrastructure, and the supply of health professionals. The agreement also highlighted the need for improved accountability and reporting to Canadians. Health indicators were developed (Statistics Canada, 2012c) (Box 1.2). The indicators are used as a performance measure of the health care system, and Health Canada periodically publishes data on themes of key concern to Canadians, such as timely access to care, quality of care, and self-reported health status and wellness.

In addition to these performance measures, in 1999 a formal Women's Health Strategy was developed to enhance the ability of the Canadian health care system to meet the unique needs of women. The strategy is no longer in effect, but Health Canada has "an internal policy that requires sex and gender considerations in the development of our policies, programs, and research activities" (personal e-mail communication, Cindy Moriarity, Health Canada Program Management Division, February, 2013).

 The nurse practitioner suggests to Elaine that she come back to visit in 3 weeks to follow up with some teaching suggestions, recheck her blood pressure, and evaluate the effectiveness of some interventions to manage stress. Elaine looks discouraged. "This is going to cost more money. I have to make sure we can do this appointment on a day I'm not working—I can't afford to miss!" How might the nurse help Elaine with these problems?

HEALTH PROMOTION AND HEALTH STATISTICS

Health promotion begins with a knowledge of the **social determinants of health,** that is, income and social status, social support networks, education and literacy, employment/working conditions, social and physical environments, personal health practices and coping skills, healthy child development, biology and genetic endowment, health services, gender, and culture (Public Health Agency of Canada [PHAC], 2012a).

One role of nursing is to help health care consumers to recognize the positive effects that being healthy can have on all aspects of their lives; another is to help them to develop strategies to improve their health. Although nursing care needs to be individualized for each client and family, it is important to be aware of the trends and patterns of health care and to be cognizant of where the client's potential fits in the pattern. This

● **BOX 1.2** Health Indicators Framework

Health Status

How healthy are Canadians? Health status can be measured in a variety of ways, including well-being, health conditions, disability, or death

Well-being	Health Conditions	Human Function	Deaths
Broad measures of the physical, mental, and social well-being of individuals	Alterations or attributes of the health status of an individual that may lead to distress, interference with daily activities, or contact with health services; it may be a disease (acute or chronic), disorder, injury or trauma, or reflect other health-related states such as pregnancy, aging, stress, congenital anomaly, or genetic predisposition	Levels of human function are associated with the consequences of disease, disorder, injury, and other health conditions. They include body function/structure (impairments), activities (activity limitations), and participation (restrictions in participation)	A range of age-specific and condition-specific mortality rates as well as derived indicators

---

Nonmedical Determinants of Health

Nonmedical determinants of heath are known to affect our health, and in some cases, when and how we use health care

Health Behaviours	Living and Working Conditions	Personal Resources	Environmental Factors
Aspects of personal behaviour and risk factors that epidemiological studies have shown to influence health status	Indicators related to the socioeconomic characteristics and working conditions of the population that epidemiological studies have shown to be related to health	Measures the prevalence of factors, such as social support, that epidemiological studies have shown to be related to health	Environmental factors with the potential to influence human health

---

Health System Performance

How healthy is the health system? These indicators measure various aspects of the quality of health care

Acceptability	Accessibility	Appropriateness	Competence
All care/service provided meets the expectations of the client, community, providers and paying organizations, recognizing that there may be conflicting or competing interests between stakeholders, and that the needs of the clients/patients are paramount	The ability of clients/patients to obtain care/service at the right place and right time, based on respective needs	Care/service provided is relevant to the clients'/patients' needs and based on established standards	An individual's knowledge and skills are appropriate to the care/service being provided

Continuity	Effectiveness	Efficiency	Safety
The ability to provide uninterrupted, coordinated care/service across programs, practitioners, organization, and levels of care/service, over time	The care/service, intervention or action achieves the desired results	Achieves the desired results with the most cost-effective use of resources	Potential risks of an intervention or the environment are avoided or minimized

Source: Statistics Canada. (2012c). *Health indicators framework.* (Catalogue no. 82-221-X). Retrieved from http://www.statcan.gc.ca/pub/82–221-x/2012002/hifw-eng.htm.

knowledge can help the nurse to assist clients in health promotion choices, anticipate potential challenges in ensuring that health care needs of clients are met, and improve the overall experience of the client and family in the health care system.

One way that nurses can promote health is by helping health care consumers understand the importance of participating in health-promoting behaviours. Some health promotion activities have diverse and wide-ranging effects on quality of life and health. An excellent example is the achievement and maintenance of good periodontal health. For women of childbearing age, good oral health is particularly important because research suggests a potential relationship between poor periodontal health and premature birth (Huck et al., 2011). For people of all ages, periodontal health is related to the potential for achieving a healthy nutritional intake and a healthy body weight.

Another important aspect of providing quality nursing care is an understanding of key statistics for specific groups. For women, such statistics include awareness of risks for specific diseases, common fertility rates, and maternal morbidity and mortality data. Knowledge of these factors can help nurses look for certain indicators or problems when working with women of certain ages or ethnic groups.

Nutritional Status and Body Weight

Many Canadian women do not have healthy nutritional practices and do not follow *Canada's Food Guide* (Health Canada, 2011b) and *Canada's Food Guide: First Nations, Inuit and Métis* available in English, Inuktitut, Ojibwe, Plains Cree, and Woods Cree languages. (Health Canada, 2011b) (see Chapters 2 and 3). About 44% of Canadian women are either overweight or obese (Human Resources and Skills Development Canada [HRSDC], 2013d), with weight gradually increasing as they age. The issue has been identified as particularly significant in Aboriginal populations, because obesity rates in these communities have been found to be substantially higher than the national average (Allen, 2009). It is important to note that obesity has been linked with infertility and increased risks during pregnancy (see Chapters 10 and 13), as well as chronic diseases such as diabetes and heart disease.

Exercise

Obesity is linked not only to nutritional intake, but also to lack of adequate physical activity—an important component of promoting a healthy lifestyle. In 2011, 51% of women were reported to be active or moderately active, with physical activity decreasing with age (HRSDC, 2013e). Exercise is important not only to achieve or maintain a healthy weight but also to reduce the risk of heart attack, obesity, other diseases, and

stress (HRSDC, 2013e) and can be an important component of a healthy pregnancy (Society of Obstetricians and Gynaecologists of Canada [SOGC], 2011a).

A variety of exercise programs can meet the needs of various population groups, from chair- and water-based exercise programs to weight lifting and aerobics to specific prenatal and postnatal exercises classes. What is important is to ensure that the client who is healthy enough to participate in an exercise program chooses the program that suits any physical limitations she may have and enhances her health status. See Chapter 2 for further details.

Prenatal Care

In the 2006 "Maternity Experiences Survey," 6,000 Canadian women were asked about their "perceptions, knowledge and practices before conception and during pregnancy, birth and the early months of parenthood" (PHAC, 2009, p. 11). The survey indicated that, overall, Canadian women had good access to prenatal care, with 94.9% initiating care in the first trimester (Fig. 1.3). All women had at least one prenatal care visit; the average number of visits was 12.9. The proportion of women who received inadequate prenatal care, defined as having four or fewer visits, varied by province and territory. However, teenage women, women with less than a high school education, and women with low income were more likely to initiate prenatal care *after* the first trimester. In general, women were able to access prenatal care as early as they wanted, although access to care varied, depending on the area of the country. The majority of women received their prenatal care from an obstetrician/gynecologist or family physician. About 7% received prenatal care from a midwife or nurse/nurse practitioner. A limitation of this study is that it explored only the number and timing of the prenatal visits, and did not reflect the content or quality of the care (PHAC, 2009).

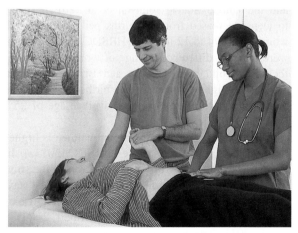

FIGURE 1.3 Prenatal care within the first trimester of pregnancy optimizes the chances for successful maternal and neonatal outcomes.

The nurse convinces Mei to let her speak with Taohua alone. Once they have privacy, Taohua says, "I'm pretty sure that I am pregnant. My boyfriend and I had unprotected sex a few times, and I've missed two periods. I don't want my family to know what's going on. I'm not sure what I want to do about this yet, and I don't need their opinions." How can the nurse respond with sensitivity but help Taohua to receive the prenatal care she needs if she decides to continue with the pregnancy?

Birth and Fertility Rates

Birth rate is defined as the number of births per 1,000 population. In the past five decades Canada has seen a dramatic decrease in birth rate, from 27.2 births per 1,000 population shortly after World War II (Canadian Encyclopedia, 2012) to an estimated 10.3 in 2012 (Indexmundi, 2012a). Age-specific **fertility rate,** adopted as a statistical measure in 2009, refers to the number of births per woman in the age category of 15 to 49 years (Statistics Canada, 2012a). Over the past 50 years, the fertility rate has dropped significantly from a high of 3.93 children per woman in 1959 to a low of 1.49 children per woman in 2000 (HRSDC, 2013b). The fertility rate for 2012 was 1.59 (Indexmundi, 2012c). To maintain the country's population at a steady state, the Canadian fertility rate must remain above 2.1 (HRSDC, 2013b).

There is a growing trend in Canada to delay pregnancy. In 2009 the average age for birth of a first child was 29.4 years, and half of all women giving birth were 30 years of age or older (HRSDC, 2013c). This trend is also occurring in Western Europe, Australia, New Zealand, and the United States (Johnson et al., 2012). Births to teens decreased from 30 births per 1,000 teenage women in 1974 to 12 in 2009 (HRSDC, 2013c). There were regional differences in age of women at birth of their first child, with Ontario and British Columbia having the highest percentage of births to women 30 and over and Nunavut having an average age of 25.1 (HRSDC, 2013c).

The fertility rate for Aboriginal women is higher than the overall Canadian rate (HRSDC, 2013a). In immigrant women, fertility rates tend to decline soon after they move to Canada, and the longer they stay, the more closely their fertility rates resemble those of Canadian-born women (Bélanger & Gilbert, 2002).

In 2011 there were more census families without children (44.5%) than with children (39.2%), a shift from 2001, when there were more couples with children (43.6%) than couples without children (40.3%) (Statistics Canada, 2012f).

Maternal Morbidity

Maternal morbidity refers to conditions outside of normal pregnancy, labour, and childbirth that negatively affect a woman's health during those times. Some of these conditions are hypertension, diabetes, and anemia. In Canada, approximately 1% of pregnancies are affected by pre-existing hypertension, 5% to 6% develop gestational hypertension without proteinuria, and 1% to 2% have preeclampsia (Ontario Midwives, 2012). Gestational diabetes develops in approximately 2% to 4% of non-Aboriginal women and up to 18% of Aboriginal women (Canadian Diabetes Association, 2012). Anemia in pregnancy can be mild, moderate, or severe, and women are treated according to their level of anemia and the possible cause. Another indicator of maternal morbidity is hospital readmission after delivery. The 30-day readmission rate for Canada in 2010 was 2% (Canadian Institute for Health Information [CIHI], 2010).

Maternal Mortality

Maternal mortality is defined as the number of maternal deaths occurring during pregnancy, childbirth, or within 42 days after delivery or termination of pregnancy (PHAC, 2011). The Canadian Perinatal Surveillance System, part of the PHAC, reported that between 2009 and 2010 the maternal mortality rate was 7.8 deaths per 100,000 deliveries. The most common diagnoses associated with these deaths were diseases of the circulatory system; other indirect causes; hypertension complicating pregnancy, childbirth, and the puerperium; postpartum hemorrhage; obstetric embolism; ectopic and molar pregnancy and abortive outcome; major puerperal infection; and antepartum hemorrhage (PHAC, 2011). The risk for death increases with increased maternal age and the stage of pregnancy. Canada has a low maternal mortality rate in comparison with countries such as India, where the rate is 200 maternal deaths per 100,000 live births (Indexmundi, 2012b).

Severe Maternal Morbidity

Although death rates are often used as a measurement of the quality of health care, in industrialized countries, maternal deaths are rare. Thus, in Canada, some researchers use severe maternal morbidity as an alternate indicator of quality of care. In 2009/10, the rate of severe maternal morbidity in Canada was 14.5 per 1,000 deliveries. The most common severe maternal morbidities include blood transfusion; postpartum hemorrhage; cardiac arrest/failure, myocardial infarction or pulmonary edema; hysterectomy; puerperal sepsis; eclampsia; uterine rupture during labour; and repair of bladder, urethra, or intestine (PHAC, 2011).

CRITICAL THINKING, ETHICALLY BASED PRACTICE, EVIDENCE-BASED CARE, AND BEST PRACTICES

Critical thinking is inherent in nursing practice; in fact, without critical thinking, there would be no professional nursing. **Critical thinking** is a higher-level, complex thought process through which competent, comprehensive decision making and problem solving can result in informed, intelligent decisions. Critical thinking is holistic: it requires more than just rote knowledge to make a decision or solve a problem. Inherent in critical thinking is an understanding of people, situations, and phenomena, along with recognizing the potential for each situation, both perceived and actualized. Mulnix (2010) surveyed critical thinking literature and found that what constitutes critical thinking varies widely. She concluded that "Critical thinking is the same as thinking rationally or reasoning well. In order to reason well, a thinker must be able to give reasons for what she believes, and these reasons must actually support the truth of the statement or belief they are claimed to support" (Mulnix, 2010, p. 14).

The term **best practice** is used in the fields of health care, education, and business. There are many definitions, but most of the definitions incorporate the idea that best practices are those in which experience and research are used to lead to a desired result. The definitions also include a commitment to use all the knowledge and technology at one's disposal to ensure success. Canadian Nurses Association (CNA) (2008) combines the concepts of best practice with standards of care that are based on the values of the profession, as articulated in the Code of Ethics for Registered Nurses.

Evidence-based practice results in better patient outcomes than care based on tradition. Within the paradigm, nurses use critical thinking to evaluate sources of evidence, transform them to meet the needs and desires of their individual clients, and evaluate the outcomes of their interventions. According to Wallen et al. (2010), "Evidence-based practice is a problem-solving approach to the delivery of healthcare that integrates the best evidence from research with a clinician's expertise and a patient's preferences and values" (p. 2768).

There are ongoing discussions regarding the term *evidence-based,* with some authors suggesting that it is too limiting, and that *evidence-informed* provides a more comprehensive view that includes practice informed by evidence and theory, leaving "ample room for clinical experience as well as constructive and imaginative judgements of practitioners and clients" (Nevo & Slonim-Nevo, 2011, para. 1). The Canadian Nurses Association, in its 2010 position statement "Evidence-informed Decision-making and Nursing Practice," made a distinction between the two terms. The concept of **evidence-informed decision-making** recognizes that "there are many factors beyond evidence—for example, available resources or cultural and religious norms—that influence decision making. Decision making in nursing practice is influenced by evidence and also by individual values, client choice, theories, clinical judgment, ethics, legislation, regulation, health-care resources and practice environments" (CNA, 2010, p 3). (Box 1.3)

Nursing practice is grounded in both informal and formal **ethical principles** or **codes**. Informal ethical codes are based on nurses' own values, general moral views, and experiences, as well as the history of the nursing profession. Registered Nurses are bound by the Canadian Nurses Association formalized Code of Ethics for use in practice and decision making (CNA, 2008). The Code provides guidance for ethical relationships, responsibilities, behaviours, and decision making and is to be used along with professional standards, laws, and regulations that guide practice. The code also informs the public and other health care professionals about nurses' commitments and responsibilities (CNA, 2008).

The ethical principles of autonomy, beneficence, nonmaleficence, and fairness or distributive justice are the basis for making ethical decisions. Autonomy is the right of the individual to make personal choices and decisions independent of the beliefs of others. Beneficence is doing good; nonmaleficence is doing no harm. The principle of justice refers to a fair distribution of benefits (including health care) and burdens within a society.

Although the Code of Ethics and the ethical principles provide guidance for nursing practice, the reality is that there are situations in which it is difficult to support them equally. Take, for example, the case of a new mother who asks the nurse for assistance in breastfeeding her 1-hour-old newborn. The nurse, a breastfeeding advocate, is aware that the client is HIV positive and that the virus can pass through breast milk to her infant. According to the SOGC, "Mothers infected with HIV, or those who continue to have risk activities associated with HIV infections, should formula feed their babies"

(text continues on page 20)

● BOX 1.3 Canadian Nurses Association Position Statement: Evidence-Informed Decision-Making and Nursing Practice

CNA Position

- Evidence-informed decision making is an important element of quality care in all domains of nursing practice and is integral to effect changes across the health-care system.[1]
- Evidence-informed decision making is a continuous interactive process involving the explicit, conscientious, and judicious consideration of the best available evidence to provide care. It is essential to optimize outcomes for individual clients, promote healthy communities and populations, improve clinical practice, achieve cost-effective nursing care and ensure accountability and transparency in decision making within the health-care system.[2]
- Evidence is information acquired through research and the scientific evaluation of practice.
  - Types of evidence include information derived from a broad range of rigorous methodologies including quantitative studies (such as randomized controlled trials, observational studies), qualitative studies (such as case studies, ethnography, phenomenology) and meta-analysis.
  - Evidence also includes expert opinion in the form of consensus documents, commission reports, regulations and historical or experiential information.[3]
- Rating systems have been developed to rank evidence; however, it is imperative to acknowledge that no level of evidence eliminates the need for professional clinical judgment or for the consideration of client preferences.[4]
- CNA believes that nurses—including clinicians, educators, researchers, administrators and policy makers—should collaborate with other health-care stakeholders to facilitate evidence-informed decision making and practice to ensure integration of the health-care system. Other key stakeholders include employers, accreditation councils, governments, patient advocacy groups, and health information agencies. These collaborative responsibilities extend to identifying and addressing the barriers and enhancing the factors within organizational structures and the health-care system that facilitate and promote evidence-informed practice.

Individual Nurses

- Are positioned to provide optimal care by having acquired competencies[5] for evidence-informed nursing practice as part of their foundational education;
- Read and critique evidence-informed literature (ie, research articles, reports) in nursing, health sciences and related disciplines;[6]
- Generate researchable questions and communicate them to their manager or clinical nurse leaders or associated researchers;
- Participate in or conduct research;[7] and
- Evaluate and promote evidence-informed nursing practice.

Professional and Nursing Specialty Associations

- Use the best available evidence as a basis for standards and guidelines;
- Lobby governments for funding to support nursing research and health information systems that include nursing care data; and
- Lobby governments for healthy public policy, regulation and legislation that are evidence informed.

Nursing Regulatory Authorities

- Use the best available evidence as a basis for standards, guidelines, and regulatory practices; and
- Support nurses to meet competencies for evidence-informed practice.

Researchers

- Identify knowledge gaps and establish research priorities in conjunction with clinicians and/or other health professionals, key stakeholders, and client groups;
- Generate high-quality evidence through research;
- Facilitate capacity building of new nurse researchers; and
- Engage in effective knowledge transfer, translation, and exchange to communicate relevant findings of the results of research to those who require the information.

Educators and Educational Institutions

- Support those graduating from basic and continuing nursing education programs to acquire competencies to provide evidence-informed nursing;
- Use and develop evidence-informed curricula by providing high-quality education in research methods, evidence collection, and analysis; and
- Promote a spirit of inquiry, critical thinking, openness to change, and a philosophy of life-long learning.

Health Service Delivery Organizations

- Reduce barriers against and enhance the factors within organizations that promote evidence-informed practice by integrating research findings and practice guidelines;
- Evaluate outcome measures through ongoing audits and formal research studies;
- Support registered nurses' involvement in research and in the transfer of research into organizational policy and practice; and
- Provide continuing education to assist nurses to maintain and increase their competence with respect to evidence-informed practice.

Governments

- Support development of health information systems that support evidence-informed nursing practice;
- Support health information institutions; and
- Provide adequate funding to support nursing research in all its phases.

(continued)

● **BOX 1.3** **Canadian Nurses Association Position Statement: Evidence-Informed Decision-Making and Nursing Practice** (continued)

National and Provincial or Territorial Health Information Institutions

- Collect, store, maintain, update, and retrieve health data in health information systems accessible to nursing and health researchers;
- Provide comprehensive, integrated, and relational systems that include nursing data and health outcomes; and
- Collect data using standardized languages to ensure that nursing data can be aggregated and compared across and between sites.

Background

The distinction between the terms "evidence-based" and "evidence-informed" is important. The concept of evidence-informed decision making builds on evidence-based health care. It acknowledges the many factors beyond evidence—for example, available resources or cultural and religious norms—that influence decision making.[8]

Evidence-informed nursing is the ongoing process that incorporates evidence from research, clinical expertise, client preferences and other available resources to make nursing decisions about clients.[9] Decision making in nursing practice is influenced by evidence and also by individual values, client choice, theories, clinical judgment, ethics, legislation, regulation, health-care resources and practice environ-

ments.[10] At the community level, evidence-informed public health is defined as "the process of integrating science-based interventions with community preferences to improve the health of populations."[11]

A variety of sources are being used by nurses to facilitate their use of evidence. These sources include systematic reviews, research studies and abstraction journals that summarize valid and clinically useful published studies.

There has also been a rapid proliferation of clinical practice guidelines for nurses to use as a source of evidence. These are defined as "systematically developed statements to assist practitioner decisions about appropriate health care for specific clinical circumstances."[12] Guidelines are based on the most rigorous research available, and when research is not available, they are grounded in expert opinion and consensus.[13]

Applied at the individual client level, guidelines provide a set of instructions containing conditional logic for solving problems or accomplishing tasks. Appropriately applied, guidelines can reduce uncertainties associated with clinical decisions, diminish variation around usual practices, demystify unfamiliar terminology, and decrease the need to search for journals and articles. It is important to evaluate the quality of the guidelines prior to implementation through the use of acceptable tools.[14]

Approved by the CNA Board of Directors October 2010
[1]Domains of nursing practice include practice, education, leadership, administration, and research.
[2](Canadian Nurses Association [CNA], 2008, p. 35; Cleary-Holdforth, 2009)
[3](Cullinset al, 2005; Lomas et al., 2005; Barton, 2009)
[4](Trammer et al., 1998; Youngblut & Brooten, 2001)
[5]Competencies are the specific knowledge, skills, judgment, and personal attributes required for a registered nurse to practise safely and ethically in a designated role and setting.
[6](CNA, 2010, p. 177)
[7](Edwards et al., 2009)
[8](Ciliska et al. 2008, p. 7.)
[9](Ciliska et al., 2001; Scott & McSherry, 2008)
[10](Dicenso et al., 2005)
[11](Kohatsu et al., 2004, p. 419)
[12](Field, 1995, p. 38)
[13](Schunemann et al., 2006)
[14](Glanville et al., 2000)

REFERENCES
Canadian Nurses Association. (2008). *Code of ethics for registered nurses.* Ottawa: Author.
Canadian Nurses Association. (2010). *The Canadian registered nurse examination prep guide.* Ottawa: Author.
Barton, A. (2009). Knowledge management and the clinical nurse specialist. *Clinical Nurse Specialist, 23*(3), 123–124.
Ciliska, D., Pinelli, J., DeCenso, A., & Cullum, N. (2001). Resources to enhance evidence-based nursing practice. *AACN Clinical Issues, 12*(4), 520–528.
Ciliska, C., Thomas, H., & Buffet, C. (2012). An introduction to evidence-informed public health and a compendium of critical appraisal tools for public health practice (Revised). Hamilton, ON: National Collaborating Centre for Methods and Tools. Retrieved from http://www.nccmt.ca/publications/8/view-eng.html
Cleary-Holdforth, L. T. (2009). Evidence-based practice: Improving patient outcomes. *Nursing Standard, 23*(32), 35–39.
Cullins, S., Voth, T., DiCenso, A., & Guyatt, G. (2005). Finding the evidence. In A. Dicenso, G. Guyatt, & D. K. Ciliska (Eds.), *Evidence-based nursing: A guide to clinical practice.* (pp. 20–43). St. Louis, MO: Elsevier/Mosby.

Dicenso, A., Ciliska, D. K., & Guyatt, G. (2005). Introduction to evidence-based nursing. In A. Dicenso, G. Guyatt, & D. K. Ciliska (Eds.), *Evidence-based nursing: A guide to clinical practice.* (pp. 3–19). St. Louis, MO: Elsevier/Mosby.
Edwards, N., Webber, J., Mill, J., Kahwa, E., & Roelofs, S. (2009). Building capacity for nurse-led research. *International Nursing Review, 56*(1), 88–94.
Field, M. (Ed.). (1995). *Committee on methods for setting priorities for guidelines development.* Washington, DC: Institute of Medicine.
Glanville, I., Schrim, V., & Wineman, N. (2000). Using evidence-based practice for managing clinical outcomes in advanced practice nursing. *Journal of Nursing Care Quality, 15*(1), 1–11.
Kohatsu, N. D., Robinson, J. G., & Torner, J. C. (2004). Evidence-based public health: An evolving concept. *American Journal of Preventive Medicine, 27*(5), 417–421.
Lomas, J., Culyer, T., McCutcheon, C., McAuley, L., & Law, S. (2005). *Final report: Conceptualizing and combining evidence for health system guidance.* Ottawa: Canadian Health Services Research Foundation.
Schunemann, H. J., Fretheim, A., & Oxman, A. D. (2006). Improving the use of research evidence in guideline development. *Health Research Policy and Systems, 4*(14). Retrieved from http://www.health-policy-systems.com/content/4/1/14
Scott, K., & McSherry, R. (2008) Evidence-based nursing: Clarifying the concepts for nurses in practice. *Journal of Clinical Nursing, 18*(8), 1085–1095.
Trammer, J., Squires, S., Brazil, K., Gerlach, J., Johnson, J., Muisiner, D., et al. (1998). *Factors that influence evidence-based decision-making. Canadian Health Action: Building on the Legacy: vol. 5. Making decisions: Evidence and information.* Sainte-Foy, QC: Multimondes and the National Forum on Health.
Youngblut, J., & Bronte, D. (2001). Evidence-based nursing practice: Why is it important? *AACN Clinical Issues, 12*(4), 468–476.
Also see:
CNA position statement: Nursing Leadership (2009)
International Council of Nurses position statement: Nursing Research (2007)
Source: Canadian Nurses Association. (2010). Retrieved from http://www.nurseone.ca/docs/NurseOne/Public%20Documents/Evidence-Informed%20decision-making%20and%20nursing%20practice.pdf.

(SOGC, 2011b, section 11). In this situation, simultaneously upholding the principles of autonomy, beneficence, and nonmaleficence *seems* impossible.

Ethical Decision Making

There are many different styles of **ethical decision making**. Some nurses are comfortable and familiar with a problem-solving method similar to the nursing process; others use ethical principles when considering ethical issues. Some nurses explore relationships and become aware of relevant values and perspectives before reaching a decision. There is no one best way to address ethical issues or to make ethical decisions. The most important aspect of making decisions is to ask questions and make the best ethical decisions possible under the circumstances.

Through the introduction of new technologies and practices, particularly in the areas of women's health and maternity nursing, the potential need for ethical decision making has increased dramatically. Situations requiring ethical decision making may be as diverse as client care decisions, application of institutional philosophical beliefs, or resource allocation. A growing number of health care institutions have formed ethics committees to assist health care clients, families, and professionals in ethically based decision making (Fig. 1.4). Gaudine et al. (2011) studied hospital ethics committees and reported that although the original focus of these committees was the resolution of clinical ethical dilemmas, most described three general functions: education about ethics and ethical decision making, ethical consultation or advice, and development or review of ethical aspects of policy. Some committees did not actually make the ethical consultation themselves; rather they tended to use independent consultants.

Advances in health care technology have brought with them numerous ethical decision-making challenges that require examination of personal beliefs, along with religious beliefs and legal boundaries. One area in which this becomes apparent is that of infertility. Nurses specializing in infertility care are frequently working with women who may have infertility based on maternal age. Is there a specific age at which infertility treatments should be denied? What about marital status? Socioeconomic status? Who should decide or be involved in the decision? Suppose a multifetal pregnancy has been achieved, but the woman wants to have only one baby, either for personal or practical reasons. What are the issues surrounding multifetal pregnancy reduction? What if the pregnancy was achieved through in vitro fertilization (IVF) and multiple embryos remain that have been frozen but are not desired by the woman or her partner and they do not wish to donate them to another infertile couple? What should happen to the embryos? Should they remain frozen in case the woman changes her mind? Should they be donated for practice? What if the woman and her partner wish to donate them for stem cell research?

All these issues are complex and controversial. To provide a legal framework for research and practice in the field of assisted reproduction, the Assisted Human Reproduction Act received royal assent in 2004 (Government of Canada, 2014). Subsequently, updated guidelines were published specifically for stem cell research (CIHI, 2010) (Box 1.4).

On the other side of fertility, that is, undesired pregnancy, the issue of personhood is also a dilemma, and one that is becoming more complex than ever with the advances in technology that have resulted in a blurring of the boundary between second-trimester abortion and fetal viability. Canada's criminal code states that a child becomes a human being when having "completely proceeded, in a living state, from the body of its mother" (Government of Canada, 2012d, p. 260).

Resolving ethical dilemmas requires the implementation of critical thinking. One of the most important aspects of applying a decision-making guideline to an ethical dilemma is that personal thoughts, beliefs, biases, and values need to be identified and acknowledged if the ethical dilemma is to be resolved appropriately and professionally. There are numerous structured decision-making strategies that have been developed specifically for, or that can be applied to, ethical decision making, including the nursing process. Murphy and Murphy (1976) developed a strategy that has been useful for health-related ethical decision making. The strategy does not include a focus on resolving the health issue. Rather, the focus is simply on deciding how to resolve the dilemma. Table 1.1 contains the steps of the Murphy and Murphy decision-making guide, along with the analogous nursing process steps.

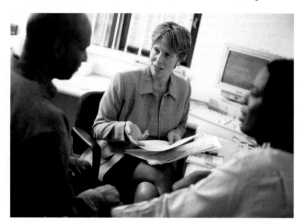

FIGURE 1.4 Nurses must carefully explain and obtain informed consent, as well as document that they have done so, to protect themselves, clients, colleagues, and employers.

● **BOX 1.4** **Embryonic Stem Cell Research**

Stem cell research holds potential to treat human disease and prevent suffering. Stem cells have the potential to provide treatments for a host of debilitating diseases including Alzheimer's, Parkinson's, diabetes, multiple sclerosis, heart disease, and spinal cord injury. Few other areas of science have generated as much excitement, scrutiny, and controversy. At the same time, their derivation and use raise ethical and social issues and legal concerns of interest to Canadians.

Canadian researchers have been pioneers in the area of stem cell research and continue to lead the way using animal models. With the introduction of these Guidelines, Canadian researchers have been able to move forward and remain at the forefront of their field while conducting their research according to explicit ethical standards.

Given the research potential and the ethical concerns inherent in human pluripotent stem cell research, CIHR convened an ad hoc Working Group on stem cell research, consisting of scientists, clinicians, philosophers and a lawyer, with national and international expertise in human reproductive tech-

nologies and stem cell research. While research on human adult stem cells was not included in the Working Group's mandate, recent scientific research has confirmed the possibility of generating stem cells with properties similar to embryonic stem cells from adult cells (eg, induced pluripotent stem cells). The Working Group considered its mandate to cover all human pluripotent cells, whatever their source, and the final guidelines are worded with that consideration in mind.

- Research undertaken should have potential health benefits for Canadians;
- Free and informed consent, provided voluntarily and with full disclosure of all information relevant to the consent;
- Respect for privacy and confidentiality;
- No direct or indirect payment for tissues collected for stem cell research and no financial incentives;
- No creation of embryos for research purposes;
- Respect individual and community notions of human dignity and physical, spiritual, and cultural integrity

Source: Canadian Institutes of Health Research. (2010). Updated guidelines for human pluripotent stem cell research, June 30, 2010. http://www.cihr-irsc.gc.ca/e/42071.html. Reproduced with the permission of the Minister of Public Works and Government Services Canada, 2013.

● **TABLE 1.1** **Comparison of Murphy and Murphy's Method of Ethical Decision Making with the Nursing Process**

Murphy and Murphy's Step	Component of the Nursing Process
1. Identify the health problem	Assessment
2. Identify the ethical problem	Assessment
3. State who is involved in making the decisions	Assessment
4. Identify your role, if any, in the decision-making process	Assessment
5. Consider as many possible alternative decisions as you can	Diagnosis
6. Consider the long- and short-range consequences of each alternative decision	Planning
7. Reach your decision	Implementation
8. Consider how this decision fits in with your general philosophy of client care	Evaluation
9. Follow the situation until you can see the actual results of your decision and use this information to help in making future decisions	Evaluation

Adapted from Murphy, M., & Murphy, J. (1976). Making ethical decisions—systematically. *Nursing, 6*(5), 13–14, p. 13.

Another method the nurse can use to gain knowledge about a situation in which ethical concerns may be raised is to view the situation from three levels: societal, institutional, and individual. By implementing this method of critical thinking, the multiple influences that affect decision making and outcomes in the specific situation will be illuminated, along with a possible direction regarding the most appropriate action for resolving the situation.

Examination has shown that Taohua, the 22-year-old from the beginning of the chapter, is pregnant. Taohua does not seem upset or surprised by this news. She says, "My aunt doesn't like my boyfriend, but I know he'll help me out. I wish she'd mind her own business, but I need her help financially right now. I'm just going to tell her nothing's wrong and let her know what's happening once Robert and I have made our decision." Think critically about the challenges that face her. What options does she have in relation to this pregnancy? What are the factors that need to be considered as she makes pregnancy-related decisions? What additional information do you need from her or from others in order to support her in her decisions?

Informed Consent

Health care consumers have a right to make informed decisions about their health care, and health care providers have an obligation to ensure that their clients are informed at a level at which active, informed decision making is possible. Although **informed consent** appears to have evolved from ethical principles, in fact, its origin is legal (Nelson-Marten & Rich, 1999). From the middle 1700s in England through the 1950s in the United States and elsewhere, there were several legal cases in which physicians were sued for not providing reasonable care—either through physical action (battery) or by not providing adequate verbal information about a medical procedure (Nelson-Marten & Rich, 1999). Since 1932, Canadian courts have required that physicians inform their patients of the nature and seriousness of treatment. In 1980, the requirement for disclosure of risks of treatment as part of informed consent was brought before the Supreme Court of Canada (Dillon, 1981). Provinces have passed legislation to address issues related to informed consent. For example, Prince Edward Island's legislation includes a "Consent to Treatment and Health Care Directives Act" that defines in detail what constitutes informed consent and the responsibilities of health care practitioners in relation to informed consent (Government of Prince Edward Island, 2010).

While the requirement for informed consent "serves the ethical goal of respecting patients' rights of self-determination . . . consent is a continuing process, not an event or signed form" (Dickens & Cook, 2004). Some ethicists believe that the emphasis on obtaining consent has overshadowed the duty of the health care provider to disclose information that will enable the client to make informed choices (Cook et al., 2003). Politi and Street (2011) proposed a collaborative decision-making model that involves "providing clear explanations, checking for understanding, eliciting the patient's values, concerns, needs, finding common ground, reaching consensus on a treatment plan, and establishing a mutually-acceptable follow-up plan" (p. 579).

Informed Consent for Health Care

Nurses are involved in two types of consent situations in clinical practice: getting consent for what nurses do and participating in the consent process for what other health care professionals do. In the first situation, when carrying out an invasive nursing procedure nurses should provide an explanation and document that the explanation was given and consent obtained. Any touching of a client requires verbal, and in some cases, written consent (Canadian Nurses Protective Society [CNPS], 1994). A nurse may assume that a client who gives permission for a specific routine procedure automatically gives permission for additional procedures. That assumption, however, may be incorrect and result in violation of the client's rights (CNPS, 1994). Encouraging the client to make an informed decision about a procedure will ensure that her rights are upheld. For example, explaining to a client about postpartum assessment, including the nurse's actions, and the benefits and risks of having the assessment completed at specific intervals, followed by an assessment of client understanding and verbal permission or denial to perform the assessment, will help ensure that the client has made an informed decision. If the client refuses, the nurse has no right or authority to proceed. Failure to obtain consent could result in professional sanctions, civil liability, and/or criminal charges (CNPS, 1994). The nurse documents the intervention very clearly in the client's chart and follow protocol in ensuring that the appropriate personnel, including the primary health care provider, are aware of the refusal to ensure the client's safety and rights. A client who has given informed consent has the right to change her mind and refuse a treatment or procedure at any time during the process, including after it has been initiated. Her decision must be shared with the health care provider who is implementing the treatment or procedure.

In the second situation, that is, when witnessing the signing of a consent form for treatment or surgery being performed by a physician, the physician (not the nurse) is responsible for provision of the information to the client. However, nurses have an ethical responsibility to inform the physician if the client does not understand the information or does not have enough information to make an informed decision. According to the CNA Code of Ethics (2008), the nurse is an advocate for the client and must provide information and support so that the client can make health care decisions.

One of the difficulties in achieving true informed consent—either verbal or written—is that many health care consumers are unaware of their basic rights in health care. Nurses are responsible for ensuring that clients understand their rights and then confirming that their rights have been upheld. Helping clients ask the questions that will get the answers they need is one way in which nurses can assist clients to participate in their care decisions. Providing informed consent is a form of personal empowerment. Barriers to informed consent are listed in Box 1.5.

Informed Consent for Research

Unlike informed consent for health care interventions, informed consent for research grew out of the ashes of

● BOX 1.5 Barriers to Informed Consent

Client-Focused Barriers

- Age, either very young or old;
- Education level, which may relate to the client's ability to process the information in the informed consent document;
- Illness, both presence and degree, which may affect the ability to process the information needed for informed consent;
- Relationship between the client and the primary health care provider, which may be construed as having coercive elements.

Process-Centred Barriers to Informed Consent

- Timing of the discussion related to the informed consent. For example, opening a discussion about a research protocol during the same meeting as receiving a devastating diagnosis will hinder informed consent;
- Time allocated for the prospective participant/subject to discuss the informed consent with the person responsible for the study;
- Reading level and the actual wording of the information in the informed consent document.

Adapted from Taylor, H. A. (1999). Barriers to informed consent. *Seminars in Oncology Nursing, 15*(2), 89–95.

the Holocaust. Among the atrocities of the Nazi regime, physicians performed horrible "experiments" involving pain, mutilation, and death on innocent men, women, and children imprisoned in the concentration camps. Following World War II, these physicians were brought to trial by the world in Nuremberg, and the need for ethically based research was brought to the awareness of the world (E. Weisel, as cited in Nelson-Marten & Rich, 1999). In Canada, researchers who conduct studies on human subjects are required to follow formal guidelines (Tri-Council Policy Statement, 2010) and undergo peer review by Research Ethics Boards. Health Canada and Public Health Agency of Canada (2010) clearly outline the requirements for informed consent for research.

Frequently, a client who is a recipient of nursing care is also approached to participate in a research study. It is imperative that the nurse as a client advocate, regardless of whether he or she is involved in the research itself or is focused on providing nursing care to the client, ensures that the client receiving health care does not feel coerced to participate in the study. The client needs to be assured that, regardless of whether she becomes or remains a study participant, the level of care she experiences will be completely independent of her

decision regarding research participation. It is of equal importance to determine that the client does indeed understand the study enough to provide true informed consent.

 As Elaine is leaving the nurse practitioner's office, she sees a flyer on the bulletin board recruiting participants for a research study on the effects of a new exercise program. Elaine points to the flyer and asks, "Does this study pay money? If I agree to participate, can we postpone starting one of these drugs you've prescribed?" How can the nurse respond?

NURSING AND WOMEN'S HEALTH RESEARCH

Historically, research relied almost exclusively on male subjects with specific cultural and racial characteristics. Women were excluded from research, particularly clinical trials. Failure to implement and consider sex and gender in research compromised its validity and the applicability of programs. The PHAC (2012b) has adopted the position that health research and intervention are about everyone's health, not solely about women's or men's health. "[This] was a transformative change that is still gaining momentum and endorsement across research areas" (PHAC, 2012b, section 1).

Developments of note in the surveillance of women's health include the Prairie Women's Health Centre of Excellence, which developed a "Profile of Women's Health in Manitoba," a comprehensive review of indicators of Manitoba women's health including health status, health services use, socioeconomic influences, health system performance, and lifestyle choices. Similar to the Manitoba review, the "Ontario Women's Health Status Report" also looks at determinants of health of Ontario women. This report looks at the physical, social, emotional, cultural, and spiritual well-being of women and provides information on the demographics, morbidity indicators, reproductive health, and health behaviours of women. It also provides information on subpopulations such as lone mothers, senior women, immigrant and visible minority women, Aboriginal women, and rural and northern women (PHAC, 2012b).

Other organizations are also addressing these issues. For example, the Women's Health Research Foundation of Canada is dedicated to the "improvement of women's health in its broadest terms–social, psychological and physical well-being" (Women's Health Research Foundation, 2013, para. 1). The Foundation has identified some of the factors influencing women's health: lack of research in women's health issues, poverty, increased burden on women as caregivers, domestic violence, marginalized women, and lack of women in policy making. As well, there are groups dedicated to the health of Aboriginal women, such as the Native Women's Association of Canada (http://www.nwac.ca/) and the Aboriginal Women's Health and Healing Research Group (2012). Because the health of women throughout the life cycle reflects racial, ethnic, and socioeconomic diversity, research should reflect the importance of understanding these differences, as well as the similarities. Understanding the responses and experiences of women throughout the life cycle is imperative for safe and effective nursing care. The very nature of nursing practice places nurses in an optimal position to be participants in research. By using critical thinking skills along with clinical expertise, theoretical knowledge, and research, nurses can make a difference in the health of their clients.

Many nurses are reluctant to use research findings as a basis for their practice. Several reasons exist for this reluctance. Comfort with evaluating research varies greatly among nurses. Research may not be easily available in a practice setting, or research may be used inappropriately to guide practice changes, for example, implementing a practice change based on a single study that additional research has not validated. Some of these objections can be eliminated through the use of systematic reviews that include the meta-analysis of research studies. The Cochrane Collaboration (http://www.cochrane.org) is an international organization focused primarily on ensuring the availability of the outcomes of health care research. Although this endeavour provides the most accurate and up-to-date studies of practice evidence available, it may not be readily accessible by many of the people in need of the information. One strategy for improving the adoption of evidence-based practice was documented by Wallen et al. (2010), who found that a mentorship program had positive effects on nurses' perceptions of research. They also identified a need for leadership support and dedicated resources to facilitate such practice. Institutional objections to the implementation of evidence-based practice may include lack of knowledge regarding research, or resource allocation that does not incorporate the time needed to seek out the relevant evidence.

Nurses can foster evidence-based practice by using practice guidelines focused on specific client needs. Implementation of these guidelines will help nurses develop more effective care because interventions have been evaluated in multiple sites by multiple

● **BOX 1.6** **Association of Women's Health, Obstetric and Neonatal Nurses (AWHONN)**

- Advances the nursing profession in the United States, Canada, and elsewhere.
- Recognized by the Canadian Nurses Association as representing perinatal, neonatal, and women's health nurses.
- Provides information based on current research and clinical practice to help nurses deliver high-quality care for women and newborns.
- Outlines general guidelines for optimal practice in its document Standards for Professional Perinatal Nursing Practice and Certification in Canada.
- Guidelines may change according to changes in research and practice.

Source: AWHONN. (2009). *Standards for professional perinatal nursing practice and certification in Canada* (2nd ed.). Washington, DC: Author.

individuals caring for different clients. And, the more effective the intervention, the more cost-effective it is for the institution, and the more likely it is that the organization will support evidence-based practice. There are a number of organizations that can help nurses access practice guidelines. One such organization is the Association of Women's Health, Obstetric and Neonatal Nurses (AWHONN) (Box 1.6). As well, the Canadian Association of Perinatal and Women's Health Nurses (CAPWHN) is accessible to nurses who work in women's health, obstetric, and newborn care (Box 1.7).

● **BOX 1.7** **Canadian Association of Perinatal and Women's Health Nurses (CAPWHN)**

- Goal is to improve health and health care of women, newborns, and families.
- Promotes excellence in nursing practice, leadership, education, and research in the areas of perinatal and women's health care.
- Facilitates networking and learning among perinatal and women's health nurses.
- Promotes evidence-based practice through standards, policies, guidelines, and programs.
- Advocates for informed choice and family-centred care.
- Collaborates with other professional groups and health-related organizations.

Source: Canadian Association of Perinatal and Women's Health Nurses. (2013). *Mission, values and goals.* Available from http://www.capwhn.ca/en/capwhn/Mission_Values_and_Goals_p2607.html.

● **BOX 1.8 The Guiding Principles of Family-Centred Maternity and Newborn Care**

Family-centred maternity and newborn care is based on the following guiding principles:

● ***Birth is a normal, healthy process.*** For most women, pregnancy will progress smoothly to the birth of a healthy, much-welcomed baby. Supported by family and friends, birth can be a time of great happiness and fulfillment. Family-centred maternity and newborn care is based on respect for pregnancy as a state of health and for childbirth as a normal physiological process. It is a profound event in the life of both a woman and her family. For some women and families, however, pregnancy may be unplanned or unwanted; complications or adverse social circumstances may occur. The birth itself may be complicated and the outcome unexpected. In these situations, in order to support the family's unique needs, family-centred care is even more critical.

● ***Pregnancy and birth are unique for each woman.*** Women have diverse experiences and needs. Women and families hold different philosophies of birth, based on their specific knowledge, experience, culture, social and family background, and belief systems. Support and care should be respectful of such factors. Some women have negative, fearful feelings about birth and are reluctant to take charge of their own care. These feelings need to be acknowledged. The approach to caring for women and families should involve adapting care to meet their needs, rather than expecting women and families to adapt to institution or provider needs.

● ***The central objective of care for women, babies, and families is to maximize the probability of a healthy woman giving birth to a healthy baby.*** No one cares more about achieving a safe and happy outcome to a pregnancy than the pregnant woman and her family. Their goal is a positive and fulfilling pregnancy, childbirth, and early postpartum period. Health care providers share this aim. Clearly, it is important to recognize each woman as an individual; each needs clear and unbiased information as to the options available to her.

● ***Family-centred maternity and newborn care is based on research evidence.*** Wherever possible, these national guidelines are based on research evidence. As already stated, if the evidence is unclear, it is noted. If a clear benefit based on strong research evidence has emerged, details are provided. If there are risks, these are noted. If no or limited research is available, it is recommended that evidence be developed. Resources for assisting with the evaluation of available evidence, and for planning and implementing research projects, include the Cochrane Library; university departments of nursing, medicine, midwifery and others;

regional perinatal centres; public health units; researchers; and consultants. Finally, one should be aware of the limitations of evidence-based practice. Much research evidence has still to be collected.

● ***Relationships between women, their families, and health care providers are based on mutual respect and trust.*** It is important for health care providers to respect and support a woman and her family. This will help her to give birth safely, with power and dignity. As well, it is crucial that a woman and her family respect and trust their health care providers. The provision of family-centred maternity and newborn care depends on such mutual respect and trust.

● ***Women are cared for within the context of their families.*** A woman's family is key when she is pregnant and giving birth. It is part of her system of care. It is up to the woman to define her family and supports; she chooses who is included or excluded. Her definition of family may include only one person, or many different people. These may be the baby's father, siblings, and grandparents; the woman's partner; the baby's aunts and uncles; the woman's friends; and so on. Family-centred care treats the family as a unit of care.

● ***In order to make informed choices, women and their families need knowledge about their care.*** Enabling a true choice among alternatives means providing information about the real options available, entering into an open dialogue that is respectful of all concerns and opinions, and providing flexible policies that accommodate planning and decision making. Sharing information is a mutual responsibility of health care providers, agencies, women, and families. The benefits and risks of all procedures need to be disclosed, as well as all the options that women and families might consider. It is not enough to expect women to bring their "choices" with them—health care providers need to provide time, support, and encouragement for exploration of the various options.

● ***Women have autonomy in decision making. Through respect and informed choice, women are empowered to take responsibility.*** Women are the primary decision makers about their care. Women and families make decisions based on many factors—the expertise of professionals being one. Health care providers can encourage and guide those women and families wishing to seek out resources for such decision making. When all relevant information has been made available to women and families for the achievement of their goals, they are guided, not directed, by the professionals they have chosen to share the responsibility for their care.

(box continues on page 26)

● **BOX 1.8** The Guiding Principles of Family-Centred Maternity and Newborn Care (continued)

● *Health care providers have a powerful effect on women who are giving birth and their families.* How a woman feels about pregnancy and childbirth is determined by at least two powerful factors: previous life experiences and the emotional support received at those times. Studies of women's satisfaction with the childbirth experience and their perceptions of the personal effects of childbirth show that satisfaction is more highly associated with the emotional care received during labour than with the birth process itself. Women remember the events of birth and their attendant feelings throughout their lives (Simkin, 1996). They remember the specific words and actions of their health care providers. Satisfaction is linked to the type of care received and the feelings of personal control and accomplishment. Health care providers must be aware of their power to influence the long-term impact of the woman's childbirth experience.

● *Family-centred care welcomes a variety of health care providers.* Women choose from a variety of health care providers of care and support during the pregnancy, birth, and early parenting periods. Health care providers need to communicate with, respect, and trust one another; to work together for the woman, her baby, and her family. Health care providers include physicians, nurses, midwives, labour companions or doulas (a lay person who provides support during labour), childbirth educators, and various others who help with physical or social needs.

● *Technology is used appropriately in family-centred maternity and newborn care.* Technology is to be used judiciously and appropriately, and only if a benefit has been demonstrated. For example, it is important that technology not be used in place of direct supportive care and observation. As well, the issue of safety should not be viewed as a reason for *unnecessary* intervention and technological surveillance; it only detracts from the experience of the mother and family.

● *Quality of care includes a number of indicators.* When measuring quality of care, it is important to monitor not only indicators such as morbidity and mortality, but also women's experience of pregnancy, birth, and postpartum care. Measuring a woman's experience during childbirth and the postpartum period is a valuable quality-assurance activity. Health care providers can use various methods to obtain feedback about staff approaches, personal sense of control, comfort and attitude in the setting, learning, preparation, and so on. Input can be obtained from regular interviews, surveys or questionnaires, and comment cards or suggestion boxes.

● *Language is important.* The style of language and choice of words used in signs, printed material, and conversation often communicate as powerfully as the information conveyed. Because words can reflect attitudes of respect or disrespect, inclusion or exclusion, and judgement or acceptance, language choices can either ease or impede communication. Such words as "guidelines," "working together," and "welcome" convey openness and an appreciation for the position and importance of families. Words such as "policies," "allowed," and "not permitted" suggest that professionals are in authority over women and families. Referring to parents and other family members as "partners," "colleagues," "joint decision makers," or "experts" acknowledges that families bring important information and insight to pregnancy and childbirth, and that families and professionals together form a team.

Source: Public Health Agency of Canada. (2000). Family-centred maternity and newborn care: National guidelines. Reproduced with permission from the Minister of Health, 2013.

SUMMARY

● Demographic and sociopolitical changes in North America over the past several decades have resulted in more diverse roles for women and their significant others, along with changes in family structure and dynamics and in fertility.

● Two diverse health care systems are found in North America. The Canadian system is supported by the federal government; in theory, it guarantees access to health care for all Canadian citizens. The US health care system is primarily for-profit and access is not guaranteed for anyone, including pregnant women. The importance of increasing health promotion activities is becoming apparent within both systems.

● Critical thinking is integral to nursing practice. It requires the ability to see beyond the obvious and view a situation from multiple perspectives. The nursing process is one method by which critical thinking can be implemented in an organized manner.

● Best practices are those in which experience and research are used to lead to a desired result. The Canadian Nurses Association combines the concepts of best practices with standards of care that are based on the values of the profession, as articulated in the Code of Ethics for Registered Nurses (CNA, 2008).

● Evidenced-based practice, through the use of evidence-informed decision making, promotes the integration and implementation of scientifically based practice into nursing and health care. It requires critical thinking skills as well as an understanding of research and the ability to access pertinent information.

- Ethical principles guide nursing practice in both formal and informal ways. Formalized nursing codes have been developed to promote ethical values within nursing. Informally, nurses practice within an informal ethical code based on unwritten values held by nurses that have been generated through moral views, experiences, and the history of the profession.
- Ethical decision making can be facilitated through the use of formal strategies.
- Informed consent in clinical practice evolved from legal auspices, despite its apparent connection to ethical principles. In research, informed consent emerged from a history of unethical practices on subjects who were forced to participate in research.
- Informed consent ensures that the client or research subject is aware of the risks and benefits of the health intervention or the research study. Written consent provides legal support for the primary health care provider responsible for the intervention or the principal investigator of the research study. Informed consent is not a mandate for the client or research subject to complete, or even to begin, the intervention or study. The client may change her mind at any time and revoke the informed consent.
- Although historically women were not included in research, it is now recognized that women need to be included in all aspects of research and that the inclusion needs to encompass women throughout the life cycle. The role that nurses have in the research process will reflect their professional experience as well as their educational backgrounds.

Questions to Ponder

1. Taohua, the young woman who came to the clinic, has decided she will continue with her pregnancy. She is still not sure what involvement her boyfriend is going to have, but she wants to move out of her aunt's home into an apartment, drop two of her classes, and get a part time job. What barriers might she face in order to access antenatal care? Why is antenatal care important? Are there any strategies you could use that would be effective in working with her to promote her health?

2. A nursing student is at the grocery when she runs into a former classmate from high school who is visibly pregnant. The two women catch up on old times for a while, and then the student asks how far along in her pregnancy the other woman is. The classmate replies "About 5 months. I'm not really sure because I haven't seen a doctor yet. I'll probably go

this month, but my mom and aunts give me lots of advice."
   - What is the nursing student's role in this scenario? What questions might she want to ask?
   - How can the nursing student help her acquaintance and begin acting as an advocate and teacher?
   - How can nurses better emphasize in the community the importance of early prenatal care?

3. Two nurses are presenting an initiative to begin incorporating more evidence-based protocols and approaches for women's health in their public health clinic. A few of the nurses seem skeptical. One nurse questions the quality of studies and findings in this area. Another nurse says that she thinks the idea is good, but that the clinic is too busy to implement this in the best way possible.
   - How might the nurses be able to confront the skepticism and reluctance shown by their colleagues?
   - How might the nurses incorporate such an initiative in an efficient and organized way that may be better received by their associates?

REFERENCES

Aboriginal Affairs and Northern Development Canada. (2010a). *Indian residential schools settlement agreement.* Retrieved from http://www.aadnc-aandc.gc.ca/eng/1100100015638/1100100015639

Aboriginal Affairs and Northern Development Canada. (2010b). *Treaties with aboriginal people in Canada.* Retrieved from http://www.aadnc-aandc.gc.ca/eng/1100100032291/1100100032292

Aboriginal Women's Health and Healing Research Group. (2012). *Canadian women's health network.* Retrieved from http://www.cwhn.ca/en/node/20083

Allen, J. (2009). *Aboriginal women and obesity in Canada: A review of the literature.* Dalhousie University, Canada: Atlantic Centre of Excellence for Women's Health. Retrieved from http://www.acewh.dal.ca/pdf/ab-obesity_lit-review_June2009rev.pdf

Association of Women's Health, Obstetric and Neonatal Nurses. (2009). *Perinatal nursing practice and certification in Canada* (2nd ed.). Washington, DC: Author.

Bélanger, A., & Gilbert, S. (2002). *The fertility of immigrant women and their daughters.* Statistics Canada, Catalogue no. 91–209-XIE, 127–153. Retrieved from http://www.statcan.gc.ca/pub/91–209-x/91–209-x2002000-eng.pdf

Canadian Association of Perinatal and Women's Health Nurses. (2011). *Joint position statement: Nurses and midwives collaborate on client-centred care.* Retrieved from http://www.capwhn.ca/en/capwhn/Joint_Position_Statement_Midwives_p3743.html

Canadian Association of Perinatal and Women's Health Nurses. (2013). *Mission, values and goals.* Retrieved from http://www.capwhn.ca/en/capwhn/Mission_Values_and_Goals_p2607.html

Canadian Diabetes Association. (2012). *Gestational diabetes: Preventing complications in pregnancy.* Retrieved from http://www.diabetes.ca/diabetes-and-you/what/gestational/

Canadian Encyclopedia. (2012). *Baby boom.* Retrieved from http://www.thecanadianencyclopedia.com/articles/baby-boom

Canadian Institute for Health Information. (2010). *Health indicators interactive tool.* Retrieved from http://www.cihi.ca/hirpt/?language=en&healthIndicatorSelection=RC_OBS

Canadian Institutes of Health Research. (2010). *Updated guidelines for human pluripotent stem cell research,* June 30, 2010.

Canadian Midwifery Regulators Consortium. (2012). *Legal status of midwifery in Canada.* Retrieved from http://cmrc-ccosf.ca/node/19

Canadian Midwifery Regulators Consortium. (2013). *Canadian model of midwifery practice.* Retrieved from http://cmrc-ccosf.ca/node/25

Canadian Nurses Association. (2008). *Code of ethics for registered nurses, 2008, centennial edition.* Retrieved from http://cna-aiic.ca/en

Canadian Nurses Association. (2010). *Position statement: Evidenced-informed decision-making and nursing practice.* Retrieved from http://www.nurseone.ca/docs/NurseOne/Public%20Documents/Evidence-Informed%20decision-making%20and%20nursing%20practice.pdf

Canadian Nurses Protective Society. (1994). Consent to treatment: The role of the nurse. *InfoLaw, 3*(2). Retrieved from www.cnps.ca

Chui, T. (2011). *Immigrant women. Women in Canada: A gender based statistical report.* Statistics Canada, Catalogue no. 89-503-X. Retrieved from http://www.statcan.gc.ca/pub/89-503-x/2010001/article/11528-eng.htm

Citizenship and Immigration Canada. (2011). *News Release—Canada welcomes highest number of legal immigrants in 50 years while taking action to maintain the integrity of Canada's immigration system.* Retrieved from http://www.cic.gc.ca/english/department/media/releases/2011/2011-02-13.asp

Cook, R., Dickens, B., & Fathalla, M. (2003). *Reproductive health and human rights: Integrating medicine, ethics, and law.* Oxford, New York: Clarendon Press.

Crompton, S. (2011). Women with activity limitations. *Women in Canada: A Gender-based Statistical Report.* Statistics Canada, catalogue no. 89-503-X. Retrieved from http://www.statcan.gc.ca/pub/89-503-x/2010001/article/11545-eng.pdf

Dickens, B., & Cook, R. (2004). Dimensions of informed consent to treatment. *International Journal of Gynaecology and Obstetrics, 85*(3), 309–314. Retrieved from http://www.ncbi.nlm.nih.gov/pubmed/15145279

Dillon, J. (1981). Informed consent and the disclosure of risks of treatment: The Supreme Court of Canada decides. *Journal of Medical Humanities, 3*(3–4), 156–162. Retrieved from http://www.springerlink.com/content/q262n2885r0635h7/

EcoKids. (n.d.). *Who are the First Nations and Inuit peoples in Canada?* Retrieved from http://www.ecokids.ca/pub/eco_info/topics/first_nations_inuit/groups.cfm

Farrao, V. (2012). Paid work. *Women in Canada.* Statistics Canada, Catalogue no. 89-503-x. Retrieved from http://www.statcan.gc.ca/pub/89-503-x/2010001/article/11387-eng.htm

Gaudine, A., Lamb, M., LeFort, S., & Thorne, L. (2011). The functioning of hospital ethics committees: A multiple-case study of four Canadian committees. *HEC Forum, 23*(3), 225–238. doi:10.1007/s10730-011-9151-z. Springer Science+Business Media B.V. 2011. Retrieved from http://link.springer.com/article/10.1007%2Fs10730-011-9151-z?LI=true

Gill, K. (2012). The health care system in the U.S. *About.com US Politics.* Retrieved from http://uspolitics.about.com/od/healthcare/tp/health_care_overview.htm

Government of Canada. (2008). *History of bilingualism in Canada.* Retrieved from http://www.pch.gc.ca/pgm/lo-ol/bllng/hist-eng.cfm

Government of Canada. (2012a). *Canadian bill of rights.* Retrieved from http://laws-lois.justice.gc.ca/eng/acts/C-12.3/page-1.html

Government of Canada. (2012b). *Canadian multiculturalism act.* Retrieved from http://laws-lois.justice.gc.ca/eng/acts/c-18.7/page-1.html

Government of Canada. (2012c). *Constitution act, 1982.* Retrieved from http://laws-lois.justice.gc.ca/eng/Const/page-15.html

Government of Canada. (2012d). *Criminal Code of Canada: Statute 223. When a child becomes a human being.* Retrieved from http://laws-lois.justice.gc.ca/PDF/C-46.pdf

Government of Canada. (2014). *Justice laws website: Assisted human reproduction act.* Retrieved from http://laws-lois.justice.gc.ca/eng/acts/A-13.4/page-1.html

Government of Prince Edward Island. (2010). *Consent to treatment and health directives act.* Retrieved from http://www.gov.pe.ca/law/statutes/pdf/c-17_2.pdf

Gushulak, B., Pottie, K., Roberts, J. H., Torres, S., & DesMeules, M. (2010). Migration and health in Canada: Health in the global village. *Canadian Medical Association Journal.* doi:10.1503/cmaj090287. Retrieved from http://www.cmaj.ca/content/early/2010/06/28/cmaj.090287.full.pdf+html

Hanson, E. (2009). *The residential school system.* Vancouver, BC: University of British Columbia. Retrieved from http://indigenousfoundations.arts.ubc.ca/home/government-policy/the-residential-school-system.html

Health Canada. (2011a). *A statistical profile on the health of first nations in Canada. Vital statistics for Atlantic and Western Canada, 2001/2002.* Retrieved from http://www.hc-sc.gc.ca/fniah-spnia/alt_formats/pdf/pubs/aborig-autoch/stats-profil-atlant/vital-statistics-eng.pdf

Health Canada. (2011b). *Eating well with Canada's food guide.* Retrieved from http://www.hc-sc.gc.ca/fn-an/food-guide-aliment/index-eng.php

Health Canada. (2012a). *Canada's health care system.* Retrieved from http://www.hc-sc.gc.ca/hcs-sss/index-eng.php.

Health Canada. (2012b). *Canada's health care system: About primary health care.* Retrieved from http://www.hc-sc.gc.ca/hcs-sss/prim/about-apropos-eng.php

Health Canada and Public Health Agency of Canada. (2010). *Requirements for informed consent documents. Science and research.* Research Ethics Board, March 2010. Retrieved from http://www.hc-sc.gc.ca/sr-sr/alt_formats/pdf/advice-avis/reb-cer/consent/document-consent-document-eng.pdf

Health Council of Canada. (2011). *Understanding and improving aboriginal maternal and child health in Canada.* December, 2011. Retrieved from http://www.healthcouncilcanada.ca/rpt_det.php?id=172

Higginbottom, G. (2013). iMOM-international migration, optimizing maternal health research. *Worldwide Universities Network.* Retrieved from http://www.wun.ac.uk/research/imom-international-migration-optimizing-maternal-health-research

Higginbottom, G., Morgan, M., Dassanayake, J., Eyford, H., Alexandre, M., Chiu, Y. et al. (2012). Immigrant women's experiences of maternity-care services in Canada: A protocol for systematic review using a narrative synthesis. *Systematic Reviews, 1,* 27. doi:10.1186/2046-4053-1-27. Retrieved from http://www.ncbi.nlm.nih.gov/pubmed/22651573

Huck, O., Tenenbaum, H., & Davideau, J. L. (2011). Relationship between periodontal diseases and preterm birth: Recent epidemiological and biological data. *Journal of Pregnancy,* Article ID 164654, 8 pages doi:10.1155/2011/164654. Retrieved from http://www.ncbi.nlm.nih.gov/pmc/articles/PMC3205685/

Human Resources and Skills Development Canada. (2013a). *Indicators of well-being in Canada. Canadians in context-aboriginal population.* Retrieved from http://www4.hrsdc.gc.ca/.3ndic.1 t.4 r@-eng.jsp?iid=36

Human Resources and Skills Development Canada. (2013b). *Indicators of well being in Canada. Canadians in context-population size and growth.* Retrieved from http://www4.hrsdc.gc.ca/.3ndic.1 t.4 r@-eng.jsp?iid=35

Human Resources and Skills Development Canada. (2013c). *Indicators of well being in Canada. Family life—age of mother at childbirth.* Retrieved from http://www4.hrsdc.gc.ca/.3ndic.1 t.4 r@-eng.jsp?iid=75

Human Resources and Skills Development Canada. (2013d). *Indicators of well being in Canada. Health—obesity.* Retrieved from http://www4.hrsdc.gc.ca/.3ndic.1 t.4 r@-eng.jsp?iid=8

Human Resources and Skills Development Canada. (2013e). *Indicators of well being in Canada. Health—physical activity.* Retrieved from http://www4.hrsdc.gc.ca/.3ndic.1 t.4 r@-eng.jsp?iid=6

Indexmundi. (2011). *Infant mortality rate.* Retrieved from http://www.indexmundi.com/g/g.aspx?c=ca&v=29

Indexmundi. (2012a). *Canada demographics 2012.* Retrieved from http://www.indexmundi.com/canada/demographics_profile.html

Indexmundi. (2012b). *Country comparison. Maternal mortality rate.* Retrieved from http://www.indexmundi.com/g/r.aspx?v=2223

Indexmundi. (2012c). *Historical data graphs per year. Total fertility rate.* Retrieved from http://www.indexmundi.com/g/g. aspx?c=ca&v=31

Johnson, J.A., Tough, S., & Society of Obstetricians and Gynaecologists of Canada. (2012). Delayed child bearing. *Journal of Obstetrics and Gynaecology Canada, 34*(1), 80–93.

Leipert, B., Delaney, J., Forbes, D., & Forchuk, C. (2011). Canadian women's experiences with rural primary health care nurse practitioners. *Online Journal of Rural Nursing and Health Care, 11*(1), 37–53. Retrieved from http://rnojournal.binghamton.edu/index. php/RNO/issue/view/3

Loppie-Reading, C., & Wien, F. (2009). *Health inequalities and social determinants of aboriginal peoples' health.* Prince George, BC: National Collaborating Centre of Aboriginal Health. Retrieved from http://ahrnets.ca/files/2011/02/NCCAH-Loppie-Wien_Report.pdf

Malott, A. M., Davis, B. M., McDonald, H., & Hutton, E. (2009). Midwifery care in eight industrialized countries: How does Canadian midwifery compare? *Journal of Obstetrics and Gynaecology Canada, 21*(10), 974–979. Retrieved from http://www.jogc. com/abstracts/full/200910_WomensHealth_7.pdf

Miller, K., Couchie, C., Ehman, W., Graves, L., Grzybowski, S., & Medves, J. (2012). *Rural maternity care.* SOGC Joint Position Paper 282, October. Retrieved from http://sogc.org/wp-content/ uploads/2013/01/gui282PP1210E_000.pdf

Mosby, I. (2013). Administering colonial science: Nutrition research and human biomedical experimentation in Aboriginal communities and residential schools, 1942–1952. *Social History, 46*(91), 145–172. Retrieved from http://muse.jhu.edu/journals/histoire_ sociale_social_history/v046/46.91.mosby.html

Mulnix, J. (2010). Thinking critically about critical thinking. *Educational Philosophy and Theory, 44*(5), 464–479. doi:10.1111/ j.1469–5812.2010.00673.x. Retrieved from http://onlinelibrary. wiley.com/doi/10.1111/j.1469–5812.2010.00673.x/full

Murphy, M., & Murphy, J. (1976). Making ethical decisions—systematically. *Nursing, 6*(5), 13–14.

Nelson-Marten, P., & Rich, B. A. (1999). A historical perspective of informed consent in clinical practice and research. *Seminars in Oncology Nursing, 15*(2), 81–88.

Nevo, I., & Slonim-Nevo, V. (2011). The myth of evidence-based practice: Towards evidence-informed practice. *British Journal of Social Work, 41*(6), 1176–1197. Retrieved from http://bjsw. oxfordjournals.org/content/early/2011/01/24/bjsw.bcq149

Ng, E., Pottie, K., & Spitzer, D. (2011). Official language proficiency and self-reported health among immigrants to Canada. Statistics Canada, Catalogue no. 82-003-X. Retrieved from http://www.statcan.gc.ca/pub/82–003-x/2011004/article/ 11559-eng.pdf

Ontario Midwives. (2012). *Hypertensive disorders of pregnancy.* Clinical Practice Guideline No. 15. June 2012. Retrieved from http://www.aom.on.ca/files/Health_Care_Professionals/Clinical_ Practice_Guidelines/No_15_CPG_HDP_062612.pdf

Parliament of Canada. (2000). *The royal commission on aboriginal peoples.* Ottawa, ON: Government of Canada. Retrieved from http://www.parl.gc.ca/Content/LOP/ResearchPublications/ prb9924-e.htm

Parliament of Canada. (2005). *Bill C-38: The civil marriage act.* Ottawa, ON: Government of Canada. Retrieved from http:// www.parl.gc.ca/About/Parliament/LegislativeSummaries/bills_ ls.asp?ls=c38&Parl=38&Ses=1

Politi, M., & Street, R. (2011). The importance of communication in collaborative decision making: Facilitating shared mind and management of uncertainty. *Journal of Evaluation in Clinical Practice, 17*(4), 579–584. Retrieved from http://onlinelibrary.wiley. com.cyber.usask.ca/doi/10.1111/j.1365--2753.2010.01549.x/ full

Public Health Agency of Canada. (2009). *What mothers say: The Canadian maternity experiences survey.* Retrieved from http:// www.publichealth.gc.ca/mes

Public Health Agency of Canada. (2011). *Maternal mortality in Canada.* Fact sheet. Retrieved from http://www.phac-aspc.gc.ca/rhs-ssg/ maternal-maternelle/mortality-mortalite/index-eng.php

Public Health Agency of Canada. (2012a). *Social determinants of health.* Canadian Best Practices Portal. Retrieved from http:// cbpp-pcpe.phac-aspc.gc.ca/public-health-topics/social-determinants-of-health/

Public Health Agency of Canada. (2012b). *The chief public health officer's report on the state of public health in Canada.* Chapter 4: Integrating Sex and Gender into Health Interventions. Retrieved from http://www.phac-aspc.gc.ca/cphorsphc-respcacsp/2012/chap-4-eng.php

Simich, L., & Jackson, B. (2010). What makes some immigrants healthy and others not? *Health Canada, Health Policy Research Bulletin, 17,* 26–29. Retrieved from http://www.hc-sc.gc.ca/sr-sr/alt_formats/pdf/ pubs/hpr-rpms/bull/2010-health-sante-migr-eng.pdf

Simpkin, P. (1996). The experience of maternity in a woman's life. *Journal of Obstetric, Gynecologic and Neonatal Nursing, 25*(3), 247–252.

Sinclair, R. (2011). *The 60's scoop. Origins Canada.* Retrieved from http://www.originscanada.org/the-stolen-generation/

Society of Obstetricians and Gynaecologists of Canada. (2011a). *Healthy eating, exercise and weight gain—before and during pregnancy.* Clinical Practice Guideline, Women's Health Information: Pregnancy. Retrieved from http://www.sogc.org/health/ healthy-eating_e.asp

Society of Obstetricians and Gynaecologists of Canada (2011b). *HIV testing in pregnancy.* Clinical Practice Guideline, Women's Health Information: Pregnancy. Retrieved from http://www.sogc.org/ health/pregnancy-hiv_e.asp#breast-feeding

Statistics Canada. (2008). *Aboriginal peoples, 2006 census.* (Release no. 5, January 15, 2008). Retrieved from http://www12.statcan. gc.ca/census-recensement/2006/rt-td/ap-pa-eng.cfm

Statistics Canada. (2011a). *Ethnic diversity and immigration.* (Catalogue no. 11-402-X). Retrieved from http://www.statcan.gc.ca/ pub/11-402-x/2011000/chap/imm/imm-eng.htm

Statistics Canada. (2011b). *Population projections by Aboriginal identity in Canada, 2006 to 2031.* (Catalogue no. 91-552-X). Retrieved from http://www.statcan.gc.ca/pub/91-552-x/91-552-x2011001-eng.htm

Statistics Canada. (2012a). *Age-specific fertility rate of females.* Retrieved from http://www.statcan.gc.ca/concepts/definitions/ fertility-fecondite02-eng.htm

Statistics Canada. (2012b). *Fifty years of families in Canada: 1961 to 2011.* (Catalogue no. 98-312-X2011003). Retrieved from http:// www12.statcan.gc.ca/census-recensement/2011/as-sa/98-312-x/98-312-x2011003_1-eng.cfm

Statistics Canada. (2012c). *Health indicators framework.* (Catalogue no. 82-221-X). Retrieved from http://www.statcan.gc.ca/pub/82–221-x/2012002/hifw-eng.htm

Statistics Canada. (2012d). *Labour force characteristics by sex and age group.* (CANSIM table 282-0002). Retrieved from http://www. statcan.gc.ca/tables-tableaux/sum-som/l01/cst01/labor05-eng.htm

Statistics Canada. (2012e). *Life expectancy at birth.* (Catalogue no. 84-537-XIE). Retrieved from http://www.statcan.gc.ca/tables-tableaux/sum-som/l01/cst01/health26-eng.htm

Statistics Canada. (2012f). *Portrait of families and living arrangements in Canada.* (Catalogue no. 98-312-X2011001). Retrieved from http://www12.statcan.gc.ca/census-recensement/2011/as-sa/ 98-312-x/98-312-x2011001-eng.cfm

Statistics Canada. (2012g). *The Canadian population in 2011: Age and sex.* (Catalogue no. 98-311-X2011001). Retrieved from http://www12.statcan.gc.ca/census-recensement/2011/as-sa/ 98-311-x/98-311-x2011001-eng.cfm

Statistics Canada. (2012h). *The Canadian population in 2011: Population counts and growth.* (Catalogue no. 98-310-X2011001). Retrieved from http://www12.statcan.gc.ca/census-recensement/2011/as-sa/98-310-x/98-310-x2011001-eng.cfm

Thomas, D. (2011). *Personal networks and the economic adjustment of immigrants.* Statistics Canada. (Catalogue no. 11-008-X). Retrieved from http://www.statcan.gc.ca/pub/11-008-x/2011002/ article/11592-eng.pdf

Tri-Council Policy Statement. (2010). *Ethical conduct for research involving humans.* Panel on research ethics. Retrieved from http:// www.pre.ethics.gc.ca/eng/policy-politique/initiatives/tcps2-eptc2/Default/

Truth and Reconciliation Commission of Canada. (2013). Retrieved from http://www.trc.ca/websites/trcinstitution/index.php?p=3

Tyson, H. (2001). A new profession dedicated to normal birth. *Birth International*. Retrieved from https://www.birthinternational.com/articles/midwifery/83-the-re-emergence-of-canadian-midwifery

Wallen, G., Mitchell, S., Melnyk, B., Fineout-Overholt, E., Miller-Davis, C., Yates, J. et al. (2010). Implementing evidence-based practice: Effectiveness of a structured multifaceted mentorship programme. *Journal of Advanced Nursing, 66*(12), 2761–2771. doi:10.1111/j.1365–2648.2010.05442.x. Retrieved from http://www.ncbi.nlm.nih.gov/pubmed/20825512

Women's Health Research Foundation. (2013). *Improving women's health through research.* Retrieved from http://www.whrfcinc.com/index.html

CHAPTER 2

Health Promotion

Marilyn K. Evans and Gayle M. Roux*

Renee is a 33-year-old married woman with a 20-month-old son. During an annual checkup, the nurse discusses with Renee nutrition, exercise, and lifestyle. Renee says, "I've lost almost all the weight I gained during my pregnancy, but I was 7 kilograms heavier than I wanted to be before I became pregnant! Now I'm so busy, I'm worried I'll never get into shape. I don't have a specific weight I want to be; I just want to be a healthy weight."

Linda, a 53-year-old single accountant, comes to the clinic complaining of hot flashes. She has not menstruated for the past 9 months. She works approximately 50 hours a week, spending at least 7 hours each day at the computer. She does not like milk but tries to eat fruits and vegetables.

Jill, 25 years old, comes to the health care facility for her first vaginal examination and Pap smear. She looks very apprehensive when the nurse begins to take her health history. The nurse asks if anything is wrong. Jill responds, "I'm really scared about what will happen during the exam."

Nurses working with such clients need to understand this chapter to promote health effectively and to address each issue appropriately. You will learn more about these clients' circumstances as the chapter continues. Before beginning, consider the following points:

- What health issues are similar among the women? What concerns are different?
- How do age, lifestyle, and other circumstances influence health and illness?

*Contributor to first U.S. edition.

● How can nurses help active and busy women prevent health-related issues from becoming sources of stress?

● How can nurses help women become motivated to manage their self-care effectively?

LEARNING OBJECTIVES

On completion of this chapter, the reader should be able to:
● Define health promotion from a multidimensional perspective.
● Discuss history-taking parameters for nutritional, social, psychological, physical, sexual, reproductive, and breast health.
● Summarize health promotion issues of special concern for Aboriginal and immigrant women.
● Describe physical examination for women across the life span, discriminating expected findings from alterations.
● Identify collaborative health promotion strategies in women throughout the lifespan.
● Explain methods of early detection of common health issues in women throughout the lifespan.
● Identify health-screening guidelines for women throughout the lifespan.
● Identify immunization recommendations for women throughout the lifespan.

KEY TERMS

alternative therapies	mammogram
body mass index (BMI)	menarche
bone mineral density	menopause
breast cancer 1 and breast cancer 2	metabolic rate
genes (*BRCA1* and *BRCA2*)	osteoporosis
breast self-examination	perimenopause
clinical breast examination	postmenopausal
complementary therapies	risk factor
health	self-management
health promotion	ultrasound
inner strength	women's health

Health promotion encompasses all areas of a woman's life. Choices related to health reflect her place in the world, including her cultural, social, and spiritual perspectives. These perspectives help form the basis for the woman's actualization of her life choices.

Nurses are in a strong position to understand the complexity of beliefs and behaviours related to health promotion and to assume leadership positions in the primary care of women and their families. Health promotion is as important as, if not more than, secondary and tertiary health care measures. Nurses have the distinct opportunity to interact with consumers in key settings, including family practice sites, communities, schools, and places of employment. They are accountable for working to reduce preventable health problems such as obesity, diabetes, intimate partner violence, and heart disease by communicating and teaching women and their families about these issues. Health promotion and disease prevention can lessen these public health epidemics and provide cost-effective approaches to community health.

As the aging population increases, economic resources for health care will become more scarce (see Chapter 24). Strategies to prevent chronic health conditions and maintain optimum functioning for women across the life span and their families are critical challenges for nurses. Nurses are obligated to be aware of current research and evolving evidence-based protocols. Translating research findings into practice helps ensure that nurses remain at the forefront of changing health promotion strategies.

In this chapter we address common health promotion issues in women, including information on healthy lifestyles, risk factors for health problems, assessment and physical examination, and early screening (and intervention) for common health problems. Important areas of focus include nutrition, exercise, psychological health, physical health, and sexual, reproductive, and breast health.

HEALTH PROMOTION

Health is one of the key concepts of nursing. Definitions of health, health promotion, and women's health have evolved based on the current philosophy that clients control their bodies and act as partners with health care providers in decision making. For this reason, nurses no longer characterize health as the absence of illness or disability. Rather, they consider **health** to be total physical, psychological, and social well-being (World Health Organization [WHO], 2006). Health is a resource for living.

Health promotion is the process that allows people to increase control over, and thus improve, health and its determinants (WHO, 2009). Choices and actions related to health promotion reflect the person's cultural, educational, social, and spiritual perspectives. In this transformative process, the nurse functions as a partner with the client and family in education, consciousness raising, and advocacy. She or he shows respect for the client's autonomy and acknowledges the dynamic relationship between the client and the environment. The goals of health promotion are to maintain and improve health. Health promotion requires highly complex professional practices that emphasize planned changes in health-related conditions that affect individuals, groups, and populations (Rootman et al., 2012).

In the past, definitions of **women's health** focused primarily on reproduction. More recently, the view of women's health has broadened to include the health of women across the lifespan, with a focus on cultural, political, environmental, and societal issues that are distinctive to women (Association of Women's Health, Obstetric, and Neonatal Nurses, 2009; Morrow et al., 2007).

Many of today's health problems are amenable to community and public health approaches. Nurses can make a difference. Sharing their concerns about issues that affect women's health is a prerequisite to changing nursing practice. Nurses should also use statistical and research information as resource material for teaching plans. For example, the continued decrease in cervical cancer incidence and mortality in Canada over the past several years has been attributed to screening programs (Dickinson et al., 2012). Evidence shows screening for cervical cancer is less frequent among recent immigrants, visible minorities, older women, and those of low income and low education (Khadikar & Chan, 2013; Lofters et al., 2010). This is just one example that demonstrates the need for increased health education and comprehensive preventive programs to improve access to and quality of health care for women of all ages (Fig. 2.1).

Nursing Approaches to Health Promotion

Nursing views women holistically. From this perspective, the individual woman, her family, and her community are a single, complex entity. Nursing within this philosophy of care provides a means for growth and change. Whether women are confronting psychological

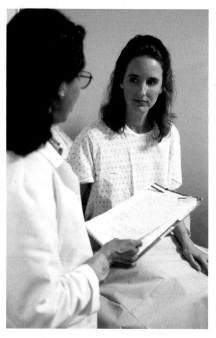

FIGURE 2.1 Screening measures and appropriate teaching are essential components of health promotion and disease prevention. Not only do women need to be encouraged to undergo routine screening, but they must also understand the importance of such examinations.

and physiologic stresses associated with substance abuse or intimate partner violence, developmental events such as menopause, or everyday decisions regarding exercise and nutrition, nurses can offer holistic approaches, support, and advocacy to improve and maintain health. Health promotion concepts include development of nursing theory in relation to empowerment, collaboration, participation, and equity (MacDonald, 2002).

Health promotion includes the complex dimensions of providing health education, marketing health messages, encouraging necessary lifestyle modifications, engaging in social and environmental changes, and incorporating the client's values. During a health history interview, nurses elicit the woman's beliefs about her health and her values as related to health behaviours and choices.

Health promotion includes both self-management strategies and interventions implemented by health care professionals. Therapies to promote and maintain health include both traditional and complementary or alternative therapies. **Complementary therapies** are nontraditional or integrative therapies that underscore or interface with traditional therapies, whereas **alternative therapies** are those used in place of traditional choices (National Center for Complementary and Alternative Medicine, 2013). Complementary/Alternative Medicine 2.1 provides a classification system with examples of common modalities.

Health Theories and Models

In many ways, the Canadian health care system remains disease-oriented. Researchers, theorists, and major public health movements have promoted a shift to valuing health promotion and fitness. In this framework, nurses form partnerships with women to blend professional therapeutic management with self-management of lifestyle and behaviour. This view conceptualizes health as an active process involving motivation, an ability to assume responsibility for health, respect for sociocultural values and economic issues, and integration of the entire person. The process is abstract and fluid. Theories evolve and are updated based on changing perspectives and research findings.

Initially, health promotion theories were criticized for being too individualistic and not designed to address broad contextual factors. For example, people may have difficulty changing behaviour not because they are "noncompliant," but because of challenges in finding access, resources, and services to support behaviours, as well as economic and cultural factors. The socioenvironmental approach to health promotion identifies factors such as housing, education, income, social support networks, social justice, health services, infrastructure, and equity that contribute to the health of an individual

or group (Mikkonen & Raphael, 2010). Using a holistic approach, nurses assist clients to promote growth toward health by focusing on strengths and facilitating clients' acceptance or overcoming of physical and sociopolitical challenges.

The educational background of nurses ideally suits them to apply theoretical concepts in clinical settings. The next section focuses on three models: the Health Promotion Model, the Transtheoretical Model, and the Theory of Inner Strength in Women. Nurses can use these and other approaches to identify assessment parameters and clinical interventions to enhance a client's strengths and promote her health. Nurses are encouraged to read further to apply techniques based on these theories to help clients and make meaningful lifestyle choices.

Health Promotion (Pender) Model

Nola Pender developed her Health Promotion Model in the early 1980s, with subsequent revisions (Pender, 1996). This model integrates nursing and behavioural sciences with a focus on health behaviours and decisions. Based on extensive research, it depicts health-promoting behaviours in relation to influences of individual characteristics and experiences, behaviour-specific cognitions and affect, commitment to a plan of action, and immediate competing demands (Fig. 2.2). Women must take responsibility for their own lifestyle choices. Nurses can assist clients to facilitate change, but only when both nurse and client explore the meaning of health promotion to the client and pinpoint the client's expectations. Nurses can use the model to shift thinking from blaming clients for weaknesses to empowering clients by building on strengths and promoting positive lifestyle changes.

Pender (1996) reports the "behaviour-specific cognitions and affect" category to contain the major motivational factors for health promotion and a focus for nursing intervention. The nurse should explore and discuss these variables with the client and family to modify health behaviours and lifestyle choices through nursing interventions. The Health Promotion Model takes an approach of partnership with the client that includes building strengths, using community resources, and fostering actualization of health potentials.

 Consider Renee, the 33-year-old with a toddler, who wants to be a healthy weight. Applying the Health Promotion Model, what information would be important to determine with her?

● COMPLEMENTARY/ALTERNATIVE MEDICINE 2.1
Classification System of Techniques With Examples

ALTERNATIVE SYSTEMS OF MEDICAL PRACTICE

- **Acupuncture:** Practitioners treat illnesses by applying needles to specific points on the body. The needles draw energy away from organs with excesses and redirect it to organs with deficits. Rebalanced energy flow relieves pain and restores health.
- **Ayurvedic medicine:** This comprehensive approach focuses on daily living in harmony with the laws of nature to achieve a clear mind, sturdy body, and peaceful spirit. Practitioners prescribe meditation, herbal therapy, yoga, and massage to maintain health or reverse disease.
- **Homeopathy:** Homeopathy means to "treat like with like." Practitioners believe that a substance that causes symptoms of illness in a healthy person may, in minute doses, also cure similar symptoms resulting from an illness.
- **Naturopathy:** This all-encompassing term refers to "natural health" modalities alone or in combination: acupuncture, herbal therapy, homeopathy, hydrotherapy, massage, nutrition, and osteopathy.
- **Traditional Chinese medicine:** This system is based on the principle of internal balance and harmony (Qi). Measures such as acupuncture, acupressure, moxibustion, exercise, advice on diet and lifestyle, and herbal medicines restore, maintain, or improve Qi.

MIND–BODY INTERVENTIONS

- **Imagery:** Negative thoughts and images can lead to illness; changing them to positive images can reverse the process. Regular use of imagery can increase relaxation, decrease pain, and facilitate healing.
- **Meditation:** A person tries to achieve awareness without thought. Meditation entails paying nonjudgmental, moment-to-moment attention to bringing about changes in perception and cognition.
- **Music therapy:** Practitioners use music to change behaviours, emotions, or physiology. Musical vibrations can help regulate a body "out of tune" and help maintain and enhance a body "in tune."

BIOLOGICALLY BASED THERAPIES

- **Aromatherapy:** Practitioners use essential oils to treat symptoms and for physiologic and psychological benefits.
- **Herbal therapies:** Practitioners use plant parts (including barks, roots, stems, flowers, leaves, fruits, seeds, or sap) as medicines.

MANIPULATIVE AND BODY-BASED METHODS

- **Massage:** Benefits of this systematic and scientific manipulation of soft tissues may include decreased stress and anxiety; enhanced mental clarity, energy, and performance; promotion of vitality, energy, and personal growth; and emotional release.
- **Tai Chi and Qigong:** Tai chi blends exercise and energy with choreographed movements performed with mental concentration and coordinated breathing. Qigong, a therapeutic Chinese practice, includes gentle exercises for the breath, body, mind, and voice. These modalities are often combined.
- **Yoga:** Yoga teaches basic principles of spiritual, mental, and physical energy to promote health and wellness. It uses proper breathing, movement, meditation, and postures to promote relaxation and enhance energy flow.

ENERGY THERAPIES

- **Bioelectromagnetic-based therapies:** Practitioners use magnetic fields to prevent and treat disease and as first aid for injuries.
- **Biofield therapies**
  - **Reflexology:** Reflexology involves massaging specific points on the hands or feet to relieve stress or pain in corresponding related body areas.
  - **Reiki:** This ancient Buddhist healing modality focuses on giving the body direct access to transcendental, universal, radiant, and light energies. Practitioners hold their hands in 12 basic positions on the client's head, chest, and back to access universal energy and help the client's body to rebalance and heal.
  - **Therapeutic touch and healing touch:** These two methods of energetic healing derive from the ancient practice of "the laying on of hands." Practitioners focus on the client's energy field to promote health.

From National Center for Complementary and Alternative Medicine. Retrieved from http://nccam.nih.gov

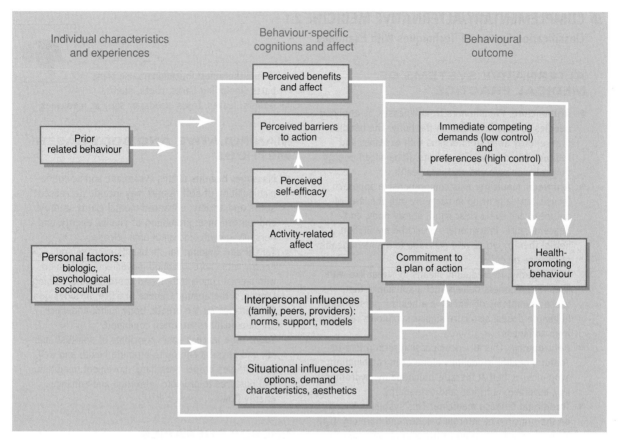

FIGURE 2.2   Pender's Health Promotion Model (Pender, 1996).

Transtheoretical Model

The Transtheoretical Model (Prochaska & DiClemente, 1983) depicts behaviour change through distinct motivational stages over time. It has been tested with lifestyle behaviours, including smoking cessation, exercise, and weight control. In this model, the stages of motivational readiness for behaviour change are as follows:

Precontemplation—not intending or not being ready to change
Contemplation—intending to change within 6 months
Preparation—actively planning change
Action—overtly making changes
Maintenance—sustaining change and preventing relapse
Relapse—expected, but desired to be transient; the person takes action again to sustain change (Prochaska et al., 1994).

This model provides a rationale for individualizing interventions based on a client's readiness for change. It continues to be researched for assessing a person's stage of change behaviour when moving from a detrimental to a healthy behaviour. Using this theory, the nurse can design intervention strategies with each client by customizing the plan of care to meet the current state of change. For example, the nurse may ask a client

who smokes, "Have you thought about quitting smoking?" If the client answers affirmatively, the nurse may continue, "What preparations have you made to help you quit?" Based on the state of readiness and desire to change, the nurse can develop effective interventions grounded in the client's experience and with a nonjudgmental approach.

Theory of Inner Strength in Women

A large body of literature explores health strengths and the interrelationship of a life-threatening or an otherwise demanding situation with the human biobehavioural response. The Theory of Inner Strength in Women (Dingley et al., 2000; Roux et al., 2002) is a gender-specific theory based on health strengths as a woman interacts with her environment during a challenging event or illness. The theory has been researched with women with breast cancer, heart disease, transplantation, and multiple sclerosis.

Inner strength is a positive healing force in healthy as well as in ill people. It underscores the desire to make changes to live as fully as possible. The middle-range theory of inner strength in women examines the woman's health needs from a model of strength as opposed to deficits. In a concept analysis of inner strength,

Dingley et al. (2000) described attributes as a component of spirituality, facet of quality of life, contributor to overcoming problems, and dimension of empowerment. A life-changing event or challenging experience initiates tapping into inner strength and its display. The essence of inner strength is an intrinsic human resource that promotes well-being and healing.

Although inner strength exists before the life-changing event, it is the *experience* of that event that often initiates the expansion and outward expression of inner strength. **Inner strength** means having the capacity to build self through a developmental process that positively moves the person through challenging events.

The four concepts of the theory of inner strength and their definitions are as follows: (1) *anguish and searching* describes the fear and searching for meaning experienced to process the challenging life event; (2) *connectedness* describes the nurturing of supportive relationships; (3) *engagement* describes the self-determinism and engaging in life possibilities; (4) *movement* describes the dimension of movement, rest, honest self-appraisal, and balance of mind and body. As women adjust to a chronic health condition, they connect with the future by reorienting themselves to a "new normal" in all life dimensions (Roux et al., 2002). This new normal encompasses responses to new activities, improved relationships, deeper understanding, different sense of purpose, and renewed spiritual connectedness.

This theory explains a process through which women can partner with health professionals to improve health outcomes. Enhancing women's inner strength is within the nurse's roles of providing care, guidance, counselling, consultation, and referral. Table 2.1 illustrates how a nurse could use the Theory of Inner Strength in Women to plan care for a woman recently diagnosed with breast cancer.

Gottlieb (2013) offers a strength-based approach to nursing practice. Nurses using this approach focus on a person's strengths rather than emphasizing problems or health deficits. Strength-based approach to care has the potential to enhance client empowerment and transformation.

HEALTH ASSESSMENT AND SCREENING

Successful assessment and screening programs for women involve many criteria and sociocultural considerations.

The first criterion for screening is that the condition has high incidence, morbidity, and mortality. An example is the need to evaluate diet, exercise, and lifestyle patterns for early detection of obesity, an epidemic that increases risks for morbidity and mortality from diabetes, heart disease, and some cancers (Centers for Disease Control and Prevention, 2012).

The second criterion is that testing is sensitive, inexpensive, and widely available. For example, practice settings can assess for alcoholism, postpartum depression, and intimate partner violence at essentially no cost by screening with easily administered, valid tools that identify high-risk women.

The third criterion is that early detection and treatment affect morbidity and mortality. Screening for cervical cancer is a good example. Some screening endeavours (eg, assessing psychological health, examining cultural beliefs about health behaviours) are

● TABLE 2.1 **Applying the Theory of Inner Strength in Women to a Client With Breast Cancer**

Theoretical Concept	Nursing Interventions
Anguish and searching: transition from shock and fear to acceptance	• Provide information about breast cancer. • Answer the client's questions. • Explain the meaning of the diagnosis to the client. • Encourage the client to voice her fears.
Movement: a realistic appraisal of one's abilities and limitations; awareness of life's possibilities	• Discuss exercise, sleep, and fatigue. Plan strategies for these areas based on the client's particular needs. • Encourage activity and balance.
Engagement: reframing circumstances to engage with life as a source of strength	• Encourage the client to put herself first and to make treatment decisions that are right for her. • Assist the client to ensure that her lifestyle includes time for reflection and relaxation. • Discuss economic and cultural concerns. • Suggest appropriate resources or referrals.
Connectedness: nurturing relationships with self, family, friends, and a Greater Source of Strength	• Assess the client's support systems. • Encourage the client to ask for help and to allow herself to experience support and caring from others. • Suggest outlets such as keeping a journal or meditating. • Assess and encourage spiritual outlets.

invaluable to the treatment and well-being of women, but outcomes may be more difficult to measure in terms of morbidity and mortality.

The fourth criterion for screening includes assessment of unique sociocultural and behavioural patterns.

This section includes information on assessment and screening for common health conditions in women, encompassing these four screening criteria.

Diet, Exercise, and Lifestyle

In 2007, Health Canada unveiled *Eating Well with Canada's Food Guide* (Health Canada, 2011), which can be individualized based on age, gender, and activity level to provide guidance on healthy nutritional choices (see Chapter 3, Fig. 3.2). A first-ever food guide tailored to Canada's Aboriginal population was released in April, 2007. It acknowledges the unique values, beliefs, traditions, and food choices among First Nations, Inuit, and Métis people (see Chapter 3, Fig. 3.3).

Nutritional education also should emphasize positive methods of cooking. For example, broiling is preferred to frying, because broiling decreases fat intake. Steaming vegetables retains more vitamins than does boiling them in water.

Although a balanced diet provides adequate vitamins and minerals, nurses give special consideration to each woman's health history, cultural practices, and developmental circumstances. For example, the woman who is over 50 needs to balance cholesterol and calcium needs by consuming low-fat dairy products for a daily calcium intake of 1,500 mg (Society of Obstetricians and Gynaecologists of Canada [SOGC], 2009). A woman with heavy menstrual periods is at increased risk for iron-deficiency anemia (MedLine Plus, 2013b). The nurse who performs a thorough health and diet history to identify nutritional risks for various stages can adapt dietary guidelines to meet special needs for specific clients (see Chapter 3).

Renee informs you that she has found a 3-day crash diet on the internet that guarantees weight loss of up to 10 pounds over 3 days. She says it is quite simple to follow and is strongly considering trying the diet but wants to know your thoughts. What might you say to her?

Overweight, Obesity, and Body Mass Index

Recent reports indicate that between 2000 and 2011, the percentage of obese Canadians has increased by almost 18%, with 25% to 30% of Canadians estimated to be obese (Gotay et al., 2013). The likelihood of progressing from overweight to obese is greater for women than for men (Le Petit & Berthelot, 2006). The Public Health Agency of Canada (PHAC) (2007) identified overweight and obesity as a major public health epidemic in Canada and globally. Health Canada and other sectors such as the Centre for Health Promotion (http://www. utoronto.ca/chp/) are actively working with various stakeholders to address the issue of obesity by promoting physical activity, healthy eating, and healthy weight. Although the terms *overweight* and *obesity* are often used interchangeably, they are distinct conditions of varying magnitude.

Body mass index (BMI) is a calculated measure of weight in relation to height (Health Canada, 2012b). It is one assessment parameter, along with height, weight, body measurements, hip-to-waist ratio, and percentage of body fat, used to determine overweight and obesity. Overweight is defined as a BMI between 25 and 30, obesity is defined as a BMI of 30 or greater, and extreme obesity is defined as a BMI of 40 or greater. Figure 2.3 depicts methods by which nurses can calculate a client's BMI and an accompanying scale for determining BMI status.

Recall Jill, the 25-year-old undergoing her first vaginal examination. As part of her evaluation, the nurse measures her height and weight. What would be Jill's BMI if she is 164 cm tall and weighs 62 kg?

Fat and Cholesterol

All fats are composed of fatty acids; their attributes are determined by the amounts and mixtures of fatty acids they contain. Fatty acids may be saturated, monounsaturated, or polyunsaturated, depending on their amount of hydrogen. *Saturated fatty acids* are found mainly in animal foods (eg, meat, poultry, butter, milk). *Monounsaturated fatty acids* are found in plant foods (eg, canola, peanut, and olive oils; nuts; avocados). *Polyunsaturated fatty acids* are found in plant foods (eg, corn and sesame oils, fish, and seafood). Through hydrogenation, polyunsaturated fatty acids can be made more saturated, resulting in a more stable semisolid form, called *trans fat* (Health Canada, 2007). *Trans fats* are in a wide range of foods, including most foods made with partially hydrogenated oils: baked goods, fried foods, and some margarine. High consumption of trans fats can lead to elevated cholesterol levels and subsequent cardiovascular and other problems (see later discussions).

Vitamins and Minerals

Vitamins and minerals are essential for life; a balanced, nutritious diet can provide them in sufficient amounts

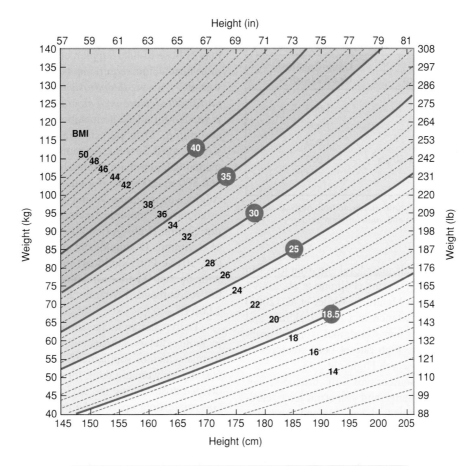

FIGURE 2.3 Measures to calculate and to interpret body mass index. From Douketis, J., Paradis, G., Keller, G., & Martineau, C. (2005). Canadian guidelines for body weight classification in adults: Application in clinical practice to screen for overweight and obesity and to assess disease risk. *Canadian Medical Association Journal, 172*(8). Retrieved from http://www.cmaj.ca/cgi/content/full/172/8/995.

(see Chapter 3). Because women do not always have the time, education, or finances to eat a balanced diet, nurses must be aware of common nutritional deficiencies in women. Two of the most important considerations are calcium and iron.

Calcium. Calcium needs vary with age (Table 2.2). Dairy products probably account for most calcium in the average Canadian diet. Concern has been raised that Canadians have an inadequate intake of calcium and vitamin D. In a nationwide survey, calcium intake by

● TABLE 2.2 **Recommendations for Calcium Intake in Women**

Demographic Group	Daily Calcium Needs (mg)
4–8 yrs	1,000
9–18 yrs	1,300
19–49 yrs	1,000
Pregnant or lactating, 19–50 yrs	1,000
50 yrs or older	1,500

From Osteoporosis Canada. (2013). Retrieved from http://www.osteoporosis.ca/osteoporosis-and-you/nutrition/calcium-requirements/

women was below the adequate level and even lower in women past the age of 50 years (Poliquin et al., 2009). In a study conducted in Manitoba, Weiler et al. (2007) found that Aboriginal women had lower calcium and vitamin D intakes than non-Aboriginal women, probably contributing to the high rate of bone fractures in Aboriginal women (Research Highlight 2.1).

Dietary calcium sources are milk products, calcium-fortified foods (orange and grapefruit juice, cereals, breads), calcium-fortified soy, almond, and rice beverages, dark green leafy vegetables, and canned salmon and sardines (with the bones) (Health Canada, 2012c). To balance calories and cholesterol, clients should opt for nonfat and low-fat dairy foods. It takes only three 300-mL glasses of milk to supply 1,000 mg of calcium. Women who need more dietary calcium may choose to take supplements. A woman can determine her calcium requirements by visiting the following website: *www.osteoporosis.ca/osteoporosis-and-you/nutrition/calculate-my-calcium/*. Because vitamin D is needed for adequate metabolism and proper calcium absorption, Osteoporosis Canada recommends that women aged 50 years or more take 1,500 mg of elemental calcium daily, preferably from dietary sources, and 800 to 2,000 IU of a vitamin D supplement daily. Adults who are under 50 and considered at high risk for osteoporosis, multiple fractures, or conditions affecting vitamin D absorption also require 800 to 2,000 IU of a vitamin D supplement daily (Osteoporosis Canada, 2013). For individuals under the age of 50 years with no risk factors affecting vitamin D absorption, the recommended vitamin D daily intake is 400 to 1,000 IU.

Daily calcium intake should not exceed 2,000 mg, including dietary sources and supplements. Most commercial calcium supplements come in pills of 200 to 500 mg. A woman taking three of these pills can take divided doses during the day or a single bedtime dose. Gastrointestinal upset is the most common side effect. Constipation, flatulence, gastric distention, and nausea also may be experienced.

Iron. Losses of iron from menstruation and the increased demands during pregnancy place women at

● **RESEARCH HIGHLIGHT 2.1** Canadian Aboriginal Women Have a Higher Prevalence of Vitamin D Deficiency Than Non-Aboriginal Women Despite Similar Dietary Vitamin D Intake

PURPOSE

Canadian Aboriginal women have high rates of bone fractures, possibly due to low dietary intake of minerals and vitamin D. This study was undertaken to estimate dietary intake of calcium and vitamin D, and to determine if there were disparities in intake between Aboriginal women and non-Aboriginal women. Serum levels of vitamin D were also measured.

DESIGN

A culturally appropriate dietary survey questionnaire was developed, validated, and administered to 183 urban-dwelling and 26 rural-dwelling Aboriginal women and 145 non-Aboriginal urban women in Manitoba, Canada.

RESULTS

Urban non-Aboriginal women had higher calcium intakes than urban Aboriginal women. The main sources for all groups were milk, cheese, yoghurt, orange juice, and breads. Canadian Aboriginal women, regardless of rural or urban residence, had lower calcium and vitamin D intake than non-Aboriginal women. The data from this study support other Canadian reports. For all women in this study, calcium intake (465 mg) from milk was well below the recommended daily intake of 1,000 to 1,200 mg for women between the ages of 19 and 45. Despite intakes of vitamin D that were within the recommended levels, all women, regardless of age or ethnic grouping, showed deficiency in their serum levels of vitamin D. Margarine and milk were key sources of vitamin D, highlighting the importance of Canada's policy of fortifying these two staple foods.

From Weiler, H., Leslie, W., Krahn, J., Steiman, P., & Metge, C. (2007). Canadian aboriginal women have a higher prevalence of vitamin D deficiency than non-aboriginal women despite similar dietary vitamin D intake. *The Journal of Nutrition, 137*(2), 461–465.

increased risk for iron-deficiency anemia (see Chapter 4). Nurses are alert to the following situations in which even a balanced diet may not supply enough iron:

- Women with very heavy menstruation
- Women on a low-calorie diet (particularly those consuming less than 1,500 calories/day)
- Pregnant women
- Vegetarians and women who do not eat red meat
- Adolescents

Iron absorption is a complex process that varies with the food combinations consumed. Eating foods high in vitamin C facilitates the body's absorption of iron. Therefore, nurses encourage vitamin C intake from fruits, fruit juices, or vegetables at meals in combination with the selected iron food source. Although moderate amounts of lean meat contribute to iron intake, consumption of meat is not essential for adequate iron. Vegetarians need to consume legumes and nuts for iron as well as protein. Breads, cereals, and pasta enriched with iron also supply a fair amount of iron for women.

Exercise

Regular exercise has many benefits, including weight control, reduced stress, improved mood, and increased bone mass. Exercise is an area of special consideration for women who work continually to control their weight. Walking, jogging, hiking, swimming, and cycling contribute to cardiovascular health, bone mass, and muscle strength, and Tai Chi and Yoga help balance and flexibility (Senter et al., 2013) (Fig. 2.4). In Research Highlight 2.2, the "First Step Program" is identified as a strategy for increasing physical activity. Nurses can emphasize the relationship between diet and exercise in the teaching plans for clients.

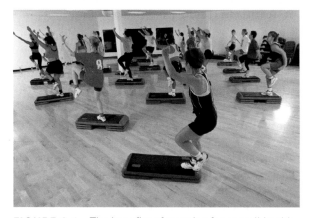

FIGURE 2.4 The benefits of exercise for overall health cannot be overestimated. In addition to assisting with weight control, exercise helps to prevent cardiovascular disease, diabetes, and other leading contributors to morbidity and mortality.

Renee wants to be a healthy weight and is busy with a 20-month-old son. What suggestions about exercise might be appropriate for Renee?

Exercise has definite effects on **metabolic rate** (a measure of energy production, or how fast the body burns calories). Factors that affect metabolic rate include sex, age, heredity, food intake, body composition, activity level, and frequent cycles of weight loss. Frequent weight loss through severe caloric restriction, followed by increased caloric intake and weight gain, seems to slow metabolic rate in many people. Commonly, this is called *starvation metabolism* or *yo-yo dieting.* It is as though the body fears starvation and becomes more efficient at conserving and storing energy. This weight-loss cycling can be discouraging and potentially harmful. Clients are advised to avoid excessive over-exercising. Like restrictive dieting, it can give the body the same starvation message.

Numerous genetic, physiologic, environmental, and psychological causes have been proposed in energy balance and weight control. Increasing evidence suggests that overweight and obesity are not simple problems, but a complex disorder of appetite regulation and energy metabolism. The *set point theory* states that some areas of the brain might control body composition. According to this theory, severe dietary restriction will cause the body to fight to maintain the set point by decreasing energy expenditure and increasing appetite. Set point is thought to be one factor controlling metabolic rate, probably through hormonal and nervous system connections. The set point is not really "set," but changes in response to diet components and calories.

Aerobic exercise burns calories, lowers the set point, and promotes good health. Other theories include fat cell theories, insulin response, and genetic theories. Health professionals are encouraged to do further reading by visiting the website of the Heart & Stroke Foundation of Canada (http://www.heartandstroke.com/site/c.ikIQLcMWJtE/b.2796497/k.F922/Heart_Disease_Stroke_and_Healthy_Living.htm). It contains position statements, BMI calculations, strategies for healthy weight, and other resources for nutrition and weight management.

Osteoporosis

Osteoporosis is a major public health problem in Canada with a high prevalence among older women. **Osteoporosis** is a condition resulting from decreased density, or thinning, of the bone. Imbalances in bone resorption (osteoclastic activity) and bone formation (osteoblastic activity) result in decreased bone density. Osteoporosis

● **RESEARCH HIGHLIGHT 2.2** **Controlled Outcome Evaluation of the First Step Program: A Daily Physical Activity Intervention for Individuals With Type II Diabetes**

BACKGROUND

Exercise is an important component in the management of type 2 diabetes; however, a substantial proportion of this population is not physically active. Physical inactivity and lack of cardiovascular fitness are predictors of death in men with type 2 diabetes. Physical inactivity may also contribute to the functional limitations or disabilities of people in this group. For instance, 50% of women and 32% of men over the age of 60 have difficulty or are unable to walk a quarter mile.

Regular physical activity can reduce the risk of coronary heart disease by as much as 55%. The American Diabetes Association endorses the public health recommendation that all adults should accumulate 30 minutes or more of moderate intensity physical activity on most days of the week.

PURPOSE

Although individuals with type 2 diabetes may know they should get more exercise, they may not be interested in formal exercise programs. Many prefer other activity options that accommodate their individual abilities, lifestyles, and preferences. The First Step Program was developed in collaboration with diabetes educators and adults with type 2 diabetes. Participants use pedometers to establish baseline levels of physical activity, set personal goals, and monitor their progress.

DESIGN

The study participants were recruited from a London, Ontario, diabetes education centre, according to the following criteria: aged 40 to 60; type 2 diabetes diagnosed more than 3 months; treated by diet alone or by oral hypoglycaemic medications; no limitations on physical activity; no documented heart conditions; not currently in an exercise program; and taking less than 8,800 steps per day, as measured by a pedometer. They were randomly assigned to either the First Step Program group or the wait-list control group. Study participants were assessed at baseline and 16 weeks later, when they were asked to return their pedom-

eters and return for a follow-up assessment at 24 weeks. Assessments included physical activity using a pedometer; anthropometric measurements; resting heart rate and blood pressure; an oral glucose tolerance test; and blood samples for determination of insulin, hemoglobin A1c (HbA1c), and plasma lipid profiles.

RESULTS

Sixty individuals (33 men, 27 women) were accepted into the study. Seven participants in the control group and six in the First Step Program (four males, two females) did not return for the 16-week assessment. The results are based on the 47 participants assessed at both baseline and 16 weeks. First Step participants increased their physical activity by approximately 3,000 steps per day from baseline, a significant difference ($p < 0.0001$) in comparison with the control group. Body weight and BMI remained constant in the two groups over the 16 weeks studied. Waist and hip measurements decreased more in the First Step group than in the control group, although the difference was not statistically significant over time. None of the remaining indicators of cardiovascular fitness, glycemia, or lipid status differed significantly over time or between groups. At the follow-up assessment at 24 weeks, steps per day for the First Step group were still higher compared to the control group, but there were no significant longer-term changes for any of the other health indicators.

This study showed that the First Step Program is an effective intervention for sedentary or insufficiently active adults with type 2 diabetes. By the end of the first phase of this study, participants were walking an additional half hour per day, an important "first step" toward a more active lifestyle. However, by 24 weeks, steps per day decreased, suggesting that additional strategies may be needed in order to sustain the behaviour change.

From Tudor-Locke, C., Bell, R., Myers, A., Harris, S., Ecclestone, N., & Lauzon, N. (2004). Controlled outcome evaluation of the First Step Program: A daily physical activity intervention for individuals with type II diabetes. *International Journal of Obesity, 28,* 113–119.

develops as a consequence of aging, with approximately 20% of women between 50 and 70 years of age being diagnosed, increasing to 30% for women aged 71 and older (Statistics Canada, 2013a). Osteoporosis may lead to fractures and is the most common of all skeletal disorders. With poor calcium intake in childhood and adolescence, osteoporosis is now considered a pediatric problem. Factors that affect bone development adversely

during childhood and adolescence include low calcium intake, poor general nutrition, sedentary lifestyle, carbonated beverage intake, and smoking.

Osteoporotic bone is weaker and more porous than normal bone, allowing fractures to happen more easily. Fractures in postmenopausal women contribute to long-term disability, frailty, and enormous expense. Bone loss in women begins around 30 to 35 years of age and proceeds at a rate of 0.75% to 1% per year until menopause; at about 5 years after menopause, the rate increases to between 2% and 3% per year (Watkins, 2010). Common fracture sites are the spine, wrists, forearms, and hips. With the exception of arthritis, osteoporosis is the leading cause of musculoskeletal disturbances in older adults (National Osteoporosis Foundation, 2013a). Women are at higher risk for osteoporosis than are men, primarily as a result of differences in bone mass and density (National Osteoporosis Foundation, 2013a).

Osteoporosis is commonly called the "silent epidemic" because early stages have no symptoms. Without improved preventive care for girls and women during the growth years and throughout the life span, osteoporosis will not be recognized until it is too late and fractures are likely. An early prediction of which clients are at risk is helpful.

Risk Factors. In simple terms, a **risk factor** is an action or behaviour that increases a person's chances of developing a condition. In complex human terms, clients have combinations of social, psychological, cultural, physical, and addictive behaviours that lead to negative results.

Risk factors contributing to osteoporosis are important to emphasize in educating and motivating women to practice preventive screening and positive lifestyle behaviours. All men and women over the age of 50 are recommended to talk with their physician or nurse practitioner about their risk factors for osteoporosis and their bone health (Canadian Medical Association, 2010). Four major risk factors for fracture include low **bone mineral density**, fragility fracture after the age of 40, age, and family history of osteoporosis. Individuals who present with major risk factors as well as a low bone mineral density are at increased risk for fractures. Bone mineral density refers to the concentration of minerals such as calcium; testing can help determine bone strength. Indicators for measuring bone mineral density in clients are included in Box 2.1. The fracture

risk assessment tool (FRAX) tool developed by WHO can be used to evaluate fracture risks and accessed by visiting the Osteoporosis Canada website (http://www.osteoporosis.ca/health-care-professionals/guidelines/).

Remember Linda, the 53-year-old accountant described at the start of the chapter. What factors in the scenario might place Linda at risk for osteoporosis?

Prevention. Because women are at increased risk for osteoporosis, nurses should teach preventive health measures. Dietary instruction on calcium intake requires special attention when developing teaching plans for girls and women because preventive measures are the primary defense. Physical activity and adequate calcium and vitamin D help build optimum bone mass (Osteoporosis Canada, 2013). Strategies identified as helpful in preventing further bone loss include increasing calcium intake; taking vitamin D supplements; maintaining adequate protein intake; avoiding excessive caffeine, soft drinks, salty foods, and alcohol; not smoking; increasing physical activity, particularly weight-bearing exercises such as walking, jogging, aerobics, dancing, stair climbing, and skating; and bone density screening for women at risk (Howe et al., 2011; National Osteoporosis Foundation, 2013b; Osteoporosis Canada, 2013).

COLLABORATIVE CARE: DIET, EXERCISE, AND HEALTHY LIFESTYLE

The nursing response to the public health epidemic of overweight and obesity involves educating clients and supporting their efforts to change behaviours through

● BOX 2.1 Indicators for Measuring Bone Mineral Density

Older Adults (Age ≥50 Yrs)	Younger Adults (Age <50 yrs)
Age ≥65 yrs (both women and men)	Fragility fracture
Clinical risk factors for menopause (menopausal women, men age 50–64 yrs)	Prolonged use of glucocorticoids
	Use of other high-risk medications
	Hypogonadism
Fragility fracture after age 40	Premature menopause (age <45 yrs)
Prolonged use of glucocorticoids	Malabsorption syndrome
Use of other high-risk medications	Primary hyperparathyroidism
	Other disorders strongly associated with rapid bone loss and/or fracture

Source: 2010 Clinical practice guidelines for the diagnosis and management of osteoporosis in Canada: Summary at http://www.cmaj.ca/content/early/2010/10/12/cmaj.100771.full.pdf+html?ijkey=edc6c6048e7d4acdc41368fe3f1e622bf5a2deac&keytype2=tf_ipsecsha

diet and exercise. Nurses should advise women to consume most dietary fat as polyunsaturated and monounsaturated fat, whereas reducing saturated and trans fats (Teaching Tips 2.1). The best results in weight management have been with nutritional programs that decrease both fat and calories and focus on exercise and remaining active (Shay et al., 2009; Wing & Phelan, 2005).

Assessment

When working with clients in the area of diet, exercise, and healthy lifestyles, the nurse performs a thorough health history and may ask the client to keep an exercise log and a diet diary that covers typical eating patterns. The client records her fat, iron, and calcium intake for 2 weeks to increase awareness of her choices. The nurse asks the client about the type, amount, and frequency of exercise, along with satisfaction with routines.

Select Potential Nursing Diagnoses

Nursing diagnoses that may apply in the area of diet, exercise, and lifestyle management include the following:

- Imbalanced Nutrition: More Than Body Requirements
- Health-Seeking Behaviours
- Deficient Knowledge
- Readiness for Enhanced Knowledge
- Readiness for Enhanced Nutrition

Planning/Intervention

Discussing concerns such as weight control, lowering cholesterol, and food preferences is essential. If the woman is allergic to milk products, she needs information about other sources of dietary calcium and calcium supplementation. Ways to balance cholesterol and calcium include consuming low-fat yogurt, skim milk, pudding made with skim milk, and low-fat cheese. Nursing Care Plan 2.1 provides a sample scenario of a client seeking to improve her health habits.

 Think back to Linda, who came to the clinic for help with her hot flashes. History taking reveals that Linda does not like milk. What other suggestions could the nurse give to ensure that Linda consumes enough calcium and vitamin D?

Controlling Fat Intake

For healthy functioning a certain amount of fat is needed in the daily diet. Experts no longer recommend following a diet low in *total* fat only; instead, they emphasize that the type of fat eaten is as important for health as the total amount consumed (Heart and Stroke Foundation of Canada, 2013a). Research indicates that a reduction in dietary saturated and trans fats may lead to lower levels of low-density lipoprotein (LDL) cholesterol and higher levels of high-density lipoprotein (HDL) cholesterol. Increased HDL cholesterol is associated with a decreased risk of high blood pressure, atherosclerosis, heart attack, and stroke. The nurse teaches the client that fats are essential for health but must be consumed in moderation. Although enjoyment of the appealing qualities and satiety of high-fat items is normal, clients should balance their intake with low-fat choices such as fresh fruits, vegetables, grains, and lean meats. Also, clients need to monitor the type of fats they consume. One type of polyunsaturated fat is omega-3, which has the health benefits of preventing clotting of blood, reducing the risk of stroke, and lowering triglycerides, a type of blood fat linked to heart disease. The best sources of omega-3 fat are coldwater fish such as mackerel, sardines, herring, rainbow trout, and salmon, as well as canola and soybean oils, omega-3 eggs, flaxseed, walnuts, pecans, and pine nuts (Heart and Stroke Foundation of Canada, 2013a). The *Eating Well with Canada's Food Guide* (Health Canada, 2011) recommends at least two servings of fatty fish with omega-3 oil (eg, char, salmon, mackerel, lake trout, herring, or sardines) every week.

Emphasizing Portion Control

Portion control is a major component of weight management. New trends in portion control that have been successful include having the woman visualize her portion in terms of a concrete object. For example, the nurse may recommend that the client take a portion of rice or vegetables the size of a tennis ball. Another example is for the nurse to show apples of various sizes so that the client fully understands what is meant by a "medium-sized" apple. The new Food Guide recommendations include reviewing the nutrition facts on food labels to help choose products that contain less fat, saturated fat, trans fat, sugar, and sodium.

Developing Exercise Routines

The client should slowly increase the intensity of her exercise routine. The nurse focuses exercise guidelines on process—a healthy lifestyle across the life span. Focusing on the end result—weight control or weight loss—can become counterproductive. Fitness and fun are more important than being thin. Nurses need to reinforce exercise measures in teaching plans that promote the idea of exercise being a life habit.

Evaluation

Nurses can conduct follow-up discussions to evaluate progress. One method they may use is to ask the client

● TEACHING TIPS 2.1   Nutrition and Weight Management

Nurses should share with clients the following points about nutrition:

- Ensure that your diet contains a variety of foods.
- Limit fat intake to 20% to 25% of daily calories. Most calories should come from grains, fruits, and vegetables.
- Monitor the *types* of fat consumed. Choose foods low in saturated and trans fats and cholesterol and moderate in monounsaturated fat:
  - Include a small amount—30 to 45 mL (2 to 3 tbsp)—of unsaturated fat each day. This includes oil used for cooking, salad dressings, margarine, and mayonnaise.
  - Use vegetable oils such as canola, olive, and soybean.
  - Choose soft margarines that are low in saturated and trans fats.
  - Limit butter, hard margarine, lard, and shortening.
- Trim fat from meat; remove skin from poultry.
- Limit intake of bacon, sausages, salami, and bologna.
- Use egg whites and egg substitutes.
- Choose fat-free or low-fat milk, yogurt, and cheese.
- Always check Nutrition Facts labels to determine saturated fat and cholesterol in prepared foods.
- When eating out, choose lean meats, limit intake of creamy sauces, and select fruit as dessert.
- Use moderate sugar and salt.
- Drink water regularly to quench your thirst. Drink more water in hot weather or when you are very active.
- Recommended servings of the food groups include the following:
  - Sparing amounts of fats, oils, and sweets
  - 6 to 7 servings of bread, cereal, rice, and pasta. Make at least half of your grain products whole grain each day. Eat a variety of whole grains such as barley, brown rice, oats, quinoa, and wild rice. Enjoy whole grain breads, oatmeal or whole wheat pasta. Choose grain products that are low in fat, sugar or salt.
  - 7 to 8 servings of fruits and vegetables
  - 2 to 4 servings of milk, yogurt, and cheese
  - 2 servings of meat, poultry, fish, dry beans, eggs, and nuts
- Obtain 1,000 to 1,500 mg/day of calcium and 400 to 800 IU/day of vitamin D. Sources of calcium include:
  - Vitamin supplement
  - Low-fat yogurt
  - Low-fat milk
  - Soy-based beverages with added calcium
  - Breakfast cereals with added calcium
  - Fruit juices with added calcium
  - Dark green, leafy vegetables
- Obtain 400 µg/day (0.4 mg/day) of folate. Sources of folate include the following:
  - Vitamin supplement (folic acid)
  - Cooked dry beans and peas, peanuts
  - Oranges, orange juice
  - Dark green, leafy vegetables: spinach, mustard greens, romaine lettuce
  - Green peas
- Obtain 18 mg/day of iron. Sources of iron include the following:
  - Vitamin supplement
  - Shellfish: shrimp, clams, mussels, and oysters
  - Lean meats, especially beef, liver, and other organ meats
  - Cereals with added iron
  - Turkey dark meat with skin removed
  - Sardines
  - Spinach
  - Cooked dry beans, peas, and lentils
  - Enriched and whole grain breads
- Obtain 25 to 30 g/day of fibre. Sources of fibre include the following:
  - Fruits
  - Vegetables
  - Whole grains
  - Cereals
  - Dried beans and peas

SUGGESTED READINGS

Eating Well With Canada Food Guide. (2007). Retrieved from http://www.hc-sc.gc.ca/fn-an/food-guide-aliment/index-eng.php

Ryan-Harshman, M. & Aldoori, W. (2006). New dietary reference intakes for macronutrients and fibre. *The Family Physician.* Retrieved August 18, 2008, from http://www.cfpc.ca/cfp/2006/Feb/vol52-feb-clinical-3.asp

Whiting, S. & Barabash, W. (2006). Dietary reference intakes for the micronutrients: Considerations for physical activity. *Applied Physiology and Nutrition Metabolism, 31,* 30–35. Retrieved from http://pubs.nrc-cnrc.gc.ca/rp/rppdf/h05-021.pdf

to complete a daily food intake and exercise diary and bring it to the nurse for evaluation. If necessary, the nurse asks the client to suggest alternatives when current plans do not seem to be working. Consultation with a dietitian, physician, or both may be initiated if the client requires additional assistance.

NURSING CARE PLAN 2.1

•

A Client Making Nutrition, Exercise, and Lifestyle Choices

 Consider Renee from the beginning of the chapter. During the interview, Renee mentions a history of heart disease and type 2 diabetes in her family. She states that she is motivated to maintain physical activity and a weight-control program. She does not smoke. Renee's BMI is 25.4. She wants to bring that number down from overweight to within normal.

NURSING DIAGNOSIS

Health-Seeking Behaviours related to weight control and exercise.

EXPECTED OUTCOMES

1. The client will verbalize areas of daily routine that may contribute to unhealthy behaviours leading to weight gain.
2. The client will identify measures that promote weight control and gradual weight loss.
3. The client will participate in an exercise routine for approximately 20 to 30 minutes three to four times each week.

INTERVENTIONS	RATIONALES
Question the client about her daily routine and activities, including child care and home demands.	This information provides a baseline to identify problem areas and develop suggestions for healthy behaviours.
Review the client's daily eating patterns, including frequency of eating and types of foods and fluids consumed. Ascertain the client's likes and dislikes.	Knowledge of current dietary patterns provides clues to nutritional status and amount and types of calories and nutrients ingested. Information about the client's likes and dislikes aids in individualizing suggestions for proper food selection.
Encourage the client to eat small, frequent meals throughout the day and not to skip meals. Provide suggestions to replace empty calories with nutritious ones.	Small frequent meals throughout the day maintain metabolism and proper insulin secretion and prevent starvation metabolism.
Reinforce the need to limit consumption of fats and to select vegetables, fruits, whole grains, legumes, fish, poultry, and lean meats low in saturated and trans fats and cholesterol. Instruct the client in methods of cooking such as broiling and steaming.	Because of the client's family history, the client should avoid intake of foods high in trans fat and cholesterol to reduce her risk. Consumption of diets high in saturated fats, elevated lipid levels, and obesity are associated with type 2 diabetes. Positive methods of cooking promote the intake of healthier, more nutritious foods.
Offer suggestions about how to incorporate healthy eating into her daily routine.	Incorporating healthy habits into the routine enhances the chances for success and adherence to the plan.
Reinforce the need for portion control; show how to estimate or visualize portions in terms of concrete objects.	This measure aids in compliance with the regimen.

(continued)

NURSING CARE PLAN 2.1 ● A Client Making Nutrition, Exercise, and Lifestyle Choices *(Continued)*

INTERVENTIONS	RATIONALES
Encourage the client to keep a food diary or log of her intake for review on the next visit.	Keeping a food diary or log helps the client to visualize the amount and types of food consumed and possible patterns of intake that need adjustment or correction.
Investigate the types of activities that the client enjoys.	Doing exercise that the client enjoys promotes adherence and increases the chances for success.
Encourage the client to exercise with someone else.	Women with exercise partners may feel safer participating in outdoor activities. Research has shown that people with partners are more likely to maintain consistent exercise patterns.
Advise the client to start slowly. Recommend a 5-min warm-up and cool-down at the beginning and end of each exercise session. Encourage her to exercise approximately three to four times a week for 20 to 30 min. If she cannot afford a health club, she may find walking to be an economical and rewarding activity.	Consistency, not speed, is the key to aerobic exercise. For women, it is very important to select an exercise that will fit easily into their schedule and responsibilities.
Emphasize the need to vary exercise routines and gradually increase intensity as tolerated.	Varying exercise decreases boredom and works different muscle groups. Increasing intensity helps strengthen muscles and increase endurance.
Instruct the client to avoid weighing herself daily; suggest that she weigh herself approximately twice a week, at the same time, and wearing approximately the same amount of clothing at each measure.	Weight fluctuates throughout the day and daily. Too frequent weighing may lead to discouragement. Improved fitness and a gradual sustained weight loss are key.

EVALUATION

1. The client reports that she is engaging in brisk walks of 1.5 to 2.5 km three times a week.
2. The client states that her energy level has increased and that she feels "healthier."
3. The client verbalizes the intake of a healthy, nutritious diet low in saturated and trans fat and cholesterol.
4. The client demonstrates a weight loss of approximately 1 kg by return visit in 3 to 4 weeks.

Psychosocial Health

Psychological health includes factors in every woman's life related to balancing work, home, stress, relationships, family, and sense of meaning and healing. In this chapter, psychological health promotion focuses on the woman, her family, and her community; it applies to all women, including those with diagnosed psychiatric conditions. Therefore, this section briefly summarizes health history and assessment parameters for psychological health promotion and common mental health concerns for women, including depression, anxiety, domestic violence, substance use, and gun safety. Chapter 5 explores these issues in more detail.

Mental Health Promotion

Mental health promotion is the process of enhancing the capacity of individuals and communities to take control over their lives and improve their mental health (PHAC, 2012a) by creating supportive environments. Positive mental health involves the ability to achieve a sense of well-being and to effectively deal with everyday challenges (PHAC, 2012a). Mental health promotion uses strategies that foster empowerment, resilience, human fulfillment, and overall well-being (Kobau et al., 2011). Canada's Centre for Addiction and Mental Health (2012), established in 1998, integrates specialized clinical care with innovative research, education, health promotion, and policy development.

Women fulfilling multiple roles often need support from health providers to ensure that they attend to their own psychological needs. Teaching Tips 2.2 provides some general strategies for nurses to communicate with their clients.

Health history questions to assess the woman's environment and mental health needs include the following:

- Do you pay attention to your inner feelings?
- How many hours of sleep do you get each night? Do you feel rested?

- What activities do you do to relax? What are your hobbies?
- Do you take at least 15 minutes out for yourself each day?
- Do you have anyone close to you in whom to confide?
- Do you have an outlet that satisfies your spiritual needs?
- Do you have anything that lifts your spirits?

Mental health promotion facilitates healing by restoring harmony and balance between mind and body. Mind–body and complementary/alternative therapies can alleviate stress-related health problems. Nursing interventions to promote psychological health include touching, listening, praying, caring, music, humour, counselling, pharmacotherapeutics, and story telling.

Depression

Physical and psychological symptoms of depression can cause significant distress and impairment to the woman and her family. Clients with depression either have a depressed mood or express a lack of interest in all or most routine activities. They develop a constellation of the following: significant weight loss, weight gain, or alterations in appetite; sleep disturbances manifested by insomnia or hypersomnia; psychomotor agitation or retardation; fatigue or loss of energy; feelings of worthlessness or inappropriate guilt; diminished ability to concentrate; poor concentration or difficulty making decisions; feelings of hopelessness; and recurrent thoughts of

---

● TEACHING TIPS 2.2   Taking Care of You—Personal Action Steps

Nurses share the following points with clients when teaching about self-care:

- Find time for yourself each day. Focus on what your body/mind is telling you. Try to take at least 15 minutes a day to do something special and relaxing for you.
- Exercise every day. It increases endorphins in the body and improves emotional and physical health. Risk for CAD almost doubles in a sedentary person. Walking 30 minutes a day, three to five times a week, is beneficial. Exercise has more cardiovascular benefits if the pace is brisk enough to elevate heart rate.
- Eat a nutritious diet. Studies have shown a connection between early and continued consumption of fruits and vegetables and reduced risk for chronic health conditions such as obesity and heart disease. Overweight women have been shown to have higher rates of morbidity and mortality than lean women.
- Get your annual examination. This is an opportunity to screen for common conditions such as hypertension, breast and cervical cancer, and depression. Most

importantly, it is also a time to address your concerns with a nurse practitioner or physician. During the annual examination, you can get answers and discuss how to modify lifestyle as necessary.
- Get enough sleep. Don't eat, exercise, or do stimulating activity right before bedtime. Have a ritual every night to promote a relaxed sleeping pattern. Sleep will allow you to be more equipped to deal with everyday stressors.
- If you are a smoker, quit smoking. Smoking does not affect just the lungs. It is associated with diseases that affect every organ in the body. Smoking affects and can harm not only the smoker but also those exposed to secondhand smoke.
- Reduce your risk for injury.
- Practice safer sex.
- Avoid violence and contact with violent people.
- Be aware of safety principles at home and when travelling.
- Always wear a seatbelt.
- Never drive under the influence of alcohol or drugs.

death. Five or more of these symptoms must represent a change in recent functioning and be present and persistent (almost every day) for at least two consecutive weeks (Mood Disorders Association of Canada, 2011). Depression can be a single episode or periodically recur, but it remains independent of life events. Loss of a loved one or a life-changing event may act as a catalyst to depression, but in the category of mood disorders, depression remains a psychiatric diagnosis distinct from grief.

Depression may occur with or without comorbid conditions. Close monitoring includes assessment for anxiety, panic disorder, posttraumatic stress disorder, substance use, or grief reactions.

Risk Factors. Depression has multiple causes. Factors associated with depression include family or personal history of depression, family or personal history of postpartum depression, poor self-concept or low self-esteem, female gender, chronic health conditions, biochemical imbalances in the brain, substance abuse, loss or death, and stressful life occurrences (PHAC, 2011a). Risk factors for suicide include previous attempts at suicide, depression, dysfunctional family, abuse, intimate partner violence, alcoholism and other substance use, and chronic illness (Hawton & van Heeringen, 2009).

Screening Tools. Depressive disorders are more common in women than in men. Screening for depression as a component of the annual comprehensive examination can enhance early detection and treatment. The Canadian Task Force on Preventive Health Care (MacMillan et al., 2005) supports screening for depression in clinical settings that have systems in place to ensure accurate screening, diagnosis, and follow-up. Although there are many screening tools used in primary care settings, the Task Force suggested that asking two simple questions (ie, "Over the past 2 weeks, have you felt down, depressed, or hopeless?" and "Over the past 2 weeks, have you felt little interest or pleasure in doing things?") might be as effective as the longer screening tools. The following are examples of depression screening tools that can be found in an internet search: *Beck Depression Inventory, Zung Self-Rating Scale, Geriatric Depression Scale, Center for Epidemiological Studies Depression Scale (CES-D).*

Health care providers follow up on all positive results on screening tests with an extensive interview, health history, and physical examination along with a full diagnostic workup. Sample tools and expanded discussions, including treatment, are found in Chapter 5.

Anxiety Disorders

Anxiety differs from fear, in that anxiety is a response to an unknown, internal, vague, or conflictual threat (Running & Berndt, 2003), whereas fear is a response to a known or definite threat. Anxiety may be temporary or a persistent health issue. When anxiety escalates beyond healthy functioning and interferes with quality of life, assessment for anxiety disorders and potential treatment are indicated.

Anxiety disorders are characterized by symptoms of physiologic arousal (eg, palpitations, sweating) and excessive worry that persist over time and interfere with normal functioning (Uphold & Graham, 2003). They are further classified as panic disorders, with or without agoraphobia; specific phobia; social anxiety disorder; generalized anxiety disorder; obsessive–compulsive disorder; and posttraumatic stress disorder (Canadian Psychiatric Association, 2006). The most common risk factors for anxiety disorders are being female, physical and mental illness, personal history of stressful or traumatic life situations or events (including past violence), family or personal history of anxiety disorders, abuse, and intimate partner violence (Canadian Psychiatric Association, 2006).

Women with potential anxiety disorders require a thorough examination and history with diagnostic testing to rule out other medical, neurologic, or endocrine disorders (Running & Berndt, 2003). Clients should be referred to a psychiatrist or psychologist for follow-up. A woman with an anxiety disorder may need pharmacologic treatment. Nonpharmacologic treatments include therapy, biofeedback, relaxation therapies, meditation, journaling, and yoga. The use of Kava for anxiety is outlined in Complementary/Alternative Medicine 2.2. Support groups and family therapy may be beneficial,

● COMPLEMENTARY/ALTERNATIVE MEDICINE 2.2
Use of Kava for Anxiety

Kava is a herb that has shown great promise in the treatment of anxiety. Results from systematic reviews of nutritional and herbal supplements for anxiety disorders indicate kava significantly decreases symptoms of anxiety (Lakhan & Vieira, 2010; Pittler & Ernst, 2000). Findings also indicate that kava have results equivalent to those of benzodiazepines, with the added benefit of fewer side effects.

The client should not take kava if she is using other substances that act on the central nervous system, such as antidepressants, alcohol, and barbiturates. As with all complementary/alternative medicine products, the nurse should urge the client to discuss the use of kava with her primary health care provider before initiating any therapy independently.

as well as establishing normal eating, sleeping, and exercise patterns tailored to the woman's lifestyle. See Chapter 5 for more information.

Intimate Partner Violence

"I really wanted the nurse to ask me about what was going on at home. He always seemed too busy. I get the feeling he didn't ask me because he did not want to deal with my problems."

Intimate partner violence refers to a real or threatened physical, sexual, emotional, or psychological abuse perpetrated against a spouse or life partner. It includes measures to control another person's actions, for example, economic control, stalking, and control of social contacts. Experiencing fear in a relationship is characteristic of abuse, regardless of whether there is physical violence. In a 2011 homicide report the rate of intimate partner homicides committed against females increased by 19%, the third increase in 4 years (Statistics Canada, 2013b).

Nurses assess clients for risks for or presence of domestic violence at each visit. Assessment Tool 2.1 presents the *SAFE* screening tool, which helps identify victims of violence. Chapter 5 provides a more detailed discussion of this important topic.

Jill starts to cry saying, "I am so scared this is really going to hurt. Could we just forget this and I'll just go home?" How might you respond?

Substance Use

Alcohol, drug, and tobacco abuse are prominent public health issues for women and their families. Consequences of addictive use of alcohol, drugs, and tobacco include liver disease, heart disease, breast and lung cancer, violence, sexual victimization, and auto accidents. Factors that may increase women's risk for substance use or dependence include genetic influences, early initiation of smoking and substance use, and victimization. Some increased risks for substance use in women compared with men may be gender-related differences in metabolism, brain chemistry, genetic risk factors, or entirely different factors still undiscovered. Because of the increased consequences of substance use in women, early assessment and treatment are the key to increasing awareness and preventing serious consequences.

Nurses assess adolescents and women for alcohol and substance use while taking their health history. Assessment Tools 2.2 to 2.4 have wide screening applicability for high-risk clients. Women and girls whose scores indicate a problem require extensive interviews and medical follow-up. The nurse provides community resources and referrals to these clients and their families.

Frequently, girls report that they initiate smoking to lose weight and maintain the weight loss. They also see smoking as part of their social image, a way to bond with peers, and a method of controlling moods. Nurses adapt smoking cessation programs for adolescents to concepts that teens view as meaningful to their development. Adolescents may be more likely to stop smoking

---

● **ASSESSMENT TOOL 2.1** **"SAFE" Questions That Can Help Identify Victims of Abuse**

STRESS/SAFETY

- What stresses do you have in your relationship with your partner?
- How do you handle disagreements?
- Do you feel safe in your relationship with (name spouse/partner)?
- Should I be concerned for your safety?

Afraid

- Are there situations in which you feel afraid?
- Have you ever been threatened or abused?
- Has your partner forced you to have sexual intercourse that you did not want?

Friends/Family

- If positive responses to items above: Ask "Are your friends/family aware that this is happening?"
- If negative responses to items above: Ask "Do you think you could tell them if it did happen?"
- Would they help you?

EMERGENCY PLAN

- Do you have a safe place to go in an emergency situation?
- If you are in danger now, would you like me to help you find a shelter?
- Would you like to talk with a social worker/counsellor to help you develop a plan?

Follow any questions answered affirmatively with additional questions to determine the following:

- How and when mistreatment occurs?
- Who perpetrates it?
- How the woman copes with it?
- What she plans to do to protect herself (and children)?

From Uphold, C. R., & Graham, M. V. (2003). *Clinical guidelines in family practice* (4th ed.). Gainesville, FL: Barmarrae Books.

● ASSESSMENT TOOL 2.2   CAGE Questionnaire for Alcoholism Screening

Have you ever felt you should **C**ut down on your drinking?
Have people **A**nnoyed you by criticizing your drinking?
Have you ever felt **G**uilty about your drinking?
Have you ever had a drink first thing in the morning (**E**ye-opener) to steady your nerves or get rid of a hangover?

Two or more "yes" answers indicate probable alcoholism. Any one "yes" answer deserves further evaluation.

Source: Ewing, J. A. (1984). Detecting alcoholism: The CAGE questionnaire. *Journal of the American Medical Association, 252,* 1905–1907.

---

if providers relate the effects to body image and attractiveness, such as bad breath, smelly clothes, and wrinkles (Teaching Tips 2.3).

Gun Safety

When examining violence as a public health promotion issue, nurses must consider gun safety as a variable. Although the use of firearms to commit homicide has been decreasing in Canada and a 2011 report shows a rate of 0.46 firearm homicides per 100,000 population, the lowest in almost 50 years, 27% of all homicides in 2011 involved firearms and most (91%) occurred in large urban settings areas (Statistics Canada, 2013b).

Most (81%) gun-related deaths in Canada were suicides, 15% were homicides, and 4% were unintentional. In 1995, gun registration became compulsory in Canada, and the rate of gun-related injuries, which had been dropping since the early 1990s, continued to decline. In 2012, the Federal Government passed Bill C-19 to end mandatory gun registration.

The Canadian Paediatric Society (2005) advocates banning firearms from homes or environments in which children and adolescents live and play. The Society recommends that firearms in homes be stored unloaded, locked, and separate from ammunition. Nurses must promote awareness of safety and specific rules of gun safety in the home. Key points for gun safety education to emphasize with girls, adolescents, parents, and grandparents are given in Teaching Tips 2.4.

Cardiovascular Health

Heart disease is a leading cause of death for Canadian women. In 2008, cardiovascular disease accounted for 29.7% of all female deaths (Statistics Canada, 2011). The incidence of cardiovascular disease in women continues to rise markedly in perimenopause and menopause. Natural and surgically induced menopause are associated with changes in serum lipid profiles, with a decline in HDL cholesterol, and an increase in LDL cholesterol. These cholesterol changes may be factors in the development of a woman's increased risk for postmenopausal heart disease (see Chapters 4, 23, and 24).

Deposits of cholesterol in plaque-laden arterial walls are the primary pathologic risk for heart disease. *Angina pectoris* occurs when the client experiences a deficit of oxygen being infused through the myocardium itself. The actual pain sensation is thought to result from a state of anaerobic physiology. *Myocardial infarction* occurs with an actual necrosis, or "death," of the myocardial cells from anaerobic insult. A clot, spasm, or atherosclerotic plaque in the coronary arteries can

---

● ASSESSMENT TOOL 2.3   Primary Screening Tools for Alcohol Problems

Halt	**Bump**	**Fatal DTs**
1. Do you drink to get **H**igh?	1. Have you had **B**lackouts?	**F**amily history of alcohol problems?
2. Do you drink **A**lone?	2. Is your drinking **U**nplanned (you drink when you said you would not or drink more than you thought)?	**A**lcoholics Anonymous attendance?
3. Do you **L**ook forward to drinking (instead of going to an event)?		**T**houghts or attempts at suicide?
4. Has your **T**olerance for alcohol increased or decreased?	3. Do you drink **M**edicinally (when depressed, sad, anxious)?	**A**lcoholism. Ever thought you might have it?
	4. Do you **P**rotect your supply (so that you will always have enough)?	**L**egal problems, such as driving under the influence or assault?
		Depression, feeling down, low, or sad?
		Tranquilizer or disulfiram use?

Source: Martin, A., Schaeffer, S., & Campbell, R. (1999). Managing alcohol-related problems in the primary care setting. *The Nurse Practitioner, 23*(8), 14–39.

● **ASSESSMENT TOOL 2.4**   **CRAFFT Substance Use Screening Tool**

This tool has been tested recently in adolescent clinic patients.

1. Have you ever ridden in a **C**ar driven by someone (including yourself) who was "high" or had been using alcohol or drugs?
2. Do you ever use alcohol or drugs to **R**elax, feel better about yourself, or fit in?
3. Do you ever use alcohol or drugs when you are **A**lone.
4. Do your family or **F**riends ever tell you that you should cut down on your drinking or drug use?

5. Do you ever **F**orget things you did while using alcohol or drugs?
6. Have you gotten in **T**rouble while using alcohol or drugs?

Two or more "yes" answers indicate a significant problem (Knight et al., 2002).

For more information, visit http://www.SAMHSA.gov/ Substance Abuse and Mental Health Services Administration (SAMHSA) is an agency of the United States Department of Health and Human Services.

cause these anaerobic conditions (Fig. 2.5). The most common cause is atherosclerosis. Contrary to common belief, many women who die suddenly of coronary heart disease have no prior symptoms. This highlights the need for preventive screening with blood pressure monitoring, lipid profiles, weight management, smoking cessation, and prevention and management of diabetes mellitus.

Risk Factors for Heart Disease

Nurses can play a key role in educating their professional peers and clients about the facts of heart disease in women. Although many of the risk factors for heart disease are similar for women and men, the following are unique characteristics related to women's heart health that nurses need to consider (Heart and Stroke Foundation of Canada, 2013b):

- The role of estrogen
- Oral contraceptives
- Pregnancy (preeclampsia, gestational diabetes)
- Menopause
- Elevated cholesterol
- High triglyceride

The major modifiable risk factors for heart disease are cigarette smoking, high cholesterol, hypertension, diabetes, physical inactivity, excessive alcohol consumption, stress, and obesity, particularly, central or abdominal obesity (Heart and Stroke Foundation of Canada, 2013b). In women with diabetes, mortality from heart disease is two to four times that of women without diabetes.

The following key points regarding gender differences in coronary heart disease have implications for nursing practice:

Age. Women tend to show signs of cardiovascular disease later than men. Between 25 and 35 years, men have three times the incidence of heart disease as women. Even though menopause decreases a woman's protection from heart disease, this biologic advantage persists until 65 to 70 years. With advanced aging, about 90% of women die of heart disease and related complications. At older ages, women who have heart attacks are twice as likely as men to die from them within a few weeks. Although rates of mortality are decreasing in Canada, death from heart disease increases dramatically for women over age 55 (PHAC, 2009).

● **TEACHING TIPS 2.3**   **Prevention of Adolescent Smoking**

Nurses share the following points with adolescent clients when discussing smoking:

- Adolescent women who smoke:
  - May have more painful menstruation
  - May stop menstruating all together
  - May have menstrual irregularity
  - Have less oxygen available to their lungs, making playing sports difficult
  - Run slower and not as far as nonsmokers
  - Have bad breath, cracked lips, sores, and bleeding in the mouth from tobacco

- Have an increased risk for ectopic pregnancies and spontaneous abortions
- Babies born to women who smoke are at an increased risk for sudden infant death syndrome (SIDS).
- Women smokers who die of a smoking-related disease lose approximately 14 years of potential life.

Know the truth. Despite all the tobacco use on TV and in movies, music videos, billboards, and magazines, most teens, adults, and athletes DON'T use tobacco!

● TEACHING TIPS 2.4   Gun Safety

Nurses share the following points with clients when teaching about gun safety:

GENERAL GUIDELINES

- Learn the characteristics of your firearm.
- Treat the firearm as if it were loaded at all times.
- Point the muzzle in a safe direction.
- Keep your finger off the trigger, unless you intend to fire it.
- Never rely on mechanical safety features to protect you or someone else.
- Keep the gun unloaded and action open until you are ready to shoot.
- Know your target and what is beyond it.
- Use only the correct ammunition for your firearm.
- Know what to do in case of a misfire.
- Wear protective eye and ear equipment.
- Keep the firearm free from obstructions and keep it well maintained.
- Do not modify your firearm.
- Do not mix guns with alcohol, drugs, or fatigue.

SAFETY FOR PARENTS AND GRANDPARENTS

If there is a gun in your home:

- When to teach the child about gun safety: when the child starts to ask questions or acts out gun play. Keep your lessons simple, but credible. Repeat, repeat, and repeat.
- Teach facts, not fear: The first rule for small children is DON'T TOUCH! Once the child is older, taking him or her to a gun range may take away the "forbidden fruit" attraction. Consider having the older child take a gun safety course.

- Distinguish between fantasy and reality. Many parents establish their home as a "no gun zone," meaning no real or pretend guns allowed. If children are allowed to play with pretend guns, teach them the difference between real and pretend. Tell them to always assume a gun is real first! They should be taught to play with their pretend guns as if they were real.
- Options for safe storage: vaults, safes, and locked metal storage boxes. Store ammunition and the firearm in separate safes. Think about gun storage from your child's point of view. Children will climb up onto areas that you think they cannot reach! Consider using trigger, action-blocking locks for additional safety.
- Practice what you preach:
  - Follow the rules you have set for your children! Remember, you are their role model!
  - Don't leave firearms lying around.

If your child encounters a gun not in your home:

- If your child discovers a gun outside the home or in the home of a friend, he or she should know the four steps of the Eddie Eagle gun safety program, including:
STOP!
DON'T TOUCH.
LEAVE THE AREA.
TELL AN ADULT.
- Discuss gun safety with other parents or family members if your child spends time in their homes. It is not enough to assume that if they do have guns in the house, they have them stored properly.

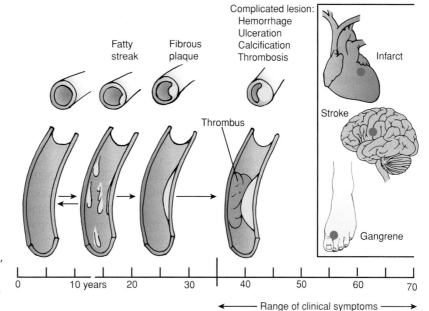

FIGURE 2.5 In atherosclerosis, the process begins with fatty streaks, which can progress to form fibrous plaque. The plaque can progress to cause hemorrhage, ulceration, calcification, or thrombosis. The result can be a myocardial infarction or a cerebrovascular accident.

Signs and Symptoms. Previously, women were not included in heart disease research and treatment, greatly compromising the known facts regarding early identification and treatment for women. Often, the signs and symptoms of heart disease in women differ significantly from those in men. However, the most common symptom in women is still chest pain (Heart and Stroke Foundation of Canada, 2013b). Women may also have unspecified pain and vague symptoms, which can lead physicians and women themselves to look for other causes. Nurses need to begin to suspect heart attack in a woman the same as they would for a man. They should ask women how the symptoms respond or change in response to exercise, extremes in temperature, and heavy meals.

Social Factors. Although heart disease affects all ages and socioeconomic strata, studies have demonstrated that people with lower education and income levels are at increased risk, even when adjustments are made for biomedical and behavioural factors. The relationship between low levels of education and risk for heart disease is stronger among women than among men. Women with lower levels of education are more likely to be of low income, unemployed, and single parents. The clustering of these risk factors among women may account for some of the differences seen in the relationships between low education and risk for heart disease (Thurston et al., 2005). Having diabetes is a greater risk factor for developing heart disease among women than among men (Canadian Diabetes Association, 2013).

Cardiovascular Preventive Health Behaviours

Clients can do many things to reduce the risk for heart disease. The first step is to increase awareness of the need to take responsibility at a young age and to develop health behaviours that will decrease cardiovascular risks as women age. Childhood is the best time to develop health behaviours, but it is never too late (Fig. 2.6).

Although heart attacks are uncommon in premenopausal women, the factors after menopause that lead to increased incidence are not exactly clear. Because women present with heart disease at different ages and with different signs and symptoms, providers may take them less seriously than their male counterparts. Women eventually may be diagnosed with heart disease when they are of advanced age, are more likely to be taking other medications, and have other conditions such as diabetes, hypertension, and osteoporosis.

Nurses, women, and the general community must recognize that women's higher risk for heart disease accompanies the years surrounding menopause; however, nurses need to emphasize that heart disease is not an inevitable consequence of aging. It is a disease process that can be influenced by lifestyle behaviours.

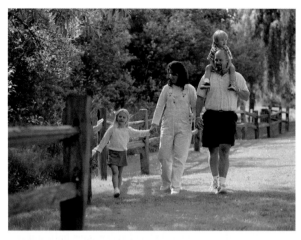

FIGURE 2.6 Families should try to instill good health and exercise habits in their children from the earliest ages. A healthy lifestyle from childhood onward helps prevent problems like cardiovascular disease, diabetes, and obesity later in life.

Diabetes Mellitus

The rising incidence of the constellation of obesity, dyslipidemia, heart disease, and diabetes in women is a critical public health issue (see Chapter 4). Diabetes is a major source of morbidity, mortality, and economic burden in Canada. Lifestyle changes can frequently prevent it. Public health education marketed toward women, weight management, exercise, control of blood glucose levels, and preventive diabetic health services can reduce the incidence of diabetes.

The classification of diabetes includes type 1 diabetes, type 2 diabetes, and gestational diabetes. Autoimmune destruction of the pancreatic islets causes type 1 diabetes. Type 2 diabetes, which is more prevalent, is a defect of insulin secretion, action, and resistance. Although type 2 diabetes was previously most commonly seen in people older than 40 years, its prevalence is increasing among children and adolescents as more of them become overweight or obese (Amed et al., 2010). Results of a Canada-wide population-based study of new-onset childhood type 2 diabetes conducted between 2006 and 2008 are alarming; a minimum national incidence rate of 1.54 new cases per 100,000 children under the age of 18 years was determined (PHAC, 2011b). The incidence of children and youth aged 18 and under with type 2 diabetes was higher among Aboriginal children and youth than among Asian, African and Caribbean, and Caucasian children and youth.

Gestational diabetes is a temporary condition that occurs in approximately 3% to 5% of pregnancies in non-Aboriginal women, but ranges from 8% to 18% in pregnant Aboriginal women (Canadian Diabetes Association, 2013). Having gestational diabetes increases a woman's risk of eventually developing type 2 diabetes (Bellamy et al., 2009). Follow-up and support programs are recommended to assist postpartum women engage in health-promoting behaviours.

Risk Factors

Risk factors for type 2 diabetes mellitus include the following:

- Hypertension (>130/80 mm Hg in adults on at least two separate occasions and measured in both arms)
- Family history (parents or siblings) of diabetes
- Overweight (BMI >25) (see Fig. 2.3)
- Abdominal obesity
- Race/ethnicity (Aboriginal, African, Latin American, Asian, Pacific Islanders)
- Sedentary lifestyle
- HDL >1 mmol/L; LDL >2 mmol/L
- History of gestational diabetes or delivery of a baby weighing more than 4,000 g
- History of impaired glucose tolerance
- Polycystic ovary syndrome

Screening

The Canadian Diabetes Association (2013) recommends diabetes screening for individuals over age 40 at least every 3 years. People presenting with any of the listed risk factors should be screened for diabetes earlier and annually. Any person presenting with frequent urination, extreme thirst, unexplained weight loss, or repeated infections should also be screened. Screening consists of a comprehensive health history and physical examination, along with taking blood glucose levels, both fasting and 2 hours postprandial. A fasting plasma glucose level less than 5.7 mmol/L and/or hemoglobin A1C less than 5.5% is within the normal range. A blood glucose level at or above 7 mmol/L and/or hemoglobin A1C at or above 6.5% supports a medical diagnosis of diabetes mellitus. Diabetes treatment goals for management of plasma glucose include a hemoglobin A1C level of less than 7, a preprandial plasma glucose level of 4 to 7 mmol/L, and a 2-hour postprandial plasma glucose level of between 5 and 10 mmol/L (Canadian Diabetes Association, 2013). See Chapter 4 for more information on the pathophysiology and management of diabetes.

Education and Prevention

Education and prevention are of great importance in decreasing incidence of diabetes in women and in promoting **self-management** practices to reduce complications when it is diagnosed. Clients take self-management decisions and actions in response to their environment and situation to improve their health status. Women need the skills, information, and community and financial resources for effective self-management.

The importance of prevention in high-risk clients is substantiated by the alarming increase in diabetes in women and in minority women. Although genetic susceptibility has a role in the development of type 2 diabetes, the current epidemic is associated primarily with particular lifestyle behaviours. Such behaviours include lack of regular exercise, consumption of diets high in saturated fat, dyslipidemia, obesity, and smoking. Moderate sustained weight loss and regular moderate to vigorous exercise can decrease the risk for developing type 2 diabetes.

The role of the nurse and other health care providers is to prevent the disease, promote early detection, and encourage preventive services to reduce short- and long-term complications. These interventions can improve client outcomes and ultimately reduce health care costs. To accomplish these objectives, providers must adopt a multifaceted management approach that consists of education, promotion of self-management, well-established communication between the providers and client, and regular feedback on the client's outcomes.

Early preventive interventions can reduce the morbidity, mortality, and economic burden of diabetes. Many preventive interventions can achieve this balance. Table 2.3 provides a quick reference of specific interventions for the prevention of selected long-term complications of diabetes.

Menstrual Health

The discipline of women's health provides a comprehensive view of the care of young girls to aging women. The menstrual cycle can serve as a developmental parameter for specific health promotion needs focused on specific age cohorts. For example, school-age girls and adolescents need information to prepare them for their bodily changes. This developmental phase highlights decision making regarding initiation of sexual activities, birth control, and peer pressure regarding sex, alcohol, and drugs. Aging women need health education on the transition of perimenopause and on prevention of specific health risks such as osteoporosis, heart disease, and diabetes. In the following section we discuss phases of the menstrual cycle and health promotion needs for women in various cohorts.

Menarche

On average, girls begin menstruating at approximately 12 years, with the age of onset ranging from 8 to 18 years (Youngkin & Davis, 2012). **Menarche**, initiation of menses, begins when the brain, ovaries, and adrenal glands are mature and when the percentage of body fat is adequate. Initial menstrual cycles are usually irregular and unpredictable because hormonal communications may be erratic. Pregnancy can occur at any time, even before a girl's first menstrual period, if she has ovulatory cycles.

The nurse's health promotion focus for girls is to provide health education on how the body functions,

● TABLE 2.3 **Recommendations to Prevent Complications of Diabetes**

Potential Complications	Recommendations
Cardiovascular disease A. Maintain BP ≤130/80 B. LDL cholesterol <2 mmol/L C. HDL cholesterol >1 mmol/L D. Total cholesterol: HDL ratio <4 E. Smoking cessation F. Plasma glucose: 　HgA1c <7% 　Preprandial plasma glucose 4–7 mmol/L 　Peak prandial glucose <10 mmol/L	Blood pressure every visit Orthostatic BP every visit Early lifestyle interventions Serum lipids yearly Smoking cessation counselling HgA1c every 3 mos SMBG several times daily before meals, peak prandial, and bedtime. The Canadian Diabetes Association recommends at least three times per day for patients with type 1 diabetes or at least four times per day for pregnant women taking insulin. Greater frequency of SMBG is needed when adding to or changing therapy
Renal disease	BP every visit Maintain BP at <130/80 mm Hg Yearly testing for microalbuminuria
Retinopathy	Annual dilated eye examination by ophthalmologist Glasses for sun protection Optimal glycemic control Optimal BP control
Foot ulcers with high potential for amputations	Yearly comprehensive foot examination by a podiatrist Visual foot inspection every visit Daily skin care Appropriate footwear
Influenza, pneumococcal disease	Yearly flu vaccine Limit exposures during high incidence times Pneumococcal vaccine at age 65 yrs or older Revaccinate if a dose was given 　≥5 yrs before 65 yrs of age

BP, blood pressure; HDL, high-density lipoprotein; LDL, low-density lipoprotein; SMBG, self-monitoring of blood glucose.

changes to expect (including breast enlargement and secondary sexual characteristics), and what happens with initiation of menses. It is also important that young girls understand the relationship between ovulation and their beginning fertility (see Chapter 6). Health education about sexual intercourse and how pregnancy occurs are essential to promote positive sexuality and safer sexual practices and to prevent unplanned adolescent pregnancies and sexually transmitted infections (STIs).

Folic acid is essential to normal cell development and the formation of major fetal structures. Many women do not consume adequate folate in their diets before they know they are pregnant. This is the time when the need for folate is most critical. For that reason, it is recommended that all adolescents and women who can become pregnant should consume a multivitamin containing 0.4 mg of folic acid daily, starting at least 3 months before becoming pregnant, in addition to eating foods that contain folate (PHAC, 2008a). Good sources of folate include dark green leafy vegetables, broccoli, peas, legumes, citrus fruits and juices, peanuts, whole grains, and some fortified breakfast cereals. In 1998, Canada began fortifying grains, pastas, and cereals with folic acid (PHAC, 2004). Imported products are not fortified. The daily recommended value is 0.4 mg; pregnant women need more (0.6 to 0.8 mg/day).

 Consider Jill, the young woman who is to have her first pelvic examination. Because this is her first experience, what information would be critical for the nurse to assess?

Perimenopause and Menopause
QUOTE 2-1

"Women may be the one group that grows more radical with age."

Gloria Steinem

Perimenopause refers to the period during which ovarian function regresses; it can last as long as 7 to 10 years. This time begins with the last menstrual cycle leading to menopause and extends to 1 year after the last menses. Thereafter, the woman is considered **postmenopausal**. Menstrual periods stop because the ovaries no longer produce progesterone and estrogen.

The simplest definition of **menopause** is the end of menstruation. Although menopause literally means cessation of menses, it is actually a process rather than a discrete, single event. Referring only to the cessation of menses is a narrow definition, and menopause is now being defined as a transition of biologic and cultural events over months to years, and not purely the single event of absence of menses (see Chapter 23).

The major source of estrogen before menopause is the ovarian follicle, which accounts for more than 90% of the body's total production. Estrogen deficiency that accompanies menopause can result in symptoms such as hot flashes, vaginal dryness, emotional changes, and weight gain. Some women experience no symptoms at all. Menopause is a gradual process and does not occur suddenly, unless it is surgically or medically induced (eg, chemotherapy, radiation).

In 2002, the Women's Health Initiative study was conducted to determine the risk-to-benefit ratio of hormone replacement therapy (HRT) in healthy postmenopausal women (Writing Group for the Women's Health Initiative Investigators, 2002). The results had a major impact on HRT decision making by women and their health care providers. A review of long-term hormone therapy for perimenopausal and menopausal women by the Cochrane Collaboration (2012) reinforced the concerns identified in 2002 (Marjoribanks et al., 2012). However, some researchers suggest HRT may be beneficial for younger menopausal women (Lobo, 2013). Current recommendations suggest that health care providers need to review the risks and benefits of hormonal therapy to a menopausal woman (SOGC, 2009). (Research Highlight 2.3).

To work most effectively, sensitively, and practically with midlife women, nurses should recognize

---

● RESEARCH HIGHLIGHT 2.3 Risks and Benefits of Estrogen Plus Progestin in Healthy Postmenopausal Women: Principal Results From the Women's Health Initiative Randomized Controlled Trial

BACKGROUND

For decades, HRT had been used routinely for perimenopausal and menopausal women. In addition to alleviating bothersome symptoms of menopause such as hot flashes and vaginal dryness, HRT also had been advised as a primary prevention measure for more serious conditions affecting postmenopausal women such as cardiovascular disease, osteoporosis, and even Alzheimer disease. Despite widespread use of HRT, however, the risk-to-benefit ratio had remained uncertain.

PURPOSE

The purpose of the Women's Health Initiative study was to assess the risk-to-benefit ratio of HRT.

DESIGN

The study was designed as a randomized controlled primary prevention trial to last 8.5 years. Eligible women were recruited from 40 participating US clinical centres over a 5-year period. Eligibility was defined as age 50 to 79 years, postmenopausal, intact uterus, probability of remaining in the area for at least 3 years, and written informed consent. An equal number of women were selected randomly to receive HRT versus placebo, respectively. HRT initially was started as equine estrogen, 0.625 mg/day, plus medroxyprogesterone acetate, 5.2 mg/day, given as a single pill, with dose adjustments permitted to allow for the treatment of side effects such as breast tenderness and vaginal bleeding. Data from each client were collected concerning incidences of breast cancer, hip fractures related to osteopenia or osteoporosis, and

coronary artery disease (CAD), including myocardial infarction, stroke, and thrombosis.

RESULTS

In 2002, 3 years before the scheduled end of the trial, the data and safety monitoring board recommended terminating the trial because of the risks for breast cancer exceeding the original boundary set to stop the study. In addition, the board also determined that overall risks of HRT exceeded its benefits. Although hip fractures decreased among those women on HRT, incidences of breast cancer, stroke, cardiovascular disease, and pulmonary embolus increased significantly.

Based on the results of the Women's Health Initiative and further studies, the current recommendation is not to initiate or continue HRT in the primary prevention of cardiovascular disease. In addition, providers must weigh the substantial risks for breast cancer and cardiovascular disease against the benefit of management of vasomotor symptoms. Currently, the management of hot flashes and other menopausal symptoms is the only recommended first-line therapy for HRT. Choosing other pharmacotherapy options for clients with osteoporosis is suggested. When prescribing HRT to treat menopausal symptoms, providers should use the lowest dose feasible along with annual reassessment. When used for menopause, optimal duration of HRT is less than 5 years.

From Writing Group for the Women's Health Initiative Investigators. (2002). Risks and benefits of estrogen plus progestin in healthy postmenopausal women: Principal results from the women's health initiative randomized controlled trial. *Journal of the American Medical Association, 288*(3), 321–333.

that menopause takes months to years: it is not merely the absence of menses. Although "perimenopause" is a correct term to use to refer to this entire change-of-life process, women themselves do not always use this term. Therefore, to avoid confusion when counselling women, it is often best to explain the change of life as a process. Nurses can teach women about the entire process, in addition to the cessation of menses, and counsel women regarding the maintenance of contraceptives. Women and their partners need advice about contraception because ovulation may be sporadic during perimenopause. Many physicians and nurse practitioners advise women 50 years or older to continue contraception for 1 year after the last period.

In Western culture, with its strong emphasis on female youth and beauty, menopause may be a difficult adjustment for some women, who may find symptoms bothersome or emotions unexpected. Nurses can assist women in dealing with this transition. Historically, the negative stereotypes surrounding "change of life" probably began when a woman's life expectancy was short. Generations ago, many women didn't live past menopause. Women who did live long enough to reach menopause were so few that they were considered old if they survived to 50 years! Naturally, menopause came to be associated with all the undesirable attributes of extreme old age. Also, when female life expectancy was low, women were valued primarily for their reproductive capacity. Today many women who are approaching menopause have had the advantage of better nutrition and higher education than did previous generations.

As nurses, conveying positive attitudes toward sexuality, sexual expression, intercourse, and the maturing adult is important. With an average life expectancy of 82.6 years, many women will live one third of their lives after menopause. Along with changes in women's rights and roles in society, many women and health care providers want to replace negative stereotypes of menopause with a realistic and positive outlook. This new viewpoint is easier to achieve as women learn more about how to live through the changes of middle age with good health and peace of mind. A woman's understanding and expectations of menopause, marital or relationship stability, financial resources, family views, physical health, and sociocultural expectations influence her adjustment to menopause. Research has shown a relationship between ethnicity, culture, and women's experience of menopause. Nurses need to acknowledge that variations exist across cultures and be prepared to discuss specific symptoms with each woman when planning care (Freeman & Sherif, 2007).

Cessation of menses frees women from menstrual periods, fear of pregnancy, and contraceptive concerns. Many women see menopause as a time of fewer child care responsibilities and increased opportunities

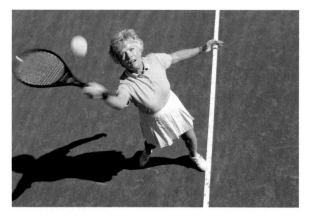

FIGURE 2.7 Many women today are using the time after menopause to pursue hobbies and activities they may not have had time to enjoy in younger years. They are also maintaining health and wellness through exercise and physical activity.

to pursue other goals (Fig. 2.7). This combination is often energizing for women seeking added dimensions to their careers or relationships. The transition to menopause often provides more leisure time as well as increased opportunities for self-expression and community involvement. Despite a strong cultural message that youth is better than age, women who maintain a positive image and value themselves adapt well to menopause.

The perimenopausal years can be eased for women if they have information about normal anticipated changes. Menopause can be used as a time to make some important health or lifestyle changes. Preventive health behaviours are suggested for aging women to decrease the incidence of chronic or fatal illnesses such as osteoporosis, heart disease, and diabetes. For further details, refer to Nursing Care Plan 2.2 and Chapter 23.

Sexual and Reproductive Health

Increasingly, experts are recognizing environmental factors and lifestyle patterns as crucial variables affecting individual, family, and public health. This is especially true in the areas of sexual and reproductive health. Lifestyle-related diseases are influenced not only by diet, smoking, alcohol consumption, and exercise, but also by emotional relationships and sexuality. Nursing care involves developing competency in conducting a thorough and sensitive health history, sexual health history, and assessment of sexual and reproductive health in women of all ages (see Chapter 6).

Participation by women in screening programs for STIs, in addition to breast and cervical cancer, is far from optimal. Because these conditions sometimes are not detected until they have reached advanced stages, many lives are lost or adversely affected when such consequences could have been prevented. Therefore, nurses

NURSING CARE PLAN 2.2

●

A Client Experiencing Perimenopause

 Recall Linda, the 53-year-old perimenopausal accountant. Further questioning reveals that Linda became aware only recently of how much time had passed since her last menstrual cycle. "I didn't realize it. Am I starting menopause? Work has been so crazy over the last several years. Where has the time gone?" Her last visit to her primary care physician was almost 5 years ago; she has gained 9 kg since then. When questioned about exercise, she states, "I hate it. Who has time for it? I can't even think about it. I realize that exercise might help me manage my stress better, but I'm so drained when I get home."

NURSING DIAGNOSIS

Deficient Knowledge related to normal body changes associated with perimenopause and menopause and healthy lifestyle.

EXPECTED OUTCOMES

1. The client will describe perimenopause and menopause and the associated normal body changes.

INTERVENTIONS	RATIONALES
Assess the client's knowledge about her body and typical changes in perimenopause and menopause.	Assessment of knowledge provides a baseline from which to develop appropriate teaching strategies.
Define perimenopause and menopause. Review the typical accompanying body changes and correlate them with what the client is experiencing.	Accurate descriptions are essential to understanding the changes. Correlating the client's signs and symptoms promotes her understanding of these events.
Assess the client's interpretation of the relationship between her womanhood and perimenopause/menopause.	Some women view menopause as a loss of female youth and beauty; others view it as a time of increased opportunities.
Emphasize that the client can use this time to make important health and lifestyle changes.	Such changes can reduce the incidence of heart disease and osteoporosis, which can be chronic or fatal.

EVALUATION

1. The client identifies typical normal body changes associated with perimenopause and menopause.

NURSING DIAGNOSIS

Ineffective Health Maintenance related to demands of work, sedentary lifestyle, and weight gain.

(continued)

NURSING CARE PLAN 2.2 ● A Client Experiencing Perimenopause *(Continued)*

EXPECTED OUTCOMES

1. The client will identify appropriate strategies to deal with body changes.
2. The client will verbalize measures that contribute to a healthy lifestyle.
3. The client will identify the required screening and examinations needed to promote health.

INTERVENTIONS	RATIONALES
Review the client's daily routine, including diet, activity level, and rest.	Knowledge of the routine aids in developing an individualized program to fit the client's lifestyle, thereby enhancing the chances for success.
Encourage exercise. Suggest aerobic, weight-bearing exercise three to four times a week for at least 20 min.	Aerobic weight-bearing exercise helps slow down bone loss, keeps weight down, and improves sense of well-being.
Recommend the Health Canada balanced diet, which consists of 45–65% complex carbohydrate, 20–25% fat, and 10–35% protein. Also encourage adequate vitamin D (400–800 IU/day) and calcium (1,200–1,500 mg/day) intake. Provide the client with a list of foods that would promote adequate intake.	A diet low in saturated fats and cholesterol reduces the client's risk for heart disease. Adequate vitamin D (400–800 IU/day) and calcium (1,200–1,500 mg/day) help prevent osteoporosis. Maintaining ideal body weight with a BMI less than 25 decreases incidence of type 2 diabetes.
Instruct the client about the need for appropriate screenings: Pap smear, mammogram, cholesterol testing, clinical breast examination, fecal occult blood and digital rectal examination, and blood pressure checks; biannual or annual dental care; annual fasting blood glucose screening (if at risk for diabetes).	Routine screenings are necessary for early detection and treatment of health problems.
Assist the client to determine her priorities. Work with her to develop a written plan for exercise, diet, and health screenings. Provide positive reinforcement for changes.	Midlife adjustment can be a time to reflect on future goals and development of new roles. Positive reinforcement promotes adherence to the plan.

EVALUATION

1. The client demonstrates appropriate self-management strategies to promote health during perimenopause and menopause.
2. The client collaborates with the health care provider to devise a healthy lifestyle plan, demonstrating healthy behaviours.
3. The client participates in setting up a schedule for appropriate screenings and examinations.

can increase health education and improve availability of screening programs for optimum sexual and reproductive health. It is particularly important that nurses put effort into reaching women in the lower socioeconomic or minority groups who have a disproportionate burden of breast and cervical cancer. Nurses must provide support, information, and a caring attitude as women make difficult and emotional health care decisions.

Sexual History and Risk Factors

Through a sexual health history, the nurse and client are better equipped to mutually identify risk factors and discuss sexual behaviours that may be placing the client at risk for STIs or pregnancy. This health history can be conducted at the annual examination with a nurse practitioner, midwife, or physician, or when the woman presents with a sexual health or contraceptive concern. Health history questions include the following objective data:

- Are you sexually active? At what age did you begin intercourse? With men? With women? With both?
- What kind of sexual activity do/did you engage in?
- How many lifetime sexual partners have you had? How many sexual partners have you had in the last year?
- What type of contraceptive do you use? Are you satisfied with this contraceptive?
- Do you use condoms? Do you use them with every sexual encounter?
- When was your last Pap smear? Have you ever had an abnormal Pap? If so, when and what treatment was performed?
- How many times have you been pregnant? Have you had any term births, preterm births, elective abortions, or miscarriages? If you have had a miscarriage, what was the gestational age? Was the cause known? Were births vaginal or cesarean? Were births normal or were there complications?
- Do you have living children? If so, what are their ages?
- Are you satisfied with your sexual relationship?

Sexual and reproductive health is not always a comfortable topic for discussion. Consequently, women, their families, and health care professionals sometimes minimize or hide the full effects of sexual health. Concerns about gynecologic problems, sexuality, and childbearing are common. With the diagnosis of any gynecologic condition or breast or cervical cancer, guilt, embarrassment, shame, and body image disturbances are common feelings. Women may also feel their personal privacy is being invaded. They may feel defensive and angry with the health care team having to treat such an innermost private part of them. Some women associate problems in the genital area with forms of punishment for real or imagined sexual expression. Health care providers can diminish shame and guilt associated with the diagnosis if they communicate an accepting and nonjudgmental approach.

Providers can discuss with the client the potential for some conditions to interfere with sexual function, since some women may feel uncomfortable asking questions or initiating a discussion on the subject of sexual activity. Nursing Care Plan 2.3 addresses these issues in more detail.

Papanicolaou Test (Pap Smear)

Regular pelvic examinations and Pap smears are the best way to assess and to detect various conditions in the reproductive system early (Nursing Procedure 2.1). The Papanicolaou (Pap) test, or smear, is a safe and inexpensive tool for the early detection of cervical cancer. Developed by the Greek physician Dr. George Papanicolaou in the 1940s, the Pap smear became a regular component of gynecologic examinations during the 1950s.

The Pap smear involves scraping the endocervix with a swab, brush, or spatula to obtain a sample of cells. Computerized analysis of the Pap smears, such as "Papnet," is now available. This technique holds promise of decreasing false-positive or false-negative Pap reports. Most women barely feel the "scraping" of the cervix during the Pap smear. Barriers to gynecologic checkups and Pap smears include fear, denial, lack of information, cultural beliefs, social status, embarrassment, absence of symptoms experienced, and lack of access to a primary care provider.

Screening Schedule and Guidelines. Recommendations regarding how frequently women should have Pap smears vary among the provinces and territories. The guidelines for cervical cancer screening were updated in 2013 (Canadian Task Force on Preventive Health Care, 2013). Screening is no longer recommended in sexually active women who are younger than 25. Asymptomatic women aged 25 to 69 (who are or have been sexually active) are to be screened every 3 years, and for women older than 69, screening is recommended if prior screening has not been adequately performed. Screening can cease in women aged 70 or older after receiving three successive negative Pap smear results. Women who have had a hysterectomy may still need a Pap test and should discuss this with their physician. Pap tests are usually continued if the hysterectomy was done to treat a precancerous or cancerous condition, but may not be necessary if the hysterectomy was done for a noncancerous (benign) condition and if the woman has no history of a cervical precancerous condition or human papillomavirus (HPV). Women who have sex with women should follow the same cervical screening recommendations as women who have sex with men. It is critical for nurses to emphasize to clients that women need health care appointments to discuss sexual questions, risk factors related to sexual behaviour, STIs, contraception, blood pressure, weight control, clinical breast examination, and any other issues of concern.

Classification of Pap Tests. In many women, cervical cells go through a series of changes. Cervical intraepithelial neoplasia is the term used to encompass all epithelial abnormalities. An older classification system described two separate entities (dysplasia and carcinoma *in situ*); this classification also influenced

NURSING CARE PLAN 2.3

●

A Client With Sexual and Reproductive Concerns

 Jill is about to undergo her first vaginal examination and Pap smear. She is nervous and scared. The nurse asks Jill to identify specifically what is frightening her most. Jill sighs and says, "I've just put off doing this for so long. I'm worried that I have a tumour or an infection. What will I do if something is wrong?"

NURSING DIAGNOSES

Anxiety related to fear and lack of information about reproductive and sexual health.

Deficient Knowledge related to vaginal examination, Pap smear, and preventive measures for reproductive health.

EXPECTED OUTCOMES

1. The client will verbalize fears and concerns openly.
2. The client will identify positive methods to cope with fears.
3. The client will identify what will happen during the examination, including possible findings.

INTERVENTIONS	RATIONALES
Use a nonjudgmental approach and establish rapport with the client. Maintain this approach throughout the visit and care of the client.	Establishing a nonjudgmental and caring relationship with the woman will enhance the therapeutic relationship, foster honesty, and communicate respect.
Provide as much privacy and comfort as possible. Explore the woman's feelings of privacy and how you can meet her needs within the scope of the examination.	Privacy communicates respect of the client's personal boundaries and comfort zone.
Perform a complete nursing assessment of the woman's sexual and reproductive history.	The data provide a baseline from which to develop a plan of care; they also give clues to potential problems.
Encourage the client to discuss the "causes" of any real or perceived problems. Communicate accurate facts; answer questions honestly. Reinforce facts. Provide brochures. Encourage the client not to blame herself if problems are found.	Information about possible causes provides clues to the client's anxiety. Facts help dispel unfounded fears, myths, misconceptions, and guilt.
Review the steps of the vaginal examination and Pap smear. Show the client the various pieces of equipment that may be used (eg, the speculum).	Providing the client with information about the procedure aids in alleviating fear of the unknown.
Instruct the client to take slow deep breaths during the examination.	Slow deep breaths aid in relaxing the client, which facilitates the examination.
Warm the speculum before insertion; drape the client appropriately.	Warming the speculum and proper draping provide comfort and privacy for the client.

(continued)

NURSING CARE PLAN 2.3 ● A Client With Sexual and Reproductive Concerns *(Continued)*

INTERVENTIONS	RATIONALES
Perform the vaginal examination and Pap smear, explaining each step before doing it (see Nursing Procedure 2.1).	Explaining what is to happen helps prepare the client for what to expect and aids in alleviating anxiety.
After the examination, openly and sensitively discuss any issues of fertility, sexual expression, body image, and safer sexual practices.	Open discussion alleviates anxiety and provides facts to promote health.
Encourage the woman to follow up with future examinations, Pap smears, and contraceptive planning as necessary. Reinforce the use of safer sexual practices.	Follow-up is important to promote positive health-seeking behaviours, empowering the client to protect her safety and health.
Provide the client with information about support services in the community. Encourage their use as appropriate.	Community services provide additional means of support in dealing with reproductive and sexual health concerns.

EVALUATION

1. The client states that her anxiety about the vaginal examination is decreased.
2. The client uses positive methods to cope with the procedures.
3. The client demonstrates knowledge of the examination and possible findings, verbalizing information and questions related to reproductive health.

treatment techniques. The newer classification system, the Bethesda system, is preferred because it indicates a neoplasia continuum and is descriptive of actual cellular changes (see Chapter 4).

What do these changes in classification mean from the client's perspective? Nurses can inform women that the changes were implemented to improve identification and treatment of changes in cervical cells before they become invasive cancer. Also, researchers are beginning to understand the pattern of changes that cervical cells undergo as a continuum over months to years. The woman needs to know that if the Pap test shows any abnormality, the physician or nurse practitioner will follow up to discover the problem. When a vaginal infection is the suspected cause of an abnormal result, the practitioner will treat the infection and then repeat the test, usually in 3 months. If an infection is not the reason, the practitioner may perform a colposcopy and biopsy.

Risk Factors for Cervical Cancer. Most risk factors for cervical cancer are ultimately related to sexual behaviour and can be identified through a sexual history. Although the exact etiology is unknown, the general cause is thought to be cellular changes in the cervix resulting from "insult" caused by viruses and multiple partners. Women with cervical cancer often report a history of cervical infections. Infections linked to cervical carcinoma are caused by herpes simplex virus 2; HPV types 16, 18, 45, and 58; HIV; and possibly cytomegalovirus. HPV 16 is linked most frequently to squamous cancers and HPV 18 to adenocarcinomas. Women whose HPV infection persists in genital skin cells are at greatest risk for subsequently developing cervical cancer. These women require close follow-up treatment and repeat Pap smears. These viruses alter the DNA of nuclei of immature cervical cells. Adolescent pregnancy, multiple sexual partners, weakened immune system, and smoking are thought to promote the process that ends in dysplasia (MedLine Plus, 2013a). In July 2006, Health Canada approved the use of HPV vaccine by girls and young adult women as a preventive measure against the majority of cervical cancers. The vaccine provides protection against HPV 16 and 18, and "low-risk" HPV types 6 and 11 which cause 90%

(text continues on page 66)

NURSING PROCEDURE 2.1
Performing a Pelvic Examination and Pap Smear

PURPOSE

To evaluate the condition of the internal female reproductive structures and to obtain specimens for cytologic screening.

ASSESSMENT AND PLANNING

- Assess client's knowledge of and previous exposure to the procedure.
- Determine the date of the client's last menstrual period. (Ideally, the Pap smear should be taken approximately 2 weeks after the first day of the last menstrual period to enhance obtaining the best specimen possible.)
- Ask the client if she has abstained from sexual intercourse and douching for the past 48 hours.
- Question the client about the use of tampons; contraceptive foams, jellies, or creams; or vaginal medications within the last 72 hours.
- Check for evidence of current vaginal bleeding, which would require rescheduling the Pap smear. (Blood cells interfere with examination of the sample.)
- Gather the necessary equipment such as:
    - Examination gloves
    - Speculum
    - Sheet or bath blanket for draping
    - Specimen collection devices such as Cytobrush and plastic spatula
    - Properly labeled specimen container (liquid-based preservative) or slide and spray fixative
    - Completed laboratory request form
    - Adequate light source
    - Water-soluble lubricant (only if not performing Pap smear)

Equipment for pelvic examination and Pap smear.

IMPLEMENTATION

1. Explain the procedure to the client and answer any questions *to help allay her anxiety.*
2. Have the client empty her bladder *to minimize discomfort during the procedure.*
3. Wash hands thoroughly.
4. Have client position herself on the examination table with her feet in stirrups or foot pedals (or flat on the examination table) so that her legs fall outward. Ask the client to move herself down on the table so that her buttocks are just past the bottom edge of the table. *This positioning ensures adequate access to the perineum.*

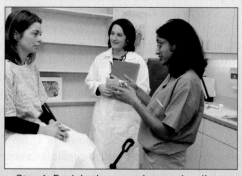

Step 1: Explain the procedure to the client.

5. Place sheet or bath blanket over the client, keeping the area over the perineum exposed *to ensure privacy and allow access to the perineum.* Adjust the light source as necessary.
6. Put on gloves.
7. Warm the speculum with warm water *to avoid chilling the client.*
8. Tell the client that you are about to touch her *to prevent startling her.*
9. Using a gloved hand, spread the labia, inspecting and palpating the area to check for abnormalities; throughout encourage the woman to take deep breaths *to aid in relaxation.*

(continued)

NURSING PROCEDURE 2.1 (CONTINUED)
Performing a Pelvic Examination and Pap Smear

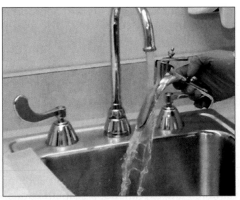

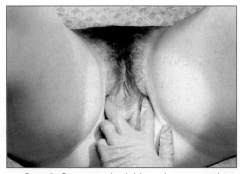

Step 9: Separate the labia to inspect and palpate the vaginal area.

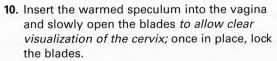

Step 7: Warm the speculum with warm water.

10. Insert the warmed speculum into the vagina and slowly open the blades *to allow clear visualization of the cervix;* once in place, lock the blades.
11. Obtain samples for Pap smear; use the Cytobrush or sterile cotton tipped applicator and swab the endocervix, using one full circular motion.
12. Use the plastic curved spatula to gently and firmly scrape the cervix os.
13. Swab the posterior fornix or vaginal pool using the opposite end of the cervical spatula or a sterile cotton-tipped applicator.
14. Immediately after collecting each specimen, place the specimen in the appropriately labelled container or the slide and spray with a fixative.
15. Unlock the blades of the speculum and remove it gently *to reduce the risk for trauma to the client.*
16. Remove the glove from the nondominant hand and place on lower abdomen; insert a lubricated gloved finger of the dominant hand into the vagina *to perform the bimanual examination.*

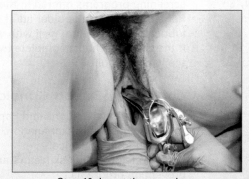

Step 10: Insert the speculum.

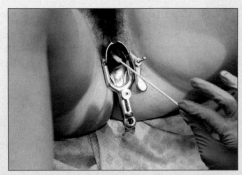

Step 11: Swab the endocervix.

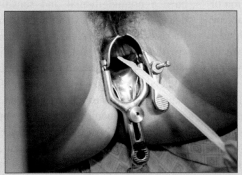

Step 12: Scrape the cervical os.

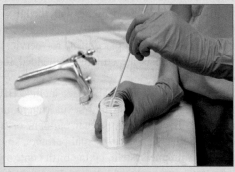

Step 14: Appropriately preserve the specimen.

(continued)

NURSING PROCEDURE 2.1 (CONTINUED)
Performing a Pelvic Examination and Pap Smear

17. On completion, remove the glove from the dominant hand and discard appropriately.
18. Assist the client to sitting position and allow her to get dressed.

EVALUATION

- The client tolerated the procedure without difficulty.
- Specimens were obtained and sent to the laboratory.

AREAS FOR CONSIDERATION AND ADAPTATION

Lifespan Considerations

- If this is the client's first experience with pelvic examination, ensure that an additional person is available to support the client and reinforce any explanations or instructions.
- Keep in mind that Pap smear recommendations vary across the country with specific screening programs offered in the provinces and territories.
- Remember that some older adult women may experience atrophic vaginitis; be sure to lubricate the speculum well with water.
- If the client has had a complete hysterectomy, obtain the specimen for the Pap smear from the vaginal pool.

Community-Based Considerations

- Most pelvic examinations and Pap smears are done on an outpatient basis as part of the routine gynecologic examination. Private offices, clinics, and community-based health centres offer this service.
- Education about the risk factors and techniques to prevent cervical cancer is key to primary prevention programs.

Equipment for Pelvic Examination and Pap Smear

- Step 1: Explain the procedure to the client.
- Step 7: Warm the speculum with warm water.
- Step 9: Separate the labia to inspect and palpate the vaginal area.
- Step 10: Insert the speculum.
- Step 11: Swab the endocervix.
- Step 12: Scrape the cervical os.
- Step 14: Appropriately preserve the specimen.

of genital warts. The National Advisory Committee on Immunization in Canada recommends immunization of females from 9 to 26 years of age with the HPV vaccine (Health Canada, 2010). The HPV vaccine is considered a complement, not a replacement, for cervical cancer screening. Pap tests are still recommended for vaccinated women.

Risk factors for cervical cancer include HPV, multiple pregnancies, having had sexual intercourse at a young age, having many sexual partners or a sexual partner who has had many sexual partners, smoking, a weakened immune system, taking birth control pills for a long time, and socioeconomic status (Canadian Cancer Society, 2013a). Most predisposing factors relate to patterns of sexual activity, which could lead to bar-

riers for early detection and treatment. Nurses need to have a nonjudgmental and sensitive approach when discussing psychosexual factors and the implications for risk for cervical cancer. Communication should convey that nurses regard sexual health as a basic component of total health and a normal physiologic function. Societal norms today differ from 40 years ago. Today, many women marry later. Divorce and remarriage are relatively frequent, and many women will have more than one sexual partner in their lifetime. Nurses should consider these changes as a social norm, not a stigma associated with a risk factor for cervical cancer. They can educate themselves and their clients regarding both sexual health and risk factors for cervical cancer. The best approach is to encourage any sexually active woman to participate in regular gynecologic checkups and Pap smears and to use safer sex practices, such as limiting sexual partners and using latex condoms.

Perineal Hygiene and Infection Prevention

Organisms, transmission, and complications of perineal infections and STIs are known and in many cases preventable. Despite efforts, however, these problems continue. The rate of STIs has increased during the past few decades; they continue to be a public health concern (PHAC, 2012b). The spread of STIs demonstrates the need to address the social determinants of disease. Nurses need to be informed regarding the pathophysiology, transmission, and social dimensions of perineal infections and STIs, and provide education and anticipatory guidance to clients of all ages at each stage of the life span. Chapter 4 discusses STIs in more detail.

In addition, some infections during pregnancy may cause additional risk to the fetus or newborn, and require special care. In the near future, widespread administration of the HPV vaccine to female adolescents before initiation of sexual activity offers the best hope for preventing cervical cancer. By immunizing adolescents against HPV, the epidemiologic profile of cervical cancer could change dramatically. The Canadian Paediatric Society (2007) states that all Canadian girls between the ages of 9 and 13 should receive the HPV vaccine and that girls at high risk for early sexual activity (eg, those who are street-involved or under the care of child welfare) be targeted for immunization. Health professionals are addressing the ethical concerns of some groups over an immunization linked to sexual activity.

Nurses can provide women with a teaching plan for perineal hygiene. The goal is to prevent organisms such as *Escherichia coli* from spreading from the rectum to the vagina and urethra. Nurses can instruct women to wash their hands before and after genital contact and after using the restroom. It also is important to instruct women to wipe the perineum from front to back each time they void or defecate, as well as after sex and during menstruation. Women prone to vaginitis should use only white, unscented toilet tissue and unscented pads or tampons. They should not use feminine hygiene or other sprays near the perineum. They should avoid tampons or pads containing deodorant or scent; if using tampons, they must be sure that the string does not slip to the rectal area. If it does, the tampon should be changed immediately.

Women are often at risk for genital infections or vaginitis because of the warm, moist vaginal environment, which promotes microbial growth. Wearing cotton underpants with a cotton crotch, especially under the panty hose, girdles, and Lycra shorts, can decrease this risk. Cotton pants are best during any exercise such as aerobics, jogging, or biking. Women should avoid nonabsorbent clothes as much as possible, especially when exercising. Showers are preferable to tub baths. Women susceptible to vaginitis and urinary tract infections should avoid bubble bath and other bath additives. If a lubricant is necessary during sexual intercourse, women can use a water-soluble lubricant such as K-Y jelly, Replens, or Astroglide (over-the-counter products). Vaseline is a less effective vaginal lubricant because it is not water soluble and may not be compatible with some contraceptives. Allowing time for sexual stimulation before intercourse (foreplay) is often the only lubrication technique necessary. Vaginal dryness may occur, however, with perimenopausal changes.

 Recall Linda, the 53-year-old with hot flashes. During the interview, she mentions that she has noticed increased vaginal dryness, especially during sexual intercourse. How can she minimize this dryness?

Douches are rarely necessary. Douching washes out the normal balance of bacteria in the vagina, increasing the risk for bacterial vaginosis (Brotman et al., 2008). Women do not need to douche, unless otherwise instructed by a health care provider. If a nurse practitioner or physician recommends douching, a solution of distilled white vinegar (15 mL per litre of water) is more economical and efficacious than commercial products. Women should avoid perfumed or flavoured douches. Vaginal deodorants, sprays, gels, or powders are not recommended for routine hygiene.

Changes in vaginal physiology or a rise in pH makes women more vulnerable to vaginal infections. The nurse should caution women that risk factors for vaginitis include pregnancy, use of high-estrogen oral contraceptives, antibiotic therapy, and uncontrolled diabetes. Women in these situations should follow the suggested techniques in addition to a protocol for care for a specific risk factor. If the woman is taking antibiotics, eating yogurt or sour cream may help prevent vaginal infections. Some women need prophylactic antifungal therapy in conjunction with antibiotic therapy. If a woman has itching, irritations, burning, sores, or odour, she should be examined to determine the exact cause. There are many different types of vaginal infections, each with different treatments (see Chapter 4).

During any treatment for vaginal infections, the woman should refrain from sexual contact or use a condom. If the woman develops irritations easily, she should check with her partner, because his soap or other personal products could be inadvertently promoting infection.

Breast Health

The outlook for breast cancer diagnosis, treatment, and survival remains promising. The most important research breakthrough, however, will be when researchers find the key to preventing breast cancer. In this section the focus is on risk factors, screening, and diagnostic testing for breast health. Detailed information on the breast cancer diagnosis, treatment, and nursing management is found in Chapter 4.

Risk Factors for Breast Cancer. The cause of breast cancer remains essentially unknown and continues to elude investigators. Although researchers have identified some clear risk factors, the significance of many is still controversial. The greatest risk factor for breast cancer is being a woman. Other strongly accepted risk factors are age and personal and family history of breast cancer.

In 1994, *breast cancer 1 and breast cancer 2 genes* (***BRCA1*** and ***BRCA2***) were discovered and found to correlate with increased risk for breast, ovarian, and other cancers. *BRCA1* is located on chromosome 17; *BRCA2* is located on chromosome 13. Mutations of *BRCA1* and *BRCA2* impair production of tumour-suppressor proteins. Although alterations in these genes may increase the risk for cancer, they certainly do not fully explain the history of breast or ovarian cancer in every family. Carriers of *BRCA1* and *BRCA2* have an estimated lifetime risk of breast cancer of 40% to 85% (Pruthi et al., 2010).

An understanding of breast health and breast cancer is important for all women. Breast cancer is the most common cancer in women. It is also one of the most treatable cancers if detected early. It is estimated that in 2013, breast cancer will represent 26% of all new cancer cases in women (Canadian Cancer Society, 2013b). The risk to Canadian women of developing breast cancer in their lifetime is reported as one in nine (Canadian Cancer Society, 2013b). Risk increases with age, meaning that if a woman lives to be 90 years old, her risk is one in eight. Nodal involvement remains the single most prognostic criterion for long-term survival. Most recent evidence indicates the 5-year survival rate for breast cancer in women as 88% (Canadian Cancer Society, 2013b) and is attributed to increased awareness, early detection, and treatment.

More than half of all women who menstruate regularly go through, at one time or another, the frightening experience of finding a breast lump. Most of these lumps are benign (Canadian Cancer Society, 2013b). Nevertheless, few conditions create as much concern for women as breast cancer. Understanding breast health, screening protocols, and options for treatment are important dimensions of women's health. Early detection and treatment remain the best hopes for improving both quality of life and survival. It is recommended that women who are identified at high risk for breast cancer be referred for genetic assessment and counselling (Christinat & Pagani, 2013). Nurses have a vitally important role as educators and advocates in

● TABLE 2.4 **Breast Cancer Screening Recommendation**

BREAST CANCER SCREENING GUIDELINES	
If You Are	**You Should**
40–49	Have a clinical breast examination by a trained health care professional at least every 2 yrs. Talk to your doctor about your risk of breast cancer, along with the benefits and risks of mammography.
50–69	Have a clinical breast examination by a trained healthcare professional at least every 2 yrs. Have a mammogram every 2 yrs.
70 or older	Talk to your doctor about how often you should be screened for breast cancer.

Source: Canadian Task Force on Preventive Health Care. (2011).

shaping the woman's and family's experiences during all aspects of breast health care and breast cancer. Women with breast cancer that is detected early are living full and productive lives.

Individualized Screening Information. Breast cancer screening programs vary among Canadian provinces and territories. The Canadian Cancer Society (2013a) provides screening guidelines. See Table 2.4.

Screening mammography and clinical breast examinations are considered the most reliable methods of finding breast cancer. Each woman must make informed choices with her health care provider regarding her individual and family risk factors and personal screening schedule choices. Nurses must communicate to women and their families that these recommendations are just those based on the generalized population of women. Individual risk factors and informed choice should still guide each woman.

Breast Self-Examination. Research indicates that routine monthly **breast self-examination** does not reduce mortality and likely increases benign biopsy rates (Canadian Task Force on Preventive Health Care, 2011). The Canadian Cancer Society (2013a) no longer recommends monthly breast self-examinations and states that there is no right or wrong way for women to check their breasts, as long as they get to know the whole area of their breast tissue—up to the collarbone, under the armpits, and including the nipples—well enough to notice changes. Women need to know the early symptoms of breast cancer and report promptly any changes or concerns to a health professional. Many women discover their own breast cancer through changes in the look and feel of their breasts. If a woman finds a change in her breasts, she should not try to diagnose it herself. There is no substitute for a practitioner's evaluation and further diagnostic tests.

The following signs and symptoms require follow-up:

- Lump
- Pain (breast cancer may or may not be painful)
- Discharge
- Skin changes
- Lymphadenopathy, with or without other symptoms
- Any change the woman finds as personally unusual

Clinical Breast Examination. **Clinical breast examination**, an important part of the Canadian Cancer Society's breast cancer detection guidelines, is a physical examination of the breasts by a trained health professional. Overall, it has a dual purpose. First, experienced professionals may find breast changes that the woman has missed, thus reinforcing the importance of women becoming familiar with their breasts by looking at and feeling them. Second, the examination is an opportunity to demonstrate and explain a thorough breast examination. The effectiveness depends on its precision, accuracy, and time spent doing the examination (Fenton et al., 2005). Controversy exists because of the lack of strong research evidence linking its effectiveness in screening for breast cancer (Fenton et al., 2005). Until new techniques and diagnostic tests provide strong research evidence as proven alternatives, clinical breast examinations and mammograms are still commonly conducted for breast cancer screening.

Mammography. Screening recommendations in Canada include a clinical breast examination every 2 years in women aged 40 to 49 years and a clinical breast examination and mammogram every 2 years in women 50 to 59 (Canadian Cancer Society, 2013a). Women aged 70 and

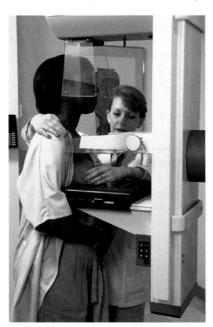

FIGURE 2.8 Mammography can help detect cancerous breast lumps and masses and is an important screening tool for women.

older should discuss with their doctor or nurse practitioner about having a mammogram. Most breast lesions are present for several years before they are palpable. Lumps that cannot yet be felt by the woman can be detected by **mammogram**, the soft tissue x-ray of the breast (Fig. 2.8). Mammography has the potential to detect breast cancer at its earliest stage of development. Although mammography has significantly increased the number of breast cancers identified, it does fail to detect some malignancies. Few diagnostic tests are 100% sensitive.

Ultrasound. Experts agree that women need regular mammograms and a clinical breast examination every 2 years after the age of 50. For women younger than 50, risk factors and informed choices will determine the schedule. There is little debate that women with special risk factors should begin routine mammograms and clinical breast examinations by their nurse practitioner or physician at approximately 35 years. Mammograms are less reliable in young women because of the density of the breast tissue. **Ultrasound** of the breast is useful to differentiate a solid or fluid structure (cyst) in the breast. Although recent statistics demonstrate that mammograms for women younger than 50 years might not dramatically affect the overall picture of breast cancer, there is a woman behind every number. Ultrasound is also used in older women after mammography to confirm or differentiate findings.

Cultural Beliefs Regarding Health Promotion Issues

In 2005, four health goals for Canadians were agreed upon by the Federal, Provincial and Territorial Ministers of Health. The health goals—basic needs, belonging and engaging, healthy living, and a system for health (PHAC, 2008b)—have implications for promoting the health of women and their families. Socioeconomic factors and cultural beliefs and practices affect the health behaviours of women, thereby influencing their access to and use of health services, confidence in practitioners and recommended prevention guidelines, and general health beliefs. Promoting the health and well-being of Canadian women involves assessing their cultural beliefs and values as well as acknowledging the diversity among women across the country. Immigrant women, newly arrived refugees, Aboriginal women, women residing in remote and rural communities, women in large urban settings, homeless and impoverished women, all present differing health care needs and access to health services.

Canada is a country characterized by the culturally diverse nature of its population. The continuing influx of new immigrants into Canada has resulted in approximately one in five women currently living in Canada being foreign-born. According to the 2006 Census, visible minority women made up 16.4% of the total female population in Canada, of which the majority are

Chinese (24.3%), South Asian (East Indian, Pakistani, Sri Lankan) (24%), or Black (15.7%) (Chui & Maheux, 2011). Non-European immigrants are more likely than Canadian-born women to experience, over time, a decline in their health status (Ng et al., 2005).

The history of colonization and marginalization of the indigenous population in the Western world has severely affected the health and well-being of Canada's Aboriginal people, the women in particular. The imposition of Western values and health care practices has led to Aboriginal women losing their economic status, language, community rights, culture, and traditional roles as healers and leaders. Aboriginal women comprise approximately 4% of the women in Canada and their number is increasing. In 2006, 60% of Aboriginal women reported being First Nations, 33% were Métis, and 4% were Inuit (Statistics Canada, 2012). The First Nations communities are spread across the country, and each has distinct values, traditions, and cultural beliefs about health. This rich diversity among Aboriginal women is reflected in the variety of health issues that need to be acknowledged in the provision of effective, sensitive, and appropriate care. Many important health promotion issues are of special concern to Aboriginal women.

Aboriginal women do not share the same level of health status experienced by other Canadian women. In comparison to non-Aboriginal women, they are at higher risk for type 2 diabetes, hypertension, obesity, heart disease, stroke, kidney disease, arthritis, HIV/AIDS, intimate partner violence, mental illness, and cervical and breast cancer (Mann, 2005). Socioeconomic factors such as poverty and unemployment, poor housing and living conditions, the cost of quality food in remote communities, marginalization, and colonialism contribute to the health condition of Aboriginal women. To address the many health needs of Aboriginal women, health services have been made more accessible to and governed by the Aboriginal people. Health care service delivery to the Aboriginal population is complex, with the federal, provincial, and territorial governments all having a role to play. There is continual movement toward First Nations and Inuit communities having control over their own health services. Health Canada's First Nations and Inuit Health Branch (FNIHB) has published a strategic plan to enhance health services and benefits that are responsive to needs and that improve health status of the Aboriginal population (Health Canada, 2012a).

Environmental Factors Related to Health Issues

Nurses need to recognize that many women, frequently and unknowingly, are exposed to unseen health threats in the environment. Table 2.5 contains a variety of environmental risks that can pose serious health concerns. For each risk, the table lists specific steps to avoid exposure and to minimize harm from exposure to a health hazard.

● TABLE 2.5 **Environmental Risks and Protective Measures**

Potential Risks	Preventive or Corrective Action
Allergies	Keep environment free of known allergens. Consider allergy-free pets. Use high efficiency particulate air (HEPA) filters. If exposure is unavoidable, consider antihistamine use.
Asbestos	Have a qualified contractor check old homes and remove any existing asbestos. Avoid handling or working with asbestos-containing materials (eg, patching compounds, ceiling tiles, pipe insulation, vinyl floors, brake shoes, clutch pads). Vigorously wash hands and shower after use of these materials.
Benzene	Avoid breathing cigarette smoke, gasoline fumes, and vehicular emissions.
Carbon monoxide	Ensure appliances are installed and operating correctly. Perform annual automobile and home heating inspections. Do not burn charcoal or operate gasoline engines in confined areas (home, garage, camper). Install detectors with audible alarms in home and garage. Avoid cigarette smoke.
Cigarette smoke	Avoid cigarette and cigar smoking and secondhand smoke.
Dioxins	These are fat soluble and cross the placenta into breast milk. They are found in meats, fish, eggs, and dairy products. Reduce fat consumption. Broil food instead of frying. Limit use of chlorine-bleached products (eg, toilet paper, tampons).
Food poisoning	Use proper hand washing technique when preparing food. Refrigerate food at adequate temperatures. Thoroughly cook meat, fish, poultry, and eggs. Disinfect countertops and utensils that come in contact with uncooked food. Wash thoroughly all fruits and vegetables to be eaten uncooked.
Hair solutions and products	Read labels carefully. Avoid direct inhalation and prolonged exposure. Use pump instead of aerosolized products.
Histoplasmosis	Avoid areas that may harbour the disease-causing fungus (eg, areas with accumulated bird or bat droppings, such as caves).
Lead	Have old homes tested before renovations. Ensure lead removal when feasible. Cover lead paint in good condition with lead-free paint or wallpaper. Pregnant women should avoid contact with lead-contaminated water, soil, and paint. Keep yard well vegetated to reduce contamination from soil. Clean floors and sills regularly with wet mop or cloth. Run faucet for 15 s before drawing drinking water.

(continued)

● TABLE 2.5 **Environmental Risks and Protective Measures** (continued)

Potential Risks	Preventive or Corrective Action
Lightning	Seek shelter during storms; avoid open fields and trees. Unplug appliances not on a surge protector. Avoid phone and water use during thunderstorms.
Mercury	Avoid eating large, long-lived fish (eg, shark, swordfish, king mackerel, tilefish). It is safe for pregnant women to eat an average of 12 oz of cooked shellfish, canned fish, or small ocean or farm-raised fish weekly.
Motor vehicle collisions	Wear seatbelts. Ensure proper airbag functioning. Children 12 yrs or younger should sit in the back. Use appropriate car seats for infants, toddlers, and young children. Use headlights and turn signals. Avoid speeding (leave early). Conduct annual automobile inspections.
Radon	Have home inspected or buy test kit from local grocery or hardware store. If radon is detected, arrange for a qualified radon-reduction contractor to visit the home. (The government hotline for info is 1-800-SOS-RADON.)
Teratogenic medications	Read warnings on medication labels carefully. Avoid ingesting or handling any medication shown to cause birth defects. Discuss risks with physician or pharmacist.
Toluene	Use toluene-containing substances (eg, glue, paint, paint thinner, nail polish, adhesives) in well-ventilated areas.
Ultraviolet (UV) radiation	Avoid sun exposure between 10 AM and 4 PM. Wear sunscreen with minimum SPF 15, using approximately 1 oz per application. Wear wide-brimmed hats, pants, and long sleeves (wear white clothing to avoid overheating). Wear sunglasses with UV protection year-round.
Viral infections	Vaccinate against infections such as rubella and hepatitis B before pregnancy. Practice strict hand washing and personal hygiene. Avoid unprotected sexual contact.
Xenoestrogens	Avoid pesticides (eat organic foods; wash fruits and vegetables thoroughly before eating). Avoid microwaving plastics and reusing plastic containers (eg, margarine or butter tubs).

Internet Resources for Environmental Health Issues

Clean Air Online

http://www.ec.gc.ca/air/

Canadian Lung Association

http://www.lung.ca/home-accueil_e.php

Canada Safety Council

http://canadasafetycouncil.org/

Environment Canada

http://www.ec.gc.ca/default.asp?lang=En&n=FD9B0E51-1

PHYSICAL EXAMINATION

With an overwhelming amount of health information available to women, nurses must focus on identifying risk factors based on the woman's health history, assessment, and physical examination. Table 2.6 discusses body systems and organ changes in relation to normal and alterations in normal across the woman's life cycle.

NURSING AND COLLABORATIVE CARE ROLES RELATED TO HEALTH PROMOTION

QUOTE 2-2

"When you cease to make a contribution, you begin to die."

Eleanor Roosevelt

Health behaviours involve complex variables and decisions. Examples include issues such as weight control, smoking cessation, obesity, and intimate partner violence. Decisions related to these areas are best made within a partnership of equity and support from health professionals.

When working with clients to make changes in the area of health promotion, nursing interventions address the following health needs:

• Social support
• Strengths of the woman and her family
• Need for culturally sensitive education and expression of questions
• Sexuality and relationship concerns
• Spirituality and psychological needs
• Financial needs

Box 2.2 represents a model for the woman making health-related decisions or lifestyle changes. The nurse focuses on a multidisciplinary model to ensure that the woman and her family have referrals to dietitians, counsellors, specialists, and community health resources, as needed. Box 2.3 provides a list of internet resources for women.

(text continues on page 75)

● TABLE 2.6 **Physical Examination Guidelines**

Considerations, Findings, and Life Cycle Perspectives	Therapeutic Interventions
Dermatologic System	
Skin should be dry, warm, and smooth. *Wrinkles* are a natural part of aging, determined mostly by genetics and sun exposure. Normal facial expressions ultimately cause crease lines. Smiling, squinting, and frowning all contract the facial muscles, causing accordion-like lines to develop. *Dry skin* increases with age, mostly from sun exposure, which thins the skin and decreases moisture retention. *Acne* may appear for the first time or worsen in midlife from hormonal fluctuations. Some women experience alopecia, but to a much lesser extent than men. *Excessive hair growth*, especially on the upper lip or along the jaw line, can result from hormones as menopause approaches.	Check sun-exposed areas well, especially head, neck, and hands. Use sunscreen with a broad spectrum that protects from ultraviolet A and B (UVA and UVB) rays. Apply enough; apply frequently; reapply immediately after swimming or every 2 h if out of the water. Apply sunscreen 15–30 min before going into the sun. Wear clothing that has been specially made to block UV rays. Avoid the sun from 10 AM to 4 PM when rays are most intense. A wide-brimmed hat will protect the client's face. Advise client to avoid cigarettes, which cause cancer *and* wrinkles. Certain medications cause a photosensitivity reaction; check adverse reactions for all medications the client uses. Add moisture to the air with humidifiers or a pan of water set on the radiator to help prevent dry skin. Instruct clients to use lukewarm water instead of hot water, which strips away natural oils, when showering. Advise clients to use nondrying soaps without abrasives or irritants. Cleansing bars and super-fatted soaps are less drying. Clients should pat, not rub, the skin dry. Instruct clients to apply moisturizer immediately after a bath or shower to retain the water absorbed.
Eyes, Ears, Nose, Throat	
Sclera may look buff-coloured at the extreme periphery. Visual acuity is fairly constant between 20 and 50 yrs. Near vision begins to blur for almost everyone. As the lens loses its elasticity, it increasingly cannot focus on nearby objects. This presbyopia becomes noticeable after 40 yrs of age (Bickley, 2013)	
Cardiovascular System	
Heart sounds: assess for regular rate and rhythm, murmurs, jugular venous pressure (JVD), carotid bruits, and pulses. *Heart rate* may be as low as 50 beats/min in a woman who regularly engages in aerobic activity. A *split S2* can be normal in women 20–30 yrs of age. The split may widen on inspiration. *Spider veins* are groups of blood vessels close to the skin surface that have dilated. They may appear on thighs, calves, and ankles as part of aging, heredity, hormonal changes, or external injuries. *Varicose veins* may result from pooled blood as veins lose elasticity and the valves malfunction.	Regular exercise, such as walking, jogging, biking, and swimming, will help prevent varicose veins. The Heart and Stroke Foundation of Canada and the Canadian Cardiovascular Congress suggest taking an aggressive approach to screening for and treating high cholesterol.
Pulmonary System	
A healthy person typically breathes effortlessly and automatically 20,000 times a day	To keep lungs healthy, instruct clients to avoid irritants, such as chemical and gas fumes, smoke, and asbestos, as much as possible. Encourage them to consider installing a particulate air filter, especially if they have asthma or respiratory problems or live with a smoker. Encourage clients to eat a diet rich in antioxidants: fruits and vegetables, carotenes (found in carrots, yellow squash), and dark leafy greens. Antioxidants may help protect against cancer. Regular aerobic exercise strengthens the muscles of breathing. Advise clients to breathe consciously: practice breathing more deeply, slowly, quietly, and regularly, working to extend each exhalation to squeeze out more air. Advise clients to alert the health care practitioner right away for a cough that lasts longer than 1 mo, frequent chest colds, shortness of breath with limited exertion, difficulty breathing, wheezing, or coughing up blood.

(continued)

● TABLE 2.6 **Physical Examination Guidelines** (continued)

Considerations, Findings, and Life Cycle Perspectives	Therapeutic Interventions
Gastrointestinal System Inspect abdomen, noting posture, contour, masses, bulging, distention, scars, venous patterns, lesions, and striae. Note the abdominal contour after asking the client to take a deep breath and raise her head. Listen for bowel sounds in all four quadrants; they should be high pitched. The skin of the abdomen is subject to the same colour variations as the rest of the body. Venous patterns may be more prominent in thin clients. Striae result from stretched tissue: obesity or pregnancy. The abdomen may be symmetrically distended from a heavy meal, obesity, or gas. No bulges should appear. Clicks or gurgles are normal. Bowel sounds may last from half second to several seconds.	Educate clients regarding diet, which greatly influences risk for colorectal cancer. A diet that is generally: ● High in fresh fruits and vegetables ● Modest in calories ● Modest in alcohol consumption ● Low in red meat and animal fat is cancer protective. Eating foods high in fibre and low in fat, exercising regularly, drinking plenty of water, and avoiding foods that cause problems can help keep the digestive system healthy. A "Western" dietary pattern is associated with: ● Higher body mass index ● Greater intake of total energy and dietary cholesterol The "prudent" pattern is associated with: ● Higher levels of vigorous leisure time physical activity ● Smaller body size ● Higher intakes of dietary fibre and folate The "Western" dietary pattern is associated with an increased risk for colon cancer in both men and women. Evidence supports the hypothesis that overall dietary intake pattern is associated with colon cancer and that the dietary pattern associated with the greatest increase in risk is the one that typifies a Western-style diet (Fung et al., 2003). Counsel the client about hepatitis B, a type of hepatitis virus that attacks and damages the liver. Advise immunizations, if appropriate.
Urologic	Educate clients about factors that contribute to infection of the urinary tract: ● Sexual activity can introduce bacteria into the urethra. ● Poor hygiene habits, such as not bathing or showering routinely, or changing underwear and sanitary pads infrequently, can introduce bacteria from the rectum into the urethra. ● Excessive use of caffeine can cause urinary irritation and diuresis. ● Excessive stress can reduce the immune response. ● Using a diaphragm may press on the bladder and cause stasis of urine. Spermicides inhibit growth of lactobacilli. ● Waiting long periods between urinations results in stasis of urine and decreases flushing of bacteria from the bladder.
Breasts Inspect breasts and nipples with the client sitting, disrobed to the waist.Look for skin changes, symmetry, contours, and retraction. Also examine her breasts with her hands over head, and hands on hips. Some difference in the size of the breasts, including the areolas, is common. Long-standing inversion of a nipple is usually normal. Normal tissue varies widely. Nodularity may increase premenstrually. A firm transverse ridge of breast tissue is often found along the lower edge of the breast, especially in large breasts. Tenderness is common premenstrually.	Educate clients about breast cancer screening, early symptoms of breast cancers. Encourage women to become familiar with their breasts by looking at and feeling them. Advising routine breast self-examination not recommended (Canadian Task Force on Preventive Health Care, 2011). Women between the ages of 40 and 49 should discuss their risk of breast cancer, along with the benefits and risks of mammography, with their doctor. Women between the ages of 50 and 69 should have a mammogram every 2–3 yrs. ● With increased risk factors, the examination should begin sooner ● Family history of a first-degree relative with breast cancer ● Menstrual history: age at menarche younger than 12 yrs, age at menopause older than 55 yrs ● Pregnancy: nulliparous ● Breast conditions such as atypical hyperplasia or lobular carcinoma *in situ* Further, counsel clients about the relationship between obesity, diet, and breast cancer: ● In premenopausal women, obesity is not associated with increased risk for breast cancer, presumably because it decreases the number of ovulatory cycles, reducing exposure to estrogen between menarche and menopause.

(*table continues on page 75*)

● TABLE 2.6   **Physical Examination Guidelines** (continued)

Considerations, Findings, and Life Cycle Perspectives	Therapeutic Interventions
	● Obesity may increase breast cancer risk because body fat is critical in the early initiation of menarche, expanding the period between menarche and menopause, thereby increasing total exposure to estrogen. ● Obese postmenopausal women show a greater risk for breast cancer. ● A positive correlation between alcohol consumption and breast cancer risk was observed in premenopausal but not in postmenopausal women. ● Isothiocyanates found in broccoli and watercress have been found to have antitumour activity in mammary tissue.
Reproductive System Women's reproductive needs vary across the lifespan, whether they are heterosexual or lesbian.	Counsel clients about various aspects of reproductive health. ● Birth control (or contraception) helps a woman plan her pregnancies. Some methods of birth control also help protect against STIs, including AIDS. The more the client knows about birth control and her own needs, the easier it will be for her to choose a method that's right for her. ● There are many methods of birth control. The birth control pill, implants, injections, intrauterine device (IUD), diaphragm, and cervical cap require a prescription. ● The most commonly used method of hormonal birth control is the birth control pill (oral contraceptive). ● If a woman has sex without any type of birth control, she may be able to use a type of backup birth control called *emergency contraception*. In this method, high doses of certain birth control pills are taken within 72 hrs (3 days) of sex without birth control. ● Most birth control failures result from not using birth control correctly each time. ● Barrier methods are some of the oldest and safest forms of contraception (birth control). These methods work by acting as barriers to keep the man's sperm from reaching the woman's egg. Some methods also may protect against certain STIs. Barrier methods are effective when used correctly and every time the client has sex. Today, barrier methods are safe and effective ways to prevent pregnancy. The diaphragm, cervical cap, sponge, and condom (male and female) act as physical barriers. ● Spermicides act as chemical barriers. The best results are achieved when spermicides are used along with a physical barrier method, such as a condom, diaphragm, sponge, or cervical cap. Use of latex condoms, especially those with spermicide, can help protect against the spread of some STIs, including HIV infection, the virus that causes AIDS. If a woman has sex without any type of birth control or if she thinks her barrier method has failed (for instance, a condom broke), she may use emergency birth control. ● The nurse counsels her client to begin good care and a healthy lifestyle before pregnancy to increase the odds that the client will have a healthy baby. ● If the client is planning to become pregnant, the nurse counsels her to have a prepregnancy checkup. ● As a part of this visit, the nurse practitioner asks the client about her medical and family history, medications she takes, any past pregnancies she has had, and her diet and lifestyle. Her answers will help her nurse practitioner decide whether she needs special care during pregnancy. ● Some women have medical conditions, such as diabetes, high blood pressure, and seizure disorders, that can cause problems during pregnancy. Instruct the client to let her primary health care provider know if a past pregnancy was complicated by diabetes, high blood pressure, premature labour, preterm birth, or birth defects. ● Folic acid, taken before pregnancy and for the first 3 mos of pregnancy, can reduce the risk for neural tube defects. ● Three types of providers offer medical care for pregnancy and birth: obstetrician-gynecologists, family practitioners, and certified midwives. Labour and delivery nurses help care for women and their babies during labour, during delivery, and right after birth.

(continued)

● TABLE 2.6 **Physical Examination Guidelines** (continued)

Considerations, Findings, and Life Cycle Perspectives	Therapeutic Interventions
	The nurse counsels the client on safe sex practices, including common STIs. ● HPV is a virus that causes warts. HPV is one of the most common STIs. ● Infection with gonorrhea and chlamydia causes two of the most common STIs. ● Gonorrhea and chlamydia often have no symptoms. When symptoms do occur, they may show up 2 days to 3 wks after infection. ● Syphilis, another STI, occurs less often, but can be serious if it is not treated. ● If the client thinks she may be at risk for gonorrhea, chlamydia, or syphilis, the nurse encourages her to see her primary health care provider to get tested. ● Pregnant women may also be offered testing for gonorrhea and chlamydia. ● Women who douche at least once a month have higher rates of bacterial vaginosis infections than women who don't douche. The nurse should counsel her clients to see their primary health care provider regularly for preventive health care. Such care includes routine tests and examinations that all women need, regardless of their sexual orientation. The nurse counsels her client about premenstrual syndrome (PMS), including educating the client on how the menstrual cycle works. ● During the menstrual cycle, estrogen and progesterone—two hormones made by the ovaries—cause changes in the lining of the uterus (endometrium). Women with PMS have symptoms in the second half of the cycle (after they ovulate on about day 14). ● As many as 85% of women who menstruate report some symptoms of PMS in the days or weeks before menstruation.
Nervous System	
Results from the Canadian population-based study (Reitsma et al., 2011) show that chronic pain is most prevalent among women (16.5% to 21.5%) and is highest among women over 65. Arthritis/rheumatism, fibromyalgia, migraine headaches, and back pain are four conditions known to be strongly related to chronic pain	Counsel clients that limiting stress, avoiding triggers, and exercising regularly can help manage chronic pain. Incorporate multidisciplinary treatment as necessary.
Psychological	
It is estimated that 12.2% of Canadians will experience major depression at some time of their lives (Public Health Agency of Canada, 2011a). A family history of depression may increase a client's risk; such clients should tell health care providers about symptoms	Counsel clients that depression is a treatable medical problem, similar to diabetes, hypertension, and heart disease.

Health Screening

As providers collaborating with other health care and community professionals, nurses must be knowledgeable regarding proper health screening for women. In educating women and conducting health screenings, nurses play a key role in preventing illness and optimizing health. As advocates for clients, nurses are obligated to help them understand and integrate the need for routine screening as a preventive strategy. Within these general guidelines, the nurse collaborating with other professionals must consider each woman's history and risk factors. Table 2.7 summarizes health screening guidelines, laboratory and diagnostic tests, and immunization recommendations for client education, referral, and clinical practice.

 Linda, the 53-year-old perimenopausal woman from the beginning of the chapter, asks how often she should have a mammogram and Pap smear. What response is appropriate?

(text continues on page 78)

● **BOX 2.2** **Nursing Interventions to Encourage Health-Promoting Behaviour Changes**

Social Support
- Give the woman time and space to adjust to the lifestyle change.
- Encourage networking with other women with a similar situation.
- Encourage women to ask for help and to allow themselves to experience others' expressions of support and caring.

Strengths of Woman and Family
- Focus on current strengths in making the decisions and lifestyle changes.
- Explore what skills and strengths work for this client and her family.

Need for Culturally Sensitive Education and Expression of Questions
- Give the information needed or requested. Offer brochures and internet resources.
- Encourage sharing of thoughts and feelings on barriers to the lifestyle change.
- Explore and clarify misconceptions or unrealistic fears.
- Provide information about any medication regimen prescribed for treatment. Include medication, dosage, side effects, and desired benefit. Review any over-the-counter medications or herbal therapies being used.
- Provide information to the client regarding risk factors, screening guidelines, and recommended diagnostic or laboratory test and follow-up plan.

Sexuality and Relationship Concerns
- Encourage the client to seek support from spouse/partner as well as others.

- Spouses or partners may not be able to fulfill all the woman's connection needs. Suggest outlets to connect with oneself, such as journaling, poetry, and meditation.

Spirituality and Psychological Needs
- Discuss the need to keep a positive outlook. Explain that relapse is expected.
- Encourage the client to do what is important to her. Promote self-nurturing activities and positive self-talk.
- Suggest journaling, music, imagery, or yoga for relaxation and to enhance health-promoting behaviours.
- Encourage release of energy through humour and playful activities.
- Encourage church activities or personal expressions and prayer with their spiritual power, as appropriate.

Financial Needs
- Discuss behaviour changes and treatment options in relation to financial circumstances.
- Discuss alternative behaviours or treatments when the client has financial burdens.

Community Resources and Collaborative Care
- Offer the resource of a support group, counsellor, or specialist, as needed.
- Offer community resources and validation of experiences with others in the community.

● **BOX 2.3** **Internet Resources for Women's Health**

http://ww2.heartandstroke.ca/
http://www.phac-aspc.gc.ca/index-eng.php
http://www.osteoporosis.ca/
http://www.womenshealthmatters.ca/
http://www.niaaa.nih.gov/
http://acsh.org/
http://www.cdc.gov/wisewoman/
http://www.cdc.gov/women/
http://www.cdc.gov/ncbddd/folicacid/index.html
http://www.youngwomenshealth.org/healthyeating.
   html

http://www.nap.edu/catalog.php?record_id=6035
http://sogc.org/
http://www.ahrq.gov/research/findings/factsheets/
   women/womenh/index.html
http://www.ncbi.nlm.nih.gov/
http://www.cwhn.ca/
http://www.motherisk.org/women/index.jsp
http://www.healthywomen.org/

● TABLE 2.7 **Health Screening for Women During the Reproductive Years**

Screening Tests	18–39 Yrs	40–49 Yrs	50–64 Yrs
General Health			
Full checkup, including height, weight, and BMI	Dependent on risk factors	Yearly	Yearly
Thyroid test	Starting at 35 yrs, then every 5 yrs; sooner if symptomatic	Every 5 yrs	Every 5 yrs
Heart Health			
Blood pressure measurement	Begin testing at 21 yrs, then every 2 yrs depending on risk factors	Every 2 yrs depending on risk factors	Every 1–2 yrs depending on risk factors
Cholesterol screening	At 20 yrs, discuss testing with health professional	Discuss with health professional	Begin testing at age 50. Every 5 yrs; more frequently with CAD, DM, obesity, or dyslipidemia
Bone Health			
Bone mineral density test	Only if significant risk factors (anorexia, multiple fractures)	Dependent on risk factors	At 65 yrs
Diabetes			
Blood glucose test	Only if significant risk factors (family history, obesity, symptomatic)	Begin testing at 40 yrs, then every 3 yrs	Every 3 yrs
Breast Health			
Breast examination	Yearly by a health care provider	Yearly by a health care provider	Yearly by a health care provider
Mammogram	Only if significant risk factors (family history, mass noted in breast)	Every 1–2 yrs depending on risk factors	Every 2 yrs
Reproductive Health			
Pap smear and pelvic examination	Screening not recommended <20 yrs. Every 3 yrs after three consecutive normal results and minimal risk factors	Every 3 yrs after three consecutive normal results and minimal risk factors	Every 3 yrs after three consecutive normal results and minimal risk factors
Chlamydia test	If sexually active, yearly until 25 yrs. Continue to perform if high risk (multiple sexual partners, recent change in partner); first prenatal visit	If high risk for contracting an STI, continue testing yearly; otherwise, according to risk factors; first prenatal visit	If at high risk for contracting an STI, continue testing yearly; otherwise, according to risk factors
STI tests	Yearly if client has multiple sexual partners, a partner with multiple sexual partners, a partner with an STI, or a personal history of STI	Yearly if client has multiple sexual partners, a partner with multiple sexual partners, a partner with an STI, or a personal history of STI	Yearly if client has multiple sexual partners, a partner with multiple sexual partners, a partner with an STI, or a personal history of STI
Colorectal Health			
Colonoscopy	Only if significant risk factors or rectal bleeding	Only if significant risk factors or rectal bleeding	Only if significant risk factors or rectal bleeding
Double contrast barium enema	Only if significant risk factors or rectal bleeding	Only if significant risk factors or rectal bleeding	Every 5–10 yrs only if not having colonoscopy every 10 yrs
Flexible sigmoidoscopy	Only if significant risk factors or rectal bleeding	Only if significant risk factors or rectal bleeding	Every 5 yrs
Rectal examination	Only if significant risk factors or rectal bleeding	Only if significant risk factors or rectal bleeding	Yearly
Fecal occult blood test	Only if symptomatic	Only if symptomatic	Every 2 yrs unless significant risk factors

(table continues on page 78)

● TABLE 2.7 **Health Screening for Women During the Reproductive Years** (continued)

Screening Tests	18–39 Yrs	40–49 Yrs	50–64 Yrs
Eye and Ear Health			
Vision examination	Examination with an eye care provider once initially between 20 and 39 yrs and then as recommended by provider	Every 2–4 yrs	Every 2–4 yrs
Hearing test	Initial examination at 18 yrs, then every 10 yrs unless hearing changes	Every 10 yrs	Dependent on symptoms and risk factors (eg, employed in a noisy workplace)
Skin Health			
Mole examination	Monthly self-examination starting by 20 yrs; every 3 yrs by a health care provider	Monthly self-examination; every year by a health care provider	Monthly self-examination; every year by a health care provider
Oral Health			
Dental examination	One to two times a year	One to two times a year	One to two times a year
Mental Health Screening	Abuse and depression screen with office visits based on risk factors and symptoms	Abuse and depression screen with office visits based on risk factors and symptoms	Abuse and depression screen with office visits based on risk factors and symptoms
Nutrition Supplements	Teens to age 18, 1,300 mg calcium; age 19–50 yrs, 1,000 mg calcium daily; pregnant or lactating, 1,000 mg calcium; vitamin D, 400 to 1,000 IU; 15 mg iron daily; 0.4 mg folic acid daily	1,000 mg calcium daily; vitamin D, 400–1,000 IU; 15 mg iron daily; 0.4 mg folic acid daily	1,200 mg calcium daily; vitamin D, 800–2,000 IU; 10 mg iron daily; 0.4 mg folic acid daily
Safety	Wear a seatbelt and bike helmet. Use smoke and carbon monoxide detectors. Wear sunscreen and UV-protected sunglasses. Practice safe sex	Wear a seatbelt and bike helmet. Use smoke and carbon monoxide detectors. Wear sunscreen and UV-protected sunglasses. Practice safe sex	Wear a seatbelt and bike helmet. Use smoke and carbon monoxide detectors. Wear sunscreen and UV-protected sunglasses. Practice safe sex

BMI, body mass index; BSE, breast self-examination; CAD, coronary artery disease; DM, diabetes mellitus; STI, sexually transmitted infection; TSH, thyroid-stimulating hormone. Information adapted from National Women's Health Information Center (NWHIC). Available at http://www.womenshealth.gov/ and the Canadian Cancer Society, www.cancer.ca.

Immunizations

The goal of immunization is the eradication of vaccine-preventable diseases and the associated negative health consequences among populations (PHAC, 2006). Immunizations are recommended for adults as well as children. Nurses collaborating with other health care providers must ensure the well-being of clients by following immunization recommendations. Figure 2.9 lists the 2006 PHAC recommendations for adult immunizations.

SUMMARY

● Health promotion for each woman is situated in a complex sociopolitical context. Health promotion strategies are an interdisciplinary activity, and the nurse is a key professional team member. The focus

of health promotion is based on the woman's own perspective.

● Health promotion includes health education, marketing the health message, lifestyle modification, engaging in social and environmental change, and encompassing the client's cultural values. In partnership with the woman, the nurse can support physical and mental health promotion strategies to improve health outcomes for the woman, her family, and the community.

● The major Canadian public health epidemics, including heart disease, obesity, diabetes, substance use, and intimate partner violence, are all amenable to change through health promotion strategies. Nurses are in a position to engage with the client in motivating and regulating health-promoting behaviours.

Prevention of infection by immunization is a lifelong process. There are a number of vaccines that all adults (≥18 years) require. There are also other vaccines that need to be tailored to meet individual variations in risk resulting from occupation, foreign travel, underlying illness, lifestyle and age.

Immunizations recommended for adults – Routine

All adults should be immunized against diphtheria, tetanus, pertussis, measles, mumps, rubella and varicella. The schedule for adults who have no record or an unclear history of prior immunization as well as for booster dosing of those who have completed a prior primary series is shown in the table below.

Adult Immunization Schedule – Routinely for All

VACCINE	DOSING SCHEDULE (NO RECORD OR UNCLEAR HISTORY OF IMMUNIZATION)	BOOSTER SCHEDULE (PRIMARY SERIES COMPLETED)
Tetanus and diphtheria given as Td; and pertussis given as Tdap	Doses 1 and 2, 4–8 weeks apart and dose 3 at 6–12 months later; one of the doses should be given as Tdap for pertussis protection	Td every 10 years; 1 dose should be given as Tdap if not previously given in adulthood
Measles, mumps, and rubella given as MMR	1 dose for adults born in or after 1970 without a history of measles or those individuals without evidence of immunity to rubella or mumps; second dose for selected groups	Not routinely required
Varicella	Doses 1 and 2, at least 4 weeks apart for susceptible adults (no history of natural disease or seronegativity)	Not currently recommended

All Canadian adults require maintenance of immunity to tetanus and diphtheria, preferably with combined (Td) toxoid and a single dose of acellular pertussis vaccine. The first priority is to ensure that children receive the recommended series of doses, including the school-leaving dose at 14 to 16 years of age, and that adults have completed primary immunization with Td. Currently, only a single dose of acellular pertussis (given as Tdap) is recommended in adulthood, because the duration of protection from Tdap has yet to be determined. For adults not previously immunized against pertussis, only one dose of Tdap is required as it is assumed that most adults will have some degree of immunity due to prior pertussis infection.

Combined measles, mumps, rubella vaccine (MMR) is preferred for vaccination of individuals not previously immunized against one or more of these viruses. Adults born before 1970 may be considered immune to measles. Adults born in 1970 or later who do not have documentation of adequate measles immunization or who are known to be seronegative should receive MMR vaccine. One additional dose of vaccine should be offered only to adults born in 1970 or later who are at greatest risk of exposure and who have not already received two doses or demonstrated immunity to measles. These people include travellers to a measles-endemic area, health care workers, students in post-secondary educational settings, and military recruits. MMR is recommended for all adults without a history of mumps or mumps immunization. MMR vaccine should also be given to all adults without a history of rubella vaccination. Female adolescents and women of childbearing age should be vaccinated before pregnancy or post-partum, unless they have documented evidence of detectable antibody or prior vaccination. In addition, it is also important that health care workers of either sex be actively immunized against rubella, because they may, through frequent face-to-face contact, expose pregnant women to rubella.

A history of chickenpox infection is adequate evidence of varicella immunity. Serologic testing should be performed in adults without a history of disease, as the majority of such adults will be immune and do not require the varicella vaccine. It is particularly important to promote varicella immunization with immigrants and refugees from tropical countries, women of childbearing age, those who are at occupational risk of exposure, including health care and child care workers, household contacts of immunocompromised persons, those with cystic fibrosis, and those susceptible adults exposed to a case of varicella. There are no data at present to guide recommendations for varicella booster dosing in adults following the primary vaccination series.

FIGURE 2.9 Adult immunization schedule. (From *Canadian immunization guide* (7th ed.). 2006. Complete guide available from http://www.phac-aspc.gc.ca/publicat/cig-gci/p03-02-eng.php).

(continued)

Immunizations for adults - Specific Risk Groups

There are several specific groups of adults for whom certain vaccines are recommended because of the presence of risk factors for disease, and these are summarized in the table below. In many cases, individual factors, and in particular the presence of underlying co-morbid illnesses, define groups that specifically benefit from certain vaccines. However, there are two commonly encountered groups of healthy adults who require assessment for a series of vaccines: health care workers and international travellers. In both of these groups, the priority should be to ensure that routinely recommended immunizations are completed and booster doses provided as indicated.

Adult Immunization Schedule - Specific Risk Situations

VACCINE OR TOXOID	INDICATION	SCHEDULE
Influenza	Adults ≥ 65 years; Adults < 65 years at high risk of Influenza-related complications, their household contacts, health care workers, and all those wishing to be protected against influenza.	Every autumn using current recommended vaccine formulation
Pneumococcal polysaccharide	Adults ≥ 65 years; Adults < 65 who have conditions putting them at increased risk of pneumococcal disease	1 dose
Hepatitis A	Occupational risk, life-style, travel and living in areas lacking adequate sanitation. Outbreak control, post-exposure immuno-prophylaxis. Patients with chronic liver disease.	2 doses, 6-12 months apart
Hepatitis B	Occupational risk, life style, post exposure immunoprophylaxis. Patients with chronic liver disease.	3 doses at 0, 1, and 6 months
Meningococcal conjugate	Young adults	1 dose
Meningococcal polysaccharide	High-risk exposure groups	1 dose

Health care workers, including hospital employees, other staff who work or study in hospitals (eg, students in health care disciplines and contract workers), other health care personnel (eg, those working in clinical laboratories, nursing homes, and home care agencies) and child care workers, are at risk of exposure to communicable diseases because of their contact with patients or material from individuals with infections, both diagnosed and undiagnosed.

Hepatitis B is the most important vaccine-preventable infectious occupational disease for health care workers. The risk of being infected is a consequence of the prevalence of virus carriers in the population receiving care, the frequency of exposure to blood and other body fluids and the contagiousness of hepatitis B virus. Hepatitis B vaccine is recommended for health care workers and others who may be exposed to blood or blood products, or who may be at increased risk of sharps injury, bites, or penetrating injuries (for example, clients and staff of institutions for the developmentally challenged). Annual Influenza immunization is recommended for all health care personnel who have contact with individuals in high-risk groups. Such personnel include physicians, nurses, and others in both hospital and outpatient settings; employees of chronic care facilities; and providers of home care, visiting nurses and volunteers. Influenza immunization of health care workers has been shown to reduce the mortality and morbidity of patients under their care in long-term settings, and to reduce worker illness and absenteeism during the Influenza season. Other vaccines may be indicated for certain workers at particularly high risk of exposure, such as laboratory workers in specialized reference or research facilities. These include but are not limited to typhoid, meningococcal, BCG, rabies, and smallpox vaccines. An individualized risk-benefit assessment is required.

International travellers represent another defined group requiring specific vaccine consideration. With travel-specific vaccines, an individualized approach is required that considers a patient's health status, risk of exposure and complications from vaccine-preventable illness, as well as location and duration of travel.

Source: *Canadian Immunization Guide,* Seventh Edition, 2006. Complete guide available from http://www.phac-aspc.gc.ca/publicat/cig-gci/index-eng.php

FIGURE 2.9 *(Continued)*

- Using health history and assessment data, nurses can base their care on a woman's unique health needs.
- Health promotion issues and risk factors are embedded in cultural beliefs and barriers for women.
- Nurses should conduct physical examinations of women to identify normal and alterations in normal for women in relation to their stage of the life cycle.
- Nursing interventions for health promotion involve collaboration with multidisciplinary professionals to implement recommended traditional and complementary therapies.
- Evidence-based health screening guidelines and immunization recommendations should be implemented in the care of women throughout their reproductive years.

Questions to Ponder

1. How can you understand and respect the relational nature of women's health beliefs and health promotion behaviours?
2. How can you provide information to women about risk factors and promote improved health-seeking behaviours?
3. What culturally sensitive health promotion interventions can you implement in your nursing practice with women?

REVIEW QUESTIONS

1. In developing a teaching plan for a woman who is going to initiate an exercise program, the nurse emphasizes that people who are successful at integrating exercise into their routine find that
   A. focusing on a long-term goal is helpful.
   B. having an exercise partner helps with motivation.
   C. exercising alone helps them to focus on the process.
   D. doing the same exercise each day helps maintain consistency.

2. When designing an exercise program with a client, it is important to consider the client's
   A. basal metabolic rate.
   B. daily caloric and calcium intake.
   C. priorities in changing her appearance.
   D. preferences regarding the type of movement she enjoys.

3. When providing counselling to a client on avoiding osteoporosis, the nurse includes
   A. limiting alcoholic beverages.
   B. increasing proteins from nonanimal sources into the diet.
   C. exercising for short periods of time a few times a day.
   D. integrating non–weight-bearing exercises into the daily routine.

4. The nurse's teaching plan for a woman experiencing osteoporosis includes the information that an important source of dietary calcium is
   A. beef.
   B. chicken.
   C. fatty fish.
   D. fresh orange juice.

5. The nurse is reviewing the laboratory results of a number of clients before the beginning of the shift. Which of these women would be *least* likely to have iron-deficiency anemia?
   A. A 27-year-old primigravida woman
   B. A 40-year-old woman with menorrhagia
   C. A 54-year-old woman who is 2 years postmenopausal
   D. A 16-year-old woman who reached menarche 6 months earlier

6. The nurse is reviewing the health history of a woman who has come to the clinic complaining of a yeast infection. A risk factor for yeast infection that the woman identified during the health history is that she
   A. has been diagnosed with osteopenia.
   B. has been breastfeeding her newborn.
   C. has difficulty controlling her diabetes.
   D. had a normal vaginal delivery 8 weeks earlier.

7. Which of the following statements, if made by an adolescent who has just received information from the nurse regarding health promotion strategies, would indicate that additional educational strategies may be needed?
   A. "I will participate in low-impact aerobic classes a few times a week."
   B. "I will make sure to eat or drink foods containing dietary calcium every day."
   C. "I will get my first Pap smear once I begin to have sex, regardless of my age."
   D. "I will become familiar with the look and feel of my breasts and report changes to my health care provider."

8. When reviewing the health history of a client diagnosed with cervical carcinoma, the nurse notes that the most likely causative agent is
   A. Candida albicans.
   B. Neisseria gonorrhoeae.
   C. Herpes simplex virus 2.
   D. HPV 18.

9. Which of the following statements, if made by a client who has just received information from the nurse regarding risk factors associated with cervical cancer, indicates a need for additional teaching?
   A. "Oral contraceptives increase my risk for cervical cancer."
   B. "Having sex before I was 16 increases my risk for cervical cancer."

C. "Multiple sexual partners increase my risk for cervical cancer."

D. "I will quit cigarette smoking because it could cause cervical cancer."

Acknowledgement

The family nurse practitioner students who contributed to the development of the original chapter are greatly appreciated: C. Bickett Cupp, C. Dufner, A. Dunn, L. Gambito, Y. Gazoni, J. Gray, V. Hamilton, T. Hedspeth, A. Hirsch, T. Markwalter, R. Grubbs, A. Schaefer, J. Shelton, J. Shepherd, E. Spiker, and W. Sweeney-Rodriguez.

REFERENCES

Amed, S., Daneman, D., Mahmud, F., & Hamilton, J. (2010). Type 2 diabetes in children and adolescents. *Expert Review of Cardiovascular Therapy, 8*(3), 393–406.

Association of Women's Health, Obstetric, and Neonatal Nurses. (2009). *Standards and guidelines for professional nursing practice in the care of women and newborns* (7th ed.). Washington, DC: Author.

Bellamy, L., Casas, J., Hingorani, A., & Williams, D. (2009). Type 2 diabetes mellitus after gestational diabetes: A systematic review and meta-analysis. *The Lancet, 373*, 1773–1779.

Bickley, L. S. (2013). *Bates' guide to physical examination and history taking* (11th ed.). Philadelphia, PA: Lippincott Williams & Wilkins.

Brotman, R., Klebanoff, M., Nansel, T., Andrews, W., Schwebke, J., Zwang, J., et al. (2008). A longitudinal study of vaginal douching and bacterial vaginosis - A marginal structural modeling analysis. *American Journal of Epidemiology, 178*(3), 188–196.

Canadian Cancer Society. (2013a). Risk factors for cervical cancer. Retrieved from http://www.cancer.ca/en/cancer-information/cancer-type/cervical/risks/?region=on

Canadian Cancer Society. (2013b). *Breast cancer statistics.* Retrieved from http://www.cancer.ca/en/cancer-information/cancer-type/breast/statistics/?region=on

Canadian Diabetes Association. (2013). *Clinical practice guidelines for the prevention and management of diabetes in Canada.* Retrieved from http://guidelines.diabetes.ca/App_Themes/CDACPG/resources/cpg_2013_full_en.pd

Canadian Medical Association. (2010). 2010 clinical practice guidelines for the diagnosis and management of osteoporosis in Canada: Summary. Retrieved from http://www.cmaj.ca/content/182/17/1864.full.pdf+html

Canadian Paediatric Society. (2005). Youth and firearms in Canada. *Paediatrics and Child Health, 10*(8), 473–477.

Canadian Paediatric Society. (2007). Paediatricians stand behind HPV vaccine for Canadian girls. News Release, September 24, 2007. Retrieved from http://www.cps.ca/media/release-communique/paediatricians-stand-behind-hpv-vaccine-for-canadian-girls

Canadian Psychiatric Association. (2006). Clinical practice guidelines: Management of anxiety disorders. *The Canadian Journal of Psychiatry, 51,* (Suppl. 2), 1S–92S.

Canadian Task Force on Preventive Health Care. (2011). *Recommendations on screening for breast cancer in average-risk women aged 40–74 years.* Retrieved from http://www.cmaj.ca/content/183/17/1991.full.pdf+html

Canadian Task Force on Preventive Health Care. (2013). *Recommendations on screening for cervical cancer.* Retrieved from http://www.cmaj.ca/content/185/1/35.full

Centers for Disease Control and Prevention (CDC). (2012). *Overweight and obesity.* Atlanta, GA: Author. Retrieved from http://www.cdc.gov/nccdphp/dnpa/obesity/

Centre for Addiction and Mental Health. (2012). *About CAMH.* Retrieved from http://www.camh.net/About_CAMH/index.html

Christinat, A., & Pagani, O. (2013). Practical aspects of genetic counseling in breast cancer: Lights and shadows. *Breast, 22*(4): 375–382.

Chui, T., & Maheux, H. (2011). *Visible minority women. Women in Canada: A Gender-based statistical report.* Retrieved from http://www.statcan.gc.ca/pub/89-503-x/2010001/article/11527-eng.pdf

Dickinson, J., Stankiewicz, A., Popadiuk, C., Pogany, L., Onysko, J., & Miller, A. (2012). Reduced cervical cancer in Canada: National data from 1932–2006. *BMC Public Health, 12,* 992. doi:10.1186/1471-2458-12-992

Dingley, C., Roux, G., & Bush, H. (2000). Inner strength: A concept analysis. *Journal of Theory Construction and Testing, 4*(2), 30–35.

Fenton, J., Barton, M., Geiger, A., Herrinton, L., Rolnick, S., Harris, E., et al. (2005). Screening clinical breast examination: How often does it miss lethal breast cancer? *Journal of the National Cancer Institute. Monographs, 35,* 67–71.

Freeman, E., & Sherif, K. (2007). Prevalence of hot flushes and night sweats around the world: A systematic review. *Climacteric, 10,* 197–214.

Fung, T., Hu, F, Fuchs, C., Giovannucci, E., Hunter, D., Stampfer, M., et al. (2003). Major dietary patterns and the risk of colorectal cancer in women. *Archives of Internal Medicine, 163*(3), 309–314.

Gotay, C., Katzmarzyk, P., Janssen, I., Dawson, M., Aminoltejari, K., & Bartley, N. (2013). Updating the Canadian obesity maps: An epidemic in progress. *Canadian Journal of Public Health, 104*(1), e64–e68.

Gottlieb, L. (2013). *Strength-based nursing care: health and healing for person and family.* New York, NY: Springer Publishing.

Hawton, K., & van Heeringen, K. (2009). Suicide. *The Lancet, 373*(9672), 1372–1381.

Health Canada. (2007). TRANSforming the food supply. *Final report of the Trans Fat Task Force.* Retrieved from http://www.hc-sc.gc.ca/fn-an/nutrition/gras-trans-fats/tf-ge/tf-gt_rep-rap-eng.php

Health Canada. (2010). *It's your health: Human papillomavirus (HPV).* Retrieved from http://www.hc-sc.gc.ca/hl-vs/iyh-vsv/diseases-maladies/hpv-vph-eng.php

Health Canada. (2011). *Eating well with Canada's food guide.* Retrieved from http://www.hc-sc.gc.ca/fn-an/food-guide-aliment/index-eng.php

Health Canada. (2012a). *First nations and inuit health strategic plan: A shared path to improved health.* Retrieved from www.hc-sc.gc.ca/fniah-spnia/pubs/strat-plan-2012/index-eng.php

Health Canada. (2012b). *Food and nutrition.* Retrieved from http://www.hc-sc.gc.ca/fn-an/nutrition/weights-poids/guide-ld-adult/bmi_chart_java-graph_imc_java-eng.php

Health Canada. (2012c). *Vitamin D and calcium: updated dietary reference intakes.* Retrieved from www.hc-sc.gc.ca/fn-an/nutrition/vitamin/vita-d-eng.php

Heart and Stroke Foundation of Canada. (2013a). *Dietary fats, oils and cholesterol.* Retrieved from http://www.heartandstroke.com/site/c.ikIQLcMWJtE/b.3484237/

Heart and Stroke Foundation of Canada. (2013b). *Women and heart disease and stroke.* Retrieved from http://www.heartandstroke.com/site/c.ikIQLcMWJtE/b.3484041/k.D80/Heart_disease__Women_and_heart_disease_and_stroke.htm

Howe, T. E., Shea, B., Dawson, L. J., Downie, F., Murray, A., Ross, C. et al. (2011). Exercise for preventing and treating osteoporosis in postmenopausal women (Review). *The Cochrane Library 2011,* (7):1–157, John Wiley and Sons. Retrieved from http://www.thecochranelibrary.com

Khadikar, A., & Chan, Y. (2013). Rate of cervical cancer screening associated with immigration status and number of years since immigration in Ontario Canada. *Journal of Immigrant and Minority Health, 15*(2), 244–248.

Knight, J., Sherritt, L., Shrier, L., Harris, S., & Chang, G. (2002). Validity of CRAFFT substance abuse screening test among adolescent clinic patients. *Archives of Pediatric Adolescent Medicine, 156,* 607–614.

Kobau, R., Seligman, M., Peterson, C., Diener, E., Zack, M, Chapman, D. et al. (2011). Mental health promotion in public health: Perspectives and strategies from positive psychology. *American Journal of Public Health. 101*(8), e1–e9.

Lakhan, S., & Vieira, K. (2010). Nutritional and herbal supplements for anxiety and anxiety-related disorders: Systematic review. *Nutrition Journal, 9*(42), Retrieved from http://www.nutritionj.com/content/pdf/1475-2891-9-42.pdf

Le Petit, C., & Berthelot, J. M. (2006). Obesity—a growing issue. *Health Reports, 17*(3), Ottawa, CA: Statistics Canada. Catalogue No 82-003-XIE.

Lobo, R. (2013). Where are we 10 years after the women's health initiative? *Journal of Clinical Endocrinology and Metabolism, 98*(5), 1771–1780.

Lofters, A., Hwang, S., Moineddin, R., & Glazier, R. (2010). Cervical cancer screening among urban immigrants by region: A population based cohort study. *Preventive Medicine, 51*(6), 509–516.

MacDonald, M. A. (2002). Health promotion: Historical, philosophical and theoretical perspectives. In L. E. Young & V. Hayes (Eds), *Transforming health promotion practice* (pp. 22–45). Philadelphia, PA: F. A. Davis.

MacMillan, H. L., Patterson, C., & Wathen, N. (2005). Screening for depression in primary care: recommendation statement from the Canadian Task Force on Preventive Health Care. *Canadian Medical Association Journal, 172*, 33–35.

Mann, M. (2005). *Gender equality consultation: Aboriginal women: An issues backgrounder.* Ottawa, CA: Status of Women in Canada. Retrieved from http://publications.gc.ca/collections/Collection/SW21-146-2005E.pdf

Marjoribanks, J., Farquhar, C., Roberts, H., & Lethaby, A. (2012). Long term hormone therapy for perimenopausal and postmenopausal women (Review). *The Cochrane Library 2012,* (7). doi: 10.1002/14651858.CD004143.pub4

MedLine Plus. (2013a). Cervical dysplasia. Retrieved from http://www.nlm.nih.gov/medlineplus/ency/article/001491.htm.

MedLine Plus. (2013b). Iron deficiency anemia. Retrieved from http://www.nlm.nih.gov/medlineplus/ency/article/000584.htm

Mikkonen, J., & Raphael, D. (Eds). (2010). *Social determinants of health: The Canadian facts.* Toronto, ON: York University School of Policy and Management. http://www.thecanadianfacts.org/

Mood Disorders Association of Canada. (2011). *What is depression?* Retrieved from http://www.mooddisorderscanada.ca/documents/Publications/%20DepressEngMasterFeb2011.pdf

Morrow, M., Hankivsky, O., & Varcoe, C. (Eds) (2007). *Women's health in Canada: Critical perspectives on theory and policy.* Toronto, ON: University of Toronto Press.

National Center for Complementary and Alternative Medicine. (2013). *Get the facts: What is complementary and alternative medicine?* Bethesda, MD: Author. Retrieved from http://nccam.nih.gov/health/whatiscam/

National Osteoporosis Foundation. (2013a). *Learn about osteoporosis.* Retrieved from http://www.nof.org/learn/detection

National Osteoporosis Foundation. (2013b). *Clinician's guide to prevention and treatment of osteoporosis.* Retrieved from http://www.nof.org/files/nof/public/content/resource/913/files/580.pdf

National Women's Health Information Center (NWHIC). Retrieved from http://www.womenshealth.gov/.

Ng, E., Wilkins, R., Gendron, F., & Berthelot, J. (2005). Dynamics of immigrants' health in Canada: Evidence from the National Population Health Survey. *Healthy today, healthy tomorrow: Findings from the National Population Health Survey.* Statistics Canada: Catalogue # 82-618-MWE2005002.

Osteoporosis Canada. (2013). *Calcium: An important nutrient that builds stronger bones.* Retrieved from http://www.osteoporosis.ca/osteoporosis-and-you/nutrition/calcium-requirements/

Pender, N. J. (1996). *Health promotion in nursing practice* (3rd ed.). Stamford, CT: Appleton & Lange.

Pittler, M. H., & Ernst, E. (2000). Efficacy of kava extract for treating anxiety: Systematic review and meta-analysis. *Journal of Clinical Psychopharmacology, 20*(1), 84–89.

Poliquin, S., Joseph, L., & Gray-Donald, K. (2009). Calcium and vitamin D intakes in an adult Canadian population. *Canadian Journal of Dietetic Practice and Research, 170*(1), 21–27.

Prochaska, J. O., & DiClemente, C. C. (1983). Stages and processes of self-change of smoking: Toward an integrative model of change. *Journal of Consulting and Clinical Psychology, 51*, 390–395.

Prochaska, J. O., Velicer, W. F., Rossi, J. S., Goldstein, M. G., Marcus, B., Rakowski, W. et al. (1994). Stages of change and decisional balance for 12 problem behaviors. *Health Psychology, 13*, 39–46.

Pruthi, S., Gostout, B., & Lindor, N. (2010). Identification and management of women with BRCA mutations or hereditary predisposition for breast and ovarian cancer. *Mayo Clinic Procedings, 85*(12), 1111–1120.

Public Health Agency of Canada. (2004). Evaluation of food fortification with folic acid for the primary prevention of neural tube defects. Retrieved from http://www.phac-aspc.gc.ca/publicat/faaf/chap3-eng.php

Public Health Agency of Canada. (2006). *Canadian immunization guide* (7th ed.). Cat: HP40-3/2006E ISBN: 0-660-19392-2 Retrieved from http://www.phac-aspc.gc.ca/publicat/cig-gci/index-eng.php

Public Health Agency of Canada. (2007). *Five year priorities for action.* Retrieved from http://www.phac-aspc.gc.ca/publicat/2007/sp-ps/SPPS-06d1-eng.php

Public Health Agency of Canada. (2008a). *Folic acid.* Retrieved from http://www.phac-aspc.gc.ca/fa-af/

Public Health Agency of Canada. (2008b). *The chief public health officer's report on the state of public health in Canada 2008.* Retrieved from http://www.phac-aspc.gc.ca/cphorsphc-respcacsp/2008/fr-rc/cphorsphc-respcacsp09-eng.php

Public Health Agency of Canada. (2009). *Tracking heart disease and stroke in Canada.* Retrieved from http://www.cps.ca/english/media/newsreleases/2007/hpv.htm

Public Health Agency of Canada. (2011a). *The human face of mental health and mental illness in Canada 2006.* Retrieved from http://www.phac-aspc.gc.ca/publicat/human-humain06/6-eng.php

Public Health Agency of Canada. (2011b). *Diabetes in Canada: Facts and figures from a public health: perspective: Chapter 5 – Diabetes in children and youth.* Retrieved from http://www.phac-aspc.gc.ca/cd-mc/publications/diabetes-diabete/facts-figures-faits-chiffres-2011/chap5-eng.php

Public Health Agency of Canada. (2012a). Mental health promotion. Retrieved from http://www.phac-aspc.gc.ca/mh-sm/mhp-psm/index-eng.php

Public Health Agency of Canada. (2012b). *Executive summary-report on sexually transmitted infections in Canada: 2009. Retrieved from* http://www.phac-aspc.gc.ca/sti-its-surv-epi/sum-som-eng.php

Reitsma, M., Tranmer, J., Buchanan, D., & Vandenkerkhof, E. (2011). The prevalence of chronic pain and pain-related interference in the Canadian population from 1994 to 2008. *Chronic Diseases and Injuries in Canada, 31*(4) Retrieved from http://www.phac-aspc.gc.ca/publicat/cdic-mcbc/31-4/assets/pdf/cdic-mcbc-31-4-ar-04-eng.pdf

Rootman, I., Dupéré, S., Pederson, A., & O'Neill, M. (Eds). (2012). *Health promotion in Canada: Critical perspectives on practice* (3rd ed). Toronto, ON: Canadian Scholar's Press Inc.

Roux, G., Dingley, C., & Bush, H. (2002). Inner strength in women: Metasynthesis of qualitative findings in theory development. *Journal of Theory Construction and Testing, 6*(1), 86–92.

Running, A., & Berndt, A. (2003). *Management guidelines for nurse practitioners.* Philadelphia, PA: F. A. Davis.

Senter, C., Appelle, N., & Behera, S. (2013). Prescribing exercise for women. *Current Reviews in Musculosketal Medicine, 6*(2), 164–172.

Shay, L., Shobert, J., Seibert, D., & Thomas, L. (2009). Adult weight management: Translating research and guidelines into practice. *Journal of the American Academy of Nurse Practitioners, 21*(4), 197–206.

Society of Obstetricians and Gynaecologists of Canada. (2009). Menopause and osteoporosis update 2009. *Journal of Obstetrics and Gynaecology Canada, 31*(1), S34–S45.

Statistics Canada. (2011). *Mortality, summary list of causes 2008.* Retrieved from http://www.statcan.gc.ca/pub/84f0209x/84f0209×2008000-eng.pdf

Statistics Canada. (2012). *First nations, métis and inuit women.* Retrieved from http://www.statcan.gc.ca/pub/89-503-x/2010001/article/11442-eng.htm

Statistics Canada. (2013a). *Bone health: Osteoporosis, calcium and vitamin D.* Retrieved from http://www.statcan.gc.ca/pub/82-003-x/2011003/article/11515-eng.htm

Statistics Canada. (2013b). *Homicide in Canada, 2011.* Retrieved from http://www.statcan.gc.ca/pub/85-002-x/2012001/article/11738-eng.htm#n8

Thurston, R., Kubzansky, L., Kawachi, I., & Berkman, L. (2005). Is the association between socioeconomic position and coronary heart disease stronger in women than in men? *American Journal of Epidemiology, 162*(1), 57–65.

Uphold, C. R., & Graham, M. V. (2003). *Clinical guidelines in family practice* (4th ed.). Gainesville, FL: Barmarrae Books.

Watkins, J. (2010). *Structure and function of the musculoskeletal system* (2nd ed.). Champaign, IL: Human Kinetics.

Weiler, H., Leslie, W., Krahn, J., Steiman, P., & Metge, C. (2007). Canadian aboriginal women have a higher prevalence of vitamin D deficiency than non-aboriginal women despite similar dietary vitamin D intake. *The Journal of Nutrition, 137*(2), 461–465.

Wing, P. R., & Phelan, S. (2005). Long-term weight loss maintenance. *American Journal of Clinical Nutrition, 82*(Suppl. 1), 222S–225S.

World Health Organization (WHO). (2006). *Frequently asked questions.* Retrieved from http://www.who.int/suggestions/faq/en/

World Health Organization (WHO). (2009). *Milestones in health promotion.* Retrieved from http://www.who.int/healthpromotion/Milestones_Health_Promotion_05022010.pdf

Writing Group for the Women's Health Initiative Investigators. (2002). Risks and benefits of estrogen plus progestin in healthy postmenopausal women: Principal results from the women's health initiative randomized controlled trial. *Journal of the American Medical Association, 288*(3), 321–333.

Youngkin, E. Q., & Davis, M. S. (2012). *Women's health: A primary care clinical guide* (3rd ed.). Stamford, CT: Appleton & Lange.

CHAPTER 3

Nutrition for Adolescent and Adult Women

Sherrill Conroy, Sylvia Escott-Stump*, and Evelyn S. Farrior*

 Sheila, 37 years old and in her third trimester of pregnancy, comes to the clinic for a routine visit. She is planning to breastfeed her newborn. During the interview, Sheila tells the nurse, "I've been trying to follow the nutritional suggestions for pregnancy that you gave me as best as I can, but I'm having trouble drinking enough milk."

 Betsy, 14 years old, is at the nurse practitioner's office for a checkup. Betsy is 1.7 m tall and weighs 52 kg; she started menstruating 3 months ago. Betsy mentions feeling uncomfortable with the changes in her body over the past year. "Every day, something new is happening," she says. "My hips and thighs are thicker than they used to be, and I'm still not used to having a chest!" During assessment of her diet habits, Betsy reports that she skips breakfast and doesn't like fish or vegetables. When the nurse asks why she doesn't eat breakfast, Betsy replies, "I don't want to get fat."

You will learn more about Sheila's and Betsy's care later. Nurses working with these clients need to understand the material in this chapter to promote good nutrition and to address issues appropriately. Before beginning, consider these points.

---

*Contributor to first U.S. edition.

● What information from these scenarios may pose concerns for each client's immediate and long-term health?

● How can nurses provide instruction that will help these clients develop and maintain healthy dietary habits?

● What nutritional issues related to pregnancy and lactation are priorities for Sheila? What nutritional issues related to adolescence are priorities for Betsy?

● What external influences might vary between these clients? How might these influences affect their feelings about food?

LEARNING OBJECTIVES

On completion of this chapter, the reader should be able to:
● Explain why nurses need to understand nutrition and why there are different recommendations for different age groups and life circumstances.
● Describe the roles of various nutrients in the maintenance of overall health.
● Identify components of nutritional assessment for women.
● Discuss individual factors that can influence food selection and how nurses can work with clients to incorporate unique preferences.
● Identify special nutritional needs and adjustments required in pregnancy, lactation, and adolescence.
● Describe collaborative care strategies related to nutrition and the pregnant teen.
● Discuss nutritional concerns of special interest to adult and older adult women.

KEY TERMS

body mass index (BMI)	macronutrients
coenzyme	macrosomia
cofactor	micronutrients
complementary proteins	nutrient density
complete proteins	nutritional assessment
dietary reference intakes (DRIs)	nutritional screening
fortified	phytochemicals
glycemic index	pica
incomplete proteins	vegan

According to the 2004 Community Health Survey of 35,000 Canadians, many people do not have a balanced diet and have nutritional challenges. More than 25% of people aged 31 to 50 consume more than 35% of their total calories from fat, the threshold beyond which health risks increase. Half of the adults surveyed did not eat the recommended daily minimum requirement of vegetables and fruit. One third of children and two thirds of adults over 30 did not have the recommended serving of milk products per day. Canadians of all ages got more than 20% of their calories from foods that are not part of the four major food groups. Between-meal snacks accounted for more calories than breakfast and about the same number of calories as lunch (Statistics Canada, 2006).

Food can supply the nutrients necessary to build and to maintain healthy bodies. Although Canada has a generous food supply, many women have an imbalanced nutrient intake as a result of lifestyle and other factors (Bartley et al., 2005; Healthy Women, 2011).

Another problem is the growing number of women who are overweight or obese (see Chapter 1) and the subsequent chronic diseases related to these states (Alberta Agriculture and Rural Development, 2011; Freedman et al., 2006; Li et al., 2006).

In this chapter we provide nutritional information and emphasize strategies to promote women's health and to assist with dietary management at various developmental stages. We review the function, recommended intake, sources, and consequences of overconsumption or underconsumption of each major nutrient. We present how nurses can assess nutritional status and assist clients to make food choices appropriate for their circumstances. Because of the correlation between good nutrition and positive gestational and postpartum outcomes, this chapter contains sections on dietary adjustments and considerations related to pregnancy and lactation (Health Canada, 2010a). We also explore nutritional considerations for adolescent, adult, and older adult females. (A comprehensive exploration of newborn nutrition is found in Chapter 21.)

NUTRIENTS

For nutritional counselling and advice to be effective, nurses need to work as partners with their clients. Nurses can facilitate women's involvement by carefully assessing nutritional requirements and dietary preferences, involving them in meal planning, answering questions, and giving thorough explanations of the reasons for nutritional recommendations (Fig. 3.1).

To do these things effectively, nurses need a general knowledge of each nutrient's contribution to health and of the recommendations found within *Eating Well with Canada's Food Guide* (Health Canada, 2011). A baseline familiarity with nutrients and their functions is essential when a client's circumstances indicate a need for dietary changes. The Food Guide provides sufficient

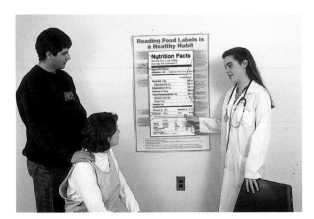

FIGURE 3.1 Involving the client in nutrition and diet planning will enhance the chances for successful outcomes.

guidelines to ensure that adequate nutrients are being consumed. Food Guide Servings are used as the units of reference for dietary recommendations for individuals, including growing women in pre- and postconception stages, during gestation, and after menopause. The Food Guide recommendations were derived from research done by Health Canada and the Canadian Food Inspection Agency. Figure 3.2 is adapted from Canada's Food Guide and is available in English, French, Arabic, Chinese, Farsi, Korean, Punjabi, Russian, Spanish, Tagalog, Tamil, and Urdu. Figure 3.3 is adapted from *Eating Well with Canada's Food Guide—First Nations, Inuit and Métis* (Health Canada, 2010c) and is available in English, Inuktitut, Ojibwe, Plains Cree, and Woods Cree. All versions can be ordered in print form, diskette, large print, audiocassette, and Braille, and can be downloaded from Health Canada's website.

Detailed and up-to-date information on nutrient values for healthy populations is provided in the **Dietary Reference Intakes** (DRIs) that have been established by Canadian and American scientists, replacing the terms **Recommended Daily Intake (RDI)** and **Recommended Nutrient Intake (RNI)**. DRIs are published as a series of reports by the U.S. National Academies. The reports can be viewed online (Health Canada, 2013b).

Macronutrients

Macronutrients are those nutrients that provide energy: carbohydrates, fats, and proteins. The recommended distribution for adults is for 45% to 65% of total energy intake to come from carbohydrates, no more than 30% to come from fat, and 10% to 35% to come from proteins (Health Canada, 2006b; Institute of Medicine [IOM], 2002).

Overconsumption of food and lack of physical activity are frequently associated with increased risk for chronic diseases such as obesity, coronary heart disease, diabetes, hypertension, and cancer (Freedman et al., 2006; Li et al., 2006; Tsai et al., 2006). An overall public health goal is to decrease the risk for such diseases (Health Canada, 2013c). When assisting clients in weight management, nurses can emphasize the need to balance energy consumed and energy expended. The amount of calories and the duration or frequency of exercise can be adjusted to promote weight loss or gain. Guidelines for physical activities that can benefit the health of individuals of any age are available from the Canadian Society for Exercise Physiology (CSEP) (2013). These guidelines, developed by CSEP and the Public Health Agency of Canada (2011b), can be downloaded from the CSEP website. The Food Guide and activity guidelines are both excellent resources for the nurse and individual clients to assess health status adjusted according to age, activity level, and gender. The Canadian Food Inspection Agency (2013) provides

Recommended Number of Food Guide Servings per Day

	Children			Teens		Adults			
Age	2–3	4–8	9–13	14–18	14–18	19–50	19–50	51+	
Sex	Both	Both	Both	Females	Males	Females	Males	Females	Males
Vegetables and fruits	4	5	6	7	8	7–8	8–10	7	7
Grain products	3	4	6	6	7	6–7	8	6	7
Milk and alternatives	2	2	3–4	3–4	3–4	2	2	3	3
Meat and alternatives	1	1	1–2	2	3	2	3	2	3

What is one Food Guide Serving?

Vegetables and fruits	Fresh, frozen, or canned vegetables 125 mL (½ cup)	Leafy vegetables cooked 125 mL (½ cup) raw 250 mL (1 cup)	Fresh, frozen or canned fruits 1 fruit or 125 mL (½ cup)	100% juice 125 mL (½ cup)	
Grain products	Bread 1 slice	Bagel ½ bagel	Flat breads ½ pita or ½ tortilla	Cooked rice, bulgur, or quinoa 125 mL (½ cup)	Cereal cold: 30 g hot: 175 mL (¾ cup)	Cooked pasta or couscous 125 mL (½ cup)
Milk and alternatives	Milk 250 mL (1 cup)	Evaporated milk 125 mL (½ cup)	Fortified soy beverage 250 mL (1 cup)	Yogurt 175 g (¾ cup)	Kefir 175 (¾ cup)	Cheese 50 g (1½ oz)
Meat and alternatives	Cooked fish, shellfish, poultry, or lean meat 75 g or 125 mL (½ cup)	Cooked legumes 175 mL (¾ cup)	Tofu 150 g or 175 mL (¾ cup)	Eggs 2 eggs	Peanut or nut butters 30 mL (2 tbsp)	

- Pregnant and breastfeeding women: add 2–3 Food Guide Servings each day
- Oils and fats: Include a small amount (30–45 mL, 2–3 tbsp) of unsaturated fat per day. This includes oil used for cooking, salad dressing, margarine, and mayonnaise. Use vegetable oils such as canola, olive, and soybean. Choose soft margarines that are low in saturated and trans fats. Limit butter, hard margarine, lard, and shortening.
- Eat at least one dark green and one orange vegetable each day.
- Choose vegetables and fruit prepared with little or no added fat, sugar, or salt.
- Have fruits and vegetables more often than juice.
- Make at least half of your grain products whole grain each day.
- Choose grain products that are lower in fat, sugar, and salt.
- Drink skim, 1% or 2% milk each day.
- Select lower fat milk alternatives.
- Have meat alternatives such as beans, lentils, and tofu often.
- Eat at least two Food Guide servings of fish each week.
- Select lean meat and alternatives prepared with little or no added fat or salt.

FIGURE 3.2 Eating Well with Canada's Food Guide. Adapted from Eating Well with Canada's Food Guide. Available online at http://www.hc-sc.gc.ca/fn-an/food-guide-aliment/index-eng.php.

a guide to food labelling and advertising that can help consumers differentiate between different brands and make informed food purchasing choices.

Carbohydrates

Sources of carbohydrates include fruits, vegetables, breads, pasta, cereals, and grains. The minimum intake level for adolescents and adults is 300 g/day (Health Canada, 2013a).

Carbohydrates come in simple and complex forms and include sugar, starch, and fibre (Harvard School of Public Health, 2013a). The digestive system breaks down sugar and starch into single molecules and converts them to glucose (blood sugar), which the body's

Recommended Number of Food Guide Servings per Day

	Childern		Teens & Adults	
	2–3 yrs	4–13 yrs	Females	Males
Vegetables and fruits	4	5–6	7–8	7–10
Grain products	3	4–6	6–7	7–8
Milk and alternatives	2	2–4	Teens 3–4 Adults (19–50) 2 Adults (>50) 3	Teens 3–4 Adults (19–50) 2 Adults (>50) 3
Meat and alternatives	1	1–2	2	3

What is one Food Guide Serving?

Vegetables and fruits	Dark green and orange vegetables 125 mL (½ cup)	Dark green and orange vegetables 125 mL (½ cup)	Other vegetables 125 mL (½ cup)	Leafy vegetables and wild plants Cooked 125 mL (½ cup) Raw 250 mL (1 cup)	Berries 125 mL (½ cup)	Fruit 1 fruit or 125 mL (½ cup)	100% juice 125 mL (½ cup)
Grain products	Bread 1 slice	Bread 1 slice	Bannock 35 g (2″×2″×1″)	Cereal cold: 30 g hot: 175 mL (¾ cup)	Cooked rice, white brown, or wild 125 mL (½ cup)	Cooked pasta 125 mL (½ cup)	
Milk and alternatives	Milk (fresh or powdered, mixed) 250 mL (1 cup)	Milk (fresh or powdered, mixed) 250 mL (1 cup)	Evaporated milk 125 mL (½ cup)	Fortified soy beverage 250 mL (1 cup)	Yogurt 175 g (¾ cup)	Cheese 50 g (1½ oz)	
Meat and alternatives	Traditional meats and wild game 75 g or 125 mL (½ cup)	Traditional meats and wild game 75 g or 125 mL (½ cup)	Fish and shellfish 75 g or 125 mL (½ cup)	Lean meat and poultry 125 g or 125 mL (½ cup)	Eggs 2 eggs	Beans (cooked) 175 mL (¾ cup)	Peanut butter 30 mL (2 tbsp)

- ● Pregnant and breastfeeding women: add 2–3 Food Guide Servings each day
- ● When cooking with or adding fat to food:
  - ● Most of the time, use vegetable oils with unsaturated fats (canola, olive, soybean oils), 30–45 mL (2–3 tbsp) per day.
  - ● Traditional fats that are liquid at room temperature (seal or whale oil, ooligan grease) also contain unsaturated fats and can be used as all or part of the 30–45 mL per day.
  - ● Limit butter, hard margarine, shortening, lard, and bacon.

FIGURE 3.3 Eating Well with Canada's Food Guide: First Nations, Inuit, and Metis. Adapted from Eating Well with Canada's Food Guide. Available online at http://www.hc-sc.gc.ca/fn-an/pubs/fnim-pnim/index-eng.php.

cells use for energy. Fibre is different from sugar and starch because the digestive system cannot break it down, and it passes through the body undigested (Harvard School of Public Health, 2013b). Fibre helps prevent constipation and decreases blood glucose and cholesterol levels (McKeown et al., 2002; Pereira et al., 2004; Slavin, 2003). Recommended intake of total fibre is 21 to 26 g/day for women (Health Canada, 2013e).

Recently, low-carbohydrate diets have been a trend for weight loss; their effectiveness over low-fat, reduced-calorie, and other types of diets remains under investigation (Saraswat et al., 2012). Other explorations related to carbohydrates are focusing on **glycemic index**, or the measure of how quickly and how high the blood sugar increases after a certain food is eaten (Thomas et al., 2007). Diets with many high–glycemic-index foods (eg, white bread, potatoes) are linked to increased risks for diabetes and heart disease (Liu & Willett, 2002; Pereira & Liu, 2003; Schulze et al., 2004; Willett et al., 2002). Other factors that influence glycemic index include fibre, fat, and acid contents; ripeness; and type of starch contained (Harvard School of Public Health, 2013b).

Fat

Fat is a concentrated source of energy and comes in several forms: saturated, monounsaturated, trans fats, polyunsaturated, and cholesterol. High intake of foods with saturated, trans fats, and cholesterol is associated with increased health risks (Harvard School of Public Health, 2013c).

Polyunsaturated fatty acids can be further subdivided based on the location of their double bonds. Omega-3 and omega-6 polyunsaturated fatty acids are essential to health and support the normal development of the brain, eyes, and nerves. Their consumption is associated with reduced risk for cardiovascular disease and increased blood levels of high-density lipoprotein (HDL) cholesterol (good cholesterol). Food sources of omega-3 fatty acids are fatty fish (salmon, tuna, sardines), fish oils, and some vegetable oils (eg, canola, soy, flax). Food sources of omega-6 fatty acids are nuts, seeds, vegetable oils, and eggs from chickens fed with enriched omega-3 and omega-6 feed.

Proteins

Proteins are made up of long chains of amino acids and are essential for building and maintaining the body. Amino acids form the structure of cells, enzymes, membrane carriers, and hormones. Recommended daily protein intake is 0.8 g/kg body weight for adult women, 1.1 g/kg body weight during pregnancy, 1.3 g/kg during lactation and lactation, and varying levels that correlate with growth needs in children and teens (Health Canada, 2006b; IOM, 2002). The newest recommendations add age-based levels for each of the nine essential amino acids and scoring procedures to account for protein quality (IOM, 2002).

Complete proteins provide all essential amino acids and are found in animal foods—meat, poultry, fish, eggs, milk, cheese, and yogurt—as well as in soybean products. Combinations of **incomplete proteins** (foods lacking one or more of the nine essential amino acids) can be selected to meet complete protein needs. Examples of foods with incomplete proteins are legumes, grains, nuts, seeds, and vegetables.

Micronutrients

Vitamins and minerals are considered **micronutrients** (Craven & Hirnle, 2009). Vitamins help regulate carbohydrate, fat, and protein metabolism and other reactions that maintain body tissues. Minerals make up bone, teeth, and structural body materials and assist with internal body processes.

Water-Soluble Vitamins

Water-soluble vitamins are eliminated with body fluids, are not stored to any extent, and require daily replacement. Consequently, their average intakes over several days should meet the recommended levels to avoid depletion. They include biotin, choline, folate, niacin (B_3), pantothenic acid, riboflavin (B_2), thiamin (B_1), pyridoxine (B_6), cobalamin (B_{12}), and vitamin C.

Biotin and Choline. Two vitamins with emerging evidence to support requirements are biotin and choline. *Biotin* is a **coenzyme** (a small organic molecule that enhances enzyme activity) in the synthesis of fat, glycogen, and amino acids. *Choline* is a precursor for acetylcholine, phospholipids, and betaine. Because adverse effects from high intake are possible, an upper limit has been established for choline (IOM, 2000a). Meats, especially liver, provide both biotin and choline.

Folate. *Folate,* an important coenzyme in nucleic and amino acid metabolism, is required to prevent megaloblastic anemia. In addition, neural tube defects in newborns are prevented when women enter pregnancy with adequate folate levels (see Chapter 11). Health Canada's recommended dietary allowance (RDA) for folate is 400 µg (0.4 mg) for women of childbearing age, with the recommendation increasing to 600 µg (0.6 mg) for pregnant women and 500 µg (0.5 mg) for lactating women (Health Canada, 2009a, 2009b). In populations where neural tube defects have been identified as a risk, women should take 0.4 to 0.6 mg daily as folic acid alone. To avoid overdose of vitamins, the higher dose of folate should not be combined with a multivitamin that is fortified with folate. Folate is present in small amounts in foods; it is often removed during processing. Thus, folate may be added to foods to prevent deficiencies or improve nutrient balance. In Canada, flour and other cereal products are **fortified** (nutrient-added) with folic acid (Health Canada, 2009b; Public Health Agency of Canada, 2004). Other sources of folate are dark green leafy vegetables and orange juice.

Niacin and Pantothenic Acid. *Niacin* (vitamin B_3) is required for the oxidation and reduction reactions of energy metabolism; thus, niacin requirements are related directly to total energy intake, as reflected in the DRIs for each age group and sex (Health Canada, 2010b). An upper limit has been established, because high intakes cause flushing and gastrointestinal distress (IOM, 2000a). Sources include meats, fish, poultry, and enriched or whole grains.

Pantothenic acid functions as a coenzyme in fatty acid metabolism. A variety of foods provide pantothenic acid: chicken, beef, potatoes, oats, cereals, tomato, liver, egg, broccoli, and whole grains.

Other B Vitamins. *Riboflavin* (vitamin B_2) functions as a coenzyme in many oxidation and reduction reactions. Food sources are organ meats, milk, breads, and fortified cereals. *Thiamin* (vitamin B_1) functions as a coenzyme in carbohydrate and branched-chain amino acid metabolism. Fortified and whole grain foods provide this nutrient.

Vitamin B_6 functions as a coenzyme in amino acid, glycogen, and sphingoid base metabolism. Foods that contain B_6 are fortified cereals, organ meats, and fortified soy-based meat substitutes. *Cobalamin* (vitamin B_{12}), an important coenzyme in nucleic and amino acid metabolism, helps prevent megaloblastic anemia. Sources include meat, fish, poultry, and fortified cereals. Supplements of B_{12} may be prescribed for those who do not eat meat, as well as those older than 50 years, who may experience decreased absorption of the nutrient.

Vitamin C. *Vitamin C* (ascorbic acid) functions as an antioxidant and in reactions that require reduced copper or iron. An upper limit has been established because excess intake of vitamin C can cause gastrointestinal distress, kidney stones, and excess iron absorption (IOM, 2000b). The need for vitamin C increases in clients who smoke (IOM, 2000b). Citrus fruits, tomatoes, potatoes, Brussels' sprouts, cauliflower, broccoli, strawberries, cabbage, and spinach are sources.

Fat-Soluble Vitamins

Fat-soluble vitamins are stored in the body. Thus, inadequate intake presents later than with water-soluble vitamins. At the same time, the danger of toxicity increases. The fat-soluble vitamins are A, D, E, and K.

Vitamin A. *Vitamin A* is required for vision, gene expression, reproduction, embryonic development, and immune function. Good sources of vitamin A are liver, dairy products, and fish. An upper limit is based on the danger of teratogenic effects and liver toxicity, mainly from preformed (or already present in body water) vitamin A (IOM, 2001). Carotene, the precursor form, is considered safe. Dark-coloured and leafy vegetables provide carotene.

Vitamin D. *Vitamin D* (calciferol) enhances calcium and phosphorus metabolism. People with adequate sunlight exposure convert a precursor compound in the skin to this vitamin. Sunlight exposure, which lessens when one lives in northern latitudes (ie, north of the 42nd parallel), enables this conversion. In Canada, all cow's milk is fortified with vitamin D. Food sources of vitamin D are fish liver oil, fatty fish (eg, salmon, herring, sardines), fortified milk products, and fortified cereals.

Vitamin E. *Vitamin E* (α-tocopherol) is an antioxidant. Toxicity is related to overuse of supplements, not overconsumption of food (Mayo Clinic, 2012a; Rosenbloom, 2013). Vegetable oils, whole grains, nuts, creamy salad dressings, and meats are food sources of vitamin E.

Vitamin K. *Vitamin K* is a coenzyme in protein synthesis related to blood clotting and bone metabolism. For those taking anticoagulant therapy, daily intake of vitamin K from all sources should remain constant. Inconsistent intake alters blood-clotting time, which can have adverse effects (Aschenbrenner & Venable, 2009; Mayo Clinic, 2012b). For example, increasing the intake of green leafy vegetables, which are high in vitamin K, during the summer growing season may need to be monitored. Other foods that provide vitamin K are plant oils and margarine.

Minerals

Minerals can be classified based on the quantity needed in the body. Macrominerals are required in large amounts; they generally make up body structures. Microminerals are needed in small amounts and serve as **cofactors** (small inorganic or organic substances that work with enzymes to promote chemical reactions). The body of knowledge about some of these elements is evolving.

Macrominerals. *Calcium* promotes blood clotting, muscle contraction, nerve transmission, bone and tooth formation, and skeletal mineralization. It is essential in the maintenance of bone mass in the pregnant woman and the attainment of bone mass in the fetus. Overconsumption can cause kidney stones, hypercalcemia, milk–alkali syndrome, and renal insufficiency. Underconsumption is largely responsible for osteoporosis in women (see Chapters 2 and 24). Dairy products (milk, cheese, and yogurt), corn tortillas, calcium-set tofu, Chinese cabbage, kale, and broccoli provide calcium. Calcium from dairy products is more bioavailable than that from other sources. Absorption is enhanced with concurrent intake of vitamin D. A woman less than 50 years requires 1,000 mg/day of calcium; after menopause, she requires 1,200 mg/day (Health Canada, 2012b).

Phosphorus plays a vital role in acid–base balance, energy transfer, and nucleotide synthesis. Foods that provide phosphorus include dairy products, meat, eggs, and some cereals and grains. Health Canada (2005) recommends a daily intake of 700 mg for adult women and 1,250 mg for adolescents or during pregnancy and lactation. *Sodium* regulates extracellular fluid volume, helps maintain acid–base balance, and functions in nerve transmission and muscle contraction. The DRI for healthy people 19 to 50 years is 1,500 mg/day (Health Canada, 2005) Overconsumption is more common than underconsumption (Health Canada, 2012a; IOM, 2013), in part due to dietary intake of processed and fast foods, which contain high levels of sodium.

Potassium regulates intracellular fluid volume, functions in nerve transmission and muscle contraction, and regulates heartbeat. This element is important in the prevention of hypertension. The adequate intake (AI) for an adult is 4,700 mg/day (Health Canada, 2005). Potassium is found in fresh fruits, particularly bananas, and vegetables.

Chloride is the major anion in extracellular fluids. With sodium and potassium, it maintains electrolyte balance. Chloride is a part of the acid in gastric juice. Salt or sodium chloride is the main food source. AI is 2,300 mg/day (Health Canada, 2005)

Sulfur functions as a part of the amino acids methionine and cysteine and as part of thiamin. A recommended intake has not been established (Health Canada, 2005).

Microminerals. *Chromium* helps to maintain normal blood glucose levels. An AI is identified, but no upper limit has been set, even though excessive consumption can lead to chronic renal failure (IOM, 2001). Meat, fish, poultry, and some cereals are food sources of chromium.

Copper is a component of enzymes in iron metabolism. Intakes above the upper limit can lead to gastrointestinal distress and liver damage (IOM, 2001). Organ meats, seafood, nuts, seeds, wheat bran cereals, whole grains, and cocoa are sources.

Fluoride hardens tooth enamel and stimulates new bone formation. Excessive intake can cause fluorosis of the skeleton and tooth enamel. Fluoridated water, beverages made with fluoridated water, and marine fish are sources. Since not all municipal water supplies are fluoridated in Canada, fluoridated toothpaste can be used for protection of tooth enamel.

Iodine regulates metabolism through production of the thyroid hormone. Excessive intakes can lead to elevated thyroid-stimulating hormone (TSH) concentrations. Food sources are seafood and iodized salt.

Iron is an essential component of hemoglobin and numerous enzymes. Anemia can result from an iron deficiency. Vegetarian diets do not provide iron in its most absorbable form; thus, vegetarians need approximately twice the DRI for iron (Cooper et al., 2006; Mangels, 2013). Excessive intakes of iron can lead to gastrointestinal distress, iron overload, or both. Meat and poultry provide the most absorbable (heme) form. Fruits, vegetables, and fortified grain products provide less absorbable (nonheme) sources.

Magnesium is a cofactor in some enzyme systems and contributes to release of cell energy and muscle relaxation. Green leafy vegetables, whole grains, nuts, meat, starches, and milk are food sources.

Manganese functions in bone formation and as a cofactor with enzymes required for amino acid, cholesterol, and carbohydrate metabolism. An upper limit is set to decrease the possibility of elevated blood concentrations and neurotoxicity. Nuts, legumes, tea, and whole grains are the food sources.

Molybdenum is a required cofactor for catabolic reactions involving sulfur amino acids, purines, and pyridines. Legumes, grains, and nuts supply this element.

Selenium functions as an antioxidant to regulate thyroid hormone action and to maintain the reduction/oxidation status of vitamin C and other molecules. The best food sources are organ meats, seafood, and plants grown in soil that contains selenium.

Zinc is a component of enzyme systems and specific proteins that regulate gene expression and assists in healing and fetal development. Fortified cereals, red meat, and some seafood are food sources. Vegetarians are at risk for zinc deficiency.

Several elements are listed in the DRIs as having no known biologic function in humans (IOM, 2001). Those elements are *arsenic, boron, nickel, silicon,* and *vanadium.* Because high intakes pose a danger of adverse effects, upper limits have been set for boron, nickel, and vanadium (IOM, 2001). Health Canada (2006a) sets the limit for organic arsenic found in apple juice and ground water at 10 µg/kg or 10 parts per billion.

Mercury is a by-product of smelting ores and of badly disposed batteries. It is harmful to young children and the fetus since it interferes with brain development. People living downstream from mines and smelters are at high risk for mercury contamination from the waters they drink and the local fish they eat. No level of mercury is safe to ingest.

 Consider Sheila, the 37-year-old woman in her third trimester of pregnancy. What if Sheila were a vegetarian? What specific nutrients might be inadequate in her diet?

NUTRITIONAL ASSESSMENT

Morbidity and mortality are closely related to behavioural choices: eating habits, exercise, smoking, drug and alcohol consumption, and stress. Choosing a healthy diet can reduce the risk for chronic disease. To address clients' health needs, nurses complete a **nutritional assessment**. The health care provider evaluates general state of health, educational background, weight history, **body mass index** (BMI) (see Chapter 2), and waist-to-height ratio—the most sensitive measurement of obesity (Weili et al., 2007). A useful tool for nurses and clients to assess BMI and height-to-weight ratio can be found at http://home.fuse.net/clymer/bmi/. A nutritionally oriented health history and physical examination are effective tools for identifying real or potential problems (Assessment Tool 3.1).

● **ASSESSMENT TOOL 3.1**   **Adult Nutritional Assessment Form**

Name: Medical Record:

Date of Birth: Age: Gender:

Physician:

Date of Assessment:

Ethnic or Cultural Background:

Notes About Family Involvement:

Current Medical Diagnoses:

Prior Medical History: _____

Weight Record:

Height: Current weight: Usual weight:

Recent weight changes:

Possible causes:

Occupation:

Activity level: Sedentary_____   Moderately active_____   Very active_____

NOTED PROBLEMS (CHECK ALL THAT APPLY)

Chewing: Swallowing: Vision: Hearing: Ambulation:

Feeding Self: Anorexia: Chronic Vomiting: Chronic Diarrhea (over 5 days):

Food Allergies: Foods not Tolerated:

Current Diet Prescribed: How Long?

Snacks Between Meals? (If yes, list what and when)

Relevant Laboratory Values:

Glucose: BUN: Albumin:

Other:

Medications With Potential Nutrient Interactions (Laxatives, Diuretics, Insulin, Coumadin, etc.):

Other:

Regular Use of Vitamins/Minerals (list):

Regular Use of any Herbs/Botanical Products (list):

Estimated Needs (To be Done by Dietitian or Dietetic Technician):

Protein _____ g/kg/day = _____   kcal/kg/day = _____ Fluid: _____ cc/kg/day = _____

Provider Name and Credentials: Date:

● **BOX 3.1** Sedentary, Low-Active, and Active Lifestyle Routines

---

Sedentary: Your typical daily routine requires little physical movement (eg, sitting for long periods, using a computer, relying primarily on motorized transportation) and you accumulate little physical activity in your leisure time.

Low-Active: Your typical daily routine involves some physical activity (eg, walking to bus, mowing the lawn, shoveling snow) and you accumulate some additional physical activity in your leisure time.

Active: Your typical daily tasks involve some physical activity and you accumulate at least 2½ hours of moderate- to vigorous-intensity aerobic physical activity each week. Moderate-to-vigorous physical activity will make you breathe harder and your heart beat faster.

Adapted from Health Canada. (2011). *Canada's Food Guide.*

Chronic problems with nausea, vomiting, diarrhea, constipation, edema, or anemia should cause concern and require more investigation. Findings may warrant laboratory testing or referrals to specialists to rule out conditions such as eating disorders that may require intervention.

Activity and exercise patterns affect overall nutritional status. Many people assume that they lead a moderately active lifestyle; however, their usual patterns are actually sedentary. Box 3.1 provides some general guidelines related to what types of activity qualify as sedentary, low-active, and active (Health Canada, 2011).

Assessing Dietary Intake

A **nutritional screening** helps identify risk factors that can be ameliorated through appropriate nutritional counselling. Once problems are identified, the diet can be adjusted to prevent or decrease the likelihood of later complications. See Research Highlight 3.1.

Women can complete a self-assessment of dietary intake and exercise patterns using *My Food Guide,* an interactive, multilingual tool that accompanies *Eating Well With Canada's Food Guide* (Health Canada, 2008b*)*. It can be individualized based on sex, age, and level of activity and is available at http://www.hc-sc.gc.ca/fn-an/food-guide-aliment/myguide-monguide/index_eng.php. A client can enter her information and receive a food plan based on the Food Servings Guide. Along with healthy nutrition choices, *My Food Guide*

● **RESEARCH HIGHLIGHT 3.1**   Introducing a Nutrition Screening Tool: An Exploratory Study in a District General Hospital

BACKGROUND

Concerns have been raised that the nutrition of clients is a neglected aspect of care. Accordingly, "nutrition screening tools" have been devised to ensure that nurses assess all clients and, as appropriate, refer them to dietitians. The tool adopted in this study was the Nursing Nutritional Screening Tool.

PURPOSE

The purpose of the study was to investigate the effects of the Nursing Nutritional Screening Tool on nutrition-related nursing documentation, client care at mealtimes, and dietitian referral.

DESIGN

This study was conducted on two similar general medical wards in a United Kingdom (UK) district general hospital, with the help of staff and clients ($n = 175$) admitted during May 1999 and January 2000. Researchers collected data over 28 days before and after introducing the screening tool on one of the wards. For both wards, in each study stage, collected data included review of clients' notes and nonparticipant observations of mealtimes. Researchers used cross-tabulations to compare frequencies of dietitian referral and documentation of weight. Nine months later, the researchers discussed the findings with ward sisters in a group interview.

RESULTS

Use of the screening tool affected the process but not the outcomes of screening. The tool increased the frequency of nutrition-related documentation: the proportion of clients with weights recorded increased on the intervention ward ($p < 0.001$) and decreased on the comparator ward. Frequency of dietitian referral decreased on both wards, but differences were statistically insignificant. No change in client care at mealtimes was observed. The nurses in charge of the wards felt that introduction of the screening tool had raised awareness of nutrition-related care.

Meeting the nutritional needs of clients is a complex aspect of nursing that may benefit from use of structured guidelines. Diverse factors that require more exploration seem to limit the potential of screening to improve care.

Adapted from Jordan, S., Snow, D., Hayes, C., & Williams, A. (2003). Introducing a nutrition screening tool: An exploratory study in a district general hospital. *Journal of Advanced Nursing, 44*(1), 12–24.

● **BOX 3.2**   **Four Steps for Better Health and Weight**

1. Eat the recommended amount and types of food each day.
2. Limit foods and beverages that are high in calories, fat, sugar, or salt.
3. Be active every day.
4. If you think you don't have time to eat well, think again.

Adapted from Health Canada. (2007). *Maintaining Healthy Habits.* http://www.hc-sc.gc.ca/fn-an/food-guide-aliment/maintain-adopt/index-eng.php

encourages daily physical activity, symbolized by physical activity graphics.

To assess usual intake, a 24-hour dietary recall, including all food groups from Canada's Food Guide, is often useful. Those clients who omit whole food groups may be at risk for nutrient inadequacies. For example, clients who do not include 7 to 10 (male and female ranges) servings of fruits and vegetables may consume low amounts of vitamins A and C in particular. Low intake of breads and cereals may place clients at risk for inadequate intake of B-complex vitamins, carbohydrates, and iron. Low intake from the protein-rich group may lead to low serum levels of zinc and iron, with poor wound healing and delayed growth. Dairy foods are rich in calcium and riboflavin, as well as protein and carbohydrate. Low levels of essential fatty acid fats may be problematic. Oils and mayonnaise are good sources of natural vitamin E, which have preventive factors against some cancers and cardiovascular disease (Fairfield & Fletcher, 2002; Rao, 2002). Box 3.2 summarizes Health Canada's Steps for Better Health and Weight.

Assessing Nutritional Status

More information about the client's nutritional status can be ascertained by performing specific physical examinations and certain laboratory tests.

Anthropometric Measurements

Anthropometric data consist of measurements pertaining to body size and composition and include height, weight, BMI, midarm circumference, and triceps skinfold thickness (Bickley, 2012). The nurse measures the client's height, with the client wearing no shoes. For weight, it is essential to actually weigh the client on a scale, rather than rely on a client's report. The nurse can then use the client's height and weight to calculate BMI (see Chapter 2).

 Betsy is 1.7-m tall and weighs 52 kg. Refer to Chapter 2 for the formula for calculating BMI. What is Betsy's BMI?

Midarm circumference helps determine skeletal muscle mass. When measuring midarm circumference, the nurse uses the nondominant arm and finds the midpoint of the upper arm between the shoulder and the elbow. He or she then marks the midarm location and positions the arm loosely at the client's side. The nurse uses a tape measure to encircle the arm at the marked position and records the circumference in centimeters.

The nurse obtains the thickness of the skinfold at the triceps or subscapular areas to estimate the amount of subcutaneous fat deposits, which is related to total body fat (Fig. 3.4). Using the same arm as for the midarm circumference measurement, the nurse grasps and pulls the client's skin apart from the muscle at the previously marked location, places the calipers around the skinfold, and records the measurement in millimeters. To calculate how much of the midarm circumference is actual muscle, the nurse multiplies the triceps skinfold measurement by 0.314. To interpret midarm circumference and triceps skinfold thickness measurements, the nurse can compare the findings with averages provided in standardized charts (Dietitians of Canada, 2010a).

Other Physical Evaluations

Additional information from the physical examination that is central to a nutritional assessment includes the client's general appearance, characteristics of skin and hair, mouth integrity, condition of teeth, ability to chew and swallow, gag reflex, joint flexibility, hand strength,

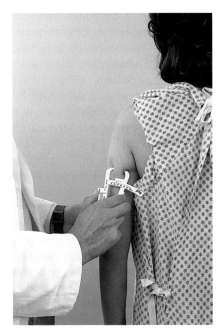

FIGURE 3.4   The nurse uses calipers to measure the client's triceps skinfold thickness.

and attention and concentration (Bickley, 2012). Abnormalities in any of these areas may have implications for overall health and require further investigation.

Laboratory Data

Common laboratory tests used in nutritional assessment include a complete blood count (CBC), especially hemoglobin, hematocrit, and number of lymphocytes; serum albumin and transferrin levels, which indicate protein status; and cholesterol, triglyceride, and lipoprotein levels.

Assessing Factors That Influence Food Choices

People tend to make food choices based on their usual patterns, most of which started in their family homes. Differences in nutrient intake, knowledge, and attitudes about diet and health can influence women's willingness and ability to choose foods for a more healthful diet (Turrell et al., 2003).

The client's *cultural or religious* background may influence the foods she likes or considers acceptable to eat. *The Food Guide* includes food serving choices that appeal to Canada's multiethnic population. The nurse should remember, however, not to make assumptions about dietary habits or preferences based solely on a client's identified ethnicity or religion.

Vegetarian diets can be healthy if planned carefully. Omission of any of the key food groups should be of concern to the practitioner. Dairy foods provide B-complex vitamins, especially riboflavin, vitamin D, calcium, potassium, protein, and other key nutrients. The meat group provides excellent sources of iron, niacin, thiamin, protein, zinc, and vitamin B_{12}. When either of these food groups is limited or severely restricted, the potential exists for nutrient deficiencies. A full nutritional assessment by a dietetics professional is suggested whenever a client states that she follows a vegetarian pattern. *A New Food Guide for North American Vegetarians,* developed by Messina et al. (2003), is useful for collaborating in food planning for and with vegetarians. Messina (2013) also maintains a website guide for planning and preparing vegetarian meals. Dietitians of Canada (2010b) provides information and guidelines for individuals who follow a vegan diet.

The nurse needs to understand the client's situation in relation to food security, that is, her resources to procure nutrition. Economic insecurity usually leads to an inability to access a nutrient supply that is predictable over time. Transportation may also be a problem, and local grocery stores may charge more for food than do supermarkets, compounding the problem. Where possible and necessary, nurses refer vulnerable pregnant or breastfeeding women, infants, and children younger than 2 years to programs that use the Canada Prenatal Nutrition Program (CPNP). The aim of this program is to reduce the incidence of unhealthy birth weight, improve the health of both infant and mother, and encourage breastfeeding. This comprehensive service includes food supplementations, nutritional counselling, support, education, referral, and counselling on health and lifestyle issues (Public Health Agency of Canada, 2011a). Nurses can also refer family members who need food to local Food Banks, social assistance programs, or farmers' markets.

One of the most influential factors related to client nutrition involves *developmental stage* and *life circumstances.* Considerations related to specific life stages are discussed in the next part of this chapter.

NUTRITIONAL VARIATIONS FOR VARIOUS GROUPS

Dietary needs, behaviours, and habits vary depending on whether a woman is just beginning to menstruate, is pregnant, is lactating, or is experiencing menopause. Her place in her family, peer group, and significant others can influence her food choices. The following sections focus on specific nutrition considerations for various developmental stages in the woman's life cycle.

Pregnancy

During pregnancy, changes must occur to ensure that gestation progresses and that both mother and fetus remain healthy (Ford, 2004). These changes involve synthesis of new tissues and hormonal variations to regulate essential processes. Nutrition has a critical role in pregnancy outcomes: maternal nutritional status at conception and throughout gestation influences not only the mother's health but also that of the fetus. Although good nutrition cannot guarantee a healthy pregnancy, it can certainly minimize problems.

Ideally, the woman's nutrition should be optimal before she becomes pregnant. Two conditions demonstrate the importance of optimal health before pregnancy: adequate folate status, which helps prevent neural tube defects, and control of blood glucose level, which improves the ability to conceive and to give birth to a healthy newborn. Even if a woman's nutritional behaviours before pregnancy were less than adequate, pregnancy can provide an excellent opportunity for nurses to teach women the importance of making sound nutritional choices and to encourage them to develop habits they will continue into the postpartum period and beyond.

QUOTE 3-1

"I always tried to follow a proper diet. Now that I am pregnant, there's so much more to consider. I'm always hungry, but some foods that I crave are not really good for me. I guess it's better to have an appetite than not, like my sister, who had morning sickness throughout her pregnancy."

A woman pregnant for the first time,
adapting to related nutrition and appetite changes

Weight Gain

One indicator of a healthy pregnancy is adequate weight gain, which is necessary to ensure optimal fetal outcomes. Suggested weight gain during pregnancy varies depending on the maternal prepregnancy BMI. For women with a normal BMI of 18.5 to 24.9, the suggested timing for weight gain during pregnancy, based on prepregnancy BMI, is 0.5 to 2 kg in the first trimester, with a steady incremental gain in the second and third trimesters—for a total pregnancy gain of 11.5 to 16 kg (Health Canada, 2010a). Extra weight gain may be beneficial to women who were underweight before pregnancy. Women who were overweight before pregnancy should gain no more than 7 to 11.5 kg, less than 0.3 kg per week. Women who are obese are advised to limit their total weight gain to 5 to 9 kg (Health Canada, 2010a).

Weight gained during pregnancy is distributed among various tissues essential to both fetus and mother. See Figure 3.5 for the components of maternal weight gain and its distribution.

Although women who were overweight before pregnancy have a decreased risk for giving birth to a small-for-gestational-age (SGA) infant, obesity is associated with an increased risk for gestational hypertension, giving birth to a baby with **macrosomia** (birth weight of ≥4,500 g), and perinatal mortality (Robinson et al., 2005; Surkan et al., 2004). Women need to be monitored closely to facilitate positive outcomes. Inquiries need to be made about the father's height-to-weight ratio before one assumes that an infant has a high birth weight; babies born to taller parents are more likely to weigh slightly over 4 kg.

Nutritional Requirements

Pregnancy requires energy to support growth and activity. The woman should follow the recommendations of the *Food Guide* for number of servings from each food group, with a total of two to three extra food servings from any food group (Health Canada, 2011). Carbohydrates are needed to spare protein and prevent formation of ketones. High levels of ketones in the blood can lead to fetal neurologic damage (Fowles, 2002). If the rate of weight gain follows the normal pattern, health care providers can assume that energy intake is ade-

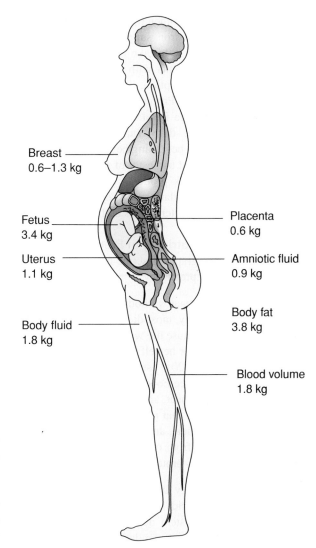

Breast
0.6–1.3 kg

Fetus
3.4 kg

Placenta
0.6 kg

Uterus
1.1 kg

Amniotic fluid
0.9 kg

Body fat
3.8 kg

Body fluid
1.8 kg

Blood volume
1.8 kg

FIGURE 3.5 Distribution and amount of maternal weight gain.

quate. Servings of milk, vegetables, and meat provide the extra protein, calcium, zinc, folate, and iron needed for successful maternal and fetal outcomes. Breastfeeding women should also increase their nutritional intake by 2 to 3 servings.

Supplements

When a woman is planning pregnancy, her primary health care provider usually prescribes a prenatal vitamin to help ensure adequate levels of nutrients essential to embryonic and fetal development (eg, folic acid). If a pregnancy is unplanned, a prenatal vitamin that includes folate should be prescribed as soon as a woman knows that she is pregnant (Health Canada, 2009c). To promote the best use of nutrients, the woman should take the supplement between meals with water or liquids other than milk or caffeinated beverages. If just an iron supplement is prescribed, bedtime is a good time to take it; the woman should not take iron supplements with antacids because the antacids decrease absorption. The Prenatal Nutrition Guidelines for Health Professionals (Health Canada, 2009a, 2009b) and the Food Guide (Health Canada, 2011) recommend a daily supplement of 400 μg (0.4 mg) of folic acid beginning before conception and continuing for the first trimester of pregnancy, as well as extra calcium (milk products food group), folate from whole grains and dark green vegetables, and iron from meats and meat alternatives and enriched grains.

Role of Specific Nutrients in Pregnancy

The following paragraphs describe nutrients of special significance during pregnancy:

Protein. Each woman's body processes protein uniquely, but generally, most dietary protein is used to form new tissue. Because the woman's body is producing tissues not only for herself but also for the growing fetus, Health Canada (2011) suggests increasing protein by an extra two to three Food Guide Servings, particularly from the milk, meat, and alternative food groups. The principal sources that provide this level of protein are dairy products, meat, and soy-based products. Getting enough energy from other sources is essential so that the body reserves protein for tissue synthesis.

Fat. Fats supply energy and essential fatty acids (linoleic and α-linolenic acids) necessary for adequate fetal brain and nervous system development and function. Although specific recommendations have yet to be established, severe lack of essential fatty acids may be associated with placental abnormalities and subsequent newborn complications (see Chapter 22).

Folate. A diet high in folate has been shown to reduce the incidence of neural tube defects. The Society of Obstetricians and Gynaecologists of Canada (SOGC) suggests that all women of childbearing age receive a daily folate supplement and that they eat folate-rich foods (SOGC, 2007). The two main forms of neural tube defect are *anencephaly* and *spina bifida* (see Chapter 22). The first condition usually results in stillbirth or early neonatal death; the second results in problems with paralysis or bowel- and bladder-control and other long-term problems. The supplementation level is much higher for the woman who has previously given birth to a child with a neural tube defect (SOGC, 2007). To avoid an overdose of vitamins, such high doses must not be combined with a multiple vitamin that also contains folic acid. In 1998, Canada began fortifying grains, pastas, and cereals with folic acid (Public Health Agency of Canada, 2004). Imported products are not fortified.

Recommended folate intakes for women with no personal health risks are as follows:

- A good diet of folate-rich foods
- Daily supplementation with a multivitamin that includes 0.4 to 1 mg for at least 2 to 3 months prior to conception and throughout pregnancy and the postpartum period, that is, 4 to 6 weeks and as long as breastfeeding continues (SOGC, 2007)

SOGC also recommends that women with specific health or lifestyle risks or a history of a previous fetus with a neural tube defect have a higher level of folate supplementation.

B Vitamins. Riboflavin, thiamin, and niacin are necessary for cellular energy production. Because energy intake increases during pregnancy, the need for these vitamins is also greater. As long as the woman's diet contains whole grains, legumes, dark green vegetables, meats, and dairy products, these nutrients probably are adequate. A diet consisting predominantly of fat and sugar necessitates B vitamin supplementation. Niacin is the one vitamin for which an upper limit has been set during pregnancy (35 mg/day; 30 mg/day for women 18 years or younger) (IOM, 2000a).

The other two vitamins necessary for protein synthesis are B_{12} and B_6. The interrelationship between B_{12} and folic acid in the synthesis of new protein is well established. B_{12} deficiency is rare during pregnancy because most women's diets usually supply an adequate level. The possible exception is the woman who is a **vegan** (a type of vegetarian who eats no meat or meat products, such as eggs or milk) or the fetus diagnosed with methylmalonic acidemia, an inborn error of metabolism. B_6 has a vital role in protein metabolism. Evidence of specific poor pregnancy outcomes related to this vitamin is lacking.

Vitamin A. The role of vitamin A in tissue development is well defined. Because the body stores vitamin A, deficiencies are rare. Two situations in which supplementation during pregnancy may be necessary are in women with HIV or anemia.

The greatest danger associated with vitamin A is that preformed (or active) vitamin A is teratogenic (causes birth defects) at high intake levels. Therefore, a pregnant woman needs to limit her intake of preformed vitamin A to less than 3,000 μg/day (IOM, 2000b). Labels of supplements need to provide information on the source of vitamin A. Carotene, the precursor to retinol, is not teratogenic.

Vitamin C. No adverse outcome has been directly associated with lack of vitamin C in the diet, and most women seem to meet the DRI of 75 (85 during pregnancy, 120 during lactation) mg/day (Health

Canada, 2010b). There is some evidence that gestational hypertension and premature rupture of the membranes is associated with a low plasma level of vitamin C (Casanueva et al., 2005). The upper limit of intake for vitamin C is 2,000 mg/day (1,800 mg/day for 18 years and under) (Health Canada, 2010b).

Vitamin K. Vitamin K is known for its role in blood clotting. The recommendation for pregnant women is 90 µg/day (Health Canada, 2010b). Infants receive an injection of vitamin K right after birth because the vitamin does not transport adequately across the placenta, and initially they do not make their own.

Iron. Iron is one nutrient required for production of heme compounds, especially hemoglobin, in red blood cells. Both mother and fetus produce red blood cells; during the last trimester, the fetus absorbs more iron to produce blood. Maternal anemia does not result in newborn anemia because the fetus removes iron from the mother. Anemia in the mother increases her risk for cardiac arrest, causes fatigue, and can result in a preterm or low-birthweight infant (Scholl & Reilly, 2000).

Anemia is common during pregnancy (Health Canada, 2009c). Although lack of folate, B_6, or B_{12} could be the cause, the most common reason is lack of iron (Scholl, 2005). One protective mechanism during pregnancy is increased absorption of iron from the diet. During pregnancy the DRI for iron increases from 18 to 27 (Health Canada, 2005) and the woman needs ferrous salt supplements. The recommended supplementation level is 16 to 20 mg/day throughout pregnancy (Health Canada, 2009c). The upper limit of 45 mg/day is not to be exceeded (Health Canada, 2009c). Supplements may cause nausea and constipation, so women may benefit from counselling on how to reduce these problems.

Diagnosis of anemia is based on hematocrit and hemoglobin levels. In Canada, 20% of women and 50% of pregnant women have iron deficiency anemia (Body and Health Canada, n.d.). Another clue that warrants a close look at these laboratory data is **pica** (eating or craving nonfood substances such as cornstarch, clay, dirt, or ice). It is not known whether pica causes anemia or anemia causes pica, but the two are closely related. With a diagnosis of anemia, the recommended supplement level may be increased (Health Canada, 2009c). Supplements may be given in divided doses to decrease side effects.

High hemoglobin levels (greater than 132 g/L) are detrimental to the mother and fetus. Failure of the blood to expand, poor circulation to the fetus through the placenta, and placental infarcts are thought to contribute to associated poor outcomes. Women with such hemoglobin levels should not use iron supplements.

Calcium. The fetus needs calcium for skeletal formation. The placental hormones of human chorionic somatomammotropin and estrogen increase bone turnover rates and maintain calcium balance by enhancing intestinal calcium absorption and decreasing urinary excretion. Increased retention of calcium throughout pregnancy helps supply the high demand needed for skeleton and tooth formation during the last trimester. The AI for pregnant women is 1,000 mg/day; 1,300 mg/day for women 18 years or younger) (Health Canada, 2012b). These levels are higher than those set by other countries, largely because the high phosphorus and protein intake in Canada causes urinary loss of calcium.

Some researchers have theorized that high calcium intake protects against hypertension in adults (Alonso et al., 2005). Some health professionals routinely recommend calcium supplements.

Other Minerals. *Magnesium* supplementation may reduce leg cramps for pregnant women with low serum levels of magnesium.

Zinc is necessary for growth and development, but conclusive evidence that zinc deficiency results in poor pregnancy outcomes is lacking. *Iron* supplementation may increase the need for zinc because iron inhibits zinc absorption.

More research is needed on *copper* needs during pregnancy. Copper deficiency is teratogenic in animals. Iron supplementation decreases absorption of copper, and Canadian diets tend to be low in copper.

Fluoride is necessary for healthy tooth formation as early as the 10th week of pregnancy. Research has not yet shown the importance of fluoride to development during pregnancy.

Phosphorus is important for bone formation; meeting the AI recommendation of 700 mg/day (1,250 mg/day if 18 or under) is not a problem for most women. Canadian diets are high in phosphorus. Calcium balance and bone formation involves phosphorus, vitamin D, calcium, and hormones. Calcium and vitamin D are the nutrients that are likely to be limiting. An upper limit has been set for phosphorus at 3,500 mg/day (Health Canada, 2005).

Sodium restriction for edema during pregnancy is not recommended. Some degree of fluid retention is expected during pregnancy, and sodium is needed to balance the electrolytes. Therefore, an intake of 1,500 mg/day is suggested (Health Canada, 2005). The only evidence we have of restriction causing problems is that women on sodium restrictions tend to deliver infants with hyponatremia.

Nutritional Deficits and Problems

Continuous dietary monitoring of pregnant women is critical; nutrients that require special emphasis include calcium, magnesium, zinc, iron, fibre, folate, and vitamins D and E (Bienz et al., 2003).

Pregnant women with poor eating habits (eg, skipping meals) or a history of eating disorders place their fetuses and infants at risk for malnutrition and its associated consequences. Women with insufficient funds to purchase foods during pregnancy; those who smoke, take drugs, or consume alcoholic beverages; those with chronic diseases (eg, diabetes, renal disease); and those with chronic anemia are at risk for poor pregnancy outcomes (Jaddoe et al., 2007; Lopez et al., 2007; Scholl, 2005). These clients need increased attention from health care providers and appropriate referrals to specialists, nutritionists, social workers, and other resources for assistance.

Isotretinoin (Accutane) is an acne medication made from vitamin A that is chemically different from over-the-counter vitamin A. It is prescribed to some nonpregnant women. It is related to preformed vitamin A, which can cause severe birth defects if levels in the mother exceed the upper limit. Women should stop using isotretinoin before becoming pregnant. In addition, all pregnant women should consume no more than 3,000 µg of vitamin A each day in the diet and supplements (Health Canada, 2010b).

Similarly, pregnant women should not use herbs and botanical supplements without first checking with their health care provider. Women using such supplements should stop immediately when they discover they are pregnant. *Motherisk,* from Toronto's Sick Kids Hospital, provides information to pregnant women about a variety of issues, including drugs and alternative health foods. See http://www.motherisk.org/prof/drugs.jsp. Canada does not produce a list of not-to-use products during pregnancy, but the American Pregnancy Association (2013) addresses the safety of using various herbs during pregnancy.

Pregnant women who experience hyperemesis gravidarum may require enteral feedings to alleviate nausea and to prevent or correct weight loss. Careful attention to recovery of lost weight is an important aspect in this group of pregnant women. See Chapter 13 for more information.

COLLABORATIVE CARE: NUTRITION IN PREGNANCY

Assessment

During the initial prenatal visit, the nurse performs a detailed nutritional assessment (see earlier discussion). The nurse and client can discuss habits and concerns for ongoing monitoring as the pregnancy progresses. During that visit and subsequent appointments, the assessment of a pregnant woman includes body weight measurement and plotting on a weight gain grid. The nurse uses this information along with other laboratory data to determine the status of the pregnant woman's nutrition (Fig. 3.6).

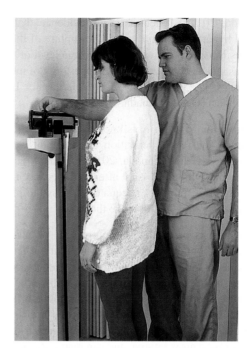

FIGURE 3.6 Monitoring the progress of weight gain in pregnancy is an essential nursing activity.

 When reviewing the client's medical record, the nurse finds that Sheila's prepregnancy weight was 65 kg, and that her BMI was 27. What would the nurse expect the client to weigh at this visit?

Select Potential Nursing Diagnoses

The following nursing diagnoses related to nutritional issues and concerns may apply to the pregnant woman:

- **Health-Seeking Behaviours** related to the desire to have a healthy baby
- **Deficient Knowledge** related to appropriate weight gain during pregnancy
- **Ineffective Health Maintenance** related to control of weight during pregnancy and appropriate food selection

Planning/Intervention

The nurse and the client discuss the relationship of weight gain to a healthy pregnancy and look at the weight gain grid with the woman's weight plotted on it. They discuss ways to manage weight gain and food intake to ensure that the client meets nutrient needs while avoiding either weight loss or excessive gain. If nutritional problems are extensive, the nurse may refer the woman to a registered dietician for in-depth assistance with food selection. See Nursing Care Plan 3.1.

NURSING CARE PLAN 3.1
●
A Teen With Nutritional Issues

 The nurse asks Betsy, the 14-year-old who mentions fear of weight gain, to provide more information about her typical diet and food preferences. Betsy mentions that she enjoys eating at fast food restaurants, consumes about two cans of carbonated soda per day, and frequently skips breakfast.

NURSING DIAGNOSES

- **Imbalanced Nutrition, Less Than Body Requirements** related to inadequate intake secondary to desire for weight control
- **Deficient Knowledge** related to importance of nutrition

EXPECTED OUTCOMES

1. The client will verbalize an understanding of nutritional needs during adolescence.
2. The client will state the rationale for taking in additional calories.
3. The client will identify appropriate nutritional choices.
4. The client will participate in developing a nutritional plan to foster growth and development.

INTERVENTIONS	RATIONALES
Assess the client's level of understanding about nutrition and nutritional requirements of adolescence.	This information provides a baseline to identify specific client needs and to develop an individualized teaching plan.
Review the nutritional needs of adolescence, describing what the needs are and why.	The client needs this basic knowledge.
Complete a 24-hr dietary recall.	Dietary recall provides information about client's typical intake during a day and helps identify eating patterns.
Ask the client about foods that she likes and dislikes; determine any cultural influences on her choices.	Knowledge of food likes and dislikes and cultural influences provides a baseline for dietary suggestions and menu planning.
Encourage client to identify foods in her diet that are nutritionally inadequate. Work with client to identify suggestions for replacing nonnutritious foods with foods that are nutritionally sound.	Client participation in evaluating her own nutrition and identifying appropriate suggestions promotes control over the situation and fosters positive self-esteem.
Arrange for consultation with dietitian about meal planning. Provide the client with menus and teaching pamphlets.	Collaborative care can ensure that diets are sound and will optimize health; printed materials can reinforce learning.
Plan with the client to keep a journal outlining her food choices and selections over the next few weeks. Schedule an appointment to monitor the client's progress within 2 wks.	The journal can provide objective evidence of the client's behaviours. Follow-up is critical to ensure that selections and behaviours are improving.

(continued)

NURSING CARE PLAN 3.1 ● A Teen With Nutritional Issues *(Continued)*

EVALUATION

1. The client expresses accurate understanding of the reasons that enhanced nutrition during adolescence is important.
2. The client commits to keeping a food journal and following the menus designed by the nurse and dietitian.
3. The client schedules and keeps her 2-week follow-up appointment and shows compliance with the recommended dietary plan.
4. The client demonstrates adequate weight gain at follow-up appointments.

NURSING DIAGNOSIS

Disturbed Body Image related to lack of understanding the difference between a healthy body and an overweight body.

EXPECTED OUTCOMES

1. The client will verbalize feelings about her maturing body and its effect on her view of herself.
2. The client will identify body changes as reflective of her developmental stage.

INTERVENTIONS	RATIONALES
Assess the client's beliefs about her current body image, developmental stage, and self-esteem. Explore with the client her feelings about her changing body.	Assessment provides a baseline from which to develop appropriate strategies for teaching and care. Exploration of client's feelings provides insight into the client's thinking to ensure planning of appropriate individualized interventions.
Communicate accurate facts and answer questions honestly; clarify any misconceptions or misinformation about weight gain and being overweight.	Clear communication helps provide accurate information to aid in alleviating fears and clarifying misinformation. Honesty promotes the development of trust in the relationship.
Question client about how her friends view her.	Adolescence focuses on the development of a sense of identity, with a strong emphasis on body image and peer influence.
Assess the client's stress level associated with her current situation and measures used to cope with similar stressful situations in the past; ask client to identify people who have been a source of support.	Identification of the client's stress level, previous coping strategies, and support people helps determine effective strategies for use in this situation.
Reassess client's view of self on next visit.	Reassessment provides information about client's progress in understanding the changes of pregnancy and her adaptation to her changing body image.

EVALUATION

1. The client states positive feelings about herself.
2. The client demonstrates acceptance of her changing body.

Evaluation

The nurse weighs the woman at the next clinic visit, plots the weight on the grid, and evaluates changes to determine the next steps to take. After being weighed, some women show signs of anxiety or depression because their weight is higher than what they normally experience. These clients may need reassurance that they can lose the weight gained during pregnancy after the baby is born.

Lactation

Breastfeeding confers important immunologic, physiologic, economic, social, and hygienic effects to the mother and infant. Infants digest and absorb human milk more efficiently than they do other forms of milk (cow's milk, goat's milk). The composition of breast milk adapts over time to meet the human infant's changing needs, whereas the composition of cow's milk or formula does not vary nor does it contain immunoglobulins (see Chapter 21).

Some researchers have indicated that asthma and associated problems are decreased in children who were exclusively breastfed (Oddy & Peat, 2003). Other researchers have reported opposite results (Flohr et al., 2011; Sears et al., 2002). Kramer and Kakuma (2012), in a Cochrane Collaboration summary of 23 independent studies, concluded that exclusive breastfeeding for 6 months, compared with breastfeeding for 3 to 4 months, resulted in lower risk of gastrointestinal infection but no reduced risks of other infections, allergic diseases, obesity, dental caries, or cognitive or behaviour problems (Kramer & Kakuma, 2012).

Breastfeeding is an ethical dilemma in mothers with HIV, which can be transmitted to infants through the breast milk. The Canadian Paediatric Society recommends that mothers with HIV should not breastfeed (Canadian Paediatric Society, 2012).

Chapter 21 provides a comprehensive discussion of breastfeeding and newborn nutrition. The following paragraphs provide a brief summary of nutritional issues during this life stage for women.

Nutrient Needs

The nutrient needs of the lactating woman are related to the energy required to produce approximately 750 mL of breast milk per day. Recommendations are for the woman to consume 400 to 500 kcal/day above the requirements for her age group (Yon & Johnson, 2005). Most nursing mothers need a total of 2,500 to 3,300 kcal/day, which should come from a varied diet to supply the vitamins and minerals recommended.

If the woman's diet is balanced and follows the Canada Food Guide, supplementation of nutrients may not be necessary. However, this decision depends on what her nutritional status was when she became pregnant, as well as the course of her pregnancy, labour, and delivery; for example, if she had hyperemesis, postpartum hemorrhage, or other complication. Fluids are important to keep the mother hydrated. A good way to ensure that a woman consumes enough fluid is to drink milk or water with every meal and every time the baby nurses. Lactating women can be encouraged to fill a sports bottle with water or another liquid and have it within reach each time they breastfeed.

 Remember Sheila, the woman in her third trimester who is planning to breastfeed her newborn. She reported that she is having difficulty drinking milk. What other suggestions could the nurse make to ensure that her calcium intake is adequate?

Counselling Issues

Health Canada (2013d) recommends that infants be breastfed exclusively for the first 6 months and that breastfeeding be sustained for up to 2 years or longer, with appropriate complementary feeding. This period maximizes the infant's benefits from breast milk and allows time for the child to transit successfully to table foods. All health care personnel should support the mother as much as possible to continue breastfeeding for as long as possible (Health Canada, 2013d).

A woman's milk supply usually remains adequate unless she is poorly nourished. Weight loss during the lactation period is not recommended because too few nutrients and calories to produce milk results in decreased quantity of breast milk (American Dietetic Association, 2001; McCrory, 2001). Women who have difficulty with a poor milk supply should rest frequently; avoid caffeinated beverages, medications, and smoking; increase fluid intake; and correct any underlying illnesses. Increasing the number of feedings per day (supply responds to demand) and not giving the infant supplemental bottles or solid food are additional ways to increase milk supply.

Nutrient Problems in Breastfeeding

Breast milk alone can meet the infant's nutrient needs in the first 6 months, with the exception of vitamin D (Kreiter et al., 2000). Health Canada (2013d) recommends 400 International Unit of vitamin D for breastfed infants. http://www.hc-sc.gc.ca/fn-an/nutrition/infant-nourisson/index-eng.php

Women can transmit alcohol, nicotine, and many drugs through breast milk to infants, and they should be discouraged from using such products. The list of drugs that transfer from the mother's breast milk to the infant and cause adverse effects is long. For many more drugs, the effects are currently unknown (Ito & Lee, 2003). Breastfeeding women can consult their practitioners for the safety of both over-the-counter medications and prescription drugs before taking them. Most drugs should not be taken during breastfeeding.

Herbs and botanical products have not been proven safe for breastfeeding mothers and their infants. Women should *not* consume kava, chasteberry, dong quai, Asian ginseng, or liquorice root during lactation. There is a danger of liver damage with kava (Health Canada, 2008a; Medline Plus, 2013). Dong quai interacts with antibiotics, St. John's wort, and blood-thinning medications to increase the danger of excessive bleeding. Asian ginseng interacts with other drugs to cause several problems: excessive bleeding with blood thinners; headache and manic behaviour with antidepressants; heart problems with digoxin; and low blood glucose levels with antidiabetic medications. Natural liquorice can increase problems with control of hypertension.

Adolescence

Sociocultural influences may affect an adolescent's eating patterns, desire for thinness, and behaviour, leading to trends such as using laxatives or diuretics to decrease weight, fasting, skipping meals, eating snacks at unusual hours, and self-induced vomiting. Teens require increased nutrients to allow for accelerated growth; nutritional deficiencies in adolescence may decrease height, lead to osteoporosis, or delay sexual maturation (Herbold & Frates, 2000).

Think back to Betsy, the teen described at the beginning of the chapter. Consider her statement, "I don't want to get fat." How might the nurse interpret this statement based on Betsy's developmental stage?

Food intake in adolescence often varies, especially during growth spurts and different stages of physical maturation. Dietary intake and body size influence age at menarche and growth patterns. Age at menarche also is related inversely to percentage of energy intake from dietary protein at 3 to 5 years and fat intake at 1 to 2 years; the percentage of energy from animal protein at 6 to 8 years influences age at peak growth (Berkey et al., 2000). These factors (body weight and protein intake) may be related to later development of diseases, including breast cancer and heart disease. Controlling weight through exercise and a balanced diet becomes important

to health in later life. Risks for breast cancer include younger age at menarche, older age at menopause, and older age at first child's birth. As body fat percentage increases, the age at menarche decreases (Freedman et al., 2003). Prevention of obesity is one strategy to reduce risks for heart disease, hypertension, and type 2 diabetes (Whitney et al., 2002). Calcium intake and exercise throughout life may help prevent osteoporosis in later life (Whitney et al., 2002).

Dietary modifications in adolescence are needed to meet ongoing or potential growth spurts and to prevent or correct anemia. Nurses can discuss unusual eating patterns, emphasizing caring and concern. In some cases, family counselling may be useful, especially if there is obesity or a tendency toward eating disorders.

More information about healthy eating during the adolescent years can be found at the Canadian Dietitians web site http://www.dietitians.ca

Nutrient Needs

Vegetarian teens may need to be encouraged to consume adequate sources of vitamin B_{12}, riboflavin, zinc, iron, calcium, protein, and energy for growth (Messina & Reed Mangels, 2001). Diets for female teens should include the following servings from *The Food Guide* (Health Canada, 2011):

- Three to four servings of milk or milk alternatives to supply calcium
- Two servings of meat or alternatives
- Six servings from the grain group
- Seven servings of fruit and vegetables

Fruit and vegetable juices are less acceptable (Health Canada, 2011); nurses can encourage teens to consume the real item for fibre and other **phytochemicals** (plant-based nutrients that may have protective health properties).

In general, teens who have healthy diets do not need vitamin and mineral supplements. Pregnant teens or those with inadequate nutrition need dietary modifications, supplements, or both. Intake of vitamins A and E, calcium, and zinc tend to be low among all teens, regardless of the use of supplements (Stang et al., 2000). Excesses of nutrients such as vitamins A and D, however, are not recommended because they may lead to toxicity.

Teen use of nonprescription medications (eg, aspirin, cold remedies), alcohol, and illegal drugs should be monitored carefully. Side effects of the use of such items may include poor oral intakes of several nutrients. Smoking tends to decrease serum levels of vitamin C.

As much as possible, the nurse supports the adolescent to make independent choices. Autonomy is part of the developmental process that teens must experience. Choices in meal planning, snacking, timing, and

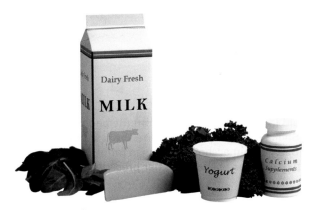

FIGURE 3.7 Calcium is very important for girls and adolescent females. Nurses, parents, teachers, and other influential adults should encourage teens to eat good sources of calcium, including milk, yogurt, cheese, and green leafy vegetables.

nutrient density (a variable used to assess the quality of a food choice) may be ways in which the teen can actively provide input. Rather than assuming that a teen will not be willing to include fruits and vegetables, the nurse can discuss the client's preferences and provide guidance about the value of specific foods to empower the adolescent while educating her about nutrition.

Because adequate calcium intake during childhood, adolescence, and early adulthood helps prevent later problems with osteoporosis, the nurse can suggest that the adolescent consume low-fat milk or milk alternative products throughout the day (Fig. 3.7). As carbonated beverages leach calcium, they should be discouraged. Some examples of healthy choices are low-fat milk at breakfast; low-fat yogurt, low-fat flavoured milk beverages, or low-fat cheese for snacks; and low-fat cottage cheese with fruit at meals or for snacks. Nondairy sources such as greens are less effective in meeting calcium requirements but can be part of the overall plan.

In addition, teens can consume other nutrient-dense foods as follows:

- Vitamin A from cantaloupe, mango, spinach, and apricots
- Vitamin C from oranges, grapefruit, citrus juices, broccoli, spinach, melon, cranberries, and strawberries
- Iron from liver, enriched rice, whole milk, raisins, low-fat red meat, and baked potatoes
- Vitamin B$_6$ from pork, bananas, potatoes, and egg yolks
- Folate from wheat germ, spinach, asparagus, and strawberries
- Zinc from meats and poultry, peanut butter, and tuna
- Omega-3 and omega-6 from eggs from chickens fed with omega-fortified feed

Vitamin B$_{12}$ is available only from meats and milk (animal foods); a true vegan diet may not suffice and cause some difficulty in learning effectively (Louwman et al., 2000). Foods acceptable to vegetarians that supply B$_{12}$ are fortified soy milk, miso (soybean paste), yeast grown on B$_{12}$ medium, and supplements. Remember to consult the food guide for vegetarians (Messina et al., 2003).

Guidance for being active is also important for this population, especially with the current inactive status of many young people. Obesity should be managed early, and family interventions are often effective.

Overall, working with teens on their nutritional intake can be rewarding and challenging. See Nursing Care Plan 3.2.

Consider Betsy, the adolescent from the beginning of the chapter. What areas would be important to assess specifically related to Betsy's nutrition?

Nutritional Concerns for Pregnant Adolescents

In general, the nutritional needs of pregnant adolescents are those for pregnancy plus those for the age group. Because growth spurts and maturation rates determine needs, the health care provider must also consider the adolescent's gynecologic age (years since start of menses). If her gynecologic age is 4 years or greater, then she is probably finished growing, and her nutritional needs will be less than those of a teen who is still growing.

Pregnancy in adolescence can pose significant dietary challenges for those adolescents who are still growing because the fetus must compete with the mother for nutrients. Height measures during pregnancy may not reflect ongoing growth because spine and postural changes during pregnancy may appear to decrease the teen's stature.

To ensure a healthy infant and mother at the time of birth, weight gain recommendations for pregnant teens need to balance concerns of both overgaining, which may result in obesity later in life, and undergaining, which may lead to low birth weight (Groth, 2007). A total gain of 11.4 to 15.9 kg is suggested. It is advisable to individualize weight gain recommendations to each teen, keeping in mind prepregnancy BMI norms (Groth, 2007). Some evidence supports gaining to the middle, but not to the top, of weight gain ranges; the concern is that high weight gain could result in excess body fat, macrosomia, need for cesarean birth, and birth asphyxia.

Energy needs vary among pregnant teens—actual needs seem related to activity level, with needs increasing with gestation. Protein intakes generally meet the

NURSING CARE PLAN 3.2

●

Nutrition for Pregnancy and Breastfeeding

 The nurse asks Sheila, the 37-year-old in her third trimester from the beginning of the chapter, about her milk intake. Sheila states, "I just don't like the taste of milk. I never have." Her weight gain has been within acceptable ranges for gestation, height, and weight. Sheila reports that she has been taking her prescribed prenatal vitamins every day.

NURSING DIAGNOSES

- **Imbalanced Nutrition, Less Than Body Requirements** related to inadequate intake of calcium rich foods.
- **Deficient Knowledge** related to nutritional needs for breastfeeding and foods high in calcium.

EXPECTED OUTCOMES

1. The client will identify the need for increased consumption of calories and fluid to promote breastfeeding.
2. The client will verbalize appropriate sources of foods to meet increased nutritional needs.
3. The client will identify options for calcium rich foods in addition to milk.

INTERVENTIONS	RATIONALES
Assess the client's knowledge of nutrition and breastfeeding.	This information provides a baseline from which to develop appropriate strategies.
Review the nutritional requirements for the current stage of pregnancy and for breast-feeding.	Ongoing education is essential to promote healthy outcomes.
Review the client's daily eating patterns, including frequency and types of foods consumed. Ascertain the client's likes and dislikes.	Knowledge of current dietary patterns provides clues to nutritional status and to the amount and types of calories and nutrients ingested. Information about likes and dis-likes aids in individualizing suggestions for proper food selection.
Discuss the need to eat 2,500 to 3,300 kcal/d, emphasizing the importance of a diet including all food groups.	Increased calories ensure an adequate pro-duction of breast milk. A varied diet ensures ingestion of necessary nutrients.
Review food sources that are high in calcium, including dairy options such as cheese and yogurt. Also instruct the client about other calcium-rich foods (eg, broccoli, sesame seeds, tofu, kale).	This information helps the client to under-stand the options available, other than milk, that can help ensure adequate calcium consumption.
Provide the client with a written list of appro-priate foods for intake.	A written list promotes learning and provides a reference source for the client.
Assess daily intake of fluid, including types consumed, amounts, and frequency.	This information gives clues to daily patterns and establishes a baseline for additional teaching and suggestions.

(continued)

NURSING CARE PLAN 3.2 ● Nutrition for Pregnancy and Breastfeeding *(Continued)*

INTERVENTIONS	RATIONALES
Encourage the client to ingest adequate fluids each day, including water. Suggest that she drink water with meals and carry water with her throughout the day.	Adequate fluid intake is essential for production of adequate breast milk.
Encourage the client to keep a diary or log of food and fluid intake for review on the next visit.	Keeping a diary or log helps the client visualize the amount and types of food and fluid consumed and possible patterns of intake that need adjustment or correction.

EVALUATION

1. The client demonstrates intake of the required amount of calories and fluid.
2. The client identifies appropriate alternative food sources for calcium with the recommended dietary plan.

---

estimated need for females who consume enough total energy to spare protein for tissue building. Because the recommended iron intake is difficult to achieve through diet alone, a supplement is recommended to prevent depletion and provide for stores. Calcium is needed to accrue bone mass and to form the fetal skeleton. If calcium intake is insufficient to meet these needs, then the calcium is absorbed from the maternal skeletal system. Diets often do not supply the needed calcium; a 600-mg supplement is prescribed. Some clinicians believe that folate should start as soon as menarche occurs and continue throughout the childbearing years (SOGC, 2007).

Often the adolescent has not consumed adequate sources of folate and enters pregnancy with a deficit that increases the danger of neural tube defects. Supplementation as soon as possible to meet needs is recommended, even though pregnancy is too late to prevent most neural tube defects.

COLLABORATIVE CARE: NUTRITION AND THE PREGNANT TEEN
Assessment

A nutritional assessment with a pregnant adolescent should include all of the following areas:

- Dietary intake
  - Source of animal or **complementary proteins** (two or more proteins that in combination supply all essential amino acids, but alone lack at least one essential amino acid)
- Vitamin C
  - Fresh fruits and vegetables
  - Fibre
  - Calcium sources
  - Iron sources
  - Empty calorie foods
  - Dietary fats
- Physical characteristics
  - Gynecologic age
  - Height and weight before pregnancy
  - Weight changes during pregnancy
  - Signs and symptoms of malnutrition
- Laboratory data
- Activity
- Medications
- Chronic diseases or infections

The results of the previous quick screening can help the provider identify important issues. Some indications of nutritional problems are identifiable by height, weight, and weight changes. The nurse assesses for sudden weight gain or loss before or during pregnancy. Dietary habits that indicate eating disorders or unusual eating patterns are another indicator requiring follow-up. The nurse should also consider unhealthy social or economic dynamics: substance use, low income, homelessness, physical violence, and psychological stress.

Select Potential Nursing Diagnoses

The following nursing diagnoses related to nutritional issues and concerns may apply to the pregnant adolescent:

- **Deficient Knowledge** related to nutrition during pregnancy
- **Situational Low Self-Esteem** related to immaturity and social situations created by the pregnancy
- **Disturbed Body Image** related to the physical changes taking place during both adolescence and the pregnancy

Planning/Intervention

Although the nutritional assessment will reveal each client's specific nutritional issues, some of the more common concerns to address with pregnant teens include excessive reliance on fast foods, which results in a diet high in fat and low in folate, and meal skipping or irregular eating. The nurse addresses the adolescent's nutritional knowledge, providing education and psychological support as necessary. Teens who show significant nutritional deficits, financial or psychosocial problems, or other high-risk factors can be referred to a dietitian and possibly to a social worker for additional information.

Evaluation

Follow-up at each visit should reveal adequate weight gain, improved food intake, and resolution of any social or psychological problems. The ideal outcome is for the adolescent to give birth to a healthy baby.

Adulthood and Older Adulthood

Leading causes of death in women include heart disease, cancer, cerebrovascular diseases, and diabetes mellitus (see Chapter 4). Osteoporosis and extremes in body weight are approaching epidemic proportions. Nutritional habits are a factor in all these illnesses. In addition, a woman's diet and nutritional habits can influence her menstrual cycles and contribute to reproductive and breast problems. Canadian dietitians have numerous resources for women's health and nutrition available at www.dietitians.ca. The following paragraphs focus on special ways for adult and older adult women to practice sound nutritional habits to promote health and prevent illness and guidance that nurses can provide in these areas.

Weight Management

When planning meals with adult and older adult women, the nurse emphasizes the nutrient density of meals. These clients have fewer natural energy requirements than found in pregnant, lactating, or adolescent women. Actual energy requirements depend on the woman's level of activity and exercise and other factors such as illness and stress. The nurse can teach them ways to avoid a sedentary lifestyle and subsequent obesity and encourage them to seek 30 to 60 minutes or more of reasonable physical activity (eg, brisk walking) most days of the week.

Bone Density Preservation

To promote adequate bone mass density, which peaks at 25 to 30 years, women should include good sources of calcium and vitamin D each day in the diet. In addition, they need sufficient but not excessive iron to prevent anemia with its resulting fatigue, irritability, and related symptoms. Chapters 2 and 24 provide detailed discussion of osteoporosis prevention and management.

Women's Health Concerns

For common complaints related to women's health, there are several reasonable nutrition-related suggestions, but insufficient evidence. The use of herbs and botanicals often increases with age to treat problems related to menstruation. See Complementary/Alternative Medicine 3.1 for more discussion.

Premenstrual Syndrome. For premenstrual syndrome (PMS), use of a low-fat vegetarian diet is associated

---

● COMPLEMENTARY/ALTERNATIVE MEDICINE 3.1
Herbal Supplements for Menstrual Problems

The use of herbs and botanicals often increases with age. Dong quai is a Chinese women's tonic for menstrual cramps and other symptoms; clients should not take it with warfarin, aspirin, or ticlopidine because dong quai has blood-thinning attributes. Nurses counsel clients to avoid use of evening primrose oil with antiseizure medications, antiepileptics, chlorpromazine, fluphenazine, and mesoridazine. If a client uses valerian as an antianxiety or sleep aid, she should not mix it with other sedatives, alcohol, and other central nervous system depressants because of the risk of additional sedation (Houghton, 1999).

See American Pregnancy Association. (2013). *Herbs and Pregnancy.* http://americanpregnancy.org/pregnancyhealth/naturalherbsvitamins.html

See SOGC (n.d.). Medications and drugs before and during pregnancy. Retrieved from http://sogc.org/publications/medications-and-drugs-before-and-during-pregnancy/

with reductions in body weight, duration, and intensity of dysmenorrhea, and duration of overall symptoms (Barnard et al., 2000). Calcium has been found to be of benefit to clients with PMS; limited evidence suggests that vitamins E and B_6 and carbohydrate supplements may be useful (Bendich, 2000). In some studies, dietary supplementation with magnesium has been found to be effective in alleviating symptoms of PMS (Quaranta et al., 2007). Other researchers have found that magnesium is no more effective than a placebo (Khine et al., 2006). Use of herbals for PMS has no supporting evidence; black cohosh in large doses may cause hypotension, vomiting, headache, dizziness, gastrointestinal distress, and limb pain. The health care practitioner may recommend a general multivitamin and mineral capsule.

Fibrocystic Breast Disease. Randomized controlled studies of caffeine restriction have failed to support nutritional interventions recommended for fibrocystic breast disease. Likewise, use of evening primrose oil, vitamin E, or pyridoxine treatments has not proven effective. Use of a low-fat (15% to 20% of kcal), adequate fibre (30 g/day) diet and soy products show some promise by reducing some markers related to this condition, but enough evidence is not available to make a recommendation without further evidence (Horner & Lampe, 2000).

Fertility Problems. The average Canadian woman has sufficient levels of body fat for reproduction. For women with fertility problems, nutritional assessment also includes caffeine intake and client weight. Dietary changes that may help enhance fertility include reducing high intake of caffeine (Homan et al., 2007). For obese women, losing weight may result in the achievement of successful pregnancy (Norman et al., 2004).

Menopause and Beyond

Nutritional needs during menopause change because of declining levels of estrogen and other hormones and because of cessation of menstrual periods, which decreases needs for extra iron. Exogenous estrogen may be a concern in the development of adenoma of the endometrium. Postmenopausal osteoporosis may lead to bone fractures. Nurses can encourage regular physical examinations for aging women to help address such concerns.

The 2006 Canadian Consensus Conference (SOGC, 2009) recommended that menopausal women receive 1,500 mg of calcium daily plus 800 IU of vitamin D to counteract osteoporosis. Researchers are examining exercise, calcium, and hormonal therapy for their roles in preventing fractures. Although some women use alfalfa, liquorice, and red clover to relieve symptoms of menopause, these supplements have not been thoroughly studied for efficacy, and health care providers should not promote their use. Black cohosh, which

some women use for menopausal symptoms, may cause undesirable side effects if taken in large doses or for a long time.

Vitamins C and E and soy may be useful to lessen hot flashes and vaginal dryness, although not yet proved. In addition, women older than 50 years must carefully select diets that provide sufficient calcium and vitamin D. Weight-bearing activity such as walking is often recommended.

SUMMARY

● Macronutrients that provide energy are carbohydrates, fats, and proteins. Nutrients that function as coenzymes are usually vitamins. Cofactors are usually microminerals; some macrominerals help form the skeleton. All these nutrients coordinate their functions to help keep the body healthy.

● If followed, the food servings in the *Eating Well with Canada's Food Guide* provide all necessary nutrients without worrying about tracking individual nutrients found in food.

● Culture, religion, and other factors influence food selection. Careful planning and choices designed to take advantage of the plusses of the cultural pattern and counteract the minuses can result in healthy, culturally acceptable meals.

● Nutritional needs of women vary with stages in life.

● Good nutrition in pregnancy is vital to positive maternal and fetal outcomes.

● Breastfeeding benefits both mother and infant.

● Pregnancy increases needs by 300 kcal/day, whereas lactation increases needs by 500 kcal/day. All other increased needs are provided when women select foods wisely. The two to three extra Food Guide Servings should provide all necessary nutrients and calories.

● Adult and older adult women need to control weight by regulating intake of energy nutrients while getting adequate folate, iron, and calcium.

Questions to Ponder

1. A 28-year-old woman who is 165 cm tall and has a prepregnancy weight of 84 kg is seeing the nurse for the first time at approximately 12 weeks' gestation. This is her first pregnancy. As a result of morning sickness, she has lost 2.2 kg and tells the nurse she is thrilled.

 • What recommendations for weight gain are appropriate for this woman based on her baseline weight?

 • What problems are associated with lack of weight gain during pregnancy?

• List some approaches to take during counselling sessions that would help this woman have a healthy pregnancy outcome.

REVIEW QUESTIONS

1. The nurse is teaching a pregnant woman of normal prepregnancy weight-for-height about appropriate weight gain during pregnancy. The nurse determines that instruction has been effective when the client states
   A. "A weight gain of about 7.3 kg per trimester is recommended."
   B. "I shouldn't gain any more than 6.8 to 9 kg for the total pregnancy."
   C. "I should eat whatever I want and not worry about my total weight."
   D. "An average weight gain between 11.5 and 16 kg is considered appropriate."

2. A client reports that she and her husband are considering starting a family within the next year. The nurse should advise the client to increase intake of folic acid
   A. immediately.
   B. if she misses her period.
   C. if pregnancy is confirmed.
   D. one week before her period.

3. The nurse is conducting a quantitative assessment of a client's food intake. Which of the following techniques would *not* be appropriate in such an evaluation?
   A. Interview of the client for recall of food intake
   B. Evaluation of foods using the *Eating Well with Canada's Food Guide*
   C. Analysis of foods eaten to determine quantities of nutrients
   D. Comparison of quantities of nutrients to DRIs

4. A nurse is working with a breastfeeding woman who has low milk production. Which of the following interventions should the nurse recommend?
   A. Increase the frequency of nursing
   B. Give the infant supplemental feedings
   C. Replace breastfeeding with formula-feeding
   D. Increase fluid intake with more caffeinated beverages

5. Your client is a postmenopausal woman recently diagnosed with diabetes mellitus who is being controlled with oral medication, diet, and exercise. Her diet should include foods that have a low glycemic index. Which of the following foods would be most appropriate for her to consume?
   A. Potatoes
   B. Seven-grain bread
   C. Lentils
   D. Watermelon

6. Assessment findings reveal an elevated total cholesterol level in a menopausal client. When assisting the client to take appropriate management measures, the nurse is correct in advising the client to consume which of the following percentages of calories from fat?
   A. 15%
   B. 20%
   C. 30%
   D. 45%

7. Following surgery, the nurse notes that an expected outcome is that the client will increase protein intake. Which of the following dietary choices would the nurse encourage?
   A. Frozen yogurt
   B. Dry cereal
   C. Apples
   D. Nachos

8. The nurse is conducting a teaching session with a group of women about iron needs. Which of the following clients would the nurse expect to have the lowest iron needs?
   A. A 15-year-old gymnast
   B. A 24-year-old pregnant woman
   C. A 38-year-old smoker
   D. A 60-year-old with arthritis

9. A client reports that she has been following a vegan diet over the past few years. When working with the client to review dietary intake and needs, which of the following sets of nutrients would the nurse expect to be potentially deficient?
   A. B_{12}, iron, zinc
   B. Vitamins A, B, and C
   C. Vitamins D, E, and K
   D. Vitamin B_6, folate, and calcium

10. Your client has difficulty drinking enough milk to provide the required intake of calcium and vitamin D to meet her nutritional needs during pregnancy. What is the adequate intake of calcium during pregnancy?
    A. 1,000 mg/day
    B. 750 mg/day
    C. 2,000 mg/day
    D. 500 mg/day

11. A client reports that she is considering smoking as a weight control strategy. Which vitamin may be lacking in people who smoke?
    A. Vitamin B
    B. Vitamin D
    C. Vitamin K
    D. Vitamin C

REFERENCES

Alberta Agriculture and Rural Development. (2011). *Canadian consumer trends in obesity and food consumption.* Retrieved from http://www1.agric.gov.ab.ca/$department/deptdocs.nsf/all/sis8438

Alonso, A., Beunza, J. J., Delgado-Rodriguez, M., Martinez, J. A., & Martinez-Gonzalez, M. A. (2005). Low-fat dairy consumption and reduced risk of hypertension: The Seguimiento Universidad de Navarra (SUN) cohort. *American Journal of Clinical Nutrition, 82*(5), 972–979.

American Dietetic Association. (2001). Position of the American Dietetic Association: Breaking the barriers to breastfeeding. *Journal of the American Dietetic Association, 101*, 1213–1220.

American Pregnancy Association. (2013). *Herbs and pregnancy* Retrieved from http://americanpregnancy.org/pregnancyhealth/naturalherbsvitamins.html

Aschenbrenner, D., & Venable, S. (2009). *Drug therapy in nursing* (3rd ed.). Philadelphia, PA: Lippincott Williams & Wilkins.

Barnard, N. D., Scialli, A., Hurlock, D., & Bertron, P. (2000). Diet and sex-hormone binding globulin, dysmenorrhea, and premenstrual symptoms. *Obstetrics and Gynecology, 95*, 245–250.

Bartley, K. A., Underwood, B. A., & Deckelbaum, R. J. (2005). A life cycle micronutrient perspective for women's health. *American Journal of Clinical Nutrition, 81*(5), 1188S–1193S.

Bendich, A. (2000). The potential for dietary supplements to reduce premenstrual syndrome (PMS) symptoms. *Journal of the American College of Nutrition, 19*, 3.

Berkey, C. S., Gardner, J. D., Lindsay Frazier, A., & Colditz, G. A. (2000). Relation of childhood diet and body size to menarche and adolescent growth in girls. *American Journal of Epidemiology, 152*, 446–452.

Bickley, L. (2012). *Bates' guide to physical examination and history taking* (11th ed.). Philadelphia, PA: Lippincott Williams & Wilkins.

Bienz, D., Cori, H., & Hornig, D. (2003). Adequate dosing of micronutrients for different age groups in the life cycle. *Food and Nutrition Bulletin, 24*(3 Suppl.), S7–S15.

Body and Health Canada. (n.d.). *Iron deficiency anemia.* Retrieved from http://bodyandhealth.canada.com/condition_info_details.asp?disease_id=274

Canadian Food Inspection Agency. (2013). *Guide to food labelling and advertising.* Retrieved from http://www.inspection.gc.ca/food/labelling/guide-to-food-labelling-and-advertising/eng/1300118951990/1300118996556

Canadian Paediatric Society. [Principal authors C. Pound, S. Unger] (2012). The baby-friendly initiative: Protecting, promoting and supporting breastfeeding. *Paediatrics and Child Health, 117*(6), 317–321. Retrieved from http://www.cps.ca/documents/position/baby-friendly-initiative-breastfeeding

Canadian Society for Exercise Physiology. (2013). *Canadian physical activity guidelines and Canadian sedentary behaviour guidelines.* Retrieved from http://www.csep.ca/english/view.asp?x=804

Casanueva, E., Ripoll, C., Tolentino, M., Morales, R., Pfeffer, F., Vilchis, P. et al. (2005). Vitamin C supplementation to prevent premature rupture of the chorioamniotic membranes: A randomized trial. *American Journal of Clinical Nutrition, 81*(4), 859–863.

Cooper, M., Cockell, K., & L'Abbé, M. (2006). Iron status of Canadian adolescents and adults: Current knowledge and practical implications. *Canadian Journal of Dietetic Practice and Research, 67*(3), 130–138.

Craven, R. C., & Hirnle, C. J. (2009). *Fundamentals of nursing: Human health and function* (6th ed.). Philadelphia, PA: Lippincott Williams & Wilkins.

Dietitians of Canada. (2010a). Promoting optimal monitoring of child growth in Canada: Using the new WHO growth charts. *Collaborative Public Policy Statement, Dietitians of Canada and Canadian Paediatric Society.* Retrieved from https://www.dietitians.ca/Downloadable-Content/Public/tcg-position-paper.aspx

Dietitians of Canada. (2010b). *Eating guidelines for vegans.* Retrieved from http://www.dietitians.ca/Nutrition-Resources-A-Z/Factsheets/Vegetarian/Eating-Guidelines-for-Vegans.aspx

Fairfield, K. M., & Fletcher, R. H. (2002). Vitamins for chronic disease prevention in adults: Scientific review. *Journal of the American Medical Association, 287*(23), 3116–3126.

Flohr, C., Nagel, G., Weinmayr, G., Kleiner, A., Strachan, D., & Williams, H. (2011). Lack of evidence for a protective effect of prolonged breastfeeding on childhood eczema: Lessons from the international study of asthma and allergies in childhood (ISAAC) phase 2. *British Journal of Dermatology, 165*(6). DOI: 10.1111/j.1365-2133.2011.10588.x. Retrieved from http://onlinelibrary.wiley.com/doi/10.1111/j.1365-2133.2011.10588.x/full

Ford, F. (2004). A guide to nutrition in pregnancy. *Practicing Midwife, 7*(11), 24, 26.

Fowles, E. (2002). Comparing pregnant women's nutritional knowledge to their actual diet intake. *The American Journal of Maternal Child Nursing, 27*(3), 171–177.

Freedman, D. M., Ron, E., Ballard-Barbash, R., Doody, M. M., & Linet, M. S. (2006). Body mass index and all-cause mortality in a nationwide US cohort. *International Journal of Obesity, 30*, 822–829.

Freedman, D. S., Khan, L. K., Serdula, M. K., Dietz, W. H., Srinivasan, S., & Berenson, G. (2003). The relation of menarcheal age to obesity in childhood and adulthood: The Bogalusa heart study. *BMC Pediatrics, 3*(1), 3.

Groth, S. (2007). Are the Institute of Medicine recommendations for gestational weight gain appropriate for adolescents? *Journal of Obstetric, Gynecologic, and Neonatal Nursing, 36*(1), 22–27.

Harvard School of Public Health. (2013a). *Carbohydrates.* Retrieved from http://www.hsph.harvard.edu/nutritionsource/carbohydrates.html

Harvard School of Public Health. (2013b). *Fiber.* Retrieved from http://www.hsph.harvard.edu/nutritionsource/carbohydrates/fiber/

Harvard School of Public Health. (2013c). *Fats and cholesterol.* Retrieved from http://www.hsph.harvard.edu/nutritionsource/fats-and-cholesterol/

Health Canada. (2005). *Dietary reference intakes. Reference values for elements.* Retrieved from http://www.hc-sc.gc.ca/fn-an/nutrition/reference/table/ref_elements_tbl-eng.php

Health Canada. (2006a). *Arsenic.* Retrieved from http://www.hc-sc.gc.ca/ewh-semt/pubs/water-eau/arsenic/index-eng.php

Health Canada. (2006b). *Dietary reference intakes. Reference values for macronutrients.* Retrieved from http://www.hc-sc.gc.ca/fn-an/nutrition/reference/table/ref_macronutr_tbl-eng.php

Health Canada. (2008a). *Health Canada advises consumers not to use life choice Ephedrine HCL and life choice Kava Kava.* Retrieved from http://www.healthycanadians.gc.ca/recall-alert-rappel-avis/hc-sc/2008/13247a-eng.php

Health Canada. (2008b). *My food guide.* Retrieved from http://www.hc-sc.gc.ca/fn-an/food-guide-aliment/myguide-monguide/index-eng.php

Health Canada. (2009a). *Prenatal nutrition guidelines for health professionals. Background on Canada's food guide.* Cat. No: H164-109/3-2009E-PDF. ISBN: 978-1-1-12209-0. Retrieved from http://www.hc-sc.gc.ca/fn-an/alt_formats/hpfb-dgpsa/pdf/pubs/guide-prenatal-eng.pdf

Health Canada. (2009b). *Prenatal nutrition guidelines for health professionals. Folate.* Cat. No: H164-109/2-2009E-PDF. ISBN: 978-1-100-12208-3. Retrieved from http://www.hc-sc.gc.ca/fn-an/alt_formats/hpfb-dgpsa/pdf/pubs/folate-eng.pdf

Health Canada. (2009c). *Prenatal nutrition guidelines for health professionals. Iron.* Cat. No: H164-109/1-2009E-PDF. ISBN: 978-1-100-12207-6. Retrieved from http://www.hc-sc.gc.ca/fn-an/alt_formats/hpfb-dgpsa/pdf/pubs/iron-fer-eng.pdf

Health Canada. (2010a). *Canadian gestational weight gain recommendations.* Retrieved from http://www.hc-sc.gc.ca/fn-an/nutrition/prenatal/qa-gest-gros-qr-eng.php

Health Canada. (2010b). *Dietary reference intakes. Reference values for vitamins.* Retrieved from http://www.hc-sc.gc.ca/fn-an/nutrition/reference/table/ref_vitam_tbl-eng.php

Health Canada. (2010c). *Eating well with Canada's food guide-first nations, inuit and métis.* Retrieved from http://www.hc-sc.gc.ca/fn-an/pubs/fnim-pnim/index-eng.php

Health Canada. (2011). *Eating well with Canada's Food Guide.* Retrieved from http://www.hc-sc.gc.ca/fn-an/food-guide-aliment/index-eng.php

Health Canada. (2012a). *Food and nutrition. Sodium in Canada.* Retrieved from http://www.hc-sc.gc.ca/fn-an/nutrition/sodium/index-eng.php

Health Canada. (2012b). *Food and nutrition. Vitamin D and Calcium: Updated dietary reference intakes.* Retrieved from http://www.hc-sc.gc.ca/fn-an/nutrition/vitamin/vita-d-eng.php#a7

Health Canada. (2013a). *Carbohydrates.* Retrieved from http://www.healthycanadians.gc.ca/eating-nutrition/label-etiquetage/table_carbohydrates-glucides-eng.php

Health Canada. (2013b). *Dietary reference intakes.* Retrieved from http://www.hc-sc.gc.ca/fn-an/nutrition/reference/index-eng.php

Health Canada. (2013c). *Diseases and conditions.* Retrieved from http://www.healthycanadians.gc.ca/health-sante/disease-maladie/index-eng.php

Health Canada. (2013d). *Infant feeding.* Retrieved from http://www.hc-sc.gc.ca/fn-an/nutrition/infant-nourisson/index-eng.php

Health Canada. (2013e). *Reference values for macronutrients.* Retrieved from http://www.hc-sc.gc.ca/fn-an/nutrition/reference/table/ref_macronutr_tbl-eng.php

Healthy Women. (2011). *Nutrition.* Retrieved from http://www.healthywomen.org/condition/nutrition

Herbold, N. H., & Frates, S. E. (2000). Update of nutrition guidelines for the teen: Trends and concerns. *Current Opinion in Pediatrics, 12,* 303.

Homan, G., Davies, M., & Norman, R. (2007). The impact of lifestyle factors on reproductive performance in the general population and those undergoing infertility treatment: A review. *Human Reproduction Update, 13*(3), 209–223. Retrieved from http://humupd.oxfordjournals.org/content/13/3/209.abstract

Horner, N. K., & Lampe, J. W. (2000). Potential mechanisms of diet therapy for fibrocystic breast conditions show inadequate evidence of effectiveness. *Journal of the American Dietetic Association, 100,* 1368–1380.

Houghton, P. J. (1999). The scientific basis for the reputed activity of Valerian. *Journal of Pharmacology, 51*(5), 505–512.

Institute of Medicine. (2000a). *Dietary reference intakes for thiamin, riboflavin, niacin, vitamin B6, folate, vitamin B12, pantothenic acid, biotin, and choline.* Retrieved from http://www.iom.edu/Reports/2000/Dietary-Reference-Intakes-for-Thiamin-Riboflavin-Niacin-Vitamin-B6-Folate-Vitamin-B12-Pantothenic-Acid-Biotin-and-Choline.aspx

Institute of Medicine. (2000b). *Dietary reference intakes for vitamin C, vitamin E, selenium, and carotenoids.* Retrieved from http://www.iom.edu/Reports/2000/Dietary-Reference-Intakes-for-Vitamin-C-Vitamin-E-Selenium-and-Carotenoids.aspx

Institute of Medicine. (2001). *Dietary reference intakes for vitamin A, vitamin K, arsenic, boron, chromium, copper, iodine, iron, manganese, molybdenum, nickel, silicon, vanadium, and zinc.* Retrieved from http://www.iom.edu/reports/2001/dietary-reference-intakes-for-vitamin-a-vitamin-k-arsenic-boron-chromium-copper-iodine-iron-manganese-molybdenum-nickel-silicon-vanadium-and-zinc.aspx

Institute of Medicine. (2002). *Dietary reference intakes for energy, carbohydrate, fiber, fat, fatty acids, cholesterol, protein, and amino acids.* Retrieved from http://www.iom.edu/Activities/Nutrition/SummaryDRIs/~/media/Files/Activity%20Files/Nutrition/DRIs/5_Summary%20Table%20Tables%201-4.pdf

Institute of Medicine. (2013). *Sodium intake in populations: Assessment of evidence. Consensus Report.* Retrieved from http://www.iom.edu/reports/2013/sodium-intake-in-populations-assessment-of-evidence.aspx

Ito, S., & Lee, A. (2003). Drug excretion into breast milk—overview. *Advanced Drug Delivery Reviews, 55*(5), 617–627. Retrieved from http://www.ncbi.nlm.nih.gov/pubmed/12706545

Jaddoe, V., Bakker, R., Hoffman, A., Mackenbach, J., Moll, H., Steegers, E. et al. (2007). Moderate alcohol consumption during pregnancy and the risk of low birth weight and preterm birth: The generation R study. *Annals of Epidemiology, 17*(10), 834–840.

Khine, K., Rosenstein, D., Elin, R., Niemela, J., Schmidt, P., & Rubinow, D. (2006). Magnesium (Mg) retention and mood effects after intravenous Mg infusion in premenstrual dysphoric disorder. *Biological Psychiatry, 59*(4), 327–333.

Kramer, M., & Kakuma, R. (2012). Optimal duration of exclusive breastfeeding. *The Cochrane Library.* DOI:10.1002/14651858.CD003517.pub2. Retrieved from http://onlinelibrary.wiley.com/doi/10.1002/14651858.CD003517.pub2/abstract

Kreiter, S., Schwartz, R., Kirkman, H., Charlton, P., Calikoglu, A., & Davenport, M. (2000). Nutritional rickets in African American breast-fed infants. *Journal of Pediatrics, 137,* 153–157.

Li, T. Y., Rana, J. S., Manson, J. E., Willett, W. C., Stampfer, M. J., Colditz, G. A. et al. (2006). Obesity as compared with physical activity in predicting risk of coronary heart disease in women. *Circulation, 113*(4), 499–506.

Liu, S., & Willett, W. C. (2002). Dietary glycemic load and atherothrombotic risk. *Current Atherosclerosis Reports, 4,* 454–461.

Lopez, L., Langini, S., & Pita de Portela, M. (2007). Maternal iron status and neonatal outcomes in women with pica during pregnancy. *International Journal of Gynecology and Obstetrics, 98*(2), 151–152.

Louwman, M. W., van Dusseldorp, M., van de Vijver, F., Thomas, C., Schneede, J. Ueland, P. et al. (2000). Signs of impaired cognitive function in adolescents with marginal cobalamin status. *American Journal of Clinical Nutrition, 72,* 762–769.

Mangels, R. (2013). Iron in the vegan diet. In *Simply vegan* (5th ed.). Vegetarian Resource Group. ISBN 13:978-0-931411-34-2. Retrieved from http://www.vrg.org/nutrition/iron.php

Mayo Clinic. (2012a). *Drugs and supplements. Vitamin E.* Retrieved from http://www.mayoclinic.com/health/vitamin-e/NS_patient-vitamine

Mayo Clinic. (2012b). *Drugs and supplements. Vitamin K.* Retrieved from http://www.mayoclinic.com/health/drug-information/DR602165

McCrory, M. A. (2001). Does dieting during lactation put infant growth at risk? *Nutrition Reviews, 59,* 18–21.

McKeown, N. M., Meigs, J. B., Liu, S., Wilson, P. W., & Jacques, P. F. (2002). Whole-grain intake is favorably associated with metabolic risk factors for type 2 diabetes and cardiovascular disease in the Framingham Offspring Study. *American Journal of Clinical Nutrition, 76,* 390–398.

Medline Plus. (2013). *Kava.* Retrieved from http://www.nlm.nih.gov/medlineplus/druginfo/natural/872.html

Messina, V. (2013). *Vegetarian diets: A dietitian's guide.* Retrieved from http://www.vegnutrition.com/index.html

Messina, V., Melina, V., & Reed Mangels, A. (2003). A new food guide for North American vegetarians. *Journal of the American Dietetic Association, 103*(6), 771–775. Retrieved from http://www.metabolicdiet.com/pdfs/veg_food_guide.pdf

Messina, V., & Reed Mangels, A. (2001). Considerations in planning vegan diets: Children. *Journal of the American Dietetic Association, 101,* 661–669.

Norman, R., Noakes, M., Wu, R., Davies, M., Moran, L., & Wang, J. (2004). Improving reproductive performance in overweight/obese women with effective weight management. *Human Reproduction Update, 10*(3), 267–280.

Oddy, W., & Peat, J. (2003). Breastfeeding, asthma, and atopic disease: An epidemiological review of the literature. *Journal of Human Lactation, 19,* 250–261.

Pereira, M., O'Reilly, E., Augustsson, K., Fraser, G., Goldbourt, U., Heitmann, B. et al. (2004). Dietary fiber and risk of coronary heart disease: A pooled analysis of cohort studies. *Archives of Internal Medicine, 164,* 370–376.

Pereira, M. A., & Liu, S. (2003). Types of carbohydrates and risk of cardiovascular disease. *Journal of Women's Health, 12,* 115–122.

Public Health Agency of Canada. (2004). *Evaluation of food fortification with folic acid for the primary prevention of neural tube defects.* Retrieved from http://www.phac-aspc.gc.ca/publicat/faaf/chap3-eng.php

Public Health Agency of Canada. (2011a). *Canada prenatal nutrition program.* Retrieved from http://www.phac-aspc.gc.ca/hp-ps/dca-dea/prog-ini/cpnp-pcnp/

Public Health Agency of Canada. (2011b). *Physical activity guidelines.* Retrieved from http://www.phac-aspc.gc.ca/hp-ps/hl-mvs/pa-ap/03paap-eng.php

Quaranta, S., Buscaglia, M., Meroni, M., Colombo, E., & Cella, S. (2007). Pilot study of the efficacy and safety of a modified-release magnesium 250 mg tablet (Sincromag) for the treatment of premenstrual syndrome. *Clinical Drug Investigation, 27*(1), 51–58.

Rao, A. V. (2002). Lycopene, tomatoes, and the prevention of coronary heart disease [review]. *Experimental Biology and Medicine, 227*(10), 908–913.

Robinson, H. E., O'Connell, C. M., Joseph, K. S., & McLeod, N. L. (2005). Maternal outcomes in pregnancies complicated by obesity. *Obstetrics & Gynecology, 106*(6), 1357–1364.

Rosenbloom, M. (2013). *Vitamin toxicity. Medscape.* Retrieved from http://emedicine.medscape.com/article/819426-overview

Saraswat, A., Jayasinghe, R., & Sweeney, A. (2012). Carbohydrate or fat-restricted diets for obesity. *Cochrane Database of Systematic Reviews.* 20120, (8). Art. No.: CD010025. DOI: 10.1002/14651858.CD010025. Retrieved from http://summaries.cochrane.org/CD010025/carbohydrate-or-fat-restricted-diets-for-obesity

Scholl, T. O. (2005). Iron status during pregnancy: Setting the stage for mother and infant. *American Journal of Clinical Nutrition, 81*(5), 1218S–1222S.

Scholl, T. O., & Reilly, T. (2000). Anemia, iron and pregnancy outcome. *Journal of Nutrition, 130,* 443S–447S.

Schulze, M. B., Liu, S., Rimm, E. B., Manson, J. E., Willett, W. C., & Hu, F. B. (2004). Glycemic index, glycemic load, and dietary fiber intake and incidence of type 2 diabetes in younger and middle-aged women. *American Journal of Clinical Nutrition, 80,* 348–356.

Sears, M. R., Greene, J. M., Willan, A. R., Taylor, D. R., Flannery, E. M., Cowan, J. L. et al. (2002). Long-term relation between breast-feeding and development of atopy and asthma in children and young adults: A longitudinal study. *Lancet, 360,* 901–907.

Slavin, J. (2003). Why whole grains are protective: Biological mechanisms. *Proceedings of the Nutrition Society, 62*(1), 129–134.

Society of Obstetricians and Gynaecologists of Canada. (2007). *Preconceptual vitamin/folic acid supplementation 2007: The use of folic acid in combination with a vitamin supplement for the prevention of neural tube defects and other congenital anomalies. Clinical practice guideline no.201.* Retrieved from http://sogc.org/wp-content/uploads/2013/01/guiJOGC201JCPG0712.pdf

Society of Obstetricians and Gynaecologists of Canada. (2009). *Menopause and osteoporosis update 2009. Clinical practice guideline #222.* Retrieved from http://sogc.org/guidelines/menopause-and-osteoporosis-update-2009-replaces-171-feb-2006-172-feb-2006/

Stang, J., Story, M., Harnack, L., & Neumark-Sztainer, D. (2000). Relationships between vitamin and mineral supplement use, dietary intake, and dietary adequacy among adolescents. *Journal of the American Dietetic Association, 100,* 905–1010.

Statistics Canada. (2006). *Canadian community health survey: Overview of Canadians' eating habits.* Catalogue no. 82-620-MWE2006002. Retrieved from http://www5.statcan.gc.ca/bsolc/olc-cel/olc-cel?catno=82-620-M2006002&lang=eng

Surkan, P. J., Hsieh, C. C., Johansson, A. L., Dickman, P. W., & Cnattingius, S. (2004). Reasons for increasing trends in large for gestational age births. *Obstetrics and Gynecology, 104*(4), 720–726.

Thomas, D., Elliott, E., & Baur, L. (2007). Low glycaemic index or low glycaemic load diets for overweight and obesity. *Cochrane Database of Systematic Reviews,* (3). Art. No.: CD005105. DOI: 10.1002/14651858.CD005105.pub2. Retrieved from http://summaries.cochrane.org/CD005105/low-glycaemic-index-or-low-glycaemic-load-diets-for-overweight-and-obesity

Tsai, S. P., Donnelly, R. P., & Wendt, J. K. (2006). Obesity and mortality in a prospective study of a middle-aged industrial population. *Journal of Occupational and Environmental Medicine, 48*(1), 22–27.

Turrell, G., Hewitt, B., Patterson, C., & Oldenburg, B. (2003). Measuring socio-economic position in dietary research: Is choice of socioeconomic indicator important? *Public Health Nutrition, 6,* 191–200.

Weili, Y., He, B., Yao, H., Dai, J., Cui, J., & Ge, D. (2007). Waist-to-height ratio is an accurate and easier index for evaluating obesity in children and adolescents. *Obesity, 15*(3), 748–752.

Whitney, E. N., Cataldo, C. B., & Rolfes, S. R. (2002). *Understanding normal and clinical nutrition* (6th ed.). Belmont, CA: Wadsworth/Thomson Learning.

Willett, W., Manson, J., & Liu, S. (2002). Glycemic index, glycemic load, and risk of type 2 diabetes. *American Journal of Clinical Nutrition, 76,* 274S–280S.

Yon, B., & Johnson, R. (2005). US and Canadian Dietary References Intakes (RNIs) for the macronutrients, energy and physical activity. *British Nutrition Foundation Bulletin, 30,* 176–181.

CHAPTER 4

Medical Alterations in Women During Adolescence and Adulthood

Robin J. Evans and Louise Aurilio*

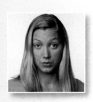 Lela, 33 years old, comes to the clinic for evaluation of vaginal discharge. She states, "It started about 2 days ago, and it seems to be getting worse. My vagina also feels sore and itchy. I've been wearing a thin sanitary pad so that the drainage doesn't get on my clothes."

 Jade, a 21-year-old woman, arrives at the clinic for a prenatal visit. Her health history reveals that she experienced menarche at 11 years old and a previous full-term pregnancy at 19 years old. Jade denies any use of drugs, alcohol, or cigarettes. Her body mass index is 23. When questioned about her family history, Jade states, "My grandmother on my mother's side just died of breast cancer. Could I be at risk now, too?"

You will learn more about Lela's and Jade's stories later. Nurses working with these clients and others like them need to understand the material in this chapter to manage care and address issues appropriately. Before beginning, consider the following points related to the above scenarios:

- Does anything about either case present any issues of immediate concern or worry? Explain your answer.

---

*Contributor to first U.S. edition.

● How might each client's circumstances influence the nurse's approach to care?

● How are the clients similar? How are they different?

● What details will the nurse need to investigate with Lela? What about Jade?

● What areas of concern would the nurse need to address with each client?

LEARNING OBJECTIVES

On completion of this chapter, the reader should be able to:
● Identify risk factors for the various alterations addressed in this chapter.
● Discuss strategies that promote and enhance the health and well-being of women experiencing health alterations.
● Review common genetic disorders with special implications for women.
● Identify common autoimmune disorders in women and their implications for childbearing.
● Describe the different types of diabetes mellitus, as well as effective prevention and management strategies.
● Describe cardiovascular and pulmonary problems addressed in this chapter and the implications of these disorders for women.
● Compare and contrast common sexually transmitted infections (STIs), including their risk factors and prevention strategies.
● Identify the different types of hepatitis and the problems posed by each.
● Summarize common benign and malignant breast disorders.
● Outline specific risk factors, treatment strategies, and collaborative care for the client with breast cancer.
● Explain disorders, infections, and cancers of the female reproductive tract.
● Discuss risks for pelvic relaxation alterations and urinary tract disorders as addressed in this chapter.

KEY TERMS

abnormal uterine bleeding	inflammatory breast cancer
amenorrhea	leiomyoma (fibroid tumour)
bacterial vaginosis	leukorrhea
BRCA1	lumpectomy
BRCA2	lymphedema
candidiasis	mastalgia
carcinoma in situ	mastectomy
cervical dysplasia	mastitis
condylomata	multiple sclerosis (MS)
cystic fibrosis (CF)	pelvic inflammatory disease
cystitis	premenstrual syndrome
diabetes mellitus	rheumatoid arthritis
dysmenorrhea	sexually transmitted infections
endometriosis	sickle cell crisis
fibroadenoma	sickle cell disease
genital herpes	systemic lupus erythematosus
hepatitis	trichomoniasis

During the past several decades, women's health has grown as a distinct specialty in the field of health care. Additionally, women themselves are becoming more active participants in their own health, demanding more information about prevention and treatment to assist them with important health-related decisions, as well as with issues of well-being and quality of life. This chapter reflects a comprehensive view of women's health beyond the traditional focus on reproduction. In this chapter, we examine STIs, problems with the reproductive organs, disorders of the breasts, as well as several alterations in other body systems that affect women in great numbers or that have different implications or manifestations in women than in men. The chapter incorporates information on illness, factors that affect health status, and trends in research, prevention, diagnosis, and collaborative care. Discussions of medical conditions that emerge during pregnancy or with dangerous implications in pregnancy are found in Chapter 13.

GENETIC DISORDERS

The field of genetics has burgeoned in recent years, largely as a result of the human genome project (see Chapter 11). Genetic disorders often influence women's reproductive capabilities and caregiver roles. Nurses must work to understand how to prevent, reduce, and overcome the adverse effects of genetic disorders in women. Additionally, women themselves need knowledge about inherent genetic risks for illness and to understand how such risks can affect their quality of life.

CYSTIC FIBROSIS

Cystic fibrosis (CF), a chronic and progressive autosomal recessive genetic disease, affects people of both sexes and of all races and ethnicities, with the highest prevalence in Caucasians of Northern European descent (American Lung Association, 2010). One in every 3,600 children born in Canada has CF (Cystic Fibrosis Canada [CFC], n.d.). Approximately 1 in 25 Canadians is a carrier of the gene for CF (CFC, n.d.). To inherit CF, a person must inherit two CF genes—one from each parent. Each time two carriers of CF conceive, there exists a 25% chance that the child will have CF, a 50% chance that the child will be an asymptomatic carrier, and a 25% chance that the child will not have CF and will not be a carrier. Although CF once was considered fatal in childhood, the median age for survival for Canadians with CF is currently estimated to be 49.7 years, and almost 60% are over the age of 18 years (Canadian Cystic Fibrosis Registry, 2012).

In CF, there is compromise of the epithelial cell function in the respiratory tract, pancreas, sweat glands, intestine, and hepatobiliary system (Chetty et al., 2011). Chronic inflammation leads to damage in the lung parenchyma and airways and excessive viscous mucus is produced (Chetty et al., 2011; CFC, n.d.). Clients with CF have exocrine pancreatic insufficiency due to blocked pancreatic ducts, which interferes with enzymes reaching the intestines to digest food (Chetty et al., 2011). Individuals need to consume large numbers of artificial enzymes with each meal and snack in order to absorb sufficient nutrition. The thick mucus in the respiratory system creates difficulties in clearing mucus and results in cycles of infection and inflammation, damaging delicate lung tissues. Many people develop chronic obstructive diffuse pulmonary disease, decreased lung volume, and shunting that result in arterial hypoxemia, possible respiratory failure, and early death.

Fifty percent of those with CF are diagnosed by the age of 6 months and 73% by the age of 2 years (Canadian Cystic Fibrosis Registry, 2012). Newborn screening is most effective as it allows for early diagnosis, leading to improved height, weight, and lung function and increased longevity (CFC, n.d.). Once symptoms are present, early damage to the lungs and digestive system may be irreversible. CF screening is part of routine newborn screening programs in Alberta, Ontario, British Columbia, Saskatchewan, Manitoba, and Nova Scotia (CFC, n.d.). If a screening test is positive, further investigation is done to rule out or confirm the diagnosis. Further tests include the sweat test, in which sweat is induced and then analyzed for the amount of salt it contains; tests for the presence or absence of intestinal enzymes; and/or more extensive genetic testing (CFC, n.d.).

Major treatment goals include clearance of secretions, control of infection, and provision of adequate nutrition. Delayed puberty and menarche often accompany CF, related to poor nutritional status, delayed growth, and chronic disease (Chetty et al., 2011). Clients with CF should be managed with a multidisciplinary approach. Antibiotics used should be evaluated for potential teratogenic effects. Preliminary studies of mucolytics do not suggest fetal transmission. Pancreatic enzymes have not been shown to be problematic in pregnancy; rather they are very helpful in maintaining nutritional status in the presence of malabsorption due to pancreatic insufficiency (Chetty et al., 2011). The pregnant woman with CF faces significant challenges related to her pulmonary status, which may be exacerbated by the pregnancy. The woman with mild to moderate pulmonary disease is not at an increased risk for morbidity during pregnancy (Chetty et al., 2011). Severe pulmonary disease increases the risk for adverse maternal and fetal outcomes, which may include preterm labour (either spontaneous or induced because of pulmonary compromise) and fetal growth restriction (Chetty et al., 2011). Women with CF should access genetic counselling and a baseline assessment of pulmonary function (Chetty et al., 2011). See Chapter 13 for considerations related to CF and pregnancy.

TAY–SACHS DISEASE

Tay–Sachs disease is an incurable, autosomal recessive metabolic disease that occurs primarily in newborns of Ashkenazi (Eastern European) Jewish descent. Approximately 80% of Jews worldwide are of Ashkenazi descent (Langlois & Wilson, 2006) and approximately 1 in 30 Ashkenazi Jews are carriers (heterozygous) of Tay–Sachs disease (Hospital for Sick Children, 2014; Langlois & Wilson, 2006).

Clients with Tay–Sachs disease exhibit a deficiency of the hexosaminidase A enzyme, normally responsible for decomposing the naturally occurring fatty substance GM2-ganglioside. Toxic buildup of GM2-ganglioside affects the cells of the nervous system. Infants may appear normal until about 3 to 6 months of age; other rare forms of the disease may occur later in life and are milder than the infantile form. Symptoms include a cherry red spot in the macular area of the retina; vision and hearing loss; progressive deterioration of both motor and mental function, beginning with mild motor weakness and occasional twitches and leading to seizures and paralysis (Genetics Home Reference, 2012; HealthLinkBC, n.d.). Infantile Tay–Sachs disease is the most common form, and there is rapid progression of the disease once symptoms appear, with death occurring by 6 years of age (Ferreia et al., 2014).

To determine carrier status, clinicians measure hexosaminidase A activity in plasma or white blood cells (WBCs); they also may use gene mutation analysis. Prenatal diagnosis by chorionic villi sampling or amniocentesis can identify affected infants. Screening for Tay–Sachs, which has been in place since the 1970s, has resulted in nearly complete eradication of the disease from the Ashkenazi Jewish population (Ferreira et al., 2014). Counselling can help couples identify options for having unaffected children. See Chapter 11 for more information on genetic counselling and screening for Tay–Sachs disease and other similar conditions.

THALASSEMIA

Thalassemia (Mediterranean or Cooley anemia) is the name given to a group of autosomal recessive disorders associated with defective synthesis of hemoglobin (March of Dimes, 2008). Clients with thalassemia have problems with the alpha or beta globin proteins in blood. As a result, red blood cells (RBCs) neither form properly nor carry sufficient oxygen, leading to potential hemolysis. The disease is associated with individuals of Chinese, Middle Eastern, Mediterranean, or African descent (Thalassemia Foundation of Canada, 2013).

Heterozygous carriers of *thalassemia minor* (thalassemia trait) usually are asymptomatic or have mild anemia with smaller RBCs. Usually, no systemic problems ensue. Clients with thalassemia minor usually have a normal life span (MedlinePlus, 2012).

Homozygous clients usually experience the more severe *thalassemia major*, a life-threatening disorder with symptoms of anemia and restricted physical and mental growth. Clients with thalassemia major are usually normal at birth but develop severe anemia and growth restriction during the first 1 to 2 years of life. They may display pronounced splenomegaly, hepatomegaly, jaundice, abnormal facial bones, infections, and cardiac problems (March of Dimes, 2008; MedlinePlus, 2012).

Diagnosis is determined through an evaluation of complete blood count (CBC). Thalassemia trait can be diagnosed by looking at the size of the blood cell and the mean corpuscular volume (MCV). Trait carriers have a low MCV reading (March of Dimes, 2008).

Hemoglobin electrophoresis is used to identify thalassemia minor (MedlinePlus, 2012; Thalassemia Foundation of Canada, 2013). Treatment consists of regular transfusions (every 2 to 3 weeks) and iron chelators such as Desferal (deferoxamine) and Exjade (deferasirox), which are available in Canada. Repeated transfusions provide needed RBCs but lead to a buildup of iron, which can cause cardiac or liver damage; chelators bind to iron, which helps the body excrete the excess iron (March of Dimes, 2008; Thalassemia Foundation of Canada, 2013).

Women with milder forms of this disorder usually have healthy pregnancies. Women with thalassemia major appear to be safe as long as the disease is well treated and there are no cardiac issues (March of Dimes, 2008).

SICKLE CELL DISEASE

Sickle cell disease (sickle cell anemia) is an autosomal recessive genetic disorder found primarily in individuals of African descent, but also in people of Mediterranean, Arabic, East Indian, and South and Central American heritage. This serious, chronic hemolytic anemia is incurable and may be fatal by midlife. Sickle cell disease results from a mutation in hemoglobin (Hb), in which sickled hemoglobin (HbS) replaces normal adult hemoglobin (HbA) and has a reduced oxygen-carrying ability. As a result, the RBCs have a decreased life span (Fig. 4.1). The sickling of RBCs leads to obstruction of small blood vessels and causes infarcts of the lungs, kidneys, spleen, and bones.

Assessment Findings

Symptoms of sickle cell disease vary. Typically, clients are healthy most of the time. The anemia causes fatigue, pallor of mucous membranes, and decreased exercise tolerance. The skin may appear grey; jaundice is common.

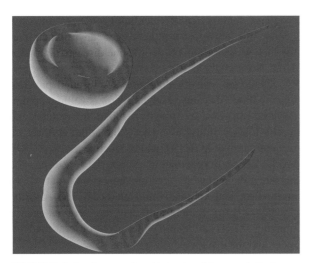

FIGURE 4.1 A normal red blood cell (*upper left*). A sickled red blood cell (*bottom*).

Clients may have frequent infections. The heart may be enlarged, leading to congestive heart failure. People with sickle cell anemia are now living longer, into their 40s, 50s, or longer (National Institutes of Health, 2012).

People with sickle cell disease are *homozygous* for the disease, carrying two genes for the disorder at the given locus on a homologous chromosome. Some people, however, have *sickle cell trait* and are *heterozygous* for the disease, carrying one affected gene and a normal gene. These individuals typically have none of the symptoms of sickle cell disease but can pass the trait on to their children (Centers for Disease Control and Prevention [CDC], 2011).

In clients with sickle cell disease, episodes of **sickle cell crisis** (sudden pain) can occur, affecting the bones, lungs, abdomen, and joints. The most common type of sickle cell crisis results from vaso-occlusion, in which sickled cells block blood flow, leading to pain and organ damage. Acute pain results as tissues become hypoxic, lasting hours to a week or more (National Institutes of Health, 2012). Precipitating factors include dehydration, viral or bacterial infections, activities in high altitudes, and changes in temperature (CDC, 2011).

Pregnant clients with sickle cell disease can experience complications such as increasing severity of the disease, increased frequency of sickle cell crisis, preterm labour, and fetal growth restriction (CDC, 2011). A woman who has early prenatal care and careful monitoring throughout her pregnancy can have a normal pregnancy (CDC, 2011). See Chapter 13 for discussion of sickle cell trait and sickle cell disease in pregnancy.

Collaborative Management

The most common problem in clients with sickle cell trait and sickle cell disease is inadequate oxygen. Thus, regular monitoring of Hb and hematocrit counts is essential. Oxygen should be administered as ordered. Clients may need to maintain bed rest to help control their metabolic requirements.

Acute painful episodes are the most common reason for seeking medical care (CDC, 2011). Thus, pain assessment and evaluation of these clients are extremely important. To promote comfort, clients with sickle cell disease can take over-the-counter medications such as acetylsalicylic acid (ASA) or ibuprofen. Those clients with severe crises may receive opioids such as morphine daily along with other analgesics (CDC, 2011).

Client teaching focuses on measures to prevent sickle cell crisis and to control the condition as much as possible. The nurse should instruct the client to avoid high altitudes and infections, and encourage her to obtain vaccines that prevent influenza and pneumonia. Adequate rest and sleep and stress reduction techniques may be beneficial. The nurse should ensure that the client maintains adequate fluid intake. See Chapter 13 for more discussion of sickle cell disease in pregnant women.

AUTOIMMUNE DISORDERS

Autoimmune disorders develop when the immune system responds inappropriately to and attacks the body's natural tissues. Although multiple theories abound, the etiology of autoimmune disorders remains unknown. Multiple environmental and genetic factors likely contribute, with the incidence of some types increasing with age. These disorders seem to occur in clusters; a client may present with more than one type.

Generally, autoimmune disorders are classified as organ-specific or systemic (Box 4.1). With organ-specific autoimmune disorders, tissue damage is localized; with

● **BOX 4.1 Common Autoimmune Disorders**

Organ-Specific

Central nervous system
    Guillain–Barré syndrome
    Multiple sclerosis
Endocrine
    Hypothyroidism
    Thyroiditis
    Type 1 diabetes
Gastrointestinal
    Ulcerative colitis
Musculoskeletal
    Fibromyalgia
    Myasthenia gravis

Systemic

Rheumatoid arthritis
Systemic lupus erythematosus

systemic autoimmune disorders, tissue damage is widespread. Regardless of classification, these debilitating and chronic disorders increase health care costs and decrease quality of life.

RHEUMATOID ARTHRITIS

Rheumatoid arthritis (RA) affects approximately 300,000 people in Canada, affecting women three times more often than men (The Arthritis Society, 2014b). Although it can occur in people of all ages, onset is most common between 25 and 50 years of age (The Arthritis Society, 2014b).

Assessment Findings

RA generally develops as inflammation, which may become symmetrical in the lining of the joints, causing erosion of bone and cartilage. It may extend to other internal organs such as the eyes, lungs, or heart (Gibofsky, 2012; The Arthritis Society, 2014b) (Fig. 4.2). Signs and symptoms can vary significantly between individuals and may include fatigue, generalized weakness, morning stiffness, joint swelling, pain, and fever (Satack et al., 2013; The Arthritis Society, 2014b). Periods of remission and exacerbation are characteristic. Because RA often affects the wrists, hands, knees, and feet, clients may have significant pain with movement.

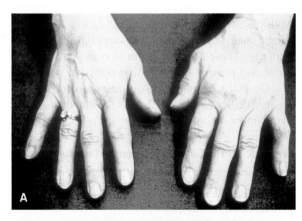

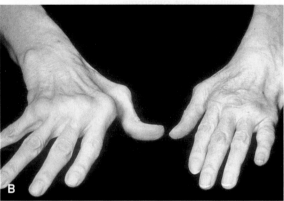

FIGURE 4.2 Joint appearance in rheumatoid arthritis. **A:** Early. **B:** Advanced.

Risk factors for RA include genetics, smoking, gender, age, or exposure to a "trigger" environment factor such as a viral infection or Lyme disease (Gibofsky, 2012; Scott et al., 2010).

Clinicians usually diagnose RA through physical examination of joints, especially for swelling or tenderness and muscle strength evaluation; medical and family history study; blood tests including erythrocyte sedimentation rate (ESR), and C-reactive protein (CRP) levels, elevated rheumatoid factor (RF) reading; the presence of anticyclic citrullinated peptide (anti-CCP) antibodies; and synovial fluid analysis (The Arthritis Society, 2014b). Radiography and magnetic resonance imaging (MRI) can identify the extent of joint involvement and the disease's progression.

Collaborative Management

Collaborative management involves a comprehensive program of drug therapy and education to prevent joint destruction. The earlier the diagnosis is made, the earlier treatment can be started; while disability associated with the disease can be reversed if arthritis is managed early enough, disability associated with joint damage cannot (Palmer & El Miedany, 2012). Nonsteroidal anti-inflammatory drugs (NSAIDs) and corticosteroids may be used to help reduce pain and inflammation. Disease-modifying antirheumatic drugs (DMARDs) such as methotrexate, leflunomide, sulfasalazine, and hydroxychloroquine, and biologic therapy agents such as abatacept and anakinra, and tumour necrosis factor inhibitors such as etanercept and infliximab can prevent joint destruction and improve comfort and functioning (Palmer & El Miedany, 2012; Scott et al., 2010). Education should focus on compliance with drug therapy, including proper administration, correct dosing, reporting of side effects, and frequent medical and laboratory follow-up. Physical therapy and acupuncture may also assist with maintenance of joint motion and muscle strength. Splinting and assistive devices are recommended to ensure joint protection. Because food allergies have been associated with RA, testing for food allergy, elimination of nonallergy food intolerances, and proper nutrition are recommended to help alleviate symptoms (Scott et al., 2010). Proper balance between rest, activity, and therapies can improve quality of life.

Nursing interventions include client education, pain management, increased range-of-motion exercises, promotion of daily activities, careful monitoring of mental functions and sleep, and assessment of psychological wellness.

MYASTHENIA GRAVIS

Myasthenia gravis is a chronic disorder characterized by fluctuating weakness of the voluntary musculoskeletal groups. It affects women more than men, usually

● TABLE 4.1 Diagnostic Tests for Myasthenia Gravis[a]

Test	Positive Finding
Blood test	Look for presence of acetylcholine receptor (AchR) or muscle-specific tyrosine kinase (MuSK) antibodies.
Repetitive nerve stimulation	Amplitude of fourth compound muscle action potential is decreased by >10% (muscle action potential is decreased)
Electromyogram	Decrementing response to repeated stimulation of hand muscles, which indicates muscle fatigue.
Edrophonium chloride (Tensilon) test. Most effective in clients with significant ptosis or restricted extra ocular movements	Unequivocal improvement of strength 1 min after IV injection

[a]Many people have negative or equivocal results. Clinical findings take precedence over negative results on confirmatory tests.

Adapted from Juel, V. C. & Massey, J. M. (2007). Myasthenia Gravis. *Orphanet Journal of Rare Diseases*, 2(44). Retrieved from http://www.ojrd.com/content/2/1/44

peaking between 20 and 30 years of age. Myasthenia gravis occurs in all races. It may be found in more than one member of a family, but it is neither inherited nor contagious. The cause is currently unknown, although it is thought that it might rest in an autoimmune process that produces antibodies directed against acetylcholine receptor sites and reduces receptors cells at the neuromuscular junction. The result is lost muscle strength (increased muscle weakness) that is usually specific to certain muscle groups as opposed to general weakness (Juel & Massey, 2007). This weakness worsens with exercise and at the end of the day. It improves with rest (Sathasivam, 2014).

Assessment Findings

The muscles most frequently affected are those that control eye and eyelid movements, chewing, swallowing, coughing, and facial expressions. The illness can change speech patterns; the voice may become faint during long conversations. It also affects upper torso muscles more than trunk and limb muscles. Weakness in the muscles that control breathing can cause dyspnea. No other indications of neurologic deficits appear. Reflexes and sensory perception remain normal, and muscle atrophy is rare. Rest usually can restore muscle strength. Weakness that is exclusive to the eyelids and extraocular muscles is classified as ocular myasthenia gravis, while generalized myasthenia gravis involves weakness extending beyond (Juel & Massey, 2007; Sathasivam, 2014).

The disease affects people differently. Certain conditions, such as emotional stress, pregnancy, menses, secondary illness, trauma, temperature extremes, injection with neuromuscular blocking drugs, surgery, and trauma, may cause exacerbations. Clients may encounter complications, such as respiratory infection, aspiration, and respiratory insufficiency, possibly necessitating hospitalization. They also may experience periods of remission.

An electromyogram, repetitive nerve stimulation, edrophonium chloride (Tensilon), and blood tests to detect abnormal antibodies can confirm myasthenia gravis (Table 4.1). Many people tested, however, have negative or equivocal results. Therefore, clinical findings always take precedence over negative conformity tests. During a test with edrophonium chloride, atropine should always be available to counteract any effects detrimental to the client.

Collaborative Management

No known cure exists for myasthenia gravis. Treatments such as medications, thymectomy, and plasmapheresis allow clients with myasthenia gravis to lead normal lives. Current treatments differ according to severity of weakness, age, sex, and degree of impairment. Ultimate goals include a return of normal muscle endurance and strength, avoidance of complications, and maintenance of quality of life, commensurate with the disease's cause.

When clients with myasthenia gravis are admitted to the hospital, management involves monitoring for respiratory infection, providing adequate ventilation and drug therapy, and observing for side effects caused by medications. An important issue is distinguishing cholinergic crisis from myasthenia crisis. Cholinergic crisis occurs when a client overdoses on anticholinesterase drugs, which will result in an increase in acetylcholine receptor sites. Clients in cholinergic crisis develop symptoms of increased weakness of the skeletal muscles, especially 1 hour after ingesting anticholinesterase: dyspnea; salivation, diarrhea, nausea and vomiting, abdominal cramps, increased bronchial secretions, sweating, and lacrimation. Myasthenia crisis occurs when the dose of medication is too low or the client forgets to take medication as prescribed. Symptoms of myasthenia crisis include muscle weakness in areas that affect swallowing and breathing, aspiration, respiratory insufficiency, and respiratory infection. Intravenous (IV) injection of edrophonium chloride (Tensilon), an acetylcholinesterase inhibitor, temporarily improves muscle contractility in women who are in myasthenia crisis.

The nurse makes accurate, detailed assessments about the client's fatigue, body area affected, and severity of affliction. Physical examination should include respiratory rate, oxygen saturation levels, arterial blood gas analysis, and pulmonary function studies. The nurse also evaluates the client's lifestyle and coping skills, swallowing, speaking volume and clarity, and coughing and gagging reflexes. Client and family education focuses on the importance of following the treatment plan, recognizing potential adverse reactions to medications, planning daily activities to avoid fatigue, investigating community resources and support groups, avoiding infections, and gaining awareness of complications of the disease and therapy. Dietary education includes information about foods that the client can chew and swallow easily. The client should schedule doses of medication so that peak action occurs during meals.

SYSTEMIC LUPUS ERYTHEMATOSUS

Systemic lupus erythematosus (SLE), a chronic inflammatory disorder of the connective tissue, affects the skin, joints, serous membranes, blood, kidneys, and central nervous system (CNS). Its effects range from mild to severe, with exacerbations and remissions. SLE affects approximately 17,000 Canadians (Lupus Canada, 2014; The Arthritis Society, 2014a). Incidence among women is nine times that among men, and usually occurs between the ages of 15 and 45 (The Arthritis Society, 2014a).

Although there is no known cause, genetics and hormones have been identified as contributing factors (Lupus Canada, 2014). While the risk of development of SLE in an identical twin is increased, siblings of an individual with SLE are usually not affected (Robinson et al., 2011). Although SLE can occur for no apparent reason, exposure to ultraviolet light (e.g., sunlight and tanning beds), pregnancy or therapeutic abortion, surgery, certain infections, and stress may trigger an episode or progression of the disease (Robinson et al., 2011).

In this disorder of immunoregulation, antibodies conflict with the client's nuclear antigens, cytoplasmic antigens, and platelets. Autoantibodies then bind with their specific antigens, resulting in an accumulation of immune complexes in blood vessel walls. Lupus vasculitis, ischemia with thickened lining of the vessels, fibrinoid degeneration, and thrombus formation ensue.

Estrogen and hormonal changes may stimulate enhanced immune reactivity, whereas antigens suppress immune reactivity, a factor that contributes to a woman's increased risk for acquiring this disorder. See Chapter 13 for more discussion of SLE and other autoimmune problems in pregnancy.

● **BOX 4.2** **Common Symptoms of Lupus**

- Fever (low grade that lasts a long time or sudden, high fever)
- Arthritis (pain may be migratory with no signs of inflammation) (all clients eventually have)
- Prolonged or extreme fatigue (most frequent symptom)
- Skin rashes
- Weight loss or gain (sudden, unexplained)
- Kidney damage
- Chest pain with shortness of breath in some positions
- Headache
- Butterfly-shaped rash across the cheek and nose
- Photosensitivity (especially during spring and summer)
- Hair loss (alopecia)
- Blood cell disorders (hemolytic anemia, leucopenia, and thrombocytopenia)
- Raynaud phenomenon (fingers turning white and/or blue in the cold)
- Seizures
- Psychosis (including hallucinations and delusions)
- Mouth or nose ulcers
- Hypertension

Adapted from Lupus Canada. (2014). Living with Lupus—questions. Retrieved from http://www.lupuscanada.org/english/living/lupus-overview.html; Robinson, M., Cook, S. S., & Currie, L. M. (2011). Systemic lupus erythematosus: A genetic review for advanced practice nurses. *Journal of the American Academy of Nurse Practitioners, 23*, 629–637; The Arthritis Society. (2014a). Lupus. Retrieved from http://www.arthritis.ca/page.aspx?pid=938c

Assessment Findings

Each affected individual usually has a unique combination and severity of symptoms (Box 4.2) with no characteristic pattern of organ or system involvement, or severity (Lupus Canada, 2014). Symptoms may include fatigue, unexplained sudden weight changes, headaches, alopecia, generalized pain, mucosal ulcers, change in finger colour when cold, and photosensitivity (Ferenkeh-Koroma, 2012; Lupus Canada, 2014; Robinson et al., 2011). Clients may also develop a characteristic butterfly-shaped rash on the face (Fig. 4.3); renal symptoms such as hematuria; fluid retention; and mild hypertension or neurologic complications, including psychosis, seizures, and neuropathies (Robinson et al., 2011; The Arthritis Society, 2014a).

Diagnosis of SLE is based on the presence of four or more of the 11 criteria listed in Box 4.3. The antinuclear antibody (ANA) must be positive for a diagnosis of SLE (Robinson et al., 2011). Clients who exhibit fewer than four of these symptoms or who demonstrate a negative ANA in the presence of other symptoms are

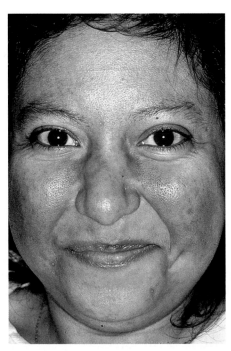

FIGURE 4.3 The characteristic facial butterfly rash of systemic lupus erythematosus.

● **BOX 4.3** **Diagnostic Criteria for Systemic Lupus Erythematosus**

- Malar rash (flat or raised erythema across cheeks)
- Discoid rash on cheeks (disc-shaped, red, raised patches)
- Photosensitivity to sunlight
- Painless ulcers of the mucosal lining of the mouth or nose
- Non-erosive arthritis of at least two joints (tenderness, swelling, or effusion)
- Renal dysfunction (proteinuria [>0.5 g/24 h or 3 g/L on urine dipstick] or cellular casts)
- Positive serum ANA
- Neurologic disorder (seizure or psychosis)
- Serositis (pleuritis or pericarditis)
- Hematologic disorders (anemia, thrombocytopenia [<100,000/mm^3], or leucopenia [<4,000/mm^3 on 2 or more occasions])
- Immunologic dysfunction (positive anti-Smith antibody, anti–double-stranded DNA, or antiphospholipid antibody)

Adapted from Ferenkeh-Koroma, A. (2012). Systemic lupus erythematosus: Nurse and patient education. *Nursing Standard, 26*(39), 49–57; Robinson, M., Cook, S. S., & Currie, L. M. (2011). Systemic lupus erythematosus: A genetic review for advanced practice nurses. *Journal of the American Academy of Nurse Practitioners, 23*, 629–637.

referred for further investigation to rule out Lyme disease, RA, scleroderma, thrombotic thrombocytopenic purpura, and other connective tissue diseases (Robinson et al., 2011).

Collaborative Management

There is no known cure or way to prevent SLE. Current treatment includes medications, nontraditional therapies, and dietary supplements. Antimalarial agents (e.g., hydroxychloroquine [Plaquenil], chloroquine [Aralen]), NSAIDs, corticosteroids, and immunosuppressive drugs (e.g., cyclophosphamide [Cytoxan], azathioprine [Imuran], methotrexate) can ease symptoms and improve quality of life (Lupus Canada, n.d.; Robinson et al., 2011).

Preventive measures are important in reducing exacerbations of SLE. Clients avoid excessive sun exposure and use sunscreen regularly to prevent rashes. The nurse encourages stress reduction modalities and exercise to prevent muscle weakness and fatigue. A well-balanced diet and avoiding alcohol are also important in preventing exacerbations. The nurse assists with strategies to protect joints to reduce pain and inflammation. In addition, the nurse can refer the client to support groups and review the benefits of dietary changes.

MULTIPLE SCLEROSIS

Multiple sclerosis (MS) is the most common neurologic disease of young adults in Canada, affecting an estimated 100,000 Canadians (Multiple Sclerosis Society of Canada, n.d.). Canada has one of the highest rates of MS in the world. It is usually diagnosed between the ages of 15 to 40 years and affects women three times more often than men. Although the cause of MS is unknown, research suggests that it results from an autoimmune process that causes progressive demyelination and scarring of nerves in the brain and spinal cord, leading to impaired transmission of nerve impulses (Multiple Sclerosis Society of Canada, n.d.).

MS cannot be definitively diagnosed, nor is there a cure at the moment (Multiple Sclerosis Society of Canada, n.d.). Four disease types can be identified. Relapsing–remitting MS (RRMS) is characterized by unpredictable, clearly defined episodes where new symptoms arise or existing ones worsen; between these episodes there is complete or nearly complete remission to pre-attack function (Multiple Sclerosis Society of Canada, n.d.). Primary progressive MS (PPMS) is characterized by a slow progression of disability without remission, although there may be periods of stability in symptoms or minor temporary improvement (Multiple Sclerosis Society of Canada, n.d.). Secondary progressive MS (SPMS) follows RRMS and is characterized by less distinct and apparent relapses and remissions, leading to increasing disability (Multiple Sclerosis Society of Canada, n.d.). Progressive relapsing MS (PRMS) is the rarest form of MS and is characterized by steadily worsening disease from initial onset with acute attacks that may or may not be accompanied by some recovery (Multiple Sclerosis Society of Canada, n.d.).

Assessment Findings

Symptoms vary from individual to individual and are often unpredictable. Symptoms may also vary from time to time in the same person, often improving during periods of remission. Visual disturbances (e.g., blurred or double vision), extreme fatigue, loss of balance, problems with coordination and speech, muscle stiffness or spasm, bladder and bowel problems, difficulty with short-term memory, and partial or complete paralysis may be experienced, depending on which part or parts of the CNS are affected (Multiple Sclerosis Society of Canada, n.d.; Nazarko, 2013).

A diagnosis of MS is typically made by ruling out other potential causes for symptoms. History and neurologic examination, together with MRI (which can reveal lesions in the CNS), evoked potentials (which records the slowing of nerve impulse conduction related to myelin damage), and lumbar puncture (used very infrequently when other tests are negative) are helpful in assisting with diagnosis (Multiple Sclerosis Society of Canada, n.d.).

Collaborative Management

Heat may increase symptoms of MS. Therefore, it is important for women to use strategies such as air conditioning, wearing cotton or cooling clothes, sleeping alone, and exercising in a pool to manage warm environments. This is especially significant for women who are pregnant; pregnancy by itself increases BMR and heat production.

Because MS is most prevalent among women, especially those in the childbearing years, women are faced with additional decisions about childbearing choices (Sponiar et al., 2007). Information about the type of MS the woman has, as well as support, are helpful for women faced with these decisions.

Immunomodulatory therapies work by targeting some aspect of the inflammatory process, focusing on prevention of inflammation. Steroids are used short term to decrease the severity and duration of MS relapses. Clinical trials have shown that these treatments actually modify the course of the disease, decreasing the frequency and severity of MS attacks, reducing the number of lesions in the brain, and slowing the progression of disability (Multiple Sclerosis Society of Canada, n.d.). Other therapies are targeted at helping with symptoms such as spasticity, bladder problems, pain, and fatigue.

Over the last few years, much media attention has been given to the research by Zamboni et al. (2009), which identified chronic cerebrospinal venous insuffi-

ciency (CCSVI) in persons diagnosed with MS. In June 2010, the MS Society of Canada and the National MS Society in the United States committed research funds to further explore the relationship between CCVSI and MS. Traboulsee et al. (2014), using catheter venography, concluded that "the hypothesis that venous narrowings have a role in the cause of MS is unlikely, since the prevalence of venous narrowings is similar in people with the disease, unaffected siblings, and unrelated healthy controls on catheter venography…The significance of venous narrowing to MS symptomatology remains unknown" (p. 143).

Complementary and alternative medicine approaches may include natural health products, herbs, homeopathic medicine, vitamins, acupuncture, massage, meditation, and prayer. It is estimated that these approaches are used by approximately 50% to 70% of Canadians with MS (Multiple Sclerosis Society of Canada, n.d.).

DIABETES MELLITUS

Diabetes mellitus, a metabolic disorder of the pancreas that affects carbohydrate, fat, and protein metabolism, affects approximately 3.6 million; over 9 million Canadians are living with diabetes or prediabetes (Canadian Diabetes Association, 2014). Because the condition is chronic, clients can experience many debilitating and life-threatening complications. Risk factors, screening, and prevention measures for diabetes mellitus are discussed in detail in Chapter 2.

Classification

The major classifications of diabetes are as follows:

- Type 1 diabetes
- Type 2 diabetes
- Gestational diabetes
- Prediabetes

In *type 1 diabetes,* the body produces no insulin. It is thought that the immune system attacks and destroys insulin-producing beta cells in the pancreas, although the cause of this is unknown. Type 1 diabetes accounts for approximately 10% of all cases of diabetes and usually develops in children and adolescents (Canadian Diabetes Association, 2014). This type of diabetes also includes those few adult clients who appear to have immune-mediated loss of pancreatic beta cells (Canadian Diabetes Association, 2014).

The number of individuals with type 2 diabetes is rapidly rising in Canada (Canadian Diabetes Association, 2014). In this type of diabetes, there is not enough insulin produced, or there is cellular resistance to its action. Type 2 diabetes typically develops in adults, although increasing numbers of children in high-risk

● TABLE 4.2 **Signs and Symptoms in Type 1 and 2 Diabetes Mellitus**

Type 1	Type 2
Short and sudden development of symptoms	Less noticeable, often "silent" symptoms
Increased thirst and urination	Frequent urination
Constant hunger	Unusual thirst
Weight loss	Weight loss
Blurred vision	Blurred vision
Extreme tiredness	Fatigue or feeling "ill"
	Frequent infections, especially vaginal, in women
	Slow healing of sores
	Tingling or numbness in the feet and hands
	Dry skin

populations are developing it (Canadian Diabetes Association, 2014). Children from populations at an increased risk for type 2 diabetes include those of Aboriginal, Arabic, Hispanic, Asian, or African descent (Canadian Diabetes Association, 2013). Obesity is a major risk factor for the development of type 2 diabetes and may be a factor in the increased development in childhood (Canadian Diabetes Association, 2013). The 2009 to 2011 Canadian Health Measures Survey found that 25% to 33% of Canadian children between the ages of 5 and 17 years were overweight or obese (Roberts et al., 2012).

Gestational diabetes first develops or is discovered during pregnancy. It usually disappears when the pregnancy is over; however, women with this condition, and their children, are at an increased risk for developing type 2 diabetes later in life (Canadian Diabetes Association, 2014). Chapter 13 discusses gestational diabetes in detail.

Individuals with prediabetes, sometimes called impaired glucose tolerance or impaired fasting glucose, have glucose levels that are higher than normal but not at the threshold for diagnosis of type 2 diabetes. Approximately 50% of these individuals will develop type 2 diabetes over time (Canadian Diabetes Association, 2014). Knowledge of the existence of pre-diabetes

is important as some of the long-term complications of diabetes have been found to begin during this time (Canadian Diabetes Association, 2014).

Assessment Findings

Table 4.2 compares the signs and symptoms of types 1 and 2 diabetes. For both types, early signs and symptoms include polyuria, polydipsia, fatigue, weight change, blurred vision, tingling and numbness in the hands or feet, nonhealing sores, and recurrent infections, especially vulvovaginitis in women (Canadian Diabetes Association, 2014).

Diagnostic testing for diabetes is relatively simple. Blood tests include a fasting blood glucose test or a 75-g oral glucose tolerance test (Table 4.3). Another method of testing is with a glucometer (Fig. 4.4), which measures capillary blood glucose from blood sampled from a finger stick or through the skin on the arm.

Collaborative Management

Treatment of all types of diabetes mellitus requires a daily commitment from the client to careful management of the condition, including healthy lifestyle patterns. Usual treatment includes a balanced combination of diet, exercise, drug therapy, frequent blood glucose

● TABLE 4.3 **Diagnostic Tests for Diabetes Mellitus**

Test	Implementation	Diagnostic Result
Fasting blood glucose	Blood specimen is obtained after 8 hours of fasting	Individuals with impaired glucose tolerance have value from 6.1–6.9 mmol/L A level of 7.0 mmol/L is diagnostic for diabetes
75 g oral glucose tolerance test	Blood sample is taken 2 hours after drinking 75 g glucose solution	Individuals with impaired glucose tolerance have range from 7.8–11.0 mmol/L Individuals with diabetes have level of ≥11.1 mmol/L
Glycosylated hemoglobin or hemoglobin A1 c	Single sample of venous blood is withdrawn	The amount of glucose stored by the hemoglobin is 7.0% in the newly diagnosed client with diabetes mellitus, in one who is noncompliant, or in one who is inadequately treated.

Canadian Diabetes Association. (2013). Clinical Practice Guidelines. Retrieved from http://guidelines.diabetes.ca/

● TEACHING TIPS 4.1 Diabetes-Related Complications

The nurse shares with the client and family the following information about diabetes mellitus:

- Up to 80% of people with diabetes will die as a result of heart attack or stroke
- Women with diabetes develop cardiovascular and cerebrovascular disease at a younger age and at a rate 5 times that of those without diabetes
- Other complications include:
  - Peripheral vascular disease
  - Congenital malformations, macrosomia

- End-stage renal disease
- Greater susceptibility to infections and illnesses
- Hypertension
- Lower-extremity amputations
- Neuropathy
- Retinopathy
- Depression

From Canadian Diabetes Association. (2014). About diabetes. Retrieved from http://www.diabetes.ca/about-diabetes

monitoring, and stress management. Health care providers educate clients and families about diabetes to enhance their understanding of the following:

- The etiology of the disorder
- Associated dietary needs
- Importance of exercise
- Relevant drug therapies and administration of insulin, as needed
- Symptoms of hypoglycemia and hyperglycemia (Box 4.4)
- Signs of infection
- Foot care

A thorough discussion of complications arising from uncontrolled diabetes is essential. Teaching Tips 4.1 provides information nurses can share with clients to help them understand the risks associated with diabetes and the reasons that aggressive prevention and management of the illness are vital.

CARDIOVASCULAR DISEASE

Cardiovascular disease (CVD) includes both heart attack and stroke. Heart disease and stroke are the leading causes of death among Canadian women. Women continue to have a lower rate of death from heart dis-

ease than men, although their risk of dying in the first year after a heart attack is higher (Turcotte, 2013).

Risk factors for CVD are often classified as modifiable and nonmodifiable (Table 4.4). Some risk factors have special significance for women. For example, the use of oral contraceptives in combination with smoking may increase the risk of stroke, especially in women who are over the age of 35 years, have pre-existing hypertension, have other risk factors for CVD, or have a problem with blood clotting. Women with hypertension are at a risk 3.5 times greater of developing heart disease than women with normal blood pressure; women who have had gestational hypertension are also at higher risk. A woman with type 2 diabetes has eight times the risk of developing heart disease than a woman without diabetes; women who have had gestational diabetes are at

● BOX 4.4 Signs and Symptoms of Hypoglycemia and Hyperglycemia

Hypoglycemia
- Anxiety
- Diaphoresis
- Dizziness
- Headache
- Hunger
- Impaired vision
- Irritability
- Shaking
- Tachycardia
- Weakness and fatigue

Hyperglycemia
- Blurred vision
- Drowsiness or increased sleep
- Dry skin
- Extreme thirst
- Frequent urination
- Nausea

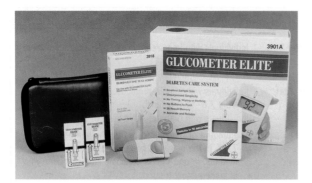

FIGURE 4.4 Clients with diabetes can take regular readings of their blood glucose level using a glucometer.

● **TABLE 4.4** **Cardiovascular Risk Factors**

Modifiable	Nonmodifiable
Hypertension	Increasing age
Smoking	Family history
Hyperlipidemia	Gender
Obesity	Ethnicity
Sedentary lifestyle	Prior stroke or transient ischemic
Diabetes	attack (TIA)
Excessive alcohol consumption	
Stress	

an increased risk for developing type 2 diabetes at a later date. Pregnancy and childbirth increase the risk of stroke by as much as 3 to 13 times, especially in the early postpartum period. Menopause can increase a woman's risk for CVD, primarily as a result of the decrease in estrogen that provides a protective effect on women's cardiovascular health, including cholesterol levels. Chapter 2 presents further discussion of measures to control risk, along with health screening.

HEART DISEASE

There are many conditions that are included in the term heart disease, such as coronary artery disease, atherosclerosis, congestive heart failure, arrhythmias, and others. Coronary artery disease is the most common form of heart disease, in which blocked or narrowed cardiac blood vessels prevent oxygenated blood from reaching the heart muscle. *Atherosclerosis,* which causes more than 90% of heart attacks, causes the heart vessels to narrow or clog as plaque or fat deposits accumulate on the inner lining of blood vessels (Heart & Stroke Foundation of Canada, 2014a). Blood flow to the heart is impeded and leads to chest pain (angina) or a myocardial infarction of the heart muscle (heart attack).

Assessment Findings

In the past, it was believed that women experience different signs and symptoms of heart attack from those of men; however, this may not be the case. The most common symptom for all clients is pain in the arm, throat, or jaw, or pain that is unusual. However, women may describe their pain differently than men (Heart & Stroke Foundation of Canada, 2014a). Other symptoms may include nausea, sweating, or shortness of breath. Clients may ignore such symptoms and may not seek immediate medical care for them.

Collaborative Management

When a woman is diagnosed with heart disease, she is informed of the risks and benefits of various medical and surgical interventions so that she can make informed decisions about her health. Treatment is based on the extent and location of occlusions. Medications used include nitrates, aspirin, and β-adrenergic receptor antagonists (β-blockers) to control hypertension and ischemic heart disease. Calcium channel blockers decrease vascular resistance and increase blood flow. Surgical interventions usually include cardiac catheterization with angioplasty or coronary artery bypass graft (Heart & Stroke Foundation of Canada, 2014a).

All clients need education and counselling about reducing modifiable risks for heart disease (see Chapter 2). Women can lower their chances by educating themselves about risk factors and making the appropriate modifications, knowing the symptoms of a heart attack, and adjusting their lifestyle and behaviours (see Chapter 2). Widespread knowledge and appropriate responses can improve women's awareness of heart disease and decrease incidence of the illness. The nurse explains that a low-fat diet and regular aerobic exercise can significantly reduce risks and can arrange for the client to consult with a dietitian about a heart-healthy diet, in addition to referring clients to smoking cessation programs.

The nurse assesses signs and symptoms of chest pain and administers prescribed drugs, as ordered. He or she encourages rest and administers oxygen to improve the available supply to the heart. The nurse teaches clients about the side effects of any drugs, and that severe, unrelieved chest pain indicates a need for immediate examination. The nurse advises the client to report changes in the usual pattern of angina.

STROKE

Stroke can result in death or serious long-term disability.

There are two major types of stroke: ischemic and hemorrhagic. Ischemic stroke, which usually involves atherosclerosis, accounts for approximately 80% of all cases and occurs if a thrombus or embolus occludes blood supply to the brain (Heart & Stroke Foundation of Canada, 2014b). A transient ischemic attack (TIA), also known as a "mini-stroke," is caused by a temporary interruption in blood supply to the brain. The symptoms are similar to those of an ischemic stroke, except that they disappear within a few minutes or hours. Hemorrhagic stroke accounts for about 20% of strokes and is caused by uncontrolled bleeding in the brain. Two main types of hemorrhagic stroke are subarachnoid hemorrhage (between the brain and skull) and intracerebral hemorrhage (deep within the brain). Both types can be caused by structural abnormalities of brain vasculature, including aneurysm, where a weakened area of a cranial blood vessel bursts, or an arteriovenous malformation, usually present at birth.

Assessment Findings

The effects of stroke are related to the area of the brain affected and the amount of damage that has occurred.

These may include motor, sensory, and cognitive deficits. Warning signs of stroke are loss of strength or numbness in the face, arm, or leg; difficulty speaking or understanding; confusion; trouble with vision; severe and unusual headache; and loss of balance, especially when in combination with any other signs. These symptoms have a sudden onset and may be temporary (Heart & Stroke Foundation of Canada, 2014b). A computed tomography (CT) scan is used to diagnose a stroke.

Collaborative Management

If a blood clot causes an ischemic stroke, the clinician uses thrombolytic agents (e.g., tissue plasminogen activator [t-PA]) within 3 hours of initial symptoms to break up the causative clot (Blakeley & Llinas, 2007; Heart & Stroke Foundation of Canada, 2014b). Antiplatelet drugs (eg, clopidogrel [Plavix], eptifibatide [Integrilin], warfarin sodium [Coumadin]) may be given to prevent recurrence. The primary goal of treatment for hemorrhagic stroke is to stop the bleeding. Usual treatment consists of drug administration to lower blood pressure, surgery to remove blood or repair damaged blood vessels, and reversal of any anticoagulants or bleeding disorder (Heart & Stroke Foundation of Canada, 2014b).

The nurse's primary focus is to accurately assess a woman for stroke. Following assessment, the nurse focuses client and family education on risk prevention and modification of lifestyle behaviours that may contribute to stroke (see Chapter 2).

SEXUALLY TRANSMITTED INFECTIONS

Sexually transmitted infections (STIs) are infections of the reproductive tract resulting from microorganisms transmitted during vaginal, oral, or anal intercourse. They pose a significant public health issue, with incidence increasing at alarming rates. Chlamydia is the most commonly reported bacterial STI in Canada, with a 72% increase between 2001 and 2010, when the rate for the general population was 277.6 per 100,000. Young women between 20 and 24 years had the highest reported rate of chlamydia, at 2,005.5 per 100,000 population Public Health Agency of Canada [PHAC], 2013h; Rotermann et al., 2013). The incidence of genital herpes in Canada is not known, because not all jurisdictions require reporting. However, the incidence and prevalence are increasing globally (PHAC, 2013d). Gonorrhea rates for young women between 15 and 19 years of age were 147 cases per 100,000 population, more than four times the national average of 33.4 cases (PHAC, 2013h). The rate of syphilis in 2010 was 5.2 per 100,000 in the general population, higher in males than females in all age groups (PHAC, 2013h). Many STIs are asymptomatic; others manifest with minor or nonspecific symptoms in early stages (Table 4.5). Consequently, many STIs are not diagnosed until the late stages, when significant damage has already resulted. Complications of STIs include infertility (see Chapter 10), high-risk and tubal pregnancy (see Chapter 13), and pelvic inflammatory disease (PID). Maternal–fetal transmission of STIs can lead to premature birth, low birth weight, or both. See Teaching Tips 4.2 and Chapters 13 and 22 for more information.

CHLAMYDIA

The causative bacterium, *Chlamydia trachomatis,* is transmitted through oral, vaginal, or anal sexual contact with an infected person, and can be transmitted from mother to neonate during childbirth (Government of Canada, 2013a). *Chlamydia trachomatis* can invade a woman's reproductive structures and urethra. Tissue irritation may be permanent despite successful eradication of the bacteria and can increase a client's risks for other STIs. Untreated infection can cause serious complications for men, women, and newborns of infected mothers.

Assessment Findings

Clients may not know that they have chlamydia, because they may be asymptomatic; more than 50% of males

---

● TEACHING TIPS 4.2 Preventing Sexually Transmitted Infections

- Abstinence is the best protection against STIs. Monogamous sexual relationships increase protection against STIs.
- Refrain from engaging in sex with anyone you suspect may have an STI.
- Know the signs and symptoms of STIs. Observe sexual partners closely for rashes and discharge.
- Use latex condoms when having vaginal, oral, or anal sex. (If you have a latex allergy, use plastic polyurethane condoms.)

- If you have an STI, your partner also must be tested and receive treatment.
- If you have an STI, do not have sex until your treatment is complete.
- Avoid wearing nylon pants, tights, and tight jeans.
- Refrain from using vaginal deodorants, perfumed soap, and bubble bath.
- Do not wear others' underwear.

	Causative Organism	Symptoms in Women	Diagnostic Testing	Treatment
Chlamydia	Bacteria: *Chlamydia trachomatis*	Frequently asymptomatic Vaginal discharge Burning on urination Bleeding between menstrual periods or after intercourse Lower abdominal pain	Urine test Cervical, vaginal, rectal, or throat swabs for culture	Doxycycline, azithromycin, erythromycin, or amoxicillin
Gonorrhea	Bacteria: *Neisseria gonorrhoeae*	Frequently asymptomatic Purulent or bloody vaginal discharge Pain or burning on urination	Cultures from the cervix, urethra, rectum, or pharynx	Cefixime or ceftriaxone
Syphilis	Bacteria: *Treponema pallidum*	May be asymptomatic Painless sores (chancres Swollen lymph glands Skin rashes Mucous lesions Mild fever Fatigue Headache Sore throat Hair loss	Examinations of blood samples	Long acting benzathine penicillin G by injection or IM procaine penicillin Doxycycline or ceftriaxone for clients with penicillin allergy
Genital herpes	Herpes simplex virus—type 2 or type 1	May be asymptomatic Itching or tingling in genital or anal areas Clusters of vesicles on erythematous background in the exocervix Fever Muscle aches Lymphadenopathy Pain on urination Pain in the legs, buttocks, or genital area	Cultures	Oral acyclovir (Zovirax) Famciclovir (Famvir) Valacyclovir (Valtrex)
Genital warts	Human papillomavirus (HPV)	May be asymptomatic Genital warts that sometimes are difficult to see on the vagina, vulva, cervix, thigh, rectum, urethra, and anus	Visual inspection Pap test Colposcopy Anoscopy Urethroscopy	May disappear without treatment in some cases Imiquimod cream Podophyllin and podofilox solutions Trichloroacetic acid (TCA) Cryotherapy Electrocautery Laser ablation
Bacterial vaginosis (BV)	*Gardnerella vaginalis* or mixed anaerobes	May be asymptomatic White or grey thin and malodourous vaginal discharge	Microscopic examination of vaginal fluid, either in stained or special lighting	Oral metronidazole or clindamycin cream
Trichomoniasis	Protozoan parasite: *Trichomonas vaginalis*	May be asymptomatic Vaginal discharge with strong odour Discomfort during vaginal sexual intercourse and urination Irritation and itching of the vagina	Physical examination or laboratory testing for parasite	Single-dose metronidazole
Candidiasis	Fungus: *Candida albicans*	May be asymptomatic Itching, burning, and irritation of the vagina Pain during urination Cottage cheese–like vaginal discharge	Gram stain and microscopic examination	Oral or suppository antifungal medications

and 70% of females have no symptoms (Government of Canada, 2013a; Mishori et al., 2012). In addition, symptoms usually occur 2 to 3 weeks after infection, although they may occur as late as 6 weeks. Symptoms may include vaginal discharge, dysuria, pain in the lower abdomen accompanied by fever and chills, dyspareunia, and vaginal bleeding after intercourse or between periods (Government of Canada, 2013a; Mishori et al., 2012). Symptoms of anal infection include rectal pain, bleeding, and discharge (Mishori et al., 2012). Individuals infected through oral sex usually have few symptoms (Government of Canada, 2013a).

The infection, usually located in the endocervix in women, can spread to the endometrium, uterine tubes, peritoneum, rectum, and urethra, and can lead to inflammation, ulceration, and scarring (Haggerty et al., 2010). Chlamydia can reside in the cervix for many years, damaging uterine tubes and resulting in PID in up to 40% of infected women (Government of Canada, 2013a; Mishori et al., 2012). Consequently, PID can lead to scarring of the fallopian tubes and subsequent problems with fertility, including ectopic pregnancy (Government of Canada, 2013a; Haggerty et al., 2010; Mishori et al., 2012). Maternal chlamydial infection can cause an infant to be born prematurely, and the newborn may have eye infections or develop pneumonia (Government of Canada, 2013a).

Diagnosis usually involves a urine test, using a nucleic acid amplification test (NAAT), which yields results within 24 hours. Cervical, vaginal, or rectal swabs may be needed for symptomatic individuals for either culture or NAAT (Mishori et al., 2012). Culture is recommended for throat specimens. Sexually active females and males under 25 years of age should be screened; all pregnant women should be screened at the first prenatal visit (PHAC, 2010a). Anyone who has been diagnosed with a chlamydial infection should be retested after 6 months.

Collaborative Management

Usual treatment of infection with chlamydia consists of doxycycline, azithromycin, ofloxacin, or erythromycin.

Sexual contacts are traced, examined, and treated with medication. The client should abstain from sexual intercourse until the sexual partner is examined or begins medication, or use condoms if the partner has not been examined or begun medication. Infected clients do not require follow-up testing, unless their sexual partners do not receive treatment.

Health care professionals screen clients for STI risk, perform comprehensive historical and physical assessment, and provide education about STIs. They recommend testing if mucopurulent vaginal drainage appears, if an STI or PID is suspected, before termination of pregnancy, before insertion of intrauterine contraceptive devices, and for all sexually active teenagers. Anyone who has more than one sexual partner, especially women younger than 25 years, should be tested routinely for chlamydia, even when no symptoms appear. Infection rates can diminish with the correct use of male latex condoms during all sexual encounters (see Chapter 8).

Think back to Lela, the young client described at the beginning of the chapter complaining of a vaginal discharge. Would the nurse suspect an STI? Why or why not?

GONORRHEA

Gonorrhea is caused by the bacterium *Neisseria gonorrhoeae* and often coexists with *C. trachomatis* infection (Mayor et al., 2012). The second most commonly diagnosed STI in Canada, it can be spread through oral, genital, or anal sex and can be spread from mother to infant. It commonly affects the cervix, urethra, rectum, and oropharynx (Fig. 4.5). Rectal infections can develop from vaginal secretions, anal sex, or both. The incubation period typically lasts 2 to 7 days (Mayor et al., 2012; PHAC, 2013e).

Assessment Findings

Many women are asymptomatic or have very mild symptoms and may be infected for several months without knowing it (Mayor et al., 2012). When symptoms occur, the most common include purulent or occasionally bloody vaginal discharge, lower abdominal pain, or dysuria. Rectal and throat infections are more likely to have a few symptoms (PHAC, 2013e). The recommended method of diagnosis is cultures from the cervix, urethra,

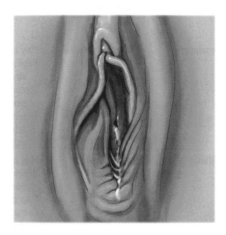

FIGURE 4.5 Gonorrhea.

rectum, and pharynx; cultures facilitate identification of appropriate antimicrobial therapy. Swabs or urine specimens may be collected for NAAT in some laboratories. The majority of cases are diagnosed by endocervical cultures. Neonates may contract gonorrhea during vaginal delivery, leading to blindness or septicemia.

Collaborative Management

Combination therapy, including treatment for chlamydia, is recommended to both improve treatment efficacy and delay antimicrobial resistance (PHAC, 2013e). Antibiotic therapy consists of a single dose of cefixime 800 mg orally. Ceftriaxone 250 mg IM is given for pharyngeal infection or PID. Azithromycin should be given as monotherapy only when cephalosporins are contraindicated. Ciprofloxacin, levofloxacin, and ofloxacin are no longer recommended drugs for treatment in Canada and are considered as an alternative treatment only if antimicrobial susceptibility testing is available and quinolone susceptibility is demonstrated or quinolone resistance is under 5% and a test of cure can be performed (PHAC, 2013e). Clients with gonorrhea should refrain from sexual activity until effectiveness of treatment has been confirmed. Sexual partners of infected clients should be contacted, screened, and treated appropriately.

SYPHILIS

Syphilis, least common among the STIs reportable in Canada, is caused by the bacterium *Treponema pallidum*. Rare in Canada prior to 2000, syphilis infection rates are increasing (PHAC, 2010a). It is more common in men and in women engaged in sex trades. Aboriginal people in British Columbia, Alberta, and Yukon are disproportionately represented, existing in the context of social and health inequities (PHAC, 2010a).

Syphilis is transmitted through oral, genital, or anal sex with an infected person, or by a pregnant woman to her fetus (PHAC, 2010a). It can also be transmitted through injection drug use or through broken skin, although this is rare. Clients with syphilis are at an increased risk for acquiring and transmitting the human immunodeficiency virus (HIV).

Maternal–fetal transmission of syphilis is high, with 70% to 100% of pregnant women with untreated primary or secondary syphilis passing the infection to their fetuses, either in utero or by contact with an active genital lesion at the time of delivery (PHAC, 2010a). The transmission is 40% with early latent syphilis, and 10% in late latent stages. The risk for fetal death is about 40% (PHAC, 2010a).

Assessment Findings

Syphilis has four stages: primary, secondary, latent, and tertiary (late).

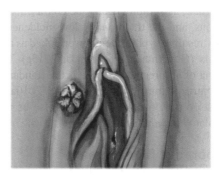

FIGURE 4.6 The painless ulcer (chancre) of primary syphilis.

- **Primary syphilis.** The initial symptoms are a painless ulcer or chancre or regional lymphadenopathy, which usually appears within 3 weeks (from 3 to 90 days) of exposure. The ulcer can occur internally, but is more frequently found on the body part that was exposed to the bacterium (Fig. 4.6). Additional ulcers may develop on the cervix, tongue, lips, and other body parts. Although the sores may disappear without treatment, syphilis is infectious in this phase and will progress to secondary.
- **Secondary syphilis.** During this stage, the client develops a skin rash, mucous lesions, condylomata, and retinitis 2 to 12 weeks (although it may be up to 6 months) after the initial ulcer. The rash may cover the soles of the feet, the palms of the hands, or the entire body. The client also may experience mild fever, malaise, headache, sore throat, hair loss, muscle and joint pain, and swollen lymph glands. Although the symptoms may again disappear without treatment, the syphilis remains infectious.
- **Latent syphilis.** During this stage, no symptoms appear, and the syphilis is usually only infectious in the early latent stage (less than 1 year).
- **Tertiary syphilis.** In the final stage, syphilis spreads to many body systems, such as the heart, eyes, brain, nervous system, bones, and joints. Clients may show signs of personality changes, dementia, blindness, neurologic disorders, and heart problems. This stage can last years to decades (Government of Canada, 2013e; PHAC, 2010a), although the client is no longer contagious. If untreated it can eventually lead to death.

Symptoms of congenital syphilis in a newborn include skin ulcers, rashes, fever, hoarse crying sounds, swollen liver and spleen, anemia, deformation, and jaundice. An asymptomatic newborn who is not treated immediately can develop serious mental and physical handicaps, which usually manifest 2 to 3 months after birth.

Syphilis is diagnosed with a simple blood test. Individuals with symptoms or who are at an increased risk for acquiring the infection should be tested. This is important, as symptoms may be confused with other conditions, and the traditionally low incidence in Canada may result in syphilis being overlooked as a possible diagnosis (Government of Canada, 2013e). Universal screening of all pregnant women is the standard of care in most jurisdictions in Canada (PHAC, 2010a). Clients who test positive for syphilis should also be tested for HIV, chlamydia, and gonorrhea.

Collaborative Management

Long-acting benzathine penicillin G by injection is the preferred treatment because of better adherence with less frequent dosing (PHAC, 2010a). Clients allergic to penicillin receive other antibiotics, usually doxycycline or ceftriaxone. Clients with congenital syphilis are treated with crystalline penicillin G for 10 days. Only benzathine penicillin G is recommended for pregnant women; there is no alternative to penicillin, so penicillin desensitization should be considered prior to treatment (PHAC, 2010a). Treatment plans should include instructional screening, with disease prevention as the ultimate goal.

GENITAL HERPES

Herpes is a highly contagious STI that can be transmitted during unprotected vaginal, anal, or oral sex even when the individual with the infection has no symptoms. It can also be transmitted to the newborn during pregnancy or childbirth. Women are at higher risk for acquiring the disease from men, than men are for acquiring it from women (PHAC, 2013d). The disease is controllable, but not curable. Although herpes simplex virus type 2 (HSV-2), also known as **genital herpes**, is primarily responsible for genital and perineal lesions, herpes simplex virus type 1 (HSV-1), associated with cold sores around the nose and lips, can also cause genital lesions.

Assessment Findings

While most individuals seroconvert within 3 to 6 weeks, approximately 60% of new HSV-2 infections are asymptomatic; 40% have symptoms. In those individuals who experience symptoms with their first episode, typical symptoms include itching or tingling in the genital and anal areas followed by clusters of vesicles on an erythematous background; these may also be present in the exocervix (PHAC, 2013d). Other symptoms may include fever, myalgia, and lymphadenopathy. Complications of first episodes of genital HSV infection may include urethritis, aseptic meningitis, and cervicitis (PHAC, 2013d). The virus incubates for 6 days with symptoms appearing 2 to 20 days following sex with an infected person and lasting up to 3 weeks (PHAC, 2013d) (Fig. 4.7). For the client whose testing indicates a pre-existing infection that was asymptomatic, symptoms experienced during the first clinically evident episode are usually less marked, last a shorter time, and

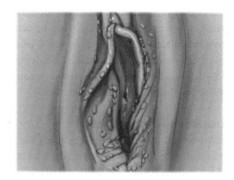

FIGURE 4.7 Ulcers in genital herpes simplex virus.

complications are less common than in those who initially present with symptoms (PHAC, 2013d).

Because no intervention prevents the development of latent sacral sensory ganglion infection, recurrences tend to occur in tissues innervated by sacral sensory nerves (PHAC, 2013d). Recurrences, which vary in frequency among individuals, tend to be characterized by milder symptoms of shorter duration. Itching, burning, tingling, or vague discomfort in the genital area may occur for a few minutes to several days before recurrence. Factors associated with recurrence include sexual intercourse, emotional stress, illness (particularly with fever), surgery, menstruation, and certain medications (PHAC, 2013d). Diagnosis is through culture.

Collaborative Management

Presently, oral acyclovir (Zovirax), famciclovir, or valacyclovir are used to treat symptoms and prevent recurrences (PHAC, 2013d). Valacyclovir may also be used to reduce transmission. Analgesia and laxatives may be used to treat symptoms. Clients should maintain cleanliness and dryness in the infected area and avoid touching lesions. Loose-fitting clothing made of natural materials such as cotton should be worn. In addition, an infected person should avoid sexual contact from the onset of prodromal symptoms until the lesions are completely healed. Clients should inform their sexual partners of the infection so they are aware of the risks of acquiring the infection. Health care personnel should screen the sexual partners of the infected client and treat them appropriately. Infected clients and partners may require counselling, including information about the disease, transmission, and potential effects on childbearing; ongoing support can prove helpful, especially if loneliness, depression, or low self-esteem is present. It is important to emphasize to clients and their partners that most transmission of genital herpes occurs during asymptomatic shedding (PHAC, 2013d). Therefore, condoms should be worn at all times, regardless of whether or not symptoms are present (Government of Canada, 2013b). It is important to remember that exposed areas of skin will still be unprotected and may require adaptations to safer

● TEACHING TIPS 4.3 Genital Herpes

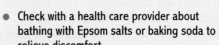

The nurse instructs clients with genital herpes infections as follows:

- Alert all past and current sexual partners of the HSV infection, even if it is inactive. Urge them to undergo appropriate screening and diagnosis.
- Tell all potential sexual partners of the infection before participating in any sexual activities with them.
- Use condoms during sexual activity, even if the infection is dormant. Refrain from sexual contact if the infection is or may be active. Condoms will not protect skin and mucous membranes that remain exposed.

- Check with a health care provider about bathing with Epsom salts or baking soda to relieve discomfort.
- Wear loose clothing and underwear that promotes air circulation.
- Thoroughly wash your hands after contact with lesions.
- Separate your personal hygiene articles (eg, towels) to avoid inadvertent use by others.
- Use a different towel to pat lesions dry.
- Have annual Pap tests.
- Reduce stress and follow other general health promotion strategies.

sex practices such as using a condom cut lengthwise or a dental dam over the female genital area during oral sex (Government of Canada, 2013b; Society of Obstetricians and Gynaecologists of Canada [SOGC], 2012).

Genital herpes increases the risk for acquiring and transmitting HIV infection. Transmission can also occur from mother to infant during a vaginal birth; cesarean birth is indicated for pregnant clients with active lesions.

The client may take oral antiviral medications episodically for 3 to 10 days or continuously to suppress the frequency of outbreaks. IV acyclovir is used when there is a severe episode of HSV-2 or when the client is immunocompromised. Clients receiving drug therapy remain infectious. See Teaching Tips 4.3 for appropriate education measures for clients with genital herpes.

HUMAN PAPILLOMAVIRUS (GENITAL WARTS)

Human papillomavirus (HPV), one of the most common STIs, is a group of more than 130 DNA viruses, acquired from direct skin-to-skin contact, that cause warts (papilloma) (PHAC, 2010a). Different types of viruses cause warts to grow on different parts of the body, such as the hands and soles. The types of viruses that cause warts on the hands and feet do not cause anogenital warts (**condylomata**). Genital warts are spread easily during oral, vaginal, or anal sex with infected people or during intimate skin-to-skin contact (Government of Canada, 2013d). HPV infection is very common, although wide variability exists between different populations; it is estimated that 70% of sexually active men and women will have at least one genital HPV infection over their lifetime (PHAC, 2010a). HPV infections are often acquired early (15 to 19 years of age); about 80% clear spontaneously within 18 months (PHAC, 2010a).

Thirteen high-risk HPV types cause abnormal results on Pap testing and can lead to cervical cancer, while other HPV types have been implicated in cancers of the skin, mouth and pharynx, and anus (PHAC, 2010a). Low-risk

viruses are associated with a low risk for cancer. It is possible to have more than one type of HPV at a time (Government of Canada, 2013d; PHAC, 2010a).

Assessment Findings

Most individuals with HPV infections are asymptomatic (Government of Canada, 2013d; PHAC, 2010a). Clients may develop condylomata on the vagina, vulva, cervix, thigh, rectum, urethra, and anus (see Fig. 4.8). The appearance of lesions may occur weeks to months after infection occurs (PHAC 2010a). Genital warts are less common in men and usually develop on the penis, scrotum, thigh, rectum, urethra, or anus (Government of Canada, 2013d; PHAC, 2010a). Warts vary in size,

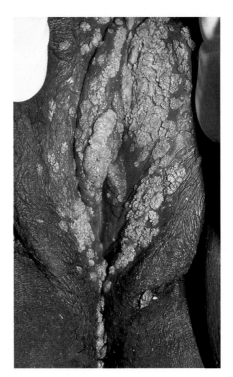

FIGURE 4.8 Genital warts.

appear flat and flesh coloured or take on a cauliflower look, occur in clusters, and can spread in large masses throughout the anal and vaginal areas. They may cause bleeding, pruritus, or discharge (PHAC, 2010a).

A health care provider usually diagnoses genital warts during a pelvic examination. Clients also may notice warts in their genital area. Sometimes warts are hard to see if they are inside the body or are very small. Because the cervix is a common place for HPV infection and almost all cervical cancers are caused by HPV, regular cervical screening using Pap tests should be available for all women within 3 years of sexual activity (PHAC, 2010a). Access to DNA testing for HPV in Canada is currently limited to a small number of jurisdictions. Colposcopy, anoscopy, and urethroscopy are additional diagnostic measures (PHAC, 2010a).

Collaborative Management

HPV is incurable. There is no way to predict whether the warts will disappear without treatment, although this appears to happen in about 80% of cases (PHAC, 2010a). Several treatments are used; options depend on the size and location of the warts. Topical methods include imiquimod cream, podophyllin and podofilox solutions (contraindicated in pregnant women), and trichloroacetic acid. Cryotherapy, electrocautery, and laser ablation may be used to remove small warts (PHAC, 2010a).

Clients need education and counselling regarding prevention and transmission of HPV. Adolescent and young women need encouragement to delay first-time sex, because younger people are at an increased risk for all STIs. Abstinence is the best way to prevent HPV infection, but it must include abstinence from skin-to-skin anogenital contact and from the use of sex toys. Risk for HPV increases as the number of sex partners increases. Education regarding the common symptoms of HPV, as well as other STIs, is important for preventing this serious infection. Partner notification recommendations that apply to other STIs are not useful in reducing HPV transmission (PHAC, 2010a). Clients should inform their sex partner(s) that they have had genital warts or an abnormal Pap test, although there is no proof that this will lower the risk to the partner (PHAC, 2010a).

Symptomatic perinatal transmission is infrequent, with clinical symptoms occurring within 2 years if it occurs. Occurrence is usually associated with anogenital and vocal-cord lesions in the newborn. Cesarean birth is not recommended, unless warts obstruct the birth canal (PHAC, 2010a).

The first prophylactic vaccine was approved in Canada in July 2006 (Pharmacology Box 4.1). Gardasil protects against four HPV types, two of which cause approximately 70% of cervical cancer cases (types 16 and 18), and the other two cause approximately 90% of anogenital warts (types 6 and 11) (Government of Canada, 2013d). It is administered IM into the deltoid muscle in a series of three doses over a 6-month period (time 0, 2, and 6 months). The vaccine is recommended for females between the ages of 9 and 45 years and males between the ages of 9 and 26 years. The vaccine is recommended even in the presence of one type of HPV as it may provide protection against other strains (Government of Canada, 2013d). The vaccine should not be given during pregnancy.

● PHARMACOLOGY 4.1   Gardasil

ACTION

Gardasil is a quadrivalent recombinant vaccine.

INDICATION

Gardasil is indicated in females aged 9 to 45 years for the prevention of HPV infections (types 6, 11, 16, and 18) and associated diseases including cervical cancer, vulvar and vaginal cancers, genital warts (condyloma acuminata), cervical adenocarcinoma *in situ* (AIS), CIN grade 1, grade 2, and grade 3, vulvar intraepithelial neoplasia (VIN) grade 2 and grade 3, and vaginal intraepithelial neoplasia (VaIN) grade 2 and grade 3. It is indicated in boys and men between the ages of 9 and 26 years for the prevention of HPV infections (types 6, 11, 16, and 18) as well as anal cancer, genital warts, and anal intraepithelial neoplasia. It is most efficacious in individuals who have not been exposed to HPV prior to the first dose and 1 month following the third dose.

DOSAGE

Three separate doses of 0.5 mL of suspension administered intramuscularly at 0, 2, and 6 months. All three doses should be given within 1 year.

POSSIBLE ADVERSE EFFECTS

Pain, swelling, and erythema at the injection site. Fever, nausea, dizziness, and diarrhea.

NURSING IMPLICATIONS

- Administer in deltoid region of the upper arm or in the higher anteriolateral region of the thigh. Do NOT administer intravenously.
- Shake well before use.

From Merck Frosst Canada. (2013). Product monograph. Retrieved from www.merck.ca/assets/en/pdf/products/GARDASIL-PM_E.pdf

A second vaccine, Cervarix, also authorized for use in Canada, provides protection against types 16 and 18, the two most common high-risk types of HPV. It is administered in three doses at 1 and 6 months after the first dose. It is approved for use in females aged 9 to 25 years (Government of Canada, 2013d).

BACTERIAL VAGINOSIS

Bacterial vaginosis develops when harmful bacteria in the vagina increase and outnumber those bacteria normally found in the vagina, leading to a change in the pH of the vagina and subsequent symptoms (Fig. 4.9). For example, *Gardnerella vaginalis* or mixed anaerobes eventually outnumber normal vaginal lactobacilli such as *Mobiluncus* and *Mycoplasma hominis*.

Bacterial vaginosis is not usually considered to be sexually transmitted (PHAC, 2010a). It is estimated to occur in 10% to 30% of pregnant women, and in 10% of women who visit family physicians (PHAC, 2010a). Predisposing factors are often absent, but it is more common in women who are sexually active, have a new sexual partner, or use an intrauterine device (IUD) (PHAC, 2010a).

Assessment Findings

Approximately 50% of clients with bacterial vaginosis are asymptomatic (PHAC, 2010a). Primary symptoms include abnormal vaginal odour and vaginal discharge. A fish-like odour may be noticeable, especially after intercourse. Vaginal discharge may be white or grey, and thin but in copious amounts.

Diagnosis involves microscopic examination of vaginal fluid, either in stained or special lighting. Classic indicators of bacterial vaginosis include decreased vaginal acidity (pH >4.5); cells from the vaginal lining coated with bacterial vaginosis organisms; odour; predominantly Gram-negative curved bacilli and coccobacilli.

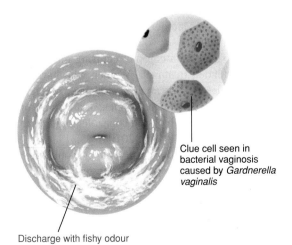

Clue cell seen in bacterial vaginosis caused by *Gardnerella vaginalis*

Discharge with fishy odour

FIGURE 4.9 Bacterial vaginosis. (From Anatomical Chart Company. [2002]. *Atlas of pathophysiology*. Springhouse, PA: Springhouse.)

Collaborative Management

Oral metronidazole or clindamycin cream is usually prescribed to treat symptomatic bacterial vaginosis. Asymptomatic bacterial vaginosis should be treated in high-risk pregnancy when there is a history of preterm delivery, prior to IUD insertion, and prior to gynecologic surgery, therapeutic abortion, or upper tract instrumentation (PHAC, 2010a). Clients in the first trimester of pregnancy should be treated with clindamycin because metronidazole is contraindicated; topical clindamycin has been associated with adverse outcomes in the newborn when used during pregnancy.

Bacterial vaginosis has been linked to premature rupture of membranes, premature labour and birth, and postpartum endometriosis. It also is associated with an increased risk for HIV infection (PHAC, 2010a). Treatment of male sexual partners is not recommended and does not prevent recurrence (PHAC, 2010a).

Recall Lela, the young woman described at the beginning of the chapter who is complaining of a vaginal discharge. What information would the nurse need to obtain to determine whether Lela is experiencing bacterial vaginosis?

TRICHOMONIASIS

The cause of **trichomoniasis** is the protozoan parasite *Trichomonas vaginalis*. Women with multiple partners are more likely to acquire the infection. Trichomoniasis is silent and asymptomatic in up to 50% of cases (PHAC, 2010a).

Assessment Findings

If symptoms do occur, they usually appear within 1 week of exposure, although they may appear as late as 6 months later. The infection is usually in the urethra or under the foreskin of uncircumcised men; symptoms include a thin, whitish discharge from the penis, and painful, difficult urination. In women, the parasites infect the vagina, urethra, bladder, or cervix (SOGC, 2012). About 50% of affected women will display symptoms including vaginal odour, vaginal discharge, dyspareunia, dysuria, and irritation or itchiness of the vagina (see Fig. 4.10).

Physical examination or laboratory testing are used to detect the parasite and confirm the diagnosis.

Collaborative Management

Both sexual partners should receive treatment together, even if no symptoms appear. Single-dose metronidazole remains the preferred regimen, although it may be prescribed twice a day for 7 days. Clients should abstain from alcohol consumption during treatment, because

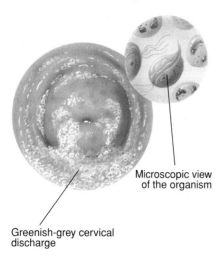

Microscopic view
of the organism

Greenish-grey cervical
discharge

FIGURE 4.10 Trichomoniasis. (From Anatomical Chart Company. [2002]. *Atlas of pathophysiology*. Springhouse, PA: Springhouse.)

the combination of metronidazole and alcohol can cause severe nausea and vomiting. To avoid recurrence, partners should not engage in sex if either has not completed treatment or while either continues to display symptoms. Condoms should be worn to prevent transmission.

Pregnant clients commonly experience recurrences of trichomoniasis, which can result in premature rupture of the membranes and preterm birth. Low birth weight and genital and lung infections in the newborn also can result.

YEAST INFECTION

Yeast infections (**candidiasis**) commonly cause vaginal irritation in women. Almost all women have *Candida albicans* in the vagina in small numbers; symptoms develop only when there is overgrowth. It is not usually considered to be sexually transmitted, although it is more common in women who are sexually active.

Overgrowth of *C. albicans* follows a disruption of the normal vaginal ecosystem. Candida or thrush can also appear in the mouth and gut. Factors contributing to yeast infection include pregnancy, use of antibiotics and corticosteroids, immunosuppression, and poorly controlled diabetes.

Assessment Findings

The most common symptoms in women include itching, dysuria, and dyspareunia. Thick or watery vaginal discharge resembling cottage cheese appears (Fig. 4.11). Up to 20% of women are asymptomatic (PHAC, 2010a).

History and physical examination are usually insufficient for diagnosis. Gram stain and microscopic examination of a swab sampling from the upper vagina or cervix may diagnose and confirm yeast forms. Home screening kits can also test for yeast infections.

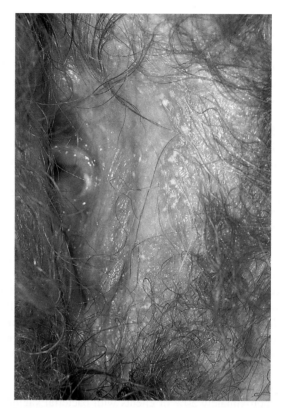

FIGURE 4.11 Overgrowth of *Candida albicans*.

Collaborative Management

Treatment is recommended only for symptomatic clients and their sexual partners. Several over-the-counter (OTC) oral and suppository antifungal vaginal medications (eg, clotrimazole, miconazole) can serve as remedies. Nevertheless, it is important for those infected to visit their clinician because some OTC products contain antihistamines that can mask the disorder. Clients with HIV are treated the same way as those who do not have HIV. However, in situations of recurrence or more severe cases, therapy may be more aggressive and longer-term.

Recurrent candidiasis is difficult to manage. Infected clients must avoid other infections and their catalysts. Those with chronic recurring infections may require extended treatment. Women who have four or more episodes in a 12-month period, have severe candidiasis, have a non-albicans species, or are compromised should be treated with oral fluconazole, topical azole, or boric acid capsules (PHAC, 2010a).

To prevent candidiasis, all women should wipe their genitalia from front to back and ensure that the genital area remains clean and dry. They also should avoid wearing nylon pants, tights, pantyhose, and tight jeans, and refrain from using vaginal deodorants, perfumed soap, and bubble bath. Moreover, when douching, using vaginal tampons, and engaging in sexual intercourse, clients should avoid vaginal trauma. Nursing Care Plan 4.1 highlights the care of a client with a yeast infection.

NURSING CARE PLAN 4.1

●

The Client With a Vaginal Infection

 Think back to Lela, the 33-year-old client who comes to the clinic for evaluation of her vaginal discharge. She reports douching daily since the discharge started. Further assessment reveals a white vaginal discharge of cottage cheese consistency. The vulva and vaginal area are red and irritated. Lela complains of burning and some pain on urination. "It's been a terrible week. First I had gone to the dentist for an abscessed tooth and he gave me a prescription for an antibiotic which I've been taking. Now this." Specimen obtained for culture reveals *Candida albicans.*

NURSING DIAGNOSES

- **Impaired Tissue Integrity** related to vaginal infection and resultant irritation and redness
- **Deficient Knowledge** related to measures to prevent infection and reduce the risk for recurrent infection

EXPECTED OUTCOMES

1. The client will experience no further vaginal irritation.
2. The client will report that redness and irritation have decreased, rating it as 3 out of 10.
3. The client will exhibit signs and symptoms of resolving infection.
4. The client will state situations that increase the risk for yeast infection.
5. The client will identify measures to maintain vaginal integrity and health.

INTERVENTIONS	RATIONALES
Assess the client's perineal area for redness, irritation, and drainage.	Assessment provides a baseline from which to develop an individualized plan of care.
Ask the client to rate her level of discomfort on a scale of 1 to 10.	Quantifying the level of discomfort helps determine measures to relieve it.
Assist the client in cleaning the perineal area with warm soap and water. Instruct her to perform frequent perineal care.	Cleaning the area removes vaginal discharge that irritates the mucosa.
Encourage the client to wipe the area using a front to back motion.	This motion prevents contamination of the vaginal area.
Discuss with the client factors that can contribute to yeast infections such as medications, douching, perfumed feminine hygiene sprays, and tight, poorly-ventilated clothing.	Knowledge of contributing factors helps the client begin measures to control them.
Instruct the client to wear cotton underwear and avoid nylon pants, tights, and jeans. Encourage her to refrain from using vaginal deodorants, perfumed soaps, and bubble baths.	Cotton underwear allows air to circulate, reducing the risk for a dark, moist environment conducive to organism growth. Nylon pants, pantyhose, tights, and tight jeans interfere with air circulation. Substances such as vaginal deodorants and soaps contain ingredients that can irritate the mucosa.
Instruct the client to avoid douching.	Douching can alter the vaginal pH, which could lead to an overgrowth of organisms.

(continued)

NURSING CARE PLAN 4.1 ● The Client With a Vaginal Infection *(Continued)*

INTERVENTIONS	RATIONALES
Encourage the client to have her sexual partner treated.	Recurrent infection can occur if the client engages in sex with an infected partner.
Administer antifungal agent as ordered; teach client about antifungal agent prescribed and how to administer.	Antifungal agents typically are used to treat symptomatic women and their infected partners.
Advise the client to monitor the amount and characteristics of her vaginal discharge. Instruct her to report an increase in drainage amount or odour, an increase in irritation, or continued burning or pain on urination.	Candidiasis can become a recurrent or chronic infection that requires extended treatment.
Arrange for a follow-up visit in 1 to 2 weeks.	A follow-up visit allows for evaluation of the infection and adherence to the treatment regimen.

EVALUATION

1. The client reports that redness and irritation have subsided, rating the discomfort at a level of 3 or less.
2. The client states that vaginal discharge has ceased.
3. The client accurately identifies situations that increase her risk for infection.
4. The client demonstrates appropriate measures to keep the vaginal area free of infection.

HUMAN IMMUNODEFICIENCY VIRUS

HIV attacks and impairs the immune system by destroying CD4+ T lymphocytes. It may lead to a chronic progressive disease, which leaves the individual prone to serious infections and cancer. The advanced stage of the disease, *acquired immunodeficiency syndrome* (AIDS), is characterized by a severely impaired immune system. Once an individual is infected, HIV can be transmitted to others through unprotected anal and vaginal sexual contact, sex toys that are used internally, from mother to baby through pregnancy and breast milk, and through sharing needles or syringes for IV drug or steroid use. Unprotected oral sex (unless there are open sores or cuts present), re-using/sharing needles for activities such as tattooing or skin piercing, and occupational exposure are considered low risk activities for the transmission of HIV, although they may be high risk activities for the transmission of other blood-borne infections (PHAC, 2010a). Because it may take years for symptoms to appear, HIV may be transmitted to others without the individuals even being aware that they are infected.

Often, HIV is associated with other STIs because it is transferred more easily with coexistent infections.

The number of Canadians with a positive HIV test has steadily decreased since 2008; the number of annual HIV cases reported for 2012 was the lowest since reporting began in 1985, although it is estimated that 24% of people living in Canada with HIV are unaware that they are infected (PHAC, 2013a, 2013f). Men who had sex with men (MSM) initially accounted for nearly all positive HIV test reports. Both the number and proportion of those exposed through heterosexual contact continues to increase and is now the second largest exposure category in men and the largest exposure category for women (PHAC, 2013f). Individuals who migrate to Canada from areas of endemic HIV also represent an increasing proportion of positive HIV tests. Cases of HIV in women continue to rise, and pregnant clients can spread the virus to their fetus (see Chap. 13).

HIV destroys CD4 cells (helper T cells), which are crucial to normal function of the immune system that helps the body ward off infection and disease. Acquired immune deficiency syndrome (AIDS) occurs when the body becomes immunocompromised to the extent that it is no longer able to fight infection (Government of Canada, 2013c).

Assessment Findings

Symptoms of HIV include lack of energy or fatigue, weight loss, frequent low-grade fevers or night sweats, skin rashes, and lymphadenopathy. Many women with HIV/AIDS experience vaginal yeast infections and other STIs, PID, and menstrual cycle changes.

HIV testing in Canada is voluntary and based on informed consent. The INSTI® HIV-1 is the rapid, point-of-care test approved for use in Canada, taking about 2 minutes to produce a result that has been shown to have 99.6% specificity (those healthy individuals correctly identified as HIV-negative using this test) (Tooley, 2010a). When the test comes back reactive it is then sent to a laboratory for confirmation (Tooley, 2010a). The enzyme immunoassay (EIA) test, which detects the presence of HIV antibodies in blood, is used for HIV testing in laboratories (Tooley, 2010a). If HIV antibodies are detected, a confirmatory Western blot test is done prior to release of the results to rule out a false positive result (Tooley, 2010a). This takes approximately 2 weeks. It takes up to approximately 3 months for the body to produce sufficient antibodies that can be detected by either the rapid test or the EIA test (Tooley, 2010b). Within this window, testing may produce a negative result, even though the individual may actually be infected with HIV. For those who test negative within that window, retesting 3 months after exposure will fully rule out HIV infection (Tooley, 2010b).

Two tests (the p24 antigen test and the HIV NAT test) have been developed to detect HIV directly; however, these are not uniformly available across Canada (Tooley, 2010b). When available, these tests are used for individuals who have had recent exposure or who are experiencing symptoms of a new HIV infection.

All pregnant women should be offered confidential HIV testing and counselling as part of routine prenatal care at their first prenatal visit (Keenan-Lindsay & Yudin, 2006). Individuals who test positive for HIV should also be screened for hepatitis B infection and immunity, hepatitis A immunity, hepatitis C infection, syphilis and other STIs, and tuberculosis, since these infections may occur concurrently with HIV.

Collaborative Management

Individuals who are asymptomatic are usually followed at 3- to 6-month intervals if no treatment is initiated. Clients with HIV/AIDS receive antiretroviral medications and supportive care during opportunistic infections. They should receive pneumococcal, hepatitis A and B, and yearly influenza vaccines. Additional treatment measures involve managing anorexia, diarrhea, weight loss, and side effects of medications.

Antiretroviral-Drug Therapy

There is no cure for HIV; however, treatment advances have improved quality and length of life. Individuals may not require treatment right away. Once the benefits of treatment outweigh the benefits of no treatment, highly active antiretroviral (HAART) therapy is started. It reduces the ability of the virus to replicate itself, increasing CD4 cell counts and reducing other symptoms. Reverse transcriptase inhibitors interfere with the viral genetic replication, while protease inhibitors inhibit the ability of HIV to leave its host. Antiretroviral drugs approved for use in Canada include nucleoside reverse transcriptase inhibitors (NRTIs) (eg, zidovudine [AZT], lamivudine [3TC], stavudine [d4T]); nucleotide reverse transcriptase inhibitors (NtRTIs) (eg, tenofovir); nonnucleoside reverse transcriptase inhibitors (NNRTIs) (eg, efavirenz, nevirapine); protease inhibitors (PIs) (eg, nelfinavir, saquinavir, ritonavir, atazanavir); and fusion inhibitors (eg, enfuvirtide/T20) (PHAC, 2013a). Other antiretroviral drugs and immune-based therapies to boost CD4 counts are still in clinical trials (PHAC, 2010a).

Opinions about when to initiate drug therapy vary. The goal of drug therapy is to suppress viral replication to the point where plasma RNA is not detectable, while minimizing toxicity in the client (PHAC, 2010a). Monotherapy and dual therapy should be avoided, as these have been associated with drug resistance (PHAC, 2010a).

Care of Opportunistic Infections

Many opportunistic infections that develop as a consequence of the weakened immunity that is secondary to HIV/AIDS are fatal. For example, HIV-positive clients are at an increased risk for Pneumocystis jiroveci (formerly carinii) pneumonia, which can lead to respiratory failure. Mechanical ventilation may be necessary, as well as deep suctioning and aerosol therapy to clear the lungs of thick sputum. Trimethoprim-sulfamethoxazole (Bactrim, Septra) taken daily or three times a week is the preferred prophylactic treatment, while dapsone, atovaquone, or aerosolized pentamidine isethionate (NebuPent) may be used as alternates. These drugs are also indicated for oral candidiasis (see earlier discussion) and Toxoplasma gondii (except for aerosolized pentamidine).

Another opportunistic infection in HIV is cytomegalovirus (CMV), which may infect the eyes, leading to blindness, as well as affecting the gastrointestinal system. Prophylactic treatment is not currently recommended (PHAC, 2010a). Instead, individuals with low CD4 counts who are at the highest risk should be aware of symptoms of CMV, including visual changes (eg, visual distortions, floaters), and should have regular fundoscopic examinations every 4 to 6 months.

Client Teaching

Nurses provide health teaching and counselling to high-risk populations about HIV/AIDS. They emphasize prevention strategies such as abstinence and safer sex (sexual activities in which body fluids are not exchanged). They encourage active injection-drug users to discontinue drug use (this may necessitate a referral to addiction treatment services); the individual who is not ready, willing, or able is provided information on harm reduction strategies (eg, not sharing needles, safer modes of drug use, needle exchange programs). Nurses encourage testing among clients with a history of risky behaviours and help clients interpret diagnostic test results and assist with ongoing monitoring in the months after potential exposure.

For clients with HIV, nurses explain the mechanisms of each drug and help clients develop a schedule for self-administration. Nurses emphasize the importance of rigidly adhering to the medication regimen to avoid contributing to drug resistance. Because many of these medications have challenging and debilitating side effects, the nurse warns clients of what to expect, while stressing the necessity of never discontinuing any prescribed drugs without first consulting the primary care provider. Women who are infected with HIV should not breastfeed. Further educational components for clients living with HIV are found in Teaching Tips 4.4.

Clients with HIV should be reminded of their ethical-legal responsibility in informing past, present, and future sexual partners about their HIV-positive status. Individuals should also inform those with whom they may engage in other risk-taking behaviours. HIV is currently reportable in all jurisdictions in Canada.

HEPATITIS

Hepatitis, an inflammation of the liver, results from different viruses that can be transmitted in a variety of ways, including sexually. This section focuses on types A, B, and C.

Hepatitis A

Hepatitis A virus (HAV) is one of the main causes of hepatitis in adults, accounting for 20% to 40% of cases. HAV is typically transmitted by exposure to water or food products contaminated with HAV (primarily from feces containing the virus) (Canadian Liver Foundation [CLF], 2012a). Those at increased risk include those living with someone newly infected with HAV, inmates in prisons or jails, injection drug users, international travellers to regions where it is common, and who have sex involving oral or anal contact (CLF, 2012a). Infected clients develop future immunity against this infection. The incubation period typically lasts 28 to 30 days, although it can range from 15 to 50 days (CLF, 2012a).

Assessment Findings

Signs and symptoms include anorexia, low-grade fever, weakness, headache, upper abdominal pain, dark urine, and jaundice. Adults often exhibit more severe symptoms than children, who may show no outward signs of the infection other than feeling unwell (CLF, 2012a). Clients with HAV neither develop chronic liver disease nor become carriers. Blood tests are used for diagnosis.

Collaborative Management

To date, there is no effective treatment. Individuals are encouraged to rest, perform safe hygiene practices (eg, hand washing after toilet use), maintain adequate hydration, and avoid alcohol and medications metabolized in the liver. Hepatitis A vaccine is the preferred method of pre-exposure immunoprophylaxis. A combination vaccine for hepatitis A and B is also available. Vaccination is recommended for people travelling to countries such as Africa, Asia, Latin America, or Eastern Europe, where HAV is common; those engaging in anal or oral sex; IV

● TEACHING TIPS 4.4   Living With HIV

For clients with HIV who are managing their conditions on an outpatient basis, the nurse emphasizes the following educational points:

- Strictly follow the medication schedule. Never omit, decrease, or increase doses without receiving approval from your primary care provider.
- Take the antiviral medications around meals. Eat small, frequent, and well-balanced meals. Drink plenty of water.
- Check your weight weekly, and report any weight loss or appetite loss promptly.
- Avoid people with infections, including colds.

- Notify the primary care provider if you show any signs of infection.
- Wash food before cooking. Do not eat any raw meat, fish, or vegetables, which may carry dangerous pathogens.
- Separate your laundry from others, especially if the bedding and clothes are soiled with body secretions.
- Avoid smoking.
- Maintain high standards of personal hygiene.
- Avoid extreme temperatures and environmental conditions.
- Rest frequently.
- Do not share needles or donate blood.

drug users; daycare and institutional workers; and people with chronic liver diseases (CLF, 2012a).

Hepatitis B

Hepatitis B virus (HBV) is the most common strain of hepatitis in the world (CLF, 2012b). Although there is no data on the incidence in Canada, it is estimated that between 0.7% and 0.9% of Canada's population has chronic HBV (PHAC, 2010b). Highly contagious, it is about 100 times more infectious than HIV (PHAC, 2010b). Modes of transmission include sexual contact and contact with blood (eg, through shared contaminated needles or personal care articles and accidental needle pricks) or body fluids. It is not spread by water, food, or casual contact. Women can also transmit HBV to their newborns during childbirth. The incubation period for HBV is 2 to 6 months.

Assessment Findings

HBV is asymptomatic in up to 50% of adults and most children (CLF, 2012b; PHAC, 2010b); adults may display fatigue, generalized aches, appetite loss, abdominal pain, and jaundice. In chronic infection, the disease may be inactive or clients may develop liver damage, liver cancer, liver failure, or death (CLF, 2012b).

Blood tests can detect immunity, or the presence of the virus (acute or chronic infection). A positive antibody test (anti-HBs) indicates immunity acquired either by a past infection from which the individual has completely recovered or successful immunization with the hepatitis B vaccine. A positive antigen test (HBsAG) indicates that the HBV is present and that the individual is infectious. If the individual has a positive HBsAG for more than 6 months, this indicates chronic (carrier) status. The risk of becoming a chronic carrier varies inversely with the age at which the infection occurs. Less than 5% of those who acquire it in adulthood become carriers (CLF, 2012b).

Collaborative Management

HBV has no cure. Treatment includes interferon and antiviral medications (CLF, 2012b). Hepatitis B immune globulin is given to anyone who has had recent contact (7 days or less) with infected blood or body fluids. HBV vaccination is available for at-risk groups. In addition, most provinces have school-based programs for children up to the age of 15 years.

Hepatitis C

It is estimated that hepatitis C virus (HCV) currently infects an estimated 242,500 Canadians, with approximately 21% of those being unaware that they have it (PHAC, 2010b). This RNA virus, first discovered in 1989, is spread by direct contact with the blood of an infected person through injection of drugs (causing at least half of the infections), tattooing and piercing with unsterile equipment, and sharing toothbrushes or razors with an infected person. The risk of getting the virus through blood transfusion is low in Canada, because of universal testing of all blood donors since 1990. However, those individuals who received blood or an organ transplant prior to July 1990 are at an increased risk of having been exposed to HCV. Infrequently, the disease is transmitted through sexual contact, usually when blood is present, and from mother to fetus during gestation. Breastfeeding does not appear to transmit HCV, unless the mother's nipples are cracked or bleeding. The incubation period for HCV is 6 to 7 weeks.

Assessment Findings

Hepatitis C is generally a silent disease, with many affected people showing no symptoms and feeling quite healthy (CLF, 2012c). When symptoms occur, they include jaundice, fatigue, abdominal pain, loss of appetite, and nausea (CLF, 2012c). Approximately 25% of people infected with HCV have a mild, brief form of the disease, and get rid of the virus completely; 75% carry the virus indefinitely (CLF, 2012c). Of those who are long-term carriers, about 25% are at an increased risk for profound fatigue, cirrhosis, liver failure, and liver cancer (CLF, 2012c).

The majority of people are unaware that they have the disease, sometimes carrying the virus for decades. Diagnosis is based on laboratory blood test analysis. Liver function studies also help determine the extent of the disease and liver functioning.

Collaborative Management

Although there is no biomedical cure for hepatitis, options are available to control the disease. Pharmacologic treatment consists of long-acting pegylated interferon and ribavirin (CLF, 2012c). Two new drugs (boceprevir and telaprevir) that are protease inhibitors have recently been approved by Health Canada for treatment in clients with genotype 1 (CLF, 2012c). Symptoms are treated with rest and supportive care. Clients should be counselled to maintain a healthy diet, get adequate rest, employ stress-reduction techniques, avoid sharing needles or syringes, use condoms, and especially to avoid alcohol. Those receiving hormonal therapy (estrogen) or oral contraceptives may be advised to discontinue use until normal liver function returns. No herbal remedies have been found to be effective (CLF, 2012c).

BENIGN BREAST DISORDERS

Women experience breast changes throughout their lives, beginning with gestation and continuing past menopause (Canadian Breast Cancer Foundation [CBCF],

2014d). In many cultures, breasts symbolize femininity and help form each woman's self-image. Throughout history, female breasts have been associated with sexuality, erotica, fashion, beauty, and art. Breasts also have associations related to their important role in nourishing babies.

Breast disorders can affect both physical and psychological health (Hill et al., 2011; Kyranou et al., 2013). They can cause problems with body image and self-esteem.

Breast assessments during routine health care visits and routine physical examination are an important part of a woman's health maintenance. Clients who practice breast awareness are in a better position to detect lumps early in their progression, which enhances rates of breast cancer detection, early treatment, and survival (CBCF, 2014a). See Chapter 2 for more information on breast health promotion and screening strategies.

Common benign breast conditions in women include pain (**mastalgia**), infections, fibrocystic changes, fibroadenoma, and nipple discharge.

BREAST PAIN (MASTALGIA)

Breast pain is usually nonspecific. It is common, occurring in almost 75% of women at some point in their reproductive lives (Parsay et al., 2009). Some causes that have been hypothesized include hormonal changes, fat necrosis, or duct ectasia (blockage and inflammation of the lactiferous ducts), breast cysts, fibrocystic breast changes, water retention, and nutritional changes; the exact cause is unknown (Canadian Cancer Society [CCS], 2014a; Parsay et al., 2009).

Assessment Findings

Clients with mastalgia usually complain of diffuse breast tenderness or heaviness. They may experience pain cyclically or continuously. Cyclic pain suggests hormonal sensitivity and often coincides with the menstrual cycle. Continuous pain is usually unilateral and may be felt specifically in one section of the breast. This type of pain is usually anatomic in nature. Both cyclic and continuous pain can be related to a mass, cyst, or thickening in the breast. All complaints and findings should be evaluated with mammogram or ultrasound.

Collaborative Management

Once cancer has been ruled out, treatment may consist of relieving the pain with NSAIDs, hormonal therapy (eg, oral contraceptives), evening primrose oil, vitamin E, tamoxifen, or danazol (CCS, 2014a; Parsay et al., 2009). Reduced intake of caffeine, chocolate, sodium, and dietary fat, as well as use of a good supporting bra, also have been found to help alleviate symptoms (CCS, 2014a).

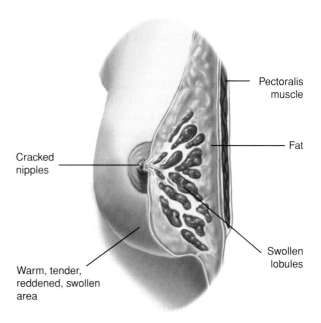

FIGURE 4.12 Mastitis.

BREAST INFECTIONS

Breast infection (**mastitis**) usually occurs in a localized area (see Fig. 4.12). Many lactating women experience mastitis (see Chapters 19 and 21). The etiology is usually staphylococci, which enter the breast through cracked or fissured nipples. Signs and symptoms include redness, pain, and tenderness on palpation.

Mastitis is usually treated with antibiotics. Lactating women are encouraged to continue to nurse. Nurses should instruct them to use a breast shield or hand pump until the pain subsides. Those with a breast abscess or purulent drainage should discard their milk and discontinue nursing until the infection clears.

Lactating women should receive breastfeeding education before beginning nursing, so they can be prepared for this potential complication. They should be aware that they should seek medical attention at the first sign of any infection. In the event that the woman does not respond to antibiotic therapy and the infection continues, she should be evaluated for inflammatory breast cancer.

FIBROCYSTIC CHANGES

Most of the changes that occur in women's breasts are benign. Many changes are age-related and include the development of excess fibrous tissue (thickening of breast tissue), cyst formation, hyperplasia of the epithelial lining of the mammary ducts, and proliferation of the primary ducts resulting in lumpy breasts (Fig. 4.13).

Assessment Findings

Pain or tenderness on a cyclic or episodic basis may result from nerve irritation caused by connective tissue

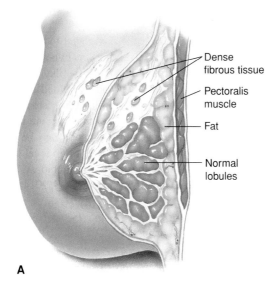

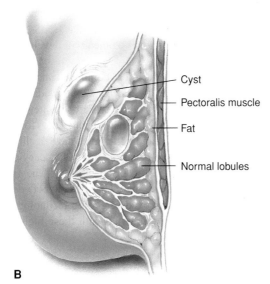

FIGURE 4.13 **A:** Fibrocystic breast changes. **B:** Breast cysts. (From Anatomical Chart Company. [2002]. *Atlas of pathophysiology.* Springhouse, PA: Springhouse.)

edema and fibrous nerve pinching. Most masses or nodular ties are bilateral and found in the upper outer quadrant (axilla area). The incidence is higher in perimenopausal women 35 to 50 years old and is related to changes and imbalances in estrogen and progestin. Most of these changes subside after menopause among women who do not receive estrogen replacement therapy (CCS, 2014a; St. Michael's Hospital, 2014).

Screening methods may include clinical breast examination, mammography, and ultrasound evaluation when the breast tissue is very dense to differentiate cystic masses from solid masses. The fluid in the cysts may be aspirated and examined for neoplastic cell changes. Most women with fibrocystic changes are not at an increased risk for breast cancer. A small percentage of women with

fibrocystic changes that result from hyperplasia, however, do appear to be at an increased risk for breast cancer (CCS, 2014a; St Michael's Hospital, 2014).

Collaborative Management

Treatment may include surgical removal of the mass, if indicated. Management consists of using good support bras and dietary and medicinal therapies. Dietary management may include restriction of sodium and caffeine (found in coffee, chocolate, and caffeinated beverages) (CCS, 2014a).

Pharmacologic management may consist of vitamin E, analgesics, danazol, diuretics, and hormone therapy. Client education is a primary nursing intervention in the care of women with mastalgia and fibrocystic breast changes. Women should be encouraged to have regular clinical breast examinations throughout their lives. Education should include reassurance that cysts do not increase risk of breast cancer and that most women experience recurrences of fibrocystic changes until menopause.

FIBROADENOMA

Fibroadenoma occurs frequently in women between 20 and 30 years of age. A **fibroadenoma** is a firm, mobile, solitary, painless breast tumour with well-defined borders (CCS, 2014a) (see Fig. 4.14). These masses are usually found during physical examination or are noted during mammography. Biopsy and tissue examination confirm the diagnosis. Screening techniques include mammography, ultrasound, and fine-needle aspiration.

Nursing care includes client education regarding procedures and tests, and reassurance about the benign

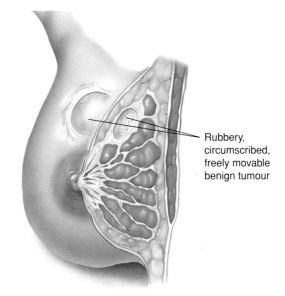

FIGURE 4.14 Fibroadenoma. (From Anatomical Chart Company. [2002]. *Atlas of pathophysiology.* Springhouse, PA: Springhouse.)

nature of these masses. Once again, women should be encouraged to be breast aware and have their health care practitioner perform regular routine clinical breast examinations as a follow-up measure.

NIPPLE DISCHARGE

Nipple discharge (fluid emission from the mammary nipple) is a common complaint that may be a manifestation of a more serious underlying disorder, such as a pituitary lesion, hypothyroidism, or substance use (Fig. 4.15). Usually, the woman reports nipple discharge to her primary health care provider, who must identify the type and rule out pathology, especially cancer (Hussain et al., 2006).

Also called *galactorrhea, physiologic discharge* results from drug therapy, endocrine problems, and neural disorders. It is bilateral and may be milky white or multicoloured and is not usually part of a disease. It requires reassurance and counselling. Treatment includes identifying the underlying cause.

Benign pathologic discharge may be related to cystic disease, intraductal papilloma, and ductal ectasia, which are related to inflammatory responses caused by stagnation of breast duct secretions and breast infections. *Intraductal papillomas* are growths in the mammary ducts that often emit a bloody discharge. They usually occur in women 40 to 60 years old. Treatment for them consists of surgical excision. *Ductal ectasia* occurs in both premenopausal and postmenopausal women and is not associated with malignancy. The discharge can be bloody, brown, cream coloured, grey, green, purulent, or white; it may be sticky, thick, or thin. It usually is painless, but some women complain of burning, itching, and pain around the nipple. Some women also experience swelling in the alveolar area. Symptoms may become more pronounced with advanced disease. Treatment consists of warm compresses, antibiotic therapy, and

close follow-up. Surgical excision of the involved ducts also may be indicated.

Pathologic discharge may be related to tumours of the pituitary gland, Addison disease, and hypothyroidism. Discharge may be bilateral and of thin, milky white colour, but generally is unilateral and is emitted from one duct orifice. The colour can be serous, pink, serosanguineous, or bloody. These lesions are small and are usually not detected on mammography. Diagnosis may be based on mammography, ductography, serum hormonal levels, cytologic examination of the discharge, and biopsy. Treatment depends on the underlying cause (CCS, 2014a).

MALIGNANT BREAST DISORDERS

Breast cancer is one of the most frightening conditions for women. Estimates are that, in 2013, approximately 5,000 Canadian women will die from breast cancer, with more than 23,800 new cases diagnosed (CCS, 2014b). One in every nine Canadian women will develop breast cancer in her lifetime (PHAC, 2013b).

Breast cancer is the most common cancer among women over the age of 20 years in Canada (CBCF, 2014a) and accounts for about 26% of all new cancer cases in women (CCS, 2014b). Incidence rates for breast cancer have stabilized and death rates have declined by 42% over the past two decades (Breast Cancer Society of Canada [BCSC], 2013; CBCF, 2014a). The largest increase in survival has been in women between 50 and 69 years old. Improved screening technology and advanced treatment are credited with these higher survival rates (CBCF, 2014b).

BREAST CANCER

Breast cancer is a malignancy that usually originates in the duct or epithelium of the lobes. One of the most lethal forms is inflammatory breast cancer, discussed at the end of this section.

Risk Factors

Risk factors associated with breast cancer include gender, increasing age, personal history of breast cancer, benign breast disorder, family history (ie, first-degree relatives), genetic predisposition (carrying mutated BRCA1 and BRCA2 genes), reproductive history, early menstruation and late menopause, hormone replacement therapy (HRT), and being overweight after menopause (CBCF, 2014a; PHAC, 2013b). Some risk factors are modifiable and can be avoided; others, such as family history, cannot.

Although certain factors have been identified as posing risk, 70% of women who develop breast cancer have no identifiable risk factor (Breast Cancer Society of Canada, 2013). Modifying lifestyle patterns by increasing physical activity, reducing excess weight, avoiding

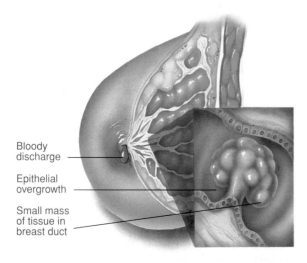

Bloody discharge

Epithelial overgrowth

Small mass of tissue in breast duct

FIGURE 4.15 Nipple discharge.

environmental factors, reducing alcohol intake and making dietary changes can help lower a woman's risk for breast cancer (CBCF, 2014b; Cummings et al., 2009). Early identification of risk factors can help women assume an active role in preventing breast cancer. Early detection of breast cancer can be lifesaving and can increase treatment options (CCS, 2014d).

Age

Age is the most important risk factor for many women. Eighty-two percent of breast cancer occurs in women older than 50 years (CBCF, 2014a). Even though the incidence of breast cancer is higher in aging women, they usually have no lymph node involvement. Although the incidence of breast cancer increases with age, approximately 18% of all new cases involve women who are under the age of 50 years; breast cancer diagnosed in younger women tends to move quickly to advanced stages (CBCF, 2014a).

Genetics

Two genes identified as associated with breast cancer are the **BRCA1** and **BRCA2** genes (see Chapter 2). Approximately 60% of women with alterations of these genes are at risk of developing breast cancer (CBCF, 2014c). This risk factor should be investigated when incidence of breast cancer in families is increased. Ovarian cancer also is associated with these genetic marker alterations (see later discussion).

A genetic predisposition to breast cancer may be suggested in the presence of

- Family members diagnosed with breast cancer prior to age 35 years
- Family members diagnosed with ovarian cancer at any age
- Multiple family members diagnosed with breast or ovarian cancer
- A male family member with breast cancer
- Family members with breast cancer in both breasts or with breast and ovarian cancer
- Ashkenazi Jewish ancestry (CBCF, 2014c)

Reproductive History

Reproductive history also contributes to the risk for breast cancer. Nulliparous women and women who have their first pregnancy after age 35 years are at an increased risk (CBCF, 2014c; PHAC, 2013b). Researchers have also established age at menarche and age at menopause as potential risk factors. Women who experience menarche before 12 years or menopause after 55 years appear to be at an increased risk (CBCF, 2014c; PHAC, 2013b). Evidence suggests that women have a lower risk of breast cancer if they breastfeed (Stuebe et al., 2009).

Other reproductive factors associated with the development of breast cancer include estrogen and diethylstilbestrol (DES) exposure. Women exposed to estrogen for a long period are at an increased risk for breast cancer. Therefore, estrogen and HRT have been called into question, with research providing evidence that these hormones place women at a greater risk for developing breast cancer (CBCF, 2014c). DES was used in the 1940s until the early 1970s to reduce spontaneous abortions in women with pregnancy complications. Recent research suggests that women who were exposed to DES may be at a higher risk for developing cancer, but there is still not enough information available to apply to daughters who may have been exposed to DES in utero (Hoover et al., 2011).

It has been reported that women with dense breasts (ie, breasts with a lot of connective and glandular tissue) are at an increased risk for breast cancer. Breast density can be measured by mammogram (CBCF, 2014c).

Oral contraceptives can lead to a small increase in the risk for breast cancer (PHAC, 2013b). However, after a number of years of not taking the pill, the woman's risk returns to approximately what it was prior to taking it (CBCF, 2014d).

Lifestyle

Being overweight increases a woman's risk for developing breast cancer, especially if the weight gain occurs in adulthood and the woman is postmenopausal (CBCF, 2014d; PHAC, 2013b). This is thought to be because of the production of estrogen in fat tissue. Increased physical activity has been associated with a decreased risk for breast cancer, although whether this is related solely to activity or in combination with other healthy behaviours is unclear. Recent research suggests that being physically active at any level of intensity combined with non-excessive weight gain throughout the childbearing and postmenopausal years may be the best preventive factor for reducing the risk of breast cancer (McCullough et al., 2012). Women who drink alcohol also may be at a slightly higher risk, with the risk increasing with greater consumption of alcohol (CBCF, 2014c; PHAC, 2013b). There is also an increased risk for women who start smoking or are exposed to secondhand smoke in adolescence (CBCF, 2014c).

Women who have been exposed to chest and breast radiation therapy are also at risk for breast cancer later in life (CBCF, 2014d; PHAC, 2013b).

 Remember Jade, the woman described at the beginning of the chapter who stated that her grandmother recently died of breast cancer. What other risk factors are present with Jade?

Assessment Findings

Signs and Symptoms

The most common sign of breast cancer is a painless breast mass, often in the upper outer quadrant. A breast mass can develop for as long as 2 years before becoming palpable. Other signs and symptoms include bloody nipple discharge, skin dimpling or thickening of the skin over the site of the lesion, nipple retraction, and bilateral difference in breast size. The lesion may be movable or fixed; lymph node enlargement in the adjacent axilla is possible.

Diagnostic Testing

Regular breast screening allows for early detection of breast cancer. Screening mammography and clinical breast examination are the most reliable methods of finding breast cancer before any symptoms develop (CCS, 2014d). In addition, being aware of how one's breasts normally look and feel allows the woman to notice any changes and have them checked by a doctor. See Chapter 2 for further discussion.

A change in the breast does not necessarily mean breast cancer; further diagnostic information is needed to determine this (CBCF, 2014e). A diagnostic mammogram examination, breast ultrasound, MRI, or biopsy may be necessary to assess for abnormal cell growth (CBCF, 2014e). Invasive diagnostic breast tests include fine-needle aspiration, core biopsy, or surgical biopsy (CBCF, 2014e).

Mammography. Diagnostic mammograms are similar to screening mammograms, although they may take longer (see Fig. 4.16 and Chapter 2).

Breast Ultrasound. Ultrasound may be used to determine whether a lump is a solid tumour or a fluid-filled cyst. It can also be used to visualize lumps that are not clear on a mammogram (CBCF, 2014e).

Fine-Needle Aspiration. A fine needle is inserted into the lump to remove fluid and cells, which are then sent to the laboratory for further analysis (CBCF, 2014e). While it can diagnose cancer, a fine-needle aspiration cannot determine whether or not the tumour is invasive.

Core Biopsy. A core biopsy removes a sample of affected breast cells and the tissue that surrounds them (CBCF, 2014e). This procedure can distinguish between invasive and non-invasive breast cancers (CBCF, 2014e). This procedure is usually done with local anaesthesia and may be done with x-ray or ultrasound guidance. Although clients may experience some temporary swelling, bleeding, minor bruising or pain, scarring is minimal, and most women can resume routine activities within 24 hours (CBCF, 2014e; Youngkin et al., 2012).

Surgical Biopsy. Surgical biopsy may include removal of all of the lump or suspicious tissue, as well as an area

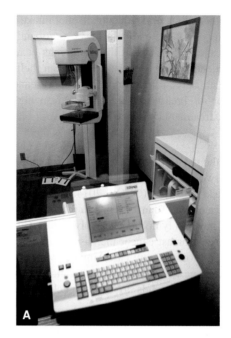

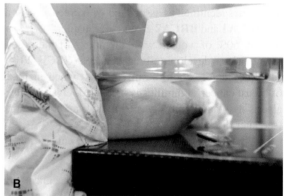

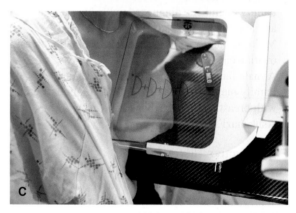

FIGURE 4.16 Mammography. **A:** Equipment. **B:** Top-to-bottom view of the breast. **C:** Side view of the breast.

of healthy tissue surrounding the lesion edges (rim), or it may include just the breast tissue that is needed for testing (CBCF, 2014e). The tissue is sent for microscopic histologic examination to check for cancer cells. The procedure may be done with either a local or general anaesthetic.

Collaborative Management

A wide range of treatment options is available to clients diagnosed with breast cancer. Providers usually suggest an individualized approach based on specific prognostic indicators. Factors that assist with clinical decisions include the overall health of the woman, the woman's personal decisions about certain treatments, lymph node status, tumour size, and metastases. Each of these factors is used to stage (Box 4.5) and grade (Box 4.6) the breast cancer. Treatment options are then offered, based on the clinical stage classification, the type of cancer, and other factors, such as overall health, her personal decision about certain treatments and if she has reached menopause (Canadian Cancer Society, 2014e). Two or more methods are often used in combination.

● BOX 4.5 Staging of Breast Cancer

Early (zero) stage: Atypical cells are localized in the breast tissue; no signs that they have spread to the lymph nodes

Stage 1: Tumour size less than 2 cm (approximately 1 inch); has not spread to surrounding lymph nodes or outside the breast

Stage 2: Divided into two groups, depending on the size of the tumour and whether or not it has spread to the lymph nodes:

- **2A:** Tumour less than 2 cm in cross section with spread to the lymph node, or tumour from 2 to 5 cm without spread to axillary lymph nodes
- **2B:** Tumour more than 5 cm in cross section (with the result of axillary lymph nodes research negative for cancer cells), or tumour from 2 to 5 cm in diameter with the involvement of axillary lymph nodes. Late (metastatic) stages of breast cancer occur when cancer cells spread to the lymph nodes and other tissues.

Stage 3: Also divided into two categories:

- **3A:** Tumour measures more than 5 cm with spread to axillary lymph nodes (local spread of breast cancer) or tumour of any size with metastases in axillary lymph nodes, which are woven to each other or with the adjacent tissues
- **3B:** Tumour (any size) with metastases into the skin, chest wall, or internal lymph nodes of mammary gland (found below the breast inside of the chest)

Stage 4: Defined by the spread of the cancer to other organs or tissues, such as the liver, lungs, brain, skeletal system, or lymph nodes near the collarbone

Source: Breast Cancer Society of Canada (2014). Stages Retrieved from http://www.bcsc.ca/p/40/l/99/t/Breast-Cancer-Society-of-Canada—Stages-of-Breast-Cancer

● BOX 4.6 Grading of Malignant Tumours

Grade	Description
GX	Grade cannot be assessed
G1	Low-grade, well-differentiated, slow-growing tumours
G2	Intermediate grade; moderately differentiated
G3	High grade; poorly differentiated; tend to grow quickly; more likely to spread
G4	High grade; undifferentiated; worse prognosis

Source: Canadian Cancer Society. (2014). About cancer. Retrieved from http://www.cancer.ca/en/cancer-information/diagnosis-and-treatment/staging-and-grading/tumour-grading/?region=on

Surgery

There are several options for surgical intervention. Breast-conserving surgery may include options such as a **lumpectomy** or wide local excision (which removes the tumour and a small amount of healthy tissue around it), partial or segmental mastectomy (which removes the tumour, some of the breast tissue around it and the lining over the chest muscles below the tumour), or a quadrantectomy which removes the tumour and about one fourth of the breast tissue (CCS, 2014f). Removal of the axillary lymph nodes is often done, either at the same time or during a later surgery, if they contain cancer. This option is used when the tumour is small enough to safely remove all the cancer and a margin of healthy tissue and is the client's choice. Radiation often follows surgery.

Mastectomy removes the entire breast or as much of it as possible. It may be recommended if the woman:

- Has had previous radiation to the chest wall or breast.
- Is pregnant.
- Has had breast conservation surgery done and the margin around the tumour is not considered clear of cancer.
- Is unable to lay flat or extend her arm during radiation.
- Has connective tissue or collagen vascular disease (eg, scleroderma, lupus).
- Has a lesion or tumour that is large in comparison to the size of the breast.
- Has cancer that occurs in more than one part of the breast.
- Has a small breast, and removal of the tumour would leave the breast very deformed or with very little breast tissue.
- Does not want radiation.
- Prefers mastectomy.

After a mastectomy, some women choose to have breast reconstruction surgery; others choose to wear

● TABLE 4.6   **Surgical Procedures for Breast Cancer**

Procedure	Description	Illustration
Lumpectomy or wide local excision	Only the tumour and a small amount of healthy tissue around it are removed.	Axillary dissection
Partial or segmental mastectomy	The tumour, some breast tissue, and the lining over the chest muscles below the tumour are removed.	
Simple or total mastectomy	All breast tissue, nipple, and some skin are removed. No lymph nodes or muscle under the breast are removed.	
Modified radical mastectomy	The entire breast, nipple, some axillary lymph nodes, and some skin are removed. The nerves and muscle under the breast are usually not removed.	

(continued)

● TABLE 4.6 **Surgical Procedures for Breast Cancer** (continued)

Procedure	Description	Illustration
Radical mastectomy	Rarely done. The breast, nipple, some axillary lymph nodes, skin, and the muscles under the breast are removed.	Pectoralis minor muscle Pectoralis major muscle

Adapted from Canadian Cancer Society. (2014). Surgery for breast cancer. Retrieved from http://www.cancer.ca/en/cancer-information/cancer-type/breast/treatment/surgery/?region=on#Mastectomy

a prosthesis. See Table 4.6 for more details about the levels of surgical procedures available for treating breast cancer.

Radiation Therapy

Radiation therapy is usually used in conjunction with breast-conserving surgery. It may be used following chemotherapy for women at an increased risk for metastasis. This type of therapy destroys any cancer cells that may remain after surgery and shrinks tumours if given before surgery (CBCF, 2014e). Women who receive radiation often experience adverse effects such as fatigue, leukopenia, discolouration (redness) of the skin, itching or peeling skin, and swelling and retraction of the breast, which usually go away within a few weeks to a few months after treatment ends (CBCF, 2014e). Radiation is not recommended during pregnancy.

Chemotherapy

Chemotherapy is used to control metastases and decrease the risk of recurrence. A multiagent approach, using more than one medication at a time, is typical. Chemotherapy is usually given in cycles every 3 to 4 weeks over 3 to 6 months (CBCF, 2014e).

Chemotherapy not only targets cancer cells but also affects normal cells. Short-term side effects include hair loss, fatigue, loss of appetite, nausea and vomiting, diarrhea, aching muscles and joints, memory disturbances, and mouth and lip sores (CBCF, 2014e). These effects gradually disappear after treatment is complete. Perimenopausal women may experience temporary or permanent infertility due to changes to their reproductive system associated with chemotherapy (CBCF, 2014e). Newer chemotherapeutic agents can help con-

trol side effects. Hair grows back after therapy is completed. Clients can be counselled to cut their hair short or to wear wigs, head coverings, and scarves during the treatment phase.

Long-term effects of chemotherapy may result in damage to the ovaries, infertility, and early menopause. Another effect is a weakened immune system, which puts the client at risk for infection. Women can receive counselling about avoiding infections and seeking medical attention promptly when they suspect one. Counselling and education also need to be provided regarding pregnancy risks. Women should avoid pregnancy during treatment because the effects of chemotherapy on the unborn child are unknown. Pregnancy after a course of chemotherapy depends on the client's age and type of drugs received.

Hormone Therapy

Hormone therapy prevents growth of cancer cells and controls metastasis and recurrence. This type of therapy is used to block the effects of estrogen when hormone receptor assays show that the breast tissue receptors are estrogen-positive (CBCF, 2014e). It is given after surgery, radiation therapy, and chemotherapy. Types of medications that may be given in hormone therapy include anti-estrogens, aromatase inhibitors, and ovarian suppressants. Tamoxifen is the most commonly used anti-estrogen. (Pharmacology Box 4.2). Other anti-estrogen medications that may be used include fulvestrant and raloxifene.

Aromatase is a natural substance that facilitates the production of estrogen in fat and other tissues in women after menopause (CBCF, 2014e). Aromatase inhibitors block the effect of aromatase, which reduces the amount of estrogen that the postmenopausal woman

● PHARMACOLOGY 4.2 Tamoxifen

ACTION

Tamoxifen is an anti-estrogen that blocks estrogen receptors on the cancer cells, thus preventing estrogen from activating the cells.

DOSAGE

20 mg daily, in divided doses, for 5 years

POSSIBLE ADVERSE EFFECTS

Hot flashes, weight gain, abnormal menstrual periods, vaginal discharge, nausea, and fatigue. Rare but serious side effects include blood clots, depression, reduced red and white blood cells and platelets, uterine cancer, and abnormal liver tests.

NURSING IMPLICATIONS

- Arrange for periodic blood counts because of the drug's effects on blood components and liver function.
- Instruct the woman to use contraception when taking tamoxifen because of possible effects on the fetus. Women should not breastfeed since it is not known if tamoxifen is excreted in breast milk.
- The client should have regular reproductive examinations because of potential effects on the reproductive system.
- Caution the client to report suspected side effects immediately.

From Ogbru, O., & Marks, J. (2012). Tamoxifen. *FDA Prescribing Information. MedicineNet.com.* Retrieved from http://www.medicinenet.com/tamoxifen/article.htm

produces. This therapy offers another option for preventing the effects of estrogen on the breast cell cancer estrogen receptors (CBCF, 2014e; Kesisis et al., 2009). Side effects of aromatase inhibitors include hot flashes, joint pain, muscle ache, fatigue, and osteoporosis.

For premenopausal women who produce most of their estrogen in the ovaries, ovarian suppression can decrease the amount of estrogen available to bind to the breast cell cancer estrogen receptors (CBCF, 2014e). This can be done by oophorectomy, radiation to the ovaries, or luteinizing hormone-releasing hormone agonists. While surgery and radiation are irreversible, the effects of medication may be reversible in some situations.

HER-2 Therapy

HER-2 therapy, or monoclonal antibody therapy, is used to strengthen and improve the immune system to fight cancer by interfering with the growth of some breast cancers (CBCF, 2014e). HER-2, a type of naturally occurring receptor, is believed to be involved in cell growth and proliferation. HER-2 positive cancers have more than the usual number of receptors and therefore tend to grow and spread more aggressively. Trastuzumab (Herceptin) binds to the HER-2 receptors and disrupts the growth of HER-2-positive cancer cells, resulting in slower growth of the cancer (CBCF, 2014e). Side effects may include fever, chills, and headache; these symptoms are usually less than those experienced with chemotherapy (CBCF, 2014e). Trastuzumab has also been associated with heart failure resulting in shortness of breath, swelling of the legs, and extreme fatigue. These symptoms require prompt medical attention.

COLLABORATIVE CARE: THE CLIENT WITH BREAST CANCER

Assessment

For all clients, health care providers identify their current knowledge level regarding being breast aware and their understanding of breast cancer and risks. When breast cancer is suspected or procedures for treatment have been established as necessary, the nurse discusses the client's medical, drug, allergy, and family history. The nurse may consider the framework that the client uses to seek and process the information as a way to facilitate information management (Loiselle et al., 2006). (Research Highlight 4.1). Further actions include taking the client's vital signs and weight, determining the location of the breast lesion, and establishing what diagnostic tests were performed before admission, if any. The nurse also reviews information the client has received about the type and extent of surgery or other treatment.

Select Potential Nursing Diagnosis

The following are examples of commonly applicable diagnoses:

- **Fear** related to situational crisis (cancer), threat to health/socioeconomic status, role functioning, interaction patterns
- **Risk for Impaired Tissue Integrity** related to surgical removal of tissues, altered circulation, edema, drainage, changes in skin elasticity, sensation, effects of chemotherapy and radiation, immunologic deficit, altered nutritional status, or anemia

● **RESEARCH HIGHLIGHT 4.1** The Searching, Processing, and Sharing of Breast Cancer Information by Women Diagnosed With the Illness

OBJECTIVE

Information-seeking has been reported to be a key strategy for women with breast cancer to cope with the demands of the illness. Few studies, however, have documented how women actually seek, process, and share cancer-related information.

DESIGN

A qualitative multiple-case design was used to examine how women diagnosed with breast cancer manage cancer-related information. The purpose of the study was to examine the process of information management from the perspective of women diagnosed with breast cancer, including women's interactions with others and the consequences of information management for adjustment outcomes. Twelve women between the ages of 43 to 88 years, at various stages of breast cancer, and from a variety of ethnic backgrounds participated in semi-structured interviews. Interpretative analysis was used to analyze the data.

RESULTS

Information management by women with breast cancer can be conceptualized as a four-component process. "Informational triggers," women's initial exposure to breast cancer-related informant and/or cancer-related events, prompted them to react and begin seeking or avoiding information. "Reactions to knowing" included information-seeking and filtering, sharing information, holding back, crying together, and sharing fears. Through "selective disclosure" women made decisions about the kinds of cancer-related information to be shared, when, and with whom; during this time they assessed whether significant others were supportive and whether they would continue to share information with them. Information outcomes for the women ranged between relieved, hopeful, supported, and distressed.

CONCLUSION

While studies have examined how women with breast cancer seek cancer-related information, the process that is used in this information seeking has not previously been studied. The process of information management was very real for this sample of women, and included four main components. The findings also highlight the intricate ways that information is managed with significant others.

From Loiselle, C. G., Lambert, S. D., & Cooke, A. (2006). The searching, processing, and sharing of breast cancer information by women diagnosed with the illness. *Canadian Journal of Nursing Research*, *38*(3), 82–104.

- **Pain (Acute)** related to surgical procedure, tissue trauma, disease process, side effects of various cancer therapies
- **Risk for Situational Low Self-Esteem** related to disfiguring surgical procedure and concern about sexual attractiveness
- **Risk for Impaired Physical Mobility** related to pain/discomfort, edema formation, neuromuscular impairment
- **Deficient Knowledge** related to breast awareness, breast cancer risks, breast disorder, prognosis, treatment, self-care, and discharge needs
- **Risk for Imbalanced Nutrition, Less Than Body Requirements** related to hypermetabolic state associated with cancer, side effects of chemotherapy, radiation, surgery, nausea
- **Anticipatory Grieving** related to loss of psychosocial well-being, perceived potential death
- **Risk for Deficient Fluid Volume** related to impaired intake of fluids, hypermetabolic state, excessive body fluid loss

- **Fatigue** related to altered body chemistry; side effects of pain, medications, and chemotherapy; overwhelming psychological/emotional demands
- **Risk for Infection** related to inadequate secondary defenses and immunosuppression, malnutrition, invasive procedures, and chronic disease processes
- **Risk for Impaired Oral Mucous Membranes** related to chemotherapy side effects, dehydration, malnutrition
- **Risk for Ineffective Sexuality Patterns** related to lack of understanding of alternative responses to health-related transitions, altered body functioning/structure, illness, medical treatment, fatigue, fear, and anxiety

Review Jade's statements at the beginning of the chapter related to her risk for breast cancer. Which nursing diagnoses might be priorities for her? How would you respond to her question about risk for breast cancer?

Planning/Intervention

Nursing goals, interventions, and outcomes depend on the client's diagnosis and treatment plan. Universal goals should include active participation in decision-making for treatment options, compliance with treatment plans, and management of the side effects of adjunct therapy.

Preventing Breast Cancer

Important strategies to prevent breast cancer include maintaining and adopting a healthy lifestyle. As discussed in detail in Chapter 2, women can reduce their risk by eating a healthy diet rich in vegetables, fruits, and whole grains; exercising daily; avoiding obesity; limiting alcohol consumption; avoiding HRT; being breast aware; and receiving screening mammograms and clinical breast examinations as recommended by health care providers (CBCF, 2014b; CCS, 2014d).

Any client at high risk needs to work with her health care provider and discuss strategies for prevention. The nurse needs to encourage anyone who detects breast changes to see a health care provider immediately for further evaluation. Nursing Care Plan 4.2 presents more information on teaching and follow-up for clients.

Assisting With Surgery

When a client needs to undergo surgical treatment for breast cancer, the nurse prepares the woman and assists with her safe recovery. When a client undergoes breast-conserving surgery, care focuses on wound management and discharge instructions. Clients also need reassurance that their skin will return to normal appearance after 1 or more months. They should be counselled to use protective clothing to prevent further damage to their skin.

NURSING CARE PLAN 4.2

●

The Client at Risk for Breast Cancer

 Recall Jade, the 21-year-old client from the beginning of the chapter. Further discussion with Jade reveals that she had planned to breastfeed her first child but had difficulty. "I became so frustrated that I decided it was better for everyone if I used the bottle." Jade reports that although she tries to exercise regularly, she really does not have time because her 2-year-old keeps her busy. Review of Jade's health history reveals that she has not seen a health professional for a clinical breast examination. "I really don't know much about my breasts."

NURSING DIAGNOSIS

• **Deficient Knowledge** related to health promotion behaviours to reduce the risk for breast cancer.

EXPECTED OUTCOMES

1. The client will identify possible risk factors for the development of breast cancer.
2. The client will verbalize the steps of being aware of her breasts.
3. The client will state warning signs of breast abnormalities to report to her health care provider.

INTERVENTIONS	RATIONALES
Assess the client's knowledge of breast cancer and associated risks.	This information provides a baseline from which to develop a teaching plan.
Explore the client's exposure to breast examination and breast cancer; correct any misconceptions or myths; allow time for questions.	Information about exposure provides additional foundation for teaching and provides opportunities to clarify or correct misinformation and teach new information.

(continued)

NURSING CARE PLAN 4.2 ● The Client at Risk for Breast Cancer *(Continued)*

INTERVENTIONS	RATIONALES
Review the health history for evidence of risk factors; teach the client measures to reduce her risk, such as increasing activity level and eating a nutritious diet. Discuss the need for breast awareness.	Identification of risk factors provides a basis for developing appropriate measures to modify risks.
Assess the client's level of comfort with touching her breasts.	Breast awareness requires touching the breasts. Discomfort or embarrassment may affect the client's ability to assess her breasts.
Teach the client about being aware of her breasts, by looking at and feeling her breasts, including up to the collarbone, under the armpits and the nipples.	Women should be aware of what is normal for their own breasts. Most women discover their own breast cancer through changes in the look and feel of their breasts.
Remind her that how or when she does this is up to her in whatever way it works for her.	Research has shown that using a particular method is not necessary.
Discuss with her the signs that may be symptomatic of breast cancer, including a painless lump in her breast; a lump in her armpit; changes in her breast size or shape; dimpling or puckering of the skin; redness, swelling, and increased warmth in her breast; an inverted nipple; or crusting or scaling on her nipple.	This will assist her to be aware of what to look and feel for and what she should report to her health professional.
Teach the client that her breast may be lumpy or tender before her period	Understanding what is normal will help her recognize changes and know what to report to her health professional.
Review with the client any possible changes in her breasts because of the pregnancy. Advise her to report these findings during her prenatal examinations.	During pregnancy, breasts increase in size; they may become tender, and sebaceous glands enlarge. Reporting these findings is important to ensure that the changes are normal and not suggestive of cancer.
Remind the client that changes are not necessarily caused by cancer but rather may be because of other health issues.	This provides reassurance and information that any changes need to be assessed by a health professional.
Arrange for follow-up visits as scheduled.	Ongoing visits provide an opportunity to evaluate the client's learning and understanding of the teaching and compliance with the procedure. It also provides opportunities for additional teaching and feedback.

EVALUATION

1. The client lists personal risk factors associated with the development of breast cancer.
2. The client discusses how she can be aware of her breasts and any changes.
3. The client states changes that she should report.

Clients are usually discharged from the health care facility soon after mastectomy. Important nursing measures thus include early discharge instructions and arrangements for home care. Common interventions for the client who has undergone mastectomy include:

- Explain care of the wound and drain or arrange for home care nursing.
- Explain why a client may experience a small amount of swelling in the arms and shoulders for the first few weeks after surgery, which then subsides.
- Explore availability of assistance from family and friends at home.
- Identify and report any signs of infection or impaired healing. Examples include drainage or a pale or dusky appearance to the skin surrounding the incision.
- Emphasize the need to continue performing arm exercises to improve muscle tone and mobility and lessen joint stiffness and swelling.
- Arrange for follow-up examinations by the surgeon.
- Teach the client the particulars of self-administration of prescribed medications.
- Explain to the client that she will likely feel numbness or tingling on the chest wall and inner side of the arm for up to 1 year after the surgery.
- Remind the client to apply cream or lotion to the skin in the incision location if it tends to be dry.
- Caution against carrying or lifting anything more than 7 kg; additionally, the client should not make repetitive or stressful movements with the affected arm.
- Alert the client not to wear tight garments around, or to sleep on the affected arm, as these could impair circulation.
- Teach the client that blood pressure measurements, infusions, injections, and so forth are contraindicated in the affected arm.

Managing Chemotherapy

The nurse assists the client receiving chemotherapy to anticipate and deal with the common side effects: nausea and vomiting, hair loss, changes in sense of taste, dermatitis, weight gain, and fatigue (Teaching Tips 4.5). Some clients also experience mild memory loss and unclear thinking, a syndrome commonly referred to as "chemo-brain." As part of patient teaching the nurse can explain the particulars of medication administration to relieve nausea and mouth sores and to boost WBC or RBC production. If alopecia is likely, the nurse may offer a list of wig suppliers or catalogues with scarves, turbans, or hats to camouflage hair loss. Such resources are available through the Canadian Cancer Society.

Managing Lymphedema

Both radiation and surgery may change the normal lymph drainage pattern, leaving clients with complications of **lymphedema** of the arm. Treatment options include arm massage, avoiding tight-fitting cuffs, jewellery, and the like, and exercising regularly (CCS, 2014d). Teaching Tips 4.6 provide more information about preventing and reducing the effects of lymphedema (CBCF, 2014e; CCS, 2014d).

Providing Client Teaching

Nursing care includes client education and counselling about the course of treatment, expected reactions, and tips for dealing with and relieving untoward effects. It is also helpful to refer the client to support programs such as Reach to Recovery or local cancer survivor and support programs in their community (Youngkin et al., 2012).

● TEACHING TIPS 4.5 Managing Adverse Effects of Chemotherapy

INFECTION

- Avoid infections.
- Avoid dental work during chemotherapy.
- Maintain a healthy diet.
- Get plenty of rest.
- Avoid large crowds and anyone with colds, infections, and contagious diseases.
- Maintain good hygiene habits (bathe daily, good oral care, wash hands frequently).
- Protect hands against cuts, burns, and irritations (use work gloves).
- Clean all cuts and wounds; keep them covered and seek medical attention immediately when infections are suspected.

NAUSEA

- Eat small meals often.
- Fast for 3 to 4 hours before treatment.
- Eat whatever you can tolerate.
- Chew food thoroughly.
- Relax during mealtime.
- Practice stress reduction techniques such as deep breathing exercises, meditation, yoga, acupuncture, and visualization strategies.

● TEACHING TIPS 4.6 Preventing Lymphedema

- Do exercises suggested postoperatively.
- Do not carry packages or handbags on the affected side.
- Avoid sunburn and burns to the affected arm or hand.
- Do not use the affected arm for blood pressure tests, blood draws, or injections.
- Avoid cuts when shaving underarms by using an electric shaver.
- Avoid infections in the affected arm, wash cuts promptly, apply antibacterial medication, and cover

with a bandage. Seek medical attention promptly at the first sign of infection.
- Wear gloves when gardening or using strong detergents.
- Avoid elastic cuffs on blouses and nightgowns or anything tight on the affected arm.
- Avoid cutting cuticles; be extremely cautious when manicuring fingernails.

INFLAMMATORY BREAST CANCER

Inflammatory breast cancer is a rare type of breast cancer in which cancer cells block lymph vessels in the skin and breast, causing inflammation. This most aggressive form of breast cancer accounts for approximately 1% to 4% of all cases; however, it kills at least 30% of clients who receive this diagnosis (CCS, 2014c). It is most common in postmenopausal women and is often misdiagnosed as mastitis. Inflammatory breast cancer progresses very quickly and aggressively and has survival rates that are much lower than other breast cancers (Robertson et al., 2010).

Assessment Findings

Symptoms of inflammatory breast cancer usually develop quite suddenly and may vary from person to person (CCS, 2014c). It usually begins with a painless change in the size or shape of the breast. Women notice a sensation of heaviness, itchiness, and mild burning. Following this initial change, the skin of the breast becomes mottled with a pink colour that progresses to a diffuse erythema. This redness usually occurs on the lower portion of the breast. Usually, no mass is palpable. The breasts then become tender and painful because the lymphatic pathways become affected. The nipple may retract and become swollen and crusted. The woman will begin to see dimpling of the skin and an orange-like skin texture/appearance in the affected area (peau d'orange) or a pink or mottled pink hue to the skin over the breasts (Robertson et al., 2010).

Collaborative Management

Clients do not usually seek attention when this process begins. Often, cases are first treated as mastitis. If a suspected case of mastitis does not respond to a 10- to 14-day antibiotic regimen, more thorough immediate investigation is necessary.

Usual treatment for inflammatory breast cancer is chemotherapy to reduce the tumour and control metastases, followed by modified radical mastectomy, radia-

tion, and/or hormonal therapy. Treatment often includes a combination of these treatments.

MENSTRUAL DISORDERS

Normally, monthly menstruation poses a few concerns for women, with cycles beginning and ending each month around the same time, lasting for an expected duration, and remaining a consistent amount and quality. Nevertheless, some women develop menstrual problems. Such problems can involve frequency, amount, or symptoms related to menstruation.

AMENORRHEA

Amenorrhea is the term used for the absence of menses during the woman's reproductive years. *Primary amenorrhea* is the term used when a woman has never experienced a menstrual cycle. It is used in the following cases:

- By 14 years of age, the adolescent has not had menses and shows no growth and development of secondary sexual characteristics.
- By 16 years of age, the adolescent has not had menses, but growth and development of secondary sexual characteristics are normal.

Secondary amenorrhea is the term used when menses are absent for three or more cycles or for 6 months or longer in women with previously established menstruation.

Etiology and Pathophysiology

The most common causes of primary amenorrhea include structural abnormalities (eg, imperforate hymen and gonadal dysgenesis), endocrine problems (eg, prepubertal ovarian failure, hypopituitarism, congenital adrenal hyperplasia, androgen insensitivity syndrome), and congenital disorders (eg, absent uterus or vagina). Eating disorders or extreme weight gain or loss can lead to primary amenorrhea, as can excessive stress or chronic illness.

Secondary amenorrhea can develop for numerous reasons. The most common and normal causes are pregnancy, lactation, and menopause. Menses also may cease as a consequence of stress, thyroid problems, endocrine tumours, excessive exercise, malnutrition, and kidney failure.

Assessment Findings

The nurse first determines whether the client is experiencing primary or secondary amenorrhea. Health history taking begins with finding out whether the client has ever had a regular menstrual pattern. If the client reports that such a pattern once existed, further follow-up is warranted to learn more about the pattern, when amenorrhea began, and what events during that time may have precipitated the problem. The nurse explores any past illnesses or hospitalizations, pregnancy history, medication history, lifestyle, nutrition, and diet.

During the physical examination, the nurse takes the client's weight and height and compares the findings with previous measurements to determine whether changes are substantial. He or she looks for any visible signs of a genetic problem or endocrine disease. The nurse takes vital signs and looks for abnormalities (eg, hypothermia, hypotension) that may indicate an eating disorder or thyroid dysfunction. If the nurse suspects primary amenorrhea in a teen, the nurse looks for characteristics of secondary sex development and performs evaluation of the reproductive tract.

Diagnostic evaluations may include karyotyping (see Chapter 11), pregnancy testing, and thyroid function tests. Ultrasound, CT scans, and laparoscopy may be ordered if a tumour is suspected as the cause. Hormonal studies may include evaluations of levels of prolactin, follicle-stimulating hormone, and luteinizing hormone.

Collaborative Management

Treatment measures vary depending on the cause. For primary amenorrhea, interventions focus on correcting the underlying problems. If necessary, estrogen therapy can be administered to induce the development of secondary sex characteristics. In cases of severe or irreversible problems, health care providers will need to focus on helping the woman accept the condition and what it means for future infertility.

DYSMENORRHEA

Dysmenorrhea (painful menstruation) is the most common gynaecologic symptom reported by women (Pinsonneault & Lefebvre, 2005). It is characterized by pain shortly before or during menstruation and can have a major impact on women's quality of life (Ju et al., 2014). *Primary dysmenorrhea* refers to pain accompanying menstruation for which no accompanying pelvic disorder or other problem exists. *Secondary dysmenor-rhea* is the term used when painful menstruation is the result of an underlying pelvic or uterine disorder.

Etiology and Pathophysiology

Increased production of prostaglandins is the main cause of primary dysmenorrhea. These levels are highest during the first 2 days of menses, when symptoms are most prevalent. Prostaglandins contribute to an increase in uterine contractions, resulting in uterine ischemia, which leads to pain (Pinsonneault & Lefebvre, 2005).

Secondary dysmenorrhea can result from numerous causes: pelvic infection, endometriosis, uterine fibroids, or congenital reproductive abnormalities.

Assessment Findings

Symptoms are more pronounced in adolescents and nulliparous women, and those women with early menarche, increased flow, a family history, or who smoke (Pinsonneault & Lefebvre, 2005). Women report sharp and intermittent suprapubic pain that may radiate to the back and legs. Pain may be accompanied by headache, nausea and vomiting, fatigue, dizziness, or other symptoms. The pain usually begins with the menses and worsens as the menstrual flow increases, improving as the amount of bleeding tapers off (Pinsonneault & Lefebvre, 2005).

The history and physical examination should enable the health care team to determine whether the dysmenorrhea is primary or secondary to better facilitate treatment. A pelvic examination is not necessary in adolescents with a history of mild to moderate dysmenorrhea who have never been sexually active (Pinsonneault & Lefebvre, 2005). With primary dysmenorrhea, the physical examination should reveal no underlying pathology contributing to the menstrual pain. With secondary dysmenorrhea, the health history may reveal fertility problems, menstrual irregularities, pelvic abnormalities, or other problems. The client will undergo a bimanual pelvic examination and laboratory testing, including blood count, urinalysis, cervical cultures for STIs, ESR, and ultrasound of the pelvis. Laparoscopy to diagnose endometriosis, PID, or pelvic adhesions is usually done when there is a strong suggestion of these conditions or when first-line therapy has failed (Pinsonneault & Lefebvre, 2005).

Collaborative Management

Treatment focuses on managing the pain and, with secondary dysmenorrhea, eliminating or controlling the underlying cause. Nonmedicinal approaches that may be used include exercise, heat, behavioural interventions, and dietary/herbal supplementation; data on the effectiveness of these remain inconclusive and controversial (Pinsonneault & Lefebvre, 2005). The client may be prescribed NSAIDs or COX-2 inhibitors. Management with oral contraceptives also is common.

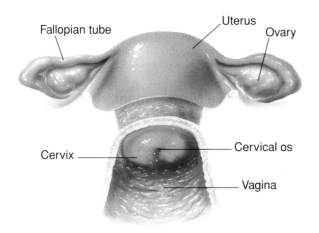

FIGURE 4.17 Abnormal uterine bleeding.

ABNORMAL UTERINE BLEEDING

Abnormal uterine bleeding is the internationally agreed term to define any variation from a woman's normal menstrual cycle and replaces terminology such as menorrhagia, metrorrhagia, and dysfunctional uterine bleeding (Singh et al., 2013). It includes changes in frequency, regularity, duration, and blood loss or menstrual flow (Maybin et al., 2013; Singh et al., 2013). The most common cause is a hormonal disturbance leading to anovulatory menstrual cycles. Abnormal uterine bleeding can be part of or overlap with other menstrual problems (see Fig. 4.17).

The client will need thorough evaluation of her health history, physical examination, and diagnostic testing to identify the cause of the abnormal bleeding. In assessment the nurse would look for symptoms of anemia or infection and explore sexual history and impact on the woman's quality of life (Singh et al., 2013). Treatment will focus on elimination or control of the cause. If no cause can be found, management efforts emphasize ways to minimize the bleeding problems so that they do not disrupt the client's lifestyle.

PREMENSTRUAL SYNDROME

Premenstrual syndrome (PMS) is defined as regular premenstrual physical or emotional symptoms that interfere with daily living and functioning at home and work. PMS occurs during the luteal phase of the menstrual cycle, when estrogen and progesterone initially rise and then fall if no pregnancy occurs. Common symptoms include anxiety, irritability, mood swings, fatigue, palpitations, crying, headaches, forgetfulness, fluid retention, weight gain, and breast tenderness (Read et al., 2014).

Despite the prevalence of PMS, much remains unknown about its cause. Several theories involve imbalances of hormones or neurotransmitters. Popular theories also include vitamin deficiency, mineral deficiency, and prostaglandin imbalance. Therefore, treatments often seek to balance levels of hormones or serotonin and to address potential lifestyle conditions. Medical treatment may include trying to balance hormones with oral contraceptives or balancing serotonin with antidepressants. Lifestyle changes that may help include decreased sodium and refined sugar content, decreased alcohol and caffeine intake, increased B vitamins and calcium, exercise, relaxation techniques, and increased rest. Aerobic exercise during the luteal phase is thought to be beneficial to decrease anxiety, depression, and anger.

REPRODUCTIVE TRACT ALTERATIONS

PELVIC INFLAMMATORY DISEASE

Infection is one of the most prevalent reproductive problems experienced by many women at some point in their lives. Infections can have serious health threats and cause significant sequelae, such as chronic pelvic pain, scarring, infertility, and PID.

PID is an infection of the internal upper reproductive tract involving any combination of the uterus (*endometritis*), fallopian tubes (*salpingitis*), ovaries (*oophoritis*), and/or pelvic peritoneum (PHAC, 2013f). There are approximately 100,000 cases of PID in Canada annually; up to two thirds of cases are unrecognized, as underreporting is quite common (PHAC, 2013f). It is estimated that 10% to 15% of women of reproductive age have at least one episode of PID (PHAC, 2013f). However, since PID is not a reportable disease in Canada, exact numbers are not known (PHAC, 2013f).

Etiology and Pathophysiology

PID develops when harmful bacteria move upward from the vagina or cervix (Fig. 4.18). Many different

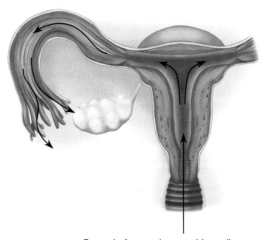

Spread of gonorrhea or chlamydia

FIGURE 4.18 Progression of pelvic inflammatory disease. A sexually transmitted infection (eg, chlamydia, gonorrhea) moves up into the uterus, progressing to the fallopian tubes and ovaries.

organisms can cause this disorder. Sexually transmitted organisms include *C. trachomatis, N. gonorrhoeae,* and, rarely, HSV, and *T. vaginalis.* Endogenous organisms may include genital tract mycoplasmas (eg, *Mycoplasma genitalium, Mycoplasma hominis,* and *Ureaplasma urelyticum*). Other organisms such as *Escherichia coli, G. vaginalis, Haemophilus influenzae,* and *Streptococcus* may also cause PID (PHAC, 2013f). Infection caused by these organisms often results in pelvic scarring and obstruction of the fallopian tubes, ectopic pregnancy, and chronic pelvic pain. The incidence of these consequences is directly related to the number of episodes of PID.

Common risk factors associated with PID are young age, history of PID or STIs, and recent IUD insertion (Caddy et al., 2014; PHAC, 2013f). Risk is increased in single, sexually active women; women who have had unprotected sex with someone with an STI; and women with more than one male sexual partner in the previous 30 to 60 days. PID often occurs during the first 5 days of the menstrual cycle. Because of the nature of PID and its consequences, accurate diagnosis and early treatment are crucial (Youngkin et al., 2012).

Assessment Findings

Symptoms can range from mild to severe, although many women are asymptomatic. The most frequent symptom is abdominal pain. Fever is present in about one third of women who present with symptoms. Other symptoms of acute PID may include bilateral lower abdominal, uterine, adnexal, and cervical motion tenderness. Minimum criteria for diagnosis of PID without a competing diagnosis (eg, pregnancy, acute appendicitis, urinary tract infection [UTI]) are lower abdominal tenderness, bilateral adnexal tenderness, and cervical motion tenderness (PHAC, 2013f).

Symptoms can be mild or subtle and include new vaginal discharge (with or without a foul odor), lower abdominal or back pain, dysuria, and pain with intercourse (SOGC, 2012). Severe symptoms include sudden and severe pelvic pain, high fever, chills, heavy vaginal discharge or bleeding, pain on movement of the cervix, feeling of abdominal fullness, and abdominal mass (when abscess is present).

Diagnosis is often difficult because the symptoms are similar to many other diseases. Health care experts have concluded that many cases of PID go undetected, which leads to serious sequelae in young women. Confirmation depends on presenting symptoms and findings from physical and pelvic examinations. Bacterial vaginal smears and cervical cultures are used to identify the causative organism. Blood analysis includes ESR, CRP, and CBC with emphasis on WBC analysis. Ultrasound may be used when pelvic abscess is suspected. A negative laboratory result or a normal ultrasound does not, however, rule out PID (PHAC, 2013f). When clients

are treated and fail to respond to therapy, a laparoscopy may be performed for further diagnostic evaluation to evaluate infertility, occlusions, and masses (Youngkin et al., 2012).

Collaborative Management

Treatment options depend on the presenting symptoms. Women with mild symptoms and suspected infection are treated as outpatients and receive antibiotic therapy with ceftriaxone and doxycycline (PHAC, 2013f). Women with an abscess or severe symptoms who do not respond to (or cannot tolerate) oral medications, or who are pregnant, are hospitalized and treated with IV antibiotics for up to 24 hours after clinical improvement (PHAC, 2013f). Laparoscopy may be performed to drain an abscess (Youngkin et al., 2012). Women must be counselled to complete all prescriptions and to receive follow-up evaluation 48 to 72 hours after starting the medication and again in 7 to 10 days. Levofloxacin and ofloxacin are contraindicated in women aged 17 years or younger, as well as in all pregnant women because of the serious side effects. In these situations, alternative medications should be used. Sexual partners also should be treated (Youngkin et al., 2012).

Nurses should educate and counsel clients about modifiable risk factors for PID, such as multiple sexual partners and sex without condoms. They should instruct clients to seek medical attention for any unusual vaginal discharge or possible signs of infection. Education also must emphasize the need for sexual partners to be treated and should include methods for decreasing risk for STIs, safer sex practices, and ways to recognize infection in partners (Gradison, 2012; PHAC, 2013f). Education programs that promote screening for STIs at the community level are essential; PID rates have declined in jurisdictions with longstanding chlamydia control programs (PHAC, 2013g).

Open discussion regarding the client's feelings and concerns about PID is important and can assist her to cope effectively with outcomes. The nurse's role for hospitalized women also includes medication administration and monitoring; comfort measures to reduce pain; assessment of status, vital signs, and characteristics of vaginal discharge (amount, colour, odour); and documentation.

ENDOMETRIOSIS

Endometriosis is a benign uterine condition in which endometrial tissue attaches to sites outside the endometrial cavity. Approximately 10% of women between the ages of 15 to 49 years are diagnosed with endometriosis (World Endometriosis Society, 2012) (see Chapter 10).

Endometrial tissue is found most commonly in and near the ovaries, the uterosacral ligaments, pouch of Douglas, and the rectovaginal septum; however, it also may appear in the stomach, lungs, bowel, spleen, and intestines. This tissue responds to hormones during the menstrual cycle and undergoes changes similar to normally sited uterine endometrial tissue. Each month, estrogen causes all the endometrial tissue, regardless of location, to bleed during menstruation, causing an inflammatory reaction leading to scarring and adhesions (Canadian Women's Health Network [CWHN], 2012a).

Although endometriosis occurs in all ethnic groups, little research has been done with women from varying ethnic groups. It is seen most frequently in women during their reproductive years and in those who report a family history (sisters and mothers), suggesting a genetic predisposition as well as women who have experienced laparoscopic assessment of infertility or pelvic pain (Wolfman, 2010). It is not usually found in women who have borne more than one child. Although endometriosis is not life-threatening, it interferes with a client's ability to work and can cause much pain and discomfort.

Etiology and Pathophysiology

Several theories have been suggested as to the cause of endometriosis, but to date it remains unknown. The most common theory is that during the menstrual cycle, some menstrual blood backs up through the fallopian tubes and bits of endometrial tissue in the fluid attach and implant in the peritoneal cavity (retrograde menstruation theory) (CWHN, 2012a; Singh et al., 2010). Other theories suggest that this disorder may be associated with an immune or hormonal problem, or that the tissue travels from the uterus to the lymphatic or blood system to reach other sites in the body (CWHN, 2012a; Singh et al., 2010).

Assessment Findings

Symptoms vary and often do not reflect the extent of this disorder. As many as one third of clients who are diagnosed with endometriosis are asymptomatic (CWHN, 2012a). Pelvic pain is the most common symptom, although the degree of discomfort is not proportionate to the severity or extent of the disease (CWHN, 2012a). Other symptoms reported include dysmenorrhea, painful defecation, lower back pain, abdominal discomfort, dyspareunia, and dysuria (Singh et al., 2010). Symptoms may be associated with menstrual cycles.

A complete history, physical examination, and pelvic examination are warranted when clients present with symptoms. Although the CA-125 assay is a marker for clients with endometriosis, it is not recommended as part of routine assessment (Singh et al., 2010). Diagnostic laparoscopy or laparotomy can be used to visually inspect and identify this disorder for definitive diagnosis (Singh et al., 2010).

Collaborative Management

Treatment often depends on the extent and location of the endometrial growths, the client's age, her desire for pregnancy, and the severity of the symptoms. Although, to date, endometriosis has no cure, several treatment options are available. The goals of management are to relieve or reduce pain, shrink or slow endometrial growths, preserve and restore fertility, and prevent or delay recurrence (The Endometriosis Network Canada, 2014). Drug therapy consists of acetaminophen or NSAIDs to reduce symptoms and relieve pain. When pain is not relieved with these medications, stronger prescriptions such as codeine products may be necessary. Hormonal therapy also is an option to interrupt or stop ovulation and menstrual cycles. Drugs used for this purpose are oral contraceptives, progesterone drugs, danazol, and gonadotropin-releasing hormone analogues (Singh et al., 2010).

An additional option is surgery. The first-line surgical treatment is conservative and aims to destroy and remove the endometrial growth and preserve reproductive functioning. This option is used in clients who fail to respond to drug therapy and desire to become pregnant. Drug therapy and conservative surgical therapy may be used together. In cases of extensive and severe endometriosis, more radical surgery may be necessary, such as hysterectomy with removal of all growths and the ovaries, although the success rate of these surgeries may be questionable (CWHN, 2012a).

The nurse's primary role is to develop a plan of care that incorporates education and counselling about endometriosis. Teaching should include reassurance that the disorder is not life-threatening. The nurse should provide information about the use of nonpharmacologic comfort measures, as well as about OTC pain relievers and hormonal drugs and their side effects. Nursing plans of care should also include psychological referrals as necessary, especially for women experiencing sexual difficulties and infertility issues.

Preoperative teaching and postoperative nursing care are required for women who undergo conservative or radical surgery. Possible adverse effects are similar to those of other surgical procedures and can include bleeding, infection, and damage to nearby organs. Postoperative discharge education includes information regarding activity, expected vaginal discharge changes (from bleeding to clear drainage), signs of infection, resumption of sexual activity, and diet.

Follow-up is important for dealing effectively with this disorder: the woman is encouraged to see her health provider routinely and to maintain a healthy lifestyle that includes a proper diet, physical activity, adequate sleep, and stress management.

LEIOMYOMAS (UTERINE FIBROIDS, MYOMAS)

One of the most common benign gynecologic tumours is a **leiomyoma (fibroid tumour)**. Leiomyomas grow from smooth muscle in the wall of the uterus (Medline-Plus, 2011) and are common in women over the age of 30 years. Approximately 20% to 25% of all women have uterine fibroids, although most women have minor or no symptoms (CWHN, 2012b).

Etiology and Pathophysiology

The etiology of these tumours is unknown. They cause the uterus to enlarge abnormally and are the most common reason hysterectomy is performed. Fibroids usually become symptomatic in women over the age of 30 years. An increased risk for fibroids is reported in women with a familial history of fibroids in close relatives, African-Canadian women, nulliparous women, women who are significantly overweight, women with early menarche, and women with high caffeine intake (Khan et al., 2014).

Fibroids are classified according to location: subserosal, intramural, or submucosal (Fig. 4.19). Leiomyomas appear to be dependent on ovarian hormones, because they grow slowly during the reproductive years and atrophy during menopause (CWHN, 2012b).

Assessment Findings

The most common symptoms are heavy, prolonged vaginal bleeding and a feeling of pressure in the pelvis; pelvic pain is rare ((Khan et al., 2014). Women may present with complaints of dysmenorrhea or dyspareunia, with large tumours causing expansion of the lower abdomen. When located in the uterine cavity, these tumours are also associated with miscarriage and infertility. During pregnancy, they typically grow and

become quite large and are associated with outcomes such as spontaneous miscarriage, preterm labor, placental abruption, premature rupture of membranes, postpartum hemorrhage, labor dystocia, and cesarean section (Vitale et al., 2013). Severe anemia can occur when women have frequent episodes of copious vaginal bleeding. Often, these symptoms are so incapacitating that women cannot participate in activities outside the home during their menstrual periods and are forced to plan their lives around their cycles. These tumours also can put pressure on surrounding organs and cause frequent urination, pelvic pressure, abdominal discomfort, and constipation (CWHN, 2012b).

A complete physical assessment with a pelvic examination may reveal an abnormally shaped uterus. Accurate diagnosis is usually made through the use of these findings (with a uterine size corresponding to 12 weeks' gestation) and a regular or trans-abdominal pelvic ultrasound or a transvaginal ultrasound.

Collaborative Management

Many treatment options are available for symptomatic fibroids. Some clients choose to treat the symptoms of discomfort and increased blood loss, rather than treating the fibroids. Iron supplements are often recommended to treat anemia related to blood loss. A diet rich in green vegetables, fruit, and fish may afford some protection against fibroids and also may help prevent constipation and hemorrhoids associated with fibroid pressure.

Hysterectomy (with or without removal of the ovaries as well) offers the definitive solution; however, other options are now available for the woman who wishes to preserve her uterus (Asch et al., 2004; CWHN, 2012b). Laparoscopic or hysteroscopic myomectomy (removal of the fibroid without removing the uterus) is one option that preserves the uterus, although there is a possibility that further treatment may be needed (Asch et al., 2004). Types include laparoscopic myomectomy, hysteroscopic myomectomy, laparotomy myomectomy, laparoscopic myomectomy with minilaparotomy, and laparoscopic-assisted vaginal myomectomy. There is a 15% rate of regrowth of the fibroids following myomectomy, and 10% of women will require a hysterectomy within 5 to 10 years (Asch et al., 2004).

One of the newest options is uterine fibroid embolization, which appears to be quickly becoming the treatment of choice for symptomatic women as an alternative to hysterectomy (WebMD, 2013). In this minimally invasive nonsurgical procedure, a catheter is placed into the artery that feeds the fibroid and small plastic particles are injected into the blood vessel, occluding it. The fibroid is thus deprived of its blood supply (CWHN, 2012b). Approximately 80% of women reported improvement of symptoms (WebMD, 2013). Side effects are rare (1% to 2%) and include infection, bleeding, and uterine

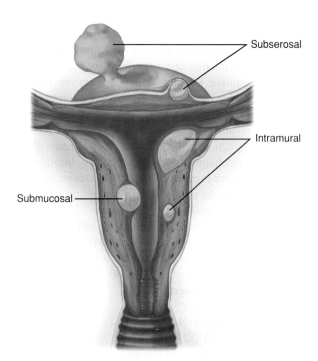

FIGURE 4.19 Leiomyomas (fibroid tumours).

Subserosal

Intramural

Submucosal

infarction (Asch et al., 2004). Long-term effects of the procedure, especially on future fertility, are still being researched (CWHN, 2012b).

A final treatment option is hormone therapy with gonadotropin-releasing hormone agonists (eg, Lupron), often used prior to surgery. These drugs (available in multiple forms including nasal spray, subcutaneous injection, and slow-release injection) reduce estrogen levels, which reduces blood flow to the fibroids, shrinking fibroids temporarily and creating a temporary menopause (Asch et al., 2004; CWHN, 2012b). These drugs should not be given for longer than 3 to 6 months because of the substantial bone loss that results (Asch et al., 2004; CWHN, 2012b). Fibroids usually regrow within 12 weeks following discontinuation of the medication (Asch et al., 2004).

POLYCYSTIC OVARY SYNDROME

Polycystic ovary syndrome (PCOS) is a syndrome the definition of which has been evolving over many years. It occurs in approximately 6% to 20% of women (Luhan et al., 2008). In order for a diagnosis of PCOS to be made, the woman must have two of three symptoms: oligo and/or anovulation; clinical and/or biochemical signs of hyperandrogenism; polycystic ovaries (Luhan et al., 2008). Other etiologies of the symptoms, such as congenital adrenal hyperplasia, androgen-secreting tumours, and Cushing syndrome, must be excluded.

Assessment Findings

Common symptoms include weight gain or obesity, infrequent or irregular periods, infertility, hirsutism (excessive growth of coarse, dark, thick hair in a male pattern distribution), acne, anxiety, depression, and elevated testosterone levels (CWHN, 2012c). PCOS is linked to insulin resistance, and these women are prone to developing impaired glucose tolerance, type 2 diabetes, gestational diabetes, and obstructive sleep apnea.

Diagnosis also should be directed to screening for possible endocrine abnormalities. Testosterone levels are assessed to detect hyperandrogenemia and rule out an androgen-secreting tumour and congenital adrenal hyperplasia. Glucose tolerance testing and assessment of lipid status is indicated. A transvaginal ultrasound may be used to assess ovarian volume.

Collaborative Management

Management focuses on addressing current needs and preventing long-term complications. Weight loss (5% to 10% of body weight) has been shown to result in return of ovulation within weeks (Vause & Cheung, 2010). Glucose intolerance is managed by diet and exercise in addition to weight control. A recent systematic review and meta-analysis suggests lifestyle interventions improve endocrine outcomes in women with PCOS

(Haqq et al., 2014). Oral estrogen antagonists, such as clomiphene citrate (Clomifene), may be used to stimulate follicular growth and ovulation. The initial regime is 50 mg/day for 5 days; estrogen levels and luteal progesterone levels must be monitored to detect ovarian hyperstimulation syndrome (Vause & Cheung, 2010). Metformin, an insulin-sensitizing agent, combined with clomiphene citrate has been shown to increase ovulation and pregnancy rates and has been used in women who are clomiphene sensitive (Vause & Cheung, 2010). Progestins or the oral contraceptive pill may be prescribed to manage menstrual dysfunction.

ENDOMETRIAL HYPERPLASIA

Endometrial hyperplasia is a benign condition in which the cells lining the uterus proliferate. It is most common in women older than 40 years and may develop into cancer. Atypical endometrial hyperplasia is thought to be a precursor of endometrial cancer; (Lacey et al., 2010; Wolfman, 2010). Heavy menstrual periods and bleeding after menopause are common symptoms. Clients at the highest risk are those who are menopausal or women at any age who take unopposed estrogen (without progesterone) (Roberts, 2014).

Diagnosis is made when the client presents with symptoms. Physical examination, including a pelvic examination, is routine. Definitive diagnosis is made with endometrial biopsy, or dilatation and curettage (D&C).

Treatment focuses on prevention of hyperplasia. Removal of the source of exogenous estrogen is often effective in simple hyperplasia. Administration of hormones (progesterone) may be useful in women for whom surgery is not indicated (Hubbs et al., 2013; Lethaby et al., 2004). The physician may recommend hysterectomy to prevent endometrial hyperplasia from developing into cancer.

UTERINE CANCER

Most uterine cancers start in the endometrium (uterine lining) (CCS, 2014i). The muscle or connective tissues of the uterus are less common sites. Uterine cancer is the fourth most commonly diagnosed cancer in women in Canada (CCS, 2014i).

Etiology and Pathophysiology

Women between 45 and 70 years of age are at the highest risk of developing uterine cancer (CCS, 2014i). Uterine cancer is more common in the Caucasian population and in women in higher-income groups. Known risk factors include the following:

- Estrogen replacement therapy
- Menstrual history
- Endometrial hyperplasia
- Being overweight or obese

- Nulliparity
- Use of tamoxifen
- Family history of cancer
- Polycystic ovarian syndrome
- Estrogen-secreting ovarian tumours

Assessment Findings

Abnormal bleeding is the most common early symptom. This may include postmenopausal bleeding, bleeding between premenopausal periods, heavy frequent bleeding at any time, and bleeding with intercourse (CCS, 2014i). Other symptoms include unusual vaginal discharge (foul-smelling or purulent), pain during intercourse, and pelvic pain. Late signs and symptoms occur with tumour growth or metastases and include pain in the lower abdomen, pelvis, back, or legs; change in bladder habits (dysuria or difficult urination); change in bowel habits; ascites, weight loss, and weakness (CCS, 2014i).

Women who are at higher-than-average risk include those who have atypical endometrial hyperplasia or who have taken tamoxifen for breast cancer. These women should have regular gynecologic examinations and an endometrial biopsy, if abnormal vaginal bleeding is experienced (CCS, 2014i). Pap tests are unreliable in detecting uterine cancer, because the tool used to obtain the sample is for detecting cervical cancer cells and does not reach inside the uterus (CCS, 2014i). Diagnostic tests are usually done when symptoms are present or there is a suspicion of uterine cancer after completing a history and physical examination. Diagnostic tests may include a CBC to assess RBCs, WBCs, and platelets; serum chemistry tests including blood urea nitrogen and creatinine to assess kidney function (in case of metastases); and alanine aminotransferase, aspartate transaminase, and alkaline phosphatase to assess liver function (in case of metastases). Definitive diagnosis is usually made after histologic examination of endometrial tissue obtained by endometrial biopsy, which can be done in a physician's office. If there is difficulty in obtaining this sample, the sample is unsatisfactory, or it is negative and symptoms persist, one or more other tests may be done. These include transvaginal ultrasound, which may be done to evaluate the thickness of the endometrium; hysteroscopic examination of the uterus to assess changes, determine the extent of the abnormality, and take tissue samples for biopsy; or a D&C to obtain further specimens for histologic examination (CCS, 2014i).

Collaborative Management

Detecting and treating uterine cancer early increase the chance of successful treatment. Early detection is facilitated by knowing and recognizing symptoms and by having regular checkups. Treatment depends on several factors, including the stage of the disease at diagnosis

● TABLE 4.7 **Endometrial Cancer Staging System**

Stage	Characteristics
I	Tumour is limited to the body of the uterus.
II	Cancer has spread from the body of the uterus to the cervix. There is no spread to lymph system or distant sites.
III	Cancer has spread beyond or outside the uterus, but remains confined to the pelvis.
IV	Cancer has spread beyond the pelvis to another part of the body.

Adapted from Canadian Cancer Society. (2014). What is uterine cancer? Retrieved from http://www.cancer.ca/en/cancer-information/cancer-type/uterine/pathology-and-staging/staging/?region=on

(Table 4.7), grade, tumour type, age, and the woman's overall health (CCS, 2014i).

There are a number of potential treatments that may be offered. Surgery may include total hysterectomy (removal of the uterus and cervix) or radical hysterectomy (removal of the uterus, cervix, upper portion of vagina, parametrial tissue and ligaments around the cervix, and nearby lymph nodes in the pelvis), bilateral salpingo-oophorectomy, and pelvic exenteration done in cases of recurrent cancer (CCS, 2014i). Radiation may be used as well as hormonal therapy. Progesterone receptor–positive tumours respond best to hormonal therapy; estrogen receptor–positive tumours are less responsive (CCS, 2014i). Chemotherapy may be used as an adjunct to other treatments or following surgery and may also be used in cases of recurrent cancer that are not responsive to hormonal therapy.

Nurses can provide emotional support and reassurance as well as education about this disease. They should counsel women on preventive lifestyle practices, such as maintenance of a healthy body weight, increased physical activity, and methods to control other medical conditions, especially diabetes and hypertension. Women who need medication to control menopausal symptoms should use combined estrogen and progesterone hormonal therapy. Oral contraceptives that are a combination of estrogen and progesterone may offer some protection to women, especially those who are anovulatory (CCS, 2014i). Women with advanced cancer will need supportive care, including pain control, nutrition counselling, information about management of symptoms and side effects, psychosocial support, and information that may include referral to local cancer support groups (CCS, 2014i).

BENIGN OVARIAN CYSTS

Ovarian cysts are fluid-filled, usually benign, growths that can vary in size from small to large (Fig. 4.20). The most common type, a functional cyst, is usually

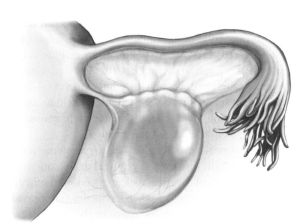

FIGURE 4.20 Ovarian cyst.

asymptomatic and disappears without treatment. Functional cysts occur when the normal development and release of an egg is disrupted; either the follicle that surrounds an ovum does not rupture to release the egg during ovulation and instead swells with fluid (*follicular cyst*), or the ovum is released from the follicle which then reseals and fills with fluid (*luteal cyst*) (Healthwise, 2013; Women's College Hospital, n.d.a). Other types of cysts are differentiated by their tissue makeup and include dermoid, cystadenoma, and endometrioma. *Dermoid cysts* form from skin precursor cells and develop when cells of the ovary not associated with reproduction itself begin to multiply; they may contain skin, hair, and bone (Women's College Hospital, n.d.a). Dermoid cysts are more likely to cause complications than functional cysts, and need to be removed. Less than 2% are malignant. A cystadenoma is non-cancerous formed from the outer surface of the ovary (Healthline, 2014). One in eight is malignant, although these are rare prior to menopause. Endometriomas occur within the ovary and are made up of endometrial tissue.

Ovarian cysts are common during the childbearing years and are generally noncancerous in this age group. Even though most cysts are benign, postmenopausal women with ovarian cysts are at an increased risk for ovarian cancer. It is imperative for these women to have cysts evaluated by their health care providers. Most clinicians will recommend surgical removal of ovarian cysts for older women (Women's College Hospital, n.d.a).

Assessment Findings
Most functional ovarian cysts cause no symptoms. When cysts become large, they can cause pelvic discomfort and pain because they tend to put pressure on nerves and other organs. Lower abdominal pain may occur in the middle of menses. Menses may be delayed or bleeding between periods may occur. A rare but serious complication is that cysts can rupture, causing pain during or after sex (Healthwise, 2013). Large cysts can

become twisted and cut off the blood vessels supplying the cyst and ovary (torsion). In such cases, the client may experience nausea, fever, and sudden severe abdominal pain (Healthwise, 2013).

Most ovarian cysts are discovered on routine pelvic examination when the health care provider palpates a swelling or mass. When this finding is seen, an ultrasound is done to identify the characteristics and location of the cyst.

Collaborative Management
Because 80% of ovarian cysts shrink and resolve on their own, the first-line treatment for childbearing women is usually a "wait and see" approach with follow-up examination in 2 to 3 months (Women's College Hospital, n.d.a). Surgical removal may be indicated when the cyst persists, has grown, causes increasing pain, or diagnostic tests indicate that it is a cyst that is unlikely to disappear on its own (eg, dermoid cyst). Surgery may involve drainage and removal of the cyst. If the cyst is so large that it has damaged the surrounding ovary, or if there is a greater risk that the cyst may be malignant, the entire ovary will be removed (Women's College Hospital, n.d.a). Oral contraceptives may be ordered for the woman to prevent ovulation and the formation of additional cysts. The low-dose formulations are not appropriate because they do not contain enough hormones to affect regression of the existing cysts.

Women need education and counselling regarding this disorder as well as reassurance that most of these cysts are benign. Standard preoperative and postoperative nursing care is required for women who undergo surgical treatment.

OVARIAN CANCER
Etiology and Pathophysiology
Women have a 1 in 68 chance of developing ovarian cancer in their lifetime, and a 1 in 95 chance of dying from it (CCS, 2014h) (Fig. 4.21). Known factors for

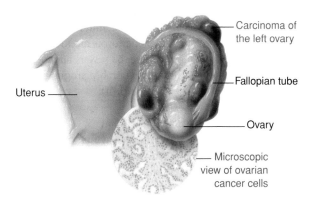

Uterus —
Carcinoma of the left ovary
Fallopian tube
Ovary
Microscopic view of ovarian cancer cells

FIGURE 4.21 Ovarian cancer. (From Anatomical Chart Company. [2002]. *Atlas of pathophysiology*. Springhouse, PA: Springhouse.)

developing ovarian cancer include a family history of other cancers, BRCA gene mutations, use of HRT, aging, Ashkenazi Jewish heritage, nulliparity, living in an industrialized country (asbestos exposure), and smoking (CCS, 2014h). Further research is needed to determine whether there is any relationship between ovarian cancer and age at menarche or menopause, obesity, diet, use of perineal talc, and tall adult stature (CCS, 2014h). Drinking coffee and the use of alcohol are not associated with ovarian cancer.

The strongest risk factor for ovarian cancer is hereditary; having one or more first-degree blood relatives who have or had ovarian cancer or having a combination of one first-degree and one second-degree relative (aunt, grandmother, niece) (CCS, 2014h). Women who have family histories of breast, colon, uterine, or pancreatic cancers are at an increased risk for ovarian cancer. Estrogen-only HRT in menopausal women increases the risk of developing ovarian cancer (CCS, 2014h). This risk is proportional to the length of time the drug is used. Women who use a combination of estrogen and progestin HRT on a daily basis may have an increased risk.

Women over the age of 50 years are at an increased risk for epithelial ovarian cancer; the highest incidence is in women aged between 60 and 79 (CCS, 2014h). Tumours with low potential for malignancy tend to occur in younger women; the median age at diagnosis is 40 years. Germ-cell tumours are more prevalent in young women, with a median age at diagnosis of 19 years. Genetic mutations are thought to be a cause of 5% to 10% of all epithelial ovarian cancers (CCS, 2014h). When ovarian cancer occurs in three or more first-degree relatives (eg, mother, sisters, daughters), or early-onset (before age 50 years) breast or ovarian cancer occurs in four or more first-degree relatives (two cases of each type), a hereditary form of ovarian cancer is suspected (CCS, 2014h). Around 85% to 95% of hereditary ovarian cancers are classified as hereditary breast-ovarian cancer syndrome. In this syndrome, the majority of the mutations are on the BRCA1 gene (on chromosome 17), with a smaller number on the BRCA2 gene (on chromosome 13). These mutations can be inherited from the father. Genetic forms are more likely to be diagnosed at an earlier age, be serous adenocarcinomas, and may have a more favourable prognosis than sporadic ovarian cancer (CCS, 2014h).

Assessment Findings

Ovarian cancer is insidious in that symptoms are usually vague, non-specific, and may not cause symptoms in the early stages. Two thirds of women have advanced disease by the time of diagnosis. As tumours begin to grow and press on other structures and organs, the woman may experience persistent or vague abdominal discomfort, with lower abdominal or pelvic pressure, distention, change in bowel habits, feeling full after a light meal, indigestion, flatulence, dyspepsia, and nausea (CCS, 2014h). Other symptoms may include fatigue, pain in the lower back or legs, frequent urination or urgency, abnormal vaginal bleeding, menstrual disorders, or dyspareunia. Later symptoms include ascites, pleural effusion, dyspnea, persistent cough, nausea and vomiting, weight loss, and constipation.

Assessment often begins when symptoms appear or after a health history and physical examination lead to a suspicion of ovarian cancer. Pelvic examination can reveal ovarian cancer when the health care provider palpates an enlargement or mass in the ovarian area. Physical examination should also include assessment of the neck, groin, and axilla for enlarged lymph nodes, and the lungs and abdomen. Blood tests may include a CBC and kidney and liver function tests. Other blood tests may include assessment for ovarian cancer tumour markers such as CA 125, beta human chorionic gonadotropin, alpha-fetoprotein, lactate dehydrogenase, and carcinoembryonic antigen. A transvaginal ultrasound may be done to identify the presence, characteristics, and location of the enlargement. An abdominal or pelvic CT or MRI may be done to estimate the size and location of masses and to assess for metastases. Other tests, including chest x-rays, mammogram, or lower GI series or barium enema, may be done to assess for metastases (CCS, 2014h). A biopsy done by laparoscopy or laparotomy will definitively diagnose ovarian cancer and may also stage the tumour (CCS, 2014h). There is currently no good screening test available to identify ovarian cancer. Women who are at a higher risk for developing ovarian cancer can have physical examinations, Pap tests, transvaginal ultrasound, and serum assessment of CA 125 done on a regular basis to detect it in an early stage, which may increase the chance of successful treatment (CCS, 2014h).

Collaborative Management

Treatment of ovarian cancer depends on the stage of the disease and the woman's general health (Table 4.8). A team approach involves many health care providers who work with the client to decide on a treatment plan. In general, treatment includes surgery, chemotherapy, and radiation (CCS, 2014h). Clients may experience preoperative and postoperative side effects and complications, as well as side effects from chemotherapy and radiation. The client may also have the option of enrolling in clinical trials, as Canada is an international leader in this area (CCS, 2014h).

Women with ovarian cancer experience many of the same problems and issues faced by women with breast cancer. They have to adapt and cope with physical, emotional, and medical challenges. Nursing support and client-to-client networks (eg, support groups)

● TABLE 4.8 **Ovarian Cancer Staging**

Stage	Characteristics
I	Growth is limited to the ovaries. Cancer cells may be on the surface of the ovaries or in fluid collected from the abdomen.
II	Growth involves one or both ovaries with pelvic extension. Cancer cells may be in fluid collected from the abdomen.
III	Growth involves one or both ovaries with metastases outside the pelvis to abdominal organs or nearby lymph nodes.
IV	Growth involves one or both ovaries with distant metastases.

Adapted from Canadian Cancer Society. (2014). What is ovarian cancer? Retrieved from http://www.cancer.ca/en/cancer-information/cancer-type/ovarian/overview/?region=on

can help improve quality of life. Nursing interventions are similar to those used for women with breast cancer and focus on teaching, counselling, giving support, and meeting the woman's physical care needs.

BENIGN CERVICAL ALTERATIONS

Cervical polyps are benign growths that may develop in the mucosa of the endocervical canal. They are usually discovered during a speculum examination and may even protrude through the cervical os. Polyps are usually bright red, small (a few millimetres to several centimetres), and may be single or multiple (Fig. 4.22).

The cause of these growths is unknown, but they are rarely cancerous. Chronic cervical inflammation may be responsible for cervical polyps. These polyps

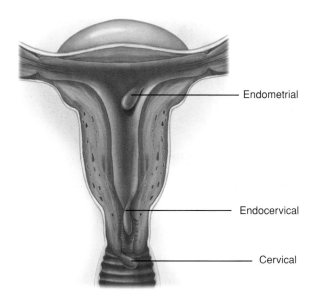

FIGURE 4.22 Endometrial, endocervical, and cervical polyps.

also have been found with endometrial hyperplasia and hyperestrogen states (Youngkin et al., 2012).

Assessment Findings

Women are usually asymptomatic, but they may have spotting between periods and after sexual intercourse, vaginal drainage (**leukorrhea**), abnormal uterine bleeding, postmenopausal bleeding, and purulent or blood-tinged vaginal discharge (Casey et al., 2011). Polyps are usually found during examination of the cervix with a speculum. They are purple-red, friable (bleed easily when touched), and prone to infection.

Collaborative Management

Surgical removal and cauterization is the usual treatment. Small polyps are excised and sent to the laboratory for tissue analysis. This is usually done as an outpatient procedure or in the office at the time of the examination and followed with cautery. Laboratory analysis is required, because polyps occasionally undergo malignant changes. Clients should receive education and counselling regarding the procedure and reassurance that most polyps are benign.

Postoperative education for women must address the need to rest the pelvic area (ie, avoid sexual intercourse) for at least 24 hours to prevent irritation and bleeding. The client will also need to inform the health care provider of any excessive bleeding or vaginal discharge. Follow-up examination and evaluation are necessary to determine the need for additional endometrial sampling.

CERVICAL DYSPLASIA

Cervical dysplasia, or cervical intraepithelial neoplasia (CIN), is a benign condition that involves abnormal changes in the cells of the cervix. Abnormal cervical cells are also called squamous intraepithelial lesions. Cervical tissue changes are classified as mild, moderate, or severe. Most cervical dysplasias are caused by the HPV (see discussion earlier in this chapter). Other risk factors include herpes virus infection, current smoking, immunosuppressant drugs, immunosuppression, a family history of dysplasia, and in women whose mothers took DES while pregnant (CCS, 2014g). Cervical dysplasia usually is asymptomatic and does not present an immediate health risk; however, it is considered a precancerous condition. Untreated cervical dysplasia can progress to cervical carcinoma in situ or invasive cervical cancer. This abnormal progression to cancer is slow and can take 10 years or longer, although in some cases the time frame may be less (CCS, 2014g). Early detection and monitoring can prevent this condition from becoming cancerous.

Assessment Findings

Routine gynecologic examinations that include Pap testing can detect dysplasia. Pap testing is the most important method of diagnosing this disorder and preventing cancer. If Pap testing indicates dysplasia, colposcopy may be done to assess the severity and location of lesions. This usually results in gradings of CIN 1 (mild dysplasia), CIN 11 (moderate dysplasia), or CIN 111 (severe dysplasia/carcinoma in situ).

Collaborative Management

Low-grade or mild dysplasia (CIN 1), usually seen in women 25 to 35 years old, is the most common type and is detected during Pap testing. High-grade moderate (CIN 11) or severe dysplasias (CIN 111) usually require treatment, because they are more likely to develop into cancer. Severe dysplasia is also referred to as **carcinoma in situ** because it is likely to become cancerous, but can be cured if treated promptly.

Treatment varies with severity and may include conization, cautery, cryosurgery, or laser treatment to remove and destroy the abnormal cells. Health care providers will require women who present with this disorder to have frequent Pap smears and gynecologic examinations to monitor for recurrences.

CERVICAL CANCER

If cervical dysplasia is not treated, the woman will develop cervical cancer (Fig 4.23). This cancer affects the lower portion of the uterus, commonly referred to as the cervical canal. Since 1972, the incidence rates for cervical cancer have steadily declined in Canada, largely due to widespread regular use of PAP test screening (PHAC, 2013c) and availability of cervical screening by cytologic sampling (Bentley, 2012).

Etiology and Pathophysiology

HPV (especially types 16 and 18) has been associated with cervical cancer and is the major risk factor for its development (Bentley, 2012). Clients who forego regular Pap testing to detect HPV or other cell abnormalities are at an increased risk for cervical cancer. Women with low income are at high risk as they are less likely to have regular Pap smears performed. Other risk factors include:

- Smoking
- Weakened immune system and immunocompromised state
- Exposure to DES in utero
- Multiple sexual partners
- First intercourse at an early age
- Having had multiple full-term pregnancies
- Age
- Oral contraceptive use (CCS, 2014g; PHAC, 2013c).

Other risk factors that are currently under study include a history of *Chlamydia* infection; a diet low in vegetables, fruits, and vitamins A, C, and E; and a family history of cervical cancer (CCS, 2014g).

Assessment Findings

Many women are asymptomatic in the early stages of cervical cancer. However, regular Pap screening has proven reliable in early identification of women with cervical dysplasia (see Chapter 2). Symptomatic women may notice and present with vague problems often associated with other conditions, such as vaginal bleeding between periods, unusually long or heavy

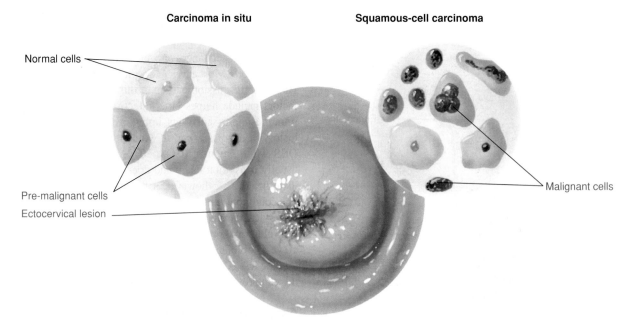

Carcinoma in situ **Squamous-cell carcinoma**

Normal cells

Pre-malignant cells

Ectocervical lesion

Malignant cells

FIGURE 4.23 Cervical cancer. (From Anatomical Chart Company. [2002]. *Atlas of pathophysiology.* Springhouse, PA: Springhouse.)

periods, bleeding after sexual intercourse, watery or increased vaginal discharge, pain during intercourse, and post-menopausal vaginal bleeding (CCS, 2014g). Clients should be advised to consult their health care provider when they have such symptoms. Later symptoms include pelvic or lower-back pain that may radiate down the leg(s); foul-smelling vaginal discharge; edema of the legs; or tiredness, lack of energy, and shortness of breath arising from anemia (CCS, 2014g).

Collaborative Management

When an abnormal Pap result is obtained, symptoms are present, or a health history or physical examination is suspicious for cervical cancer, further diagnostic tests are indicated. A CBC (to assess for anemia) or serum chemistry levels (to assess renal and liver function) are done. A biopsy will be done using colposcopy, endocervical curettage, or cervical conization to further analyze the abnormal cells and to confirm the presence of cancer cells (CCS, 2014g). A chest x-ray, CT scan, MRI, or IV pyelogram may be done to assess progression of the cancer. Secondary prevention for cervical cancer involves identifying women with CIN and conducting cytology evaluation, visual tests, and tests for HPV infection (Bentley, 2012).

Treatment varies and depends on the size and stage of the tumour, personal factors such as the woman's age and desire to have future pregnancies, and her overall health (Table 4.9). Treatments most frequently used include surgery, radiation, and chemotherapy (CCS, 2014g). Surgery may include cervical conization (cone biopsy) to remove abnormal cervical tissue; radical trachelectomy where the cervix and pelvic lymph nodes are removed; or total or radical hysterectomy. Pelvic exenteration, where the cervix, uterus, vagina, ovaries,

● TABLE 4.9 **Cervical Cancer Staging**

Stages	Characteristics
0 (carcinoma in situ)	Cancer is found in the first layer of cells lining the cervix only.
I	Cancer is found in the cervix only, beneath the top layer of cells.
II	Cancer has spread beyond the cervix to nearby tissues such as the upper part of the vagina or next to the cervix.
III	Cancer has spread to the lower third of the vagina or pelvic wall. May block the ureter. May have spread to nearby lymph nodes.
IV	Cancer has spread to the bladder, rectum, or other parts of the body.

Adapted from Canadian Cancer Society. (2014). What is cervical cancer? Retrieved from http://www.cancer.ca/en/cancer-information/cancer-type/cervical/overview/?region=on

Fallopian tubes, and nearby lymph nodes are removed, may be used to treat cervical cancer that recurs following treatment. The cone biopsy is done using loop electrosurgical excision procedure, cold-knife excision, or laser excision (CCS, 2014g).

PELVIC RELAXATION ALTERATIONS

Muscles of the pelvic floor support the abdominal and pelvic organs, and the ligaments, muscles, and connective tissues support the pelvis itself. Sometimes these structures become stretched or damaged. The most common causes of pelvic support problems are multiparity, vaginal delivery of large infants, chronic coughing or straining from constipation, surgery, aging, obesity, and menopause (Siegel, 2010). Pelvic floor dysfunction is expected to be more frequent because of the increasing aging population of women.

Organs affected may include the urethra, bladder, small intestine, rectum, uterus, and vagina. The vaginal wall weakens and descends, and the pelvic organs begin to protrude into the vaginal canal. The most common disorders associated with these changes are cystocele, rectocele, and uterine prolapse (Youngkin et al., 2012) (Fig. 4.24). All these disorders are discussed in detail in Chapter 19.

URINARY TRACT DISORDERS

Bacteria in the urinary tract can result in infections. The points where the ureters attach to the bladder act as one-way valves, preventing backflow of urine into the ureters and toward the kidneys, preventing the ascent of infectious organisms; the act of urination also assists in preventing infection by clearing microbes out of the body. In spite of this, at times a UTI may occur. *Escherichia coli,* a normal flora in the bowel, is a common causative organism in healthy women. Women are more susceptible to UTIs than are men, in part because of a shorter urethra and its close proximity to the vaginal and anal areas; sexual activity also places women at risk. Women who are pregnant also seem to be more susceptible (National Kidney and Urologic Diseases Information Clearinghouse, 2012).

CYSTITIS AND URINARY TRACT INFECTIONS

Cystitis is an infection of the bladder. Bacterial growth in a woman's urinary tract is related primarily to fecal organisms that move from the perineum to the urethra and bladder (National Kidney and Urologic Diseases Information Clearinghouse, 2012). Organisms are deposited at the periurethral opening, often because of

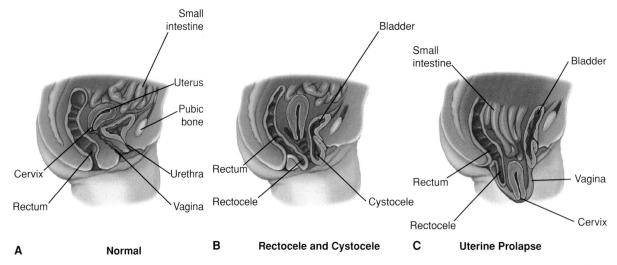

FIGURE 4.24 **A:** Normal appearance and positioning of the uterus. **B:** Rectocele and cystocele. **C:** Uterine prolapse.

fecal contamination, and move up through the urethra, often through sexual intercourse and urethral manipulation during oral sex or masturbation (Umeed, 2012). The relationship between vaginal intercourse and cystitis has led to the colloquial terminology of "honeymoon cystitis." Women should be advised that voiding after intercourse helps decrease rates of infection. Use of diaphragms and spermicide, sexual activity, pregnancy, menopause, catheter use, and a history of UTIs all increase the risk for cystitis (see Chapter 8) (Shah & Goundrey-Smith, 2013; Sheerin, 2011; Umeed, 2012).

UTIs can occur throughout the woman's lifetime, but aging is associated with increased prevalence. Factors contributing to higher rates in older women may include alteration in vaginal flora, changes in urinary tract structure, or the existence of comorbidities such as type 2 diabetes, bladder emptying problems, concurrent diseases, bowel incontinence, and poor nutrition (Shah & Goundrey-Smith, 2013; Sheerin, 2011).

Assessment Findings

Health care providers decide whether a woman's presenting symptoms are vaginal or urinary. When a UTI is suspected, the health care provider determines whether it is a lower or upper UTI. Common presenting symptoms include burning on urination; a frequent and intense urge to urinate, often with little urine to pass; pain in the back or lower abdomen; cloudy, dark, or bloody urine with an unusual smell; fever; and chills (Shah & Goundrey-Smith, 2013; Sheerin, 2011).

Diagnostic testing includes a complete health history and physical examination, as well as a urine dipstick test for nitrites, leukocytes, erythrocytes, and protein; urinalysis; and urine culture and sensitivity (Shah & Goundrey-Smith, 2013; Sheerin, 2011).

Collaborative Management

Treatment goals are to eradicate the invading bacteria; thus, antibiotics are often prescribed. Two of the most common types used are trimethoprim or nitrofurantoin (Shah & Goundrey-Smith, 2013). They are typically prescribed for 3 days in the case of uncomplicated cystitis; up to 7 to 10 days for pregnant women (Sheerin, 2011). Women are counselled to complete the entire prescription (National Kidney and Urologic Diseases Information Clearinghouse, 2012). Women are also counselled to wipe the perineum from front to back to prevent contamination with fecal bacteria.

Increasing fluid intake is controversial and should be discussed with the health care provider. Drinking cranberry juice had been thought to decrease recurrent UTIs, especially in older women (Jepson & Craig, 2009), but a more recent Cochrane review (Jepson, et al., 2012) concluded that it was less effective than previously thought; as a result it is no longer recommended. Some health care providers also suggest applying estrogen topical cream to the urinary meatus, although this has also produced inconsistent results (Sheerin, 2011). Recurrences must be treated promptly and thoroughly to prevent development of an upper UTI (kidney infection).

INTERSTITIAL CYSTITIS

Interstitial cystitis is a chronic and painful inflammatory bladder disorder that primarily affects women during their reproductive years (Women's College Hospital, n.d.b). Ninety percent of cases affect women; it is relatively uncommon, affecting approximately one person in 3,000 (Women's College Hospital, n.d.b). The condition is often one of the underlying causes of chronic pelvic pain and seriously affects women's quality of life by interfering with the ability to work, maintain a home, attend to family responsibilities, and engage in sexual relations (Women's College Hospital, n.d.b).

Interstitial cystitis does not appear to be directly caused by an infection, although it is often initially diagnosed as a bladder infection. It is most common in women with other chronic conditions, such as irritable bowel syndrome, RA, fibromyalgia, asthma, allergies, and SLE (Women's College Hospital, n.d.b).

Assessment Findings

Symptoms of interstitial cystitis may vary between individuals and even for the same individual. Women with interstitial cystitis experience pain that increases with bladder filling and decreases with urination or that presents as constant pain in the bladder, abdomen, lower back, vagina, or thighs (Women's College Hospital, n.d.b). Urinary frequency and urgency may also be present. Symptoms are often worse just prior to the onset of menses.

There is no definitive diagnostic test for interstitial cystitis. On physical examination, the health provider may note lower abdominal tenderness. Laboratory testing of the urine reveals no infection; microscopic examination of the urine may show RBCs when the bladder is overdistended.

Collaborative Management

The goal of treatment is to alleviate and relieve symptoms; there is no complete cure (Women's College Hospital, n.d.b). Women must take an active role in the management of the problem and understand that healing may take a long time. Pharmacologic agents are used to treat most symptoms. Inflammation and pain are relieved with NSAIDs. Anticholinergic drugs can relieve bladder spasms. Pentosan polysulfate sodium, which has demonstrated effectiveness in restoring the bladder lining, is also used to treat interstitial cystitis.

Another treatment option is regular weekly drug instillations into the bladder using dimethyl sulfoxide (DMSO). Transcutaneous electrical nerve stimulation (TENS) may be used to relieve pain.

Nursing interventions include education, counselling, and support. Clients need to undergo lifestyle changes, follow bladder-training programs, use stress reduction strategies, and increase physical activity to manage symptoms. Avoidance of caffeine and artificial sweeteners, alcohol, and tobacco can also help. Dietary changes that have proved helpful in alleviating symptoms include restriction of salt, sugar, yeast, acidic foods, and the amino acids tyrosine and tryptophan.

URINARY INCONTINENCE

Urinary incontinence means the inability to control urination (involuntarily loss of urine). This is common in women and may be attributable to pregnancy, child-birth, menopause, and the structures of the female urinary tract. For detailed discussion of this problem and its treatment, see Chapter 24.

SUMMARY

- Women's health care is moving from focusing only on those conditions that affect the breasts and reproductive organs to emphasizing those conditions with greater prevalence in women, different courses and manifestations in women, or both.
- CF, Tay–Sachs disease, thalassemia, and sickle cell disease are genetic disorders in women that can have an impact on outcomes in pregnancy.
- In autoimmune disorders, the body attacks its own tissues. Examples of such conditions with high prevalence in women include RA, myasthenia gravis, SLE, and MS.
- Incidence of diabetes mellitus is growing at alarming rates.
- Heart disease and stroke are the leading causes of death in Canadian women. Preventive measures can do much to avert these problems.
- Common STIs include chlamydia, gonorrhea, syphilis, genital herpes, and HPV. Bacterial vaginosis, trichomoniasis, and yeast infections may be transmitted sexually. Preventive measures can be taken to avoid all these problems; once they occur, rapid screening and management are necessary to preserve fertility and control the transfer of the problem to others.
- HIV and hepatitis are viral illnesses that are transmitted in a number of ways. These diseases often pose chronic difficulties for affected clients and may be transmitted to newborns.
- Common benign breast disorders include mastalgia, infections, fibrocystic changes, and fibroadenomas.
- A diagnosis of breast malignancy can be threatening to a client's sense of womanhood and emotionally devastating. Nevertheless, breast cancer is one of the most treatable forms of cancer, and new management modalities are being created every day.
- Screening tools for breast cancer include mammography and clinical breast examination. Diagnostic testing for breast cancer can include mammography, ultrasound, MRI, or breast biopsy.
- Treatment of breast cancer may involve surgery, radiation therapy, chemotherapy, hormonal therapy, or HER-2 therapy, or a combination of these approaches. Nursing measures focus on cancer prevention, assisting with any treatments and their side effects, and providing client teaching about expected side effects and their management, resources for assistance, and long-term outcomes.
- Menstrual disorders are common complaints for women and may develop chronically or episodically

throughout a woman's childbearing years. Examples include amenorrhea, dysmenorrhea, dysfunctional uterine bleeding, and PMS.

- PID and endometriosis are two reproductive tract problems that often require aggressive management because they have long-term consequences for a woman's fertility.
- Problems of the female reproductive tract can be benign or malignant disorders. Examples of benign conditions include leiomyomas, PCOS, endometrial hyperplasia, ovarian cysts, cervical polyps, and cervical dysplasia. Malignancies include cancers of the uterus, ovaries, and cervix.

REVIEW QUESTIONS

1. A 30-year-old client is suspected of having systemic lupus erythematosus. Which of the following assessment findings would the nurse be least likely to expect to see for this client?
   A. Butterfly-shaped facial rash
   B. Elevated erythrocyte sedimentation rate
   C. Positive antinuclear antibody titre
   D. Multiple-joint inflammation and swelling
2. After teaching a group of young women about chlamydia, which statement by the group indicates that the nurse's teaching was successful?
   A. Chlamydia can be detected early on because of a characteristic vaginal discharge.
   B. A painless ulcer forms on the area of the body that was exposed to the organism.
   C. Infertility can occur if the infection damages the fallopian tubes.
   D. An injection of penicillin is commonly used to treat the infection.
3. The nurse is assessing a woman with HIV. Which of the following T4-cell count values would make the nurse suspect that the client has AIDS?
   A. 725/mm^3
   B. 550/mm^3
   C. 375/mm^3
   D. 195/mm^3
4. Which of the following pharmacologic agents would the nurse expect the health care provider to prescribe for a woman diagnosed with genital herpes?
   A. Azithromycin
   B. Ofloxacin
   C. Metronidazole
   D. Acyclovir
5. Which of these topics should the nurse include in preparing a presentation about breast cancer for a local women's group?
   A. Breast cancer is the most lethal type of cancer for women.
   B. Knowing one's own breasts is important.

C. Most women who get breast cancer have a family history of it.
   D. Women younger than 40 years are at the highest risk for breast cancer.
6. The nurse is preparing a client who has undergone a mastectomy of her right breast for discharge from the hospital. Which statement, if made by the client, indicates the need for additional teaching?
   A. I'll immediately report any tingling on the inner side of my right arm.
   B. I'll ask my husband for help if a package feels heavy.
   C. I won't allow any blood pressures to be taken in my right arm.
   D. I should avoid sleeping on my right side.
7. A young client comes to the health clinic for an evaluation. During the visit, she asks, "When I get my period, sometimes I get cramps that can really hurt. What causes this?" Which of the following responses, if made by the nurse, would be most appropriate?
   A. You probably have an underlying infection that is causing the pain.
   B. An increase in a hormone makes the uterus contract more, causing pain.
   C. It's absolutely normal to have cramps with your period.
   D. I will get you a prescription to help with the pain.
8. Which of the following symptoms would the nurse expect to assess when caring for a 45-year-old woman diagnosed with uterine leiomyoma?
   A. High fever with complaints of pain on cervical movement
   B. Dysmenorrhea and irregular vaginal bleeding
   C. Abnormal bleeding in menopause with pelvic pain
   D. Abnormal vaginal bleeding and reports of pelvic pressure
9. When teaching a client with cervical dysplasia about this disorder, the nurse would emphasize the importance of which of the following?
   A. Regular Pap smears
   B. Yearly CA-125 testing
   C. Strict condom use
   D. Frequent perineal hygiene
10. Which of the following instructions should the nurse not include in a teaching plan for an older woman diagnosed with cystitis?
   A. Be sure to urinate after you engage in sexual intercourse.
   B. If your symptoms reappear, call the office as soon as possible.
   C. You will take medication for 5 days and then stop.
   D. Try drinking cranberry juice during the day.

REFERENCES

American Lung Association. (2010). Cystic fibrosis. In *State of Lung Disease in Diverse Communities.* 41–44. Washington, DC: Author

Asch, M., Lefebvre, G., & Vilos, G. (2004). SOGC clinical practice guidelines: Uterine fibroid embolization (UFE). *Journal of Obstetrics and Gynaecology Canada, 28*(10), 899–906.

Bentley, J. (2012). SOGC clinical practice guidelines: Colposcopic management of abnormal cervical cytology and histology. *Journal of Obstetrics and Gynecology Canada, 34*(12), 1188–1202.

Blakeley, J. O., & Llinas, R. H. (2007). Thrombolytic therapy for acute ischemic stroke. *Journal of the Neurological Sciences, 261*(1-2), 55–62.

Breast Cancer Society of Canada (BCSC). (2013). Breast cancer statistics. Retrieved from http://www.bcsc.ca/p/46/l/129/t/Breast-Cancer-Society-of-Canada—Statistics

Caddy, S., Yudin, M. H., Hakim, T., & Money, D. M. (2014). Best practices to minimize risk of infection with intrauterine device insertion. *Journal of Obstetrics and Gynaecology Canada, 36*(3), 266–274.

Canadian Breast Cancer Foundation (CBCF). (2014a). Breast cancer in Canada, 2013. Retrieved from https://www.cbcf.org/central/AboutBreastCancerMain/AboutBreastCancer/Pages/BreastCancerinCanada.aspx

Canadian Breast Cancer Foundation (CBCF). (2014b). Reduce your breast cancer risk. Retrieved from https://www.cbcf.org/central/AboutBreastHealth/PreventionRiskReduction/ReduceYourRisk/Pages/default.aspx

Canadian Breast Cancer Foundation (CBCF). (2014c). Family cancer history and genetics. Retrieved from https://www.cbcf.org/central/AboutBreastHealth/PreventionRiskReduction/risk_factors/Pages/family_history.aspx

Canadian Breast Cancer Foundation (CBCF). (2014d). Normal breast changes. Retrieved from https://www.cbcf.org/central/AboutBreastHealth/Breast-Awareness/NormalChanges/Pages/default.aspx

Canadian Breast Cancer Foundation. (2014e). How is breast cancer diagnosed. Retrieved from https://www.cbcf.org/central/AboutBreastCancerMain/Diagnosis/Pages/default.aspx

Canadian Cancer Society (CCS]. (2014a). Benign breast conditions. Retrieved from http://www.cancer.ca/en/cancer-information/cancer-type/breast/pathology-and-staging/benign-conditions/?region=bc

Canadian Cancer Society (CCS). (2014b). Breast cancer statistics. Retrieved from http://www.cancer.ca/en/cancer-information/cancer-type/breast/statistics/?region=on

Canadian Cancer Society (CCS). (2014c). Inflammatory breast cancer. Retrieved from http://www.cancer.ca/en/cancer-information/cancer-type/breast/pathology-and-staging/malignant-tumours/inflammatory-breast-cancer/?region=on

Canadian Cancer Society (CCS). (2014d). Screening for breast cancer. Retrieved from http://www.cancer.ca/en/prevention-and-screening/early-detection-and-screening/screening/screening-for-breast-cancer/?region=on

Canadian Cancer Society (CCS). (2014e). Supportive care for breast cancer. Retrieved from http://www.cancer.ca/en/cancer-information/cancer-type/breast/supportive-care/?region=nu

Canadian Cancer Society (CCS). (2014f). Treatment for breast cancer. Retrieved from http://www.cancer.ca/en/cancer-information/cancer-type/breast/treatment/?region=bc

Canadian Cancer Society (CCS). (2014g). What is cervical cancer? Retrieved from http://www.cancer.ca/en/cancer-information/cancer-type/cervical/overview/?region=bc

Canadian Cancer Society (CCS). (2014h). What is ovarian cancer? Retrieved from http://www.cancer.ca/en/cancer-information/cancer-type/ovarian/overview/?region=on

Canadian Cancer Society (CCS). (2014i). What is uterine cancer? Retrieved from http://www.cancer.ca/en/cancer-information/cancer-type/uterine/overview/?region=on

Canadian Cystic Fibrosis Registry. (2012). 2012 Annual Report. Toronto, ON: Cystic Fibrosis Canada. Retrieved from http://www.cysticfibrosis.ca/wp-content/uploads/2014/03/Canadian-CF-Registry-English-FINAL-FOR-WEB1.pdf

Canadian Diabetes Association. (2013). Clinical practice guidelines. Retrieved from http://guidelines.diabetes.ca/ScreeningAndDiagnosis/Screening

Canadian Diabetes Association. (2014). About diabetes. Retrieved from http://www.diabetes.ca/about-diabetes

Canadian Liver Foundation. (2012a). Hepatitis A. Retrieved from http://www.liver.ca/liver-disease/types/viral_hepatitis/Hepatitis_A.aspx

Canadian Liver Foundation. (2012b). Hepatitis B. Retrieved from http://www.liver.ca/liver-disease/types/viral_hepatitis/Hepatitis_B.aspx

Canadian Liver Foundation. (2012c). Hepatitis C. Retrieved from http://www.liver.ca/liver-disease/types/viral_hepatitis/Hepatitis_C.aspx

Canadian Women's Health Network (CWHN). (2012a). Endometriosis. Retrieved from http://www.cwhn.ca/en/node/40779

Canadian Women's Health Network (CWHN). (2012b). Fibroids. Retrieved from http://www.cwhn.ca/en/node/40783

Canadian Women's Health Network (CWHN). (2012c). Polycystic ovarian syndrome (PCOS). Retrieved from http://www.cwhn.ca/en/node/44804

Casey, P., Long, M., & Marnach, M. (2011). Abnormal cervical appearance: What to do, when to worry? *Mayo Clinical Proceedings, 86*(2), 147–151.

Centers for Disease Control and Prevention (CDC). (2011). Sickle cell disease (SCD). Retrieved from http://www.cdc.gov/ncbddd/sicklecell/index.html

Chetty, S. P., Shaffer, B. L., & Norton, M. E. (2011). Management of pregnancy in women with genetic disorders: Part 2: Inborn errors of metabolism, cystic fibrosis, neurofibromatosis type 1, and turner syndrome in pregnancy. *Obstetrical & Gynecological Survey, 66*(12), 765–776.

Cummings, S., Tice, J., Bauer, S., Browner, W., Cuzick, J., Ziv, E., et al. (2009). Prevention of breast cancer in postmenopausal women. *Journal of National Cancer Institute, 101*(6), 384–398.

Cystic Fibrosis Canada (CFC). (n.d.). About CF. Retrieved from http://www.cysticfibrosis.ca/about-cf/what-is-cystic-fibrosis/?lang=en

Ferenkeh-Koroma, A. (2012). Systemic lupus erythematosus: Nurse and patient education. *Nursing Standard, 26*(39), 49–57

Ferreia, J., Schreiber-Agus, N., Carter, S., Klugman, S., Fregg, A., & Gross, S. (2014). Carrier testing for Ashkenazi Jewish disorders in the prenatal setting: Navigating the genetic maze. *American Journal of Obstetrics and Gynecology,* February 5. doi:10.1016/j.ajog.2014.02.001. [Epub ahead of print]

Genetics Home Reference. (2012). Conditions: Tay-Sachs Disease. U.S. National Library of Medicine. Retrieved from http://ghr.nlm.nih.gov/condition/tay-sachs-disease

Gibofsky, A. (2012). Overview of epidemiology, pathophysiology, and diagnosis of rheumatoid arthritis. *America Journal of Managed Care, 18*, S295–S302.

Government of Canada. (2013a). Chlamydia. Accessed from http://healthycanadians.gc.ca/health-sante/sexual-sexuelle/chlamyd-eng.php

Government of Canada. (2013b). Genital herpes. Accessed from http://healthycanadians.gc.ca/health-sante/sexual-sexuelle/herpes-eng.php?_ga=1.185294379.301514305.1399164236

Government of Canada. (2013c). HIV/AIDS. Retrieved from http://www.healthycanadians.gc.ca/health-sante/disease-maladie/hiv-vih-eng.php?utm_source=aids_13&utm_medium=banner_link&utm_campaign=hpfeaturebox

Government of Canada. (2013d). Human papillomavirus (HPV). Retrieved from http://healthycanadians.gc.ca/health-sante/sexual-sexuelle/hpv-vph-eng.php

Government of Canada. (2013e). Syphilis. Retrieved from http://healthycanadians.gc.ca/health-sante/sexual-sexuelle/syphilis-eng.php?_ga=1.176363303.301514305.1399164236

Gradison, M. (2012). Pelvic inflammatory disease. *American Family Physician, 85*(8), 791–796.

Haggerty, C. L, Gottlieb, S. L., Tayolor, B. D., Low, N., Xu, F., & Ness, R. B. (2010). Risk of sequelae after *Chlamydia trachomatis* genital infection in women. *The Journal of Infectious Diseases, 201*(S2), S134–S155. doi:10.1086/652395

Haqq, L., McFarlane, J., Dieberg, G., & Smart, N. (2014). Effect of lifestyle intervention on the reproductive endocrine profile in women with polycystic ovarian syndrome: A systematic review and meta-analysis. *Endocrine Connections*. Retrieved from http://www.endocrineconnections.com/content/3/1/36.full.pdf+html

Healthline. (2014). What are ovarian cysts? Retrieved from http://www.healthline.com/health/ovarian-cysts

HealthLinkBC. (n.d.). Tay Sachs Disease. Retrieved from http://www.healthlinkbc.ca/healthtopics/content.asp?hwid=nord9

Healthwise. (2013). Functional ovarian cysts. BCHealthGuide. Retrieved from http://www.healthlinkbc.ca/healthtopics/content.asp?hwid=hw181644

Heart & Stroke Foundation of Canada. (2014a). Heart disease. Retrieved from http://www.heartandstroke.com/site/c.ikIQLcMWJtE/b.3484021/k.7C85/Heart_Disease.htm

Heart & Stroke Foundation of Canada. (2014b). Stroke. Retrieved from http://www.heartandstroke.com/site/c.ikIQLcMWJtE/b.3483933/k.CD67/Stroke.htm

Hill, J., Holcombe, B., Clark, L., Boothby, M. R., Hincks, A., Fisher, J., et al. (2011). Predictors of onset of depression and anxiety in the year after diagnosis of breast cancer. *Psychological Medicine, 41*(7), 1429–1436. doi:10.1017/S0033291710001868

Hoover, R., Hyer, M., Pfeiffer, R., Adam, E., Bond, B., Cheville, A., et al. (2011). Adverse health outcomes in women exposed in utero to diethylstibestrol. *New England Journal of Medicine, 365*(14), 1304–1314.

Hospital for Sick Children. (2014). Ashkenazi Jewish screening panel. Molecular genetics library. Retrieved from http://www.sickkids.ca/pdfs/Paediatric%20Laboratory%20Medicine/info-sheets/56249-AJ%20Screening%20Panel_OMG1620D_02.pdf

Hubbs, J., Saig, R., Abaid, L., Bae-Jump, V., & Gehrig, P. (2013). Systemic and local hormone therapy for endometrial hyperplasia and early adenocarcinoma. *Obstetrics & Gynecology, 121*(6), 1172–1180.

Hussain, A. N., Policarpio, C., & Vincent, M. T. (2006). Evaluating nipple discharge. *Obstetric and Gynecologic Survey, 61*(4), 278–283.

Jepson, R. G., & Craig, J. C. (2009). Cranberries for preventing urinary tract infections. *Cochrane Database of Systematic Reviews, 1*, Art. No.: CD001321. doi:10.1002/14651858.CD001321.pub4.

Jepson, R. G., Williams, G., & Craig, J. C. (2012). Cranberries for preventing urinary tract infections. *Cochrane Database of Systematic Reviews, 10*, Art. No.: CD001321. doi:10.1002/14651858.CD001321.pub5

Ju, H., Jones, M., & Mishra, C. (2014). The prevalence and risk factors of dysmenorrhea. *Epidemiologic Reviews, 36*(1), 104–113.

Juel, V. C., & Massey, J. M. (2007). Myasthenia gravis. *Orphanet Journal of Rare Diseases, 2*, 44. Retrieved from http://www.ojrd.com/content/2/1/44

Keenan-Lindsay, L., & Yudin, M. H. (2006). SOGC Clinical practice guideline: HIV screening in pregnancy. *Journal of Obstetrics & Gynaecology of Canada, 28*(12), 1103–1107.

Kesisis, G., Makris, A., & Miles, D. (2009). Update on the use of aromatase inhibitors in early-stage breast cancer. *Breast Cancer Research, 11*, 211. Retrieved from http://breast-cancer-research.com/content/11/5/211

Khan, A., Shehmar, M., & Gupta, J. (2014). Uterine fibroids: Current perspectives. *International Journal of Women's Health, 6*, 95–114.

Kyranou, M., Paul, S. M., Dunn, L. B., Puntillo, K., Aouizerat, B. E., Abrams, G., et al. (2013). Differences in depression, anxiety and quality of life between women with and without breast pain prior to breast cancer surgery. *European Journal of Oncology Nursing, 17*(2), 190–195. Retrieved from http://dx.doi.org/10.1016/j.ejon.2012.06.001

Lacey, J., Sherman, M., Rush, B., Ronnett, B., Ioffe, O., Duggan, M., et al. (2010). Absolute risk of endometrial carcinoma during 20 year follow-up among women with endometrial hyperplasia. *Journal of Clinical Oncology, 28*(5), 788–792.

Langlois, S., & Wilson, R. D. (2006). Carrier screening for genetic disorders in individuals of Ashkenazi Jewish descent. SOGC Clinical Practice Guideline No. 177. *Journal of Obstetrics and Gynaecology of Canada, 28*(4), 324–343. Retrieved from http://sogc.org/guidelines/carrier-screening-for-genetic-disorders-in-individuals-of-ashkenazi-jewish-descent/

Lethaby, A., Suckling, J., Barlow, D., Farquhar, C. M., Jepson, R. G., & Roberts, H. (2004). Hormone replacement therapy in postmenopausal women: Endometrial hyperplasia and irregular bleeding. *Cochrane Database of Systematic Reviews, 4*, Art No:Cd000402. doi:10.1002/14651858.CD000402.pub2

Loiselle, C. G., Lambert, S. D., & Cooke, A. (2006). The searching, processing, and sharing of breast cancer information by women diagnosed with the illness. *Canadian Journal of Nursing Research, 38*(3), 82–104.

Luhan, M., Chizen, D., & Pierson, R. (2008). Diagnostic criteria for polycystic ovary syndrome: Pitfalls and controversies. *Journal of Obstetrics and Gynecology Canada, 30*(1), 671–679.

Lupus Canada. (2014). Living with Lupus—questions. Retrieved from http://www.lupuscanada.org/english/living/lupus-overview.html

Lupus Canada. (n.d.). Lupus fact sheet: Lupus medications. Retrieved from http://www.lupuscanada.org/pdfs/LupusMedications.pdf

March of Dimes. (2008). Thalassemia. Retrieved from http://www.marchofdimes.com/baby/thalassemia.aspx

Maybin, J., Munro, M., Fraser, I., & Critchley, H. (2013). Re-definition and re-classification of menstrual disorders. *Obstetrics, Gynaecology & Reproductive Medicine, 23*(11), 331–336.

Mayor, M. T., Roett, M. A., & Uduhiri, K. A. (2012). Diagnosis and management of gonoccoccal infections. *American Family Physician, 86*(10), 931–938.

McCullough, L. E., Eng, S. M., Bradshaw, P. T., Cleveland, R. J., Teitelbaum, S. L., Neugut, A. I., et al. (2012). Fat or fit: The joint effects of physical activity, weight gain, and body size on breast cancer risk. *Cancer, 118*(19), 4860–4868. doi:10.1002/cncr.27433

MedlinePlus. (2011). Uterine fibroids. Retrieved from http://www.nlm.nih.gov/medlineplus/ency/article/000914.htm

MedlinePlus. (2012). Thalassemia. Retrieved from http://www.nlm.nih.gov/medlineplus/ency/article/000587.htm

Mishori, R., McClaskey, E. L., & WinklerPrins, V. J. (2012). *Chlamydia trachomatis* infections: Screening, diagnosis and management. *American Family Physician, 86*(12), 1127–1132.

Multiple Sclerosis Society of Canada. (n.d.). About MS. Retrieved from http://mssociety.ca/en/information/default.htm

National Institutes of Health. (2012). What is sickle cell anemia? Retrieved from http://www.nhlbi.nih.gov/health/health-topics/topics/sca/

National Kidney and Urologic Diseases Information Clearinghouse. (2012). Urinary tract infections in adults. Retrieved from http://kidney.niddk.nih.gov/KUDiseases/pubs/utiadult/index.aspx

Nazarko, I. (2013). Multiple sclerosis: Offering care tailored to the person's needs. *British Journal of Healthcare Assistants, 7*(12), 594–599

Palmer, D., & El Miedany, Y. (2012). Treat-to-target: A tailored treatment approach to rheumatoid arthritis. *British Journal of Nursing, 22*(6), 308–318.

Parsay, S., Olfati, F., & Nahidi, S. (2009). Therapeutic effects of vitamin e on cyclic mastalgia. *The Breast Journal, 15*(5), 510–514. doi:10.1111/j.1524-4741.2009.00768.x

Pinsonneault, O., & Lefebvre, G. (2005). SOGC clinical practice guideline: Primary dysmenorrheal consensus guideline. *Journal of Obstetrics & Gynaecology of Canada, 27*(12), 1117–1130.

Public Health Agency of Canada (PHAC). (2010a). Canadian guidelines on sexually transmitted infections. Retrieved from http://www.phac-aspc.gc.ca/std-mts/sti-its/cgsti-ldcits/index-eng.php

Public Health Agency of Canada (PHAC). (2010b). Hepatitis B—Get the facts. Retrieved from http://www.phac-aspc.gc.ca/hcai-iamss/bbp-pts/hepatitis/hep_b-eng.php

Public Health Agency of Canada (PHAC). (2013a). At a Glance—HIV and AIDS in Canada; Surveillance report to Dec 31st, 2012. Retrieved from http://www.phac-aspc.gc.ca/aids-sida/publication/survreport/2012/dec/index-eng.php

Public Health Agency of Canada (PHAC). (2013b). Breast Cancer. Retrieved April 11, 2013, from http://www.phac-aspc.gc.ca/cd-mc/cancer/breast_cancer-cancer_du_sein-eng.php

Public Health Agency of Canada (PHAC). (2013c). Cervical Cancer. Retrieved from http://www.phac-aspc.gc.ca/cd-mc/cancer/cervical_cancer-cancer_du_col_uterus-eng.php

Public Health Agency of Canada (PHAC). (2013d). Genital Herpes Simplex virus (HSV) infections. Canadian Guidelines on Sexually Transmitted Infections, Section 5. Retrieved from http://www.phac-aspc.gc.ca/std-mts/sti-its/cgsti-ldcits/section-5-4-eng.php

Public Health Agency of Canada (PHAC). (2013e). Gonococcal infections. Canadian Guidelines on Sexually Transmitted Infections, Section 5. Retrieved from http://www.phac-aspc.gc.ca/std-mts/sti-its/cgsti-ldcits/section-5-6-eng.php#toc361210443

Public Health Agency of Canada (PHAC). (2013f). HIV/AIDS Reports & Publications. Retrieved from http://www.phac-aspc.gc.ca/aids-sida/publication/index-eng.php

Public Health Agency of Canada (PHAC). (2013g). Pelvic inflammatory disease. Canadian Guidelines on Sexually Transmitted Infections. Retrieved from http://www.phac-aspc.gc.ca/std-mts/sti-its/cgsti-ldcits/section-4-4-eng.php

Public Health Agency of Canada (PHAC). (2013h). The chief public health officer's report on the state of public health in Canada, 2013: Infectious disease—The never-ending threat. Retrieved from http://www.phac-aspc.gc.ca/cphorsphc-respcacsp/2013/sti-its-eng.php

Read, J., Perz, J., & Ussher, J. (2014). Ways to cope with premenstrual change: Development and validation of a premenstrual coping measure. *BMC Women's Health, 14*(1), 1–15. doi:10.1186/1472-6874-14-1

Roberts, H. (2014). Hormone therapy in postmenopausal women and risk of endometrial hyperplasia: A Cochrane review summary. *Maturitas, 77*(1), 4–6.

Roberts, K. C., Shields, M., de Groh, M., Aziz, A., & Gilbert, J. (2012). *Overweight and obesity in children and adolescents: Results from the 2009–2011 Canadian Health Measures Survey.* Ottawa, ON: Statistics Canada. Retrieved from http://www.statcan.gc.ca/pub/82-003-x/2012003/article/11706-eng.htm

Robertson, F. M., Bondy, M., Yang, W., Yamauchi, H., Wiggins, S., Kamrudin, S., et al. (2010). Inflammatory breast cancer: The disease, the biology, the treatment. *Cancer: A Cancer Journal for Clinicians, 60*(6), 351–375.

Robinson, M., Cook, S. S., & Currie, L. M. (2011). Systemic lupus erythematosus: A genetic review for advanced practice nurses. *Journal of the American Academy of Nurse Practitioners, 23*, 629–637. doi:10.1111/j.1745-7599.2011.00675.x

Rotermann, M. Langlois, K. A., Severini, A., & Totten, S. (2013). Prevalence of *Chlamydia trachomatis* and herpes simplex virus type w2: Results from the 2009 to 2011 Canadian Health Measures Survey. Retrieved from http://www.statcan.gc.ca/pub/82-003-x/2013004/article/11777-eng.htm

Satack, R. J., Sahni, M., Mallen, C. D., & Raza, K. (2013). Symptom complexes at the earliest phases of rheumatoid arthritis: A synthesis of the qualitative literature. *Arthritis Care & Research, 65*(12), 1916–1926. doi:10.1002/acr.22097

Sathasivam, S. (2014). Diagnosis and management of myasthenia gravis. *Progress in Neurology and Psychiatry, 18*(1), 6–14. doi:10.1002/pnp.315

Scott, D. L., Wolfe, F., & Huizinga, T. W. (2010). Rheumatoid arthritis. *Lancet, 376*(9746), 1094–1108.

Shah, C., & Goundrey-Smith, S. (2013). Managing the symptoms of urinary tract infection in women. *Journal of Community Nursing, 27*(4), 88–92.

Sheerin, M. S. (2011). Urinary tract infection. *Medicine, 39*(7), 384–389.

Siegel, A. (2010). *Female pelvic relaxation: A primer for women with pelvic organ prolapsed. Bergen Urological Associates.* Hackensack, NJ: Hackensack University Medical Center. Retrieved from http://pelvicrelaxation.com/Female_Pelvic_Relaxation_BKLT__10v3.pdf

Singh, S., Best, C., Dunn, S., Leyland, N., & Wolfman, W. L. (2013). Abnormal uterine bleeding in pre-menopausal women. *Journal of Obstetrics and Gynaecology Canada, 35*(5eSuppl), S1–S28.

Singh, S. S., Casper, R., Laberge, P., & Leyland, N. (2010). SOGC clinical practice guidelines: Endometriosis: Diagnosis and management. *Journal of Obstetrics and Gynaecology Canada, 32*(7), S1–S26.

SOGC. (2012). STIs-STDs. Retrieved from http://www.sexuality-andu.ca/stis-stds

Sponiar, M., Sharpe, L., Butow, P., & Fulcher, G. (2007). Reproductive choices of women with multiple sclerosis. *International Journal of MS Care, 9*(1), 9–12.

St. Michael's Hospital. (2014). CIBC breast centre: Benign breast conditions. Retrieved from http://www.stmichaelshospital.com/programs/breastcentre/benign.php

Stuebe, A., Willet, W., Xue, F., & Michels, K. (2009). Lactation and incidence of premenopausal breast cancer: A longitudinal study. *JAMA Internal Medicine, 169*(15), 1364–1371.

Thalassemia Foundation of Canada. (2013). Disease: About thalassemia. Retrieved from http://www.thalassemia.ca/disease-treatment/disease-2/

The Arthritis Society. (2014a). Lupus. Retrieved from http://www.arthritis.ca/page.aspx?pid=938

The Arthritis Society. (2014b). Rheumatoid arthritis. Retrieved from http://www.arthritis.ca/page.aspx?pid=982

The Endometriosis Network Canada. (2014). Physician fact sheet. Retrieved from http://endometriosisnetwork.com/physician-endo-sheet/

Tooley, L. (2010a). A rapid approach to community-based HIV testing. CATIE. Canada's Source for HIV and Hepatitis C Information. Retrieved from http://www.catie.ca/en/pif/spring-2010/rapid-approach-community-based-hiv-testing

Tooley, L. (2010b). Detecting HIV earlier: Advances in HIV testing. CATIE. Canada's Source for HIV and Hepatitis C Information. Retrieved from http://www.catie.ca/en/pif/august-2010/detecting-hiv-earlier-advances-hiv-testing

Traboulsee, A. L., Knox, K. B., Machan, L., Zhao, Y., Yee, I., Rauscher A., et al. (2014). Prevalence of extracranial venous narrowing on catheter venography in people with multiple sclerosis, their siblings, and unrelated healthy controls: A blinded, case-control study. *The Lancet, 383*(9912), 138–145. doi:10.1016/S0140-6736(13)61747-X

Turcotte, M. (2013). Women and health. Women in Canada: A Gender-based Statistical Report. Statistics Canada 89–503-X. Retrieved from http://www.statcan.gc.ca/pub/89-503-x/2010001/article/11543-eng.htm

Umeed, M. (2012). Take home messages in the management of cystitis. *Practice Nurse, 42*(12), 13–16.

Vause, T. D., & Cheung, A. P. (2010). SOGC clinical practice guidelines: Ovulation induction in polycystic ovary syndrome. *Journal of Obstetrics and Gynecology Canada, 32*(5), 495–502.

Vitale, S., Tropea, A., Rossetti, D., Carnelli, M., & Cianci, A. (2013). Management of uterine leiomyomas in pregnancy: Review of literature. *Updates Surgery, 65*(3), 179–182. doi:10.1007/s13304-013-0198-z.

WebMD. (2013). Uterine fibroid embolization. Healthwise Incorporated. Retrieved from http://www.webmd.com/women/uterine-fibroids/uterine-fibroid-embolization-ufe

Wolfman, W. (2010). SOGC clinical practice guidelines: Asymptomatic endometrial thickening. *Journal of Obstetrics and Gynecology Canada, 32*(10), 990–999.

Women's College Hospital. (n.d.a). Gynecological health. Retrieved from http://www.womenshealthmatters.ca/health-centres/pelvic-health/

Women's College Hospital. (n.d.b). Interstitial cystitis. Retrieved from http://www.womenshealthmatters.ca/health-centres/pelvic-health/interstitial-cystitis/

World Endometriosis Society. (2012). Facts about endometriosis. Retrieved from http://endometriosis.ca/Facts-about-endometriosis.pdf

Youngkin, E. Q., Davis, M. S., Schadewald, D., & Juve, C. (2012). *Women's health: A primary care clinical guide* (4th ed.). Upper Saddle River, NJ: Pearson Prentice Hall.

Zamboni, P, Menegatti, E., Galeotti, R., Malagoni, A. M., Tacconi, G., Dall'Ara, S., et al. (2009). The value of cerebral Doppler venous haemodynamics in the assessment of multiple sclerosis. *Journal of the Neurological Sciences, 282*(1-2), 21–27. doi:10.1016/j.jns.2008.11.027

WEB RESOURCES

Canadian Cancer Society, http://www.cancer.ca

Canadian Association of Midwives, http://www.canadianmidwives.org/

Society of Obstetricians and Gynaecologists of Canada (SOGC), http://www.sogc.org and http://sexualityandu.ca

Canadian Diabetes Association, http://www.diabetes.ca/

Heart and Stroke Foundation of Canada, http://www.heartandstroke.com

Canadian Nurses Association, http://www.cna-aiic.ca/en

Canadian Association of Perinatal and Women's Health Nurses (CAPWHN), http://www.capwhn.ca/en/capwhn/About_CAPWHN_p3185.html

CATIE. Canada's Source for HIV and Hepatitis C Information, http://www.catie.ca/

Centers for Disease Control and Prevention (CDC), http://www.cdc.gov

Canadian AIDS Society, http://www.cdnaids.ca/

Canadian Breast Cancer Foundation, http://www.cbcf.org

Canadian Women's Foundation, http://www.canadianwomen.org

Canadian Federation for Sexual Health, http://www.cfsh.ca

Canadian Liver Foundation, http://www.liver.ca

Breast Cancer Society of Canada, http://www.bcsc.ca

Canadian Cystic Fibrosis Foundation, http://www.cysticfibrosis.ca

Arthritis Society of Canada, http://www.arthritis.ca

Lupus Canada, http://www.lupuscanada.org

Multiple Sclerosis Society of Canada, http://www.mssociety.ca

Thalassemia Foundation of Canada, http://www.thalassemia.ca/

CHAPTER 5

Mental Health Concerns for Women in Adolescence and Adulthood

Deborah Salyzyn and Faye Gary*

 Gladys, a 35-year-old multigravida in her 23rd week of pregnancy, comes to the emergency room (ER) accompanied by a male friend. She reports difficulty sleeping, periodic dizziness, and late-day swelling in her feet. She states, "Sometimes, I hear voices telling me to 'watch out for the baby inside...it might just jump out at any minute.'" The nurse notes that Gladys seems easily distracted and frequently looks away, making some statements irrelevant to the conversation at hand and appearing annoyed. She murmurs, "My friend and I are in a hurry to move things along."

 Dina, a 30-year-old multigravida, is making her first visit to the neighbourhood prenatal clinic at 6 months' gestation. She and her husband moved to Canada approximately 12 years ago. Although she classifies herself and her husband as Arabic, she states that she frequently tells people that she is white for fear of rejection and prejudice, including from health care professionals. She has two children younger than 5 years. She works approximately 60 hours a week at a local bakery. She reports that her unemployed husband has difficulty keeping a job because of his "hot temper."

*Contributor to first U.S. edition.

Nurses working with such clients need to understand this chapter to manage care and address issues appropriately. Before beginning this chapter, consider the following points related to the above scenarios:

● How will the nurse working with both clients tailor care to best suit the needs of the women and their families?

● What aspects of teaching do these women require? What issues are similar for the women? What issues are different?

● What mental health issues or concerns might be relevant for each of these women?

● How might each client's current situation affect her health literacy? What factors might be important to assess?

LEARNING OBJECTIVES

On completion of this chapter, the reader should be able to:
● Describe conceptual models of mental health and illness pertinent to women's health care.
● Discuss common psychiatric disorders in women, including signs and symptoms, treatment, and pertinent nursing issues.
● Explore the societal problems of suicide and intimate-partner violence.
● Discuss the therapeutic benefits and potential side effects of psychotropic medications to manage psychiatric disorders, particularly in the care of pregnant or lactating women.
● Discuss the nurse's responsibilities for overall health care when a pregnant or lactating woman has past or current mental illness.
● Describe a health literacy plan for women with mental illness.

KEY TERMS

anorexia nervosa
attachments
bingeing
bulimia nervosa
dysthymic disorder
intimate-partner violence

learned helplessness
mental health literacy
postpartum blues
postpartum pinks
postpartum depression

This chapter provides information about mental health and illness in women throughout adolescence and adulthood. The content has a special focus on pregnant or lactating women facing mental health challenges. The discussions in this chapter are pertinent to all health care settings and based on the assumption that all health professionals, especially nurses who provide health services to women and their children, are in a unique position to assist families.

Encounters between nurses and women experiencing mental health challenges abound. Common examples include the following (Schatzberg & Nemeroff, 2009; Usher et al., 2005):

- A woman experiencing her first episode of mental illness
- A woman experiencing an exacerbation of signs and symptoms of an established mental illness
- A woman who uses psychotropic medications needing consultation for family planning
- A woman using psychotropic drugs who conceives and likely needs her medications throughout the gestation
- A woman who plans to breastfeed but is at risk for postpartum mental illness and needs psychotropic drugs to prevent or treat her condition

Early identification and prompt and efficient treatment remain the cornerstones of quality health care. The information in this chapter is designed to assist nurses in providing such care.

The chapter is divided into four sections. The first section summarizes common conceptual models in mental health. The second section covers major psychiatric and social problems affecting women. It discusses risk factors and common conditions for women of all age groups and circumstances. A special emphasis is placed on pregnant or lactating women. The third section explores psychopharmacologic treatment and its related risk-to-benefit ratio during pregnancy or lactation. The fourth section provides recommendations germane to nursing management and nursing interventions for women experiencing psychosocial health concerns.

CONCEPTUAL MODELS IN MENTAL HEALTH CARE

This section briefly reviews psychoanalytic, behavioural, sociocultural, feminist, and biologic conceptual models of mental health. Those desiring more content on these theoretical foundations should consult psychiatric–mental health nursing textbooks.

Psychoanalytic Models

Psychoanalytic models explore unconscious motivations and seek to explain behaviours related to these shielded motivations. Although many of their tenets have been called into question over time, they can be useful for understanding women's mental health because of their focuses on the motivations for behaviours, the way in which attachments are formed in early life, and developmental progression of the personality. Two important theorists of this model are Sigmund Freud and Erik Erikson.

Freud

Freud postulated that the mind was divided into two parts: the small conscious segment, and the much larger *unconscious* part. The powerful and driving unconscious mind contains hurtful memories, forbidden desires, and other repressed experiences, or things that a person has pushed from awareness. Unconscious material seeks expression, which may be reflected in a woman's dreams or fantasies; according to Freud, it also may lead to irrational and maladaptive behaviour (Brenner, 1957; Mohr, 2012).

Freud also proposed a topography of the mind, consisting of the id, ego, and superego.

- The entirely selfish *id* consists of instinctual drives (ie, aggression and sexuality). It demands immediate gratification, regardless of external constraints. The id supplies all the power for the other two subsystems.
- The *ego* emerges during childhood and controls the id by supplying mechanisms for reality testing, judgement formation, and other functions essential to daily living. The ego enables the person to meet the id's demands, but in a way that allows her to function normally in society.
- The *superego*, which develops gradually, regulates and sanctions behaviour by providing a conscience for decision making. It provides a way of distinguishing right from wrong. Freud postulated that attachments in early life lay the foundation for future relationships.

Attachments are those significant relationships between an infant or child and his or her caregivers. Optimal attachments provide security, trust, warm and affectionate exchanges, satisfaction of physical and emotional needs, and psychological and physical comfort (Fig. 5.1) (Zeanah et al., 2008).

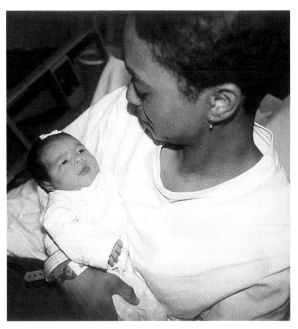

FIGURE 5.1 Attachments in early life provide lifelong foundations for each person's sense of security, trust, affection, and comfort.

Erikson

Erikson built on the concepts of attachment and its consequences, focusing on physiologic and cognitive influences on child development (Mohr, 2012). His approach is grounded on the *epigenetic principle,* dominant in embryology (see Chapter 11), that human development proceeds in an organized, sequential, and defined manner. His framework emphasizes the particular tasks that a person should master at each specific stage if growth and development are to continue without tension and conflict (Sadock & Sadock, 2007) and those elements that can help or hinder the person on the road to task achievement (Table 5.1).

 Consider Dina, the 30-year-old Arabic woman from the beginning of the chapter. Using Table 5.1, at which of Erikson's stages would the nurse expect Dina to be? What tasks would be of chief concern?

Behavioural Models

Behavioural models emphasize that all behaviour is learned from the environment through timed reinforcement and gradual conditioning. Many psychological therapies are based on behavioural models; examples include substance use treatments, management of hallucinations, and enhancement of school performance.

Learned helplessness, a behavioural theory proposed by Seligman (1975), deserves comment. Seligman posited that negative thought patterns, as often observed in depressed and suicidal clients, are learned. A client's perception of her control over her life affects how she feels about herself and her ability to act. Low self-esteem, negative self-concept, and self-critical commentary typically are evident in the thought processes of those with depression as well as in victims of intimate-partner violence (Al-Modalial, 2012; Cyranowski et al., 2012; Seligman, 1975).

Sociocultural Models

Heterogeneous societies include numerous cultural groups. Acculturation occurs when continuous interactions among the different groups change the original cultural patterns of all the groups involved over time. Nurses working with culturally diverse populations must understand the perspective of the client, who may be struggling with his or her cultural identity. They also need to always consider the relationship between the client's culture and the health care issue requiring attention.

Feminist Models

Feminism and feminist movements have helped raise awareness in some societies that tradition, history, and necessity largely have dictated women's various roles and functions. Demographic realities such as diversity among women, socioeconomic differences, health and education disparities, and environmental factors require in-depth thinking about, and perhaps the repositioning of, feminist theory (Hale, 2002).

Feminist models shed light on the contextual variables in a woman's life. They include the building of knowledge related to such concepts as power and powerlessness, egalitarianism, self-determination, and control over reproduction.

One feminist theorist is Carol Gilligan, who studied moral development and its differences in girls and women. Gilligan stressed that women often emphasize the effects of caring on human relationships, which tend to be different from a male focus on individual rights and rules. She emphasized that neither approach was necessarily right or wrong, and that both viewpoints needed to be considered, not one at the expense of another. Gilligan also diverged from feminist colleagues who posited that no differences exist between men and women. According to Gilligan, moral and psychological tendencies are gender oriented, and Western societies traditionally have limited women by valuing "male" morality over female (Gilligan, 1993).

Biologic Models

Biologic models that explain mental illness are based on relatively recent findings indicating a link between mental disorders and neurochemical alterations and imbalances in the brain. Biologically oriented treatments for mental illness did not begin until the 1940s, when researchers discovered that some drugs could reduce the intensity and frequency of hallucinations and other devastating psychiatric symptoms. In recent years, scientists have given additional attention to the promise of neurotransmitters in the treatment of mental disorders. For example, increased levels of dopamine have been implicated in schizophrenia. Consequently, researchers have developed drug therapies to decrease the effects of dopamine on the disease process (Schatzberg & Nemeroff, 2009). Use of drugs to treat psychiatric disorders is the major focus of the third section of this chapter.

COMMON PSYCHIATRIC CHALLENGES IN WOMEN

This section introduces readers to major psychiatric and social problems in women. It contains detailed presentations on common psychiatric illnesses, suicide, and intimate-partner violence. Most of this section is relevant to women across the life span. The effects of disorders on pregnant or lactating women receive special focus. Although the risk for untreated mental illness

● TABLE 5.1 **Erikson's Developmental Stages**

Stage	Approximate Age Range	Description	
Basic trust vs. mistrust	Birth to 18 mo	The person experiences a reliable or unreliable world in which needs are met or unmet	
Autonomy vs. shame and doubt	18 mo–3 yr	The person learns about body and thought control and confronts realities about how to satisfy others and self	
Initiative vs. guilt	3–5 yr	The person struggles with wanting to take over relationships with loved ones and exclude others from their affection	

(table continues on page 180)

● TABLE 5.1 **Erikson's Developmental Stages** (continued)

Stage	Approximate Age Range	Description	
Industry vs. inferiority	5–13 yr	Major concerns relate to self-identify, peers, and academic demands. The person begins to understand the nature of work and should learn skills associated with goal attainment	
Identity vs. role confusion	13–21 yr	The person deals with many new growth phenomena; additional demands at school and home related to self-management, identity, and career choices; and independence	
Intimacy vs. isolation	21–40 yr	The person is concerned with developing mature attachments and making commitments. Being in love has responsibilities; decision making could have far-reaching consequences into midlife	
Generativity vs. stagnation	40–60 yr	The person focuses on a vocation and career and experiences continued growth and development through intellectual and emotional stimulation. Attachments to others should be evident; needs for intimacy, belonging, and a sense of self ought to be solidified	

(continued)

● TABLE 5.1 **Erikson's Developmental Stages** (continued)

Stage	Approximate Age Range	Description
Ego integrity vs. despair	60 yr to death	The person engages in reflective self-appraisal, with the outcome being a sense of accomplishment or despair/anguish about the previous years. The person must accept responsibilities and decisions related to life's outcomes

during pregnancy has not been documented definitively, certain negative associations have been established. For example, untreated schizophrenia is linked to increased perinatal deaths; untreated depression may contribute to low-birth-weight infants; and maternal stress can cause elevated maternal serum concentrations of cortisol, which may be deleterious to fetal brain development (Grote et al., 2010; Patel & Prince, 2006; Poggi-Davis & Sandman, 2010; Schatzberg & Nemeroff, 2009).

Depression and Related Disorders

Clients with depression have either a sad, depressed mood or a loss of interest or inability to derive pleasure from previously enjoyed activities. Symptoms include recurrent suicidal thoughts, appetite changes, lack of concentration, faulty decision making, feelings of worthlessness, poor energy, sleep problems, substance use, and social withdrawal. These symptoms cause significant distress or impair functioning nearly every day for at least 2 weeks. Typically, episodes last many weeks or months, followed by periods of normal mood and behaviour.

Dysthymic disorder differs from major depression in terms of intensity and duration. Its course can be persistent or intermittent. The client with dysthymic disorder has a sad or irritable mood and feelings of inadequacy, guilt, anger, and difficulty experiencing joy and elation on most days for at least 2 years. During this time, no more than 2 months pass without symptoms; however, the client has no manic or depressive episodes (Public Health Agency of Canada [PHAC], 2012). The chronic nature of dysthymic disorder often manifests as a lifelong struggle, which can cause significant distress (Mohr, 2012). Negative feelings, lack of energy, and

pessimism impair occupational functioning and interrupt activities of daily living.

Both depression and dysthymia are more prevalent in women than in men (Hales et al., 2008). Genetics, reactions to stress, interpersonal relationships, and other factors may contribute to this disparity. Other possible risk factors that lead to the greater preponderance of depression and dysthymia in women include the following:

* Hormonal influences (eg, premenstrual syndrome, pregnancy, postpartal adjustments) (Kornstein et al., 2005)
* Financial disparities or poverty
* Insufficient social support
* History of sexual or physical abuse
* Traditional caretaking roles of women in caring for elderly or sick family members (Pinquart & Sorensen, 2006)
* Chronic medical conditions (Farr et al., 2011)

As discussed in Chapter 2, nurses should incorporate assessment of a woman's mental health into the overall assessment of her physical and reproductive health. Each health care appointment provides an opportunity to screen for depression and dysthymic disorder. A brief mental health history assessment can help prevent or identify these serious problems (Lolak et al., 2005; Perfetti et al., 2004).

Evidence has shown that women with depressive disorders respond best to combined treatment with psychotherapy and psychopharmacology (Mazure et al., 2002). The most common antidepressants used are the selective serotonin reuptake inhibitors (SSRIs). Examples of SSRIs include citalopram (Celexa), fluoxetine

(Prozac), sertraline (Zoloft), and paroxetine (Paxil) (Schatzberg et al., 2010). Other commonly prescribed classes of drugs for depressive disorders include cyclic antidepressants and monoamine oxidase inhibitors.

Pregnancy

The reported prevalence of depression in pregnancy varies widely. Approximately 7% to 20% of pregnant women experience a depressive disorder, a rate similar to that among nonpregnant women (Bowen & Muhajarine, 2006; Mian, 2005). Depression in pregnancy is associated with compromised prenatal care, insufficient nutrition, and poor overall health. If a woman becomes depressed during pregnancy, her chances of experiencing postpartum depression (PPD) increase (Toohey, 2012). Extreme stress during pregnancy leads to elevated maternal serum concentrations of cortisol, which are detrimental to fetal brain development. Infants and children born to women with untreated depression could experience complications and long-range problems (Field, 2011; Pawlby et al., 2009).

General guidelines for treatment of depression during pregnancy have been difficult to establish. As much as possible, the health care provider should avoid prescribing antidepressants for women during the first trimester, when organogenesis occurs. If symptoms are severe (eg, mood lability, disorganization, inability to care for self, cognitive deficits) or the woman has a history of chronic relapse without medication, then the primary health care provider should consider medication. Fluoxetine (Prozac) in the smallest dosage that will control florid symptoms is one potential agent (Hales et al., 2008). Other options include tricyclic and tetracyclic antidepressants. Although these drugs are considered relatively safe, the literature has not yet substantiated these findings. They may cause perinatal toxicity near the end of pregnancy, resulting in maternal urinary retention (Schatzberg et al., 2010) (see Chapter 13). Results from a recent systematic review and mean analysis revealed significant association between antepartum antidepressant exposure and neonatal tremors and respiratory distress (Grigoriadis et al., 2013). In light of conflicting evidence regarding potential risks, others suggest that treatment decisions need to consider the effects of untreated antepartum depression against potential adverse effects on the fetus (Ross et al., 2013).

Postpartum

Postpartum depressive and anxiety disorders can affect mother, infant, and other family members. Depending on the extent of the problem, the client may require attention from a health care provider. Support from partner or spouse, family, and friends is key in helping the woman regain and strengthen her sense of stability (Fig. 5.2).

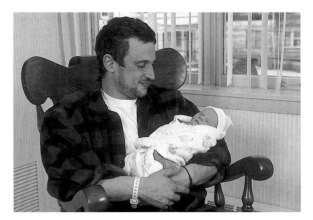

FIGURE 5.2 Support from others can assist the new mother to avoid or to manage symptoms of postpartum "blues" or depression.

Postpartum Blues. Postpartum blues ("maternity blues") is a mild condition of short duration that affects approximately 30% to 75% of all women who give birth (Seyfried & Marcus, 2003). Symptoms include tearfulness, moodiness, irritability, and anxiety. They worsen progressively over the first 3 to 4 days postpartum and improve by approximately the 12th postpartum day. Unlike PPD and postpartum psychosis, postpartum blues typically resolves without professional intervention.

During prenatal teaching and before discharge from the health facility following childbirth, nurses should caution women and their support people about postpartum blues. Health care professionals might not see clients before or while symptoms emerge, since most clients return home 2 to 3 days after birth. Hence, teaching and enhancing the health literacy of the client and her support people are essential roles for nurses in maternal and child health settings (Hales et al., 2008). Nurses should teach clients the early signs and symptoms of postpartum blues and give clear instructions about how to access treatment should the need arise (Hales et al., 2008). See Teaching Tips 5.1 for more information.

Postpartum Pinks. Postpartum pinks ("the pinks") is a less known condition of mild euphoria developing after childbirth and lasting anywhere from several hours to days (Heron et al., 2005). Like the postpartum blues it should resolve spontaneously without treatment. If the euphoric state continues, or becomes extreme in nature, it may indicate a more serious mood problem requiring treatment by a mental health specialist (Ross et al., 2005).

Postpartum Depression. PPD may develop anytime within the first year after delivery (Ross et al., 2005). Clients typically complain of being tired; they are irritable and find care for themselves and the newborn difficult. The infant is likely to experience a poor quality of mothering and be exposed to behavioural, emotional, and cognitive deficits because of the mother's

● TEACHING TIPS 5.1   Postpartum Blues

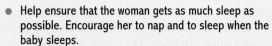

The nurse teaches the client about to give birth or who has recently given birth the following information related to mood changes that frequently develop in the early postpartal period:

- Feeling sad, anxious, tired, and irritable in the days and weeks after giving birth is normal. The combination of fluctuating hormone levels and sleep deprivation is challenging alone, in addition to providing constant care for a helpless and utterly dependent human being. Many women find the adjustment to motherhood (whether with a first or subsequent baby) difficult. Talk about your feelings with a supportive person.
- Plan for and ask for help with child care, chores, cooking, and errands. Use this assistance to rest and find some time for yourself apart from taking care of the baby. Try reading, taking a bath, or getting out of the house for a short walk and some fresh air.
- Keep a journal of your feelings to explore your frustrations and concerns. As time moves on, you can reread your entries to see how you have progressed and what has changed.
- Accept that you will have days in which you cannot get anything done other than caring for your baby. Let go of the "supermom" myth. Set small goals, and don't be shy about asking others to help you.
- If your feelings do not improve with time, talk with your doctor about how you feel.

The nurse teaches the client's partner or spouse as follows:

- Help ensure that the woman gets as much sleep as possible. Encourage her to nap and to sleep when the baby sleeps.
- Assume responsibility for some feedings (of either pumped breast milk once nursing is well established or formula). Sharing feedings not only gives the mother a break but promotes your bonding with the infant.
- See that the new mother has opportunities to spend time outside the house, even for brief breaks. Arrange babysitting so that you and she can spend some time together without the baby.
- Help make arrangements for you, family, friends, paid help, and volunteers to assume duties and household chores. People can assist with tasks from cleaning and cooking, to writing thank-you notes, to caring for older children and pets.
- Each day, ask the new mother what is most important and with what she needs your help specific to baby care. She needs to be in control of the situation as much as possible, even if it means mainly giving orders for some time!
- Remember to praise the woman and encourage her repeatedly if she feels she is not doing a "good job" as a mom. Love and admiration from her significant other will likely mean more to her than all the kind words of other people combined.

depression. If a woman has a low social support, history of depression, anxiety symptoms, or depression during pregnancy, her odds of experiencing PPD are increased (Davey et al., 2011; Lanes et al., 2011). PPD is also reported to be associated with a prepregnancy history of physical or sexual abuse (Silverman & Loudon, 2010). Women without adequate support from others are also at risk (Negron et al., 2013).

The woman with PPD loses pleasure in things that once brought satisfaction. She typically feels tired, down, guilty, hopeless, and worthless; in some cases, she has thoughts of death or suicide. The Edinburgh Postnatal Depression Scale (EPDS) has shown to be an effective self-report measurement scale to identify postpartum women with depressive symptoms (Cox et al., 1987; Registered Nurses Association of Ontario [RNAO], 2005).

A multimodal treatment approach is best. Interpersonal therapies typically are helpful with their focus on transitional roles, new demands, and expectations that the woman must confront. Individual, group, family, and couple therapies are examples of interpersonal interventions. Evidence indicates new mothers are highly receptive to counselling and support for post-

partum depressive symptoms (Segre et al., 2010). Furthermore, recognition of women's social circumstances may enhance their emotional well-being following birth (Yelland et al., 2010). Appropriate psychopharmacologic treatment administered under the supervision of a knowledgeable primary care provider or mental health specialist may be indicated (Fitelson et al., 2011). See Chapter 19 for more information.

Postpartum Anxiety. Anxiety symptoms may begin during pregnancy or in the postpartum period (Ross et al., 2005). If a woman has experienced prior difficulties with anxiety, the pregnancy or postpartum period may be a time of symptom exacerbation. Women may experience a variety of symptoms, including excessive anxiety or worry, irritability, restlessness, fatigue, trouble concentrating, and physical symptoms (eg, headaches, muscle tension, gastrointestinal upset) (Ross et al., 2005).

In some cases, women may develop intrusive and persistent thoughts and/or images of harm coming to the baby, or of themselves causing harm to their baby (eg, dropping the baby on the stairs, throwing the baby, injuring the baby with a knife). These thoughts are distressing to the woman, and may be accompanied by excessive checking of the infant or avoidance behaviours such as not carrying the baby on the stairs, or locking away knives (Bennett & Indman, 2006).

It is important that nurses routinely ask postpartum women about these symptoms. One approach is to say, "It's common for some women to have scary thoughts or images after childbirth. Have you experienced any scary thoughts or images?" This approach may be viewed as reassuring, and can make it easier for the woman to discuss any distressing symptoms.

As with depression, a multimodal treatment approach is best. Cognitive behavioural therapy (CBT), teaching breathing techniques and relaxation therapies, as well as psychoeducation are useful for improving coping strategies and for symptom reduction. In addition, women may require pharmacologic intervention, which may include antianxiety or antidepressant medication (Ross et al., 2005).

Postpartum Psychosis. In this most severe disorder, the client develops psychotic symptoms: hallucinations, delusions, and feelings of unreality. Postpartum psychosis affects approximately 1 to 2 in 1,000 women (Ross et al., 2005). These clients usually require hospitalization and are at risk for suicide, infant neglect, self-neglect, failed reality testing, and poor judgement. They need several therapies, including supportive therapy, individual and group therapies, and medication. Pharmacologic treatment usually involves several classes of medications, including antipsychotics and antidepressants (Schatzberg et al., 2010).

Nurses need to understand and educate others regarding this severe disorder. Family, particularly the client's partner or spouse, can play an important role in the detection of PPD and should be involved in planning care. As a consequence, partners and other family members need to be informed about the signs and symptoms of PPD (Ross et al., 2005). The partners and spouses of women with postpartum psychosis need support and understanding from immediate and extended family members and friends (MacKey et al., 2000). See Chapter 19 for more information.

Older Women and Depression

Epidemiologic studies suggest that the risk for depression does *not* increase as women enter perimenopause and beyond (Hales et al., 2008). The current thinking is that women who experience depression later in life may have had previously neglected signs and symptoms of depression, vasomotor symptoms, or other health-related and socioeconomic problems that were troublesome stressors (Mazure et al., 2002).

Nurses caring for women across all settings must be aware that distinguishing depression from other psychiatric conditions, such as dementia and cognitive decline, can be difficult as women age. Physical health problems may precipitate depression. Contributing factors also may include side effects from medications to treat physical problems, pain, and compromised activities of daily living (Mazure et al., 2002). For more information on psychological health in menopausal and older women, see Chapters 23 and 24.

Suicide

Suicide is a serious public health problem in Canada. In 2009, 3,890 individuals committed suicide, that is, 11.5 suicide deaths per 100,000 population. The rate of suicide in females (5.3) is lower than in males (17.9) (Statistics Canada, 2012b). Approximately 90% of all people who commit suicide have been diagnosed with a mental illness, primarily depression or alcoholism. Hence, if a woman has a mental disorder, especially depression or alcoholism, health care providers must be alert at all times to her risk for suicide.

Clients who are suicidal display common characteristics. One core element is a sense of hopelessness. Another is desperation, or a feeling that life is too difficult and that change is unlikely. Guilt, too, is dominant and associated with self-hatred. Feelings of shame and humiliation also are common. Some clients elect suicide as a reaction against shame or humiliation related to past or current overwhelming events (Hales et al., 2008). An example might be sexual abuse, child abandonment, or prostitution.

Suicide and its implications present difficult challenges for health care providers. Completed suicides cause enormous pain and suffering for millions of Canadians who endure the loss of a loved one. When the nurse suspects that a woman is experiencing tremendous stress or feeling hopeless, he or she should complete a suicide assessment of the client. Clinical scales useful for promptly and effectively identifying suicidal clients include the modified SAD PERSONS scale, the revised Beck Depression Inventory, the Beck Anxiety Inventory, the Beck Hopelessness Scale, and the Beck Scale for Suicidal Ideation (BSS). Positive results on any of these scales should prompt the nurse to refer the client to a mental health specialist.

 Dina, the young Arabic woman pregnant with her third child, states, "I feel so alone. I don't speak English well. I'm worried about my baby and my two young children, money, and my husband's temper. Sometimes I wonder if it is worth trying to carry on." How would the nurse interpret Dina's statements? What questions might the nurse ask Dina?

● **BOX 5.1   Common Manifestations of Anxiety**

- Diarrhea
- Dizziness, lightheadedness
- Hyperreflexia
- Hypertension
- Nausea and vomiting
- Palpitations
- Restlessness
- Tachycardia
- Tingling in the extremities
- Tremors
- Upset stomach
- Urinary frequency, hesitancy, urgency

Anxiety, Stress, and Anxiety Disorders

Anxiety needs to be differentiated from fear. Anxiety alerts a person to impending danger, but the source of that danger is unknown. Thus, anxiety is internal, vague, conflictual, and insidious. With fear, the danger is known, identifiable, and sudden (Sadock & Sadock, 2007).

Anxiety presents with many symptoms expressed in two ways. First, the client becomes aware of associated physiologic sensations, such as sweating and palpitations (Box 5.1). Second, the client experiences nervousness, fright, or upset. Others observe that she is experiencing anxiety even if the client herself is unaware of it. Anxiety also affects thinking, perception, and learning.

Anxiety disorders are among the most common psychiatric illnesses, affecting one in four people at any given time (Sadock & Sadock, 2007). Their prevalence decreases with increased socioeconomic status (Sadock & Sadock, 2007). Recent studies have implicated anxiety in the etiology and exacerbation of numerous physiologic problems, including heart disease.

Many disorders, reactions to medications and other substances, and exposure to real trauma and stressors can cause signs and symptoms of anxiety disorders. Examples include cardiac disease, thyroid disorders, lupus, blood disorders, and the effects of caffeine or nicotine. Herbal medicines, decongestants, steroids, and appetite suppressants can induce anxiety. Violent events in a woman's past, such as rape or sexual assault, increase her chances of experiencing anxiety problems (Schatzberg et al., 2010; Schatzberg & Nemeroff, 2009). The health care team must rule out such problems before establishing a diagnosis of an anxiety disorder.

COLLABORATIVE CARE: THE CLIENT WITH ANXIETY

When working with clients with anxiety, nurses may find it useful to conceptualize the level of anxiety (Mohr, 2012; Peplau, 1963):

- *Mild.* The client experiences and manages tension related to activities of daily living. She sees, hears, and is aware of environmental stimuli. This level of anxiety acts as a motivator, helping the woman to accomplish tasks.
- *Moderate.* The client's attention focuses on immediate concerns. What she hears, sees, and perceives is compromised.
- *Severe.* The client's perceptual field is restricted significantly, narrowing her awareness. The intent is to relieve or reduce anxiety to a more reasonable or comfortable level, at which functioning can be restored.
- *Panic.* The client experiences awe, dread, and terror. Even when directed by others, she may be unable to follow simple commands. She experiences increased motor activity, loses the capacity to think and reason, and could become a danger to herself and others.

Assessment

The nurse should ask the client if she is anxious or worried or has experienced such feelings lately. If the client answers positively, the nurse should continue to discuss feelings and use observation and interview techniques to gauge whether the client has had or is having the signs and symptoms of anxiety presented in Box 5.1. The nurse should suspect an anxiety disorder when the client shows evidence of anxiety that she cannot dismiss, reports anxiety that interferes with her daily life, or both.

The nurse should ask the client about worrying, obsessive thinking, repetitive activity, specific phobias, and exposure to trauma. If the client's responses to any of these questions are affirmative, the nurse should elicit details about the behaviour or response.

If a pregnant client experiences anxiety, an especially important aspect of assessment is to determine associated risks to the fetus. The nurse should take necessary action to prevent the client from harming herself or her fetus. Teaching about the woman's changing body and the growing fetus, alcohol and nicotine use during pregnancy, nutrition, rest, family support, and self-care are some areas for discussion.

Select Potential Nursing Diagnoses

Three major nursing diagnoses are associated with anxiety disorders (Mohr, 2012):

- Anxiety
- Ineffective coping
- Ineffective breathing pattern

Other nursing diagnoses may apply, based on the client's specific circumstances.

Planning/Intervention

The nurse should plan interventions based on the client's level of anxiety. Also, he or she should determine

● TEACHING TIPS 5.2 Controlling Breathing

The nurse instructs the client how to perform a slow-breathing exercise to help deal with symptoms of anxiety. Although such exercises have variations, a common approach to use is to:

1. Hold the breath and count to 5.
2. On 5, breathe out, slowly and calmly saying the word *relax*.
3. Then breathe in for 3 seconds and out for 3 seconds, saying the word *relax* with each exhalation.

4. After 1 minute, hold the breath for 5 seconds again and then continue breathing using the 6-second cycle (3-second inhalation, 3-second exhalation).
5. Continue until hyperventilation is under control and all symptoms have subsided.

Adapted from Mohr, W. K. (2012). *Psychiatric mental health nursing* (8th ed.). Philadelphia, PA: Lippincott Williams & Wilkins.

whether the level is appropriate to the client's specific situation and consider whether the client's thought patterns seem logical and rational.

To help the client meet established goals, the nurse should display the hallmarks of the therapeutic relationship: trust, empathy, respect, and calmness. He or she should help the client identify those thoughts and behaviours related to anxiety, as well as effective coping strategies to deal with them. Therapeutic questioning techniques and reflective listening can make the client feel understood and supported.

A quiet environment is important. The nurse should provide facts to negate any misconceptions. By doing so, the client can objectively appraise her situation. If the client is breathing rapidly, the nurse should assist with slow or controlled breathing exercises. See Teaching Tips 5.2.

The nurse should encourage a healthy lifestyle that can help limit or control stress (see Chapter 2). Examples of suggestions include getting sufficient aerobic exercise, eating a well-balanced diet (see Chapter 3), and minimizing the use of alcohol, tobacco, drugs, and caffeine.

Coping strategies help determine the client's overall mental health status. Moreover, constructive or useful coping mechanisms help protect the client and give her direction for problem solving. The nurse should assist the client to identify maladaptive coping strategies (eg, alcohol use) and to replace them with positive techniques. Two common examples of positive coping strategies are the use of relaxation and reliance on problem solving (Mohr, 2012).

Relaxation

Regular use of relaxation techniques can reduce autonomic arousal, which in turn decreases oxygen demands, heart rate, blood pressure, and metabolic rate. Common methods of relaxation include visualization, meditation, yoga, progressive muscle relaxation, and hypnosis (Complementary and Alternative Medicine 5.1). The nurse and client should together identify the most acceptable method; the nurse can then teach the selected technique or refer the client to a professional who can do so.

Problem Solving

The nurse also may assist the client to develop or enhance problem-solving skills. In this way, the client learns to replace avoidance and worry with clear and effective thought and reflection. Problem-solving skills may include learning to first identify the specific problem, as well as all possible solutions, followed by identifying the pros and cons of each solution, and ultimately arriving at one solution or a combination of solutions that best addresses her circumstances and helps eliminate the original conundrum. Importantly, the client devises a way to implement the solution. After doing so, she also reviews the effectiveness of her solution.

● COMPLEMENTARY/ALTERNATIVE MEDICINE 5.1
Visualization

Visualization can be an effective technique to manage anxiety. The client starts by practicing techniques such as focused breathing or progressive muscle relaxation. Another person, an audiotape, or the woman herself may then guide the client to imagine a calm and peaceful environment where she can work through a problem or stress. The client may choose to focus on an inspirational person, event, or deity to provide guidance and wisdom.

Thus, even when the client's actions do not completely resolve the original problem, she learns how to connect feelings, thoughts, and actions, rather than allowing anxiety to paralyze and overwhelm her.

Evaluation

Successful care is based on the client's report of improved feelings and observable changes in behaviour. Examples of positive outcomes include the following:

- The client reports use of one or more relaxation techniques.
- The client reports decreased anxiety or panic.
- The client uses problem-solving techniques in difficult situations (Mohr, 2012).

Schizophrenia

Schizophrenia, a debilitating psychiatric disorder affecting approximately 1% of the population, occurs in all societies and among people of all socioeconomic levels (Sadock & Sadock, 2007). The peak age of onset in women is 25 to 35 years (Robinson, 2012), which coincides with the woman's optimal childbearing years. The number of women diagnosed with schizophrenia who become pregnant is increasing (Vigod et al., 2012). Factors associated with this trend include deinstitutionalization (placement of people with psychiatric illnesses in the community rather than in long-term health care facilities), psychopharmacologic agents with fewer side effects, and improved perinatal care strategies for women with chronic illness (see Chapter 13).

No one theory explains the cause of schizophrenia; biologic, environmental, and psychosocial etiologies have been posited. Women with schizophrenia present with various clinical symptoms, experience the illness in numerous ways, and respond to treatment and rehabilitation diversely. Table 5.2 reviews the subtypes of schizophrenia.

Assessment Findings

This chronic, complex, and potentially devastating illness has a plethora of signs and symptoms. Prominent characteristics include numerous changes in mood, cognition, perception, motivation, interpersonal relations, and motor function (APA, 2013; Sadock & Sadock, 2007; Schatzberg et al., 2010). Each group of symptoms can change in intensity, wax and wane, or become stable with treatment.

Mood Changes. The client experiences anxiety, depression, tension, and irritation. She may isolate herself and withdraw from events and people. One example is *blunted affect,* in which the person appears emotionless. Another example is *anhedonia,* in which the client seems to experience continuous apathy and cannot experience joy or happiness.

Cognitive Changes. The cognitive changes of schizophrenia can make life strange and difficult for the woman. Disordered thoughts make up the core component of the condition. The client loses the capacity to

● TABLE 5.2 **Subtypes of Schizophrenia**

The five subtypes of schizophrenia demonstrate the variety in symptom formation and expression related to the condition (Sadock & Sadock, 2007):	
Subtype	**Characteristics**
Paranoid	Preoccupation with one or more delusions Frequent hallucinations (usually auditory) Organized speech and behaviour, with appropriate affect
Disorganized	Disorganized speech Disorganized behaviour Flat and inappropriate affect
Catatonic	At least two of the following: ● Motor immobility with *waxy flexibility* (allowing others to move the limbs, but then holding them for hours in the position in which they are placed) or stupor ● Purposeless but excessive motor activity not influenced by external stimuli and demand ● *Negativism* (resistance to all instructions or guidance) ● Maintenance of a rigid posture that continues even with attempts by others to move or reposition the client ● Mutism Peculiar movements such as posturing and excessive grimacing Strange speech patterns
Undifferentiated	Delusions, hallucinations, and disorganized speech, but no symptoms that meet the predetermined criteria for paranoid, disorganized, or catatonic
Residual	No prominent delusions, hallucinations, disorganized speech, or disorganized or catatonic behaviour Negative signs, odd thought content and form, and unusual perceptual experiences

concentrate. Sometimes, health care providers confuse this symptom with intellectual impairment or another organic disorder. On the contrary, the client's energy and interest are centred elsewhere.

Objective observations of cognitive changes are evident in speech and written communication. The client's conversation may shift from one topic to another irrelevantly and sometimes incoherently. The client may make up new words and phrases with no meaning to others but highly significant for her. For example, a woman, upset with her nurse, makes this statement: "The nurse is meaquous and has vinlengenge, and she will get a hyptismytous statement from me about her behaviour."

Disturbances in thought content manifest themselves primarily through delusions or false beliefs. The woman expresses her ideas and interpretations about stimuli in a manner different from those of others in the same environment. Delusions are the most frequently observed phenomena in this category.

Perceptual Changes. Hallucinations in schizophrenia can affect any of the five senses. In addition, nurses should be aware of kinesthetic hallucinations (altered bodily states affecting different organ systems). Among clients of childbearing age, the nurse might encounter those who think they are pregnant but are not. Conversely, nurses may also encounter women who are pregnant but who state, emphatically, that they are not and attribute accompanying physical changes to some other process. Some might deny any changes whatsoever.

Clients with schizophrenia also can misinterpret things in the environment. For instance, they may perceive a string on the clinic floor to be a snake. Such a phenomenon is referred to as an *illusion*.

Physical Changes. During the early stage of schizophrenia, clients might present with sweaty palms, dilated pupils, and mild tachycardia. Other changes may include psychomotor activity (eg, restlessness), which often occurs in those who have been taking psychotropic medications over an extended period.

 Gladys says she hears voices. What evidence would the nurse identify as suggesting that Gladys is experiencing disturbances in thought perception and content? What strategies might a nurse initially use to engage effectively with Gladys?

Interpersonal Disturbances. Various behaviours in schizophrenia can be bizarre and inappropriate for social norms. For example, a client might interrupt conversations, mutilate body parts with knives, bang her head repeatedly, or attempt suicide. She might pick her nose in public, cough over others, introduce inappropriate topics, or laugh about things that typically provoke sadness and remorse in others.

Disturbances in Motor Function. The client might no longer interact with others. With *catatonia* (Table 5.2), the client becomes rigid and unresponsive to the environment. This rare condition is an extreme response to crisis, such as when a woman with schizophrenia experiences a miscarriage or stillbirth.

Collaborative Management

Primary assessment for schizophrenia includes interviewing and direct observation. The interview focuses on signs and symptoms, degree of impaired thought processes, risk for injury or violence toward self or others, and available support. If the client's reports are unreliable because of the severity of the illness, a family member or friend may be called on to supply pertinent information about the client's health history.

Treatment for clients with schizophrenia requires collaboration from all members of the health care team, as well as the client, family, and other support people. Nursing Care Plan 5.1 highlights the care of a pregnant woman with schizophrenia. The team individualizes the plan for the particular client's needs, strengths, and limitations.

In the early stages of treatment, health care providers should focus on improving the client's sense of reality. The nurse should involve the woman in conversations and activities about real events, particularly in the event of hallucinations and delusions. The nurse should not engage in arguments about such content. Rather, he or she should gently introduce doubt and attempt to shift the client's focus to other activities (eg, taking a walk, looking at a magazine).

Because the client's language can be confusing and disorganized, the nurse should listen and try to clarify meaning. He or she should be alert for any behaviour or speech that indicates mounting aggression or agitation. Such manifestations usually require an emergency response.

One of the most difficult aspects of schizophrenia for clients is the social isolation it tends to impose. The chronic and inconsistent nature of the illness, even when controlled with medication, can make forming and maintaining friendships and social outlets difficult. By using therapeutic communication, the nurse can model behaviours to help the client improve social skills and learn ways to build rapport with others.

The nurse should assess the knowledge of the woman's family regarding schizophrenia. Relatives may require teaching about the illness, its symptom management, the necessity of following the therapeutic regimen, signs of relapse, and lifestyle accommodations. Schizophrenia imposes not only enormous physical and psychological difficulties, but also challenges relative

NURSING CARE PLAN 5.1

●

The Pregnant Client With Psychoses

 Recall Gladys, the 35-year-old client from the beginning of the chapter. Further assessment reveals slightly elevated blood pressure and pulse; history of cigarette smoking, approximately 1 pack/day for the past 15 years; and client reports that something is aggravating her. Review of the health history reveals remissions and exacerbations of schizophrenia over several years. Assessment of pregnancy status indicates that gestation is progressing normally; however, the client has not yet received any prenatal care. The physician assigned to the case prescribes chlorpromazine (Thorazine) to manage the client's schizophrenic symptoms.

NURSING DIAGNOSES

- **Disturbed Sensory Perception, Auditory** related to hearing voices
- **Disturbed Thought Processes** related to underlying schizophrenia and hallucinations
- **Risk for Injury** related to auditory hallucinations and medication therapy and possible associated extrapyramidal side effects and dystonic reactions

EXPECTED OUTCOMES

1. The client will verbalize an accurate interpretation of her environment.
2. The client will report fewer episodes of hearing voices.
3. The client will use appropriate measures to deal with voices.
4. The client will experience minimal to no adverse effects of drug therapy.

INTERVENTIONS	RATIONALES
Use active listening, knowledge, and skills; accept the client as she presents herself. Develop a trusting relationship with her	Listening helps elicit more information to use during overall treatment. Avoiding approaches that the client does not understand or cannot implement facilitates trust. The therapeutic relationship allows the client to attain basic health goals for herself and the fetus
Determine the intensity and frequency of hallucinations and whether they have ever been commanding	Close observation of the client's behaviour provides information about how she is responding and the degree to which hallucinations control her behaviour
Review changes and sensations associated with pregnancy. Discuss hallucinations with the client and help her gain control over them. Request that the client take notice of the frequency, duration, and intensity of the sensations	Knowledge about pregnancy's physical progression helps the client understand the changes and sensations that she experiences. Teaching her to identify reality from sensations could help her feel "in charge", enhance her health literacy, and empower her to take control of the situation
If the client is hearing voices, do not argue about whether the experience is real	Arguing could increase the client's anxiety, disrupt the therapeutic relationship, and decrease the chances that she will return to the clinic

(continued)

NURSING CARE PLAN 5.1 ● The Pregnant Client With Psychoses *(Continued)*

INTERVENTIONS	RATIONALES
Communicate understanding of the client's feelings and sensations as real. Provide reality testing, assuring the client that the fetus is not talking to her or threatening to jump out	Honest, clear communication fosters trust, promotes the therapeutic relationship, and enhances the effectiveness of the interventions
Assess the client for drug and alcohol use; include over-the-counter medications and herbal preparations	Substances can alter sensory, perceptual, and cognitive functioning and can have deleterious effects on both mother and fetus
Assist client with referral to mental health services	Mental health services aid in providing necessary therapy to treat the underlying disorder
Administer drug therapy as prescribed; instruct the client in the specifics of the drug regimen, including the need to comply with therapy	Antipsychotic drug therapy is a primary mode of treatment. Compliance with therapy is essential to control the client's signs and symptoms

EVALUATION

1. The client verbalizes a realistic view of her environment, stating that the fetus is not communicating with her.
2. The client reports that episodes of hearing voices have decreased to approximately once per week.
3. The client uses appropriate strategies to deal with voices.
4. The client demonstrates no signs and symptoms of extrapyramidal effects or dystonic reactions.

NURSING DIAGNOSIS

Deficient Knowledge related to prenatal care and underlying schizophrenia

EXPECTED OUTCOMES

1. The client will verbalize understanding of teaching and instructions.
2. The client will return for scheduled follow-up appointments.
3. The client will identify danger signs and symptoms that need to be reported immediately.

INTERVENTIONS	RATIONALES
Assess the client's knowledge about pregnancy, labour, and birth	This information provides a baseline from which to develop an individualized plan of care based on the client's needs
Instruct the client in prenatal care measures, including strategies to promote optimal fetal growth and development and methods to cope with common discomforts of pregnancy. Review the progression of pregnancy and signs and symptoms of labour, including true and false labour and danger signs and symptoms to report	Adequate knowledge of care measures enhances the client's sense of control over the situation, thereby promoting a positive self-image

(continued)

NURSING CARE PLAN 5.1 ● The Pregnant Client With Psychoses *(Continued)*

INTERVENTIONS	RATIONALES
Instruct the client in her medication regimen; teach her the signs and symptoms of adverse effects to report immediately	Adherence to the medication regimen is key. Prompt reporting of adverse effects minimizes the risk for injury
Create a written schedule of follow-up appointments; stress the need to keep them	A written schedule serves as a reminder for the client and reinforces what is discussed
Have the client repeat teaching information	Repeating information aids in determining the effectiveness of teaching
Assist with referral to social services as appropriate	Social service referral can help meet the client's needs and ensure follow-up

EVALUATION

1. The client states that she understands the teaching and instructions.
2. The client adheres to the schedule of follow-up visits.
3. The client states which signs and symptoms are dangerous and need to be reported immediately.

to employment, finances, social support, and ability for self-care. The client's support from others is pivotal, particularly in terms of helping her to follow the treatment plan and to assist with monitoring for signs of relapse or exacerbation.

Eating Disorders

Eating disorders include extremely problematic eating behaviours and are often first seen during adolescence or early adulthood, affecting women more than men (Statistics Canada, 2012a).

Pregnant women with a history of eating disorders seem to be at high risk for birth and neonatal complications (Kouba et al., 2005).

Several theories exist about the etiology of eating disorders; most researchers believe that they result from complex interactions among biologic, environmental, and sociocultural factors. Other contributors include family functioning style and stress.

Assessment Findings

Anorexia nervosa is characterized by disturbed body image, extreme fear about being fat, and emaciation. The primary indicators are refusal to eat and weight below 85% of normal for age and height (APA, 2013). Despite objective evidence, women with anorexia nervosa view their extremely thin bodies as fat. Preoccupation with

food and dieting may extend to fixating on particular body parts that these clients see as "defective"; obsession with cooking for others; and extreme exercise. Women with anorexia tend to be compliant, obedient perfectionists, and achieving in school, sports, employment, and other objectively measured endeavours. Physiologic consequences of self-starvation are severe and often life threatening. They include hypotension, bradycardia, hypothermia, chronic constipation, and electrolyte imbalances. Many of these clients experience amenorrhea (cessation of menstruation).

Bulimia nervosa is characterized by the consumption of extreme amounts of food (*bingeing*), with subsequent behaviours to eliminate the excess calories (*purging*). Many women with bulimia binge and purge secretly; their weights may be normal. Clients with bulimia consume incredible calories in short periods (2,000 to 3,000 per episode), a behaviour called **bingeing**. To prevent associated weight gain, they induce vomiting, use laxatives, exercise obsessively, or employ a combination of these methods. Like their counterparts with anorexia, typical clients with bulimia are high achievers. Physiologic complications include changes in heart rate and rhythm, gastric dilation, menstrual irregularities, and electrolyte imbalances. The tooth enamel of these clients frequently becomes eroded from frequent contact with gastric fluids, leading to excessive cavities.

Collaborative Management

Treatment of eating disorders is often difficult (Mohr, 2012). Many of these clients deny their problems. Most require a combination of therapies: individual and group psychotherapy, behavioural therapy, cognitive-behavioural therapy, and family therapy. Medications are not usually a primary treatment measure. However, antidepressants, antianxiety drugs, lithium, and anticonvulsants have been reported useful.

The client requires a thorough physical examination. The nurse should obtain weight, history of previous high and low weights, and chronology of recent weight fluctuations. He or she should determine the rate of weight loss or gain and any associated circumstances. The nurse also should ask the client to describe typical food and fluid intake, any problems related to elimination (eg, constipation, diarrhea), and whether she regularly menstruates. He or she should ask the client about types of exercise, difficulty sleeping, and energy level. In addition, laboratory and cardiac testing can be done to look for electrolyte abnormalities and cardiac dysfunction.

Interventions focus largely on measures to restore nutritional balance. Other measures are geared toward encouraging realistic thinking processes, improving the client's self-esteem and body image, and assisting the client to develop effective coping and problem-solving strategies. In extreme cases of self-starvation, the client is hospitalized and receives intravenous or enteral feedings until nutritional balance is restored.

Intimate-Partner Violence

Intimate-partner violence is a real or threatened physical, sexual, emotional, or psychological abuse perpetrated against a spouse or life partner; it includes measures to control another person's actions. Women who experience intimate-partner violence are at risk for depression, anxiety, eating disorders, alcoholism, post-traumatic stress disorder, and numerous other maladies (Coker et al., 2005).

According to Statistics Canada, (2013b), in 2011 the overall rate of intimate-partner violence against women was 542 per 100,000 women, almost four times higher than the rate for men. However, due to underreporting of violence, this is considered a conservative estimate of the number of women who experience it. Intimate-partner violence has been reported to start, escalate, or temporarily end during pregnancy, and is experienced by 1.5% to 17% of all pregnant women (SOGC, 2005). Such violence places the fetus at risk for low birth weight and other detrimental conditions, such as brain damage and broken limbs (Boy & Salihu, 2004; Curry & Harvey, 1998). Younger women, aged 15 to 24 years, are at most risk for being subjected to violence (Statistics Canada, 2013b).

Intimate-partner violence occurs in both heterosexual and homosexual relationships; the overwhelming majority of cases are perpetrated by men against women. Thus, the following discussions focus on heterosexual relationships.

Cycle of Intimate-Partner Violence

The woman in a violent relationship is conflicted. On the one hand, she is satisfied with and accepts the good aspects of her partner and does not want to lose him. On the other hand, she must endure abuse to remain with him. Nurses who have researched the interpersonal components of intimate-partner violence have proposed that it is a dynamic process with several phases: binding, enduring, disengaging, and recovering (Landenburger, 1998). The long process from binding to recovery is not linear but involves a series of triggers, maintenance behaviours, disturbances in identity, and eventually, the regaining of identity and recovery.

Binding Phase. During this phase, the woman believes that the support and love of her partner can fill her dreams for romance and commitment. She makes concerted efforts to satisfy the partner and to do what will make him happy. There may be warning signs, however, characterized by disconcerting behaviours. Nevertheless, the woman overlooks them and continues to try to please her partner.

Enduring Phase. Violence begins to dominate more of the relationship. The woman continues to highly value the relationship while enduring the violence. Frequently, she blames herself, thinking that her own behaviour justifies the partner's reaction. She begins to lose her identity; her self-esteem wanes. The partner treats her as if she were an object or invisible, except when he needs her to satisfy his needs. The conflict intensifies: if she tries to leave, the partner might kill or harm her; if she stays, the partner might kill her, she might kill herself, or she might kill herself and her partner.

Disengaging Phase. This phase begins when the woman identifies with other women who are experiencing or have experienced violence. Conflict abides, but this time it is related to struggles over loyalty to the relationship and loyalty to self. The woman is likely to be amenable to professional help and might actually seek counselling or report to others that she is unsafe. She begins to communicate with herself about the violent situation, thinking that if she remains in the relationship, she will not survive. When feelings of empowerment begin to emerge, the woman actually might become frightened and overwhelmed.

Recovering Phase. The woman will need to readjust to life away from the violent partner and regain balance. At this point, she is focused on self-survival and the continued existence of any children. Moreover, the woman is aware that her experiences of violence have influenced her attitudes toward and behaviours in the world. Her recovery will continue, as she struggles to derive meaning from the experiences and search for meaning in her new existence. This process can take years. It also requires the help of supportive and informed professionals, family members, and friends.

 Suppose that Dina reports that her husband has hit her on numerous occasions. She states, "I've really been pushing him to find a job lately so that we'd have more money, especially when the baby comes. I guess he's been under a lot of stress." Dina is in which phase of the process?

Collaborative Management

The Registered Nurses Association of Ontario Best Practice Guideline (2012) pertaining to woman abuse suggests that routine universal screening helps to identify effective interventions and validates that woman abuse is a health care concern (Assessment Tool 5.1). The guideline further recommends that screening be implemented for all females 12 years of age and older. Screening for intimate-partner violence should be part of prenatal assessment (SOGC, 2005). When a nurse suspects that a client is experiencing violence, he or she performs an assessment to detect this problem. Some validated tools to use for screening are the Abuse Assessment Screen (AAS), the Abuse Assessment Screen-Disability (AAS-D), and the Woman Abuse Screening Tool (WAST) (RNAO, 2012) (Assessment Tool 5.2).

Time is a persistent problem in such cases; however, screening can be simple. Two basic questions are, "Has a past or current partner ever caused you to be afraid?" and "Has a past or current partner ever physically hurt you?" (Hinderliter et al., 1998). Nursing Care Plan 5.2 highlights the care of a woman experiencing intimate-partner violence.

Landenburger (1998) has developed interventions for each phase of intimate-partner violence:

- **Binding:** The woman, at this time, does not perceive herself as abused and is not willing to use this concept to define her predicament. The nurse should help the client identify what she wants for herself; however, he or she must tell the client that she is being abused. The nurse should assist the woman to identify those behaviours exhibited by the partner that are abusive. The nurse also should help the woman strengthen her self-esteem and self-concept.

- **Enduring:** In cases of intimate-partner violence, psychological and physical violence can become the essence of the relationship. The good sense of self that the woman once experienced slips away. The nurse should help the client understand that the violence will not end and that the partner will continue to blame her for the situation. The nurse should support the client to deal with shame about the violence and help her move beyond covering for her partner. In these ways, the woman can realize that she is confronted with danger and needs intervention and support.

- **Disengaging:** At this time, the woman constantly deals with her feelings of fear and shame. The nurse should reinforce that the partner can be dealt with within the legal, health care, and social systems. The nurse should assist the client to realize that she can successfully leave the partner. Careful assessment of the client's safety is essential; the nurse should outline strategies to ensure a safe departure. Together, the nurse and client should consider safe places, shelters, and housing with family members. The focus is on helping the client to achieve a sense of self-worth and to realize that she has an identity, is competent to care for herself, and is worthy of the help that she has and will receive.

- **Recovering:** During this phase, the woman assumes control of her own life. She needs employment and perhaps therapy to sort out the nature and components of the previous relationship. With time, she must assign the violence that she experienced to the source (her partner) and let go of feeling like she caused the violence. Then, the woman needs to perceive the abusive partner as a person once, but no longer, in her life. The nurse can help the woman work through feelings of worthlessness, self-doubt, depression, and vulnerability, lest she become involved in another violent relationship.

Nurses who provide care for women should always be aware of local resources in the community from which women can receive help. The National Clearing House on Family Violence number is 1-800-267-1291 or (613) 957-2938. The Assaulted Women Helpline (AWHL) is 1-866-863-0511. Other strategies for assisting clients are outlined in Box 5.2.

Substance Use

Substance use contributes significantly to rates of morbidity and mortality. Problems with alcohol and drugs contribute to physical illnesses such as cardiovascular disorders, liver disease, and infections. They are also associated with intimate-partner violence, crime, and accidents. Commonly used drugs include alcohol, marijuana, cocaine, heroin, hallucinogens, and amphetamines.

(text continues on page 199)

● **ASSESSMENT TOOL 5.1**   **Intimate-Partner Violence Documentation Form**

INTIMATE-PARTNER VIOLENCE DOCUMENTATION FORM

Explain to Client: The majority of what you tell me is confidential and cannot be shared with anyone without your written permission. However, I am required by law to report information pertaining to child abuse and gunshot wounds or life-threatening injuries.

STEP 1—Establish total privacy to ask screening questions. Safety is the first priority. Client must be alone, or if the client has a child with her, the child must not be of verbal age. ONLY complete this form if YOU CAN assure the client's safety, privacy, and confidentiality.

STEP 2—Ask the client screening questions.

"Because abuse is so common, we are now asking all of our female clients:

Are you in a relationship in which you are being hurt or threatened, emotionally or physically?
____Yes   ____No

Do you feel unsafe at home?"
____Yes   ____No

If both screening questions are NO in STEP 2, and you are not concerned that the client may be a victim, sign and date the form in the signature block directly below. Provide information and resources as appropriate.

Signature _____ Title _____ Date _____

If both screening answers are NO and you are concerned that the client may be a victim, go to STEP 5. If the client answers YES to either question, proceed to STEP 3 below. Sign and date the signature block on the back of the form after completing STEP 6.

STEP 3—Assess the abuse and safety of the client and any children

Say to client: "From the answers you have just given me, I am worried for you."

"Has the relationship gotten worse, or is it getting scarier?"   ____Yes ____No

"Does your partner ever watch you closely, follow you, or stalk you?"   ____Yes ____No

Ask the following question in clinic settings only. Do not ask in home settings:

"If your partner is here with you today, are you afraid to leave with him/her?"   ____Yes ____No

"Is there anything else you want to tell me?" _____

_____

_____

_____

Name: _____

ID No: _____

Date of Birth: _____

DH 3202, 2/03
Stock Number: 5744-000-3202-2

(continued)

● **ASSESSMENT TOOL 5.1   Intimate-Partner Violence Documentation Form** *(Continued)*

"Are there children in the home?" ____Yes ____No

If the answer to the question above is "yes," say to client: "I'm concerned for your safety and the safety of your children. You and your children deserve to be at home without feeling afraid."

"Have there been threats of abuse or direct abuse of the children?" ____Yes ____No

STEP 4—Assess client's physical injuries and health conditions, past and present

Observations/Comments/Interventions:

STEP 5—If both screening answers are NO, and you ARE CONCERNED that the client may be a victim:

a. Say to the client: "All of us know of someone at sometime in our lives who is abused. So, I am providing you with information in the event you or a friend may need it in the future."

b. Document under comments in Step 6.

STEP 6—Information, referrals, or reports made

Yes No
____ ____ 1. Client given domestic violence information including safety planning
____ ____ 2. Reviewed domestic violence information including safety planning
____ ____ 3. Provincial and local hotline numbers
____ ____ 4. Client called hotline during visit
____ ____ 5. Client seen by advocate during visit
____ ____ 6. Report made. If yes, to whom: _____

Comments

Signature _____ Title _____ Date _____

● **ASSESSMENT TOOL 5.2** **Woman Abuse Screening Tool (WAST)**

1. In general how would you describe your relationship...
   [ ] a lot of tension [ ] some tension [ ] no tension
2. Do you and your partner work out arguments with...
   [ ] great difficulty [ ] some difficulty [ ] no difficulty
3. Do arguments ever result in you feeling put down or bad about yourself?
   [ ] often [ ] sometimes [ ] never
4. Do arguments ever result in hitting, kicking, or pushing?
   [ ] often [ ] sometimes [ ] never
5. Do you ever feel frightened by what your partner says or does?
   [ ] often [ ] sometimes [ ] never
6. Has your partner ever abused you physically?
   [ ] often [ ] sometimes [ ] never
7. Has your partner ever abused you emotionally?
   [ ] often [ ] sometimes [ ] never
8. Has your partner ever abused you sexually?
   [ ] often [ ] sometimes [ ] never

Adapted from Brown, J., Lent, B., Schmidt, G., & Sas, S. (2000). Application of the women abuse screening tool (WAST) and WAST-short in the family practice setting. *Journal of Family Medicine, 49,* 896–903.

NURSING CARE PLAN 5.2

●

The Client Who is Being Abused

Recall Dina, the 30-year-old multipara in her sixth month of gestation. During the visit, Dina complains about feeling tired. She says that she thinks that she needs vitamins and, maybe, some food vouchers. At one point in the interview, she quietly mentions a concern about her husband hitting her. She states, "I've thought about leaving him, but I have no money."

Further assessment reveals frequent awakening during the middle of the night with the inability to return to sleep; intermittent crying during the day; and decreased appetite with a failure to gain weight over the past 2 months. "I don't know if I have the strength to take care of two small children and a new baby. I'm worried about everything. Sometimes I wonder if it is worth trying to carry on."

NURSING DIAGNOSES

- **Ineffective Coping** related to current life stressors, overwhelming demands of situation, and lack of support
- **Situational Low Self-Esteem** related to feelings of inferiority secondary to cultural background and current life stressors
- **Risk for Injury** (self and fetus), related to husband's episodes of violence, failure to gain weight in pregnancy, and difficulty sleeping
- **Fear** related to husband's violent episodes

EXPECTED OUTCOMES

1. The client will identify stressors affecting her life.
2. The client will identify positive methods for dealing with current stressors.
3. The client will verbalize at least one positive aspect of herself by the end of the visit.
4. The client will identify possible sources of support and assistance.
5. The client (and fetus) will remain safe.
6. The client will identify appropriate measures to deal with husband's violent episodes.

(continued)

NURSING CARE PLAN 5.2 ● The Client Who is Being Abused *(Continued)*

INTERVENTIONS	RATIONALES
Assess the client's level of understanding about pregnancy and its associated changes, intimate-partner violence, and the effects of stress on herself and her fetus	This information provides a baseline for identifying specific client needs and developing an individualized plan
Discuss with the client her concerns, feelings, and perceptions related to pregnancy, her family (including her husband's violent episodes), and how they are affecting the current family situation	Discussion provides opportunities to emphasize positive aspects of the current situation; verbalization of concerns aids in establishing sources of stress and problem areas to address
Inquire about methods used to cope with past stressful situations; encourage the client to use positive methods that were successful; provide additional suggestions for ways to cope with the current situation	Use of past successful methods enhances the chance of current success. Additional suggestions to deal with the current situation aid in relieving stress associated with outside variables and events, provide more options, and thereby promote a greater feeling of control
Review with the client measures to ensure a healthy pregnancy, including the need for adequate nutrition, sleep, and rest	Pregnancy places added demands on the woman's body; adequate nutrition, sleep, and rest are essential for fetal growth and development
Arrange for the client to speak with nutritionist to aid in meal planning	Adequate nutritional intake is necessary for optimal fetal growth and development as well as for prevention of complications that would compound the client's current stress
Review with the client known behaviours associated with intimate-partner violence; help the client correlate the husband's behaviours with them; assist the client to acknowledge that she is being abused.	Identification of known behaviours provides a base for comparison, giving support to the fact that the client is being abused. Acknowledging the reality of the abuse is a first step in stopping it
Assist the client to identify her desires and goals for her own life	Identification of client's wishes is important in developing strategies appropriate for her
Provide the client with accurate facts and communicate openly; answer questions honestly	Open, honest communication promotes trust and helps to correct any misconceptions or misinformation
Review and reinforce the client's positive attributes about herself and her abilities; reinforce with the client that husband's violent episodes are not "her fault"	Targeting positive attributes provides a foundation for enhancing self-esteem and aids in the realization that the client has an identity, can care for herself and her children, and is worthy of assistance
Assist the client in measures to promote her safety; help her develop a plan for leaving the partner, including strategies for safe departure. Provide suggestions for storing resources such as money, clothing, and keys in a safe place and for places to go such as shelters or houses of friends	The client's safety is paramount. Preplanning aids in minimizing risks and enhances the chances of a successful, safe departure

(continued)

NURSING CARE PLAN 5.2 ● The Client Who is Being Abused *(Continued)*

INTERVENTIONS	RATIONALES
Discuss with the client available community services. Inquire about any friends or family who could help	Additional support can alleviate the stress of the client's current situation and provide her with options should problems arise
Assist with referral to social services for additional support in areas such as finances	Social services can provide additional mechanisms for support and guidance
Provide the client with emergency contact numbers, with instructions to call at any time	Having emergency contact numbers readily available promotes safety
Institute a referral to a public health nurse; arrange for a follow-up visit within 1 week	Follow-up with public health nurse and return visits aids in evaluating the effectiveness of interventions and changes in the client's situation. Such measures provide an opportunity for additional teaching, support, and guidance

EVALUATION

1. The client accurately identifies the multiple stressors affecting her life.
2. The client demonstrates at least two positive coping strategies for dealing with stressors.
3. The client identifies positive attributes in herself.
4. The client states that she will use available sources of support.
5. The client and fetus exhibit no further evidence of injury, with the client's pregnancy progressing without incident.
6. The client implements strategies to protect herself and children from further violence.

● BOX 5.2 **Protecting Safety in Intimate-Partner Violence**

- Identify safe retreats for the client when the potential for violence exists. If she cannot escape, alert her to avoid rooms where no exit is possible and rooms that may hold weapons (eg, kitchen).
- Alert the client to memorize phone numbers of people who can help during violent episodes. Advise her to develop a code with phone contacts to alert them to the need for assistance.
- Give the client contact information for one or more domestic shelters. Such shelters house women and children for 1 to 2 months and provide food and counselling for employment, finances, and new residences.
- Explain how to obtain a *peace bond* (a document that forbids contact between the abuser and victim

for a specified period) or a *temporary restraining order* (a legal document that requires the abuser to avoid all contact with the victim).
- Encourage the client to press charges against the abuser.
- Suggest that police or a friend photograph physical injuries for use in future court cases.
- Offer phone numbers of community mental health therapists available for crisis intervention and family counselling.
- Recommend discussing personal safety with employer security.

For additional information on Safety Plans, visit www.shelternet.ca

Causes

Substance use often starts with experimentation, progresses to psychological and physical dependence, and finally becomes an addiction. Some people use drugs in a dysfunctional effort to cope with psychosocial stressors or other disorders. For example, many women with depression or anxiety turn to alcohol or drugs to mitigate the effects of their primary psychiatric illness. That is to say, these women use substances to "self-treat" their depression. Potentially, however, the reverse is also true. Women who use substances may become depressed because of their use.

Concerns Related to Pregnancy

Use of drugs, alcohol, or both during pregnancy poses serious risks, regardless of the reasons for use. Among such dangers are premature labour, abruptio placentae, stillbirth, and numerous other complications (Mazure et al., 2002). Alcohol-related teratogenic effects put the fetus at risk for various disorders. *Fetal alcohol spectrum disorder* includes the problems of mental retardation, microcephaly, hypoplastic philtrum and maxilla, and attention deficit hyperactivity disorder during childhood (see Chapter 22) (Hales et al., 2008). Maternal use of cocaine causes intrauterine growth restriction and organ malformations. Moreover, preterm labour, abruptio placentae, and numerous other conditions are likely because of cocaine's ability to constrict normal blood flow. Research indicates there are subtle effects on the growth and development of infants and young children who have been exposed to cocaine prenatally, warranting follow-up care for early identification of any adverse health outcomes (Schiller & Allen, 2005).

Much like cocaine, heroin has potentially devastating fetal effects. Withdrawal symptoms for mother, infant, or both include irritability, poor feeding, respiratory complications, tremulousness, and other neuropsychological difficulties. Heroin use is linked to sudden infant death syndrome (SIDS). Women can be treated with methadone; those who receive treatment will have a better chance of having a positive pregnancy outcome than those women who are not treated (Hales et al., 2008).

Collaborative Management

Initiating treatment is one of the most difficult hurdles. Clients rationalize or deny their addiction, or blame other people or external circumstances for their habits. Often, they must "hit bottom" before getting help. Clients in recovery need to learn new methods of coping with stressors, repair relationships, and develop interests and activities to fill the time once devoted to alcohol or drugs.

Many clients benefit from treatment plans that involve abstinence, counselling, and peer support. Twelve-step programs are free and provide specific guidelines for becoming and remaining free from substance use. Frequent attendance at meetings where members share their experiences and discuss topics related to recovery is essential.

 Think back to Gladys, the woman at the beginning of the chapter who reports hearing voices. What if she states, "With all this commotion, I could really use a drink." How should the nurse respond?

PSYCHOPHARMACOLOGIC THERAPY DURING PREGNANCY OR LACTATION

The use of pharmacologic agents to manage psychiatric problems during pregnancy and lactation poses challenges for both health care providers and clients (Davanzo et al., 2011). Such agents can be detrimental to fetal or newborn development and health; some of these medications are totally contraindicated during pregnancy. At the same time, many women who stop taking these medications when they are trying to conceive or after they become pregnant suffer relapses or exacerbations of their conditions. In some cases, maternal health or safety is compromised because of a lack of psychotropic medication, which, in turn, also can compromise fetal and newborn health.

Primary health care providers must always remember that medicating a pregnant woman is a serious undertaking requiring great caution. A basic assumption is that all psychotropic medications cross the blood–placenta barrier during pregnancy. Placental transport occurs through simple diffusion; the amount of diffusion is linked to the drug's molecular size, amount of protein binding, polarity, lipid solubility, and frequency and duration of exposure. For the most part, a drug's safety during pregnancy is based on outcomes from monitoring therapeutic plasma levels of nonpsychotropic medications (Schatzberg & Nemeroff, 2009). Even though the mother and fetus share the same blood circulation, fetal characteristics could increase the fetus's risk for exposure to the psychotropic medication, resulting in increased drug concentrations in the developing central nervous system. Potential outcomes are increased cardiac output, augmented blood–brain barrier permeability, decreased plasma protein and plasma-binding activity, and reduced hepatic enzyme activity (Schatzberg & Nemeroff, 2009).

The use of psychotropic agents during lactation also requires special attention. First, the newborn hepatic system is still evolving after birth and does so with great variability among infants. Delay of hepatic development is likely among premature and low-birth-weight infants. Second, the neonate's glucuronidation and oxidation systems are immature. The potential for high serum concentrations and metabolites of any drug needs careful and deliberate clinical consideration (Schatzberg & Nemeroff, 2009). Third, glomerular filtration and tubular secretions in neonates are 30% to 40% and 20% to 30% lower, respectively, than those in adults.

SickKids Motherisk has published important information on drugs and other chemicals in breast milk (Moretti, 2013). Knowledge about a drug's specific risk classification is helpful in making determination about the safety of its use in pregnancy or lactation (Box 5.3).

Determining Risks and Benefits

The health care provider and client need to evaluate the risks and benefits of maternal drug therapy during pregnancy or lactation, even though, to date, little empirical research exists to inform clinicians (Schatzberg & Nemeroff, 2009). Limited large-scale epidemiologic studies addressing the adverse effects of untreated mental illness among pregnant or lactating women leave many questions unexplored, among which are the potential adverse effects of psychopharmacologic treatment and the short-term and long-term outcomes for the infant. The nurse should be alert to mental illness during pregnancy or lactation. It is important to be especially cautious for psychotic disorders, such as schizophrenia and schizoaffective disorders (a subtype of schizophrenia that involves features of a thought disorder and mood disturbances), and depression, all of which are likely to worsen during pregnancy.

The U.S. Food and Drug Administration (FDA) has not approved psychotropic agents for the treatment of mental illness during pregnancy or lactation. The FDA has, however, developed a classification system for clinicians to use as a guide when prescribing medications (Table 5.3). Current research has helped with the creation of three categories of somatic risk to the fetus

● **BOX 5.3 Risk–Benefit Assessment for Lactation**

The information is divided into three sections: what is known, what is being considered, and what is unknown.

Known Knowledge

● Breastfeeding is beneficial for the infant.
● All professional organizations consider breastfeeding to be the best form of nutrition for the infant.
● Less than 60% of women plan to breastfeed during the puerperium.
● Approximately 5% to 17% of all nursing women take a prescription drug during their breastfeeding activities.
● Approximately 12% to 20% of nursing mothers smoke cigarettes.
● The postnatal period is a high-risk time for onset or relapse of psychiatric illness.
● All psychotropic medications with scientific data available are considered to be excreted in breast milk.

Increasing Data

● Untreated maternal mental illness has an adverse effect on mother–infant attachment and later infant development.
● The adverse effects of psychotropic agents on infants are limited to case reports.
● The nursing infant's daily dose of psychotropic agents is less than the maternal daily dose.
● Psychotropic medications are excreted into breast milk with a specific time course, allowing the minimization of infant exposure with continuation of breastfeeding.

Unknown

● The long-term neurobehavioural effects of infant exposure to psychotropic medications through breastfeeding are unknown.

Adapted from Schatzberg, A. F., & Nemeroff, C. B. (2004). *The American Psychiatric Publishing textbook of clinical pharmacology* (3rd ed.). Washington, DC: American Psychiatric Publishing.

● TABLE 5.3 **U.S. Food and Drug Administration (FDA) Use-in-Pregnancy Ratings**

Category	Interpretation
A	Controlled studies show no risk: adequate, well-controlled studies in pregnant women have failed to demonstrate risk to the fetus
B	No evidence of risk in humans: either animal findings show risk, but humans do not; or, if no adequate human studies have been done, animal findings are negative
C	Risk cannot be ruled out: human studies are lacking, and animal studies are either positive for fetal risk or lacking as well. However, potential benefits may justify the potential risk
D	Positive evidence of risk: investigational or postmarketing data show risk to the fetus. Nevertheless, potential benefits may outweigh risks
X	Contraindicated in pregnancy: studies in animals or humans, or investigational or postmarketing reports, have shown fetal risk that clearly outweighs any possible benefit to the patient

or newborn with the use of psychotropic agents during pregnancy or lactation (Altshuler et al., 1996):

1. Teratogenicity and organ malformation
2. Neonatal toxicity
3. Neurobehavioural and developmental teratogenic effects (Schatzberg & Nemeroff, 2009)

Clearly, all these outcomes would be deleterious to the infant and the family.

Commonly Used Agents for Psychiatric Disorders

National trends suggest that people are receiving more psychopharmacologic treatment and less psychotherapy or interpersonal therapy for psychiatric disorders, although nonpharmacologic treatments remain important. Family therapy, individual therapy, cognitive therapy, relaxation therapy, and so forth are viable options and should be considered appropriate. Nevertheless, an additional resource is medication. The intent of the following discussion is to acquaint nurses with the options in treatment and at the same time to alert all health providers to the potential dangers associated with the agents.

Antidepressants

The marketing of effective antidepressants with few side effects and enhanced therapeutic benefits is one major reason for the shift away from nonpharmacologic treatment modalities for the various types of depression (Olfson et al., 2002). For pregnant or lactating women, however, management of mood disorders may require exclusive reliance on nonpharmacologic methods, such as psychotherapy, for the safety of both mother and fetus.

Tricyclic Antidepressants. Tricyclic antidepressants have been on the market for some time. No clear-cut relationship has been established between their maternal use and congenital malformations (Eberhard-Gran et al., 2005). It is not yet established clearly if these drugs affect woman or infant during labour.

The AAP Committee on Drugs (2001) has suggested that clinicians proceed with caution, because support for the use of tricyclic antidepressants for lactating women is not clearly documented. Agents such as amitriptyline (Elavil), desipramine (Norpramin), and trazodone (Desyrel) are known to reach a peak in breast milk 4 to 6 hours after dosing. Should the infant develop health problems, the pediatrician might consider obtaining a blood sample to determine the level of medication in the infant's system. If the mother with depression experiences psychotic symptoms, including hallucinations, delusions, or a sense of unreality, her provider should consider antipsychotic medications (Schatzberg & Nemeroff, 2009).

Monoamine Oxidase Inhibitors (MAOIs). MAOIs are listed in the FDA's C category, indicating that providers cannot rule out their risks and that human studies are lacking to provide the needed evidence to support or rule out definitively their use during pregnancy or lactation. Therefore, MAOIs should not be used in pregnancy or during lactation (Schatzberg et al., 2010). Use of MAOIs also requires dietary restrictions associated with preventing hypertensive crisis, which could be dangerous during pregnancy and lactation (Schatzberg & Nemeroff, 2009). Dangerous foods are beer, red wine, aged cheese, smoked fish, brewer's yeast, beef and chicken livers, yogurt, bananas, soy sauce, chocolate, caffeine-based beverages, and raisins (Schatzberg et al., 2010).

Selective Serotonin Reuptake Inhibitors (SSRIs). Breastfeeding mothers can be treated for depression relatively safely with SSRIs. The drug sertraline (Zoloft) is considered a safe choice for these women (Davanzo et al., 2011). Traces of this drug enter the breast milk, but little evidence is shown in the infant's body.

Paroxetine (Paxil) is also a choice for use in lactating women because it is not detectable in breast milk or nursing infants. Fluoxetine (Prozac) and citalopram (Celexa) are known to enter the mother's breast milk, but in small amounts (Berle & Spigset, 2011). Breast milk will contain different levels of SSRIs, as determined by the time between the mother taking the medications and the infant's actual nursing (Schatzberg & Nemeroff, 2009).

Mood Stabilizers

Mood stabilizers are another group of psychotropic agents used to treat mental illness, particularly bipolar disorder. Lithium carbonate (Carbolith, Duralith) is the major mood stabilizer; however, lithium is contraindicated during pregnancy and lactation (Schatzberg et al., 2010). The main alternatives to lithium in pregnancy and lactation are anticonvulsant drugs. Commonly used examples are carbamazepine (Tegretol), valproic acid (Depakene), and clonazepam (Rivotril). Evidence suggests that these drugs do pose teratogenic risks (Hunt & Morrow, 2005).

Anxiolytics

Anxiolytics are a commonly used class of drugs. Benzodiazepines are the most frequently prescribed drugs for anxiety disorders; this class of drugs can accumulate in the fetus if given to the mother for a prolonged period. The half-life of benzodiazepines is longer in infants than in adults (Schatzberg & Nemeroff, 2009). These drugs should not be withdrawn abruptly from the mother; they should be tapered significantly before birth, if at all possible, to prevent infant withdrawal. Research data regarding this class of drugs are scarce, but clinicians have posited that benzodiazepines produce infant withdrawal syndromes that can last as long as 3 months (Eberhard-Gran et al., 2005).

Because such limited data are available about the use of anxiolytics during pregnancy and lactation, the clinician always uses caution when prescribing any medications for the expectant mother. During lactation, benzodiazepines administered to the woman in small doses are considered relatively safe; this class of drugs has a low milk-to-maternal serum ratio (Schatzberg & Nemeroff, 2009).

Antipsychotics

Antipsychotic drugs are used to manage schizophrenia and other thought disorders in women. Most antipsychotic medications fall in the FDA's C category of drugs, indicating that they are associated with rare anomalies, such as fetal jaundice and anticholinergic effects at birth (Schatzberg et al., 2010). The risk of administering these drugs is related to teratogenesis, and during the

first trimester, the woman and infant are at risk. Again, it is assumed that all psychotropic drugs, to some degree, cross the placenta, predisposing the infant to potential problems (Usher et al., 2005). Three antipsychotics, haloperidol (Haldol), perphenazine (Trilafon), and chlorpromazine (Thorazine), have received attention from researchers, who have determined no direct link between these agents and major congenital malformations (McKenna et al., 2005; Schatzberg & Nemeroff, 2009).

Aside from teratogenic risks, several antipsychotic drugs pose potential problems for the woman, including extrapyramidal side effects and neuroleptic malignant syndromes (Schatzberg et al., 2010; Schatzberg & Nemeroff, 2009). Table 5.4 outlines the extrapyramidal

● TABLE 5.4 **Antipsychotic-Induced Side Effects**

Condition Induced by the Psychotropic Medication	Side Effects
Akathesia: a continuous, observable restlessness	• Fidgety movements • Swinging of the legs and arms • Foot-to-foot rocking when standing • Pacing • Inability to sit or stand still for more than a few minutes
Dystonia: abnormal postures and muscle spasms	• Torticollis: abnormal positioning of the head and neck • Trismus: spasms of the jaw muscles • Laryngeal: pharyngeal spasm, which may impair swallowing or breathing • Macroglossia: slurred or thick speech because of enlarged tongue • Protrusion of the tongue that is not under voluntary control • Oculogyric crisis: eyes are positioned upward, downward, or to the side • Abnormal positions: the limbs or trunk in abnormal positions
Parkinsonism: involuntary movements	• Parkinsonian tremor: rhythmic, intermittent oscillating movements, which may be unilateral or bilateral and affect the head, mouth, tongue, or limbs • Muscular rigidity: extreme firmness and tensing of muscles, which may affect all skeletal muscles or discrete muscle groups • Lead pike-like rigidity or cogwheel rigidity: forms of resistance • Akinesia: decreased spontaneous motor activity, such as expression in facial gestures, speech, and other body movements
Tardive dyskinesia	• Involuntary movements of the tongue, jaw, trunk or extremities, which persist for 4 wk or more and include activities such as jerky, choreiform movements; athetoid movements; rhythmic movements; typically, the condition is irreversible but treatable with varying degrees of therapeutic response
Neuroleptic malignant syndrome	• Triad of rigidity, hyperthermia, and autonomic instability • Elevated serum creatinine kinase activity • Risk factors include being young, pre-existing neurologic disability, physical illness, dehydration, and rapid advance of dosage
Sedation	• Most common side effect, most evident during the initial phase of treatment • May cause daytime drowsiness beyond initial treatment
Anticholinergic and antiadrenergic effects	• Dry mouth, blurred vision, constipation, tachycardia, and urinary retention, which range from mild to other complications such as ileus of the bowel and others • Impaired memory and cognition, confusion, delirium, somnolence, and hallucinations • Tachycardia related to anticholinergic effects as well as postural hypotension
Weight gain	Slightly less than 50% of clients experience weight gain
Ophthalmologic effects	Pigmentary retinopathies and corneal opacities can occur with administration of antipsychotics over time

Adapted from Schatzberg, A. F., & Nemeroff, C. B. (2009). *The American Psychiatric Publishing textbook of clinical pharmacology* (4th ed.). Washington, DC: American Psychiatric Publishing; and American Psychiatric Association. (1997). Practice guideline for the treatment of patients with schizophrenia. *American Journal of Psychiatry, 154*(4), 1–62.

side effects and neuroleptic problems associated with antipsychotics.

 Suppose Gladys is started on chlorpromazine (Thorazine). She comes to the clinic for a visit 2 weeks later. During the visit, the nurse notices akathesia. What behaviours might the nurse observe?

NURSING CARE AND MENTAL HEALTH AND ILLNESS IN WOMEN

Nurses have many opportunities to ensure that women are knowledgeable about their own health as well as health-related concerns linked to pregnancy, lactation, and aging. The discussions in this section describe some basic roles and functions of nurses in these practice areas as related to women experiencing alterations in mental health and illness.

Discussing Informed Consent

Many risks are associated with psychotropic medications; these risks usually increase when a woman is pregnant or lactating. One major nursing responsibility is to ensure that the woman and her family (when appropriate) are knowledgeable about the risks of using psychotropic medications during pregnancy and lactation; this is also true for aging clients (Bonari et al., 2005). A thorough discussion of the risks versus the benefits of medications is essential. Exploring and discussing other available treatment alternatives to medications is also essential (Usher et al., 2005). See Chapter 2.

Documenting Risks Versus Benefits

Another important nursing responsibility is to document potential risks if an illness is untreated, including risks to the woman and the fetus and, eventually, to the infant as well (Schatzberg & Nemeroff, 2009). The nurse should discuss these concerns with the woman and her family. Critical decisions must be based on scientific knowledge, the client's clinical history, cultural considerations, and personal preferences. It may be helpful, if the woman is pregnant or lactating, to include the pediatrician in the discussion, because maternal medication decisions may affect the infant.

Promoting Community and Psychosocial Interventions

The current approach to treatment for women with mental illness is to maintain them in the community

as much as possible. Many women with chronic and severe mental illness are sexually active, and motherhood is either a present or future reality for them. These women require integrative mental health and physical health services, including information about sexual health, pregnancy prevention, and prenatal health. They also might need added help and support to care for children appropriately. Several community-focused interventions exist, including case management, rehabilitation, self-help groups, and day hospitalization.

Teaching Stress Management

Most women face stress daily. Both happy and unhappy events have stress-related consequences. Planning for an extensive vacation or getting married can produce the same stress as caring for an ill relative or having financial difficulties. The plethora of obligations and responsibilities that women confront daily can produce stress in their lives (Fig. 5.3). Each type of stress causes reactions within the psyche and human body. The body typically responds with "fight or flight" strategies. Common physical reactions to stress include increased blood pressure, palpitations, tense muscles, poor or excessive appetite, and disturbed sleep. As stress increases, so do the hormones that the stress produces. Ever-present stress is not congruent with a healthy immune system, and the body reacts with colds, fatigue, sluggishness, and other warning signs. Common symptoms of stress also include being short-tempered, feeling tired

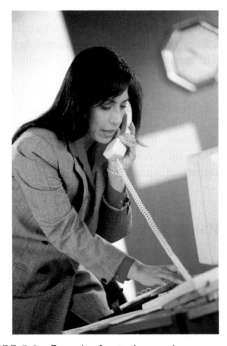

FIGURE 5.3 Everyday frustrations and pressures can accumulate and compromise the mental health of women of all ages. Effective stress management techniques can assist clients to avoid some triggering factors for psychiatric problems.

frequently, eating too much or too little, sleeping too much or too little, changes in the menstrual cycle, forgetfulness, anxiety, frustration, irritability, difficulty concentrating, angering easily, crying easily, and sleep disturbances. Heart disease, diabetes, irritable bowel syndrome, depression, urinary tract infections, and asthma are some illnesses linked to stress.

Effective ways to manage stress require behavioural changes. Women must make it a priority to stay healthy and to take care of their bodies. Specific strategies such as prioritizing responsibilities, taking time to relax, exercising, becoming involved in a social support system, and having a healthy perspective on life are a few simple but powerful strategies to improve quality of life. A regular sleep routine is extremely helpful; going to bed and getting up at the same time every day is a good habit to develop. Chapter 2 discusses health promotion strategies that are beneficial to all components of the woman's life: physical, spiritual, emotional, and psychological.

Assisting With Access to Health Care

The nurse is responsible for helping clients to obtain access to the mental health care system. Doing so, however, can be challenging. Mental health clinics are typically open from 9 AM to 5 PM and closed on weekends. After hours, people with mental illness and experiencing crisis must go to emergency departments, urgent care centres, or walk-in clinics for service.

Approximately 20% of Canada's population lives in rural, isolated, and northern communities (Statistics Canada, 2013a). Rural dwellers have few opportunities for adequate mental health services. Geography and long-distance travel make access to mental health services challenging (Canadian Institute for Health Information, 2006).

Language and culture can also serve as barriers to mental health care. Women of visual minority groups bear the greatest burden of most health and mental health disorders. Evidence indicates that immigrant women have limited knowledge regarding mental illness and low participation rate in health promotion pro-

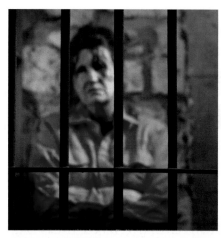

FIGURE 5.4 The number of women with mental illness and incarcerated is increasing steadily in Canada. With the push away from hospitalization and toward community-based psychiatric care, prison is the only housing alternative for some women with chronic and persistent psychiatric disorders.

grams, particularly maternal health services (Ganann et al., 2012). Mental health systems in the public domain may lack the necessary resources required to serve some ethnic minorities, in part because clients may not speak one of the two official languages and the culture of clients may not be Eurocentric. Newly arrived female immigrants are at high risk for developing mental health problems if the conditions surrounding their resettlement include previous stressful experiences, family upheaval, prejudice, discrimination, low socioeconomic status, isolation, and lack of social support (Macdonnell et al., 2012; O'Mahony et al., 2013).

There may be times when nurses need to visit jails, women's shelters, and other facilities to provide services to women and their children. In some communities, jails are the "new psychiatric hospitals," serving thousands of people who are incarcerated and mentally ill. Women who are incarcerated and mentally ill need special attention from nurses and other health care providers (Fig. 5.4).

● **TEACHING TIPS 5.3** Improving Clinician–Client Communication

Nurses should consider the following steps to improve communications with women regarding mental health and to promote mental health literacy:

● Provide written information at the appropriate reading level for the client.
● Use easy-to-follow layouts and simple pictures, especially diagrams that clarify written concepts and instructions.

● Focus discussions on desired behaviours and outcomes, not on medical terms, facts, and jargon.
● Ensure that information is culturally and personally meaningful and relevant to the woman.

Adapted from Doak, L. G., & Doak, C. C. (Eds.) (2003). *Pfizer principles for clear health communication* (2nd ed.). Potomac, MD: Pfizer Inc.

● **BOX 5.4** **Sample Health Literacy Approach**

- Make the client comfortable; offer milk, juice, or water.
- Ask the client to update her address and to share two telephone numbers of people who would know how to get in touch with her, in case she moves to another location.
- Schedule the next clinic appointment with her; write the time on the large envelope used to store the health materials given to the client.
- Include the telephone number of the clinic, the nurse's name, and the clinic's name.
- Encourage the client to phone the clinic if she feels ill or experiences an increase in any of the symptoms of which she complained (eg, swollen feet, difficulty sleeping).
- Draw out and illustrate as much health literacy content as possible during this contact (eg, smoking, high blood pressure). Give the client copies of all materials used for teaching.
- Succinctly teach the client about her blood pressure and methods of controlling it; give her a colourful pamphlet with pictures that explains high blood pressure.

- Demonstrate feet elevation; assist the client to elevate the feet during the teaching.
- Offer a referral to the smoking cessation program located at the clinic; explain to the client the potential dangerous effects of cigarette smoking on her infant and herself.
- Discuss nutrition; give simple, matter-of-fact written information about foods that she should be eating.
- Discuss the current stage of pregnancy and present to her the physiologic changes that will occur over the next 2 months.
- Schedule a psychiatric consult for further evaluation; underscore the major concern about the voices and the thoughts about the fetus's threatening behaviours.
- Discuss the necessity of rest. Review with the client basic strategies that would help increase her chances of rest.
- Make a preliminary plan for the client's labour and delivery, and orient her to the facility while she is at the clinic. Provide the names of clinic personnel to increase the sense of belonging and connectedness.

Promoting Health Literacy: A Critical Role for Nurses

Mental health literacy means knowledge and beliefs about mental illness that help the person to recognize, manage, and prevent such disorders. This information assists women to provide self-care, facilitates treatment compliance, and provides a sense of control over personal well-being.

A client's health literacy can be viewed as the currency she needs to negotiate with the nation's complex health system. Health literacy is a resource for everyday living and defined as "the ability to access, understand, evaluate, and communicate information as a way to promote, maintain, and improve health in a variety of settings across the life-course" (Rootman & Gordon-El-Bihbety, 2008, p. 11). Health care providers need to be mindful that 4 out of 10, or approximately 9 million Canadians struggle with low literacy (Canadian Institute of Health Research [CIHR], 2003). An estimated 55% of Canadians aged 16 to 65 lack the minimum level of health literacy needed to manage their health information needs on their own (Canadian Council on Learning, 2007). Most health-related materials are written at the 10th-grade level or above. Literacy problems incur heavy economic costs, estimated to be around $4 billion annually in Canada (CIHR, 2003). Health systems also have a highly specialized language. A woman could accurately understand familiar concepts and written material, but struggle to grasp content and information with new vocabulary and concepts, as in health care. Teaching Tips 5.3 provide steps to help nurses improve communication with clients and consumers.

As the demands for self-care are placed continually on women, problems with health literacy are expected to increase. It is not unusual for nurses to be in situations in which a woman needs help to understand information about prescribed medications, or about scheduled appointments. Research indicates many adult Canadians lack the capacity to obtain and understand health information and to make informed health decisions such as consent to treatment (Canadian Council on Learning, 2007). Given these findings, it is clear that nurses will need to discuss and explain those components that other providers may previously have taken for granted, erroneously assuming that clients understood and could comprehend without assistance. Nursing Care Plan 5.1 and Box 5.4 present more information related to health literacy in the care of a client experiencing hallucinations.

SUMMARY

- When caring for pregnant or lactating women, the nurse has many responsibilities and obligations. When a woman is at risk for or develops a mental illness, the nurse's responsibility expands.
- Nurses and other clinicians must recognize the unique characteristics of the woman, her culture, and her wishes.

- Psychological, physiologic, and psychopharmacologic treatments should address the woman's specific needs at the particular time in her life that she seeks or needs care.
- Nurses who provide health care to women and children are uniquely positioned to query the woman about violence in her relationship. Assessment tools should be available to aid in getting important information quickly.
- Engaging the woman in her care will enhance the level of care that she receives and is likely to increase her level of health literacy.

Questions to Ponder

1. Provide a synthesis of the theories used to explain mental health and illness. Select one theory, and detail its strengths and limitations for providing a framework for your clinical practice. Does it account for variables such as poverty, violence, access to care, ethnicity, race, and socioeconomic status? If not, how do these factors influence your plan of care, and to what extent is the theory helpful to you?

2. Of the psychiatric disorders presented, develop a grid that portrays the signs, symptoms, and predominant behaviours associated with each of the disorders. List the reasons for treating or referring the woman for special care. Determine the desired outcomes for treating the woman and the potential deleterious consequences for not treating her. Include the fetus or child in all comments. Can you create a scenario in which the woman with a serious mental disorder should not be treated? Why? Why not?

3. What would the nurse need to know when assessing a woman for suicide? Outline the major components for determining whether the woman is actively suicidal, and develop a plan of action that will address her immediate needs, future mental health and maternal health care, and other family needs.

REVIEW QUESTIONS

1. The nurse has just completed discussing stress management techniques with a client. Which of the following statements, if made by the client, would indicate the need for further information?
   A. "I will begin to practice some relaxation techniques regularly."
   B. "I need to eat a diet high in protein and yellow or orange vegetables."
   C. "I plan to exercise several times a week for at least 3 minutes each time."
   D. "I will schedule some time during the week to work on my hobbies."

2. Which of these interventions should the nurse perform *first* when caring for a client experiencing intimate-partner violence?
   A. Help the client to formulate a realistic escape plan.
   B. Share with the client that she is being abused.
   C. Document with pictures the client's physical injuries.
   D. Provide the client with the location of a local battered women's shelter.

3. A 24-year-old client is being treated as an outpatient for anorexia nervosa. Assessment reveals that the client's height is 172 cm and she weighs 45 kg. She describes eating certain foods only on specific days of the week and cutting food into cubes before eating. Which of the following expected outcomes is most appropriate for this client?
   A. The client will learn to identify situations that trigger anxiety.
   B. The client will gain 1.5 kg per week until she reaches 63.5 kg.
   C. The client will acknowledge that she looks ill and is emaciated.
   D. The client will eliminate ritualistic behaviours within 1 month.

4. The nurse is teaching an expectant couple about psychoactive medications in pregnancy. Which of the following statements from the couple indicates successful teaching?
   A. "The drugs help the symptoms of mental illness, but may lead to other problems."
   B. "The drugs act solely on specific target sites and pose limited risks."
   C. "The effects of drugs on the fetus are usually minimal."
   D. "Drug therapy has limited effectiveness for psychiatric problems."

5. A nurse is assessing a 42-year-old client who was brutally beaten and raped by her ex-husband. The client has fractures, lacerations, and bruises. She states, "This has happened before." The client cooperates with the examination and shows little emotion. The nurse attributes the client's affect to which of the following explanations?
   A. The client may have an underlying psychological problem.
   B. The client is handling the assault well emotionally.
   C. The client may be struggling internally to regain control.
   D. The client is concerned about her physical injuries at this time.

6. A client who has been diagnosed with general anxiety disorder shares with the nurse, "I'm worried about my finances. I'm afraid I will go bankrupt."

Which of the following responses would be most therapeutic for the nurse to use in this situation?

A. "Do you have extra health insurance coverage?"

B. "You think that you will lose all your money."

C. "Has there been a change in your life recently?"

D. "It sounds as if you have managed your money responsibly."

7. A client with depression who recently lost her job shares with the nurse, "I think that my family would be better off without me. I am only a burden to them." Which of these possible responses by the nurse would be appropriate?

A. "Does your family share your feelings?"

B. "Have you considered career counselling?"

C. "Are you thinking about hurting yourself?"

D. "When did you first start to feel like a burden?"

8. The community nurse is reviewing the health assessment form of a client who is to receive a follow-up home visit later in the day. Which of this information would suggest that the woman may be experiencing PPD?

A. The client is a primipara.

B. The client is 5 weeks postpartum.

C. The client has shared that she feels tired all the time.

D. The client has shared that she had no newborn experience before giving birth.

9. Which of the following observations by the nurse would suggest that the plan of care developed for a client who has been diagnosed with a mood disorder was successful?

A. The client has a strong social support network.

B. The client follows a healthy, well-balanced diet.

C. The client is dressed in a clean, coordinating outfit.

D. The client is exercising on average three times a week.

10. Which of the following outcomes in a client with schizophrenia best supports the effectiveness of the care plan?

A. The client is taking her medications and attending therapy sessions.

B. The client reports that she no longer has hallucinations.

C. The client has resumed work and attends community centre social functions.

D. The client no longer believes that she has special powers.

REFERENCES

Al-Modalial, H. (2012). Psychological partner violence and women's vulnerability to depression, stress and anxiety. *International Journal of Mental Health Nursing, 21*(6), 560–566.

Altshuler, L., Cohen, L., Szuba, M., Burt, V. K., Gitlin, M., & Mintz. J. (1996). Pharmacologic management of psychiatric illness during pregnancy: Dilemmas and guidelines. *American Journal of Psychiatry, 153*, 592–606.

American Psychiatric Association. (2013). *Diagnostic and statistical manual of mental disorders* (5th ed.). Arlington, VA: American Psychiatric Publishing.

Bennett, S., & Indman, P. (2006). *Beyond the blues: A guide to understanding and treating prenatal and postpartum depression.* San Jose, CA: Moodswings Press.

Berle, J., & Spigset, O. (2011). Antidepressant use during breastfeeding. *Current Women's Health Reviews, 7*, 28–34.

Bonari, L., Koren, G., Einarson, T. R., Jasper, J. D., Taddio, A., & Einarson, A. (2005). Use of antidepressants by pregnant women: Evaluation of perception of risk, efficacy of evidence-based counseling and determinants of decision making. *Archives of Women's Mental Health, 8*(4), 214–220.

Bowen, A., & Muhajarine, N. (2006). Antenatal depression. *Canadian Nurse, 102*(9), 26–30.

Boy, A., & Salihu, H. M. (2004). Intimate partner violence and birth outcomes: A systematic review. *International Journal of Fertility and Women's Medicine, 49*(4), 159–164.

Brenner, C. (1957). *An elementary textbook of psychoanalysis.* New York: Doubleday Anchor Books.

Canadian Council on Learning. (2007). *Health literacy in Canada.* Ottawa, ON, Canada. Retrieved August 19, 2008, from http://www.cpha.ca/en/portals/h-l/h-l2.aspx

Canadian Institute for Health Information. (2006). *How healthy are rural Canadians? An assessment of their health status and health determinants.* Retrieved May 31, 2013, from http://www.phac-aspc.gc.ca/publicat/rural06/index.html

Canadian Institute of Health Research. (2003). *Literacy and health in Canada: What we have learned and what can help in the future? A research report.* Retrieved May 31, 2013, from http://www.nald.ca/library/research/lithlthe/2.htm

Coker, A. L., Smith, P. H., & Fadden, M. K. (2005). Intimate partner violence and disabilities among women attending family practice clinics. *Journal of Women's Health, 14*(9), 829–838.

Cox, J. L., Hlden, J. M., & Sagovsky, R. (1987). Detection of postnatal depression: Development of a 10-item Edinburgh Postnatal Depression Scale. *The British Journal of Psychiatry, 150*, 782–786.

Curry, M., & Harvey, S. (1998). *Stress related to domestic violence during pregnancy and infant birth weight.* Thousand Oaks, CA: Sage Publications.

Cyranowski, J., Schott, L., Kravitz, H., Brown, C., Thurston, R., Joffe, H. et al. (2012). Psychological features associated with lifetime comorbidity of major depression and anxiety disorders among a community sample of mid-life women: The SWAN mental health study. *Depression and Anxiety, 29*(12), 1050–1057. doi:10.1002/da.2012.issue-12/issuetoc

Davanzo, R., Copertino, A., Minen, F., & Alessandro, A. (2011). Antidepressant drugs and breastfeeding: A review of the literature. *Breastfeeding Medicine, 2*, 89–96.

Davey, H., Tough, S., Adair, C., & Benzies, K. (2011). Risk factors for sub-clinical and major postpartum depression among a community cohort of Canadian women. *Maternal and Child Health Journal, 15*(7), 866–875. doi:10.1007/s10995-008-0314-8

Eberhard-Gran, M., Eskild, A., & Opjordsmoen, S. (2005). Treating mood disorders during pregnancy. Safety considerations. *Drug Safety, 28*(8), 695–706.

Farr, S., Hayes, D., Bitsko, R., Bansil, P., & Dietz, P. (2011). Depression, diabetes, and chronic disease risk factors among US women of reproductive age. *Preventing Chronic Disease, 8*(6), 1–9. Retrieved from www.cdc.gov/pcd/issues/2011/nov/10_0269.htm

Field, T. (2011). Prenatal depression effects on early development: A review. *Infant Behaviour and Development, 34*(1), 1–14.

Fitelson, E., Kim, S., Baker, A. S., & Leight, K. (2010). Treatment of postpartum depression: Clinical, psychological and pharmacological options. *International Journal of Women's Health, 3*, 1–14.

Ganann, R., Sword, W., Black, M., & Carpio, B. (2012). Influence of maternal birthplace on postpartum health and health service use. *Journal of Immigrant and Minority Health, 14*, 223–229.

Gilligan, C. (1993). *In a different voice: Psychological theory and women's development.* Cambridge, MA: Harvard University Press.

Grigoriadis, S., Vonderporten, E., Mamisashvili, L., Eady, A., Tomilson, G., Dennis, C. et al. (2013). The effect of prenatal antidepressant exposure on neonatal adaptation: A systematic review and meta-analysis. *Journal of Clinical Psychiatry, 74*(4), e309–e320. doi:10.4088/JCP.12r07967

Grote, N., Bridge, J., Gavin, A., Melville, J., Iyengar, S., & Katon, W. (2010). A meta-analysis of depression during pregnancy and the risk of preterm birth, low birth weight and intrauterine growth restriction. *Archives of General Psychiatry, 67*(10), 1012–1024. doi:10.1001/archgenpsychiatry.2010.111

Hale, B. (2002). Shifting the frame: Teaching feminist psychologics. *Transformations: A Resource for Curriculum Transformation and Scholarship, 13*(1), 61–72.

Hales, R. E., Yudofsky, S. C., & Gabbard, G. O. (2008). *The American Psychiatric Publishing textbook of clinical psychiatry* (5th ed.). Washington, DC: American Psychiatric Publishing.

Heron, J., Craddock, N., & Jones, I. (2005). Postnata euphoria: Are 'the highs' an indicator of bipolarity? *Bipolar Disorders, 7*(2), 103–110. doi:10.1111/j.1399-5618.2005.00185.x

Hinderliter, D., Pitula, C., & Delaney, K. R. (1998). Partner violence. *American Journal for Nurse Practitioners, 2*, 32–40.

Hunt, S. J., & Morrow, J. I. (2005). Safety of antiepileptic drugs during pregnancy. *Expert Opinions on Drug Safety, 4*(5), 869–877.

Kornstein, S. G., Harvey, A. T., Rush, A. J., Wisniewski, S. R., Trivedi, M. H., Svikis, D. S. et al. (2005). Self-reported premenstrual exacerbation of depressive symptoms in patients seeking treatment for major depression. *Psychological Medicine, 35*(5), 683–692.

Kouba, S., Hallstrom, T., Lindholm, C., & Hirschberg, A. L. (2005). Pregnancy and neonatal outcomes in women with eating disorders. *Obstetrics & Gynecology, 105*(2), 255–260.

Landenburger, K. (1998). *Exploration of woman's identity—clinical approaches with abused women.* Thousand Oaks, CA: Sage Publications.

Lanes, A., Kuk, J., & Tamin, H. (2011). Prevalence and characteristics of postpartum depression symptomatology among Canadian women: A cross-sectional study. *BMC Public Health, 11*, 302. doi:10.1186/1471-2458-11-302

Lolak, S., Rashid, N., & Wise, T. N. (2005). Interface of women's mental and reproductive health. *Current Psychiatry Report, 7*(3), 220–227.

Macdonnell, J. A., Dastjerdi, M., Bokore, N., & Khanlou, N. (2012). Becoming resilient: Promoting the mental health and well-being of immigrant women in a Canadian context. *Nursing Research and Practice, 2012,* 576586. doi:10.1155/2012/576586.

MacKey, M., Williams, C., & Tiller, C. (2000). Stress, pre-term labour and birth outcomes. *Journal of Advanced Nursing, 32*(3), 666–674.

Mazure, C., Keita, G., & Blehar, M. (2002). *Summit on women and depression: Proceedings and recommendations.* Washington, DC: American Psychological Association.

McKenna, K., Koren, G., Tetelbaum, M., Wilton, L., Shakir, S., Diav-Citrin, O. et al. (2005). Pregnancy outcome of women using atypical antipsychotic drugs: A prospective comparative study. *Journal of Clinical Psychiatry, 66*(4), 444–449.

Mian, A. I. (2005). Depression in pregnancy and the postpartum period: Balancing adverse effects of untreated illness with treatment risks. *Journal of Psychiatric Practice, 11*(6), 389–396.

Mohr, W. K. (2012). *Psychiatric mental health nursing* (8th ed.). Philadelphia, PA: Lippincott Williams & Wilkins.

Moretti, M. (2013). *Drugs usually contraindicated during breastfeeding. SickKids Motherisk.* Retrieved May 31, 2013, from http://www.motherisk.org/prof/breastfeeding.jsp

Negron, R., Martin, A., Almog, M., Balbierz, A., & Howell, E. (2013). Social support during the postpartum period: Mothers' views on needs, expectations, and mobilization of support. *Maternal and Child Health Journal, 17*(4), 616–623.

Olfson, M., Marcus, S., Druss, B., Elinson, L., Tanielian, T., & Pincus, H. (2002). National trends in the outpatient treatment of depression. *Journal of the American Medical Association, 287*(2), 203–209.

O'Mahony, J., Troung-Donnelly, T., Raffin-Bouchal, S., & Este, D. (2013). Cultural background and socioeconomic influence of immigrant and refugee women coping with postpartum depression. *Journal of Immigrant and Minority Health, 15*, 300–314.

Patel, V., & Prince, M. (2006). Maternal psychological morbidity and low birth weight in India. *British Journal of Psychiatry, 188*, 284–285.

Pawlby, S., Hay, D., Sharp, D., Waters, C., & O'Keane, V. (2009). Antenatal depression predicts depression in adolescent offspring: Prospective longitudinal community-based study. *Journal of Affective Disorders, 113*, 236–243.

Peplau, H. (1963). A working definition of anxiety. In S. Burd & M. Marshall (Eds.), *Some clinical approaches to psychiatric nursing* (pp. 323–327). New York: Macmillan.

Perfetti, J., Clark, R., & Fillmore, C. M. (2004). Postpartum depression: Identification, screening, and treatment. *Wisconsin Medical Journal, 103*(6), 56–63.

Pinquart, M., & Sorensen, S. (2006). Gender differences in caregiver stressors, social resources, and health: An updated meta-analysis. *Journals of Gerontology. Series B, Psychological Sciences and Social Sciences, 61*(1), 33–45.

Poggi-Davis, E., & Sandman, C. (2010). The timing of prenatal exposure to maternal cortisol and psychosocial stress is associated with human infant cognitive development. *Child Development, 81*(1), 131–148. doi:10.1111/i.1467-8624.2009.01385.x

Public Health Agency of Canada. (2012). *A report on mental illnesses in Canada.* Retrieved from http://www.phac-aspc.gc.ca/publicat/miic-mmac/chap_2_e.html

Registered Nurses Association of Ontario. (2005). *Interventions for postpartum depression.* Toronto, ON: Registered Nurses Association of Ontario.

Registered Nurses Association of Ontario. (2012). *Women abuse: Screening, identification and initial response.* Toronto, ON: Registered Nurses Association of Ontario.

Robinson, G. (2012). Treatment of schizophrenia in pregnancy and postpartum. *Journal of Population Therapeutics and Clinical Pharmacology, 19*(3), e380–e386.

Rootman, I., & Gordon-El-Bihbety, D. (2008). *A vision for a health literate Canada: Report of the expert panel on health literacy.* Ottawa, ON: Canadian Public Health Association.

Ross, L., Dennis, C., Robertson Blackmore, E., & Stewart, D. (2005). *Postpartum Depression: A guide for frontline health and social service providers.* Toronto, ON: Centre for Addictions and Mental Health.

Ross, L., Grigoriadis, S., Mamisashvili, L. Vonerporten, E., Roerecke, M., Rehm, J. et al. (2013). Selected pregnancy and delivery outcomes after exposure to antidepressant medication: A systematic review and meta-analysis. *JAMA Psychiatry, 70*(4), 436–443. doi:10.1001/jamapsychiatry.2013.684

Sadock, B., & Sadock, V. (2007). *Kaplan and Sadock's synopsis of psychiatry.* Philadelphia, PA: Lippincott Williams & Wilkins.

Schatzberg, A., Cole, J., & DeBattista, C. (2010). *Manual of clinical psychopharmacology* (7th ed.). Washington, DC: American Psychiatric Publishing.

Schatzberg, A. F., & Nemeroff, C. B. (2009). *The American Psychiatric Publishing textbook of clinical pharmacology* (4th ed.). Washington, DC: American Psychiatric Publishing.

Schiller, C., & Allen, P. J. (2005). Follow-up of infants prenatally exposed to cocaine. *Pediatric Nursing, 31*(5), 427–436.

Segre, L., O'Hara, M., Arndt, S., & Beck, C. (2010). Screening and counseling for postpartum depression by nurses: The women's views. *MCN. The American Journal of Maternal Child Nursing, 35*(5), 280–285.

Seligman, M. (1975). *Helplessness: On depression, development, and death.* San Francisco, CA: Freeman & Co.

Seyfried, L. S., & Marcus, S. M. (2003). Postpartum mood disorders. *International Review of Psychiatry, 15*(3), 231–242.

Silverman, M., & Loudon, H. (2010). Antenatal reports of pre-pregnancy abuse is associated with symptoms of depression in the postpartum period. *Archives of Women's Mental Health, 13*, 411–415. doi:10.1007/s00737-010-0161-7

Society of Obstetricians and Gynecologists of Canada. (2005). *Intimate partner violence consensus statement.* Retrieved May 31, 2013, from http://sogc.org/guidelines/intimate-partner-violence-consensus-statement/

Statistics Canada. (2012a). *Health state description for Canadians. Section D-eating disorders.* Retrieved June 25, 2013 from http://

www.statcan.gc.ca/pub/82-619-m/2012004/sections/sectiond-eng.htm

Statistics Canada. (2012b). *Suicides and suicide rate, by sex and by age group*. Retrieved May 31, 2013, from http://www.statcan.gc.ca/tables-tableaux/sum-som/l01/cst01/hlth66a-eng.htm

Statistics Canada. (2013a). *Canada's rural population since 1851: Population and dwelling counts, 2011 CensusCat. No. 98-310-X2011003.*

Statistics Canada. (2013b). *Family violence in Canada: A statistical profile, 2000.* Ottawa, ON>: Statistics Canada, Canadian Centre for Justice Statistics, Cat. No. 85-224-XIE, 11.

Toohey, J. (2012). Depression during pregnancy and postpartum. *Clinical Obstetrics and Gynecology, 55*(3), 788–797. doi:10.1097/GRF.0b013e318253b2b4

Usher, K., Foster, K., & McNamara, P. (2005). Antipsychotic drugs and pregnant or breastfeeding women: The issues for mental health nurses. *Journal of Psychiatric and Mental Health Nursing, 12*(6), 713–718.

Vigod, S., Seeman, M., Ray, J., Anderson, G., Dennis, C., Grigoriandis, S. et al. (2012). Temporal trends in general and age-specific fertility rates among women with schizophrenia (1996–2009): A population-based study in Ontario, Canada. *Schizophrenia Research, 139,* 169–175. doi:10.1016/j.schres.2012.05.010, Epub 2012 Jun 1.

Yelland, J., Sutherland, G., & Brown, S. (2010). Postpartum anxiety, depression and social health: Findings from a population-based survey of Australian women. *BMC Public Health, 10,* 771. doi:10.1186/1471-2458-10-771, Retrieved from http://www.biomedcentral.com/1471-2458/10/771

Zeanah, C. H., Satfford, B., Boris, N. W., & Scheeringa, M. (2008). Infant development: The first 3 years of life. In: A. Tasman, J. Kay, & J. Lieberman (Eds.), *Psychiatry* (3rd ed., *Vol. 1,* Chapter 8). New York: Wiley.

CHAPTER 6

Sexuality and Reproduction

Viola Polomeno, Robin J. Evans, and Vi Wilkes*

Rochelle, 42 years old, brings her 14-year-old daughter, Kendra, to the facility for a yearly examination. Kendra is wearing makeup, platform shoes, and other items that make her appear several years older. While Kendra is getting changed in the examination room, Rochelle quietly states, "These teenage years are tough. I know girls my daughter's age are already having sex. I just hope Kendra isn't."

Patti is a 54-year-old married woman who has made an appointment to discuss problems related to fatigue and a "personal sexual issue." During the interview, the nurse asks Patti to describe her concerns. Patti looks down and quietly responds, "My sex life with my husband just isn't what it used to be. We haven't had sex for several months because I no longer enjoy it. Frankly, it's really become painful. Do you have any suggestions about what might help us?"

You will learn more about these stories later in this chapter. Nurses working with these clients and others like them need to understand the material in this chapter to manage care and address issues appropriately. Before beginning, consider the following points.

- What behaviours and approaches from nurses are especially important when dealing with the aspects of sexuality for clients?
- What other information from both clients is needed to fully address the concerns?
- How might age and developmental stage be influencing Kendra's scenario? What about Patti?
- How would the nurse need to modify care when working with a parent and child together? What about when working with a husband and wife?

*Contributor to first U.S. edition.

On completion of this chapter, the reader should be able to:
- Discuss issues related to sexuality and reproduction across the life span.
- Summarize assessment factors related to the anatomic, physiologic, and psychological aspects of sexuality development in both genders across the life span.
- Identify the effects of historical, sociocultural, and economic issues on sexuality and reproduction.
- Discuss the aspects of sexuality for clients along the sexual orientation continuum.
- Discuss ethnosociocultural rites of passage associated with sexual and reproductive milestones.
- Identify nursing strategies to promote positive sexual and reproductive outcomes.

KEY TERMS

adolescence	menarche
androgen	menopause
androgyny	menstrual cycle
andropause	menstrual phase
conception	nocturnal emissions
corpus luteum	ovulation
cultural identity	proliferative phase
dyspareunia	pseudohermaphroditism
estrogen	puberty
gender	rites of passage
gender constancy	secretory phase
gender identity	sex compatibility
gender role development	sexual orientation
hermaphroditism	stigma
masturbation	testosterone

Development of sexuality is an important part of each person's psychosocial identity, integrated sense of self, reproductive capacity, and ability to fulfil role functions in society. Although sexuality is separate and different from reproduction, the two concepts are inherently linked. Nevertheless, sexual behaviour and function are separate from reproductive function in that reproduction is not the aim of all sexual activity. Engagement in sexual activity is often for pleasure (Berman, 2005; Meston & Buss, 2007).

The purpose of this chapter is to differentiate and discuss manifestations of sexuality and reproduction within a sociocultural and economic perspective. A historical overview is first presented to situate the nurse in regard to the domain of sexuality. Male and female sexual anatomy, development, and responses are presented. Sexual orientation and sexual and reproductive rites of passage are explored. Understanding of the issues in this chapter will assist the nurse to appreciate the sexual and reproductive needs of individuals, design nursing care plans that address client needs, and promote sexual and reproductive health for all women and families.

HISTORICAL OVERVIEW OF SEXUALITY

Significant developments associated with sexuality date back to the late 1920s.

- The intrauterine device was developed in 1928.
- Latex condoms were distributed in the 1930s and were useful during the Second World War.
- Antibiotics were discovered and used in sexually transmitted infections (STIs) in the 1940s.
- The first oral contraceptive pill was developed by Gregory Pincus and Min Chueh Chang in 1953.

- Alfred Kinsey published two research reports on sexual behaviour in the human male and the human female (Kinsey et al., 1948, 1953).
- Masters and Johnson published their research on the human sexual response in 1966 (Masters & Johnson, 1966).
- Shere Hite published her reports on female and male sexuality, overturning some of the facts previously presented by Kinsey and Masters and Johnson, particularly in relation to women attaining orgasm through sexual intercourse (Hite, 1976, 1981).

The women's movement that started at the beginning of the nineteenth century had a major impact on improving women's condition through obtaining the right to vote and legal equality between men and women. This eventually led to women's rights for contraception and abortion. In 1969, contraception was legalized in Canada and homosexuality was decriminalized. In 1989, the Supreme Court of Canada struck down abortion legislation, leaving Canada without abortion legislation to this day. The outbreak of AIDS in the 1980s helped promote sexual education in many spheres of society, especially in the school system from the elementary level up to the university one. Canada has been at the forefront of legalizing same-sex marriage, adoption of children by gay and lesbian parents, and promoting other sexual rights.

Sexuality in Canada and abroad has been influenced by two declarations published by the World Association of Sexology. The Hong Kong Declaration of Sexual Rights was adopted at the 14th World Congress of Sexology (see http://www.worldsexology.org/resources/declaration-of-sexual-rights/). In this declaration, sexuality is an integral part of every human being, sexual rights are universal rights, and since health is a fundamental human right, sexual health must be a basic human right (World Association for Sexual Health, 2013a). This was followed by the 2005 Montreal Declaration "Sexual Health for the Millennium," which was adopted at the 17th World Congress of Sexology (World Association for Sexual Health, 2013b). In this declaration (http://www.worldsexology.org/resources/millennium-declaration/), all levels of society from government to the private sector are urged to develop plans of action to prioritize sexual health interventions, address systemic and structural barriers, and monitor progress.

SEXUAL AND REPRODUCTIVE DEVELOPMENT ACROSS THE LIFE SPAN

Sexual development and reproductive development are closely aligned, demonstrating their interdependence in forming the mature sexual being. The sections that follow emphasize the anatomic, physiologic, and psychological aspects of sexual and reproductive development.

Understanding the concept of **gender identity**, that is, a person's sense of maleness or femaleness, acceptance of the roles associated with that gender, and internalization of the gender and gender roles (Witchel & Azziz, 2011) is essential to the discussion in the rest of the chapter. Physiologic and genetic factors determine whether a person is biologically male or female; however, many other factors contribute to gender identity. Children proceed through predictable stages in which they achieve **sex compatibility** or comfort with a certain sex (gender role development), affirm their gender identity (labeling themselves male or female), adopt the stereotypical roles or behaviours associated with that gender (gender role behaviour), and express an attitude of gender superiority (Zucker, 2009, 2010). By the time most children are 6 or 7 years old, they have been socialized by parents, peers, and others to assume and accept the gender identity and roles that match their biologic gender. Nevertheless, some children, regardless of biologic sex determination, identify with the opposite sex and adopt its associated sexual behaviours.

Recall Kendra described at the beginning of the chapter. What findings would provide some evidence that Kendra has adopted a female gender identity?

It is important to note that a conflict over gender identity is *not* the same as homosexuality. Although gay men and lesbian women are attracted sexually to people of the same sex, they recognize and accept themselves as men or women. They have no desire to change their gender or assume behaviours and roles commonly associated with the opposite sex. Those with conflicted gender identity may be attracted sexually to people of the same sex, the opposite sex, or both. There are males who identify with and may wish to become females, and females who identify with and may wish to become males.

Conception Through Infancy

Genes determine the gender of the fetus. An ovum always has an X chromosome; a sperm can have an X or a Y chromosome. When a sperm with an X chromosome fertilizes an ovum, a female (XX) is produced. Similarly, when a sperm with a Y chromosome unites with an ovum, a male is produced (XY).

While in utero, three distinct stages occur, each of which is marked by increasing and rapid cell division and differentiation (Fig. 6.1). The pre-embryonic (also called germinal) stage of a fertilized ovum (zygote) lasts from gestational days 1 to 14, the embryonic stage from

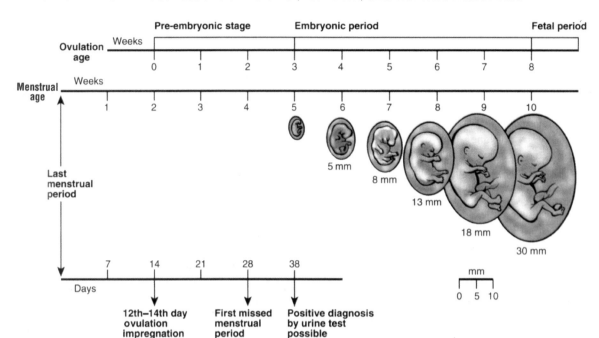

FIGURE 6.1 Stages of in utero development: pre-embryonic, embryonic, and fetal. The fetal period continues until the birth of the baby, normally at approximately gestational week 40.

gestational day 15 to the end of gestational week 8, and the fetal stage from the beginning of gestational week 9 until birth. Chapter 11 discusses the associated genetic processes and fully outlines pre-embryonic, embryonic, and fetal development in detail.

In Utero Sex Organ Differentiation

Initially, the zygote shows no physical characteristics specific to either gender. The anatomic rudiments of the genetically determined sex organs begin to differentiate in the embryo at approximately gestational day 14 (coinciding with the start of the embryonic stage). Clinicians can distinguish gender with high-resolution ultrasound as early as the first trimester (Efrat et al., 2006; Krone et al., 2000). Figure 6.2 depicts the differentiation of both external and internal genitalia from the embryonic stage to birth.

Female. In an embryo with normal XX sex chromosomes, the ovaries begin to develop between gestational weeks 11 and 12. The ovaries give rise to oocytes by gestational week 16; hormone-producing cells and associated ovarian tissues also begin to emerge by this time. It is important to note that in biologically female organisms, the sex organs differentiate independently of hormonal influences. External genital structures emerge and their development progresses even in cases of ovarian impairment or absence. Thus, an embryo with only one sex chromosome of X is considered, and has the sexual characteristics of, a female. She will be infertile in adulthood due to a lack of ovarian function and, subsequently, produces no ova for fertilization.

Male. Because the male embryo has X and Y chromosomes, an extra step is necessary for the development of the sex organs. The sequence of events is as follows.

1. The maternal placenta secretes human chorionic gonadotropin (hCG) hormone during pregnancy.
2. The hCG stimulates the secretion of testosterone from the testes.
3. Testosterone stimulates the development of additional male sex organs starting at approximately 8 weeks' gestation.

An embryo with a compromised Y chromosome and inhibited testosterone production will have female external genitalia, but no ovarian development, and will be infertile. With normal XY sex chromosomes and testosterone production, the testes begin to grow, and cells begin to organize to form the seminiferous cords, which are the basis for the seminiferous tubules. Testosterone secretion leads to the development of several ducts that later become the vas deferens, epididymis, and seminal vesicles. From 29 to 32 weeks' gestation, the testes descend into the fetal scrotum in response to increased secretion of testosterone (Sadler, 2012). Each newborn male testis is approximately 1.5 to 2 cm long and 1 cm wide, remaining this size until right before puberty (Bickley, 2009).

Variations in Normal Gestational Development

Hermaphroditism is a condition in which a person has both ovarian and testicular tissues. Sometimes the

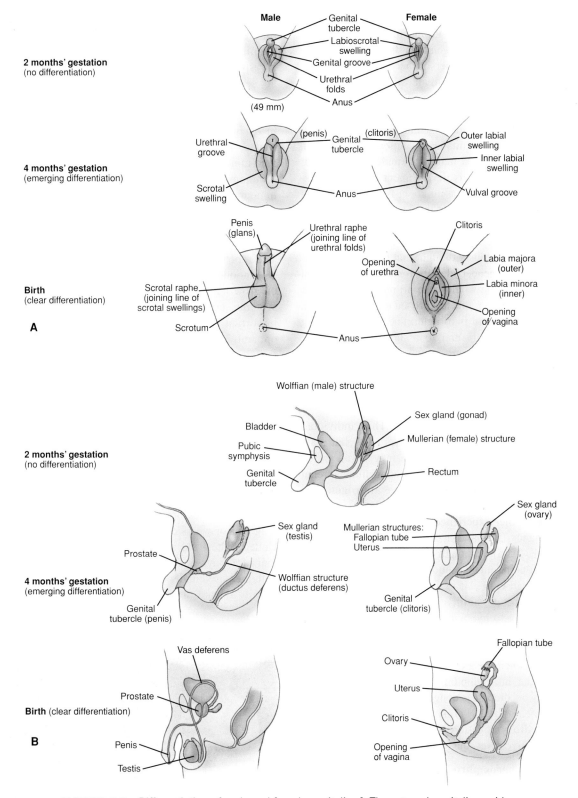

FIGURE 6.2 Differentiation of male and female genitalia. **A:** The external genitalia are identical until gestational week 7, when differentiation begins. By birth, the genitalia clearly indicate whether the infant is a boy or girl (except in rare cases of gender ambiguity). **B:** The same process of differentiation occurs in the internal genitalia.

external genitalia are ambiguous; in many cases, they present as female. In **pseudohermaphroditism**, the appearance of the outer genitalia fails to match the internal sex organs. The person may have ambiguous genitalia, male-appearing genitalia with internal ovarian tissue, or female-appearing genitalia with internal testicular tissue (Sadler, 2012). Other terms used to describe this condition are ambiguous genitalia or intersex.

When external genitalia are ambiguous at birth, identifying the baby as male or female is difficult or may be impossible. This development prompts investigation and testing; sex assignment is usually consistent with the internal rather than the external organs. The genital malformation may be corrected surgically; replacement hormones may also be required (Sanghavi, 2008). It was previously thought that this would facilitate a consistent gender identity for the child and that optimally, he or she would have no recollection of the experience. However, this has proven untrue (Sanghavi, 2008). The goal now is to determine the "underlying metabolic abnormality and to assign a gender more compatible with the future sexual satisfaction" (Sanghavi, 2008, p. 13) of the individual, recognizing that the gender chosen may not be the same as that chosen by the person later in life (Bomalaski, 2005).

Female Pseudohermaphroditism. This individual has ovaries and female chromosomes (XX) but male external genitalia. The condition may result when the fetus has autosomal recessive congenital adrenal hyperplasia or is exposed to excessive **androgen** (any steroid hormone with masculinizing effects), such as when the mother experiences an ovarian tumour during pregnancy (Bomalaski, 2005; Kousta et al., 2010; Lean et al., 2005). Although congenital adrenal hyperplasia results in female pseudohermaphroditism, it can also appear in males. It is potentially life-threatening because of the possibility of mineralocorticoid deficiency leading to hyponatremia, hyperkalemia, dehydration, and circulatory collapse (Bomalaski, 2005).

Early diagnosis of female pseudohermaphroditism is possible when the external genitalia are ambiguous or the infant has symptoms of adrenal crisis, which commonly accompanies congenital adrenal hyperplasia (Witchel & Azziz, 2011). A neonatal screening blood test, 17-hydroxyprogesterone, can provide early detection; in positive cases, the level is elevated.

Male Pseudohermaphroditism. These children have a sex chromosome genotype of XY; however, their external genitalia appear female. The condition is frequently associated with inadequate testosterone production or metabolism, or through an androgen receptor defect (Bomalaski, 2005). Inadequate testosterone production is most commonly a result of an inborn error in androgen biosynthesis (Bomalaski, 2005). Inadequate

metabolism is secondary to 5α-reductase deficiency; this results in normal testosterone production and an inability to produce dihydrotestosterone (DHT), which is responsible for the development of the male secondary sexual characteristics (Bomalaski, 2005).

Tumours that accompany these conditions can complicate management. Wilms tumour is common in clients with Denys–Drash syndrome (Majumdar & Mazur, 2013; McTaggart et al., 2001). Other associated tumours are gonadoblastoma, dysgerminoma, and seminoma (Majumdar & Mazur, 2013). Gonadectomy, tumour excision, and chemotherapy may be necessary components of treatment.

Childhood

The reproductive system is essentially at rest during childhood. Physiologic and psychological tasks focus on growth and development of other body organs and systems, cognition, and language. Nevertheless, an important task of childhood related to sexual development is socialization to the gender role. Gender role development typically begins in accordance with ethnic, cultural, religious, and societal norms and expectations.

The toddler stage is from approximately 12 to 36 months. By 24 months, toddlers can identify anatomic and visual differences between males and females. Gender identity begins to be established; however, the concept of gender constancy does not occur until the child is 5 or 6 years old (Berger, 2011; Zucker, 2010). **Gender constancy** means that the child understands that gender does not change if a person has short or long hair or wears dresses or pants. In Canada and the United States, old stereotypes of "acceptable" behaviours for boys and girls are becoming less important with increased understanding that activities do not necessarily dictate or belong to either gender (Fig. 6.3).

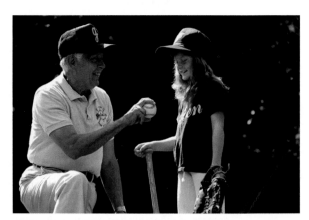

FIGURE 6.3 Expectations related to gender roles for children have changed and are continuing to evolve. Girls are increasingly participating in sports, with involvement from parents and extended family.

Androgyny, that is, flexibility regarding stereotypical masculine and feminine roles, has increased in Western society as it has become clearer that both sexes can have masculine and feminine attributes.

Stereotyped beliefs about sex roles can contribute to anxiety and guilt in children who do not meet such expectations. For example, peers may ostracize a boy in school if he does not play in team sports such as soccer, hockey, football, baseball, and basketball. Parents and peers may exert pressure on the child to conform to these gendered stereotypes. Some parents believe children who engage in behaviours commonly associated with the opposite sex may become gay or lesbian; parents also may fear criticism from friends and relatives.

Stereotyped sex role behaviours can be traced to historical, cultural, social, and religious influences. The more traditionally stereotypical the masculine and feminine roles are in a culture, the more that parents, schools, churches, and peers will enforce those stereotypical behaviours (Lobel et al., 2001). See Research Highlight 6.1.

Pubescence and Adolescence

Adolescence begins with a growth spurt that leads to puberty, that is, the maturation of the primary sex organs. The timing varies among individuals of both sexes. Teens have to cope with this physical growth and change and are usually anxious and sensitive about their physical appearance. They worry about their height, weight, skin, and hair and may be quick to find fault with themselves (Public Health Agency of Canada [PHAC], 2005).

At **puberty** reproduction becomes physically possible. Experts differ on the average age of the onset of puberty. Generally, it starts between 8 and 14 years, depending on ethnicity, sex, health, nutrition, genetics, and activity level (Pinyerd & Zipf, 2005). **Adolescence** is the developmental stage that begins with puberty and lasts 8 to 10 years (Berger, 2011). Tasks associated with adolescence include developing relationships, preparing for careers, and participating in family life (see Chapter 5).

Those going through puberty and adolescence are often preoccupied with sexual issues and concerns as a result of increased hormones and changes in body appearance and functioning. **Masturbation** (self-manipulation of the genitals for sexual pleasure) is common and normal for both boys and girls during this time. In addition, some adolescents periodically engage in sexual activity with same-sex partners, even if they do not consider themselves homosexual or engage in homosexual behaviour later in life. Dating activity prepares teens for mature relationships and helps them learn social skills they will need upon entering young adulthood.

Adolescents often feel conflicted about sex. On one hand, peers and internal feelings are pushing them toward physical relationships (Boyce et al., 2006). On the other hand, parents and society are pulling them back, asking them to delay sexual gratification until they have reached maturity and are accountable for the

---

● **RESEARCH HIGHLIGHT 6.1**   Children's Gender-Related Inferences and Judgments: A Cross-Cultural Study

OBJECTIVES

The authors studied the effects of culture on gender specificity and gender flexibility. The authors assumed that there is no justifiable reason for children to hold role and sex behaviour stereotypes; they posited that the strength and rigidity of the culture maintain these stereotypes. There were several hypotheses, one of which was that children would associate feminine activities with females and masculine activities with males, and that differences would be based on known characteristics of the culture.

DESIGN

The study sample included 542 third-grade and fifth-grade Israeli, Taiwanese, and Chinese students. The authors developed and administered a questionnaire to the children about activities, occupations, and emotional traits stereotypical for male and female.

RESULTS

The more traditional the culture, the more strongly the children associated with male and female stereotypical activities, occupations, and emotional traits. The Taiwanese children held stronger, more rigid, and more traditional stereotypes of characteristics of masculine and feminine roles, activities, and emotional traits.

CONCLUSION

The strength of the study favors the possibility that culture defines many activities as being typically feminine or masculine.

From Lobel, T. E., Gruber, R., Govrin, N., & Mashraki-Pedhatzur, S. (2001). Children's gender-related inferences and judgments: a cross-cultural study. *Developmental Psychology, 37*(6), 839–846.

consequences. Satisfactory relationships are built on self-confidence, self-esteem, trust in and concern for the partner, open communication skills, and dexterity. Preteens and adolescents are still developing these skills required for satisfactory, positive, and mature sexual relationships.

 Recall Rochelle and Kendra from the beginning of the chapter. Rochelle states, "Kendra has all these magazines in her room that talk about boys, dating, and sex. And she's been talking a lot about this boy at school who is 16 years old. I remember what I was like at her age. But I was a late bloomer and things are so different now." How can the nurse respond to Rochelle?

In 2005, 43% of Canadian youth aged 15 to 19 reported that they had had sexual intercourse at least once (Statistics Canada, 2008). This had decreased from 1996/1997, when 47% had reported intercourse. In 2005, 8% of youth aged 15 to 19 indicated that they had had intercourse before the age of 15, down from 12% in 1996/1997 (Statistics Canada, 2008). Fewer females reported intercourse prior to the age of 15; the proportion of males did not change significantly (Statistics Canada, 2008). Young Canadians are engaging in intercourse with fewer partners compared with previous generations, yet there is a proportion that continues to have multiple partners (Boyce et al., 2003, 2006). The preferred method of contraception amongst grade 9 and 11 students was condom use: 75% to 80% of grade 9 students and 64% to 75% of grade 11 students reported being protected from STIs by condom use at last intercourse (Boyce et al., 2006). However, for grade 11 females, the tendency was for less condom use as the use of the pill increased. The 2006 survey conducted by the Canadian Association for Adolescent Health found that 24% of sexually active adolescents between the ages of 14 and 17 did not use a condom the last time they had intercourse (PHAC, 2006). In 2005, there were 61,482 teen pregnancies in Canada (Statistics Canada, 2008). In 2003, Nunavut reported the highest adolescent pregnancy rate, at 98 per 1,000 women under 20 years. This was more than three times the national average, which was 27 per 1,000, while Prince Edward Island had the lowest rate at 20 pregnancies per 1,000 (Statistics Canada, 2006a, 2006b). While the national rate rose just slightly from 27.9 per 1,000 teens to 28.2, four provinces experienced significant increases between 2006 and 2010; teen pregnancy rates, for women aged 15 to 19, jumped by nearly 40% in New Brunswick, nearly 36% in Newfoundland, more than 17% in Nova Scotia, and 15% in Manitoba (Bielski, 2013). Abortion was the most frequent pregnancy outcome among adolescents in Ontario, Québec, and British Columbia (McKay, 2004, 2006).

These statistics make it clear that many people begin sexual activity at an early age. Many youth are at risk for unwanted pregnancy, STIs, interrupted schooling, delayed careers, changes in career or educational goals, and lowered social and economic status. These risks pose potential and actual costs to society in terms of lost wages, increased health care costs, and increased use of public assistance programs. Sex education for parents is most effective before children enter puberty. Such education requires discussion of the changes inherent in puberty, along with the consequences of unprotected sex and methods of contraception (see Chapter 8).

Nurses can play important roles in teaching related to sexual activity for teens and their families by identifying the existing knowledge base of each involved individual, supplementing the knowledge as appropriate, and identifying and promoting strategies uniquely individualized to each situation. For example, the nurse might assist the adolescent to explore the consequences of sexual activity and the effects on the teen's personal life in the home, school, and community. The nurse will also consider, when appropriate, encouraging adolescents and their parents or other adult caretakers to communicate about sexual issues. This may require that the nurse assists the parents or caretakers not only in learning information, but also in ensuring that important strategies are culturally and religiously specific and will promote positive interactions with their adolescents. Nursing Care Plan 6.1 addresses some of these issues of adolescence and sexuality.

Teaching Tips 6.1 provides suggestions on how parents can talk with their teen about sex. A number of resources provide guidance and suggestions for parents to discuss sex with their children (Alberta Health Services, 2014; Kaufman, 2011; PHAC, 2012). Box 6.1 presents definitions of sexuality, sexual health, and sexual health education; the philosophy contained in the guidelines; and principles underlying the philosophy.

Male Pubescent Changes

Anatomy and Physiology. The major organs of the male sexual and reproductive system are the penis, scrotum, testes, prostate gland, and seminal vesicles (Fig. 6.4). The penis is composed of the shaft and glans. The shaft contains the urethra, which allows urine to flow from the bladder. The glans is cone shaped and covered with loose skin called the *foreskin* or *prepuce*. In men who are circumcised, removal of the foreskin exposes the glans.

The scrotum is a loose sac that contains the testes. It is within the testes that sperm and testosterone are

(text continues on page 222)

NURSING CARE PLAN 6.1

●

A Family With Concerns Related to Adolescent Sexual Activity

Recall Kendra, a 14-year-old, whose mother voices concerns about her potential sexual behaviour. Kendra's history reveals that she experienced menarche at 12 years old. She reports that her menstrual cycle is somewhat irregular, ranging in frequency from every 28 to 35 days and lasting anywhere from 3 to 6 days. She states that her flow is heaviest on the first day but then gradually subsides.

During the physical examination, Kendra states, "I've been dating this boy who is about 2 years older than me for a few months now. Some of my friends have had sex with their boyfriends. I really like him a lot. I'm afraid that he'll break up with me if I don't sleep with him."

NURSING DIAGNOSES

- **Decisional Conflict** related to participation in sexual activity and fear of loss.
- **Deficient Knowledge** related to consequences of engaging in unsafe sex.

EXPECTED OUTCOMES

1. The client will identify information necessary to make an informed decision about sexual activity.
2. The client will identify the positive and negative aspects of engaging in sexual activity.

INTERVENTIONS	RATIONALES
Assess the client's beliefs about her developmental stage, self-esteem, and current body image. Explore her feelings about herself and her peers.	These data provide a baseline from which to develop appropriate strategies for teaching and care. Exploration of feelings provides insight into the client's thinking to ensure appropriate planning of individualized interventions.
Question the client about her understanding of the menstrual cycle, sexual activity, pregnancy, and STIs. Communicate accurate facts and answer questions honestly; clarify any misconceptions or misinformation.	Clear communication helps provide accurate information to aid in alleviating fears and clarifying misinformation. Honesty promotes the development of trust in the relationship.
Review the developmental changes common during adolescence, including the search for identity and independence from parents and strong influence of peers.	Adolescence focuses on the development of a sense of identity, emphasizing body image and peer influence. An understanding of developmental changes helps to promote understanding of the client's feelings as normal.
Teach the client about safer sex practices and contraceptive methods as appropriate. Provide the client with written material and appropriate internet resources for adolescents.	Knowledge of safer sex practices and contraception help reduce risks for pregnancy and STIs should she decide to engage in sexual activity. Written material and access to appropriate internet sites promote learning and allows for later review and reference.

(continued)

NURSING CARE PLAN 6.1 ● A Family With Concerns Related to Adolescent Sexual Activity *(Continued)*

INTERVENTIONS	RATIONALES
Explore with the client the consequences of sexual activity and how it might affect her life at home, at school, and in the community.	Exploration of the consequences helps to promote awareness in teens who are self-focused and present oriented and believe that "it won't happen to me."
Ask the client to identify person(s) with whom she can openly discuss her concerns, fears, and beliefs, such as her mother, a teacher, an older sibling, or a friend.	Open discussion of fears and concerns aids in reducing anxiety and promotes clear decision-making.
Offer nonjudgmental support throughout the client's care.	Nonjudgmental support fosters trust and promotes effective decision-making.

EVALUATION

1. The client makes an informed decision about engaging in sexual activity based on sound rationales.
2. The client demonstrates understanding of the consequences of unprotected sexual activity.
3. The client employs safer sex behaviours.

● **TEACHING TIPS 6.1** **How Parents can Talk to Their Teen About Sex**

Get a game plan. Talk things over with your partner/spouse if you have one, to help you clarify issues and the messages you want to give. Choose a time when you both are relaxed and have time to talk. Find a regular time to be with each of your children so that there are built-in opportunities for discussion and sharing.

Know what values you want to be part of your family rules. Share your beliefs with your teen. The values you live by and the discussions you have are important. Encourage your son/daughter to set his/her own limits. Stress the importance of being able to clearly communicate to a partner and being respected by him/her.

Respect each other's privacy. Make it clear that you want to discuss information, choices, and opinions—not their sexual experiences. You also do not have to share your personal experiences unless you are comfortable doing so and can use them as a teachable moment.

Listen. Try to listen calmly, even when there is a difference of opinion. If you really listen to your child, you'll learn a lot about what he/she is thinking. Your child will also feel heard, and that goes a long way toward building his/her self-esteem. Be willing to stop, and to discuss the topic again later if the discussion gets too heated.

Talk about the facts and more. Teens also want to know about relationships, decision-making, alternatives to sexual intercourse, how to talk openly and honestly about sex with others, contraception, safer sex, sexual orientation, and sexual assault. Talk about violence, assault, and date rape with your teen. If your teen discloses assault, remember to be supportive and let him/her know that he/she is not to blame.

Know you don't have to have all of the answers. Sometimes we are not ready for questions or challenges. It's all right to say, "That's a good question. I need to think about my answer for a while"; or "I don't know, but give me a day or two to find out." At other times, you may need to reconsider a response you've given earlier by saying, "I thought about what we talked about yesterday and I want to change something I said."

Get ready to blush and laugh. Don't be afraid to say you're embarrassed or uncomfortable. Often just saying so will make you and your teen more comfortable. Use your sense of humor in these situations. A little laugh can release a lot of tension.

Adapted from The Canadian Federation for Sexual Health. (Updated 2008.). *How do I talk to my teen about sex?* Retrieved from http://www.cfsh.ca/Your_Sexual_Health/How_to_Talk_about_Sex/with-teens.aspx (Adapted from *information prepared by the Sexuality Education Resource Centre in Winnipeg & Brandon MB*)

● **BOX 6.1** **Canadian Guidelines for Sexual Health Education**

Sexuality is a central aspect of being human throughout life and encompasses biologic sex, gender identities and roles, sexual orientation, eroticism, pleasure, intimacy, and reproduction.

Sexual health is a state of physical, emotional, mental, and societal well-being related to sexuality. It is not merely the absence of disease, dysfunction, or infirmity.

Sexual health education is concerned with the well-being of individuals. It recognizes that individuals have responsibilities, and are affected by each other and by the social environment in which they live. Sexual health education is one important aspect of health promotion. Sexual health education is a broadly based, community-supported activity that requires full participation of the educational, medical, public health, social welfare, and legal systems in our society. It involves the individual's personal, family, religious, and social values in understanding and making decisions about sexual behaviour and implementing those decisions.

Philosophy of Sexual Health Education

The expression of human sexuality and its integration in an individual's life involves an interplay between personal desires, the needs and rights of others, and the requirements and expectations of society. Effective sexual health education should be provided in an age-appropriate, culturally sensitive manner that:

– is respectful of individual choices and focuses on the self-worth and dignity of the individual.
– helps individuals to become more sensitive and aware of the impact of their behaviour on others. It stresses that sexual health is an interactive process that requires respect for self and others.
– integrates the positive, life-enhancing, and rewarding aspects of human sexuality while also seeking to reduce and prevent sexual health problems.
– is based on a life span approach that provides information, motivational support, and skill-building opportunities that are relevant to people at different ages and stages in their lives.
– is structured so that changes in behaviour and attitudes happen as a result of informed individual choice. They are not forced upon the individual by an external authority.
– does not discriminate on the basis of race, ethnicity, gender, sexual orientation, religious background, or disability in terms of access to relevant information.

– provides accurate information to reduce discrimination based on race, ethnicity, gender, sexual orientation, religious background, and disability.
– encourages critical thinking about gender-role stereotyping.
– recognizes the importance of gender-related issues in society, the increasing variety of choices available to individuals, and the need for better understanding and communication to bring about positive social change.
– recognizes and responds to the specific sexual health education needs of particular groups, such as adults, seniors, people who are physically or developmentally disabled, children and adults who have experienced violence, and marginalized populations such as Aboriginal people, immigrants, gay, lesbian, bisexual, and transgendered people as well as youth and street youth.
– provides sexual health education within the context of the individual's moral beliefs, ethnicity, sexual orientation, religious backgrounds, and other such characteristics.

Guiding Principles

Accessibility—It should be accessible to all people.

Comprehensiveness—It is a shared social responsibility that requires the coordinated effort of individuals, organizations, agencies, and governments.

Effectiveness of educational approaches and methods—It incorporates the key components of knowledge acquisition, development of motivation and personal insight, development of skills that support sexual health, and development of the critical awareness and skills needed to create an environment conducive to sexual health.

Training and administrative support—It is presented by well-trained individuals who receive strong administrative support from their agency or organization.

Planning, evaluation, updating, and social development—It achieves maximum impact when it is planned carefully in collaboration with intended audiences, evaluated on program outcomes and participant feedback, updated regularly, and reinforced by an environment that is favourable to sexual health.

Adapted from Public Health Agency of Canada. (2008). *Canadian guidelines for sexual health education.* Ottawa: Minister of Health. Retrieved from http://sexualityandu.ca/teachers/making-the-case-for-school-based-sexual-health-education

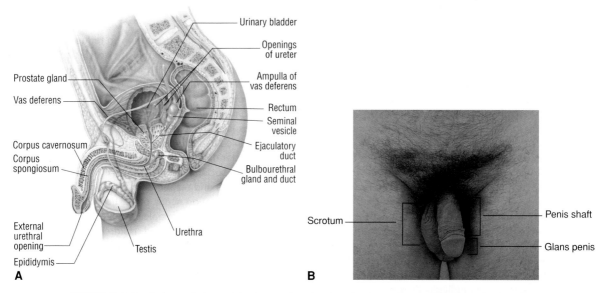

FIGURE 6.4   **A**: Lateral view of the internal male reproductive system. **B:** The external male genitalia. (**A** from The Anatomical Chart Company. [2001]. *Atlas of human anatomy.* Springhouse, PA: Springhouse.)

produced (Fig. 6.5). The prostate gland and seminal vesicles produce and store most of the seminal fluid. Together, the seminal fluid and the spermatozoa form semen, which is discharged during male orgasm.

Sperm develop in the seminiferous tubules in the testes. The process of sperm maturation is complex. The testes form approximately 120 million sperm per day; along with the epididymis and vas deferens, they are capable of storing sperm for 1 month (Hall, 2011).

During fertilization, approximately 120 million sperm cells mix with fluid from the seminal vesicles, prostate gland, and vas deferens. The man ejaculates this mixture through the penis to deposit sperm into the woman's vaginal canal, where they travel through the cervix and uterus up to the fallopian tubes and the released ovum. Only one sperm fertilizes the female ovum to create a new organism.

Box 6.2 describes pubescent physical changes in boys. The testes enlarge first, followed by growth of facial, axillary, and pubic hair, followed by enlargement of the penis. Approximately 1 year after the penis begins to grow, the adolescent male begins to experience **nocturnal emissions** (ejaculation of semen during sleep). The first nocturnal emission, commonly referred to as a "wet dream," is considered the hallmark of male puberty.

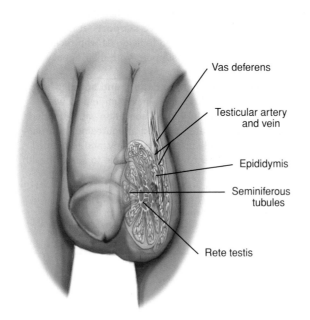

FIGURE 6.5   Internal testicular structures.

● BOX 6.2   Physical Changes in Male Puberty

- Enlargement of the testes and scrotum (first major event)
- Appearance of facial, axillary, and pubic hair (second major event)
- Enlargement of the penis (third major event)
- Thickening of larynx and deepening of voice
- Thickening of skin over body
- Roughening of scrotal skin
- Deeper pigmentation of scrotum
- Excessive secretion of the sebaceous glands
- Increase in long bone width and length

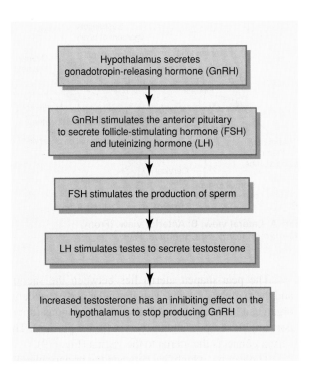

FIGURE 6.6 Summary of male reproductive hormones.

Male Hormones. Hormones are responsible for the maturation of the sexual organs (Fig. 6.6). **Testosterone** is the major androgen responsible for development and maintenance of male sex characteristics, muscle mass, and bone density. Testosterone is also found in females, but only in small amounts. Essentially, the hypothalamus controls the onset of puberty by secreting gonadotropin-releasing hormone (GnRH), which in turn stimulates the anterior pituitary gland to secrete luteinizing hormone (LH). LH then stimulates the testes to produce testosterone and follicle-stimulating hormone (FSH), which stimulates the production of sperm. Secretion of GnRH coincides and is coordinated with the growth spurt of adolescence, specifically, growth of the long bones (Hall, 2011). The timing of the increase in GnRH and testosterone production is executed carefully in the male body, so that he attains a maximum height before closure of the epiphyses of the long bones, in turn, stopping growth.

Any significant secretion of testosterone during preadolescence causes premature closure of the epiphyses. In such cases, these males are sexually precocious and short in stature.

Female Pubescent Changes

Anatomy and Physiology. External female genitalia include the mons pubis, labia majora, labia minora, clitoris, urethral meatus, Skene and Bartholin glands, and the vaginal orifice (Fig. 6.7). Collectively, these parts are called the *vulva*.

The mons pubis consists of fatty tissue that covers the bony prominence called the symphysis pubis. The labia majora surround the external genitalia; the labia minora lie on either side of the vaginal opening. Stimulation of the *clitoris* is generally responsible for female orgasm. The Skene and Bartholin glands provide some lubrication.

The internal genitalia include the ovaries, fallopian tubes, uterus, and vagina (Fig. 6.8). The ovaries are two almond-shaped bodies, one on each side of the woman's pelvic cavity. The ovaries hold ova (female sex cells) and secrete estrogen and progesterone. The narrow fallopian tubes are approximately 11.4 cm long and extend laterally along the sides of the uterus. They end with finger-like projections near, but not touching, the ovaries. Each month, the ovaries release a single ovum, which travels into the uterus by way of the fallopian tubes. If a male sperm fertilizes the ovum, the ovum implants in the uterus and develops progressively into a zygote, embryo, and fetus. If the ovum is not fertilized, the ovum and

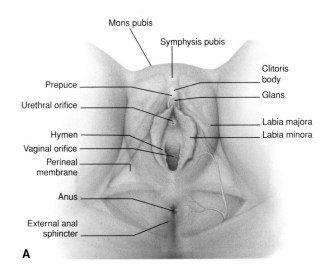

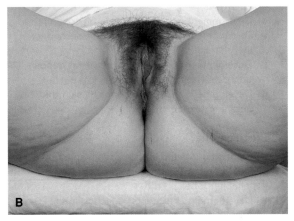

FIGURE 6.7 **A, B:** The external female reproductive system.

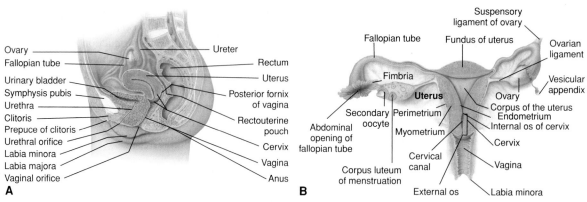

FIGURE 6.8 Internal female reproductive organs. **A**: Lateral view. **B**: Anterior view. (From The Anatomical Chart Company. [2001]. *Atlas of human anatomy*. Springhouse, PA: Springhouse.)

preparatory lining (endometrium) are expelled as the female menstrual period. Box 6.3 reviews the major hormonally dependent changes of puberty in females.

Unlike male sperm, ova are not replenished. At birth, the two ovaries of the female newborn contain approximately 2,000,000 ova. By puberty, this number has declined to 300,000 to 400,000 ova, and by menopause, the number of ova is very small (Hall, 2011). Women in developed countries can expect to release 400 ova and have approximately 400 menstrual cycles over their reproductive lives (Cunningham et al., 2010). In contrast, women in developing countries experience fewer menstrual cycles because of many factors including poor nutrition, many pregnancies, and prolonged lactation periods (Critchley et al., 2001).

The pear-shaped uterus lies between the sacrum and the symphysis pubis. This muscular and expandable organ can be divided into three parts: the fundus (upper portion), the corpus, and the cervix (lower portion). The cervix connects the uterus to the vagina (Fig. 6.9).

The vagina, which lies between the urinary bladder and rectum, serves as a passageway from the uterus to the vulva. The walls of the vagina stretch during sexual intercourse and the birth of a baby.

The breasts (mammary glands) are directly influenced by estrogen and progesterone. They are the primary organs of lactation. Each breast consists of fatty and glandular tissue (Fig. 6.10). The lobes of the breasts drain through ducts that open on the nipple. The round areola surrounds the nipple; its colour depends on the

● BOX 6.3 Physical Changes in Female Puberty

Estrogen

- Increase in size of external genitals at puberty
- Development of mature ovaries, uterus, and fallopian tubes
- Development of the breasts
- Growth of long bones and closure of the epiphyses
- Development and maintenance of bone matrix
- Development and maintenance of secondary sex characteristics
- Development and maintenance of fat deposition patterns
- Development and maintenance of skin thickness and texture

Progesterone

- Preparation of the uterus for implantation
- Development of secretory function of the fallopian tubes
- Development of secretory function in the breasts

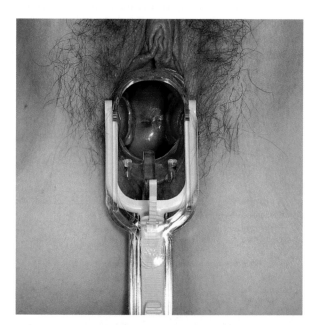

FIGURE 6.9 Appearance of the normal cervix in a multipara.

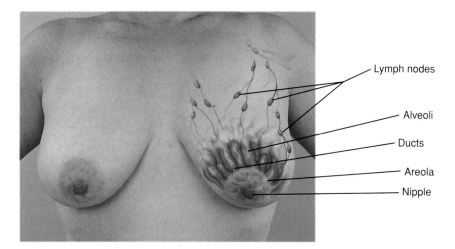

Lymph nodes

Alveoli

Ducts

Areola

Nipple

FIGURE 6.10 Anatomy of the breasts.

rest of the woman's pigmentation. Breast size varies, not only among different clients, but also in the same client at different parts in her life.

Menstrual Cycle. The menstrual cycle is characterized by rhythmical fluctuations in the secretion of female hormones; more accurately called the "female monthly sexual cycle," it is more commonly referred to as the "menstrual cycle" (Hall, 2011). These hormones control both the release of the unfertilized ovum at ovulation and the preparation of the uterus for the fertilized ovum. The menstrual cycle lasts an average of 28 days, but it can vary from 21 to 40 days. It starts with the first day of menstruation (day 1) and ends the day before the beginning of the next period (approximately day 28) (Fig. 6.11). From **menarche** (the first ovulation and menstrual period) to **menopause**, the menstrual cycle continues.

Figure 6.12 summarizes the role of hormones in the menstrual cycle. The **proliferative phase** (estrogen phase) of the menstrual cycle lasts from approximately day 5 to day 13. The hypothalamus secretes GnRH, which stimulates the anterior pituitary to secrete both FSH and LH. FSH causes several follicles to grow on both ovaries. At a given size, the follicles secrete **estrogen** (the primary female hormone), which stimulates further follicular growth and sensitivity to LH. Secreted estrogen is also responsible for the increased proliferation of epithelial cells in the endometrium (uterine lining), which thickens in preparation for a fertilized ovum (Hall, 2011). Together, the secretion of estrogen and LH and follicular growth continues until one follicle achieves full maturation. At that time, the other follicles begin to atrophy. Secretion of LH increases, stimulating the secretion of progesterone in larger quantities than of estrogen.

Ovulation occurs with rupture of the mature follicle and release of its ovum, as estrogen secretion diminishes and progesterone secretion increases, usually at approximately day 14 of the menstrual cycle. Sexual intercourse within 72 hours of ovulation has the potential to result in pregnancy. Methods of contraception (see Chapter 8) and interventions in cases where a couple experiences difficulty conceiving (see Chapter 10) are related to identifying ovulation and avoidance of, or recommendation of, intercourse at this time, depending on the desired outcomes.

The **secretory phase** (progesterone phase) is under the control of progesterone and lasts from approximately day 15 to day 28 of the menstrual cycle. Shortly after ovulation, the ruptured follicle remains. Granulation cells surround the empty follicle and fill with fluid (luteinize) to form a mass called the **corpus luteum**. The corpus luteum secretes a large amount of progesterone and a smaller amount of estrogen. Progesterone increases blood supply to the endometrium and adds nourishing and secretory glycoprotein and lipid deposits to the endometrial lining, making it receptive to implantation (Hall, 2011).

If a sperm does not fertilize the ovum during ovulation, the **menstrual phase** occurs on day 1 of the new cycle and lasts until approximately day 4. The plush endometrial lining that developed in anticipation of a fertilized ovum is sloughed off as a bloody discharge through the vaginal canal. The withdrawal of progesterone and estrogen acts as a positive feedback mechanism to the hypothalamus to secrete GnRH. Secretion of GnRH begins the proliferative phase, reinitiating the menstrual cycle.

Studies show that the withdrawal of progesterone is responsible for uterine desquamation and repair; it also activates the inflammatory process of vasoconstriction, white blood cell invasion, and the complement cascade (Critchley et al., 2001). Activation of these processes may explain some of the discomfort that some women experience during menstruation.

Adulthood

Experts in sexual behaviour have categorized phases of sexual arousal and orgasm. Identifying and using

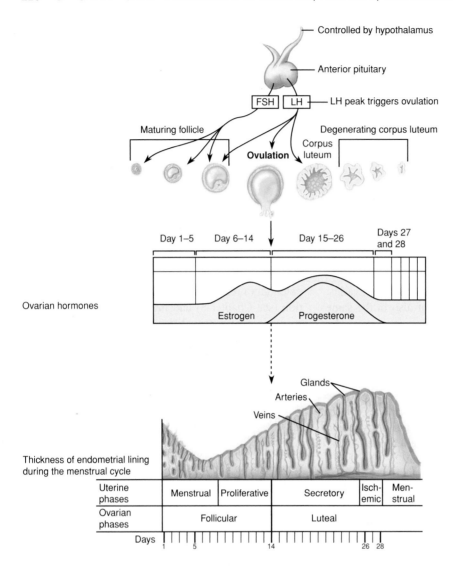

FIGURE 6.11 The 28-day (average) menstrual cycle.

categorical phases enable sexual behaviourists to describe normal function and disorders. Most attempts at establishing these phases are adaptations of the original sexual response cycle studies conducted by Masters and Johnson in 1966 (Levin, 2002).

Male Sexual Response

The physiology of the male sexual response consists of penile erection, lubrication, ejaculation of semen through the internal urethra, and resolution.

- Both psychogenic stimulation from the brain and physical stimulation of the glans penis can result in erection of the penis.
- Upon sustained stimulation of the penis through intercourse or other mechanisms, the internal urethra ejects a fluid that lubricates the receptacle and further heightens sexual arousal.
- Ejaculation of semen occurs at the climax (orgasm) in spasms that originate in the sympathetic nervous

system. The impulses travel from the reflex arc located at L1 and L2 to the genital organs (Hall, 2011).

- Resolution occurs after ejaculation, as the penis returns to normal size and sexual excitement disappears. Unlike in women, who are capable of multiple orgasms within a short period, vasocongestion returns to baseline much faster in men; therefore, men have limited capacity for multiple orgasm (Mah & Binik, 2001; McMahon, 2011).

Female Sexual Response

The sexual response phases discussed earlier for males (desire, excitement, plateau, orgasm, and resolution) are also appropriate classifications for female sexual response. Because of male and female anatomic differences, however, females are capable of having sexual intercourse without experiencing the sexual response phases.

The female sexual response can be described from an anatomic and physiologic perspective. Stimulation

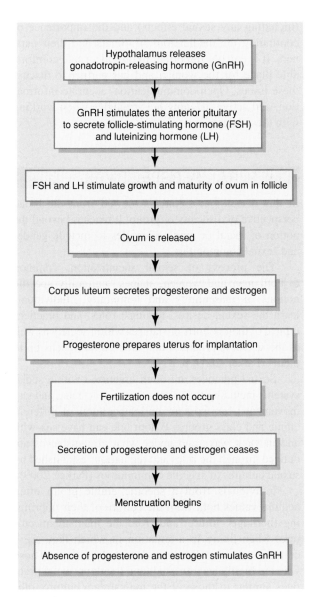

FIGURE 6.12 Summary of female reproductive hormones.

of the external genitalia, specifically the labia majora, labia minora, and clitoris, can cause sexual arousal. Once aroused, genital vasocongestion results from stimulation of the reflex arc located at S1 and S2. Lubricating fluid is caused by a combination of increased blood flow to the microcirculation of the vagina, leading to increased hydrostatic pressure and movement of a plasma transudate through and between the cells of the vaginal epithelium, and secretion of mucus from the Bartholin glands; this lubrication allows penetration of the vagina without pain (Hall, 2011; Salonia et al., 2010). Rapid firing of nerve impulses exceeds the threshold, resulting in orgasm (Salonia et al., 2010). Presently, no scientific evidence can explain orgasm, but it is known that vaginal and uterine contractions characterize orgasm and that degree of intensity var-

ies by person and with each occurrence (Salonia et al., 2010).

During resolution, sexual excitement decreases and the neurons return to the normal state. Women have a longer resolution phase than men. For this reason, women can have a second orgasm (or more) if stimulation continues.

Relationship Between Timing and Fertility

Conception is more likely to occur in the presence of female orgasm, which may assist in the promotion of fertilization (Hall, 2011). This may be related to the spasms of the female reproductive tract that occur during orgasm, facilitating movement of the sperm upward toward the ovum. Oxytocin released during orgasm causes uterine contractions which may also assist in the upward movement of the sperm (Hall, 2011). Widely accepted research has shown that fertilization should occur within a few hours and no longer than 1 day following ovulation; the majority of pregnancies occur during the 2 days preceding or the day of ovulation (Cunningham et al., 2010).

Middle and Older Adulthood

Menopause occurs on average in Canadian women at approximately 52 years of age, but it can happen at any time between the ages of 42 and 56 (Canadian Women's Health Network, 2007) (see Chapter 23). Clinically, a woman is considered menopausal if she has gone for 1 year or more without a menstrual period; however, symptoms of menopause and irregular menstrual cycles can last for 2 years or longer (Buckler, 2005). Cessation of menses before 40 years is considered premature and requires clinical investigation.

Menopause results in a decreasing supply of estrogen; consequently, women may experience a thinning of the vaginal wall and increased vaginal dryness (Katz, 2007). These changes often make sexual intercourse painful (called **dyspareunia**) which may lead to a loss of sexual arousal and decreased frequency of intercourse (Katz, 2007). Both FSH and LH decrease, and the ova are either depleted or fail to mature. As a result, women cannot conceive naturally after menopause.

The nurse counsels women that the end of the menstrual periods does not always coincide with the end of ovulation. Although female hormones have decreased to the point of suppressing the proliferative phase of the menstrual cycle, they may still be present in sufficient quantities to produce ovulation. Thus, women experiencing menopause can still become pregnant. The nurse should advise women that a blood test for FSH level can determine ovarian function and whether menopause has begun. Once ovarian failure has been established, the woman has reached menopause, and pregnancy is not a possibility.

Similarly, **andropause** (decreased production of androgens in men), also known as *male menopause*, occurs as early as 40 years as a result of the decrease in testosterone that accompanies aging. Because of decreased testosterone, aging men experience delays in achieving erections (DeLamater & Friedrich, 2002). With less testosterone, fewer sperm are produced. The testes become less firm, ejaculation is less forceful, pubic hair thins, and scalp hair thins or is lost. Unlike women, who can no longer reproduce naturally when menopause is fully established, men continue to produce sperm and can reproduce for a lifetime.

 Recall Patti, the 54-year-old woman who describes problems having sex with her husband. What areas of assessment would the nurse likely focus on relative to Patti's age and potential physiologic changes?

In the past, society tended to assume that older people did not engage in sexual activity. More recent research, however, has shown that sex continues well past menopause and andropause. Both men and women are known to have satisfactory, active sex lives well into older age. Maintenance of sexuality in older adulthood is an integral part of mental and physical health, self-esteem, and self-worth (Health Canada, 2006).

Sexual health histories should be done routinely with older clients, in addition to providing health information and teaching about safer sex practices and risky sexual behaviour. A thorough sexual history helps identify problems in sexual relationships. Examples of these problems include dyspareunia (painful sexual intercourse) related to decreased estrogen levels and resulting vaginal dryness in women, erectile dysfunction in men, and psychological problems such as feelings of rejection when the spouse or partner no longer desires sexual intercourse. See Nursing Care Plan 6.2.

As people age, sexual expression may need to be adapted as physical limitations and capabilities appear. As men age, the force and frequency of penile erections often decrease, the time to achieve effective erection increases, and the erection does not last as long. Nurses can explain these normal phenomena and make suggestions for adaptation.

Medications prescribed to treat illnesses can cause sexual dysfunction. Examples include antihypertensive drugs, insulin, and some antidepressants. Men may decide to not take these medications because of the fear of, or actual experience of, sexual dysfunction. Nurses can assist by explaining the side effects (including any sexual effects) and the importance of continuing the medications to clients and their partners. It is equally important to provide a safe comfortable place for the woman and her partner to discuss these issues. Open communication, accurate information, and active listening are strategies when working with these clients.

CULTURAL PERSPECTIVES

In this discussion, culture is viewed from the broad perspective of a society or group. It reaches beyond the notion of racial or ethnic identities to include gender and sexual communities.

The process of sexual socialization, common to both men and women, shapes "culturally specific notions of masculinity and femininity....Individuals learn the sexual desires, feelings, roles, and practices typical of their cohorts or statuses within society as well as the sexual alternatives that their culture opens up to them" (Parker, 2009, p. 257).

Sexual practices are often organized within social systems including the young; feminist, lesbian, and gay movements; sex workers; and subcultures of different ethnic and class groups. Whom one can have sex with and in what ways and under what circumstances are defined through the rules and regulations established by sexual cultures of specific communities (Parker, 2009).

Individuals from a specific ethnic group often acquire values both from the culture of their upbringing (heritage culture) and from the mainstream culture, when living in a situation in which they are a cultural minority (Meston & Ahrold, 2010). Those who are highly acculturated tend to adopt sexual practices similar to those of the mainstream culture; others may not, especially if they have maintained strong ties to their heritage culture (Meston & Ahrold, 2010). Therefore, it is important for the nurse to assess culturally influenced attitudes and behaviours, which includes assessment of the client's own individual beliefs and traditions. Some individuals may endorse conservative sexual behaviours including variations in age at first sexual encounter, frequency of intercourse, and number of partners. This conservatism can extend to sex education, health screening, and comfort with these and similar topics. Other clients may relate more closely to a mainstream sexualized culture and are more comfortable with these discussions. Nurses keep these considerations in mind when working with clients, particularly when discussing topics such as the perceived consequences of risky sex, multiple partners, violence, the importance of routine breast and cervical screening tests, birth control, pregnancy, and other sexually oriented topics.

NURSING CARE PLAN 6.2

●

The Client With Pain During Intercourse

 The nurse asks Patti how sexual problems have affected her marital relationship. Patti states that her husband has been patient, but the lack of intimacy is causing a strain. She also says that her husband thinks it is his fault. "He thinks I no longer find him attractive. That isn't true. It just hurt so much the last few times we had sex, that I'm afraid to do it anymore."

Assessment of Patti's sexual history reveals that she went through menopause approximately 2 years ago and that the problems with sex started around the same time. During discussion of sexual activity, Patti mentions that she wishes her husband would spend more time on foreplay, but that she's embarrassed to talk about this with him. "I don't want him to feel criticized. He's such a good man, and I know he wants me to be happy."

NURSING DIAGNOSIS

Sexual Dysfunction related to physiologic or psychological issues.

EXPECTED OUTCOMES

1. The client will understand the cause of the sexual dysfunction and take measures to treat it.
2. The client will indicate resumption of a satisfying sexual relationship and adapt to altered function (if necessary).

INTERVENTIONS	RATIONALES
Refer the client for a comprehensive physical evaluation.	Nurses must look for physical causes of pain during intercourse and make sure that there is no underlying problem that needs to be addressed.
Explain the age-related changes associated with menopause, including vaginal atrophy and resulting irritability and dyspareunia.	Understanding normal changes in aging may help the client realize that her experience is not uncommon or necessarily a reflection of her marital sexual relationship. Her knowledge can also assist her to communicate effectively about the problems with her husband.
Discuss possible treatment modalities with the client. Include information about estrogen tablets or creams, as well as over-the-counter moisturizers and lubricants.	Such modalities can provide the lubrication and protection against irritation needed to ensure a pleasurable sexual experience.
Discuss alternative methods for sexual expression. Explore personal values and cultural beliefs about sexual activity, and suggest methods for sexual gratification that are consistent with the client's beliefs.	The client can engage in activity other than vaginal intercourse with her spouse. Both partners may achieve orgasm through methods such as mutual masturbation or oral–genital stimulation.

(continued)

NURSING CARE PLAN 6.2 ● The Client With Pain During Intercourse *(Continued)*

INTERVENTIONS	RATIONALES
Instruct the client on techniques of clear and honest communication. Encourage her to express her feelings to her spouse. Model effective listening and how to elicit feedback.	Improved communication abilities will foster greater emotional intimacy and help prevent misunderstandings and resentment.
Encourage the client to engage in cuddling and caressing with her husband.	Physical and emotional intimacy can strengthen their overall relationship.

EVALUATION

1. The client verbalizes understanding possible causes of the pain during sex and takes steps to treat it.
2. The client reports beginning to engage in pleasurable sexual behaviours again with her husband.

SEXUAL PRACTICES AND BEHAVIOURS

A total of 76,275 positive HIV tests have been reported to the Public Health Agency of Canada (PHAC, 2013). The number of adult (≥ age 15) HIV cases reported in Canada decreased in 2012, which saw the lowest number of annual cases since reporting began in 1985 (PHAC, 2013). The proportion of cases in women remained relatively constant at 23.1%; diagnosis in women occurs at a younger age than in men (PHAC, 2013). Incidence is tracked through exposure categories. By creating such categories, health professionals can identify and work with the groups at greatest risk for exposure to HIV/AIDS. However, it is important to note that surveillance data only tracks the number of people tested and diagnosed; the data do not represent the total number of people infected or the number of those newly infected, nor do all provinces and territories collect consistent data (PHAC, 2013).

- *Gay men:* Men who have sex with men (MSM) continue to be the group most affected by HIV/AIDS in Canada, accounting for an estimated 63.6% of all reported new HIV infections in 2012.
- *Injection drug users:* Injection drug users were estimated to account for 11.9% of the new infections in 2012 in men and 29.8% in women.
- *Heterosexual contact with person at risk:* This category accounts for 6.4% of men and 28.8% of women with positive HIV test reports in 2012. *Heterosexual*

contact with someone with no identified risk: 10.3% of men and 18.6% of women fell into this category in 2012.
- *Heterosexual contact among people born in a country where HIV is endemic:* This category accounts for 3.3% of adult males and 18.1% of adult females.

Sexual behaviours can pose risks for contracting other STIs and for having unplanned pregnancies. Table 6.1 shows potential outcomes of sexual practices.

● TABLE 6.1 **Potential Outcomes of Sexual Practices**

Sexual Practice	Potential Outcomes
Unprotected anal sex	Sexually transmitted infections HIV/AIDS Hepatitis B and C Anal fissures and abscesses Colitis, enteritis, gastrointestinal disturbances Scabies, pubic lice
Unprotected vaginal sex	Sexually transmitted infections HIV/AIDS Hepatitis B and C Unplanned pregnancy Scabies, pubic lice
Unprotected oral sex	Sexually transmitted infections Urethritis HIV/AIDS Hepatitis B and C

● TEACHING TIPS 6.2   Safer Sex Options for Physical Intimacy

TEACHING POINTS

A common nursing role is educating clients in a variety of health care settings (hospitals, clinics, and community groups) about the prevention of STIs. The following is a listing of guidelines for safer sex that the nurse may wish to share with clients.

Safer Sexual Activities

- Massage
- Hugging
- Dry kissing
- Masturbation
- Hand-to-genital touching (hand job)
- Mutual masturbation
- Body rubbing
- Erotic books and movies
- All sexual activities when both partners are monogamous, trustworthy, and known by testing to be free of HIV

Possibly Safer Sexual Activities

- Wet kissing with no broken skin, cracked lips, or damaged mouth tissue
- Vaginal or rectal intercourse using latex or synthetic condom correctly
- Oral sex on a man using latex or synthetic condom

- Oral sex on a woman using a latex or synthetic barrier such as a female condom, dental dam, or modified male condom, especially if she does not have her period or a vaginal infection with discharge
- All sexual activities when both partners are in a long-term monogamous relationship and trust each other

Unsafe Sexual Activities in the Absence of HIV Testing, Trust, and Monogamy

- Any vaginal or rectal intercourse without a latex or synthetic condom
- Oral sex on a man without a latex or synthetic condom
- Oral sex on a woman without a latex or synthetic barrier such as a female condom, dental dam, or modified male condom, especially if she is having her period or has a vaginal infection with discharge
- Semen in the mouth
- Oral–anal contact
- Sharing sex toys or douching equipment
- Blood contact of any kind, including menstrual blood, or any sex that causes tissue damage or bleeding

From Mohr, W. K. (2012). *Psychiatric–mental health nursing: Evidence-based concepts, skills, and practices* (8th ed.). Philadelphia, PA: Lippincott Williams & Wilkins.

The key to avoiding potential outcomes is the practice of safer sex. Safer sex is called "safer" rather than "safe," because no method is 100% safe other than total abstinence. Teaching Tips 6.2 provides information on safer sex options for physical intimacy.

One major risk factor for sexual health concerns is having multiple sexual partners. Health care professionals encourage clients to maintain monogamous sexual relationships to reduce their risks for health problems. They advise clients to ask about previous relationships and the possibility of having acquired an STI in order to screen sexual partners for disease. It is important to note that heterosexual, lesbian, and bisexual women should be screened. The desired outcomes are to reduce the risk for HIV/AIDS and other STIs to the client and the client's contacts (see Chapter 4).

SEXUAL ORIENTATION AND GENDER IDENTITY

While the terms sex and gender are often used interchangeably, they are not exactly the same. The term **sex** typically describes one's status as male or female; this is predominantly determined at birth by the appearance of external genitalia. The term **gender** refers to "the trait characteristics and behaviors culturally associated with one's sex...a person's subjective judgments and inferences about sex including stereotypes, roles, presentation and expressions of masculinity and femininity" (Diamond et al., 2011, p. 630).

Sexuality

Sexual orientation refers to an "individual's patterns of sexual, romantic, and affectional arousal and desire for other persons based on those persons' gender and sex characteristics" (Dillon et al., 2011, p. 650). In the past, the most common terms used were heterosexuality and homosexuality; more current terms of gay, bisexual, straight, pansexual (sexual attraction regardless of gender), asexual (no sexual attraction), or the contemporary notion of queer may or may not be used by individuals, suggesting that some terms may hold meaning for some while not for others (Glover et al., 2009; Hammack & Choler, 2011). Within the sexual orientation continuum, heterosexuality is the assumed norm and dominant culture from birth. Sexual orientation and identification is a much more fluid process in females, who are more likely to experience nonexclusive attractions and relationships beginning in adolescence (Glover et al., 2009).

Gender identity represents a "person's sense of self as a boy/man or a girl/woman" (Diamond et al., 2011, p. 630). Gender influences how parents treat children, dress them, and the names they give them; it is typically presumed to align directly with biologic sex. Gender identity begins to develop and is transformed through parental influences, particularly in the early years when activities are often linked to gender and parents contribute to the child learning about gender. Differences in toy preferences appear as early as the first year of life; by the age of 5 children often have some sense of their gender identity (Bussey, 2011).

Gender identity continues to develop throughout life, also influenced by peers, media, and the educational system (Bussey, 2011). These influences may include such things as modeling of gender roles, gender-segregated play, media emphasis on portrayal of women engaging in domestic duties, and as sex objects (Bussey, 2011).

According to the 2003 Statistics Canada Canadian Community Health Survey (Steele et al., 2009), the first time data was collected about sexual orientation, 0.7% of Canadian women identified as lesbian or gay among the 18- to 59-year age group; 0.9% identified as bisexual. This survey found differences for Canadian women in health status and health risk behaviours correlated with sexual orientation (Steele et al., 2009; Veenstra, 2011). Women who self-identified as bisexual reported an increased rate of hypertension, more likely to have been diagnosed with an STI, and reported poor to fair personal and mental health (Steele et al., 2009). Lesbian women were more likely to have considered suicide than heterosexual or bisexual women. Lesbian and bisexual women were more likely to report smoking and risky drinking habits than heterosexual women. Overlapping, multilevel forms of stigma, and discrimination also present barriers to health and well-being and may account for such behaviours (Logie et al., 2011) (Research Highlight 6.2).

The term **transgender** is a "broad category typically used to denote any individual whose gender-related identification or external gender presentation conflicts in some way with their birth sex, and who therefore violates conventional standards of unequivocal 'male' or 'female' identity and behavior" (Diamond et al., 2011, p. 630). Contemporary perspectives view the primary dilemma as a conflict between psychological gender and assigned sex. The normal, healthy endpoint to this conflict is presumed to be a stable, unambiguous identity that is either all male or all female, typically achieved through physical transformation resulting in an alignment of psychological gender and biologic sex. This is more commonly the case for transsexual individuals, who seek to transform their physical appearance through clothes, makeup, hormones, or sex reassignment surgery in order to align with their psychological self; a change in legal sex status may also occur. However, this is only one subset of the transgender population. There is increasing evidence that this simplistic view fails to appreciate the complexity and diversity of this population, some of whom may identify as both male and female, or neither. Typically, there is a continuum of outcomes that result from their experiences; some may achieve a singular outcome whereas others may experience an

● **RESEARCH HIGHLIGHT 6.2** HIV, Gender, Race, Sexual Orientation, and Sex Work: A Qualitative Study of Intersectional Stigma Experienced by HIV-Positive Women in Ontario, Canada

OBJECTIVES

The authors studied the experiences of stigma and discrimination and coping methods among marginalized HIV-positive women in five cities in Ontario, Canada.

DESIGN

Fifteen focus groups were held with 104 marginalized HIV-positive women. Thematic analysis was used to analyze the data from these focus groups.

RESULTS

The authors found that these women experienced multiple types of stigma: HIV-related stigma, sexism and gender discrimination, racism, homophobia and transphobia, and sex work stigma. Multilevel coping strategies highlighted included resilience, social networks, and challenging the stigma.

CONCLUSION

This study expands on previous conceptualization of HIV-related stigma, suggesting that it is also experienced on the basis of sexual orientation, female gender, and transgender identity. In addition, the multiple levels of stigma and multilevel coping strategies to challenge stigma are highlighted.

From Logie, C. H., James, L., Tharao, W., & Loutfy, M. R. (2011). HIV, gender, race, sexual orientation, and sex work: a qualitative study of intersectional stigma experienced by HIV-positive women in Ontario, Canada. PLoS Medicine, 8(11), e1001124. doi:10.1371/journal.pmed.1001124

outcome that includes multiple and shifting identities (Diamond et al., 2011).

An important association exists between experiences with violence and sexual orientation, as well as risky health behaviours such as substance use and suicide, and risky sexual behaviours (Bontempo & D'Augelli, 2002). In 2011, Canadian police services reported that 18% of hate crimes were motivated by sexual orientation (Statistics Canada, 2013). Violence may include bullying, cyberbullying, verbal insults, social exclusion, and physical assault (Berlan et al., 2010; Bontempo & D'Augelli, 2002). Bullying experiences, both victimization and perpetration, are more likely among sexual minority females than heterosexual females; this is different from the experience of males (Berlan et al., 2010). However, cyberbullying is an issue for young adolescent girls across the continuum of sexuality. Therefore, health care providers routinely inquire about sexual orientation and experiences with bullying, interpersonal violence, and abuse. In addition, screening for depression, suicidal thoughts, and involvement in high-risk behaviours is implemented.

 Recall Patti, the woman who reports that she is having pain during intercourse. What if, instead, Patti had reported that she secretly had always been attracted to other women and no longer wanted to pretend with her husband? How might the nurse change her approach to the client's problem?

The openly lesbian, gay, bisexual, transgendered, and queer (LGBTQ) person often is a visible subject of scrutiny by the general population. Others judge the stigmatized LGBTQ person based on stereotypes. As stigmatized people, LGBTQ persons may feel compelled to "hide," "pass as straight," or "come out" and face the full effects of that choice, regardless of whether they are fully ready to do so. Once LGBTQ people have "come out," their relationships with all segments of society may change. Because society tends to assume that everyone has a heterosexual orientation, LGBTQ people may face judgment on two planes: as a person and as a sexual person. Many LGBTQ people have difficulty integrating their sexual self into their overall self because they are viewing themselves through the eyes of the heterosexual community.

One strategy that some heterosexual people use in an attempt to show acceptance of LGBTQ people, ironically, has the opposite effect. For example, in some cases, heterosexual people act as though there is nothing different about the lesbian woman, or they avoid the issue altogether. The strategy of accepting the lesbian woman without acknowledging her sexual orientation is paramount to setting up a power base to control the issue. By ignoring a friend's sexual orientation, the heterosexual person has, in essence, placed a restriction of silence on the relationship. The lack of discussion permits denial of the friend's sexual orientation. Thus, seeming blindness to sexual orientation (as well as to ethnicity, race, age, disability, or gender) does not equate with acceptance and lack of prejudice.

Nursing Care

Because lesbian and bisexual women access health care less frequently than heterosexual women, they may experience poorer health status. For example, lesbians and bisexuals participate less frequently in breast and cervical cancer screening, smoke more, and consume higher amounts of alcohol than heterosexual women (Seaver et al., 2007; Tjepkema, 2008).

Lesbian and bisexual women have identified preferences specific to the care provided to them (Seaver et al., 2007; Tjepkema, 2008). These preferences include clinicians who have specific knowledge about lesbians/bisexuals and are therefore able to provide information specific to them; a provider–client relationship where disclosure is encouraged in a nonheterosexist, nonjudgmental atmosphere; sufficient time for disclosure of information about their sexuality; assurance that information about their sexuality would be treated confidentially; settings with information available in waiting rooms that pertains specifically to lesbians/bisexuals; and an option to identify sexual orientation on intake forms (Seaver et al., 2007; Tjepkema, 2008).

COLLABORATIVE CARE: SEXUAL ORIENTATION

Nurses and other health care professionals address differences in sexual orientation to identify health issues specific to the person. It is important for nurses to view sexual orientation as part of the client's psychosocial and biologic makeup. Each person presents with unique and individual needs as a result of identification as lesbian, gay, bisexual, queer, or heterosexual. For example, the nurse approaches the collaborative care of all clients with an appreciation and respect for each client's worth and dignity and with a nonjudgmental attitude (Durham & Lashley, 2009; Seaver et al., 2007; Tjepkema, 2008). Health care professionals provide support to clients by assisting them through periods of disclosure to others and simply by accepting them and valuing them for who they are.

Assessment

The nurse completes a sexual history on all clients. Because sex is a sensitive issue for many, the nurse may begin by asking the client to agree to answer the questions in the sexual history. Privacy and confidentiality are essential. The health professional conveys to the client the importance of the sexual history in identifying risks and planning care. The nurse asks questions professionally and with concern. See Assessment Tool 6.1 for appropriate questions to ask in a sexual, nonreproductive history in any setting.

The nurse uses the assessment in evaluating risks to sexual health, as well as overall physical, psychological, and social consequences of such risks. Along with the client, the nurse integrates the findings in developing appropriate client-centred interventions.

Select Potential Nursing Diagnoses

Some potential nursing diagnoses are as follows:

- **Ineffective Sexuality Patterns** related to possible transmission of disease
- **Deficient Knowledge** about sexual orientation and lack of information about protection from STIs
- **Anticipatory Grieving** related to loss of psychosocial well-being
- **Ineffective Health Maintenance** related to lack of information about acquisition and transmission of disease
- **Ineffective Sexuality Patterns** related to fear of acquiring an STI and impaired relationship with significant others
- **Impaired Social Interaction** related to sociocultural dissonance
- **Sexual Dysfunction** related to ineffective or absent role model and conflicting values
- **Risk for Powerlessness** related to low self-esteem
- **Risk for Infection** related to high-risk behaviour and lack of knowledge about safer sex methods
- **Risk for Situational Low Self-Esteem** related to decreased power and control over environment
- **Risk for Suicide** related to low self-esteem, isolation, fear, and powerlessness

Planning/Intervention

When assisting a client to deal with issues of sexuality, the nurse tailors planning, interventions, and goals to the client's specific circumstances.

Related nursing interventions for clients focus on the following strategies.

- Determine high-risk behaviours for health problems; discuss findings with the client.
- Provide safer sex education.
- Encourage monogamous relationships; explain the dangers and risks associated with multiple sexual partners.
- Provide information about community resources and support groups geared toward clients' specific needs.
- Refer the client to a counsellor, if appropriate.
- Offer support if the client is facing family issues related to her sexuality.
- Encourage the client to discuss any episodes of bullying, violence, or abuse.
- Provide referrals for spiritual counselling, if desired.
- Screen the client for depression or suicidal thoughts.
- Refer the client for appropriate medical screening and laboratory tests for STIs.

Evaluation

The nurse evaluates the effectiveness of interventions for specific goals based on each client's particular concern. Possible desired outcomes for the client dealing with issues related to sexuality include the following.

- The client verbalizes behaviour considered "high risk" for STIs, the types of STIs that can result from high-risk behaviour, and understanding of how STIs are acquired and transmitted.
- The client verbalizes strategies for safer sex.
- The client identifies positive and negative aspects of sexuality and designs a plan to manage threats to psychological well-being.
- The client verbalizes names and phone numbers of relevant support groups.

● ASSESSMENT TOOL 6.1   **Appropriate Questions in a Sexual (Nonreproductive) History**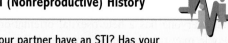

- Are you now in or have you been in a sexual relationship?
- Is your relationship with a person of the same sex or opposite sex?
- Are you having sexual intercourse in this relationship?
- Is the sexual intercourse vaginal-penile, anal, oral, or manual?
- Do you prefer relationships with men, women, or both?
- Are you worried about STIs such as HIV?
- Have you ever had an STI?

- Does your partner have an STI? Has your partner had an STI in the past?
- Have you had multiple sexual partners?
- How many partners have you had in the past year?
- Do you use contraception? If so, what kind?
- Do you use condoms or other protection during sex?
- Does your partner use protection or contraception?
- Does your partner have multiple sex partners?
- Are you happy with your sexuality?
- Have you experienced intimate partner violence?

- The client identifies a role model that may be of assistance to them.
- The client identifies positive aspects of sexuality and specific individual talents and abilities that contribute to the improvement of the community to which he or she belongs.
- The client verbalizes no suicidal ideation.

SEXUAL AND REPRODUCTIVE RITES OF PASSAGE

The concept of **cultural identity** includes "religion, rites of passage, language, dietary habits, and leisure activities" (Bhugra et al., 1999, p. 245). **Rites of passage** are traditions, often ceremonious, that mark specific points or milestones in a human life. They have the positive function of demonstrating that the culture has accepted a person as part of the community; thus, they are associated with a strong sense of belonging. Rites of passage go beyond celebrations. For example, a baby shower is a celebration; it is not a rite of passage, however, because it does not signify a transformation, is not a tradition embraced by one specific culture, has not been passed down for generations, is not associated with standard symbolic dress or ritual, and is not required for acceptance into a culture.

An example of a rite of passage is the Vision Quest that may be held by the Algonquin and Sioux Nations and nations on the Interior Plateau (Royal Canadian Mounted Police [RCMP], 2010). The person who embarks on a Vision Quest goes to a sacred location and fasts for 4 days while seeking a vision to provide direction in life. Preparation is made throughout the preceding year. Parents or elders may advise a youth to take a Vision Quest. The elder may then interpret the vision. Another rite of passage involving First Nations is the Naming Ceremony. Different from the birth name, which normally identifies a person for legal purposes, the name given to a child or adult in the naming ceremony is a traditional one that has particular significance to the individual, reflecting his or her personality or perhaps a particularly noteworthy deed (RCMP, 2010).

Female Genital Mutilation/Female Circumcision

The term "female genital mutilation" refers to all procedures in which parts or all of the female genitalia are removed or injured for nonmedical reasons (World Health Organization [WHO], 2008). The procedure has been reported to occur in all parts of the world, but is most prevalent in areas of Africa, some countries in Asia and the Middle East, and among some immigrant communities in North America and Europe (WHO, 2008). It is estimated that between 100 million and 140 million girls and women have undergone female genital mutilation, and 3 million girls are at risk for the procedure each year. There are a variety of cultural reasons suggested for this practice, such as reduction of promiscuity, better chances for marriage, or perceived preservation and proof of virginity (Vissandjee et al., 2003). There are no known health benefits; rather, the procedure is harmful, painful, and causes immediate and long-term consequences (Perron & Senikas, 2012). "Seen from a human rights perspective, the practice reflects deep-rooted inequality between the sexes, and constitutes an extreme form of discrimination against women" (WHO, 2008, p. 1). A number of international organizations and local communities have, for decades, worked toward elimination of this practice, resulting in a slow reduction of its prevalence.

Under the Criminal Code of Canada, female genital mutilation is considered an "aggravated assault," punishable by imprisonment for up to 14 years, unless it is performed by a medically qualified person for (a) the benefit of the physical health of the person or for the purpose of that person having normal reproductive functions or normal sexual appearance or function or (b) the person is at least 18 years of age and there is no resulting bodily harm (Ontario Human Rights Commission, 2000, p. 13).

Those who support female circumcision and immigrate to countries that ban or oppose the practice sometimes change their perceptions after leaving their countries of origin. However, many immigrants to the West still believe in female circumcision and either find a practitioner who will perform the procedure or return females to their home countries for the procedure (Vissandjee et al., 2003).

Concern has arisen among Western health care professionals about female genital mutilation, especially those in Canada (Perron & Senikas, 2012). Canadian and American health professionals are being approached to perform the procedures, thus putting them in the position of considering the procedure from an ethical decision-making model. They may believe that, even though it may be illegal and regardless of whether they agree with it, if they were to perform the procedure, the client would at least suffer fewer complications (WHO, 2008).

Male Circumcision

Male circumcision originated with native West African tribes more than 5,000 years ago (Chessler, 1997). It is a rite of passage in some cultures; for example, the Jewish faith requires the circumcision of all healthy males on the eighth day after birth. The Jewish procedure is done by a *mohel*, a ritual expert, outside the hospital during a celebration (the *bris*) with many relatives and friends. In the Muslim faith, circumcision is a religious obligation; however, the ritual differs from that practiced by Jews. Muslim boys are required to be circumcised sometime before adulthood, and the ceremonies are often held for a group of boys circumcised at the same time (Miller, 2002).

In Canada, male circumcision as a medical procedure is often performed unrelated to religion or culture. By 2005, the rate had decreased from 20% to 9.2% (Circumcision Reference Library, 2006). In the Canadian Maternity Experiences Survey, about one-third (31.9%) of the women reported having their male baby circumcised (Public Health Agency of Canada, 2009). This proportion varied widely among provinces and territories.

A medical rationale for circumcision has been that it promotes cleanliness and prevents smegma (whitish collection of dead cells) from accumulating under the foreskin (Dennington et al., 2013; Miller, 2002). Other medical rationales for circumcision have included prevention of HIV, penile cancer, cervical cancer in women, urinary tract infections, and masturbation. These rationales have been challenged. Multiple physical consequences include infection, hemorrhage, decrease in size of penis, excessive removal of foreskin, eventual impaired growth, and urinary retention (Dennington et al., 2013).

The Canadian Paediatric Society's (CPS) neonatal circumcision policy (currently under review) states that there is no medical indication for male neonatal circumcision (CPS, 1996). All provincial health insurance plans have removed nontherapeutic male neonatal circumcision from the schedule of covered procedures due to the lack of benefit to health (Circumcision Reference Library, 2006).

SUMMARY

- Development of the sexual self is an important part of a person's identity, integrated sense of self, ability to reproduce, and ability to fulfil role functions.
- The human germ cell goes through three stages before birth: pre-embryonic (gestational days 1 to 14), embryonic (gestational day 15 through gestational week 8), and fetal (end of gestational week 8 to birth).
- The internal sex organs determine the infant's gender; however, in some cases, gender is ambiguous.
- Hermaphroditism and female and male pseudohermaphroditism are examples of variations in normal sexual development.
- Gender constancy does not occur in children until approximately 7 years.
- Origins of sex role behaviour can be traced to historical, cultural, social, and religious influences.
- During fertilization, the man ejaculates approximately 120 million sperm cells in a fluid from his penis, but only one sperm fertilizes the female ovum for a single birth.
- The male hormone testosterone is responsible for the development of male sex characteristics, development and maintenance of muscle mass, and bone density.
- The menstrual cycle depends on the female hormones of gonadotropin, LH, FSH, estrogen, and progesterone.
- The menstrual cycle is divided into three phases: proliferative, secretory, and menstrual. Ovulation occurs between the proliferative and secretory phases.
- Conception is more likely when sexual intercourse occurs within 72 hours of ovulation.
- Female menopause is established after 1 year of no menstrual bleeding. Menopause is associated with the inability to conceive.
- Men and women often remain sexually active into old age.
- Sexual intercourse and unwanted pregnancies are community health concerns in Canada.
- Because the sexual self is an integral part of the self, the nurse conducts a sexual history on all clients who seek or need care regardless of disease process, sexual orientation, and age.
- Female genital mutilation is recognized internationally as a violation of women's and children's rights. The Canadian Paediatric Society is currently revising its policy about male circumcision.

Questions to Ponder

1. A 6-year-old boy undergoes surgery for a ruptured appendix. During the operation, surgeons discover that the boy has two functional ovaries. Because the boy has had male external genitalia from birth (except for smaller than usual testes), the parents have raised the child as a boy. Health care professionals refer the family to a psychologist for counselling.
   - What are some gender issues that the family will have to consider?
   - Should a sex assignment as female be made and surgery to construct a vagina be planned? If so, why? If not, why?

REVIEW QUESTIONS

1. Molly is a 3-year-old girl who plays with Michael, a 3-year-old boy who lives next door. One day, Michael brings his toy trucks and railroad cars to Molly's house for Molly to see. While Michael is there, Molly intently plays with Michael's dump truck. She pretends that she is driving and hauling dirt. Molly's mother, Jill, sees this and is concerned that Molly seems so interested in playing with the

trucks, because this is a "boy" activity. Which of the following is the probable rationale for Jill's concern?

A. Jill is afraid that Molly will get hurt playing with toys that boys like.

B. Jill is worried that Molly will try to keep the trucks and Michael will be upset.

C. Jill is worried that Molly will lose interest in all her other toys.

D. Jill is concerned that Molly is showing early signs of lesbian traits.

2. The nurse discusses with Jill her concerns about her daughter's interest in trucks. Which of the following is the most appropriate advice for the nurse to offer?

A. Jill should continue to watch for more signs of male gender-specific behaviour.

B. Jill should not worry because behaviour is not gender specific until school age.

C. Jill should take Molly to a child psychologist as soon as possible.

D. Jill should quietly put Michael's toys out of sight.

3. The nurse is working with a group of children of various ages. Which of the following children would the nurse expect to show the most androgyny?

A. A 3-year-old boy

B. A 4-year-old girl

C. A 6-year-old boy

D. A 7-year-old girl

4. Mary, 50 years old, has not had a menstrual period for 14 months. She asks the nurse if she is considered menopausal. Which response from the nurse would most accurately describe Mary's sexual reproduction status?

A. Mary has reached menopause and cannot conceive.

B. Mary has not reached menopause and may still conceive.

C. Mary has reached menopause, but may still conceive.

D. Mary has not reached menopause, but she can no longer conceive.

5. The nurse is working with a client who has been found to have premature testosterone production and secretion. Which of the following would the nurse expect to find in the client's history and medical record?

A. Learning disabilities

B. Aggressive behaviour in school

C. Short stature

D. Feminization

6. During a routine visit, a client mentions that her male partner has been recently experiencing erectile dysfunction frequently, even though he has no previous history of this problem. Which of the following responses from the nurse would be most appropriate?

A. Has your partner recently begun taking any new medications?

B. How do you feel about this problem?

C. How much exercise has your partner been doing lately?

D. Have you tried engaging in any new sexual practices?

7. A nurse educator is teaching a group of nurses the best approaches for educating families with teenagers about sexual issues. Which of the following interventions would the nurse be most likely to advocate?

A. Teach all families the necessity of providing their teens with birth control.

B. Discuss high-risk behaviours that can lead to sexually transmitted infections.

C. Reassure teens with possible minority sexual orientation that they are too young to know.

D. Inform parents that they must discuss sexual issues even if teens are embarrassed.

REFERENCES

Alberta Health Services. (2014). *The parent's role*. Retrieved from http://parents.teachingsexualhealth.ca/education/parents-role

Bazemore, P., Wilson, W., & Bigelow, D. (2005). *Homosexuality*. Retrieved from http://www.emedicine.com/Med/topic3359.htm

Berger, K. S. (2011). *The developing person through the life span* (8th ed.). New York, NY: Worth Publishing.

Berlan, E. D., Corliss, H. L., Field, A. E., Goodman, E., & Austin, S. B. (2010). Sexual orientation and bullying among adolescents in the growing up today study. *Journal of Adolescent Health, 46,* 366–371.

Berman, J. (2005). Physiology of female sexual function and dysfunction. *International Journal of Impotence Research, 17,* S44–S51.

Bhugra, D., Bhui, K., Mallett, R., Desai, M., Singh, J., & Leff, J. (1999). Cultural identity and its measurement: A questionnaire for Asians. *International Review of Psychiatry, 11,* 244–249.

Bickley, L. S. (2009). *Bates' guide to physical examination and history taking* (10th ed.). Philadelphia, PA: Lippincott Williams & Wilkins.

Bielski, Z. (2013, January 29). Why teen pregnancy is on the rise again in Canada. *The Globe and Mail.* Retrieved from http://www.theglobeandmail.com/life/health-and-fitness/health/why-teen-pregnancy-is-on-the-rise-again-in-canada-and-spiking-in-these-provinces/article7927983/

Bomalaski, M. D. (2005). A practical approach to intersex. *Urologic Nursing, 25*(1), 11–23.

Bontempo, D. E., & D'Augelli, A. R. (2002). Effects of at-school victimization and sexual orientation on lesbian, gay, or bisexual youths' health risk behavior. *Journal of Adolescent Health, 30,* 364–374.

Boyce, W., Doherty, M., Fortin, C., & MacKinnon, D. (2003). *Canadian youth, sexual health and HIV/AIDS study.* Toronto, ON: Council of Ministers of Education, Canada.

Boyce, W., Doherty-Poirier, M., MacKinnon, D., Fortin, C., Saab, H., King, M., et al. (2006). Sexual health of Canadian youth: Findings from the Canadian youth, sexual health and HIV/AIDS study. *The Canadian Journal of Human Sexuality, 15*(2), 59–68.

Buckler, H. (2005). The menopause transition: Endocrine changes and clinical symptoms. *Journal of the British Menopause Society, 11*(2), 61–65.

Bussey, K. (2011). Gender identity development. In S. J. Schwartz, K. Luyckx, & V. L. Vignoles (Eds.), *Handbook of identity theory and research* (pp. 603–628). New York, NY: Springer.

Canadian Paediatric Society. (1996). Neonatal circumcision revisited. *Canadian Medical Association Journal, 154*(6), 769–780. Retrieved from http://www.cps.ca/en/documents/position/circumcision

Canadian Women's Health Network. (2007). *Menopause.* Retrieved from http://www.cwhn.ca/en/faq/menopause

Chessler, A. J. (1997). Justifying the unjustifiable: Rite v. wrong. *Buffalo Law Review, 45*, 555–613.

Circumcision Reference Library. (2006). Canadian circumcision statistics. Retrieved from http://www.cirp.org/library/statistics/Canada/

Critchley, H. O., Kelly, R. W., Brenner, R. M., & Baird, D. T. (2001). The endocrinology of menstruation: A role for the immune system. *Clinical Endocrinology, 55*, 701–710.

Cunningham, F., Levano, K., Bloom, S., & Hauth, J. (2010). *Williams obstetrics* (23rd ed.). New York, NY: McGraw-Hill.

DeLamater, J., & Friedrich, W. N. (2002). Human sexual development. *Journal of Sex Research, 39*(1), 10–14.

Dennington, G. C., Hodges, F. M., & Milos, M. F. (Eds.) (2013). *Genital cutting: Protection children from medical, cultural, and religious infringements.* New York, NY: Springer. Retrieved from http://download.springer.com/static/pdf/641/bok%253A978-94-007-6407-1.pdf?auth66=1380338599_ba0d9abd6eed3e4015f30bc27305ba6b&ext=.pdf

Diamond, L. M., Pardo, S. T., & Butterworth, M. R. (2011). Transgender experience and identity. In S. J. Schwartz, K. Luyckx, & V. L. Vignoles (Eds.), *Handbook of identity theory and research* (pp. 629–647). New York, NY: Springer.

Dillon, F. R., Worthington, R. L., & Moradi, B. (2011). Sexual identity as a universal process. In S. J. Schwartz, K. Luyckx, & V. L. Vignoles (Eds.), *Handbook of identity theory and research* (pp. 649–670). New York, NY: Springer.

Durham, J. D., & Lashley, F. R. (2009). *The person with HIV/AIDS nursing perspectives.* New York, NY: Springer.

Efrat, Z., Perri, T., Ramati, E., Tugendreich, D., & Meizne, I. (2006). Fetal gender assignment by first-trimester ultrasound. *Ultrasound in Obstetrics & Gynecology, 27*(6), 619–621.

Glover, J. A., Galliher, R. V., & Lamere, T. G. (2009). Identity development and exploration among sexual minority adolescents: Examination of a multidimensional model. *Journal of Homosexuality, 56*, 77–101. doi:10.1080/00918360802551555

Hall, J. (2011). *Guyton and Hall textbook of medical physiology* (12th ed.). Philadelphia, PA: W. B. Saunders.

Hammack, P. L., & Gohler, B. J. (2011). Narrative, identity, and the politics of exclusion: Social change and the gay and lesbian life course. *Sexuality Research and Social Policy, 8*, 162–182. doi:10.1007/s13178-011-0060-3

Health Canada. (2003). *Canadian guidelines for sexual health education.* Ottawa, ON: Minister of Public Works and Government Services Canada.

Health Canada. (2006). *Seniors and aging-sexual activity.* Retrieved from http://www.hc-sc.gc.ca/hl-vs/alt_formats/pdf/iyh-vsv/life-vie/seniors-aines-eng.pdf

Hite, S. (1976). *The Hite report: A nationwide study on female sexuality.* New York, NY: MacMillan.

Hite, S. (1981). *The Hite report: A nationwide study on male sexuality.* New York, NY: Alfred Knopf.

Katz, A. (2007). When sex hurts: Menopause-related dyspareunia. *American Journal of Nursing, 107*(7), 34–39. doi:10.1097/01.NAJ.0000279264.66906.66

Kaufman, M. (2011). *Sex education for children: 8 tips for parents.* Retrieved from http://www.aboutkidshealth.ca/En/HealthAZ/FamilyandPeerRelations/Sexuality/Pages/Sex-Education-for-Children-8-Tips-for-Parents.aspx

Kinsey, A. C., Pomeroy, W. B., & Martin, C. E. (1948). *Sexual behaviour in the human male.* Philadelphia, PA: W. B. Saunders.

Kinsey, A. C., Pomeroy, W. B., Martin, C. E., & Gebhard, P. H. (1953). *Sexual behaviour in the human male.* Philadelphia, PA: W. B. Saunders.

Kousta, E., Papathanasiou, A., & Skordia, N. (2010). Sex determination and disorders of sex development according to the revised nomenclature and classification in 46,XX individuals. *Hormones, 9*(3), 218–231.

Krone, N., Wachter, I., Stefanidou, M., Roscher, A. A., & Schwarz, H. P. (2000). Mothers with congenital adrenal hyperplasia and their children: Outcome of pregnancy, birth, and childhood. *Clinical Endocrinology, 55*, 523–529.

Lean, W. L., Deshpande, A., Huston, J., & Grover, S. R. (2005). Cosmetic and anatomic outcomes after feminizing surgery for ambiguous genitalia. *Journal of Pediatric Surgery, 40*(12), 1856–1860.

Levin, R. J. (2002). The physiology of sexual arousal in the human female: A recreational and procreational synthesis. *Archives of Sexual Behavior, 31*(5), 405–411.

Lobel, T. E., Gruber, R., Govrin, N., & Mashraki-Pedhatzur, S. (2001). Children's gender-related inferences and judgments: A cross-cultural study. *Developmental Psychology, 37*(6), 839–846.

Logie, C. H., James, L., Tharao, W., & Loutfy, M. R. (2011). HIV, gender, race, sexual orientation, and sex work: A qualitative study of intersectional stigma experienced by HIV-positive women in Ontario, Canada. *PLoS Medicine, 8*(11), e1001124. doi:10.1371/journal.pmed.1001124

Mah, K., & Binik, Y. M. (2001). The nature of human orgasm: A critical review of major trends. *Clinical Psychology Review, 21*(6), 823–856.

Majumdar, I., & Mazur, T. (2013). Management of infants born with disorders of sex development. In P. M. Conn (Ed.) *Pediatric endocrinology* (pp. 423–439). New York: Springer. Retrieved from http://download.springer.com/static/pdf/34/bok%253A978-1-60761-395-4.pdf?auth66=1380317198_eb663157c6454823a4cceba8f5910bf7&ext=pdf

Masters, W. H., & Johnson, V. E. (1966). *Human sexual response.* Philadelphia, PA: Lippincott.

McKay, A. (2004). Adolescent sexual and reproductive health in Canada: A report card. *The Canadian Journal of Human Sexuality, 13*(2), 67–81.

McKay, A. (2006). Trends in teen pregnancy in Canada with comparisons to U.S.A. and England/Wales. *The Canadian Journal of Human Sexuality, 15*(3–4), 157–161.

McMahon, C. G. (2011). Disorders of ejaculation and male orgasm. In I. Incrocci, I. Goldstein, & R. Rosen (Eds.), *Cancer and sexual health* (pp. 235–238). New York: Springer.

McTaggart, S. J., Algar, E., Chow, C. W., Powell, H. R., & Jones, C. L. (2001). Clinical spectrum of Denys-Drash and Frasier syndrome. *Pediatric Nephrology, 16*, 335–339.

Meston, C. M., & Ahrold, T. (2010). Ethnic, gender, and acculturation influences on sexual behaviors. *Archives in Sexual Behavior, 39*, 179–189. doi:10.1007/s10508-008-9415-0

Meston, C. M., & Buss, D. M. (2007). Why humans have sex. *Archives in Sexual Behavior, 36*, 477–507.

Miller, G. P. (2002). Circumcision: Cultural-legal analysis. *Virginia Journal of Social Policy & the Law, 9*, 497–585.

Ontario Human Rights Commission. (2000, revised in 2009). *Policy on female genital mutilation (FGM).* Retrieved from http://www.ohrc.on.ca/en/policy-female-genital-mutilation-fgm

Parker, R. (2009). Sexuality, culture and society: Shifting paradigms in sexuality research. *Culture, Health & Sexuality, 11*(3), 251–266.

Perron, L., & Senikas, V. (2012). *Policy on female genital cutting/mutilation.* Ottawa, ON: SOGC. Retrieved from http://sogc.org/wp-content/uploads/2013/01/gui272PS1202E.pdf

Pinyerd, B., & Zipf, W. B. (2005). Puberty–timing is everything! *Journal of Pediatric Nursing, 20*(2), 75–82.

Public Health Agency of Canada. (2005). *The parent-teen relationship: Life through a teenager's eyes.* Retrieved from http://publications.gc.ca/collections/Collection/H72-22-17-1995E.pdf

Public Health Agency of Canada. (2006). *2004 Canadian sexually transmitted infections surveillance report: Pre-release.* Ottawa, ON: Surveillance and Risk Assessment Division, Centre for Infectious Disease Prevention and Control, Public Health Agency of Canada.

Public Health Agency of Canada. (2009). *What mothers say: The Canadian maternity experiences survey.* Ottawa, ON.

Public Health Agency of Canada. (2012). *"Talk to me" - Sexuality education for parents.* Retrieved from http://www.phac-aspc.gc.ca/publicat/ttm-pm/index-eng.php

Public Health Agency of Canada. (2013). *At a glance – HIV and AIDS in Canada: Surveillance report to December 31st, 2012*. Retrieved from http://www.phac-aspc.gc.ca/aids-sida/publication/survreport/2012/dec/index-eng.php

Royal Canadian Mounted Police (RCMP). (2010). *Native spirituality guide*. Retrieved from http://www.rcmp-grc.gc.ca/pubs/abo-aut/spirit-spiritualite-eng.htm

Sadler, T. W. (2012). *Langman's medical embryology* (12th ed.). Baltimore, MD: Lippincott Williams & Wilkins.

Salonia, A., Giraldi, A., Chivers, M. L., Georgiadis, J. R., Levin, R., Maravilla, K. R., et al. (2010). Physiology of women's sexual function: Basic knowledge and new findings. *The Journal of Sexual Medicine, 7*(8), 2637–2660. doi:10.1111/j.1743-6109.2010.01810.x

Sanghavi, D. (2008). Somewhere between a boy and a girl. *Ambulatory Pediatrics, 8*(1), 1530–1567.

Seaver, M. R., Freund, K. M., Wright, L. M., Tjia, J., & Frayne, S. M. (2007). Healthcare preferences among lesbians: A focus group analysis. *Journal of Women's Health, 17*(2), 215–225.

Statistics Canada. (2006a). *Pregnancy outcomes 2003*. Ottawa, ON: Statistics Canada.

Statistics Canada. (2006b). *Induced abortion statistics 2003*. Ottawa, ON: Statistics Canada.

Statistics Canada. (2008). *Teen pregnancies*. Ottawa, ON: Statistics Canada. Retrieved from http://www.statcan.gc.ca/tables-tableaux/sum-som/l01/cst01/hlth65a-eng.htm

Statistics Canada. (2013). Police-reported hate crimes, 2011. *The Daily*. Retrieved from http://www.statcan.gc.ca/daily-quotidien/130711/dq130711a-eng.htm.

Steele, L. S., Ross, L. E., Dobinson, C., Veldhuizen, S., & Tinmouth, J. M. (2009). Women's sexual orientation and health: Results from a Canadian population-based survey. *Women & Health, 49*(5), 353–367. doi:10.1080/03630240903238685

Tjepkema, M. (2008). Health care use among gay, lesbian and bisexual Canadians. *Health Reports, 19*(1), 53–64. Retrieved from http://www.statcan.gc.ca/pub/82-003-x/82-003-x2008001-eng.pdf

Veenstra, G. (2011). Race, gender, class, and sexual orientation: Intersecting axes of inequality and self-rated health in Canada. *International Journal for Equity in Health, 10*(1), 3. doi:10.1186/1475-9276-10-3

Vissandjee, B., Kantiebo, M., Levine, A., & N'Dejuru, R. (2003). The cultural context of gender identity: Female genital excision and infibulation. *Health Care for Women International, 24*, 115–124.

Witchel, S. F., & Azziz, R. (2011). Congenital adrenal hyperplasia. *Journal of Pediatric and Adolescent Gynecology, 24*(3), 116–126.

World Association for Sexual Health. (2013a). *Declaration of sexual rights*. Retrieved from http://www.worldsexology.org/resources/declaration-of-sexual-rights/

World Association for Sexual Health. (2013b). *Montreal Declaration–Sexual health for the millennium*. Retrieved from http://www.worldsexology.org/resources/millennium-declaration/

World Health Organization. (2008). *Eliminating female genital mutilation: An interagency statement*. Retrieved from http://whqlibdoc.who.int/publications/2008/9789241596442_eng.pdf

Zucker, K. J. (2009). The DSM criteria for gender identity in children. *Archives of sexual behavior*. Published online. Retrieved from http://link.springer.com/article/10.1007/s10508-009-9540-4/fulltext.html#CR63

Zucker, K. J. (2010). The DSM diagnostic criteria for gender identity disorder in children. *Archives of Sexual Behavior, 39*, 477–498.

CHAPTER 7

The Family

Viola Polomeno, Robin J. Evans, Rebecca Cahill*, and Thelma Sword*

 Olivia and her husband Tyler have been married for 3 years. They have shared many activities together, such as skiing, camping, and travelling. The couple has just found out that they are going to have their first child. Olivia and Tyler are excited about the baby. During a regular prenatal visit to the health clinic, Olivia confides to the nurse, "I'm feeling a bit overwhelmed by the pregnancy. And Tyler seems happy about the baby coming, but lately, he seems a bit distant from me."

 Jacob and Rachel, a couple who have undergone 5 years of unsuccessful infertility treatments, have arranged for a private adoption of a female baby born to a young, single girl. They have been in contact with the biologic mother almost daily during the pregnancy. When the biologic mother goes into labour, she calls Jacob and Rachel to attend the birth of their new daughter. Rachel chooses to be present in the delivery room; Jacob goes to the health care facility, but remains outside in the waiting room.

You will learn more about these families later in this chapter. Nurses working with these clients and others like them need to understand the content of this chapter to manage care and address issues appropriately. Before beginning, consider the following points related to the above scenarios:

- Does anything about either case present any issues of immediate concern or worry? Explain your answer.
- Which type of family structure or arrangement is depicted for each couple? How are these structures similar? How are they different?
- What areas would the nurse need to assess with Olivia and Tyler? With Rachel and Jacob?

The **family** represents the unit of interrelationships from which a person functions in society. Definitions of family and current family structures have evolved to include new variations and configurations. A basic understanding of theoretical foundations of family and family dynamics assists in providing direction to nursing care. Every area of nursing needs to recognize and address the issues that families face today. This is especially true in maternity and women's health care because the family as a whole is the target of health care delivery.

In this chapter we present theories of family that apply directly to the nursing care of women and their families. The focus is on contemporary families in the 21st century. Adoption issues are addressed from both domestic and international perspectives. The chapter closes with a section on collaborative care when working with families.

DEFINITIONS OF FAMILY

Several definitions of family exist. Some basic definitions include the following:

● "Two or more individuals who depend on one another for emotional, physical, or financial support or a combination of these" (Stanhope et al., 2011, p. 7)
● "The basic unit in society traditionally consisting of two parents rearing their children; also, any of various social units differing from but regarded as equivalent to the traditional family" (Merriam Webster, 2014a)
● Who they say they are (Wright & Leahey, 2013)

See Nursing Care Plan 7.1.

Theories of Families

No single theory or conceptual model adequately describes the complexity of a family's structure, function, and processes. In this chapter we explore a number of family theories, including Systems Theory, Friedman's Systems Theory, the McGill Model, and the Calgary Family Model. In Chapter 1 you have already encountered the *Guiding Principles of Family-Centred Maternity and Newborn Care*.

The systems theory of families has been around for a significant number of years, evolving from von Bertalanffy's General Systems Theory (von Bertalanffy, 1968). In the context of this theory, the family is viewed

NURSING CARE PLAN 7.1

●

The Family in Transition

Recall Olivia and Tyler from the beginning of the chapter. The nurse prompts Olivia to provide more information about her feelings of being overwhelmed and that her husband is becoming "distant" since she became pregnant. Olivia states, "Sometimes I feel like such a wimp. I find myself asking Tyler for help with things that I never would have before I was pregnant. He's really not used to this. Sometimes, he ignores me and says I'm behaving like a child. He tells me he wonders what will happen when a real baby is around. I'm not sure what's happening. What kind of mother will I be?"

NURSING DIAGNOSIS

Anxiety related to changes in responsibilities, roles, relationships, and family structure secondary to pregnancy

EXPECTED OUTCOMES

1. The couple will identify problem issues and areas of concern.
2. The client will state areas in which she needs assistance.

INTERVENTIONS	RATIONALES
Assess the client's level of understanding about pregnancy and changes	Assessment provides a baseline to identify specific client needs and to develop an individualized plan
Discuss with the client her concerns, feelings, and perceptions related to pregnancy and its possible effects	Discussion provides opportunities to highlight positive aspects of the current situation; verbalization of concerns aids in establishing sources of stress and problem areas that need to be addressed
Communicate accurate facts; answer questions honestly	Open and honest communication promotes trust and helps clear up any misconceptions or misinformation
Discuss the physiologic and psychological changes of pregnancy (see Chapter 12), including their basis and measures to cope with them	Adequate knowledge of possible changes and measures to cope with them helps to alleviate concerns related to the unknown
Include the client's partner in the discussion about pregnancy, both partner's needs, and necessary adaptations	The participation of both partners increases feelings of control over the situation and promotes sharing and support
Encourage the couple to communicate clearly and openly about events, issues, or concerns	Clear communication is essential for sharing information
Provide the couple with information about support groups, websites, and other sources of appropriate information	Shared experiences and knowledge of similar situations can aid in preparing the couple for what to expect
Investigate sources of available support, such as extended family, friends, and community; encourage the couple to use these sources	Additional sources of support are helpful in reducing anxiety and stress

(continued)

NURSING CARE PLAN 7.1 ● The Family in Transition *(Continued)*

INTERVENTIONS	RATIONALES
Continue to assess the client's and partner's adaptation and functioning at subsequent visits	Continued assessment aids in monitoring progress of the situation and provides opportunities to address concerns that may arise as the pregnancy progresses

EVALUATION

1. The couple identifies realistic measures to cope with the demands of pregnancy and the family.
2. The couple develops a workable plan that promotes healthy functioning of both partners, the fetus/newborn, and overall family.

as a system, a microcosm of our world (Satir, 1988). **System** is interpreted as a unit in which the whole is greater than the sum of its parts. The following basic principles of systems apply to families.

- Systems have boundaries.
- Boundaries may be open or closed.
- Systems need rules to function.
- Interrelationships occur with interchangeable causes and effects.
- Communication feedback must occur within the system.

Systems operate within the larger environment; whatever affects the system as a whole affects each of its parts. For example, when one member of the family has a change in health, each family member, as well as the family as a unit, is affected. Friedman et al. (2003) challenge nurses to view families as units and to provide appropriate assessments of the family as a whole.

 Consider the family system of Olivia and Tyler, who are expecting their first child. Obviously, the family unit will change with the birth of the baby. How might the family system already be changing during the pregnancy?

The McGill model of nursing initially proposed the family as the unit of care, rather than the individual, theorizing that problems related to health are a phenomenon of the family (Gottlieb & Gottlieb, 2007). Gottlieb and Gottlieb expanded this notion to include both the individual (within the family context) and the family unit as the focus of nursing care. Whether or not the nurse provides care for the family as a unit, the nurse is "family minded and many nurse patient interactions are, at the very least, considered through a family lens where relevant and appropriate" (Gottlieb & Gottlieb, 2007, p. E54–E55). This includes creating conditions so that the individual and family are part of a collaborative partnership with health care providers. The individual and family are the central focus of care. Power is shared and open, and respectful relationships are established and maintained. Health care providers are nonjudgmental, accept the individual and family, and are self-aware and reflective (Gottlieb & Gottlieb, 2007).

Wright and Leahey define the family as whomever the individual(s) indicates is their family (Wright & Leahy, 2013). They first used the term "family systems nursing" in 1990, distinguishing it from family nursing in that it focused "simultaneously on the individual, the family, and the larger systems, attending to interaction, reciprocity and relationships (Moules et al., 2012, p. 264). Wright and Leahey (2013), who developed the Calgary Model, explain that "family-centered care is achieved responsibly and respectfully by relational practices consisting of collaborative nurse–family relationships together with sound family assessment and intervention knowledge and skills" (p. 1). Although some of these theoretical perspectives were developed in the mid-1960s, they remain applicable to families today. Nursing can integrate the concepts associated with these theories to guide nursing practice in the care of families.

Friedman's Theory

Friedman's systems theory focuses on family nursing (Friedman et al., 2003). It stresses a key interrelational characteristic of the family system—the whole is greater than the sum of its parts. Friedman identifies specific activities or functions of the family as the basis for wholeness. Family function is the family's purpose with respect to individual, family, other social systems, and society (Hanson, 2006). The major func- tions of families described by Friedman et al. (2003) include affective, socialization, reproductive, eco- nomic, and health care functions. Families carry out these functions through different roles within a wide range of cultural settings, as discussed next and in Table 7.1.

● TABLE 7.1 **Friedman's Family Functions**

Function	Description	Image
Affective	Support and respect with affirmation occurs within the family.	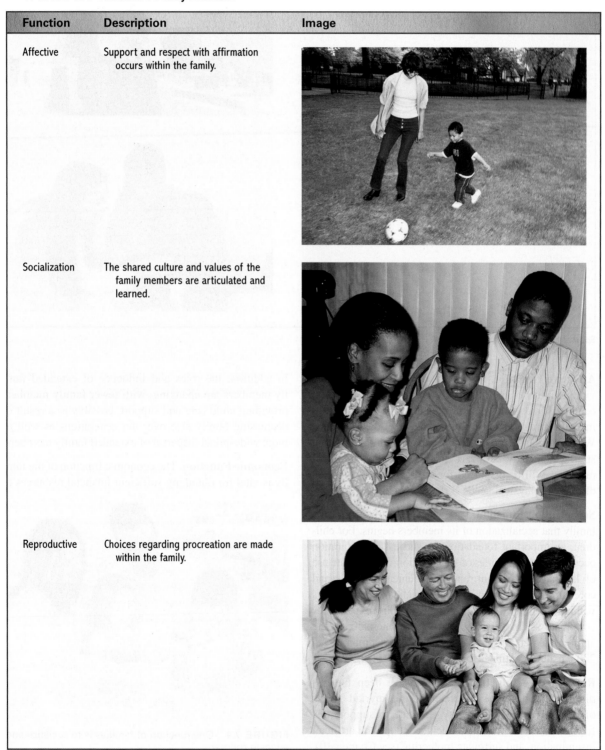
Socialization	The shared culture and values of the family members are articulated and learned.	
Reproductive	Choices regarding procreation are made within the family.	

(table continues on page 246)

• TABLE 7.1 **Friedman's Family Functions** (continued)

Function	Description	Image
Economic	Financial resources hold the family together.	
Health care	Provisions for the physical necessities of life are made.	

Source: www.cwhn.ca; in French, www.rcsf.ca

Affective Function. The affective function represents a vital activity for the family. In a rapidly changing 21st century society, the person depends on the family to meet the affection and emotional needs of the members. With families in poverty and experiencing significant stress, there may be a risk that the affection needs of members will be displaced for the more basic function of meeting physical needs (Friedman et al., 2003).

Socialization Function. It is within the structure of the family that socialization of its members begins. For children, an important foundation for successful maturation occurs with the activities of socialization. Appropriate use of language, behaviour, and communication skills and core family values are part of the socialization that occurs within the family. The child's many learning experiences contribute as this lifelong process of "internalizing the appropriate set of norms and values" (Friedman et al., 2003, p. 402) continues for family members (Fig. 7.1).

Reproductive Function. Families have been the traditional structure for procreation; the myriad forms of families in today's society continue to support this function, which may also include adoption, artificial insemination, and surrogate mothering (see Chapter 10).

In addition, the roles and influence of extended family members are changing, with fewer family members providing child care and support, possibly as a result of decreasing family size over the generations as well as more widespread dispersal of extended family members.

Economic Function. The economic function of the family is vital for obtaining sufficient financial resources to

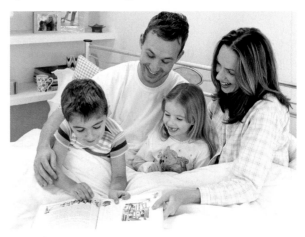

FIGURE 7.1 One function of families is to socialize and educate children.

meet material needs even though it has changed over the years (Friedman et al., 2003). Historically, the head of the family was the sole support for the family, providing the needed financial resources. In today's society, many women work outside the home; two-income families are common and often necessary for economic stability. Although children in Canada typically do not work to provide economic support for the family, employment as they become teenagers may assist them to enjoy luxuries and "extras." There is also a wide range of community resources available to assist families in meeting those needs they may not be able to meet independently (Hitchcock et al., 2010).

Health Care Function. The essentials needed to keep the family healthy may include food, clothing, and shelter, as well as health care itself. Health care practices of families may be diverse. Home remedies, complementary therapies or healers, for example, may be used; this use may be culturally based in some instances and not in others. The family may or may not be aware of health prevention activities or their availability in their community. Despite such diversity, families support the health and well-being of their members. Nurses working with families strive to gain an understanding of each family's health beliefs, decision-making activities, and knowledge about health in order to provide the most appropriate family-centred care. When family rituals are interrupted or functions are jeopardized, the nurse

identifies resources to the individual and family to assist in resolution of the issues and to limit disruptions.

The Calgary Family Intervention Model

The Calgary Family Intervention Model (CFIM) is a companion model to the Calgary Family Assessment Model that is presented later in this chapter (see Assessment Tool 7.1). The CFIM, the first family intervention model to emerge within nursing, is a strengths-based, resiliency-oriented model (Wright & Leahey, 2013). Thus, the CFIM is an organizing framework for conceptualizing the intersection between a particular domain of family functioning and the specific intervention offered by the nurse. The elements of the CFIM include interventions, domains of family functioning, and fit or effectiveness. There must be a fit between the domain of family functioning (cognitive, affective, and behavioural) and a nursing intervention. Interventions are designed to promote, improve, or sustain family functioning in any or all three domains, but a change in one domain can affect the other domains (Wright & Leahey, 2013). The most profound changes occur within the family's belief system. One nursing intervention can influence all three domains of family functioning at the same time.

Promoting or effecting change within the family system involves specific nursing interventions. Nurses choose the appropriate intervention to facilitate the change to occur. Specific interventions can vary for

---

● **ASSESSMENT TOOL 7.1** **Components of the Calgary Family Assessment Model**

STRUCTURAL ASSESSMENT

Internal

- Family composition
- Gender
- Sexual orientation
- Rank order or birth order of children
- Subsystems in the family
- Boundaries

EXTERNAL

- Extended family
- School
- Church
- Health care systems

CONTEXT

- Ethnicity
- Race
- Social class

- Religion
- Environment

DEVELOPMENTAL ASSESSMENT

- Stages of the family
- Associated tasks

FUNCTIONAL ASSESSMENT

Instrumental

- Activities of daily family living

Expressive

- Communication patterns
- Problem solving
- Roles of family members
- Influence and power of different members over other members
- Family beliefs
- Alliances

each family, but the same intervention can be used for several families and for different problems. The CFIM assists in determining the domain of family functioning that needs to be changed and the most useful intervention to effect change in that domain (Wright & Leahey, 2013).

Intervention Questions. One of the simplest, yet most powerful, interventions is the use of interventive questions (Wright & Leahey, 2013). Questions may be linear or circular. Linear questions are investigative, exploring a family's perceptions of a problem. An example of this would be: "When did you notice that your wife was having contractions?" Linear questions are used to gather information about problems that the family is dealing with. Circular questions seek to reveal explanations about the problems and to obtain information about relationships amongst family members, beliefs, ideas, events, and values. Circular questions tend to facilitate behavioural change. There are different types of circular questions that can be used for each of the three family functioning domains. A *difference* question explores differences between people, relationships, time, ideas, and beliefs: "Who in the family is the most concerned about Angela's blood test results?" (affective domain). *Behavioural effect* questions explore the effect of the behaviour of a family member on the family: "What do you do when your husband does not visit your daughter in the hospital?" (behavioural domain). *Hypothetical and future-oriented* questions explore family options and alternative actions: "What do you think will happen if these skin grafts continue to be so painful for your daughter?" (cognitive domain). *Triadic* questions are posed to a third person about the relationship between two other people: "What does your mother do that encourages your father to be less stressed about her condition?" (affective domain).

Other Interventions. Nursing interventions are helpful for change within the family functioning domains. Examples of interventions for the *cognitive domain* include the following:

• Commending family and individual strengths
• Offering information and opinions

Examples of interventions for the *affective domain* are as follows:

• Validating or normalizing emotional responses
• Encouraging the telling of illness narratives
• Drawing family support

Finally, nursing interventions for the *behavioural domain* are as follows:

• Encouraging family members to be caregivers and offering caregiver support

• Encouraging respite
• Devising rituals

The Calgary Model is useful for both assessment and intervention in different family circumstances. Questions can be used for both data collection and for therapeutic intervention; family interviews are part of the underlying framework. Nurses can become skilled in interviews with families that are experiencing difficult circumstances, facilitating dynamics between family members, and promoting change. The Calgary Model utilizes hypotheses rather than nursing diagnoses to explore problems in the three family functioning domains and to guide the family interview. Cooperation and collaboration are characteristic of this model and replace the more linear concepts of resistance and noncompliance.

FAMILIES IN CANADA

In Canada, no "norm" exists for a family. Today's families reflect a growing diversity that encompasses variations in living arrangements, structures, gender and number of family members, racial and ethnic backgrounds, sexual orientation, and family member roles. In keeping with this, Statistics Canada has changed the categories for which data are collected and has expanded the definition of families over the years so that in the 2011 Canadian census, **census families** are defined as "a married or common-law couple, with or without children, or a lone parent living with at least one child in the same dwelling. Couples can be of the opposite sex or of the same sex" (Statistics Canada, 2012a, p. 17). The change to this definition has evolved over time. In 1981, data were first collected for common-law unions. In 2001 the census family was expanded to include same-sex common-law couples, children in a census family who were previously married, grandparents and grandchildren living in the same dwelling without the presence of a middle generation (skip-generation families), and a child and his/her lone parent (middle generation) living in a three-generation household (Statistics Canada, 2012b). In 2006, same-sex married couples were counted for the first time, and in 2011, stepfamilies were counted in the census (Statistics Canada, 2012a). Table 7.2 provides a summary of variations in family structure.

Nuclear Families

Although the view of the family has changed dramatically over the years, the more traditional concept of a family composed of a married mother and father and their children remains (Fig. 7.2). The term "nuclear family" has traditionally referred to such a family group (Merriam Webster, 2014b).

● TABLE 7.2 **Family Types**

Type of Family	Definition/Description	2011 Census
Census family	Married or common-law couple, opposite or same sex, with or without children, or lone parent living with at least one child in the same dwelling (Statistics Canada, 2012a)	Almost 3.7 million couple families counted (Statistics Canada, 2012a)
Nuclear family	Married mother and father and their child/children (Merriam Webster, 2014b)	Declining number of married census families, but remains the predominant family structure. From 2006–2011, the increase in common-law couple families was more than four times the increase in married couple families.
Common-law family	Unmarried mother and father and their child/children	Data first collected in 1981 2011—more common-law couple families than lone-parent families
Lone parent family, single-parent family, one-parent family	Family headed by an adult not currently living with a spouse or partner, with her/his child/children	Comprise 16.3% of all census families (1.5 million) - 31.5% never legally married - 17.7% widowed - 50.8% divorced or separated - 80% headed by women (Statistics Canada, 2012b)
Same-sex common-law or married family	Male or female same-sex couple	Same-sex marriages legalized in 2005 (Statistics Canada, 2007a). About 9.4% same-sex couples had children living with them (Statistics Canada, 2012a). More common in female same-sex couples than male same-sex couples
Blended family, stepfamily, remarried family, reconstituted family	Couple family where there is at least one child whose birth or adoption preceded the current relationship (Statistics Canada, 2012a)	First counted in 2011 census. Represent 12.6% of all families counted (Statistics Canada, 2012a).
Simple stepfamily	All children are biologic or adopted children of only one of the partners	Represent 7.4% of couples with children
Complex stepfamily		Represent 5.2% of couples with children
Extended family	Child lives with at least one parent and at least one other person who is not a part of the census family	
Skip-generation family	Grandparents and grandchildren living in the same dwelling without a middle generation	30,005 households in Canada (Statistics Canada, 2012a)
Multigenerational family	At least three generations, relatives or non-relatives, or both	
Extended kin network family	Two or more households that live in close proximity and share social support, responsibility, goods, and services	Slightly more prevalent than in 2001 (Statistics Canada, 2012c)

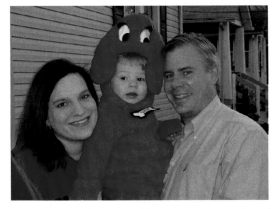

FIGURE 7.2 The nuclear family refers to a married couple with their biologic child or children.

Canada is experiencing a decline in the number of married census families, although this category remains the predominant family structure (Statistics Canada, 2012a). Over the 10-year period from 2001 to 2011, couples with children living at home fell as a share of all census families (Fig. 7.3). This gap has increased steadily over the years (Statistics Canada, 2012a, 2012b). The proportion of children aged 14 and under who lived with married parents, while still the highest, fell between 2001 and 2011, while the proportion living with common-law parents increased; the proportion of children aged 14 and under living in lone-parent families increased only slightly over the same 10-year period (Statistics Canada, 2012a).

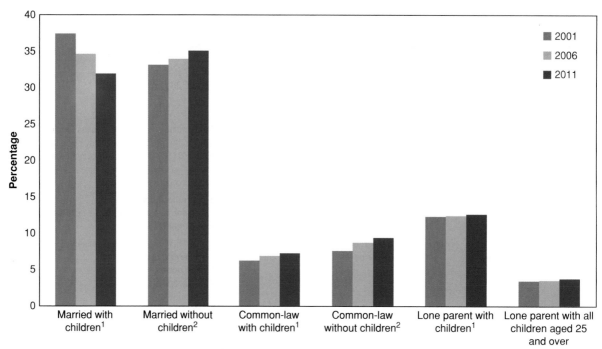

Census families by presence of children

Notes:
1. Refers to at least one child aged 24 and under present in the home.
2. Includes families with all children aged 25 and over.
Sources: Statistics Canada, censuses of population, 2001 to 2011.

FIGURE 7.3 Married-couple families without children is the largest family structure in 2011. (Adapted from Statistics Canada publication, Portrait of Families and Living Arrangements in Canada – Families, Households and Marital Status, 2011 Census of Population, Catalogue 98–312-X2011001 page 9.)

Families with Same-sex Parents

For the first time, the census of 2006 counted same-sex married couples (Fig. 7.4), reflecting the legalization of same-sex marriages for all of Canada as of July 2005 (Statistics Canada, 2007a). In the 2011 census, a total of 64,575 same-sex couples was reported, representing 0.8% of all couples in Canada (Statistics Canada, 2012a). Just under half of the same-sex couples were

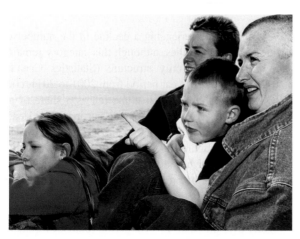

FIGURE 7.4 A family headed by lesbian parents.

female (Statistics Canada, 2012a). The number of same-sex married couples tripled between 2006 and 2011; the number of opposite-sex married couples increased by 2.9% in the same time period. The number of common-law couples experienced a more modest increase with less disparity: 15% for same-sex couples and 13.8% for opposite-sex couples (Statistics Canada, 2012a). In 2011, 45.6% of all same-sex couples in Canada lived in the three largest census metropolitan areas, Montréal, Toronto, and Vancouver.

Single-parent Families

These families may include men or women who are separated, divorced, widowed, or who have chosen to live alone. Between 2001 and 2006, growth was higher for male lone-parent families (+16.2%) than for female lone-parent families (+6%) (Statistics Canada, 2012b). One explanation for the faster gain among lone-parent families headed by men is that fewer mothers are granted sole custody following a divorce (Fig. 7.5).

Blended Families

In a **blended family**, children from a previous marriage or relationship become part of a new family. This structure

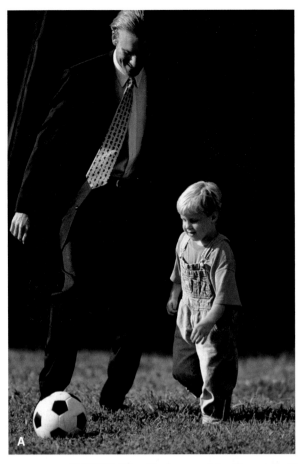
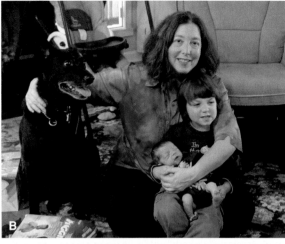
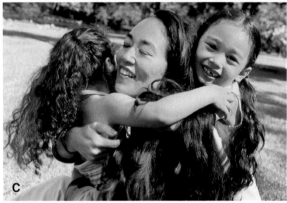

FIGURE 7.5 Single-parent families are led by adults who are not currently living with a spouse. The head of the household can be the father **(A)** or the mother **(B)** and **(C)**.

also may be referred to as *stepfamilies, remarried families*, or *reconstituted families* (Clark, 2007). Additional children may result from the new relationship, blending all the individuals into one family (Fig. 7.6).

Stepfamilies can be classified as either simple or complex. In a simple stepfamily, all children are the biologic or adopted children of one and only one married or common-law partner. A complex stepfamily includes any of the following:

• At least one child of both parents and at least one child of only one parent
• At least one child of each parent and no children of both parents
• At least one child of both parents and at least one child of each parent

Across Canada, as a share of couples with children, stepfamilies were highest in the province of Quebec (16.1%) and lowest in Ontario (11.0%). Among the census metropolitan areas, the proportion of stepfamilies was highest for Trois-Rivières (18.7%), Saguenay (18.5%), and Sherbrooke (18.4%). The proportion was lowest in the two most populous census metropolitan

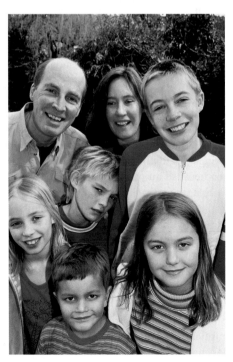

FIGURE 7.6 A blended family.

areas of Toronto (7.8%) and Vancouver (8.4%) (Statistics Canada, 2012a).

Extended Families

An **extended family** is one in which a child lives with at least one parent and at least one other person who is not a part of the census family. Often, extended families are **multigenerational**, and may be a temporary arrangement because of illness, divorce, adolescent pregnancy, and older family members who need assistance. A variation of the extended family is the **extended kin network** family, where two or more households share social support, responsibility, goods, and services. They are most common in Nunavut (10.6%), possibly due to housing shortages, high cost of living, cultural preference, or a combination of these factors (Statistics Canada, 2012c). They are also more common in municipalities that surround the city of Toronto and in Surrey and Abbotsford in British Columbia, reflective of higher proportions of immigrants in these areas relative to the rest of Canada (Statistics Canada, 2012c).

According to the 2011 census, 8% of persons aged 80 and above live with relatives (Statistics Canada, 2012a). 4.8% of all children under the age of 15 live with at least one grandparent, most commonly in a multigenerational household that also includes their parents or a lone parent; this increased from 3.3% in 2001 (Statistics Canada, 2012a).

Whether they live within a multigenerational home or not, grandparents provide a wide range of support to their children and grandchildren, including child care, housework, transportation, and financial support (Mei et al., 2013). Extended family ties may be highly regarded in some cultures (Fig. 7.7) and grandparents may spend a significant amount of time providing unpaid care work and transmission of cultural values and traditions.

Grandparents as Primary Caregivers

In the 2011 census, 0.5% (30,005) of households in Canada were considered skip generation (Statistics Canada, 2012a). In these households, grandparents have primary parenting responsibilities for their grandchildren because no parent is present (Fig. 7.8). Some factors that precipitate the need for grandparents to parent their grandchildren include alcohol and substance use by biologic parents, divorce, abuse and neglect of children, incarceration, teenage pregnancy, and death of biologic parents (Bundy-Fazioli et al., 2013; Edwards & Ray, 2010; National Council on Aging, 2008; Rosenthal & Gladstone, 2007). Because the events themselves are major stressors, in addition to the emotional stress experienced by the grandparents in relation to this changing role, children in these families may have increased mental or physical health needs (Edwards & Ray, 2010).

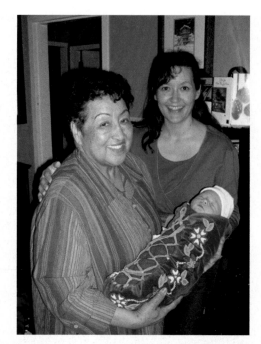

FIGURE 7.7 Aboriginal grandmothers often are the most respected members of their families.

Grandparents with primary parenting responsibilities face unique challenges. As a group, they have more physical and mental health challenges, poverty, and impoverished living conditions as well as a lack of social support than their noncaregiving peers (Bundy-Fazioli et al., 2013; Hayslip & Kaminski, 2005; Mei et al., 2013). The addition of caregiving responsibilities disrupts life,

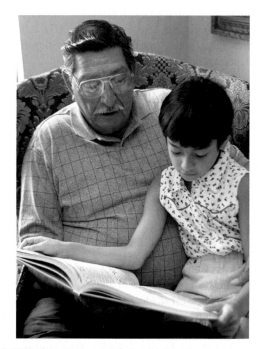

FIGURE 7.8 This grandfather is the primary caregiver of his granddaughter.

increasing risks for role overload and role confusion, and marital conflict (Bundy-Fazioli et al., 2013; Edwards & Ray, 2010). The transition to a full-time parental role is an emotional challenge, both in relation to the reason for becoming the primary caregiver and the emotional toll taken by their relationship with their adult children (Bundy-Fazioli et al., 2013; Edwards & Ray, 2010).

Despite the challenges, benefits have been noted (Edwards & Ray, 2010; Hayslip & Kaminski, 2005; Rosenthal & Gladstone, 2007). Grandparents often show positive levels of physical activity and self-care, caregiver satisfaction, improved health habits, and are able to foster positive emotional well being in the face of adversity (Bundy-Fazioli et al., 2013). Grandparents themselves report that the experience gives them a feeling of contribution and having a "second chance" at parenting. Children raised by grandparents have been found to have fewer behavioural problems in school than their peers (Hayslip & Kaminski, 2005).

Family Roles

A role can be considered a consistent behaviour that occurs in a particular situation (Wright & Leahey, 2013). Family members assume various roles within the family that affect the functioning of the family as a unit. Roles may be based on a variety of expectations. Roles are not constant, in part influenced by each person's interactions with other family members.

The roles of women and men have changed over the past decades. Women typically work outside the home; the number of employed women with children has increased from 39.1% in 1976 to 72.9% in 2009 (Farrao, 2010). As mothers' roles in the family change, fathers' roles have expanded, with increased participation in the care of children (Fig. 7.9). Other roles emerge as families change. For example, grandparents may need care within the family or grandparents may provide care for their grandchildren. Alternatively, other

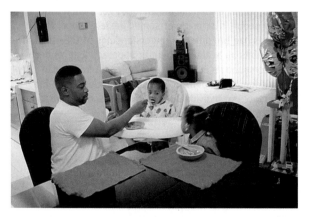

FIGURE 7.9 Many of today's fathers are taking active roles in child care, with some dads providing the predominant child care while mothers work outside the home.

situations such as the absence of a parent through death or divorce, parents at work, dysfunction of a parent due to mental illness or substance use or others, may lead to children assuming roles and responsibilities normally assigned to the parents (Byng-Hall, 2008).

Family Values

Family values refer to the "moral and ethical principles traditionally upheld and transmitted within a family, [such] as honesty, loyalty, industry, and faith" (Dictionary.com Unabridged, n.d.). Cultural perspectives enhance these common ideas. Family dynamics have the potential for constant change. The basic values of the family anchor the family in society. "As families grow and change over time, so too do their values" (Hitchcock et al., 2010, p. 631).

Family Decision Making

One essential task of the family is decision making, which combines the use of power and communication. Good communication within the family lays the foundation for effective decision-making strategies. Traditionally, parents take on the role of decision makers. Allocating power on a daily basis between parents effectively distributes decision-making responsibilities. Families with open and honest communication strategies within the family can foster greater joint problem solving among family members (Friedman et al., 2003; Wright & Leahey, 2013). Cultural values and beliefs are foundational elements for how decision making will be handled within any given family. Often, even the communication of the decision is overshadowed by the cultural framework of the family.

CULTURAL PERSPECTIVES

Nurses are responsible for incorporating cultural competencies into all phases of the nursing process and in all domains of nursing practice (Canadian Nurses Association [CNA], 2010). The influence of culture on family dynamics cannot be overlooked or ignored. Nurses need to be culturally sensitive and competent as they provide care to women and families. Historically, **cultural competence** included attaining cultural knowledge, having an open attitude, and implementing appropriate clinical skills (Callister, 2001). However, as time has passed, the concept of cultural competence has undergone changes. Campinha-Bacote (2011) suggests that "cultural competence is viewed as an expansion of patient-centered care" (p. 1, para 1). Gregory et al. (2010) believe there has been a shift from culture as a fixed, static understanding to a "notion of culture as a dynamic process understood contextually through historical, social, political, and economic lenses" (p. 1). In a position statement, the

CNA addresses cultural competence and cultural safety: "While cultural competence is an important concept, it can sometimes overlook systemic barriers, which make it inadequate to fully address health-care inequities. Cultural safety, however, 'promotes greater equity in health and health care...[as it addresses the] root cause of health inequities.'" (CNA, 2010, p. 3).

Understanding different cultures from the perspective of **cultural relativism** will guide nursing interactions and perceptions during caregiving. Purnell and Paulanka (2008) define cultural relativism as "the belief that the behaviours and practices of people should be judged only from the context of their cultural system" (p. 352). A difficulty arises when the nurse is assumed to be responsible for prior knowledge of the client's cultural beliefs. This understanding develops during assessment; the best source of information regarding specific cultural practices is the client and her family.

It is paramount to avoid stereotyping clients based on their ethnic or religious cultural groups. Many clients and families follow only some or few of the typical customs of their cultural groups. For example, some people of Jewish descent follow Kosher dietary laws, whereas others do not. Within families, there may be generational differences in approaches to customs such as food preferences and health beliefs. See Research Highlight 7.1.

Canada is increasingly multicultural. The 2011 census enumerated 6,775,800 foreign-born residents in Canada, representing almost one in five (20.6%) of the total population (Statistics Canada, 2011). Between 2006 and 2011, around 1,162,900 foreign-born people immigrated to Canada. These recent immigrants made up 17.2% of the foreign-born population and 3.5% of the total population in Canada. Asia (including the Middle East) was Canada's largest source of immigrants during the past 5 years, although the share of immigration from Africa and Caribbean, Central, and South America increased slightly. The vast majority of the foreign-born population lived in four provinces: Ontario, British Columbia, Quebec, and Alberta, and most lived in the nation's largest urban centres (Statistics Canada, 2011).

When these figures are combined with the many second- and third-generation Canadian-born citizens, the ever increasing need for culturally competent nursing care is evident. With each opportunity to learn from clients and families, nurses become increasingly conscious of the unique customs and beliefs that people from various cultural and ethnic groups may or may not follow. Learning to view the behaviour of clients and families from an understanding of their adherence, or nonadherence, to their cultural background is an important initial step in delivering culturally sensitive care.

Remembering to include cultural components in a family assessment offers additional opportunities for focusing on the client's culture. Boyle (2008) suggests including the following areas in a cultural assessment:

- Family/kin system
- Social life
- Language and traditions
- Value orientation and cultural norms
- Religion
- Health beliefs and practices
- Political systems

● RESEARCH HIGHLIGHT 7.1   Meanings of Food, Eating, and Health in Punjabi Families living in Vancouver, Canada

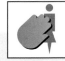

PURPOSE

In comparison to Caucasian families, South Asians living in western countries are at increased risk for developing diet-related chronic diseases. In this study, researchers explored the meanings of food, health, and well being in families of Punjabi heritage living in Vancouver, Canada.

DESIGN

Using a qualitative design, researchers interviewed 39 members of 12 families of Punjabi Sikh origin (ages 13 to 70 years). They also observed participants' grocery shopping trips and family meals. Transcripts were analyzed using constant comparative analysis, and themes were generated.

RESULTS

Elders' use of traditional Indian foods contrasted with young people's inclusion of some "western" food. Participants had two different understandings of the effect of food habits on health: a scientific approach that connects food components to chronic disease and a traditional knowledge about food. Women paid attention to the food preferences of individual family members, demonstrating concern for their psychosocial well-being.

NURSING IMPLICATIONS

These findings provide insight into cultural influences on health behaviours.

From Chapman, G., Ristovski-Slijepcevic, S., & Beagan, B. (2011). *Health Education Journal, 70*(1), 102–112. doi: 10.1177/0017896910373031

The literature and the internet can provide vast resources for increasing cultural knowledge and competence. Research that has been done with various cultural and socioeconomic groups can help nurses better understand how cultural differences and similarities may affect a family's responses to life transitions. See Research Highlight 7.2.

FAMILIES GROWING THROUGH ADOPTION

Canada's history of adoption legislation is complicated. In 1873, New Brunswick was the first province to pass an adoption law. In that era, Canadian families were fluid, often including near or distant relatives and nonrelatives; many children lived in a "wider environment of care" well beyond the nuclear family (Strong-Boag, 2006, p. 3). It was not uncommon for a child to be given by the birth family to another family, if the birth family was unable to provide for the child. In 1896, Nova Scotia passed an Adoption Act, and legislation appeared across the nation within the next few years. Most Acts included provisos for "in camera proceedings, sealed records, concealed illegitimacy, and restricted power of consent [promising] a clean slate" (Strong-Boag, 2006, p. 31). Confidentiality was intended to protect the privacy rights of the birth parents, particularly to shield the birth mother from the stigma of the "unwed mother" and "illegitimacy," the child from social ridicule, and the adoptive parents from the stigma of infertility.

As the 20th century began, bureaucracy demanded that citizens keep track of personal records. Although the law required births to be registered, many were not, particularly those that were "illegitimate"; many of those children were "adopted" by family members. Even in the early 1990s, it was estimated that 10% of adoptions by relatives never came to the attention of the adoption services (Strong-Boag, 2006). Adoptions—legal or otherwise—were viewed as something to be hidden; there were efforts to "cancel the child's past" (Strong-Boag, 2006, p. 3). Records of adoptions may or may not have been kept, may have been falsified or lost, and were not comparable across jurisdictions, governments, and agencies. The results of all of these irregularities have contributed to difficulty for those adoptees who wish to trace their biologic and genetic histories.

Many adopted children were unaware of their nonbiologic connection to their adoptive parents, often times until later in adulthood. Family stories abound in which a mother took her unwed daughter's newborn as her own, or a middle-aged man discovered that he was born out of wedlock and that the father who raised him was not his biologic father. In the 1960s, young women who became pregnant out of wedlock were sent to homes for unwed mothers, away from public scrutiny (Strong-Boag, 2006). An unwed mother was perceived as "good" when she gave up her "blue-ribbon baby" to be available for adoption into a "normal home setting" (Strong-Boag, 2006, p.8). Babies who were white and female were particularly in demand by potential adopters, while boys, older children, Aboriginal or black babies, and children in sibling groups or with disabilities faced a more uncertain future.

In 1938, the Supreme Court of Canada confirmed that adoption, custody, guardianship, and child protection were provincial responsibilities (Strong-Boag, 2006). Adoption legislation developed at different paces across the country. Although legislation was updated and expanded between 1945 and 1970, society persisted in its support of the rights of the "natural" family (Strong-Boag, 2006). In some provinces a new birth certificate could be issued with a new name and a new place of birth, as requested by adopters, further muddying the waters for connections to be made between adoptees and their birth parents. Closed, sealed records prevented access to any information about biologic parent(s) or health.

Between 1970 and the 1990s, adoption became a significant public concern, as issues surfaced such as: fetal alcohol spectrum disorder; decreased availability of babies from unwed mothers who tended to keep and raise their babies rather than giving them up for adoption from the developing world where more children tend to be available for adoption; adoption of Aboriginal children and the redress movement; and the desire of gay and lesbian couples for equal access to adoption (Strong-Boag, 2006). Adoption Acts were modified and expanded to try to regulate adoptions. Children's rights were prominent in these revisions, as legislators attempted to apply the Canadian Bill of Rights. Some legislation shifts recognized the birth parent's desire to maintain contact with the child after adoption (Strong-Boag, 2006).

From 1970 until the end of the 20th century, Canadian legislation allowed for increased access to information and openness to a "changed world where alternatives to the heterosexual nuclear family were increasingly presumed legitimate" (Strong-Boag, 2006, p. 51).

Open Adoptions

While the secrecy that once accompanied adoption is becoming less common, a new generation of "late discoverers" is now coming to light—offspring who have only recently discovered that they were either adopted or conceived using donor insemination (Riley, 2013).

To help promote positive approaches to adoption, nurses working with both birth and adoptive parents need to be sensitive to the language used when discussing this topic. Table 7.3 suggests positive adoption language that nurses may want to use when working in these circumstances.

Birth or Biologic Parents

The decision to place a child for adoption is difficult for many birth parents who have to sort through many realities as they make this choice: available resources and support for raising the child, their own emotional pain and suffering, and the child's best interests. When considering their options, many birth parents seek guidance from

● TABLE 7.3 **Positive Adoption Language**

Negative Language	Positive Replacement
Real parents	Birth parents
Natural parent	Biologic parents
Own child	Birth child
Adopted child	My child
Illegitimate	Born to unmarried parents
Give up	Terminate parental rights
Give away	Make an adoption plan
Keep	Parent
Adoptable child; available child	Waiting child
Begetter	Biologic father
Reunion	Making contact with
Adoptive parent	Parent
Foreign adoption	International adoption
Adoption triangle	Adoption triad
Disclosure	Permission to sign a release
Track down	Search
An unwanted child	Child placed for adoption
Child taken away	Court terminated
Handicapped child	Child with special needs
Foreign child	Child from abroad
Is adopted	Was adopted

trained professionals to assist with the complex decision making involved. Once they make the decision to place their child for adoption, the next decision is whether to go through a public or private adoption agency, and whether to have an open or closed adoption. Those who opt for an open adoption may have continued contact with the adoptive parents throughout the later parts of pregnancy; at times the adoptive parents may be present for the birth.

Preadoptive Parents

Preadoptive parents also have special needs to consider. Sometimes, adoption is the first choice for people to add children to their families. Other couples decide to adopt after being diagnosed with infertility (see Chapter 10). Issues surrounding infertility involve loss that requires grieving.

Because of the highly charged and complex issues, it is important that all preadoptive parents be psychologically and emotionally ready for any challenges they may face both during the adoption process and from society, their relatives, or their other support systems. Enlisting the help of a professional who is trained in adoption-related issues may be helpful to assist these parents to be ready for the road ahead.

Once parents have chosen to adopt, they face a multitude of decisions. Preadoptive parents will need to consider the benefits and risks of domestic versus

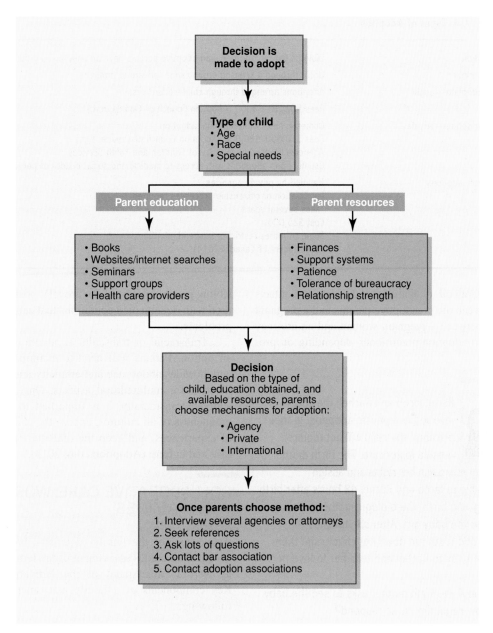

FIGURE 7.10 Decision tree for adoption.

international adoption, adopting a child of a different race, adopting an older child, and using a public or private agency. Information from a knowledgeable professional can be helpful in these circumstances.

Figure 7.10 outlines a model that parents can use in the decision-making process.

Types of Adoption

In general, there are three basic types of adoption: public domestic, private domestic, and international (Table 7.4). Because agency adoptions are regulated by province and territory, each with individual guidelines, regulations, and requirements, potential adoptive parents will want to seek advice from a professional who is knowledgeable about adoption law.

Domestic Adoptions

Domestic adoptions occur through a licensed organization that does all necessary legal, administrative, and social work to ensure that processes are handled efficiently and in the child's best interests. A tax credit is offered by the Federal government. Some provinces may also offer tax credits.

All agencies require a home study, an in-depth application, and an interview process conducted by a social worker. While the requirements vary across provinces, a home study generally includes interviews; references, police, and background checks; and home visits (Adoption Council of Canada, n.d.).

Private adoption agencies exist only in Alberta, British Columbia, Manitoba, Ontario, and Québec

● TABLE 7.4 **Types of Adoption**

Open adoption	Biologic parent, adoptee, and adoptive parents have an ongoing association
Domestic adoption	Occur through a licensed organization, private or public
Domestic adoption—public	Adoptions arranged through child welfare system
	Fees from $0–$3000 (Adoption Council of Canada, n.d.)
Domestic adoption—private	Domestic and/or international adoption
	Fees $10,000–$20,000 (Adoption Council of Canada, n.d.)
	Agencies licensed by Ministry of Children and Youth Services
	Usually open adoptions with access to medical and social history of parents
International adoptions	Handled by private agencies
	Immigration or citizenship processes required
	Takes several years
	Cost $25,000+
	Some countries restrict or suspend adoptions
	(Government of Canada, 2014)

(Adoption Council of Canada, n.d.). Initial contacts may be between the preadoptive parents and a pregnant woman or between a pregnant woman and an attorney or a licensed adoption practitioner, depending on provincial laws.

 Recall Jacob and Rachel, the couple involved in a private adoption. In their province, the child will not require outside foster care. The birth mother will initially relinquish her rights and assign guardianship to Jacob and Rachel 48 hours after birth.

After giving birth, the biologic mother asks to briefly see the baby girl. After she touches the newborn and tears run down her cheek, she then hands the baby to Rachel and tells her to love her daughter.

Imagine if the birth mother asks to see the baby again. How might the nurse respond?

International Adoptions

International adoptions are those in which the adoptive parent(s) and child are from two different countries; they are handled through a licensed private agency, which manages all aspects of the adoption. Although complex, international adoptions are gaining popularity as the number of newborns available for adoption in Canada continues to decrease; more children are available overseas.

Special Circumstances with Adoption

Some children are labelled as "special needs" and are particularly hard to place (AdoptiveParents.ca, n.d.), for example, children with physical or health problems; children older than 5 years; minority children; children with a history of abuse, neglect, or emotional problems; sibling groups; children who are HIV positive; and children with documented conditions that can lead to future problems.

Transracial or transcultural adoption also may be an option. Parents will need to examine their beliefs and attitudes about race and ethnicity and their current lifestyle for multicultural aspects. Once parents have adopted transracially, it is important to celebrate the uniqueness of all cultures, expose the child to a variety of experiences, and keep the dialogue open regarding race and culture (Adoption.com, 2013).

COLLABORATIVE CARE: WORKING WITH FAMILIES
Assessment

Assessment of the family requires a broad approach because it includes assessment of the family as a whole as well as assessment of the individual members. Key components of a family assessment include the following:

- Family structure and function
- Roles, tasks, and responsibilities of each member
- Family developmental stage
- Family dynamics, power, and decision making
- Family support systems
- Health beliefs and practices
- Culturally related issues
- Community interactions

Family assessment data typically reveal strengths, weaknesses, and stressors. Learning about the family's established support systems and past successful coping strategies provides valuable information for planning care. In addition, although families may already have some knowledge of available community resources, the nurse may be able to recommend further sources of support based on the assessment process.

Structure and Function

Ideally, the nurse completes a family assessment using a tool that provides cues about the family's specific details and needs. Skills in interviewing and observation assist the nurse with family data collection. The Friedman Family Assessment Model and the Calgary Family Assessment Model are two widely used assessment tools. Friedman's model assesses family strategies within the dimensions of system maintenance, coherence, system change, and individualization (Denham, 2003). It has a short and a long form. Sections of the short form are as follows:

• Identifying data
• Developmental stage of the family
• Environmental data
• Family structure
• Family functions
• Family stress, coping, and adaptation (Friedman et al., 2003)

The Calgary Model includes structural, developmental, and functional categories for assessment (Assessment Tool 7.1). It emphasizes the identification of strengths and resources. Repeated use of a family assessment tool assists nurses to refine their skills.

Nurses use assessment tools to organize data about a family visually and to map relationships. Examples include genograms and family maps. The **genogram** (Assessment Tool 7.2) uses visual links and other symbols to represent family relationships. In essence, it depicts a family tree (Diem & Moyer, 2005). Most genograms include the parents, siblings, and children over three generations. They can depict structural and functional patterns, relationships, and significant life events.

Ecomaps are family maps (Assessment Tool 7.3). Whereas the genogram illustrates relationships within the family, the ecomap depicts the family's relationship to the larger community (Kennedy, 2010). After the assessment is completed, the nurse refers to the ecomap while evaluating the family's external support systems.

Roles and Tasks

As discussed earlier, family roles can be informal or formal as members perform tasks within a given situation within the family. Formal roles are expected roles; for example, father as income earner, mother as homemaker. Informal roles hold a significant place in the family dynamics. Examples may include encourager, harmonizer, blocker, follower, martyr, scapegoat, or

● **ASSESSMENT TOOL 7.2 Sample Genogram**

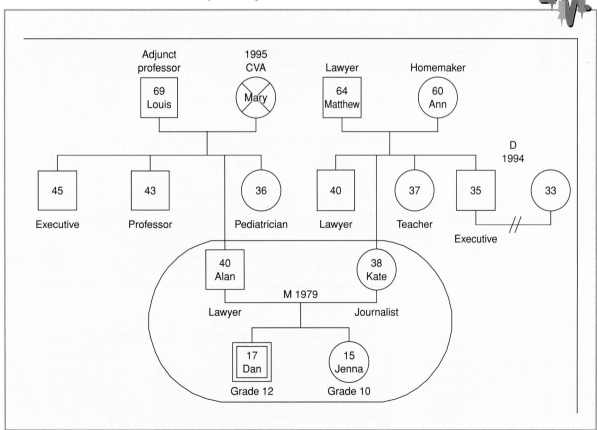

● **ASSESSMENT TOOL 7.3** **Sample Ecomap**

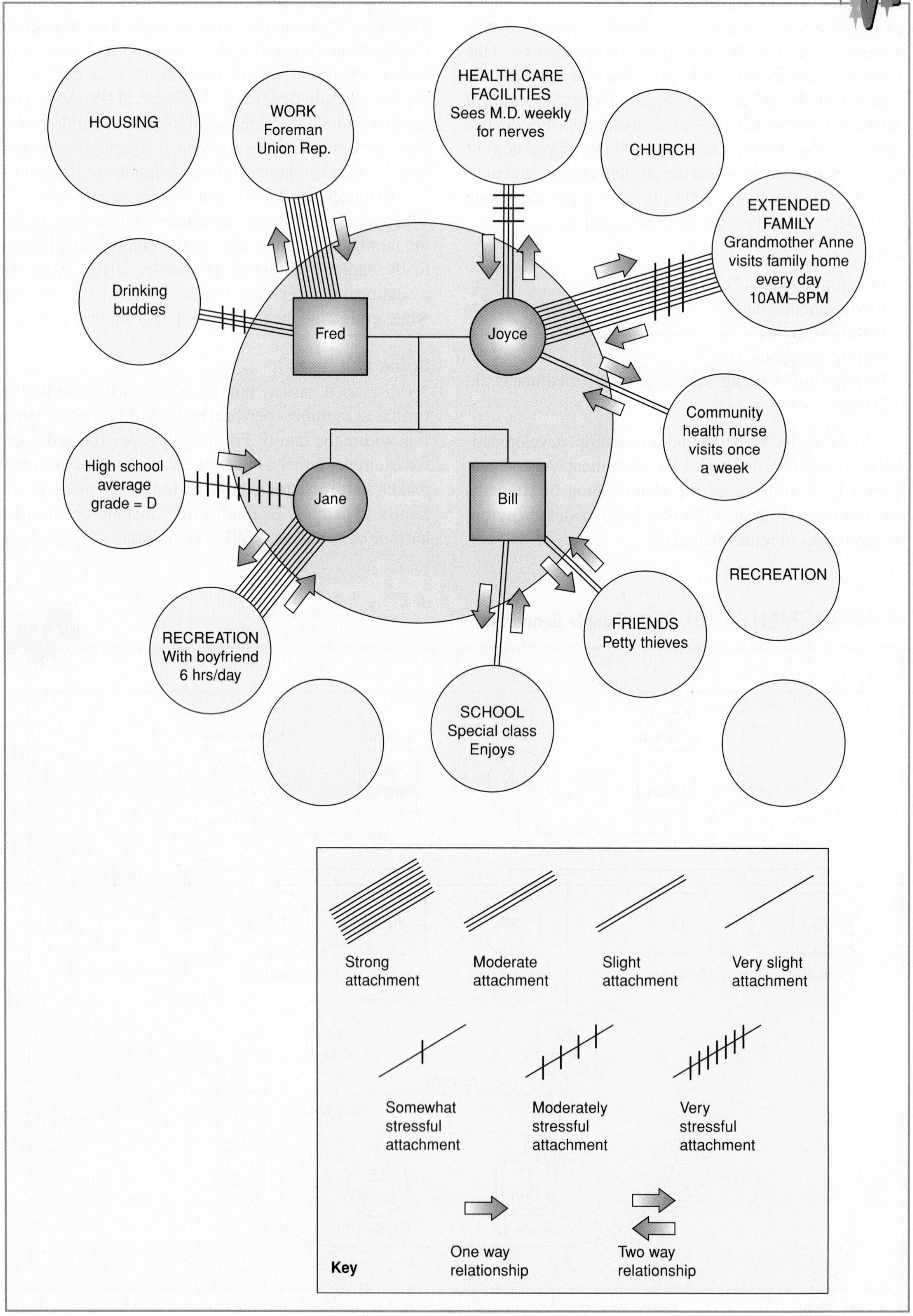

Key

| Strong attachment | Moderate attachment | Slight attachment | Very slight attachment |

Somewhat stressful attachment

Moderately stressful attachment

Very stressful attachment

One way relationship

Two way relationship

go-between (Clark, 2007). The nurse notes the presence of these formal and informal roles as part of the assessment process.

Gathering information about the family's place in the life cycle also assists the nurse with assessing roles and tasks. Sometimes, during completion of a genogram, information about family tasks and roles flows naturally from the discussion. The nurse's understanding of systems and developmental theories provides a framework for seeking information about family roles and tasks as part of the interviewing process of the assessment. With the birth of a child, the family may be required to reassign roles and tasks.

Dynamics and Communication Patterns

Communication patterns and level of anxiety are core elements in assessing family dynamics. Communication has many levels, and family members naturally develop their own way of interacting. Verbal and nonverbal communication patterns within the family should be considered, "as should the listening ability of the family members" (Clark, 2007, p. 328). The nurse assesses family dynamics in interaction with family members. Assessing communication style is one of the first steps in assessing family dynamics (Maurer & Smith, 2009). What is the family style?

- Receptive (open to suggestions)
- Distancing (has difficulty connecting to resources)
- Resistive (denies or disagrees with suggestions)
- Rigid (has a fixed way of dealing with problems)
- Ordered (clearly spells out roles and communication)
- Dependent (prefers to look to others for direction)

(Cooley, as cited in Maurer & Smith, 2009.)

In the course of this assessment, the level of anxiety within the family should become clear. If anxiety is high, future assessment may need to focus on family coping. All these assessments will produce more data if a family meeting can be part of the entire process.

Family as Part of the Community

The concept of health literacy is increasingly important in health care. Nurses have an important role in helping families become health literate, that is, "placing one's own health and that of one's family and community into context, understanding which factors are influencing it, and knowing how to address them" (Sorenson et al., 2012, p. 1). Assessing the family within the community is best accomplished with a home visit. Home visits include an assessment of the home environment for safety issues that need to be addressed. When a home visit is not possible, the detailed information from the ecomap provides a basic assessment of the family's role within the community. The nurse remembers that

some families who belong to a resource-rich community still have difficulty accessing and connecting with the needed resources and does whatever is possible to assist them to do so.

Family Culture

In addition, the nurse completes a family cultural assessment to have full information about the family's norms, beliefs, and culturally related health care practices. Gaining insight into culturally influenced perspectives on health care is a valuable component of understanding the family dynamics in any given situation (Boyle, 2008; Rozzano, 2003).

Select Potential Nursing Diagnoses

Determining a family diagnosis may be new to some nurses who are more familiar with arriving at diagnoses for individual clients. Some commonly applicable family diagnoses include the following:

- Deficient Knowledge
- Impaired Verbal Communication
- Risk for Impaired Parent/Infant/Child Attachment
- Risk for Caregiver Role Strain
- Compromised Family Coping
- Disabled Family Coping
- Health-Seeking Behaviours
- Interrupted Family Processes
- Readiness for Enhanced Family Processes
- Impaired Home Maintenance Management
- Impaired Parenting
- Ineffective Family Therapeutic Regimen Management
- Parental Role Conflict

Although the nurse is responsible for determining appropriate family diagnoses based on the specific assessment data, he or she confirms with the family members that this diagnosis correctly addresses the problems identified.

Planning/Intervention

Planning involves forming the desired outcomes (goals) and choosing interventions to help meet them. Outcomes need to be realistic, specific, and measurable.

When planning care and intervening, the nurse works in partnership with family members. Together, they establish a plan to address the family's observed and verbalized needs (Nursing Care Plan 7.2). Planning is also a time for the nurse to empower family members to become part of the solution to their own problems.

While working with the family, the nurse makes them aware of various community resources available. Although communities vary in the availability and provision of such resources, the nurse collaborates with a social worker to connect families to local support.

NURSING CARE PLAN 7.2

●

A Family Growing Through Adoption

 Think back to Jacob and Rachel, the couple at the beginning of the chapter who are adopting a baby girl. The birth mother has relinquished the baby to the couple. Jacob and Rachel are holding their daughter closely, pointing out some of her features. They state, "She is so beautiful, really a dream come true. We have to learn so much about caring for her."

Six hours after the birth, you check on the birth mother who tearfully states that she knows she is making a good decision but would like to hold the baby for a while to say goodbye. After informing Jacob and Rachel of this request, they agree to honor it. They state, "Do you think she has changed her mind?"

NURSING DIAGNOSIS

Readiness for Enhanced Parenting related to new role as parents and limited knowledge of newborn care

EXPECTED OUTCOMES

1. The couple will identify areas of needed information about newborn care.
2. The couple will identify basic newborn care measures.

INTERVENTIONS	RATIONALES
Assess the parents' level of understanding about newborn care	Assessment provides a baseline to identify specific client needs and to develop an individualized teaching plan
Explore the couple's exposure to newborn care; clear up any misconceptions or myths; allow time for questions	Information about exposure provides additional foundation for teaching and provides opportunities to clarify or clear up misinformation and teach new information
Provide the parents with teaching materials related to newborn care in various forms, such as in writing or via videos	Teaching materials in various formats enhances learning; written materials can be used as a reference at home
Demonstrate newborn care measures; allow parents to participate in care, offering anticipatory guidance and suggestions; have parents return demonstrate care measures, such as bathing, feeding, and diapering (see Chapter 20)	Participation enhances learning; return demonstration allows for evaluation of that learning
Encourage the use of en face positioning and close cuddling during feeding; instruct parents in newborn's cues and appropriate responses	Proper positioning during feeding and appropriately responding to cues promotes the development of trust in newborn
Investigate availability of community/public health resources for support; if necessary, arrange for a home health care follow-up	The birth of a newborn brings about many changes in the family unit. Community/public health resources and follow-up provide additional support and assistance if needed

(continued)

NURSING CARE PLAN 7.2 • A Family Growing Through Adoption *(Continued)*

EVALUATION

1. Parents demonstrate beginning independence with newborn care.
2. Parents exhibit ability to identify and respond to newborn cues.

NURSING DIAGNOSIS

Fear related to possible change in birth mother's decision

EXPECTED OUTCOMES

1. The couple will state an understanding of the rationale for the birth mother's request.
2. The couple will report decreased fear that birth mother may change her mind.

INTERVENTIONS	RATIONALES
Explain the underlying reason for the birth mother's request	Explanation helps in providing factual, concrete information to allay misconceptions and fears
Inform the couple that the birth mother's request is part of the grieving process	Grieving requires knowledge of the person. Allowing the birth mother to know the newborn as a person facilitates this process
Gently remind the couple that the birth mother can still change her mind	Legally, the birth mother has a specified time in which to make her decision. Knowledge of this by all parties is crucial
Ensure open, honest communication	Such communication promotes trust and enhances the nurse–client relationship
Provide emotional support to the couple as they cope with the situation; enlist the aid of other relatives if appropriate	Additional support promotes positive coping

EVALUATION

1. The couple states that their fears about a change in decision are decreased.
2. The couple demonstrates behaviors that indicate incorporating the newborn into their family unit.

In choosing interventions necessary to meet desired outcomes, the nurse considers both the actions and the support needed to implement the actions. Priorities should be clear if the nurse remains focused on the desired outcome. The nurse involves the family by providing choices of possible interventions that would meet the desired outcome and explaining the pros and cons of potential interventions.

Evaluation

Evaluation of the outcomes of the planned interventions is necessary to determine the success of the plan. Whenever possible, family members participate in the follow-up evaluation. Doing so with the nurse will provide additional learning about what worked for the family and what did not seem helpful.

SUMMARY

- Many definitions of family are found in the literature, but nurses acknowledge that families are individually defined.
- System theory views a family as greater than the sum of its members.
- Families have roles and tasks, values, methods of decision making, patterns of communication, and unique cultural aspects.
- Culture may influence families during the childbearing and childrearing stages. Nurses ask each client and family about specific cultural beliefs and practices.
- Using the nursing process of assessment, planning and intervention, and evaluation, nurses can provide family-centred care.

Questions to Ponder

1. Think about your experiences in the clinical setting in working with families. What experiences do you have in which you worked well with a family? Can you identify factors that positively influenced that situation?
2. Think of an experience in which working with a family was difficult. Have you learned anything new that you could apply to that situation?
3. Think of a personal situation in which your family had contact with the health care system. In your personal situation, assess the use and effectiveness of the nursing process.
4. What is your family like? Think about all the cultural groups with whom you personally identify. How have your personal experiences with family and culture influenced your view of other families?

REVIEW QUESTIONS

1. Understanding that the health status of one family member affects the other family members is reflected in
   A. communication theory.
   B. systems theory.
   C. family functional theory.
   D. cultural theory.
2. The nurse is working with a married couple that has two biologic children, one child from the father's previous marriage, and one child from the mother's previous relationship. The nurse identifies the family structure as a/an
   A. nontraditional family.
   B. compound family.
   C. blended family.
   D. extended family.

3. In assessing family dynamics, the nurse collects information about the family processes. Which of the following questions might best provide data about family processes?
   A. "Who makes the decisions in the family?"
   B. "Tell me about your family illnesses."
   C. "Describe how the children are disciplined."
   D. "What recreational activities do you do as a family?"
4. Which of the following examples illustrates healthy family communication?
   A. Verbal messages go through a third party for interpretation.
   B. Family members freely discuss problems with each other.
   C. Family members seldom share thoughts and feelings with each other.
   D. Expressed verbal messages rarely match internal feelings.
5. A couple dealing with infertility asks the nurse to explain the difference between an open and a closed adoption. Which of the following responses, if made by the nurse, is most correct?
   A. In an open adoption, the birth mother retains the right to visit the child.
   B. In a closed adoption, the adopted child never knows the identity of the biologic parents.
   C. In an open adoption, parental satisfaction is higher for both biologic and adoptive parents.
   D. In a closed adoption, the birth parents and adoptive parents do not exchange identifying information.
6. All of the following adoptive children would be considered "special needs" except
   A. an infant born with a severe heart defect.
   B. a group of triplets.
   C. a child 6 years of age.
   D. a 6-month-old.

REFERENCES

Adoption.com. (2013). *Prepare for a transracial adoption*. Retrieved from http://transracial.adoption.com/interracial/prepare-for-transracial-adoption.html

Adoption Council of Canada. (n.d.). FAQs. Retrieved from http://www.adoption.ca/faqs

AdoptiveParents.ca. (n.d.). An adoption resource guide for Canadians. Retrieved from http://www.adoptiveparents.ca/

Boyle, J. S. (2008). Culture, family and community. In: M. M. Andrews & J. S. Boyle (Eds.), *Transcultural concepts in nursing care*. (5th ed., pp. 261–296). Philadelphia, PA Lippincott Williams & Wilkins.

Bundy-Fazioli, K., Fruhauf, C. A. & Miller, J. L. (2013). Grandparents caregivers' perceptions of emotional distress and well-being. *Journal of Family Social Work, 16*(5), 447–462. doi:10.1080/105 22158.2013.832461

Byng-Hall, J. (2008). The significance of children fulfilling parental roles: Implications for family therapy. *Journal of Family therapy, 30*, 147–162.

Callister, L. C. (2001). Culturally competent care of women and newborns: Knowledge, attitude and skills. *Journal of Obstetric,*

Gynecologic, and Neonatal Nursing (JOGNN), 30(2), 209–215.

Campinha-Bacote, J. (2011). Delivering patient-centered care in the midst of a cultural conflict: The role of cultural competence. *Online Journal of Issues in Nursing, 16*(2), 5. Item Number: 2011167230. Retrieved from http://gm6.nursingworld.org/MainMenuCategories/ANAMarketplace/ANAPeriodicals/OJIN/TableofContents/Vol-16-2011/No2-May-2011/Delivering-Patient-Centered-Care-in-the-Midst-of-a-Cultural-Conflict.aspx

Canadian Nurses Association. (2010). *Position statement: Promoting cultural competence in nursing.* Ottawa: CNA-AIIC. Retrieved http://www.cna-aiic.ca/sitecore%20modules/web/~/media/cna/page%20content/pdf%20en/2013/09/04/16/27/6%20-%20ps114_cultural_competence_2010_e.pdf

Clark, M. J. (2007). *Community health nursing* (5th ed.). Upper Saddle River, NJ: Pearson Prentice Hall.

Denham, S. A. (2003). Familial research reveals new practice model. *Holistic Nursing Practice, 17*(3), 143–151.

Dictionary.com Unabridged. (n.d.). *Family values.* Retrieved from Dictionary.com website: http://dictionary.reference.com/browse/family values

Diem, E., & Moyer, A. (2005). *Community health nursing projects: Making a difference.* Philadelphia, PA: Lippincott Williams & Wilkins.

Edwards, O. W., & Ray, S. L. (2010). Value of family and group counseling models where grandparents function as parents to their grandchildren. *International Journal for the Advancement of Counselling, 32*(3), 178–193. doi:10.1007/s10447-010-9098-9

Farrao, V. (2010). *Paid work. Women in Canada.* (Statistics Canada Catalogue no. 89-503-x). Retrieved from http://www.statcan.gc.ca/pub/89–503-x/2010001/article/11387-eng.pdf

Friedman, M. M., Bowden, V. R., & Jones, E. G. (2003). *Family nursing: Research, theory, and practice.* (5th ed.). Upper Saddle River, NJ: Prentice Hall.

Gottlieb, L. N., & Gottlieb, B. (2007). The developmental/health framework within the McGill model of nursing. *Advances in Nursing Science, 30*(1), E43–E57.

Government of Canada. (2014). *Adopt a child.* Retrieved from http://www.cic.gc.ca/english/immigrate/adoption/index.asp

Gregory, D., Harrowing, J., Lee, B., Doolittle, L., & O'Sullivan, P. S. (2010). Pedagogy as influencing nursing students' essentialized understanding of culture. *International Journal of Nursing Education Scholarship, 7*(1). doi: 10.2202/1548-923X.2025. Retrieved from http://www.degruyter.com/view/j/ijnes.2010.7.1/ijnes.2010.7.1.2025/ijnes.2010.7.1.2025.xml

Hanson, S. M. H. (2006). *Family health care nursing: Theory, practice, and research.* (3rd ed.). Philadelphia, PA: F. A. Davis.

Hayslip, B., & Kaminski, P. L. (2005). Grandparents raising their grandchildren: A review of the literature and suggestions for practice. *Gerontologist, 45*(2), 262–269.

Hitchcock, J. E., Schubert, P. E., Thomas, S. A., & Bartfay, W. J. (2010). *Community health nursing: Caring in action-First Canadian edition.* Toronto: Nelson Education.

Kennedy, V. (2010). Ecomaps. *MAI Review, 3,* 1–12.

Maurer, F. A., & Smith, C. M. (2009). *Community/public health nursing practice: Health for families and populations.* St. Louis, MO: Elsevier.

Mei, Z., Fast, J., & Eales, J. (2013). *Gifts of a lifetime: The contributions of older Canadians.* Final Report. Edmonton: University of Alberta and Seniors Association of Greater Edmonton.

Merriam-Webster. (2014a). Family. Accessed from http://www.merriam-webster.com/dictionary/family

Merriam-Webster. (2014b). *Nuclear family.* Accessed from http://www.merriam-webster.com/dictionary/nuclear%20family

Moules, N. J., Bell, J. M., Paton, B. I., & Morck, A. C. (2012). Examining pedagogical practices in family systems nursing: Intentionality, complexity and doing well by families. *Journal of Family Nursing, 18*(2), 261–295. doi:10.1177/1074840711435508

National Council on Aging. (2008). *"Grandparenting" today.* Ottawa: Government of Canada. Retrieved from http://publications.gc.ca/collections/collection_2011/sc-hc/H71-4-1-18-3-eng.pdf

Purnell, L. D., & Paulanka, B. J. (2008). *Transcultural health care: A culturally competent approach.* (3rd ed.). Philadelphia: F. A. Davis.

Riley, H. (2013). Exploring the ethical implications of the late discovery of adoptive and donor-insemination offspring status. *Adoption and Fostering, 37*, (2), 171–187. doi: 10.1177/0308575913490496

Rosenthal, C. J., & Gladstone, J. (2007). *Grandparenthood in Canada.* Ottawa: The Vanier Institute of the Family.

Rozzano, L. (2003). Culture perspective. *Holistic Nursing Practice, 17*(1), 8–10.

Satir, V. (1988). *The new peoplemaking.* Mountain View, CA: Science and Behavior Books.

Sorenson, K., Van den Broucke, S., Fullam, J., Doyle, G., Pelikan, J., Slonska, Z., et al. (2012). Health literacy and public health: A systematic review and integration of definitions and models. *BioMed Central Public Health, 12*(80), 1–13. http://www.biomedcentral.com/content/pdf/1471-2458-12-80.pdf

Stanhope, M., Lancaster, J., Jessup-Falcioni, H., & Viverais-Dresler, G. A. (2011). *Community health nursing in Canada.* (2nd Canadian Ed). Toronto: Elsevier Canada.

Statistics Canada. (2007a). *2006 Census: Families, marital status, households and dwelling characteristics.* Ottawa: Statistics Canada, The Daily, September 12, 2007. Retrieved from http://www.statcan.ca/Daily/English/070912/d070912 a.htm

Statistics Canada. (2011). Immigration and ethnocultural diversity in Canada. *National Household Survey, 2011.* Catalogue no. 99–010-X2011001. Retrieved from http://www12.statcan.gc.ca/nhs-enm/2011/as-sa/99-010-x/99-010-x2011001-eng.pdf

Statistics Canada. (2012a). *Portrait of families and living arrangements in Canada – Families, households and marital status, 2011 Census of population.* Catalogue no. 98–312-X2011001. Ottawa: Statistics Canada. Retrieved from http://www12.statcan.gc.ca/census-recensement/2011/as-sa/98-312-x/98-312-x2011001-eng.pdf

Statistics Canada. (2012b). *Fifty years of families in Canada: 1961-2011 - Families, households and marital status, 2011 Census population.* Catalogue no. 98-312-X2011003. Ottawa, ON: Statistics Canada. Retrieved from https://www12.statcan.gc.ca/census-recensement/2011/as-sa/98-312-x/98-312-x2011003_1-eng.cfm

Statistics Canada. (2012c). *Canadian households in 2011: type and growth.* Catalogue no. 98-312-X2011003. Ottawa: Statistics Canada. Retrieved from http://www12.statcan.gc.ca/census-recensement/2011/as-sa/98-312-x/98-312-x2011003_2-eng.pdf

Strong-Boag, V. (2006). *Finding families finding ourselves; English Canada encounters adoption from the nineteenth century to the 1990s.* Don Mills, ON: Oxford University Press.

von Bertalanffy, L. V. (1968). *General system theory.* New York: George Braziller.

Wright, L. M., & Leahey, M. (2013). *Nurses and families: A guide to family assessment and intervention.* (6th ed.). Philadelphia, PA: F. A. Davis.

SPECIAL REPRODUCTIVE AND HEALTH CONCERNS

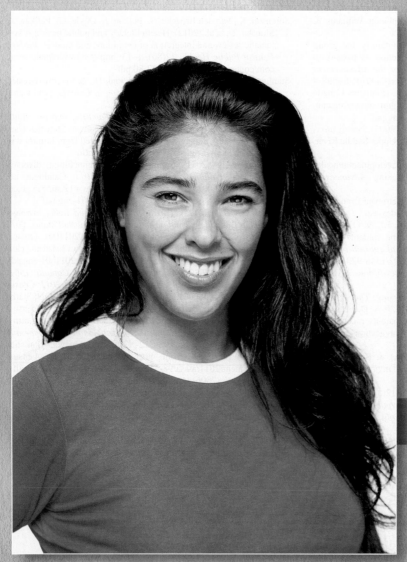

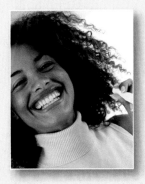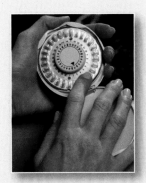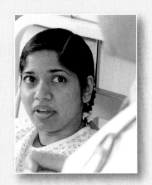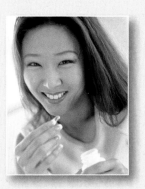

n Unit 2 we explore important topics associated with reproductive health, although not specifically related to the process and act of childbearing itself. We describe those issues and concerns that contribute to an environment in which women feel empowered to control the timing and circumstances that best promote healthy gestation. We also discuss ways for health care providers to assist clients with effectively preventing, responding to, and managing the consequences of unexpected reproductive outcomes. Examples of topics covered in this unit include contraception, abstinence, voluntary pregnancy termination, infertility, and alternative childbearing arrangements. The section also contains detailed explorations of genetics and embryonic/fetal development, focusing on problems that can develop or manifest during these phases and associated contributing factors. We review significant preventive and diagnostic screening tests and interventions that prospective parents can take to optimize family health.

CHAPTER 8

Fertility Control and Contraception

Melanie Basso and Eileen Scaringi*

Veena, 26 years old, comes to the clinic for information about contraception. She reports that she's been having sexual intercourse occasionally for 4 years and has usually used condoms. She has been with more than one partner during the 4 years she has been sexually active. She wants to explore options other than condoms so that she can feel "more control over avoiding pregnancy."

During a scheduled health maintenance visit, Kenya, 19 years old, mentions that she will be married in 4 months to Darrell. The client says that she and her fiancé are both virgins and are planning to wait until their wedding night to have sexual intercourse. The couple follows strict religious beliefs that do not permit contraception. "We'd like to have children some day, but I really would like to avoid pregnancy until I finish college," Kenya reports. She mentions that she has heard about natural family planning and wonders if the nurse can provide more information.

You will learn more about Veena's and Kenya's stories throughout this chapter. Nurses working with such clients need to understand the material in this chapter to manage care and address issues appropriately. Before beginning this chapter, consider the following points related to the above scenarios:

- Does anything about either situation present any issues of immediate concern? Are there areas for which the nurse must obtain more information? Explain your answers.
- How might the ages of the clients involved influence the nurse's approach to care?

---

*Contributor to first U.S. edition.

● What health-related areas can the nurse investigate with Veena? What about with Kenya?

● What measures can the nurse take to approach the clients with sensitivity and adequate information? How can the nurse ensure understanding of concepts taught?

LEARNING OBJECTIVES

On completion of this chapter, the reader should be able to:
● Describe a brief history of contraception and social forces that have helped to shape its development and availability.
● Explain the mechanism of action, effectiveness, contraindications, correct usage, side effects, and danger signs for specific contraceptive methods.
● Identify appropriate teaching for women about emergency contraception.
● Discuss natural family planning methods.
● Describe surgical methods of limiting fertility.
● Elicit a thorough health history for clients seeking contraception, taking into consideration sexual orientation and cultural beliefs.
● Identify appropriate counselling measures for barrier, hormonal, surgical, and intrauterine methods of contraception.

KEY TERMS

abstinence
bilateral tubal ligation
cervical cap
combined oral contraceptives
continuous or extended hormonal contraception
contraception
contraceptive sponge
diaphragm
emergency contraception
female condom
fertility awareness methods

intrauterine device (IUD)
lactational amenorrhea method
male condom
natural family planning
pelvic inflammatory disease (PID)
sexually transmitted infections
transdermal contraceptive patch
typical use failure rate
vaginal contraceptive ring
vasectomy
withdrawal

S ince ancient times, women and men have sought to control their fertility (Box 8.1).
Contraception means any method used to prevent pregnancy. The introduction of the oral contraceptive in Canada in the early 1960s ushered in a new era of fertility control and contributed to an increased sense of sexual freedom for women, who had new opportunities to determine when, how often, and with whom they would become pregnant. Birth control methods continue to evolve; examples of recently developed devices include the contraceptive patch and the vaginal contraceptive ring.

Society has traditionally placed contraceptive responsibility, along with child nurturing, on women. Until recently, except for the male condom, withdrawal, and vasectomy, currently available contraceptive methods have been female focused. Research in clinical trials on hormonal male contraceptives using a combination of testosterone and progestins is promising and has shown to be effective for spermatogenesis suppression as well

● **BOX 8.1** **Brief History of Contraception**

2000–1000 BCE. Ancient Egyptian writings discuss vaginal pessaries and mixtures to insert into the vagina to prevent conception.

500–600 BCE. Biblical writings discuss withdrawal.

500 BCE. Aristotle suggests covering the cervix with cedar oil to prevent pregnancy.

100–200 CE. The Talmud describes the insertion of sponges soaked with vinegar or wine to prevent pregnancy.

150 CE. Roman mythology describes the use of a goat bladder as a condom.

1200–1300. The Roman Catholic Church approves only "natural methods" of contraception.

1583. The writings of Fallopius describe linen "sheath" or condom.

1725–1798. Casanova writes about condoms made from animal intestines and cervical caps made from lemons.

1800–1900. Rubber condoms are introduced, along with the cervical cap, diaphragm, and sponges with spermicide.

1882. It becomes a crime to sell or advertise birth control in Canada. The maximum penalty is 2 years in prison.

1882. The first birth control clinic, located in Holland, opens.

1909. The IUD is introduced.

1916. Margaret Sanger opens the first birth control clinic in the United States. Canadian women seek information from her on how to prevent pregnancy.

1930. A. R. Kaufman, a prominent birth control advocate, sets up the Parent Information Bureau in Kitchener, Ontario.

1960s. The birth control pill becomes available in Canada, but is limited to therapeutic use, such as regulation of menstrual cycles.

1969. Birth control is legalized in Canada.

1997. Health Canada approves Depo-Provera.

2002. Health Canada approves Mirena.

2004. Health Canada approves NuvaRing and Ortho Evra.

as reversible, and safe. Current studies are searching to find the best combination of hormones that are efficacious while minimizing adverse events (Wang & Swerdloff, 2010). In this chapter we provide a historical and social context for fertility control. We explore various methods of fertility control, including barrier, hormonal, intrauterine, behavioural, and surgical methods. We describe collaborative care measures for the client seeking information about contraception and family planning. Nurses must be able to provide teaching and assistance to men and women seeking a method best suited to their needs

and lifestyles, while ensuring adequate understanding of the mechanisms, benefits, and risks of the different methods.

HISTORICAL PERSPECTIVES

In ancient times, options for limiting pregnancy were few and included prolonged lactation, ingested and inserted plant extracts (McLaren & McLaren, 1997), and, in some cultures, infanticide. Withdrawal of the penis before ejaculation was another widely used method; some cultures today continue to rely on it as a primary mechanism of birth control. Magical rites, formulas, and potions also were common methods, along with douching, positioning, and moving the body violently (Bullough & Bullough, 1994; McLaren & McLaren, 1997; Schenker & Fabenou, 1993).

Early Egyptian writings discuss vaginal insertion of a mixture of crocodile dung, honey, and gum-like substances for the prevention of pregnancy. These writings also describe an occlusive vaginal pessary, a forerunner to the modern diaphragm. Aristotle recommended covering the cervix and vagina with cedar oil. The Bible describes withdrawal (*coitus interruptus*), and Hippocrates mentions an intrauterine device (IUD) in his writings. The Hebrew Talmud details the insertion into the vagina of a sponge soaked in vinegar or wine, while the Romans may have used goat intestines as a barrier in their efforts to prevent pregnancy (Bullough & Bullough, 1994; McLaren & McLaren, 1997).

In 1583, Gabriele Fallopius, an Italian anatomist for whom the fallopian tubes are named, first described a linen "sheath" or condom. During this time, the primary use of the condom was not as a contraceptive, but as a way to combat syphilis. In the 18th century, Casanova described the use of a lemon half as a cervical cap and also wrote about condoms made from animal intestines. Such condoms, however, were expensive and had to be washed for reuse. In the 19th century, mass-produced rubber condoms became available, as did the cervical cap, diaphragm, and sponge with spermicide.

Organized religion has often shaped social policies toward contraception. Jewish and Christian religions have interpreted the Biblical narrative describing withdrawal as a prohibition against wasting semen. In the 13th century, the Roman Catholic Church put forth its policy of only "natural methods" of fertility control, that is, sex only during a "safe" period, and intercourse without ejaculation; this doctrine remains in force today. The Protestant tradition followed similar prohibitions against contraception, which were manifested as vigorous legislation against "obscenity."

In 1882, it was a crime to provide or advertise birth control in Canada. The maximum sentence was 2 years' imprisonment. Women were desperate to control their fertility, but physicians who provided information were faced with losing their medical licenses (McLaren & McLaren, 1997). Although much of society did not approve of the use of birth control, people were using a variety of methods to prevent pregnancy and space children, and between 1871 and 1937, Canada's birth rate declined from 6.8 to 2.6 (McLaren & McLaren, 1997). After Margaret Sanger opened the first birth control clinic in the United States in 1916, Canadian women turned to her for contraceptive information. She later formed the American Birth Control League, the forerunner of Planned Parenthood.

The rhythm method was first accurately described in the 1920s by two physicians who identified the relationship between ovulation and menstruation. They determined that ovulation occurred in the middle of the menstrual cycle and not during menstruation (as was previously believed), vastly improving the effectiveness of this contraceptive method. The social acceptability of a "natural" method of family planning was cause for concern to the Roman Catholic Church, which publicly banned the rhythm method in the 1930s (McLaren & McLaren, 1997).

Charles Knowlton's *The Fruits of Physiology,* published in 1933, recommended douches made of sodium bicarbonate, alum, zinc phosphate, sodium chloride, vinegar, rose leaves, or raspberry leaves or roots to prevent pregnancy. Although it was postulated in 1919 that ingestion of progesterone would prevent pregnancy, it was not until the 1940s that Russell Marker overcame the difficulty of the large quantity of hormone needed by synthesizing the steroid from Mexican yams.

Although contraception in the 1930s was available on a limited basis to the upper and middle classes, the promotion of contraception to the poorer classes had an unexpected ally in people who espoused eugenics, the belief that the population would be smarter and healthier if certain types of people did not produce offspring. They saw birth control as a way to limit the growth of the "lower classes" (McLaren & McLaren, 1997).

At the same time as the eugenics movement, A. R. Kaufman, a prominent birth control advocate, set up the Parents' Information Bureau in Kitchener, Ontario in 1930. His goal was to provide affordable birth control to poor women, which he accomplished primarily by paying for the contraceptives himself. The Bureau was successful in its mission, sending nurses and social workers into the homes of the poor across Canada, mainly in Ontario and Western Canada. A landmark decision in 1937 brought support from the Canadian Medical Association, and by 1957, over 3,000 doctors were cooperating with the Kaufman movement (McLaren & McLaren, 1997).

The first combined oral contraceptive (COC) pill was introduced in Canada in the 1960s; initial beliefs about the proposed contraceptive pill projected that the purpose of the pill was only to regulate menstruation, which would allow women to use the rhythm method with more success to space their children. The Roman Catholic Church condemned all methods of artificial birth control, sanctioning only the rhythm method. But a prominent Canadian theologian "made stained glass windows rattle around the Roman Catholic world when he said the Pill 'does not interfere with the performance of the sexual act and its use is morally indistinguishable from the rhythm method'" (O'Malley et al., 2001). "The pill" has been credited with initiating a sexual revolution, as oral contraceptives provided highly effective protection against unwanted pregnancy. Support for legalization of birth control in Canada was slow to occur, but finally in 1969, "the pill" was legalized (O'Malley et al., 2001).

The first trials for oral contraception with progesterone were done in Puerto Rico. After discovering that estrogen acted as a "contaminant," it was removed from the pill. When pregnancy rates increased, 150 µg of estrogen was readded. Subsequently, the dose of estrogen has been decreased with each new generation of oral contraceptives, which currently contain as little as 20 µg. Progesterone-only formulations are available today for women who prefer or who cannot tolerate the estrogen.

Since the legalization of contraception, Canada has experienced a revolution in contraceptive devices such as extended hormonal contraceptive pills, hormone release skin patches, vaginal contraceptive rings, and injections (Black, 2006). Much research has been done to evaluate methods of contraception over time. A review of contraceptive choices that are available in Canada has been published that outlines the many choices available, as well as the characteristics, adherence, and approaches to counseling for the various methods (Fisher & Black, 2007).

TYPES OF CONTRACEPTIVE METHODS

Table 8.1 provides an overview of the various methods of contraception discussed in this chapter. These methods can be classified as barrier, hormonal, intrauterine, behavioural, and surgical.

Barrier Methods

Barrier methods rely on mechanical devices to prevent sperm from entering the female reproductive tract. Some of them also provide protection against **sexually transmitted infections (STIs)**. Barrier methods include male and female condoms, diaphragms, and cervical caps.

Male Condom

Until the early 1900s, the **male condom** was one of the few widely available methods of contraception. Today, male condoms are available in latex, natural membrane

(text continues on page 276)

● TABLE 8.1 Summary of Contraceptive Methods

Method	Mechanism of Action	Typical Use Failure Rate	Best Candidates	Noncontraceptive Benefits and Advantages	Side Effects and Disadvantages	Contraindications
Barrier Methods						
Male condom	Encases the penis to hold ejaculate and prevent sperm from entering female reproductive tract	15%	Those looking for an over-the-counter product Cooperative male partners	Latex and polyurethane forms protect against STIs	May be perceived as interruptive of sex	Latex allergy (may use natural membrane or polyurethane)
Female condom	Provides a barrier between the penis and female reproductive tract	21%	Women willing to accept 21% failure rate	Controlled by woman Protects against STIs	Difficult to insert	Severe vaginal prolapse
Diaphragm (with spermicide)	Covers the cervix to prevent sperm from entering; spermicide kills sperm	16%	Women comfortable inserting device into vagina	May be inserted 6 hr before sex Protects against some STIs	Needs to be professionally fitted	Frequent UTIs Allergy to spermicide
Cervical cap (with spermicide)	Covers the cervix to prevent sperm from entering; spermicide kills sperm	16–32%	Women comfortable inserting device into vagina	May be inserted 6 hr before intercourse and can be left in for 24 hr	Needs to be professionally fitted No STI protection	Latex allergy Cervical infection
Contraceptive sponge	Blocks cervix from sperm, traps sperm; releases spermicide to kill sperm	17–24%	Women comfortable inserting device into vagina; those looking for an over-the-counter product controlled by the woman	May be inserted up to 24 hr before intercourse Does not need reinsertion or replacement within 24-hr period for subsequent acts of intercourse	No STI protection	Allergy to spermicide
Spermicide	Reduces mobility of sperm and blocks penetration into cervix	29% (Varies depending on use with or without other methods)	Women at low risk for HIV Women comfortable inserting spermicide into vagina	Foam immediately effective Some bacterial STI protection	May have unpleasant taste Film and suppositories require 15 min to become effective	Spermicidal allergy
Hormonal Methods						
Combined oral contraceptives	Prevent ovulation and sperm penetration at cervix	8%	Women who can remember to take a pill each day	Lower risk for ovarian and endometrial cancer Decreased acne and dysmenorrhea	Nausea Headaches BTB No STI protection	History of breast cancer or DVT Migraines with focal/neurologic changes CAD Smokers older than 35 yrs
Continuous or extended combined hormonal contraceptives	Prevent ovulation and sperm penetration at cervix	8%	Women who do not wish to have breakthrough bleeding on a monthly basis	Taken for 63–84 d with 7 hormone-free days for bleeding to occur	Nausea Headaches BTB No STI protection	History of breast cancer or DVT Migraines with focal/neurologic changes CAD Smokers older than 35 yrs

(table continues on page 274)

● TABLE 8.1 **Summary of Contraceptive Methods** (continued)

Method	Mechanism of Action	Typical Use Failure Rate	Best Candidates	Noncontraceptive Benefits and Advantages	Side Effects and Disadvantages	Contraindications
Contraceptive patch	Prevents ovulation and sperm penetration at cervix	8%	Teenagers who can-not remember a pill each day	Patch is changed once a week	Breast tenderness Nausea Headaches BTB No STI protection	Same as combined oral contraceptives
Vaginal contraceptive ring	Prevents ovulation	8%	Women who cannot remember a pill each day	Removed in 21 d; new ring inserted 7 d later	Vaginitis Vaginal discharge Other combined oral contraceptive side effects; no STI pro-tection	Same as combined oral contraceptives
Progestin-only pills	Prevents sperm penetration at cervix	8%	Women who cannot take estrogen (breastfeeding women)	No estrogen-related side effects	BTB Amenorrhea Ovarian cysts Headaches	Breast cancer Liver disease Impaired absorption Certain medications
DMPA	Suppresses ovulation Prevents sperm penetration at cervix	3%	Women who cannot take estrogen	Decreased risk for endometrial cancer, PID, and ectopic pregnancy May decrease seizures Reduces sickle cell crises	Irregular bleeding Amenorrhea Slow return to fertility Weight gain No STI protection Clinic visits every 70–90 d	History of breast cancer, MI, or stroke Liver disease
Intrauterine Methods						
Copper IUD	Inhibits sperm motility Destroys sperm	<1%	Women at low risk for STIs Women who cannot take hormones	Cost effective Decreased risk for ectopic pregnancy	Heavier bleeding, dysmenorrhea No STI protection	Women at risk for STIs Allergy to copper Cervicitis
Levonorgestrel IUD (Mirena)	Prevents sperm penetration at cervix Thins endometrium Suppresses ovulation	<1%	Women who desire a long-acting, highly effective method	Decreased menstrual flow and dysmenorrhea Decreased risk for ectopic pregnancy	Irregular bleeding Amenorrhea No STI protection Ovarian cysts	Women at risk for STIs Breast cancer Liver disease
Behavioural Methods						
Abstinence	Not having sexual intercourse	Not available	Those who wish to refrain from sexual intercourse	Guarantees avoidance of pregnancy and STIs	Difficult to maintain	None

Method	Mechanism	Effectiveness	Advantages	Appropriate candidates	Disadvantages	Not appropriate for
Natural family planning/fertility awareness method	Abstaining or using a barrier method or withdrawal during fertile period	25%	Woman more aware of her cycle	Those who are motivated and understand the monthly cycle; Women with regular cycles	Must be committed to abstain or use other methods during fertile time; No STI protection; Requires training	Women with irregular cycles
Withdrawal	Prevents deposit of sperm into vagina	27%	Method readily available	Women willing to accept an increased risk for pregnancy	Requires great self-control; sperm may be released before ejaculation; No STI protection	Men who cannot withdraw before ejaculating
LAM	Lactation inhibits ovulation	1–2%	Facilitates postpartum weight loss; Decreases risk for breast cancer	New mothers who are exclusively breast-feeding a baby 6 mos old or less and have not had a menses	No STI protection; Pregnancy can occur prior to menses resuming; breast-feeding must be frequent and regular	Infant older than 6 mo; Return of menses; Women with blood-borne disease or taking drugs contraindicated in breastfeeding
Surgical Methods						
Surgical sterilization	Female: occludes fallopian tubes; Male: occludes vas deferens	<1%	Female: decreased risk for ovarian cancer; Male: easier, less expensive, and more effective than female	Those wishing to have no (or no more) children	Surgical risks (greater for female); Possible regret; No STI protection	Those unsure of a permanent method

BTB, breakthrough bleeding; CAD, coronary artery disease; COC, combined oral contraceptives; DMPA, depomedroxyprogesterone acetate; LAM, lactational amenorrhea method; PID, pelvic inflammatory disease; STI, sexually transmitted infection.

Adapted from: Hatcher, R. A., Trussell, J., Stewart, F., Cates, W., Stewart, G., Guest, F., et al. (2004). *Contraceptive technology* (18th ed.). New York: Artent Media and Fisher, W., & Black, A. (2007). Contraception in Canada: A review of method choices, characteristics, adherence, and approaches to counselling. *Canadian Medical Association Journal, 176*(7), 953–961.

Canadian updates from: Black, A., Francoeur, D., & Rowe, T. (2004a). Canadian contraception consensus: SOGC clinical practice guidelines, No. 143, part 1. *Journal of Obstetrics and Gynaecology Canada,* Retrieved from http://www.sogc.org/guidelines/public/143E-CPG1, Black, A., Francoeur, D., & Rowe, T. (2004b). Canadian contraception consensus: SOGC clinical practice guidelines, No. 143, part 2. *Journal of Obstetrics and Gynaecology Canada,* Retrieved from http://www.sogc.org/guidelines/public/143E-CPG2, Black, A., Francoeur, D., & Rowe, T. (2004c). Canadian contraception consensus: SOGC clinical practice guidelines, No. 143, part 3. *Journal of Obstetrics and Gynaecology Canada,* Retrieved from http://www.sogc.org/guidelines/public/143E-CPG3

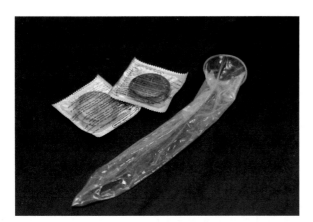

FIGURE 8.1 Male condoms are available in various colours, textures, and sizes.

(usually sheep intestine), and polyurethane forms. They come in various sizes and colours, with or without lubricants or spermicides, and with or without a reservoir tip (Fig. 8.1). The type of lubrication on condoms varies. Some are not lubricated at all, some are lubricated with a silicone substance, and some have a water-based lubricant. Lubrication makes the condom easier to put on and more comfortable to use and helps prevent condom breakage. Condoms are also available textured and flavoured. No prescription is needed for condoms.

Latex and polyurethane condoms protect against the transmission of STIs, including HIV. Natural membrane condoms do not protect against virus transmission (ie, HIV and human papillomavirus [HPV]); however, some clients prefer them because they facilitate increased male sensitivity during intercourse.

Mechanism of Action and Effectiveness. Condoms work by containing ejaculate and its estimated 300 million sperms, preventing them from entering the female reproductive tract and, subsequently, preventing conception. The condom provides a physical barrier to prevent direct genital contact. Couples choose this method because of its lack of side effects, ease of use and its availability when needed (Fisher & Black, 2007). **Typical use failure rates** (rates at which the method fails to prevent pregnancy, factoring in incorrect and inconsistent use, as well as failure despite correct application and use with every act of intercourse) range from perfect use at 2% to 7% to 15% (Fisher & Black, 2007; Hatcher et al., 2004). Condoms used with spermicide (see the next section) decrease the likelihood of pregnancy, especially in the event of slippage or breakage of the condom. A new condom must be used for each episode of intercourse. The primary benefit of condom use is the prevention of human immunodeficiency virus (HIV) and other STIs.

Contraindications and Side Effects. Some clients may have an allergic reaction to latex. Primary symptoms of latex allergy include genital irritation or burning.

Clients with latex allergy can use natural membrane or polyurethane condoms, as well as other contraceptive options discussed in this chapter.

Client Teaching and Collaborative Interventions. Some clients may not understand correct placement or use of condoms. One method by which nurses can educate them is to demonstrate correct use with a model of a penis or a similarly shaped object. The nurse can ask the client for a return demonstration on the model to validate understanding, provided the client is comfortable doing so. If a model penis is unavailable, a banana can be used instead.

As discussed earlier, latex and polyurethane condoms protect against STIs, but natural membrane condoms contain microscopic holes through which virus particles may pass. Thus, clients seeking use of condoms for STI prevention require instruction about using latex or polyurethane types. There is also a role for male condoms in preventing viral transmission of diseases such as herpes simplex virus (HSV), hepatitis B, and HPV (Myer, 2010).

Before use of condoms, the client, partner, or both should check them for date of expiration and to be sure that the packaging is intact. If a condom feels sticky or very dry, it shouldn't be used, as the package has probably been damaged. Condoms should appear to be in good condition; they can deteriorate if not stored properly and are affected by both heat and light. To be used correctly, the condom must be placed over the erect penis before any genital contact is made with the partner (Fig. 8.2). Application of the condom before the penis enters the vagina is critical because the penis may release a few drops of semen before ejaculation, even if the man is unaware that this has happened. Although this ejaculate consists mostly of semen from the Cowper's and prostate glands, it also contains some sperm, making this fluid potentially fertile. The fluid could also contain virus particles.

The client or partner should place the correct side of the condom on the glans (tip) of the penis and unroll the condom down the shaft while holding onto the tip of the condom, to provide a reservoir for the ejaculate. If the condom is placed inside out, the couple should discard and replace it with a new one. If the condom-covered penis is placed into the partner's mouth or anus, a new condom should be applied before vaginal intercourse to ensure that it is intact and free of bacteria. For extra protection, clients may choose to wear two condoms.

After ejaculation, the man should hold the condom in place at the base of the penis while removing the penis from the vagina or other orifice. He should pull down on the tip of the condom while sliding the condom down the shaft, to prevent spillage of the ejaculate. Latex condoms should be used only with water-based lubricants because petroleum- or oil-based products (eg, Vaseline or cold cream) can weaken the latex and increase the risk for

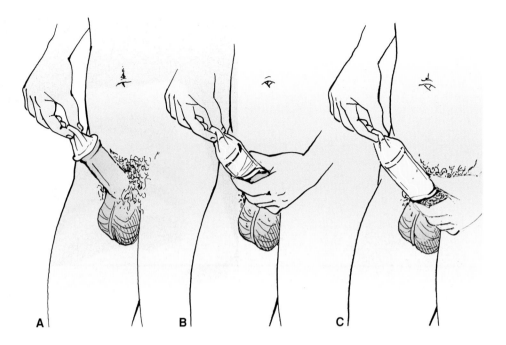

A   B   C

FIGURE 8.2 The client places the condom over the erect penis before making any genital contact with the partner. Some space should be left at the tip of the condom to contain the ejaculate.

breakage. Use of a water-based lubricant (eg, KY Jelly, Astroglide, water, saliva) with condoms is acceptable.

Female Condom

The **female condom**, introduced in Canada in 1994 (Hardwick, 2002), consists of a barrier of polyurethane inserted into the vagina and an outer ring that extends to cover the labia (Fig. 8.3). The composition of the female condom may provide protection from and for the labial tissues, which are a common site for HSV and HPV infections. Female condoms also protect against other STIs, including HIV (Hatcher et al., 2004). They are easily obtainable as they do not require a prescription and they are not made of latex, which is an advantage as some women may have latex allergies.

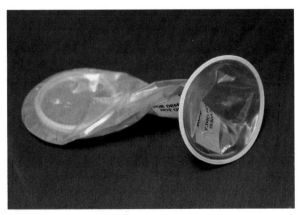

FIGURE 8.3 The female condom.

Mechanism of Action and Effectiveness. Like male condoms, female condoms work by containing ejaculate during sexual intercourse and provide protection from direct genital contact. The smaller of the two polyurethane rings in the closed end of the condom should be inserted as deep as possible into the vagina, leaving the larger ring at the open end outside the vagina.

The female condom can be inserted up to 8 hours before intercourse; it must be left in place until after intercourse is completed. More recent research indicates that the female condom may be washed out and reused (Planned Parenthood of America, 2013). The failure rate is 5% with perfect use and up to 21% with typical use (Fisher & Black, 2007).

Contraindications and Side Effects. The only contraindication to use of the female condom is difficulty with insertion, which may result from a woman's discomfort with touching herself or an inability to follow the instructions. Female condoms may produce noise during intercourse, which some clients find distracting or undesirable; use of water-soluble lubricant may minimize this problem. They protect against STIs only with correct use. Some clients find the appearance of the female condom unusual; its use may be problematic for male partners who are not used to the appearance of this device.

Client Teaching and Collaborative Interventions. Clients who choose the female condom need instruction about insertion, which can be challenging. The woman should compress and guide the condom into the vagina

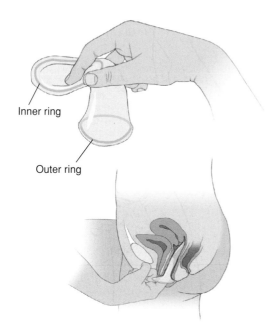

FIGURE 8.4 The client should compress and guide the inner ring of the female condom into the vagina with the outer ring resting against the vulva.

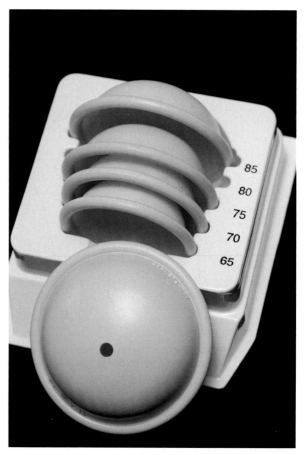

FIGURE 8.5 The diaphragm covers the cervix to prevent sperm from entering the female reproductive tract.

with the inner, small ring, until the outer ring rests against the vulva (Fig. 8.4). To avoid inserting the penis outside the condom, one partner should manually insert the penis into the vagina during sexual intercourse. Also, one partner should hold the outer ring in place during intercourse to prevent the condom from slipping. The nurse should advise clients that male condoms should not be used at the same time because the resultant friction may cause slippage.

Diaphragm

The **diaphragm** consists of a dome and flexible ring, which is sized from 50 to 100 mm (Fig. 8.5). Diaphragm domes may be made of either latex or, if a woman has a latex allergy, silicone diaphragms are available. Available types of rings include arching, flat spring, and coil spring, which are designed to fit variations in pelvic anatomies. Diaphragms are available only with a prescription. They must be used with spermicidal cream or jelly. Diaphragms must be fitted properly by a health care provider (Fisher & Black, 2007).

Mechanism of Action and Effectiveness. The diaphragm is placed into the vagina to cover the cervix so that sperm cannot enter for fertilization. Use of spermicidal foam and jelly increases effectiveness. The failure rate for diaphragms with spermicide with perfect use is 6%, and with typical use ranges from 16% to 20% (Fisher & Black, 2007). Diaphragms may provide some protection against STIs but provide no protection against HIV (Fisher & Black, 2007).

Contraindications and Side Effects. Women with a history of frequent urinary tract infections (UTIs) are not good candidates for diaphragms. The spermicides used with diaphragms can cause a change in vaginal flora and increase the risk for UTIs (Black et al., 2004c). Other contraindications include spermicidal allergy, latex allergy, and inability to insert and remove the device from the vagina. Clients with latex allergy who wish to use a diaphragm should choose the silicone diaphragm. Clients should be informed that silicone diaphragms are more expensive.

Client Teaching and Collaborative Interventions. Clients who choose diaphragms must be fitted for them by a health care provider to ensure appropriate type and size. Before use, the client should hold the diaphragm dome side down while placing a tablespoon of spermicidal cream or jelly in the dome. She should also place additional spermicide around the ring. To correctly insert a diaphragm, the client should hold the diaphragm dome side down between the thumb and middle finger, squeeze the edges together, and place the diaphragm into the vagina (Fig. 8.6A). The diaphragm should fit snugly between the symphysis pubis and beneath the cervix,

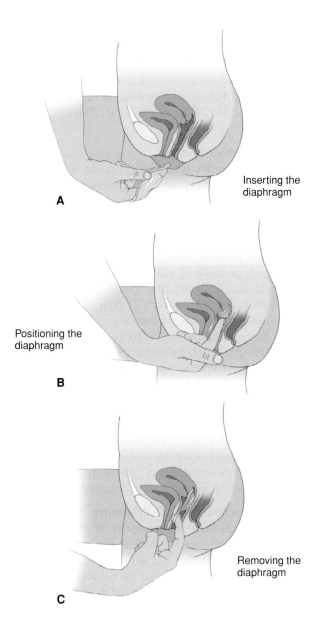

A

Inserting the
diaphragm

Positioning the
diaphragm

B

Removing the
diaphragm

C

FIGURE 8.6 A: To insert the diaphragm, the client holds the dome side down between thumb and middle finger. She squeezes together the edges and places the device into the vagina. **B:** To check for correct insertion, the client reaches inside her vagina to feel for the cervix and make sure that the diaphragm is covering it. **C:** For removal, the client hooks her finger above the diaphragm's ring and pulls it out.

while covering the cervix and touching the lateral vaginal walls (Youngkin & Davis, 2004). The woman may find insertion easier if she is lying down or standing with one foot on the toilet. After insertion, she must check to feel that the diaphragm is covering the cervix (see Fig. 8.6B). To help the woman locate the cervix, the nurse should tell her that the cervix feels like the tip of the nose. The nurse should allow the client private time to practice inserting and removing the diaphragm.

The diaphragm should remain in place 6 to 8 hours after intercourse. The nurse should instruct the client not to douche after use and to wait 3 hours after removal for any douching. If intercourse is repeated, the woman should leave the diaphragm in place and insert additional spermicide into the vagina. There is some evidence that diaphragm use during menstruation may increase the risk for toxic shock syndrome (Options for Sexual Health, 2012). Caution should also be given to users that the risk of toxic shock syndrome increases when wearing a diaphragm for greater than 24 hours (Fisher & Black, 2007). To remove the diaphragm, the client should hook a finger above the ring and pull it out (see Fig. 8.6C). After removal, the client should wash the diaphragm with mild soap and water only, dry it, and store it in the case. The nurse should advise against the use of any powders or oil-based lubricants with a diaphragm, because these substances may weaken the integrity of the latex dome (Options for Sexual Health, 2012). Diaphragms may be dusted with plain cornstarch, but must be washed prior to use.

Before each use, the client should verify that the diaphragm is intact by filling the dome with water and inspecting for leaks. The presence of leaks indicates the need for replacement of the diaphragm and use of an alternate method of contraception until the new diaphragm is ready and fitted. The client should replace the device a minimum of every 2 years (Hatcher et al., 2004). Women should visit a health care provider annually for assessment of the fit of the diaphragm. After a pregnancy, or any weight change of 10 pounds gain or loss, the diaphragm should be refitted (Hatcher et al., 2004; Options for Sexual Health, 2012).

Veena described wanting to feel "more control over avoiding pregnancy." Would a diaphragm be an appropriate contraceptive option for the nurse to suggest?

Cervical Cap

The **cervical cap** consists of a firm rubber cap with a rim sized to fit over the cervix (Fig. 8.7). Cervical caps are available in 22, 25, and 31 mm sizes, the internal diameter of the cap. Cervical caps are no longer made in Canada. A health care provider can fit a woman for a cervical cap, but then she must purchase one online or at certain family planning clinics (Society of Obstetricians and Gynaecologists of Canada [SOGC], 2012).

Cervical caps must be used with spermicidal jelly. Health care providers must write a prescription for the woman to obtain a cervical cap.

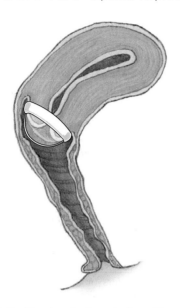

FIGURE 8.7 The rim-sized cervical cap fits over the cervix. It requires concomitant use of spermicide.

Mechanism of Action and Effectiveness. The cervical cap differs from the diaphragm in that a seal forms over the cervix, with the rim of the cap holding the mechanism in place. Failure rates range from 9% with perfect use to 16% with typical use for nulliparous women, and from 26% to 40% for multiparous women (Options for Sexual Health, 2012). The reason for such a high failure rate in multiparas is because pregnancy and childbirth cause the cervix to become softer and more pliable. This renders the cervical cap less capable of remaining in place.

Contraindications and Side Effects. Spermicide allergies, as well as an unevenly shaped cervix, are contraindications to use of the cervical cap. Women who are uncomfortable with touching their bodies would not be good candidates for the cervical cap, which requires insertion and removal directly into and from the vagina.

Client Teaching and Collaborative Interventions. The prescription-only cervical cap must be fitted by a health care provider. The client fills one third of the cap with spermicidal jelly or cream (Black et al., 2004c). If the cap is filled more than that, it becomes too slippery to handle. She should then insert the cap into the vagina over the cervix. After insertion, the client should gently try to dislodge the cap to ensure that the suction is intact; she should do this again after one minute. No additional spermicide is necessary for repeated acts of intercourse over the next 24 hours.

Clients should not use the cap with any petroleum-based products in the vagina, as they may weaken the device's structural integrity. The client should leave the cervical cap in place at least 6 hours but no longer than 24 hours after intercourse. She should not use it during menstruation or with any vaginal or cervical bleeding.

Removal is achieved by applying firm, pulling pressure on the rim or strap to break the suction. Following removal, the client should clean the cap with mild soap and water and dry it. The cervical cap does not protect against STIs. It is recommended that women have a follow-up Pap test after 3 months of use, then return to normal yearly screening (Black et al., 2004c; Hatcher et al., 2004).

Contraceptive Sponge

The **contraceptive sponge** fits over the woman's cervix and releases spermicide to prevent fertilization by absorbing and trapping sperm. The sponge ensures that the spermicide remains close to the cervix.

Mechanism of Action and Effectiveness. The sponge acts as a physical barrier between the cervix and the sperm. It is made of polyurethane, which traps and absorbs semen. Finally, the sponge regularly releases the built-in spermicide over a 24-hour period. The typical use failure rate ranges from 9% to 16% for nulliparous women and 20% to 32% for parous women (Fisher & Black, 2007; Options for Sexual Health, 2012).

Contraindications and Side Effects. Women who are uncomfortable with touching their bodies are not good candidates for the sponge. Some women find that correct insertion and removal are difficult. The device may cause irritation or allergic reactions to spermicide. Finally, all users must be cautioned not to leave the device in place for more than 24 hours because doing so can increase the risk for toxic shock syndrome.

Client Teaching and Collaborative Interventions. The client can insert the sponge up to 24 hours before intercourse. She does not need to remove or replace it to engage in more than one act of intercourse. The client needs to wait 6 hours after the last act of intercourse before removing the sponge, but she should not leave the sponge in place for more than 24 hours. The client should not use the sponge during menstruation. On its own, the contraceptive sponge is not a very effective contraceptive method, and should not be used without another form of contraception. They do, however, provide good secondary protection when used with condoms. Some women find it difficult to remove the sponge, or forget to take it out all together. Some may be allergic to the spermicide. By itself, the sponge will not protect against STIs (Options for Sexual Health, 2012). The sponge does not require a prescription. To insert the sponge, the client should hold the unpackaged device in one hand with the "dimple" side up and make sure that the loop is dangling under the sponge. Then the client needs to wet the sponge thoroughly with clean water, which will activate the spermicide. The client should squeeze the wet sponge gently until it becomes sudsy, but stop before she squeezes it dry. Next, the client should fold the sides upward until the sudsy sponge looks narrow and long, with the loop beneath dangling from one end of the fold to the other. The client should then point the folded end of the sponge toward the vagina for insertion, sliding the sponge into the vaginal opening as far as she can. Once the sponge is in place, the client should check to make sure that her cervix is not exposed and that she can still feel the string loop.

To remove the sponge, the client should wait at least 6 hours after the last act of intercourse. She should reach into the vagina with her finger to find the string loop. Then she should bear down and push the sponge toward the vaginal opening, while hooking the finger around the string loop or grasping the sponge between her thumb and forefinger. Once the sponge is used, it should be discarded.

Spermicidal Products

Spermicidal foam, cream, film, suppositories, and jelly are available over the counter. As already discussed, they are frequently used in conjunction with other barrier devices; diaphragms and cervical caps require their use for optimal effectiveness. The active ingredient in most spermicides is nonoxynol-9.

Spermicides act as a barrier at the cervix and decrease sperm motility on contact. The typical use failure rate of spermicide alone is between 6% and 21% (SOGC, 2012). When used with other barrier contraceptive devices, effectiveness increases. If used alone, spermicide does not protect against STIs.

Spermicide allergy is a contraindication for use. Symptoms may include genital irritation or burning. Clients may perceive the drainage of the foam or suppository from the vagina as messy or unappealing. When used during oral sex, partners may report an unpleasant taste.

To allow enough time for the spermicide to dissolve and coat the vagina, the client should insert film and suppositories at least 15 minutes, but not longer than 1 hour, before intercourse. Spermicidal foam is effective immediately after placement in the vagina. The couple should complete intercourse within 60 minutes of spermicidal insertion. For repeated acts of intercourse, they should use additional spermicide. The nurse instructs women using spermicide not to douche or bathe for at least 6 hours after intercourse.

Women at high risk for contracting HIV should not use spermicides, either alone or as part of another method, because repeated and high-dose use of the spermicide nonoxynol-9 has been associated with increased risk of vaginal lesions, which may increase the risk of acquiring HIV infection (Centers for Disease Control and Prevention, 2002; SOGC, 2012). The popular spermicide called nonoxynol-9 does not protect people from STIs as previously thought. Studies are ongoing in an attempt to prove the efficacy of microbicides in the interruption of the transmission of sexually transmitted diseases in general and HIV in particular. Microbicides are pharmacologic agents and chemical substances that are capable of killing or destroying microorganisms that commonly cause human infection. The use of microbicides could offer both primary protection, in the absence of condoms and secondary protection, if a condom breaks or slips off during intercourse. Research has not yet proven that microbicides are safe and effective in reducing the risk of HIV transmission during sexual activity with an infected partner, but it is ongoing and promising (Hillier, 2013).

Hormonal Methods

Hormonal methods of contraception have two variations. Combined methods use both estrogen and progestin, a synthetic form of progesterone. Progestin-only methods are prescribed for women who cannot take estrogen.

Combined hormonal methods have multiple mechanisms of action, including suppression of ovulation, thickening of cervical mucus, and thinning of the endometrium. Oral contraceptives have a number of noncontraceptive benefits that increase their desirability as an option (Fisher & Black, 2007). Combined hormonal methods include the COC, the transdermal contraceptive, and the vaginal contraceptive ring.

Progestin-only methods provide highly effective contraception and may be a good choice for breastfeeding women, smokers older than 35 years, hypertensive women, and those at risk for thromboembolic events. These methods include progestin-only pills such as depomedroxyprogesterone acetate (DMPA or Depo-Provera). Levonorgestrel injectables, which are subdermal contraceptive implants (the Norplant system), are no longer available in Canada. Mirena is an intrauterine system that combines the mechanisms of progestin with an IUD (see Intrauterine Methods).

Combined Oral Contraceptives

COCs rely on administration of estrogen and progestin together to control fertility. Most COCs are low dose and contain 20 to 35 µg of ethinyl estradiol. The progestins found in the majority of COCs are norethindrone, levonorgestrel, desogestrel, or norgestimate. Progestin provides the main mechanism for contraception (Black et al., 2004b), whereas estrogen stabilizes the endometrium to decrease breakthrough bleeding. The risk for thromboembolic events with the use of COCs has been the topic of much research. Current research indicates that for normal healthy women with no risk factors for venous thromboembolism, there is no increase in risk for deep vein thrombosis (DVT) when COCs are used (Reid, 2010). Furthermore, there is no increased risk of myocardial infarction (MI) and stroke events for healthy women (Fisher & Black, 2007).

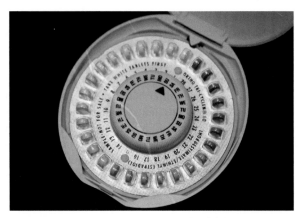

FIGURE 8.8 A sample pack of combined oral contraceptives.

● **BOX 8.2** **Contraindications to Use of Combined Oral Contraceptives**

- Migraines with focal neurologic symptoms
- Coronary artery disease or cerebral vascular disease
- Diabetes with retinopathy/nephropathy/neuropathy
- Hypertension (systolic ≥160 mm Hg or diastolic ≥100 mm Hg)
- Liver disease (cirrhosis)
- Breast or endometrial cancer
- Deep vein thrombosis (current or past history)
- Unexplained vaginal bleeding

Types. Various COCs are available by prescription, including biphasic and triphasic (dosages of estrogen or progestin vary) and monophasic (dosages are constant). They come in 28-day packs, which include 21 active pills and 7 placebos, and 21-day packs, which contain only active pills (Fig. 8.8). Alternatively, extended cycle regimes are also available (see Continuous or Extended Hormone Contraception).

Mechanism of Action and Effectiveness. COCs prevent pregnancy primarily by suppressing ovulation, thickening cervical mucus, decreasing tubal motility, and thinning the endometrium. Suppression of the hypothalamus—pituitary–ovarian axis prevents ovulation because the exogenous hormones provide negative feedback to the hypothalamus' secretion of gonadotropin-releasing hormone. This in turn suppresses pituitary secretion of follicle-stimulating hormone (FSH) and luteinizing hormone (LH). Without proper circulating levels of FSH and LH, the ovaries will not develop a follicle and release an egg.

Without follicular development and its accompanying surge in estrogen production, the cervical mucus fails to thin as is normal before ovulation. As a result, penetration of the mucus by the sperm becomes difficult. Without normal FSH or LH stimulation, the thinner endometrial lining decreases the ability of a fertilized egg to implant. The thinner lining also leads to decreased menstrual flow for most women. COCs have a typical user failure rate ranging from 1% to 8% (Fisher & Black, 2007).

Contraindications and Side Effects. Side effects associated with taking COCs are discussed with women and may include irregular bleeding or spotting, breast tenderness, nausea, and headache (Fisher & Black, 2007). Reid (2010) and his colleagues reviewed the literature on the use of oral contraceptives and the risks of venous thromboembolism. Conclusions from this review indicate that venous thromboembolism in healthy women

who take oral contraceptives is a rare event; the risk increases from 5 in 10,000 to 9 to 10 in 10,000 (Reid, 2010). To put things in perspective, the risks of venous thromboembolism for women in pregnancy is 29 in 10,000 and increases to 300 to 400 in 10,000 in the immediate postpartum period.

Women who wish to use COCs must be carefully screened for several contraindications, listed in Box 8.2. Users should not be pregnant, less than 6 weeks postpartum, or breastfeeding. Research indicates that modern oral contraceptives have lower doses of estrogen (ethinyl estriol) and carry a lower risk of venous thromboembolism than their earlier ancestors, which contained much higher levels of estrogen. Women with risk factors for venous thromboembolism, such as obesity, smoking, and hypertension, should be counselled to choose an alternate form of contraception or consider the progestin-only pill (Fisher & Black, 2007).

Women with a family history of breast cancer have not been found to have an additional risk for breast cancer when taking oral contraceptives (Burkman et al., 2004). Women with a current history of breast cancer should consider nonhormonal options for contraception first, such as IUD or barrier methods (Black et al., 2004b; McNaught & Reid, 2006). Women with renal, kidney, or adrenal disease should not take Yasmin, which contains a progestin called drospirenone that may increase potassium levels in their body (Archer, 2001; Options for Sexual Health, 2012). Drospirenone may help clients with premenstrual symptoms, water retention, and bloating resulting in monthly weight gain (Foidart, 2005; Krattenmacher, 2000; Options for Sexual Health, 2012).

Less serious side effects include breakthrough bleeding, breast tenderness, headaches, and nausea. Often, these side effects decrease after 1 to 2 months of use. Taking the pill in the evening or with food may help alleviate nausea. Some women gain weight while taking COCs, but average weight gain is no different than in women taking placebos (Hatcher et al., 2004). There has been no demonstrated infertility following any length of use.

Potentially beneficial side effects include decreased acne; lighter and shorter menstrual flow and thus a decreased risk for anemia; and decreased dysmenorrhea (Black et al., 2004b; Burkman et al., 2004; Fisher & Black, 2007). A reduced risk for endometrial and ovarian cancer has been documented (Burkman et al., 2004; Grimes, 2001; Gross & Schlesselman, 2003). In addition, there is a lower risk for colorectal cancer (Fisher & Black, 2007) ovarian cysts, and benign breast disease (Hatcher et al., 2004).

Client Teaching and Collaborative Interventions. The nurse should instruct the client to start the COCs as prescribed, on either the first day of her menstrual period or the first Sunday within her menstrual period. The client should use a backup method of contraception for the first week. If the woman has been instructed to take COCs continuously (monophasic only), she will skip the placebo pills and start a new pack. Otherwise, she may expect a menstrual period during the placebo week. The nurse should encourage women to take the placebos to maintain the scheduled dosing and as a reminder to start a new package. Occasionally, women do not have a menstrual flow; a pregnancy test is indicated if they have missed any pills or taken any late during that pack.

The client needs to take the pill at the same time each day, within 2 to 3 hours. Otherwise, she may experience breakthrough bleeding or pregnancy. For one missed or late pill, the nurse should instruct the client to take the pill as soon as she remembers and continue to take one pill daily until the end of the pack (Guilbert et al., 2008). If the missed pill was at the beginning of the pack, the health care provider may offer her emergency contraception (discussed later in this chapter) (Guilbert et al., 2008; Hatcher et al., 2004). The client may choose to take missed pills 12 hours apart to avoid nausea. For two missed pills, the woman should take a pill every 12 hours until her regimen is caught up, and be offered emergency contraception, again using a backup method for 1 week.

With three or more missed pills, the nurse should instruct the woman to contact her primary health care provider (Guilbert et al., 2008). She may be offered emergency contraception and counselled to use a backup method of contraception until her next menses, when she would start a new pack of pills. As with any restart, a week of backup contraception is advised.

There is controversy about whether the concurrent use of antibiotics decreases the efficacy of COCs (Black et al., 2004b). Current research advises that additional contraceptive precautions are no longer required when using combined hormonal contraception (CHC) with antibiotics (Faculty of Sexual & Reproductive Healthcare Clinical Guidance, 2012). Herbal preparations

containing St. John's wort may lead to decreased effectiveness (Redmond & Self, 2002) and require backup contraception with concurrent use.

The nurse instructs women to monitor for dangerous side effects. A helpful mnemonic is ACHES (Box 8.3).

A woman just starting or restarting COCs will be given 3 months of the pills and instructed to return to her health care provider, before refills are needed, for assessment of blood pressure and evaluation for side effects. See Teaching Tips 8.1.

Transdermal Contraceptive Patch

The **transdermal contraceptive patch** (Evra) has been available in Canada since January 2004. It is a 4×4 cm beige patch that sticks to a woman's skin and continuously releases 20 μg of ethinyl estradiol and 150 μg of the progestin norelgestromin (the primary metabolite of norgestimate) per day (SOGC, 2012). The patch provides an alternative delivery system of estrogen and progestin (Fig. 8.9). The woman applies the patch to clean, dry skin on the first day of her menstrual period. The patch may be placed on the buttocks, abdomen, or upper outer arm, but not on the breasts. The patch is changed every 7 days for 3 weeks. The patch is either not worn in the fourth week to allow for menstruation, or else may be worn continuously to avoid menses. The

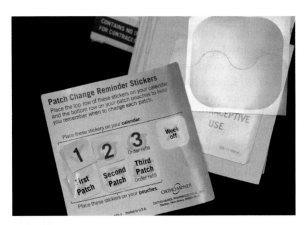

FIGURE 8.9 The client changes the transdermal contraceptive patch weekly. She can apply it to the arms, trunk, or buttocks, but not the breasts.

● TEACHING TIPS 8.1 Starting Oral Contraceptives

For a woman starting oral contraceptives for the first time, the nurse carefully reviews the following information:

- *How to start:* Depending on the prescription, the woman may begin taking the first active hormone pill on the first day of menses or on the Sunday after menses begins. She may request to start on a Sunday because then her menstrual flow would occur only on weekdays. It is important for her to understand to start on the first Sunday of her menses (she may still be bleeding), not to wait for the Sunday after menses ends. Have a sample pack available so that the woman can see how to remove the pill from the packaging. Allow time for questions. Advise the client to use a backup method of contraception for the first week. Discuss alternatives for backup method; advise her to always have her choice available.
- *How to take the pill:* The woman needs to take the pill at the same time each day (within 2 to 3 hours). Ask her when she thinks she will take it: does she wake up or go to bed at a consistent time? If not, she may want to set a watch timer at, for example, noon to remind her. To help her remember to take the pill, she might choose to put the pack next to her toothbrush or something else that she uses every day (eg, deodorant). Counsel her regarding common side

effects: nausea, breakthrough bleeding, and breast tenderness. If she experiences nausea, she can take the pill with food or at a different time of day (switching from morning to evening would constitute a late pill and necessitate backup for 7 days). Breakthrough bleeding is worse in smokers. Women should be counselled to quit smoking while using oral contraceptives, or to choose another method.
- *What to do if she misses pills:* For one missed or late pill, the client should take the pill as soon as she remembers and use backup contraception for 7 days thereafter. If the missed pill was at the beginning of the pack, the health care provider may offer her emergency contraception (Guilbert et al., 2008; Hatcher et al., 2004). The client may choose to take missed pills 12 hours apart to avoid nausea. For two missed pills, the woman should take a pill every 12 hours until she is caught up, and be offered emergency contraception, again using a backup method for 1 week. With three or more missed pills, the woman should contact her primary health care provider.
- Danger signs include abdominal pain, chest pain, headaches, eye problems (blurred or lost vision), and severe leg pain.

---

patch is changed weekly. The transdermal contraceptive patch requires a prescription.

Mechanism of Action and Effectiveness. The mechanisms of action and effectiveness of the transdermal contraceptive are the same as for COCs; it works by stopping the ovaries from releasing an egg and by thickening the cervical mucus, making it difficult for sperm motility. It can cause endometrial atrophy, which makes implantation more difficult (SOGC, 2012). Typical failure rates for the patch are about 3% (Fisher & Black, 2007). Patch users have significantly better compliance (correct and consistent use) than pill users (Hatcher et al., 2004). Studies also have shown a slightly higher failure rate in women who weigh more than 90 kg (Black et al., 2004b; Fisher & Black, 2007). Although it is not understood why heavier women have a higher risk for pregnancy, theories include decreased absorption or decreased hormone levels resulting from increased blood volume (Contraceptive Technology Update, 2002; SOGC, 2012).

Contraindications and Side Effects. Contraindications and side effects of COCs also apply to users of the transdermal contraceptive. In addition, users of the patch may experience skin reactions at the application site. Rotation of the application site is encouraged.

Research (Cole et al., 2007) has shown that users of the contraceptive patch have small but increased risk

of developing clots in their legs and lungs compared with women who use traditional contraceptive pills. There is a warning on the label that the patch delivers a higher dosage of estrogen than do birth control pills. Other independent personal factors can also exacerbate the chance of developing blood clots, such as smoking, obesity, physical inactivity, and surgery.

Client Teaching and Collaborative Interventions. Ortho Evra is prescribed in boxes of three transdermal patches. The client should start the patch on either the first day of the next menstrual period or the first Sunday within the next menstrual period. If she applies the patch within 5 days of the onset of menses, the woman needs no backup contraception. One week from the day of original application, she should remove the patch and apply a new one. She will not apply a patch on the fourth week and will experience withdrawal bleeding (have a menstrual period). If the health care provider prescribes a continuous patch regimen (9 weeks of continual dosing), the client starts a new box every 3 weeks.

Studies have shown effective adhesiveness of the patch with showering and even daily swimming (Zacur et al., 2002). To promote adhesion, the client should press the patch firmly if it seems to be releasing from the skin. If the patch will not adhere, the client should remove the current patch and apply a new patch for the rest of that week.

If the woman applies the patch 1 to 2 days late, it remains effective. If she is more than 2 days late in applying a new patch, she should start a new package when her menstrual flow begins or on the first Sunday within her next menstrual flow. The client should use backup contraception until she has applied the new patch, if used within the first 5 days of menses (Guilbert et al., 2008).

The nurse should counsel the client to monitor for ACHES (see Box 8.3). Women just starting or restarting use of the transdermal contraceptive should return to their health care provider after 3 months for assessment of blood pressure and evaluation for side effects. Women are counselled that the patch does not protect against sexually transmitted diseases.

The client should be careful not to apply the patch to any area on which she uses lotions, makeup, moisturizers, or creams. She also should avoid application to any red or irritated skin area, as well as to sites with open sores, abrasions, or cuts. If the skin at the application site becomes mildly irritated (a normal side effect), the client can remove the current application and apply a new patch to a new location (Fisher & Black, 2007).

If a patch becomes loose, the client should remove it and replace it with a new one. She does not need additional contraception if she is certain that the patch has been detached for 24 hours or less. If the patch has been loose for more than 24 hours or if the client is unsure of how long it was detached from the skin, she should remove it and apply a new one (Guilbert et al., 2008). She also will need to begin a new 4-week cycle, with a new day 1 and a new day for changing the patch. For the first week of the new cycle, the woman needs to use backup contraception, such as a condom with spermicide.

A client who wants to discontinue use of the patch as part of her plans for conception should first discuss this situation with her health care provider. The provider guides the client in decision making involving the best timing for attempting pregnancy. He or she may recommend that the woman use nonhormonal contraception until her natural menstrual cycles are regularly established to better facilitate the dating of any pregnancy that ensues.

Vaginal Contraceptive Ring

The vaginal contraceptive ring (NuvaRing) is available in Canada. This 2-in (54 mm) flexible ring contains estrogen and progestin, which are released slowly over 21 days (Fig. 8.10). The mechanism of action is suppression of ovulation, thickening of cervical mucus, and thinning in the lining of the uterus. The typical use failure rate is 8%, similar to that of COCs (Black et al., 2004b; Fisher & Black, 2007; Stewart & Barnhart, 2002). The vaginal contraceptive ring requires a prescription.

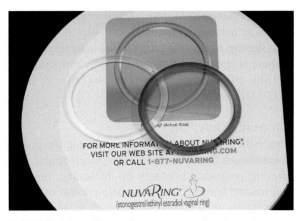

FIGURE 8.10 The vaginal contraceptive ring releases estrogen and progestin slowly over 21 days to suppress ovulation.

Contraindications for the vaginal contraceptive ring are the same as those for COCs (Hatcher et al., 2004; SOGC, 2012). Some users may experience vaginitis or vaginal discharge (Veres et al., 2004). Women also may experience headache, nausea, weight gain, or breast pain (Fisher & Black, 2007). This device may not be acceptable to users who are not comfortable inserting and removing the ring from the vagina.

The client compresses the ring between two fingers and inserts the ring up into the vagina. Clients may find insertion easier while standing with one leg up, squatting, or lying down. The woman should insert the ring during the first 5 days of her menstrual period. She uses a backup method of contraception for the first 7 days and should remove the ring after 3 weeks, which will result in withdrawal bleeding. After 7 ring-free days, the client should insert a new ring.

If the client leaves a ring in up to 35 days, she may remove it and insert a new ring after 7 days without concern for pregnancy. If the client leaves a ring in place for longer than 35 days, she should use a backup method of contraception until she has a menses, when she may reinsert a new ring. She also should use a backup method for the first 7 days (Guilbert et al., 2008).

The client should not remove the ring for intercourse; however, she can remove the ring for up to 3 hours without decreasing contraceptive efficacy. The client should not douche and may use any necessary vaginal medications.

In rare cases, the ring may be expelled spontaneously, related to intercourse, tampon removal, or straining during bowel movements. An essential teaching item is for the nurse to remind the woman that she should always have an extra ring available in case the ring is lost. The woman and partner usually cannot feel the ring during intercourse. Studies indicate that the ring does not hinder sexual comfort for women or their partners (Novak et al., 2003; SOGC, 2012).

The woman using the vaginal contraceptive ring needs to monitor for ACHES (see Box 8.3). Women just starting or restarting the vaginal contraceptive ring require assessment of blood pressure and evaluation for side effects after 3 months of use (Fisher & Black, 2007; Hatcher et al., 2004).

Progestin-Only Pills

Progestin-only pills, also known as minipills, provide a continuous dose of progestin (no placebo pills). They prevent pregnancy primarily by thickening the cervical mucus; however, they also help prevent ovulation. In addition, they inhibit implantation by thinning the endometrium. The typical use failure rate is 8%, but effectiveness approaches 100% in women with perfect use (Fisher & Black, 2007).

Contraindications include unexplained vaginal bleeding, pregnancy, history of breast cancer, and liver disease (McNaught & Reid, 2006). Gastrointestinal disease that interferes with absorption (active colitis), as well as certain medications (eg, rifampin, certain anticonvulsants, St. John's wort, griseofulvin), because they increase hepatic clearance, are also contraindications. It was previously thought that there is an interaction with orlistat (Xenical), a prescription weight-loss medication, but this has been disproven for women taking progestin-only pills (Faculty of Sexual and Reproductive Healthcare Clinical Guidance, 2012). Breakthrough bleeding is a common side effect in women taking progestin-only pills, as are amenorrhea, ovarian cysts, and headaches (Fisher & Black, 2007).

The client should begin her pills as prescribed, on the first 5 days of menses, immediately postpartum, or after the 6-week postpartum examination if she has not resumed sexual relations. She should use a backup method of contraception for 7 days. It is very important for the user to take the pill at the same time each day, within 2 to 3 hours. If she takes a pill late, she may experience breakthrough bleeding or pregnancy. A woman who takes a pill more than 3 hours late should use backup protection for 48 hours. She may also be offered emergency contraception if she has had intercourse in the past 3 to 5 days (Guilbert et al., 2008; Hatcher et al., 2004), As well, she should continue to take one pill daily at the same time each day.

Recent evidence exists to dispel the belief that broad-spectrum antibiotics decrease the effectiveness of progestin-only pills (Faculty of Sexual and Reproductive Healthcare Clinical Guidance, 2012). Progestin-only pills are not gut flora–dependant and therefore are not affected by courses of antibiotics. The nurse should advise women with vomiting and diarrhea to take additional contraceptive precautions during periods of illness with these symptoms because of the risks of contraceptive failure.

Depomedroxyprogesterone Acetate (DMPA or Depo-Provera)

DMPA had been available internationally for 25 years and was approved for use in Canada in 1997 (Black, 2006). This injectable progestin is given intramuscularly into the deltoid or gluteus maximus muscle every 11 to 13 weeks.

DMPA prevents pregnancy by suppressing ovulation through inhibition of the secretion of pituitary gonadotropins, thickening the cervical mucus, thinning the endometrium, and slowing tubal motility. It has a typical use failure rate of 3% (Fisher & Black, 2007; Hatcher et al., 2004). Contraindications for use include pregnancy (known or suspected), unexplained vaginal bleeding, and women with current breast cancer (Black, 2006; Fisher & Black, 2007; McNaught & Reid, 2006). DMPA does not contain estrogen, so it is a good choice for women who are breastfeeding, are over 35 and are smokers, have a history of clotting disorders, have hypertension, or who experience migraines (Black, 2006). Relative contraindications include women with a history of ischemic heart disease, or liver disease (SOGC, 2012). A common side effect of DMPA is irregular bleeding; users also experience weight gain at an average of 2.5 kg in the first year (Fisher & Black, 2007; Hatcher et al., 2004). Other side effects include amenorrhea, breast tenderness, headaches, tenderness at the injection site, mood disturbances, and decreased libido (Black, 2006; Hatcher et al., 2004; SOGC, 2012). In addition, women may experience amenorrhea for many months and nonovulatory cycles for more than 1 year after cessation of DMPA, with an average return to fertility 9 to 10 months after the last injection (Black, 2006; Hatcher et al., 2004).

Women begin DMPA during the first 5 days of a menstrual period or immediately postpartum. If given at any other time in the menstrual cycle, DMPA takes 2 weeks to become effective. Breastfeeding women may choose to wait 6 weeks until their milk supply is established, because high doses of exogenous progesterone may interfere with the stimulus for milk synthesis (Hatcher et al., 2004). Women starting DMPA should use backup contraception for the first 7 days. Women can expect irregular menstrual bleeding for the first year of use. Amenorrhea is also likely and is not harmful, but women need to monitor for symptoms of pregnancy.

Women should return for their next injection in 11 to 13 weeks. It is helpful for the nurse to provide a calendar that lists the next visit (Freeman, 2004). If the next injection is scheduled at 12 weeks, this would provide a 1-week "grace period" if the woman misses her appointment. If a woman is more than 90 days past the last injection, the nurse may counsel her to return during her next menses to receive her next injection. Because of the length of time it may take for menses to resume, clinicians may choose to give an injection without a menses if they are certain the woman is not pregnant.

Long-term effects of DMPA on bone mineralization resulted in a warning by the United States Food and Drug Administration (FDA) in 2004. Product information inserts now include information about the potential risks for long-term use on bone demineralization, and recommend the use of calcium and Vitamin D supplementation (Robinson, 2005). Regular exercise will assist in maintaining bone density and preventing weight gain (see Chapter 2). The nurse should also offer DMPA users advice on healthy nutrition. To monitor for allergic reactions, the nurse may ask women to wait in the office for 20 minutes after injection. Women who experience heavy bleeding require screening for cervical infection, cancer, pregnancy, and anemia. Clinicians may advise the use of ibuprofen, 800 mg three times a day for 3 days, estrogen daily for 5 days, or the addition of COCs for 1 to 2 months to control bleeding (Hatcher et al., 2004). A woman considering pregnancy within 1 year may not be an ideal candidate for Depo-Provera because there is an average 10-month delay in return to fertility. DMPA does not provide any protection against STIs.

 Veena, the 26-year-old woman seeking contraceptive options, verbalizes an interest in combined hormonal contraceptive methods, but states, "I'm terrible with remembering to take pills." What alternatives could the nurse suggest?

Intrauterine Methods

IUDs are plastic T-shaped objects inserted into the uterus for contraception (Fig. 8.11). Several models of IUDs were available in the 1970s until studies showed that certain types, including the Dalkon Shield, increased risks for uterine perforation and **pelvic inflammatory disease (PID)**. Currently, two types of intrauterine contraceptives are available in Canada: the copper IUD (Flexi-T and Nova-T), which are made of copper and plastic and work by preventing implantation. The second intrauterine system, known as IUS (Mirena), is made of plastic and contains a small amount of progesterone (Black et al., 2004b; Fisher & Black, 2007).

A physician, midwife, or nurse practitioner inserts the IUD during the woman's menses, midcycle, or immediately postpartum. Expulsion is least likely if insertion occurs at midcycle. The health care provider performs a bimanual examination with a speculum in place (see Chapter 2). He or she then places the IUD, contained inside an insertion tube, into the uterine cavity and then withdraws the tube and then cuts the string

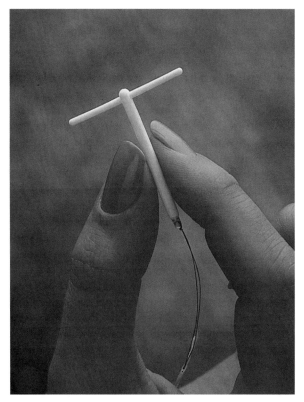

FIGURE 8.11 Intrauterine devices (IUDs) are inserted by a health care provider directly into the uterus.

to approximately 2.5 cm. The client may feel some discomfort or cramping during the procedure.

Use of IUDs is not advised in nulliparous women. Pregnancy that occurs with an IUD in place must be carefully assessed due to the risks of ectopic pregnancy.

Women should monitor for serious side effects with IUDs, using the mnemonic PAINS:

- **P**eriod late or abnormal spotting (indicating a possible pregnancy)
- **A**bdominal pain or pain with intercourse (indicating a possible infection)
- **I**nfection exposure (to any STI) or abnormal vaginal discharge (any new discharge or change in discharge)
- **N**ot feeling well, fever, chills
- **S**tring missing, longer or shorter

Women should check to ensure that the string is still in place after each menses. They should also check after insertion for any problems, because these devices come with a 3-month warranty. If the woman changes sexual partners, she should combine a barrier method such as latex condoms to protect against STIs.

Copper IUD

The copper IUD prevents fertilization by creating a hostile uterine environment in which copper ions inhibit sperm motility and an inflammatory endometrial process phagocytizes the sperm. It provides 5 years of contraception with a 0.8% typical use failure rate (SOGC, 2012). Use is appropriate for breastfeeding women.

Contraindications to the copper IUD include women who are not in a monogamous relationship (at risk for STIs), are HIV positive, are pregnant, or have undiagnosed vaginal bleeding, cervicitis, pelvic infection, recent endometritis, suspected uterine or cervical cancer, or an allergy to copper. Side effects of the copper IUD include increased menstrual flow and dysmenorrhea, anemia, risk for uterine perforation, and a vasovagal reaction with insertion or expulsion. For these reasons, women who normally experience heavy menstrual flow and dysmenorrhea are not good candidates for the copper IUD.

In most countries, the copper IUD is the most popular IUD. Its very low failure rate makes its effectiveness comparable to that of surgical sterilization.

Advantages to use of the copper IUD generally outweigh the risks for women who have never given birth and are younger than 20 years of age. These devices can be safely inserted at any point in the menstrual cycle, as long as the provider feels reasonably confident that the client is not pregnant.

Mirena

Mirena thickens the cervical mucus, impairs sperm migration, and alters the endometrium to prevent implantation. It also inhibits ovulation. Mirena provides 5 years of contraception and has a 0.1% typical use failure rate (Fisher & Black, 2007; Hatcher et al., 2004). Contraindications for the Mirena IUD are the same as for with the copper IUD (except allergy to copper), breast cancer, undiagnosed vaginal bleeding, and liver disease. Mirena users may experience irregular bleeding or amenorrhea, expulsion, uterine perforation (rare), ovarian cysts, headaches, or breast tenderness. They are at decreased risk for ectopic pregnancy and often have decreased flow and decreased dysmenorrhea. Mirena also may be used in the treatment of endometriosis, menorrhagia, or uterine fibroids.

Behavioural Methods

Some women, for personal or religious reasons, choose not to use devices or hormonal methods for contraception, but still wish to avoid pregnancy. Health care providers may instruct such clients about behavioural methods of controlling their pregnancy status.

Abstinence

Abstinence means not engaging in vaginal intercourse. Some people also include refraining from anal and oral sex as part of abstinence. Abstaining from vaginal intercourse is the most reliable method of contraception because it provides no opportunity for sperm to enter the woman's reproductive tract to fertilize an ovum. It can also help control the spread of many STIs.

Those who follow abstinence do so for various reasons. For some people, it coincides with religious, cultural, or ethical beliefs. Others simply wish to take no chances of becoming pregnant. Abstinent clients may participate in other forms of sexual behaviour that they consider "safe" or "acceptable." Examples include kissing, masturbation, sexual fantasy, and oral sex.

Fertility Awareness and Natural Family Planning

Fertility awareness methods of contraception focus on determining a woman's time of ovulation. Some fertility awareness methods rely on the use of barrier devices if a couple engages in vaginal intercourse during the fertile period. **Natural family planning** relies on sex only during nonfertile periods and abstinence during the determined period of fertility. For both methods, clients may choose to follow the rhythm (calendar) method, the cervical mucus ovulation detection method, the symptothermal method, or the Standard Days method (SOGC, 2012). All have a typical use failure rate of 25%.

Clients who choose natural family planning must be highly motivated to abstain from intercourse during the fertile days. They must also be capable of understanding the concept of fertile days and tracking daily temperature. If using the cervical mucus ovulation detection or symptothermal method, the client must be comfortable with checking her cervical mucus. Breastfeeding, recent childbirth, or pregnancy loss may affect signs of fertility and thus make these methods harder to use. There are no side effects to fertility awareness methods (Fig. 8.12).

 At the start of the chapter, you met Kenya, a 19-year-old seeking information about natural family planning. What assessment data are critical to ascertain when developing her teaching plan?

Rhythm (Calendar) Method. The rhythm (calendar) method requires the client to track the length of her menstrual cycles. The nurse should explain that ovulation takes place 12 to 16 days before the start of the next menstrual flow. The first day of the fertile time cannot be predicted with perfect accuracy, but may be estimated by tracking six menstrual cycles and subtracting 18 from the shortest cycle (day 1 or first day of menses to day 1 or first day of next menses). The last day of the fertile period would be the longest cycle length minus 11. To prevent conception, the client should use a barrier method or abstain from intercourse on the first day of fertility through the last day of the fertile period. Thus, a woman with a longest cycle of 35 days and a

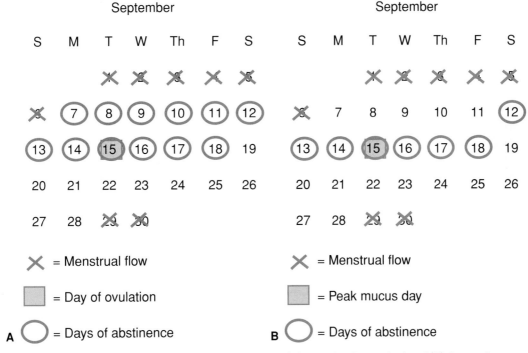

FIGURE 8.12 Sample logs kept by clients using (**A**) the calendar method and (**B**) the cervical mucus ovulation detection method. For both methods, the days circled in red indicate times when the client should abstain from intercourse or use a barrier method if engaging in intercourse to minimize chances of conception.

shortest cycle of 30 days would use a barrier method or abstain from day 12 (30 minus 18) to day 24 (35 minus 11). Women with irregular cycles cannot accurately predict ovulation; therefore, they are not good candidates for the calendar method.

Cervical Mucus Ovulation Detection Method. The nurse should teach clients who want to use this method about the changes in cervical mucus that occur around ovulation. At this time, a woman's vaginal discharge may become clear and stretchy (indicating fertile mucus). The nurse should teach the client to check at the introitus with her fingers or tissue paper for the appearance and character of mucus each morning for several months. Women must have abstained from sexual intercourse for 24 hours to make the test interpretable. To prevent pregnancy, clients should use a barrier method or abstain from intercourse at the first appearance of fertile mucus through the third day after the last appearance of fertile mucus.

Basal Body and Symptothermal Methods. The basal body temperature method is based on the woman's temperature changes around the time of ovulation. Following the postovulation elevation of progesterone, basal body temperature will rise in the luteal phase of the cycle by approximately 0.5°C with ovulation. The client needs to take her temperature every day at approximately the same time, usually when she first awakens, and definitely before getting out of bed or eating, which may alter the temperature. Use of a digital or basal body thermometer is advisable. A basal body thermometer is specially calibrated with a smaller range and thus larger and easy-to-read numbers. The client also should document if she overslept or was ill, which may affect her temperature. If tracking basal body temperature, the client should abstain or use a barrier method until 3 consecutive days of elevated temperature have passed (Hatcher et al., 2004).

As the temperature drop may not always occur, the symptothermal method, which combines basal body temperature with cervical mucus changes, provides more accuracy in predicting the fertile period. Women using the symptothermal method mark the beginning of the fertile period with the appearance of fertile mucus and the end of the fertile period with the fourth day after an elevated temperature. See Nursing Care Plan 8.1 for more information.

Standard Days Method. Women with menstrual cycles that last 26 to 32 days can use this method, which relies on the use of a standard definition of fertility that identifies day 8 to 19 as fertile days. During these days, a couple should abstain or use a barrier method of contraception. Another method of tracking standard days is through the use of cycle beads (fertility necklace) consisting of different-coloured beads. The various colours represent the first day of the cycle (red bead), nonfertile days (6 brown beads), fertile days (12 white beads), and more nonfertile days (13 more brown beads)

NURSING CARE PLAN 8.1

●

The Client Interested in Natural Family Planning

Recall Kenya from the beginning of this chapter. Assessment reveals menarche at age 12 years, with menstrual cycles every 30 to 31 days, lasting an average of 4 to 5 days. Kenya states, "Sometimes I get mild cramps on the first day, but then they disappear." She describes her flow as moderate with some small clots occasionally. "Darrell and I are hoping that we can use natural family planning. But neither of us is too sure what it involves."

NURSING DIAGNOSIS

Deficient Knowledge related to natural family planning (NFP) methods and their use

EXPECTED OUTCOMES

1. The client will identify methods for NFP.
2. The client will choose a contraceptive method of NFP that is realistic for her.

INTERVENTIONS	RATIONALES
Assess the client's level of understanding about NFP. Involve the partner in the discussions	Assessment provides a baseline to identify specific client needs and to develop an individualized teaching plan for both members of the couple
Explore the client's knowledge about NFP methods; correct any related misconceptions or myths; allow time for questions	Understanding the client's existing knowledge about this method allows the nurse to build on current information and gives opportunities to clarify or correct misinformation
Explore with the client her values and beliefs about use of a barrier method of contraception	Further knowledge of personal values and beliefs helps guide appropriate suggestions for the couple. Fertility awareness methods may involve use of a barrier method
Assess the client's level of comfort with touching her sexual organs and ability to do so	Some NFP methods require obtaining a sample of cervical mucus from the vaginal area to determine fertility. Discomfort with doing so may prohibit use of such methods
Teach the client about the various natural family planning methods, including the mechanism of action, degree of effectiveness, advantages and disadvantages, and steps of use for each	Information about each method provides a foundation from which the client can make an informed decision
Encourage the client to bring her partner to each visit to continue discussion of methods	Participation from the client's partner provides support and enhances the chances for a successful experience
Review menstrual cycle and ovulation; instruct client and partner in how to determine fertile period	NFP methods rely on determining ovulation and fertile periods

(continued)

NURSING CARE PLAN 8.1 ● The Client Interested in Natural Family Planning *(Continued)*

INTERVENTIONS	RATIONALES
Assess the client's and partner's degree of motivation for abstaining from sexual intercourse during fertile days.	Couples choosing NFP methods must be highly motivated to abstain from intercourse during fertile periods
Teach the client and partner how to use the method correctly; have couple return demonstrate/verbalize steps; provide reinforcement and reinstruction as necessary	Correct use of method enhances success

EVALUATION

1. The client states that she is comfortable with her choice of NFP method.
2. The client and partner verbalize steps for correct use of method chosen.
3. The client and partner state that they are motivated to achieve success with the method chosen and know how to implement the method.

(Fig. 8.13). The client moves a band forward by one bead each day, abstaining during the white beads, and moving the band to the red bead on the first day of the next menses (Arevalo et al., 2002).

Withdrawal

Withdrawal, or *coitus interruptus,* is the removal of the penis from the vagina before ejaculation to prevent the introduction of sperm into the vagina. This type of contraception is used by up to 9% of Canadian women (Black et al., 2004c). With a typical use failure rate of 27%, it has no contraindications or side effects (Hatcher et al., 2004; SOGC, 2012). Nevertheless, the man must be able to predict ejaculation and to control the urge to remain in the vagina. Before intercourse, the man should urinate to remove any sperm that may be present from a previous ejaculation; before insertion, he should wipe the penis clean of any pre-ejaculatory fluid.

Lactational Amenorrhea Method

The **lactational amenorrhea method** is appropriate for breastfeeding mothers in the first 6 months after childbirth, provided they have no menstrual periods and that their infants are breastfeeding exclusively (see Chapter 21). This method relies on suppression of ovulation due to the hormonal effects of breastfeeding. The method becomes less effective with the appearance of menses, supplementation with formula, or introduction of solids.

This method has no side effects; studies have shown that breastfeeding reduces the risk for breast cancer (Collaborative Group on Hormonal Factors in Breast Cancer & Beral, 2002) and facilitates postpartum weight loss (Hatcher et al., 2004). The typical use failure rate is 2% (Hatcher et al., 2004).

Lactational amenorrhea method suppresses ovulation because breastfeeding continually releases prolactin, which inhibits the FSH and the LH cycle. This

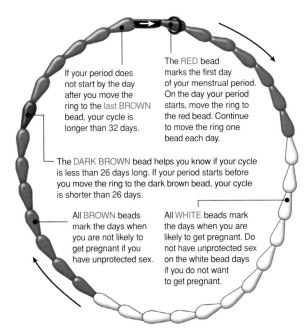

FIGURE 8.13 Fertility (cycle) beads can be used with the Standard Days method of fertility awareness.

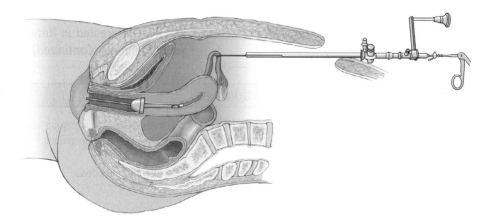

FIGURE 8.14 In tubal ligation, a section of each fallopian tube is removed, and the remaining ends are clipped, banded, or cauterized.

method is effective only if she is breastfeeding exclusively. In addition to instructing the woman not to supplement nursing with formula, juice, water, or food, the nurse also should inform the client that the baby should not use a pacifier. It is also important for the mother to breastfeed during the night, ideally between 2 and 4 AM. All these provisions give the baby adequate time at the breast, which maintains prolactin stimulation and prevents ovulation. In addition to any supplementation, the woman should not count on this method after the appearance of a menses or after 6 months postpartum.

Permanent Sterilization

If a client has made the decision not to have any or additional children, the couple may choose a permanent surgical method of contraception. The female method is called **bilateral tubal ligation**. The male method is called **vasectomy**.

Tubal ligation is done under general anaesthesia and interrupts the fallopian tubes to prevent the sperm and the ovum from meeting. Tubal ligation may be performed in three different time frames; postpartum (within 7 days); postabortion; or after decision to have this procedure separate from any pregnancy (Black et al., 2004c). The procedure involves removing a section of each tube and ligating the remaining ends through clips, bands, or cautery (Fig. 8.14). A transcervical approach involves the placement under hysteroscopy of a device consisting of two concentric metal coils into the fallopian tubes (Black et al., 2004c). Failure rates vary from 0.8% to 3.7%, with younger women experiencing higher failure rates (Hatcher et al., 2004).

The client must sign a consent form 30 days before tubal ligation. The procedure is not readily reversible; therefore, it is important to ascertain that the woman is sure in her decision. One study has shown regret after 14 years in 40% of women younger than 30 years having tubal ligation (Hatcher et al., 2004). Research has

shown that women who have had a tubal ligation are at lower risk for ovarian cancer (Hankinson et al., 2012). Potential complications include wound infection, bladder or vessel damage, hemorrhage, and death.

Male sterilization, or vasectomy, involves ligation or cauterization of the vas deferens, preventing delivery of sperm (Fig. 8.15). This procedure is safer than tubal

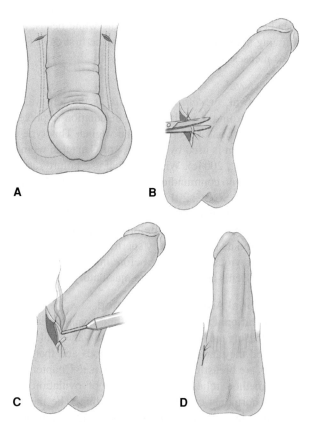

A   B

C   D

FIGURE 8.15 **A:** Vasectomy involves ligation or cauterization of the vas deferens to prevent delivery of sperm. **B:** The surgeon cuts through the vas deferens. **C:** The ends of the vas deferens are cauterized and **(D)** sutured.

ligation, as it does not require general anaesthetic and provides a typical use failure rate of 0.15% (Hatcher et al., 2004). Possible side effects include hematoma, bruising, wound infection, or adverse reaction to local anaesthesia. Vasectomy has not been shown to interfere with sexual function. Men should also return for two sperm counts of zero before depending on the vasectomy for contraception.

Both vasectomy and tubal ligation are considered permanent. Even though vasectomy reversal is possible, the nurse can counsel men and their partners to consider this option carefully to prevent regret.

Essure Micro-Inserts

This system is an irreversible nonsurgical birth control method in which a small flexible device is inserted into a woman's fallopian tubes. The device remains permanently in the tubes, and the body's connective tissue grows over the insert, blocking the tubes and preventing pregnancy. The device does not become effective for 90 days and requires a pelvic x-ray with injection of dye to confirm that the fallopian tubes are blocked. Another method of birth control must be used until the confirmatory tests have been completed. Women who have had the Essure procedure have reported little discomfort and have returned to normal activity more quickly compared with women who have had a tubal ligation (Duffy et al., 2005). The third generation of Essure micro-inserts was approved by Health Canada in 2007. New clinical trials are under way for the next-generation procedure that uses more advanced technology to eliminate the 90-day waiting period to confirm permanent birth control. The new procedure requires a simple noninvasive transvaginal ultrasound, immediately following the insertion, to confirm the success of the procedure, but is not yet readily available.

Emergency Contraception

Nurses may counsel all women at risk for unplanned pregnancy regarding **emergency contraception** in the event of rape or contraceptive failure (eg, condom breakage, missed pills, failure to use method). Previously called the "morning-after pill," this method has been renamed emergency contraception to reflect its effectiveness up to 5 days after intercourse and the inclusion of the copper IUD, which can be inserted up to 7 days after intercourse.

Emergency contraception prevents pregnancy through two methods: the administration of hormones that delay ovulation and may prevent implantation or thicken cervical mucus (see Table 8.2), or through a postcoital insertion of the copper IUD to prevent implantation. Emergency contraception does not abort an established pregnancy. There are three hormonal preparations available in Canada. Plan B and NorLevo both contain levonorgestrel 750 µg. The woman takes two pills (750 µg each) as a single dose. Next Choice consists of two tablets of levonorgestrel 750 µg, which are taken 12 hours apart (Dunn & Guilbert, 2012). The Yuzpe method, available since the 1970s, contains 50 µg ethinyl estradiol and 250 µg of levonorgestrel, and two doses are taken 12 hours apart. Emergency contraception is effective for preventing pregnancy 75% to 89% of the time (Black et al., 2004a; Dunn & Guilbert, 2012). Rates improve if the method is given as soon as possible after unprotected intercourse, ideally in the first 24 hours. Postcoital insertion of an IUD has 100% effectiveness (Hatcher et al., 2004). Two antiprogestin preparations (RU486 and ulipristal acetate) have been shown to be highly effective as emergency contraceptives, but neither is approved in Canada (Glasier et al., 2010).

The only contraindication to the use of emergency contraception with the levonorgestrel method is a previously established pregnancy or undiagnosed vaginal bleeding. Also, women who should not use hormonal contraception for emergency contraception include those who have acute migraines or a history of deep venous thrombosis or pulmonary embolism, as studies have not included women who had contraindications to oral contraceptives (Black et al., 2004c). Side effects to the use of either type of hormonal contraception include nausea and vomiting, although Plan B and NorLevo have significantly fewer GI effects. Gravol may be taken to help control nausea. For side effects of the copper IUD, see Intrauterine Methods.

When it is established that the woman is not pregnant (through determination of recent menses or negative

● TABLE 8.2 **Dosages of Emergency Contraception**

Brand	Dose: Take up to 120 h after Unprotected Intercourse, Repeat in 12 h, Pills Per Dose	Ethinyl Estradiol (µg/Dose)	Levonorgestrel (µg/Dose)
Plan B	2	0	750
NorLevo	2	0	7,500
Next Choice	2	0	750
Ovral	2	50	250

pregnancy test), the copper IUD may be inserted by an appropriate health care provider. Women should be aware that emergency contraception is available and effective up to 5 days after unprotected intercourse (Dunn & Guilbert, 2012). The sooner it is provided, the more effective it is at preventing pregnancy. Hormonal emergency contraception is available in Canada without a prescription and can be obtained from a physician, a walk-in clinic, or birth control clinic. Women need to continue to use a method of contraception until their next menses. They may experience an early or delayed menses from delayed ovulation and should obtain a pregnancy test if no menses occurs in 2 to 3 weeks. Emergency contraception is not suitable as a continuous method of contraception; thus, women need to be informed of other methods.

Continuous or Extended Hormonal Contraception

Continuous or extended hormonal contraception has both contraceptive (preventing pregnancy) and noncontraceptive (decreasing the frequency of menstruation) benefits. Combined hormonal contraceptives, originally designed for cyclical use, have been found to be effective for continuous or extended use, with a typical use failure rate of 8%. CHC can be given orally (pill), vaginally (ring), or through the skin (patch). Benefits for women who, for quality-of-life reasons, choose to suppress menstruation for extended periods of time, are increasingly reported (Guilbert et al., 2007). A typical regimen varies between 63 days of hormone administration, followed by 7 hormone-free days, and 84 days of hormones followed by 7 hormone-free days. The side effects, similar to the cyclical counterparts, seem to lessen in intensity and frequency with use of the extended formulation. Convenience and increased compliance with contraceptive regimen are some of the advantages of this method. This regimen does not provide protection against STIs. An extended cycle regimen called Seasonale is now available in Canada that provides women with a 91-day cycle, resulting in four periods per year. This is achieved with 84 active days of therapy followed by 7 days of placebo (SOGC, 2012).

A newer version of menstrual-suppression contraception is Anya, a continuous-use contraceptive approved by Health Canada since 2010. This pill is taken 365 days per year and completely suppresses menstruation as well as the withdrawal bleeding normally experienced with traditional birth control pills. Discussion is required to ensure that women are comfortable with long-term suppression of menstruation with the continuous use of hormones (Repta & Clarke, 2011). Today's birth control pills contain far less estrogen and progestin than the ones from two generations ago, but there may be a longer-term risk of prolonged exposure and blood clots.

COLLABORATIVE CARE: THE CLIENT SEEKING FERTILITY CONTROL

Nurses who provide care to women about fertility control, family planning, and contraception have an opportunity to teach important information that will assist them with decision making. Nurses take a detailed history, listen to each woman's needs and concerns, and provide the detailed education and follow-up necessary for a woman to make the best choice for her and to successfully use the selected methods (Freeman, 2004).

Assessment

Assessment Tool 8.1 presents questions that can guide health history taking necessary for education about fertility control. Before initiating any teaching, the nurse obtains the client's full medical, sexual, and family history, ascertaining the client's sexual orientation, desire for pregnancy or its prevention, and any beliefs that may influence decisions guide the discussion. The need for protection against STIs is an indication for use of condoms, perhaps in addition to other methods focusing primarily on avoiding pregnancy. The client also may choose abstinence or one of the Fertility Awareness Methods or Natural Family Planning, and nurses should be able to provide guidance to women choosing these methods.

Because of the intimate nature of the questions asked, it is imperative for nurses to provide a nonjudgemental atmosphere in which clients feel free to share information. It helps to begin the interview with less intimidating questions, including past medical history or menstrual history, and to normalize the situation by letting clients know that the nurse asks all women these questions in order to provide the best information for the individual client (Fig. 8.16) in the most respectful way.

The nurse should not make assumptions about a client's level of sexual activity, or that she has had freedom in her relationships to choose effective contraceptive methods. For example, for some women, intimate partner violence precludes her from having control over her access and use of contraceptive methods. Understanding that a woman may have a history of intimate partner violence or may be currently experiencing it will assist the nurse to provide contraceptive counselling that meets the individual woman's needs and circumstances. The Association of Women's Health, Obstetrical and Neonatal Nurses (AWHONN) advises that questioning

● ASSESSMENT TOOL 8.1   **Fertility Control and Planning**

MENSTRUAL HISTORY

- How old were you when you had your first period?
- What day did your last menstrual period start?
- Was it a normal period?
- How often do you have a menstrual period?
- How many days are there from the first day of one menstrual period to the first day of the next period?
- How many days do you bleed?
- Do you have cramping with your periods? If so, what do you take for them?

FAMILY, MEDICAL, AND OBSTETRIC HISTORY

- Have you or anyone in your family ever had a heart attack or stroke? If so, at what age?
- Have you or anyone in your family ever had breast cancer?
- Have you or anyone in your family ever had a blood clot or clotting disorder?
- Have you ever had the following:
  - High blood pressure?
  - Migraine headaches? If so, do you have any visual changes (blurred vision, seeing spots) or changes in sensation (numbness or tingling in your hands or feet) with these headaches?
- Have you had any unexplained vaginal bleeding?
- Do you have varicose veins?
- Have you ever had a urinary tract infection? If so, how many have you had?
- Are you allergic to any medications? To latex? To spermicides?
- Have you ever had a sexually transmitted infection (STI)?
  - Gonorrhea
  - Chlamydia
  - Syphilis
  - Herpes
  - Genital warts
  - Trichomoniasis
- Have you ever had pelvic inflammatory disease (PID)?
- Have you ever been pregnant? If so, what were the outcomes (live birth, abortion, miscarriage)?
- Do you have plans to become pregnant? If so, when?

SEXUAL HISTORY

- Have you ever had sexual intercourse (vaginal/anal/oral)?
- What do you do to protect yourself from HIV or other infections? What do you do that may be putting you at risk for HIV or other infections?
- How many partners have you had in your lifetime?
- How many partners do you have now? How many have you had in the last 3 to 6 months?
- Are your partners male or female or both?
- Do you ever use alcohol or drugs in connection with sexual activity? Do you ever exchange sex for drugs, shelter, or money?
- Have you ever been forced to have sex?
- Do you enjoy sex? Do you have orgasms? Do you or your partner have any questions or concerns about sex?
- When was the last time you had vaginal intercourse?
- (If partner is male):
  - Did you use anything to prevent pregnancy?
  - Are you seeking to become pregnant at this time?
  - How often do you have vaginal intercourse?

INTIMATE PARTNER SCREEN

- Are you afraid of your partner or someone important to you?
- Within the last year, have you been hit, slapped, kicked, or otherwise physically hurt by anyone? By whom? How often?
- Are you in a relationship where you are treated badly?
- Have you been forced to engage in sexual activities? If yes, by whom? How many times?

SOCIAL/CONTRACEPTIVE HISTORY

- Do you smoke or chew tobacco?
- Do you have any cultural or religious beliefs that influence your view of birth control.
- What birth control methods (eg, birth control pill, Depo-Provera, condoms), if any, have you used before? Did you like or dislike the methods (if any)? Did you have any problems with those methods?
- What methods of birth control are you considering?
- What is important to you in a birth control method?
- Do you have any concerns or questions about birth control?

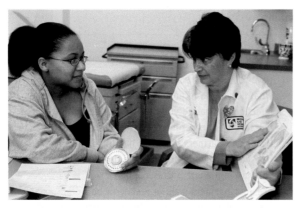

FIGURE 8.16 As with all issues related to sexuality, the nurse shows sensitivity and shapes the interaction according to the client's comfort level and responses when discussing family planning, contraception, and prevention of sexually transmitted infections.

for intimate partner violence should occur with each client encounter (see Chapter 5).

Think back to Veena, the 26-year-old from the beginning of the chapter who wants to explore options for contraception. What areas should the nurse address during assessment to assist Veena in making an informed choice?

The nurse must take time to listen to the woman and ask questions about how she feels and what she knows about contraception. It is important to clear up any misinformation and misperceptions she may have received from the media, peers, or others. The information provided by the nurse should be practical, easy to understand, and provided in multiple formats to encourage understanding. For example, a woman receiving contraceptive counselling can hear it from the nurse and also be given a written pamphlet or an approved website where she can get more information or reinforce what she already knows.

The nurse needs to be aware of and recognize any personal biases that can influence his or her approaches to counselling. Canadian women have the right to expect contraceptive services that are provided with dignity and respect and that recognize their age, ability to understand information, cultural and ethical values as well as their needs for both contraception and protection from STIs. Women have the right to choose a method that is safe and acceptable to them. See Research Highlights 8.1 and 8.2.

Potential Nursing Diagnoses

• **Health-Seeking Behaviours** related to contraception
• **Risk for Infection** related to sexual behaviours
• **Deficient Knowledge** related to methods and use of contraception

---

● **RESEARCH HIGHLIGHT 8.1** Women's Knowledge, Beliefs, and Information Needs in Relation to the Risks and Benefits Associated With Use of the Oral Contraceptive Pill

PURPOSE

The goal of this study was to identify knowledge, beliefs, and information needs about oral contraceptive pills among Australian women.

DESIGN

1200 women's names and postal addresses were randomly selected from among each of the 150 Australian electorate regions. All women between the ages of 18 and 50 were eligible. Prior or current use of oral contraceptive pills (OCP) was not a criterion for inclusion. Informed consent was obtained from all participants. Women were sent a study package that included a question regarding current and previous contraceptive practices. From among the OCP users, women were assessed with regard to their knowledge of the risks, benefits, and side effects of OCPs, their rating of the importance of information about OCPs, as well as how they would prefer to receive information about OCPs.

RESULTS

1,200 study packages were mailed to women; 42 were returned due to incorrect addresses. Of the 1,158 packages, 305 were returned (26%). Of the women surveyed, 93% reported using OCPs at some time in their lives. 65% of women responded that they wanted to have up to date information on OCPs. Almost 76% of respondents said they wanted information via the internet, with an information booklet coming in a close second as a means of obtaining information. This study informs nurses on women's health information needs surrounding contraception and helps to inform communication and education strategies aimed at providing contraceptive information to women.

Source: Phillipson, S., Wakefield, C., & Kasparian, N. (2011). Women's knowledge, beliefs and information needs in relation to the risks and benefits associated with use of the oral contraceptive pill. *Journal of Women's Health, 20*(4), 635–642.

● **RESEARCH HIGHLIGHT 8.2**   Contraceptive Use and Attitudes Among Female College Students

PURPOSE

The goal was to examine contraceptive attitudes and demographic characteristics from among female college students who use contraceptives all the time, those who use them intermittently, and those who do not use contraceptives at all.

DESIGN

One hundred and twenty racially diverse female college students between the ages of 18–44 who were sexually active in the past 3 months were given the "Contraceptive Attitude Scale," which is both a contraceptive-use tool and a demographic tool. A quantitative comparative descriptive design was used. Participants were divided into three groups: consistent contraceptive users, intermittent contraceptive users, and contraceptive nonusers.

RESULTS

Of the study participants, 46.7% used contraception, and 53.3% did not. The preferred methods of contraception used were, in order of preference, condoms, the pill, withdrawal, the patch, and Depo-Provera. Age was a significant factor in contraception use: women over 35 years old were less likely to use contraception of any kind. Younger women preferred condoms. The researchers also found that students with higher Contraceptive Attitude scores were more likely to be consistent contraceptive users. This study has implications for nurses who provide contraceptive information to women to avoid unintended pregnancy. Nurses can assist women to make informed decisions about contraceptive use through education about the various contraceptive options, the reliability of various methods, as well as the need for protection against sexually transmitted diseases for women not in monogamous relationships.

Source: Bryant, K. (2009). Contraceptive use and attitudes among female college students. *Association of Black Nursing Faculty in Higher Education, 20*(1), 12–16.

- **Effective Therapeutic Regimen Management** related to method of contraception
- **Ineffective Therapeutic Regimen Management** related to nonuse of contraceptive method, lack of appropriate knowledge of how to use method of contraception, or unpleasant or problematic side effects of the method

Planning and Intervention

Methods of planning and intervention relate directly to the contraceptive method chosen. Specific measures are discussed under Client Teaching and Collaborative Interventions for each contraceptive choice that are presented earlier in this chapter. After obtaining a detailed client history, the nurse can present available options and proceed to discussion on appropriate or desired methods. Factors that influence the method choice include medical contraindications, cost, tolerability of side effects, ability to use the method, partner involvement, individual beliefs and values, cultural background, and plans for future fertility (Hatcher et al., 2004; Youngkin & Davis, 2004). Once the woman has decided on the methods of contraception that she desires and that are safe for her, the nurse should clarify proper use of the methods. It also is suggested that the nurse counsel the woman regarding emergency contraception and ensure that the woman has decided on a backup method of contraception. Written information is valuable to reinforce teaching, much of which may be new to the woman. It also helps to have a sample of the method, such as a condom, diaphragm, or pill pack. See Nursing Care Plan 8.2 for more information.

Evaluation

Follow-up is very important and the woman should be able to call the nurse for further information in the event of a question or problem. After the woman has used a method for 3 months, it is helpful to schedule a follow-up appointment to assess for side effects and danger signs and provide further teaching, if necessary. The nurse should verify correct use at each follow-up visit as well. The woman must understand the potential side effects of each method, and if she experiences any side effects, the nurse provides advice on how to mitigate or reduce the negative effects. The woman should be informed of any potential dangerous side effects and, if they occur, should seek medical assistance immediately.

NURSING CARE PLAN 8.2

●

A Client Seeking Information About Contraceptives

 Recall Veena, 26 years old, who is exploring options for contraception. Veena's health history indicates no major medical problems, including no STIs. Her weight is appropriate for her height, and her menstrual cycle is normal (every 29 days), with occasional cramping.

NURSING DIAGNOSIS

Health-Seeking Behaviours related to contraceptive alternatives

EXPECTED OUTCOME

The client will verbalize that she understands various contraceptive alternatives, how they work, and their benefits and risks.

INTERVENTIONS	RATIONALES
Take measures to protect the client's privacy and to facilitate a relaxed atmosphere of trust. Close the door or curtain to the examination area. Minimize distractions. Assure the client that information provided will be kept confidential	A client who feels comfortable and accepted and that the nurse is maintaining privacy is more likely to be frank about concerns related to sexuality and reproduction
Discuss the mechanisms of action, use, reliability, costs, and side effects of different contraceptive methods that she is interested in exploring	Accurate information facilitates the client's decision making about the best choice for her needs

EVALUATION

1. The client expresses understanding of the methods discussed.
2. The client verbalizes interest in three methods discussed with the nurse.

NURSING DIAGNOSIS

Decisional Conflict related to contraceptive alternatives.

EXPECTED OUTCOME

The client will choose one of the methods identified by the follow-up appointment in 4 weeks.

INTERVENTIONS	RATIONALES
Discuss the client's lifestyle and how the three possibilities she identified interact with her goals for contraception	Assessing the client's goals may help the nurse and client further narrow the choices

(continued)

NURSING CARE PLAN 8.2 ● A Client Seeking Information About Contraceptives *(Continued)*

INTERVENTIONS	RATIONALES
Continue to discuss the mechanisms of action, use, reliability, costs, and any side effects of the three potential options. Explore those factors that seem most important to the client (eg, finances, possible physical effects)	Additional information should help the client further narrow her options. Understanding her priorities may give clues about which factors are most important in determining the best choice
Provide brochures and other information about the three options for the client to read at home. Direct the client to reliable websites that can assist with information gathering	The client may feel less pressured to decide and may be able to think more clearly with additional time; having backup information available at home can assist her as she chooses
Review and discuss the ongoing need for safer sex practices (see Chapter 6)	The client is making a contraceptive choice based on a desire to avoid pregnancy; however, many contraceptives do not protect against STIs. The client still may need to use condoms to protect against STIs, depending on her choice of contraceptive
Reinforce the necessity of ongoing follow-up care, regardless of the actual method chosen	Ongoing health maintenance is essential to evaluate the client's compliance and satisfaction with the chosen method. It is also necessary to detect any related problems or complications

EVALUATION

1. The client verbalizes that she will examine the information provided in the next few weeks.
2. The client schedules a follow-up appointment.
3. The client chooses to use an appropriate method of contraception for herself and returns to the clinic at the follow-up appointment for appropriate instruction and related care.

SUMMARY

- Throughout history, humans have sought to control fertility. Contraceptive methods have become easier to use and are more available; several options have emerged since the first oral hormonal contraceptive in 1960s.
- Contraceptive methods are often more oriented toward use by the female. Currently, more male-oriented hormonal contraceptive options are undergoing research.
- Barrier devices of contraception include male and female condoms, diaphragm, cervical cap, contraceptive sponge, and spermicide. These mechanisms work by providing physical obstruction between sperm and the woman's reproductive tract. Male and female condoms have the additional benefit of helping prevent STIs.

- Hormonal methods of contraception can be based on oral medications that combine delivery of progestin and estrogen, or that use progestin only. The various types of medications work to suppress ovulation, thin the endometrium, and thicken cervical mucus to create a hostile environment for fertilization to occur.
- Combined methods of hormonal contraception include COCs, the transdermal contraceptive patch, and the vaginal ring.
- Progestin-only methods of hormonal contraception include progestin-only pills, and Depo-Provera injections.
- IUD are inserted into the woman's uterus by a primary care provider. They release copper or hormones that create an environment that prevents implantation of the fertilized ovum.

- Behavioural methods include abstinence, fertility awareness, withdrawal, and lactational amenorrhea. These approaches require motivation for behaviour control and a keen understanding of the woman's monthly cycles on the part of users.

- Surgical methods include bilateral tubal ligation for women and vasectomy for men. These permanent forms of sterilization are appropriate only for those clients who are definite about their decisions to have no or no more children.

- Emergency contraception is available for women up to 7 days after unprotected intercourse. Options include hormonal emergency contraception, and the insertion of a copper IUD. All women at risk for unintended pregnancy should be counselled on emergency contraception and how to obtain it if needed.

- Nurses providing teaching and interventions for fertility control and contraception should obtain the client's complete health history, including past medical history, family history, menstrual history, and sexual history to provide appropriate assessment and planning.

- For each contraceptive device or approach, the nurse should understand and be familiar with its mechanism of action, advantages, disadvantages, side effects, contraindications, and effectiveness to provide adequate guidance for individual clients.

Questions to Ponder

1. On a follow-up visit to the clinic, Veena has not yet chosen a contraceptive method she feels comfortable with and has continued to have intercourse with a male partner who is sometimes reluctant to use condoms. Until she decides which method would give her more control over avoiding pregnancy, are there additional issues that need to be addressed?

2. Kenya and her partner Darrell have reconfirmed their intent to use the natural family planning method. What are the four methods they could use to identify when Kenya is fertile so that they can avoid intercourse during that time? What is the use failure rate for these methods?

3. A 16-year-old female client presents for an annual examination. She is currently sexually active with male partners and uses no method of contraception, but states that she is not interested in pregnancy at this time. After you discuss the available methods of contraception, she is unsure if she wants to use any method because she does not want to experience any potential side effects.

   - What questions do you want to ask to understand why this teenager may be hesitant about using contraception?

   - What attitudes can this woman expect from you as a nurse providing care?

   - How can you best assist this teenager to make the right decision for her?

4. A 24-year-old woman comes to your birth control clinic for advice regarding contraception. She states that although she does not want to become exposed to STIs, her male partner will not agree to use a condom. He has told her he "does not have a disease."

   - How can you best provide support to this client?

   - What are some options that you can explore with her to support her wish not to become exposed to STIs?

   - What other resources might you discuss with her at this time?

5. A 40-year-old recently divorced woman indicates that she is beginning to date again. She is concerned about contraception, which she has not used for 20 years. She has read some articles about STIs and is wondering if she needs to be concerned.

   - What advice can you give about contraception?

   - What other concerns might she have about dating?

   - What might you discuss with her about STIs?

REVIEW QUESTIONS

1. A 28-year-old client comes to the physician's office to explore various methods of birth control. Upon reviewing the client's history, which of the following should the nurse identify as a contraindication for COCs?
   A. Fibrocystic breast changes
   B. A history of deep vein thrombosis
   C. Smoking
   D. Irritable bowel syndrome

2. A client calls the clinic and says that she had sex without birth control recently and wants to use "morning-after pill." In preparing a response, the nurse should include that the latest it can be used effectively is
   A. 24 hours after unprotected intercourse
   B. 48 hours after unprotected intercourse
   C. 72 hours after unprotected intercourse
   D. 120 hours after unprotected intercourse

3. The nurse is teaching a client who has begun using COCs about problems to report immediately and advises the client to remember the acronym ACHES. The nurse knows that teaching has been effective when the client reports that ACHES stands for
   A. **A**bnormal periods, **C**hest pain, **H**eadaches—severe, **E**ye problems—blurred or changes in vision, **S**evere leg pain
   B. **A**bnormal periods, **C**lotting with periods, **H**eadaches—severe, **E**ye problems—blurred or changes in vision, **S**evere leg pain

C. **A**bdominal pain, **C**hest pain, **H**air loss, **E**ye problems—blurred or changes in vision, **S**evere leg pain

D. **A**bdominal pain, **C**hest pain, **H**eadaches—severe, **E**ye problems—blurred or changes in vision, **S**evere leg pain

4. The nurse is teaching a couple about correct condom use. Which of the following statements if made by the man indicates that he needs more instruction?

A. "I'll be sure to put on the condom before making any contact with my partner's genitals."

B. "I will make sure that when I am wearing the condom, it is tight against the glans of my penis."

C. "To remove the condom, I'll slide it down while holding the top and pulling the tip, with my penis still erect."

D. "I will make sure that we use a brand new condom every time we engage in sexual activity."

5. The nurse is caring for a client who reports using spermicide as her regular method of contraception. Which statement, if made by the client, should indicate to the nurse that further education is needed?

A. "Spermicides protect against HIV."

B. "Spermicide is a method the woman controls."

C. "Spermicide can be inserted 15 minutes before sex."

D. "Spermicides are available without a prescription."

6. The nurse is preparing a teaching plan on noncontraceptive benefits of COCs. Which of the following should NOT be included in the teaching plan?

A. Reduced risk for endometrial cancer

B. Decreased acne

C. Prevention of HIV

D. Decreased dysmenorrhea

7. A client is just starting Depo-Provera injections. The nurse is preparing to schedule a follow-up appointment for her. The most optimal appointment time would be in

A. 3 months

B. 4 months

C. 6 months

D. 12 months

8. A client in her last trimester of pregnancy who intends to breastfeed her baby asks the nurse which contraceptive options will be available to her. Which of the following responses from the nurse is most correct?

A. Lactational amenorrhea method, progestin-only pills, Depo-Provera

B. COCs, copper IUD, progestin-only pills

C. Copper IUD, vaginal contraceptive ring, diaphragm

D. Condoms, spermicides, contraceptive patch

9. When teaching a client about the correct use of a diaphragm for contraception, the nurse should make the following statement:

A. "You must remember to remove the diaphragm immediately after intercourse."

B. "You should not use your diaphragm while you are menstruating."

C. "Remove the diaphragm to add spermicide when you have sex more than once at a time."

D. "You will need to replace your diaphragm every 5 years."

10. The nurse is assisting a client with placement of the transdermal contraceptive. Which alternative sites can the nurse and client choose for placement?

A. On the client's abdomen or buttocks

B. On the client's abdomen, buttocks, or upper arm

C. On the client's abdomen, buttocks, or upper torso

D. On the client's buttocks only

REFERENCES

Archer, D. (2001). Evaluation of a new oral contraceptive progestogen, drospirenone with ethinyl estradiol (Yasmin). *Contraceptive Technology Update, 22*(Suppl 9), 1–4.

Arevalo, M., Jennings, V., & Sinai, I. (2002). The Standard Days method: A new method of family planning (research notes). *Sexual Health Exchange, 2002*(2), 6–8.

Black, A. (2006). Canadian contraception consensus—update on Depot Medroxyprogesterone acetate (DMPA): SOGC clinical practice guidelines, No. 174. *Journal of Obstetrics and Gynaecology Canada,* 305–308. Retrieved from http://www.sogc.org/guidelines/documents/JOGC

Black, A., Francoeur, D., & Rowe, T. (2004a). Canadian contraception consensus: SOGC clinical practice guidelines, No. 143, part 1. *Journal of Obstetrics and Gynaecology Canada,* Retrieved from http://www.sogc.org/guidelines/public/143E-CPG1

Black, A., Francoeur, D., & Rowe, T. (2004b). Canadian contraception consensus: SOGC clinical practice guidelines, No. 143, part 2. *Journal of Obstetrics and Gynaecology Canada.* Retrieved from http://www.sogc.org/guidelines/public/143E-CPG2

Black, A., Francoeur, D., & Rowe, T. (2004c). Canadian contraception consensus: SOGC clinical practice guidelines, No. 143, part 3. *Journal of Obstetrics and Gynaecology Canada,* Retrieved from http://www.sogc.org/guidelines/public/143E-CPG3

Bullough, V. L., & Bullough, B. (1994). A brief history of population control and contraception (symposium: Overpopulation & contraception). *Free Inquiry, 14*(2), 16–23.

Burkman, R., Schlesselman, J. J., & Zieman, M. (2004). Safety concerns and health benefits associated with oral contraception. *American Journal of Obstetrics and Gynecology, 190*(S4), S5–S22.

Centers for Disease Control and Prevention. (2002). Nonoxynol-9 spermicide contraception use: United States, 1999. *Journal of the American Medical Association, 287*(9), 2938–2940.

Cole, J., Norman, H., Doherty, M., & Walker, A. (2007). Venous thromboembolism, myocardial infarction, and stroke among transdermal contraception users. *Obstetrics and Gynecology, 109*(2), 339–346.

Collaborative Group on Hormonal Factors in Breast Cancer, & Beral, V. (2002). Breast cancer and breastfeeding: Collaborative reanalysis of individual data from 47 epidemiological studies in 30 countries, including 50,302 women with breast cancer and 96,973 women without the disease. *Lancet, 360*(9328), 187–195.

Contraceptive Technology Update. (2002). Does weight play a role in effectiveness (of Ortho Evra contraceptive patch)? *Contraceptive Technology Update, 23*(7), 81–83.

Duffy, S., Marsh, F., Rogerson, L., Hudson, H., Cooper, K., Jack, S., et al. (2005). Female sterilization: A cohort controlled comparative study of ESSURE versus laparoscopic sterilization. *BJOG: An International Journal of Obstetrics and Gynaecology, 112*(11), 1522–1528.

Dunn, S., & Guilbert, E. (2012). Emergency contraception. *Journal of Obstetrics and Gynaecology Canada, 34*(9), 870–878.

Faculty of Sexual & Reproductive Healthcare Clinical Guidance. (2012). *Drug interactions with hormonal contraception.* Royal College of Obstetricians & Gynaecologists Clinical Effectiveness Unit, pp. 7–9. Retrieved from http://www.fsrh.org/pdfs/CEUguidancedruginteractionshormonal.pdf

Fisher, W., & Black, A. (2007). Contraception in Canada: A review of method choices, characteristics, adherence, and approaches to counselling. *Canadian Medical Association Journal, 176*(7), 953–961.

Foidart, J. M. (2005). Added benefits of drospirenone for compliance. *Climacteric, 8*(S3), 28–34.

Freeman, S. (2004). Nondaily hormonal contraception: Considerations in contraceptive choice and patient counseling. *Journal of the American Academy of Nurse Practitioners, 16*(6), 226–238.

Glasier, A. F., Cameron, S. T., Fine, P. M., Logan, S. J., Casale, W., Van Horn, J., et al. (2010). Ulipristal acetate versus levongestoral for emergency contraception: Randomized non-inferiority trial and meta-analysis. *Lancet, 375*(9714), 555–562.

Grimes, D. A. (2001). Health benefits of oral contraception: Update on endometrial cancer prevention. *Contraception Report, 12*(3), 4–7.

Gross, T. P., & Schlesselman, J. (2003). The estimated effect of oral contraceptive use on the cumulative risk of epithelial ovarian cancer. *Obstetrics and Gynecology, 83*(3), 419–424.

Guilbert, E., Black, A., & Dunn, S. (2008). Missed hormonal contraceptives: New recommendations. *Journal of Obstetrics and Gynaecology of Canada, 30*(11), 1050–1062.

Guilbert, E., Boroditsky, R., Black, A., Kives, S., Leboeuf, M., Mirosh, M. et al. (2007). Canadian consensus guideline on continuous and extended hormonal contraception, SOGC clinical practice guideline. *Journal of Obstetrics and Gynaecology of Canada, 29*(7 Suppl 2), S1–S32.

Hankinson, S. E., Hunter, D. J., Colditz, G. A., Willett, W. C., Stampfer, M. J., Rosner, B., et al. (2012). *A pocket guide for managing contraception.* Tiger, GA: Bridging the Gap Foundation.

Hardwick, D. (2002). The effectiveness of a female condom intervention on women's use of condoms. *Canadian Journal of Human Sexuality, 11*(2), 63–77.

Hatcher, R. A., Trussell, J., Stewart, F., Cates, W., Stewart, G., Guest, F., et al. (2004). *Contraceptive technology* (18th ed.). New York: Ardent Media.

Hillier, S. (2013). *Overview of products in development-topical.* Presentation at the Forum for Collaborative HIV Research Meeting on Future of PrEP and Microbicides. Washington, DC. Retrieved January 7, 2013, from http://rhrealitycheck.org/article/2013/01/16/first-trial-proposed-candidate-microbicide-women-living-with-hiv/#sthash.zf065tOB.dpuf

Krattenmacher, R. (2000). Drospirenone: Pharmacology and pharmacokinetics of a unique progestogen. *Contraception, 62*(1), 29–38.

McLaren, A., & McLaren, A. (1997). *The bedroom and the state: The changing practices and politics of contraception and abortion in Canada, 1880–1997* (2nd ed.). Toronto, ON: Oxford University Press.

McNaught, J., & Reid, R. (2006). Progesterone-only and non-hormonal contraception in the breast cancer survivor: Joint review and committee opinion of the Society of Obstetricians and Gynaecologists of Canada and the Society of Gynecologic Oncologists of Canada. *Journal of Obstetrics and Gynaecology of Canada, 179,* 616–626.

Myer, L. (2010). Barrier methods. In: Karim S. & Karim Q. (Eds.). *HIV/AIDS in South Africa* (2nd ed.). Cape Town, South Africa: Cambridge University Press; 183–201.

Novak, A., de la Logeb, C., Abtezc, L., & van der Muelen, E. (2003). The combined contraceptive vaginal ring, NuvaRing®: An international study of user acceptability. *Contraception, 67*(3), 187–194.

O'Malley, M., Wood, O., & Foulkes, A. (2001). The birth control pill. CBC News Indepth: Genetic and Reproduction. Retrieved July 2, 2001, from http://www.cbc.ca/news2/background/genetics_reproduction/birthcontrol_pill.html

Options for Sexual Health. (2012). Retrieved from https://www.optionsforsexualhealth.org/

Planned Parenthood of America. (2013). Retrieved from www.plannedparenthood.org

Redmond, A., & Self, T. (2002). Oral contraceptives and drugs that compromise their efficacy. *Journal of Critical Illness, 17*(8), 306–308.

Reid, R. (2010). Oral contraceptives and the risk of venous thromboembolism: An update. *Journal of Obstetrics and Gynaecology of Canada, 252,* 1192–1197.

Repta, R. & Clarke, L. (2011). "Am I going to be natural or am I not?": Canadian women's perceptions and experiences of menstrual suppression". *Sex Roles: A Journal of Research, 68*(1–2), 91–106.

Robinson, K. (2005). Depo-Provera: New concerns—same issues? *Association of Women's Health Obstetric and Neonatal Nurses Lifelines, 9*(3), 214–217.

Schenker, J., & Fabenou, V. (1993). Family planning: Cultural and religious perspectives. *Human Reproduction, 8*(6), 969–976.

Society of Obstetricians and Gynaecologists of Canada. (2012). Birth control. Sexuality and U. Retrieved from http://www.sexualityandu.ca/birth-control/birth_control_methods_contraception/non-hormonal-methods

Stewart, F. H., & Barnhart, K. T. (2002). The vaginal contraceptive ring: Efficacy, cautions and frustrations. *Contraceptive Technology Reports, 23*(2), SSSI–SSS9.

Veres, S., Miller, L., & Burington, B. (2004). A comparison between the vaginal ring and oral contraceptives. *Obstetrics and Gynecology, 104*(3), 555–563.

Wang, C., & Swerdloff, R. S. (2010). Hormonal approaches to male contraception. *Current Opinion in Urology, 20,* 520–584.

Youngkin, E. Q., & Davis, M. S. (2004). *Women's health: A primary care clinical guide* (3rd ed.). Stamford, CT: Appleton & Lange.

Zacur, H., Hedon, B., Mansour, D., Shangold, G., Fisher, A., & Creasy, G. (2002). Integrated summary of Ortho Evra™ contraceptive patch adhesion in varied climates and conditions. *Fertility and Sterility, 77*(2), 32–35.

WEB RESOURCES

www.managingcontraception.com
www.arhp.org (Association of Reproductive Health Professionals)
www.sexualityandu.ca
www.itsyoursexlife.com/
www.womenshealthmatters.ca
www.wontgetweird.com
www.optionsforsexualhealth.org
www.familyplanning.net
www.contracept.org

CHAPTER 9

Voluntary Pregnancy Termination

Luisa Ciofani and Judith A. Lewis*

Patti, a single 24-year-old client with a 3-year-old daughter, comes to the physician's office for a checkup. She says that she's been very tired, nauseous, and just "not feeling herself." Examination reveals that Patti is 9 weeks pregnant. Patti is shocked by the news and cries inconsolably. She states, "Another baby? What will I do?"

Gina, 44 years old, is recovering from an abortion she underwent after an amniocentesis at 16 weeks' gestation revealed severe congenital anomalies in the fetus. During a follow-up discussion with the nurse, Gina, visibly exhausted, states, "This was the hardest decision I ever had to make."

You will learn more about Patti's and Gina's stories later in this chapter. Nurses working with women undergoing pregnancy termination need to understand the material in this chapter both to manage care and to address issues which affect the client and the health care provider(s). Before beginning, reflect on the following points related to the above scenarios:

• What is your initial reaction to the circumstances presented in each case? Do you have different responses to each client for any reason? Explain your answer.
• How are the clients similar? Different?
• How might each client's particular situation influence the nurse's approach to her care?
• How might the nurse's values influence his or her ability to care for the client?
• What other details should the nurse investigate with Patti? What about with Gina?
• What measures can the nurse take to explore the topic so that he or she is sensitive to a client's needs, but also provides appropriate and accurate information?

*Contributor to first U.S. edition.

Voluntary (or induced) **abortion** is the planned or intended termination of an established pregnancy. An abortion may be performed at any point in the pregnancy, but is performed most frequently prior to viability. The term abortion is used interchangeably with pregnancy termination and therapeutic abortion. **Viability** is commonly considered as the end of the second trimester, or 24 weeks' gestation. Viability is a medical, not a legal, term. The point of viability may vary according to the availability of specialized technology and care as well as individual practices surrounding the limits of viability, usually described as 22 to 26 weeks (Canadian Paediatric Society & Fetus and Newborn Committee, 2012). Pregnancies that end due to a variety of physiologic reasons are discussed in Chapter 13. This chapter focuses on voluntary termination of pregnancy, more commonly referred to as **voluntary abortion**.

Abortion is one of the most controversial procedures in health care, yet a frequent phenomenon in Canada as well as the United States and internationally. Nurses in various settings are often in positions to provide information to pregnant women about available pregnancy options, resources, and counselling for access to abortion services. Understanding the health-related, religious, sociopolitical, ethical, and legal issues associated with voluntary abortion will help nurses provide appropriate care for their clients.

HISTORICAL PERSPECTIVES

Evidence has shown that, throughout history, humans have attempted to control family size (Riddle, 1992).

During some periods and in various locations, large families with many children were desired, whereas at other times the preferred family size was smaller. Historically, ways of controlling family size have included abstinence, primitive contraception usage (see Chapter 8), and voluntary abortion. Although abortion has been practiced for centuries, it has been used considerably less frequently than contraception in limiting family size.

In ancient times, women who wanted to induce abortion tried to do so by a variety of activities, including carrying heavy loads, jumping, walking, and horseback riding. They also ingested diuretics or laxatives and took sitz baths with poultices containing various materials (eg, old olive oil, iris oil, ox bile, linseed). Other means of inducing abortion included inserting suppositories composed of agents such as myrtle and wallflower into the vagina (Riddle, 1992).

During the Middle Ages, knowledge of antifertility measures existed in classical texts, but it is unclear how much of this information would have been available or known to the average citizen. Church fathers, however, did speak against the use of contraception and abortion. This leads one to believe that these topics may not have been safe to discuss. Although medieval writings contain a great deal of material about herbal remedies, there are no references to any abortifacient qualities.

The first reference to abortion law in England appeared in the 13th century; abortion was allowed until quickening, the first perception of fetal movement, at which time it was believed the soul entered the body. The passage of the Ellenborough Act of

1803 made abortion a capital offence for British subjects when terminating a pregnancy after quickening. Terminating an earlier pregnancy carried lesser penalties. In 1837, the Ellenborough Act was extended to include abortions carried out at any time (Dunsmuir, 1998). This development marked the beginning of the criminalization of abortion. In 1852, Dr. Pascoe of Cornwall, England, was convicted for administering oil of savin to a woman who aborted: such convictions made physicians reluctant to become involved with matters concerning abortion. The first Canadian criminal law on abortion was passed in 1869. The statutes were meant to protect the fetus, but were also concerned about the health of the mother at a time when abortions were medically unsafe and often performed by nonphysicians.

In the 1960s, the women's movement and the availability of oral contraceptives encouraged many women to expect and to demand control over their reproductive capacity. Many women without access to safe, aseptic, abortions performed by physicians resorted to "back-alley" abortions, those performed in unclean and unsafe conditions. Women who sought these abortions, or attempted to self-induce abortions, often experienced significant morbidity and mortality resulting from infection, hemorrhage, or other complications (Boston Women's Health Book Collective, 2011). Many of these procedures resulted in injuries significant enough to jeopardize or ruin the woman's reproductive future. Although there are anecdotal accounts of these activities, reliable data do not exist, as a result of the shame and secrecy surrounding these procedures. *If These Walls Could Talk* (Cher & Savoca, 1996), a Hollywood film depicting the struggles faced by women experiencing unintended pregnancies in 1952, 1974, and 1996, presents a powerful portrayal of the dangers that women seeking to terminate their pregnancies faced before abortion services became legal. The book *No Choice: Canadian Women Tell Their Stories of Illegal Abortion* (Childbirth by Choice Trust, 1998) describes Canadian women's personal stories of illegal abortion.

Throughout history, prevention of pregnancy has been more socially acceptable than termination (Riddle, 1992). In 1995, the United Nations stipulated that abortion should not be promoted as a method of family planning, but rather it should be seen as an alternative to contraception failure or neglect (United Nations Population Fund [UNFPA], 1995). The World Health Organization (2012) released the second edition of *Safe Abortion: Technical and Policy Guidance for Health Systems.* This update reviews the evidence in favor of providing abortion care services in order to address the universal need for safe induced abortion worldwide.

RELIGIOUS PERSPECTIVES

The number of unintended pregnancies remains high in a context where many reliable contraception methods are available. In addition to knowledge about contraceptive options, factors that might contribute to an individual's or a couple's use (or nonuse) of contraceptives may be cultural or religious. Basic knowledge regarding religious teachings about the acceptability and use of contraception may be helpful when counselling individuals or couples. An individualized approach is necessary; an individual or couple may identify with a particular faith, but may not adhere to all the beliefs of that faith (Srikanthan & Reid, 2008). Abortion counselling, therefore, not only requires acknowledgement of a client's religious faith, but also an exploration of the meaning of pregnancy and beliefs about voluntary abortion. Discussion of acceptable contraceptive options must also consider the method of action of the selected contraceptive, which may be seen as inducing an abortion in the user and may thus be determined to be unacceptable.

CURRENT LEGAL AND POLITICAL CLIMATE

The earliest Canadian law related to abortion dates back to 1869; it was based on an 1861 British law. This law was challenged by the medical and legal communities in Britain because it did not make any provisions for the mother's health, so in 1938, the British Medical Association set up a special committee to consider medical issues related to abortion. The law was subsequently revised; abortions became legal if they were done to protect the life and health of the mother. As a commonwealth country at the time, this law became applicable in Canada.

The Criminal Code of Canada was amended in 1969 to include the provision for an abortion to be offered by a physician if a therapeutic abortion committee (composed of three physicians) certified that continuing the pregnancy was detrimental to a woman's physical or emotional health. Once approved, the procedure had to be performed in an accredited hospital. This strategy created wide variation in access across the country on two levels. Interpretation of the endangerment posed by the pregnancy on the life or health of the mother varied across the country. Regional disparities in accessing therapeutic abortion committees created inequity in women's ability to obtain legal therapeutic abortion in a timely manner. Women who lacked financial or personal resources were often denied needed procedures, whereas affluent or "well-connected" women had little difficulty obtaining access to abortion services. This led, in 1975, to the establishment of a Committee on the Operation of the Abortion Law whose mandate was to assess if therapeutic abortions were available equitably across Canada. The 1977 Badgley report concluded that "the procedures set out for the operation of Abortion Law are not working equitably across Canada" (Dunsmuir, 1998, Section D).

In 1973, the United States Supreme Court deemed abortion a fundamental right under the United States constitution in the case of *Roe v. Wade*. In 1982, the Charter of Rights and Freedoms came into effect in Canada and in 1983, Dr. Henry Morgentaler challenged the Canadian abortion law. Dr. Morgentaler, who had been performing illegal abortions since 1973, appealed to the Supreme Court of Canada. In 1988, the law was struck down because the system regulating access to therapeutic abortions was deemed to be unconstitutional and in violation of the *Canadian Charter of Rights and Freedoms*. Abortion became decriminalized. Since this time, the Canadian Parliament periodically attempted to frame a new law, but was unsuccessful in passing it through the House of Commons and the Senate.

There is currently no abortion law in Canada. Nonetheless, access to abortion is not equally available to women across the country, particularly for those who live outside of large urban centres, or who live in Prince Edward Island where induced abortions are not performed (Canadian Institute for Health Information [CIHI], 2011). Attempts have been made to indirectly curtail access to abortion by introducing legislative changes in both Canada and the United States (Boston Women's Health Book Collective, 2011). Examples include Bill C-537, the Protection of Conscience Rights in the Health Care Profession, Bill C-484, the Unborn Victims of Crime Act in Canada (Arthur, 2008; Palmer, 2008), and House Bill 2 in Texas (Tomlinson, 2013).

Canadian statistics reflect that 92,524 induced abortions were performed in 2011, down from 93,755 performed in 2009 (CIHI, 2011, 2013). Less restricted access to emergency contraception is hypothesized to have reduced the need for elective termination of pregnancy, but no data exist in Canada to support this. Since 2007, the CIHI has been responsible for the Therapeutic Abortions Database. Not all provinces provide information in the same manner, data about induced abortions performed in clinics is submitted voluntarily, and abortions performed outside hospitals and publicly funded clinics are not captured; these factors make it difficult to analyze trends. Access to provincial data from year to year also varies (CIHI, 2013). In a 2011 review of international trends of legal abortion, Canada was deemed to have incomplete data for the 2008 analysis, but com-

plete data for the 2003 analysis (Sedgh et al., 2012). Comprehensive reporting and collating of data would provide a clearer national perspective.

In the United States, 2011 data reveals that 69% of women who have abortions are economically disadvantaged, 58% are in their 20s and 88% have their abortions in the first 12 weeks of pregnancy. In 2008, teen pregnancies (ages 15 to 19) reached the lowest level in 40 years. The improved use of contraceptives among teens was identified as key to this reduction (Guttmacher Institute, 2011, 2012).

From an international perspective, the previously observed substantial decline in abortion rates has stalled and the proportion of unsafe abortions has increased (Sedgh et al., 2012). Even in Canada, significant barriers remain that compromise access to abortion. These include health professionals who refuse to provide referrals for abortions, the lack of hospitals (particularly outside large urban centres) that provide abortion services, the refusal of provincial and territorial governments to fund abortion services, and the general decrease in physicians trained to perform abortions (Kaposy, 2010; Sethna & Doull, 2007). See Research Highlight 9.1.

NURSING PERSPECTIVES, ROLES, AND RESPONSIBILITIES

For most individuals, feelings and beliefs about abortion are intensely private and based on personal ethical systems rather than scientific evidence. These beliefs span an entire range of possibilities. At one end of the continuum is abortion on demand from conception until the onset of labour; at the other end is a total ban on abortion from the moment of conception, regardless of the reason. Each individual is entitled to his or her beliefs; therefore ethical dilemmas may be present for nurses and other health care workers with regard to client choices related to a termination of pregnancy. Based on the principle of respect for autonomy, the clinician's role is to assist the client with decision making (Canadian Nurses Association, 2008). To meet the ethical challenges of practice, nurses must understand how ethical principles translate into practice (Cappiello et al., 2011).

Unintended pregnancy and its outcome are socially and politically controversial. As a core competency, clinicians caring for women with unintended pregnancy, or working with clients whose pregnancy outcome choice may be different from their own, must be able to identify personal beliefs that might interfere with the performance of clinical duties (Simmonds & Likis, 2011). In addition to providing care that is free of bias and judgement, core competencies when caring for women with unintended pregnancy include ensuring confidentiality

● **RESEARCH HIGHLIGHT 9.1** **Far From Home? A Pilot Study Tracking Women's Journeys to a Canadian Abortion Clinic**

PURPOSE

To describe the journey that women travel to access an abortion clinic in metropolitan Toronto.

METHODS

The researchers developed a questionnaire in consultation with clinic staff and an advisory panel. The questionnaire underwent one revision midway through the study. Women presenting for an abortion were asked to provide details about their journeys to accessing an abortion.

RESULTS

The overall response rate was 81%. Women chose the clinic because of the clinic's good reputation, a doctor's referral to the clinic, knowledge of someone who had already been to the clinic, or close proximity to their residence. Respondents who first contacted other clinics encountered a lack of available appointments, expensive fees, and concerns about their safety because of antiabortion protesters. The most frequently handwritten comment reflected that women were unable to access an appointment within the necessary timeframe. Women who reported incomes of less than $30,000 travelled greater distances, as much as 1,000 km, more than distances travelled by wealthier women. This study supports the idea that geographical distance may be a barrier to accessing abortion, and creates an additional burden for women who need this service.

NURSING IMPLICATIONS

Nurses need to keep in mind that clients may be travelling significant distances to access abortion services and may need additional support when separated from their support systems. More research is needed to determine the extent of women's travel and the health, political, and legal implications of these journeys.

From Sethna, C., & Doull, M. (2007). Far from home? A pilot study tracking women's journeys to a Canadian abortion clinic. *Journal of Obstetrics and Gynaecology Canada, 27*(8), 640–647.

and recognizing the unique needs of vulnerable (eg, adolescent) and special needs (eg, survivors of violence) women (Simmonds & Likis, 2011). It is relevant to note that since personal and professional beliefs are dynamic, nurses must continue to assess their values on an ongoing basis (Cappiello et al., 2011). Assessment Tool 9.1 provides an exploration of counselling options for the woman facing an unintended pregnancy.

Early diagnosis of pregnancy allows more time to make a decision, since early abortion is a safer option. Nurses will care for a woman with an unintended pregnancy in a variety of encounters. Professional responsibilities for nurses and other health care providers include appropriate assessment, assisting and supporting women by offering counselling about pregnancy options, and provision of referral and care coordination (Davis, 2006). Contextual issues such as a woman's age, geographical location, financial resources, and gestation will affect her options (Simmonds & Likis, 2011). Many women struggle with the decision to have an abortion, and those who reach this conclusion do so for a variety of reasons (Finer et al., 2005). It is appropriate to provide clients with information on options available as well as abortion counselling when the woman makes the decision to terminate the pregnancy. It is *never* appropriate to make it evident that one option is more acceptable to the nurse than any other. Clients make many decisions that are different from what the nurse may make under the same circumstances. The nurse's responsibility to clients deciding on the outcome of a pregnancy is the same as with clients deciding on whether to have a surgical procedure, adhere to a medication regimen, or make any other health-related decision. Women concerned about the safety of abortion can be reassured that it is a very safe procedure and markedly safer than childbirth (Raymond & Grimes, 2012).

Decision-Making Process

A client may elect to terminate a pregnancy for one or multiple reasons, including concerns about maternal health, genetic conditions affecting the fetus, rape, incest, and personal circumstances (Finer et al., 2005). The reasons may be intensely personal and may be as varied as women themselves. For a client with a chronic medical condition, a contraceptive failure that has resulted in pregnancy may place her own life in jeopardy. A client who becomes pregnant when in a relationship complicated by intimate-partner violence may select abortion so that she does not have permanent ties to the male partner with whom she would share offspring (Simmonds & Likis, 2011). The woman who knows that she or her partner is a carrier of a genetic condition may seek prenatal genetic diagnosis with the goal of terminating those pregnancies that would result in affected children (see Chapter 11). The woman who is a victim of rape or incest may wish to terminate any resultant pregnancy because of the trauma associated with the event that resulted in conception.

● **ASSESSMENT TOOL 9.1** **Decision Tree of Pregnancy Options**

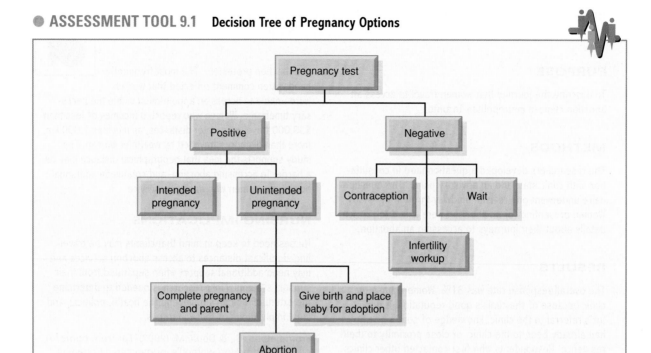

A four-topic framework for approaching unintended pregnancy adheres to the ethical principles of autonomy, respect, beneficence, and justice (Jonsen et al., 2006). Using the framework, which includes consideration of medical indications, patient preferences, quality of life (of the mother and/or fetus) and contextual factors, the nurse can collect data, provide information to respond to questions or address learning needs, and review alternatives such as termination, parenting the child, or adoption (see Chapter 7). Nursing Care Plan 9.1 highlights the care of a client considering elective abortion.

Some clients reach a decision in conjunction with, or have support from, their partners; not all women, for various reasons, can do so. Even though a client needs to know that she can confer with her partner, ultimately she is the one who must provide informed consent. The client has the autonomy to make this decision for herself. An exception is in those provinces or territories that require parental consent when the client is a minor or, in the absence of parental consent, judicial sanction. In those provinces or territories where parental consent is required, the age at which this is required varies.

Consider Gina, the 44-year-old woman described at the beginning of the chapter who had an abortion. Based on the information provided, what factors may have influenced her decision?

Methods of Voluntary Abortion

Methods of voluntary abortion available to the woman depend largely on gestational age. Although most abortions performed in North America are surgical, a growing number of women are choosing medical terminations when offered the option (Davis, 2006). Most abortions in Canada are performed in hospitals because there is no financial cost for the woman. Abortions in clinics may be fully, partially, or not covered.

First-Trimester Methods

Vacuum Aspiration. Most first-trimester abortions are performed by vacuum aspiration or suction curettage (Davis, 2006) (Fig. 9.1). The client may visit the clinic or doctor's office the day before the procedure for insertion of a laminaria tent. **Laminaria tents** are small cones of dried seaweed that, when exposed to moisture, expand, thus passively dilating the cervix. The clinician inserts the laminaria during examination with a speculum. A tampon or a piece of gauze is then inserted to hold the

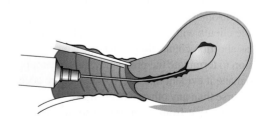

FIGURE 9.1 Vacuum extraction.

NURSING CARE PLAN 9.1

●

The Client Considering an Abortion

 Recall Patti from the beginning of this chapter. She states, "There is no way I can have another baby. I can't afford it. My daughter can't be put through this. I broke up with her father a month ago, and he'll never support me through another pregnancy. He'll just say it's my fault and that he's glad to be rid of me." She sobs. "I never thought I'd have to consider an abortion. How am I going to make it through?"

NURSING DIAGNOSES

- **Decisional Conflict** related to uncertainty about abortion and lack of available support
- **Ineffective Coping** related to anxiety about abortion, situational crisis, and inadequate social support

EXPECTED OUTCOMES

1. The client will identify areas of stress related to her current situation.
2. The client will make an informed decision about her pregnancy by the next visit.
3. The client will begin to demonstrate positive coping mechanisms.

INTERVENTIONS	RATIONALES
Assist the client in problem identification; encourage her to explain her personal circumstances and describe what she has been considering	Assessment provides a baseline to identify specific client needs and to develop an individualized plan of care
Assess the client's level of understanding about available options, including abortion	Explore her beliefs related to her options Determine how her context affects her options
Communicate facts and answer questions; clarify any misconceptions or misinformation	Clear communication helps provide accurate information to aid in alleviating fears and clarifying misinformation
Provide the client with a chance to discuss any concerns, fears, or worries about her situation; encourage the client to share her feelings	Communication can reveal sources of stress and any problematic areas that need to be addressed; sharing of feelings aids in promoting positive coping
Ask the client about available support systems (eg, family, friends)	Identifying such supports helps to establish sources of assistance
Assist the client to identify possible areas for support. Provide her with information about support groups, websites, and other avenues for education and assistance	Shared experiences and knowledge of similar situations for others can help the client prepare for what to expect and to realize that she is not alone
Ask the client about measures used to cope with previous stressful situations; determine which measures were successful. Reinforce use of successful strategies; instruct the client in simple relaxation techniques, as appropriate	Identifying previous coping strategies helps to determine effective strategies for use in this situation. Simple relaxation techniques provide one means of positive coping

(continued)

NURSING CARE PLAN 9.1 ● The Client Considering an Abortion (Continued)

INTERVENTIONS	RATIONALES
Provide the client with information (oral, written, and electronic) related to her options and choices; encourage the client to review material before the next visit.	Nurses are responsible for providing the client with appropriate information so that she is able to make an informed choice, active participation promotes feelings of control; focusing on one aspect reduces the risk for feeling overwhelmed
Encourage active participation and review a timetable for decision making. Identify different aspects of the decision that need to be considered	
Assist the client with scheduling a return visit in 1 week	Follow-up is necessary to determine the client's decision and to proceed with the provision of or referral for care. Coordination of care may be indicated

EVALUATION

1. The client states she is satisfied with her decision, and has developed strategies for follow-through.
2. The client exhibits behaviours congruent with her decision.
3. The client verbalizes areas of concern related to her situation.
4. The client reports using relaxation techniques for times when she feels stressed.

tent in place. Alternatively, the health care provider may apply prostaglandin gel to the cervix to soften it or may have the client self-administer 400 μg of misoprostol, orally or vaginally, 4 to 12 hours prior to the procedure (Davis, 2006).

Just before the vacuum aspiration procedure, the client may elect to take a mild sedative. Local anaesthesia in the form of a lidocaine paracervical block is common. The health care provider performs a bimanual examination to document the size of the uterus. He or she cleanses the cervix, which is held by a *tenaculum* (a surgical instrument used to grasp and stabilize the cervix). The health care provider inserts a thin plastic catheter through the cervix; this catheter is connected to a vacuum aspirator or syringe. The aspirator or syringe then evacuates the contents of the uterus. During the procedure, the nurse supports the woman, explains the process, and informs her that she will likely experience mild to moderate cramping.

After the aspiration, the health care provider ensures that the uterine contents have been completely removed. The client is monitored for 1 to 2 hours following the procedure to ensure that her vital signs are stable and that she is not experiencing excessive blood loss. Women are informed to expect bleeding similar to that of a heavy menstrual period in duration and intensity, and are advised to avoid the use of tampons while actively bleeding and sexual activity until the bleeding ceases. Other teaching measures include instructing the client to contact a health care provider if she has an elevated temperature, excessive cramping or tenderness, or excessive bleeding. Resumption of menses is expected to occur 4 to 6 weeks after the procedure.

Some health care providers request the client to schedule a return visit, at which time a pelvic examination and pregnancy test are performed to ensure that the voluntary abortion has been successful. As appropriate, instruction about and a prescription for contraceptives may be offered. Discussion of risk-reduction strategies for avoiding sexually transmitted infections and recurrent unintended pregnancy is imperative at any follow-up appointment (Davis, 2006).

Medical Abortion Methods

Methotrexate and Misoprostol. A combination of two medications is most commonly used in medical abortions up to 9 weeks' gestation: mifepristone (also known as RU-486) and misoprostol. In Canada, however, mifepristone is not available, and no medication is currently indicated for medical termination of pregnancy.

Consequently, misoprostol alone, or in combination with methotrexate, is commonly used off-label for this purpose (Davis, 2006). Methotrexate is cytotoxic and has been used as a chemotherapeutic agent for many years. It is also used to treat unruptured ectopic pregnancies, rheumatoid arthritis, choriocarcinoma, and psoriasis. It is a folic acid antagonist; prolonged or recurrent use of methotrexate may predispose women to future pregnancies complicated by a neural tube defect. Misoprostol is a prostaglandin-based drug that is lethal to proliferating trophoblastic tissues and leads to abortion by blocking folic acid in fetal cells, preventing them from dividing. Used together in early-voluntary abortion (at gestational ages less than 49 days), methotrexate and misoprostol have a 90% success rate (Davis, 2006).

Treatment regimens vary, but at least two visits to the health care provider are required. Typically, at the initial visit, the client receives an injection into the gluteal muscle, or an oral dose of methotrexate. The client should be advised to avoid foods that contain folic acid such as green vegetables, and sexual intercourse (Davis, 2006). Researchers disagree about the optimal timing for insertion of misoprostol, which is dispensed in tablet form. The provider gives the woman 800 μg of misoprostol and instructs her to insert it high into the vagina 5 to 7 days after the administration of methotrexate, using a tampon to hold it in place for 12 hours or until active vaginal bleeding begins. If bleeding does not occur, or there is no tissue passed within 24 hours, an additional 800 μg is again inserted (Davis, 2006). Some providers may prefer that the client return to the office or clinic to have the provider insert the drug rather than administering it herself. Providers should give all women undergoing this procedure an appropriate analgesic in preparation for discomfort. See Teaching Tips 9.1 for more information.

Alternatively, misoprostol may be used alone. In this case, 800 μg is administered high in the vagina by the client every 24 or 48 hours either until abortion occurs or three applications (a total of 2,400 μg) are administered (Davis, 2006). This method results in a complete abortion in up to 93% of cases.

All clients are required to return to the clinic 3 to 7 days after administration of misoprostol to ensure that the abortion has been complete. Some clients require a surgical abortion by vacuum aspiration if the medical procedure is not effective in terminating the pregnancy (see previous discussion).

Acetaminophen alone can control most discomfort, although some providers combine a narcotic with the acetaminophen. Blood loss is proportional to the length of gestation, but typically is less than 100 mL. Contraindications to a medical abortion include suspected ectopic pregnancy, renal failure, and concurrent use of steroids or anticoagulant therapy.

 Think back to Patti, the single woman who has just found out that she is 9 weeks pregnant. Patti makes an informed decision to have an abortion, which is scheduled for next week. Which options would be available for her? What factors might affect her choice?

Second-Trimester Methods

Dilatation and Evacuation (D&E). This procedure is similar to a first-trimester vacuum aspiration but requires greater cervical dilatation, because of the increased volume of uterine contents, and forceps extraction of the products of conception (Fig. 9.2). Dilatation is accomplished with serial administration of osmotic dilators (ie, laminaria tents): several are placed the day prior to the procedure if less than 18 weeks' gestation; 10 to 13 dilators are placed over 2 days prior to the procedure if 18 weeks' gestation or more (Davis, 2006). Alternatively, misoprostol may be administered between 14 and 16 weeks' gestation. This procedure is often more uncomfortable, so sedation is typically administered prior to the procedure. Many providers use this procedure through 20 or more weeks' gestation.

● **TEACHING TIPS 9.1 Self-Insertion of Misoprostol**

The provider instructs the client as follows:

- Insert the medication at bedtime or some other time when you can lie down and rest.
- Eat sparingly or lightly because of the possibility of nausea.
- Drink sufficient fluids to maintain hydration and avoid postural hypotension.
- Insert the medication deep into the vagina with clean hands; remain supine for at least 30 minutes.

- Expect cramping and bleeding to begin within 12 hours.
- Take acetaminophen with or without codeine every 4 hours as needed for cramping; notify the health care provider if the bleeding is heavy enough to soak through four sanitary napkins in less than 2 hours.

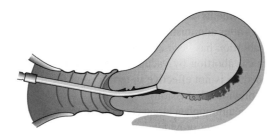

FIGURE 9.2 Dilatation and extraction (D&E).

For women who undergo diagnostic amniocentesis for genetic anomalies, results may not be definitive before 16 weeks and therefore may be a reason for a delayed decision to terminate the pregnancy.

Induction of Labour With Misoprostol and Oxytocin. When an abortion is required in the second trimester, most commonly after a diagnosis of fetal anomaly, induction of labour may be carried out using misoprostol for cervical ripening and oxytocin for subsequent induction of labour. Vaginal misoprostol may be used for cervical ripening, at doses of 25 µg every 4 to 6 hours to prevent excessive uterine stimulation, which may occur at higher dosages. Once the cervix is favourable, induction of labour with oxytocin infusion can proceed, with 50 units in 500 mL of 5% dextrose and normal saline administered over 3 hours, followed by 1 hour of rest. If labour has not commenced, a second solution with an additional 50 units of oxytocin is administered over an additional 3 hours with 1 hour of rest following. This pattern is repeated until either labour begins or a maximum concentration of 300 units in 500 mL is reached (Davis, 2006).

Amnioinfusions. Infusions of hypertonic solutions such as saline or urea are now rarely used. Typically, the health care provider inserts laminaria tents the day before or just prior to the procedure. The woman is asked to empty her bladder before the procedure to avoid inadvertent injury to that organ. The client then undergoes an amniocentesis, at which time amniotic fluid is withdrawn and a similar amount of hypertonic solution is infused. Intra-amniotic installation of prostaglandins may also be an effective technique, but may require repeat injections, and cause significant gastrointestinal effects. The combination of prostaglandin and hyperosmolar urea leads to lower failure rates, limits the need for repeat administration of prostaglandin injections, and the risk of expulsion of a live fetus is significantly reduced (Davis, 2006). The goal of the infusion procedure is to stimulate uterine contractions and expulsion of the uterine contents. In some cases, intravenous oxytocin is used to facilitate contractions and to shorten the time between medication administration and abortion.

 Remember Gina, the 44-year-old woman who had an abortion for severe fetal physical and congenital abnormalities. Which type of abortion procedure was most likely performed?

Care Post Procedure

Abortion is a safe procedure (Davis, 2006). Rates of medical complications of abortion are low when compared with the medical risk of pregnancy and childbirth (Raymond & Grimes, 2012). Complications may include hemorrhage, infection, complete or partial perforation of the uterus, and incomplete abortion. Many providers encourage return visits to ensure that no complications exist as well as to review contraceptive use, and risk-reduction strategies to promote safer sex (Davis, 2006).

Nursing implications include the following:

- Ensure that women who are Rh-negative receive anti-D immune globulin following the procedure (see Chapter 18).
- Teach women to recognize the abatement of early signs of pregnancy (nausea, swollen breasts) and to identify and report warning signs:
  - Fever
  - Chills
  - Abdominal pain
  - Abdominal tenderness
  - Excessive or prolonged bleeding
  - Foul-smelling vaginal discharge
  - Lack of menses by 6 weeks after the procedure
  - Unresolved grief affecting ability to perform activities of daily living

For some clients experiencing mid to late second-trimester abortion, there is the possibility of lactation. Nurses should prepare women for this possibility and encourage them to have a tight-fitting bra and nursing pads available. When lactation occurs, some clients find it especially distressing. Nurses can help by providing anticipatory guidance so that the client is not surprised or frightened if she begins to lactate.

No evidence has demonstrated that first-trimester abortions affect future fertility or pregnancy risks. Although some women experience sadness and show signs of stress during and after the procedure, others report relief. Psychological and emotional sequelae will vary with the client (Broen et al., 2005). Nursing Care Plan 9.2 highlights the care of a client after an abortion.

The client may be fertile almost immediately after undergoing an abortion. The nurse should offer the client information about contraception, as appropriate (see Chapter 8). Several contraceptive methods can be

NURSING CARE PLAN 9.2

●

The Client Recovering From Abortion

 Gina, the 44-year-old woman from the beginning of the chapter, has undergone a dilatation and evacuation procedure. She is awake, alert, and able to tolerate food and fluids. Her vital signs are within acceptable parameters. She has moderate vaginal bleeding and is complaining of only mild cramping at present. She states, "I feel like it was the right choice for me, my husband, and my family. But it's hard not to consider what might have been."

NURSING DIAGNOSES

- **Grieving** related to the loss of the fetus
- **Anticipatory Grieving** related to the loss of an unknown future and possibilities

EXPECTED OUTCOMES

1. The client will verbalize feelings about the loss.
2. The client will begin to demonstrate acceptance of the loss.
3. The client will recognize that the grief process is unique to her and her situation.
4. The client will be able to identify the signs and symptoms of unresolved or pathologic grief.

INTERVENTIONS	RATIONALES
Explore with the client the meaning of the loss of the fetus to her and to her family; encourage her to openly verbalize her feelings and concerns	Exploration and encouraging verbalization of feelings provide the client with a safe outlet and allows the nurse to educate the client about the grief trajectory
Review the client's reasons for her decisions	Such review helps to minimize any misconceptions and questions related to her decision and may aid in lessening any feelings of guilt
Assess the client for possible feelings of guilt associated with her decision to abort	Guilt may affect her ability to progress through the grieving process
Reassure the client that her feelings are common; encourage participation in support groups, as appropriate	Normalization, when appropriate, helps reduce anxiety and fear. Support groups promote sharing of feelings with others who have had similar experiences
Encourage the client to include her spouse and other family members in visits and discussion of feelings	Participation of other relatives promotes sharing and provides support for one another. Sharing of feelings promotes positive coping
Provide the client and family with information about the grieving process and stages of grief. Identify behaviours that would indicate unresolved or pathologic grief	Information about grieving provides a basis for the client and her family to understand what is happening to them

(continued)

NURSING CARE PLAN 9.2 ● The Client Recovering From Abortion *(Continued)*

INTERVENTIONS	RATIONALES
Allow the client (and family members) time to cry; use appropriate methods to help them express feelings comfortably (eg, role-playing, activity, drawing)	Expression of feelings is essential to progress through the grief and mourning process
Arrange for a follow-up visit with the client	A follow-up visit allows time to reassess and evaluate the client's progress

EVALUATION

1. The client continues to state that she made the correct decision and demonstrates acceptance of the decision.
2. The client demonstrates positive methods of coping.
3. The client demonstrates acceptance and resolution of the loss by resuming her activities of daily life.

started immediately; insertion of an intrauterine device may be performed as soon as termination of the pregnancy is confirmed. Because some contraceptive methods take time to become effective, a backup method of contraception is advised until the woman has had her first postabortion menses. Teaching women to use emergency contraception as a backup when contraceptives fail or are not used will assist in avoiding recurrent unintended pregnancy.

CONCLUSION

Presently, Canada does not have an abortion law. Although this prevents the restriction of abortion services, abortion access is not protected, therefore resulting in inequities across the country. Geographical area and access to providers willing to perform abortions also vary significantly across the country.

The decision to terminate a pregnancy may not be easy. However, it may be the best option for the woman with an unintended pregnancy when the woman's life circumstances do not support having a child, for the woman who is a victim of rape or incest, or when carrying a fetus with a diagnosis of significant congenital anomaly. From a public health perspective, an abortion performed in Canada today is safe and effective.

SUMMARY

- Women have sought ways to control family size since the beginning of recorded history.
- Women may elect to terminate a pregnancy for a variety of reasons.
- Religious and cultural considerations may affect women's utilization of abortion services.
- Individuals often have strong feelings about abortion that are based as much in faith traditions as they are in scientific knowledge.
- Medical and surgical procedures are options for first- and second-trimester abortions.

Questions to Ponder

1. Iona, 27 years old, comes to the clinic for confirmation of a positive home pregnancy test. She is afraid that her husband of 5 years will become physically violent if she has another baby. She states that they cannot afford to support the children they already have and that he has threatened to "kill her" if she ever gets pregnant again.
   - What is your reaction to this scenario?
   - What options are available to the client?
   - What preventative measures need to be considered to ensure Iona has the supports necessary?

2. George and Susan have received the results of their prenatal genetic screen, which reveal that their 18-week fetus has Tay–Sachs disease (see Chapter 4). One previous child affected with Tay–Sachs disease died at 35 months after a long period of suffering. George and Susan also have a 3-year-old unaffected child. They state that watching another child suffer from this genetic condition is more than they could bear.
   - What is your reaction to this scenario?
   - What options are available to the client/couple?
   - Is this scenario similar to the previous one? Why or why not?

3. Caroline is 17 years old and had sexual intercourse with her boyfriend of 3 months. She has come to the clinic because she believes she is pregnant and wants an abortion. She underwent an abortion last year when she became pregnant after her first sexual encounter.
   - What are your feelings about these circumstances?
   - What considerations would be appropriate when counselling Caroline?

REVIEW QUESTIONS

1. A nurse who believes abortion is unacceptable under all circumstances should
   A. Share her beliefs with clients.
   B. Share beliefs with clients, if asked.
   C. Keep her personal beliefs to herself.
   D. Never work in women's health.

2. Which of the following is an example of a surgical abortion?
   A. Misoprostol
   B. Methotrexate
   C. Dilatation and evacuation
   D. Insertion of laminaria tents

3. Which of the following should the nurse do prior to providing care to a client considering an abortion?
   A. Explore personal beliefs, values, and biases related to abortion rights.
   B. Present information on what the nurse believes the client needs.
   C. Insist that a partner be present at the counselling session.
   D. Share decision-making responsibilities with the client.

4. After teaching a client who is scheduled to undergo a vacuum aspiration, which client statement indicates the nurse's teaching has been successful?
   A. "The physician will give me an injection into my buttocks and a suppository several days later."
   B. "I'll get some pills from the physician 1 day and then come back to the clinic in about 2 days for some more pills."
   C. "I'll get a local anaesthetic and then the physician will use a small catheter to remove what's in my uterus."
   D. "The physician will do an amniocentesis, take out some fluid, and replace it with a strong salt solution."

5. Which of the following would the nurse include in the discharge teaching plan for a client undergoing a dilatation and evacuation?
   A. Use tampons for any vaginal bleeding
   B. Resume sexual activity in 24 hours
   C. Notify the care provider of any temperature elevations
   D. Use a moderately strong narcotic analgesic for pain

6. A woman who has had an abortion is Rh-negative. Which of the following would the nurse expect to administer?
   A. Prostaglandin
   B. Laminaria
   C. Methotrexate
   D. Anti-D immune globulin

REFERENCES

Arthur, J. (2008). Arguments against Bill C-537 "Protection of conscience rights in the health care profession." Retrieved from http://www.arcc-cdac.ca/action/c-537.html

Boston Women's Health Book Collective. (2011). *Our bodies, ourselves.* New York: Simon & Schuster.

Broen, A. N., Moum, T., Bødtker, A. S., & Ekeberg, O. (2005). The course of mental health after miscarriage and induced abortion: A longitudinal, five-year follow-up study. *BMC Medicine 3*, 18.

Canadian Institute for Health Information. (2011). Quick Stats: Induced abortions reported in Canada in 2009. Retrieved from http://www.cihi.ca/cihi-ext-portal/pdf/internet/ta_09_alldatatables 20111028_en

Canadian Institute for Health information. (2013). Induced abortions reported in Canada in 2011 (Data file). Retrieved from http://www.cihi.ca/CIHI-ext-portal/pdf/internet/TA_11_ALLDATA BLES20130221_EN

Canadian Nurses Association. (2008). *Code of ethics for registered nurses.* Ottawa, ON: Canadian Nurses Association.

Canadian Paediatric Society, & Fetus and Newborn Committee. (2012). *Position statement: Counselling and management for anticipated extremely preterm birth.* Ottawa, ON: Canadian Paediatric Society.

Cappiello, J., Beal, M. W., & Gallogly-Hudson, K. (2011). Applying ethical practice competencies to the prevention and management of unintended pregnancy. *Journal of Obstetric, Gynecologic, and Neonatal Nursing, 40*, 808–816.

Cher, & Sovoca, N. (1996). *If these walls could talk* [Motion picture]. New York: HBO NYC Productions.

Childbirth by Choice Trust. (1998). *No choice: Canadian women tell their stories of illegal abortion.* Toronto, ON: Childbirth by Choice Trust.

Davis, V. J. (2006). *SOGC clinical practice guideline # 184: Induced abortion guidelines.* Ottawa, ON: Society of Obstetricians and Gynaecologists of Canada.

Dunsmuir, M. (1998). *Abortion: Constitutional and legal developments.* Government of Canada. Retrieved from http://dsp-psd.pwgsc.gc.ca/Collection-R/LoPBdP/CIR/8910-e.htm

Finer, L. B., Frohwirth, L. F., Dauphinee, L. A., Singh, S., & Moore, A. M. (2005). Reasons U.S. women have abortions: Quantitative and qualitative perspectives. *Perspectives in Sexual and Reproductive Health, 37*(3), 110–118.

Guttmacher Institute. (2011). *In brief: Facts on induced abortion in the United States.* Retrieved from www.guttmacher.org

Guttmacher Institute. (2012). *U.S. Teenage pregnancies, births and abortions, 2009: National trends by age, race, ethnicity.* Retrieved from www.guttmacher.org

Jonsen, A., Siegler, M., & Winslade, W. (2006). *Clinical ethics: A practical approach to ethical decisions in clinical medicine.* New York: McGraw-Hill.

Kaposy, C. (2010). Improving abortion access in canada. *Health Care Analysis, 18,* 17–34.

Palmer, R. (2008). *Canada abortion debate rekindled a bill passes.* Reuters Canada. Retrieved from http://ca.reuters.com/article/domesticNews/idCAN0625185820080306

Raymond, E. G., & Grimes, D. A. (2012). The comparative safety of legal induced abortion and childbirth in the United States. *Obstetrics & Gynecology, 119*(2), 215–219.

Riddle, J. M. (1992). *Contraception and abortion from the ancient world to the renaissance.* Cambridge, MA: Harvard University Press.

Sedgh, G., Singh, S., Shah, I. H., Ahman, E., Henshaw, S. K., & Bankole, A. (2012). Induced abortion: Incidence and trends worldwide from 1995 to 2008. *The Lancet, 379*(9816), 625–632.

Sethna, C., & Doull, M. (2007). Far from home? A pilot study tracking women's journeys to a Canadian abortion clinic. *Journal of Obstetrics and Gynaecology Canada, 27*(8), 640–647.

Simmonds, K. E., & Likis, F. E. (2011). Caring for women with unintended pregnancies. *Journal of Obstetric, Gynecologic, and Neonatal Nursing, 40,* 794–807.

Srikanthan, A., & Reid, R. L. (2008). Religious and cultural influences on contraception. *Journal of Obstetrics and Gynaecology Canada, 30*(2), 129–137.

Tomlinson, C. (2013). Texas house passes abortion bill; Senate next stop. Texas: Associated Press. Retrieved from http://bigstory.ap.org/article/texas-house-vote-abortion-restrictions

United Nations Population Fund (UNFPA). (1995). International conference on Population and Development - ICPD - Programme of Action. Retrieved from http://www.unfpa.org/public/home/publications/pid/1973

World Health Organization. (2012). *Safe abortion: Technical and policy guidance for health systems* (2nd ed). Retrieved from http://apps.who.int/iris/bitstream/10665/70914/1/9789241548434_eng.pdf

WEB RESOURCES

http://www.apctoolkit.org/
http://www.guttmacher.org
http://www.canadiansforchoice.ca/
http://www.morgentaler25years.ca/
http://www.nursingstudentsforchoice.org/
http://www.prochoice.org/
http://www.prochoiceactionnetwork-canada.org/abortioninfo/history.shtml

CHAPTER 10

Fertility Challenges

Jean Haase, Elisha Ogglesby, Judith A. Lewis*, and Jennifer J. Black*

Ted and Joan have been undergoing preliminary evaluation for infertility. The couple has been married for 5 years; they have been trying to get pregnant for the past 2 years. Ted is 39, and Joan is 37. Their medical histories are negative for any major medical problems.

Stacy, 42 years old, was married for the second time 1 year ago. She is visiting the examiner for a routine reproductive examination. Before they begin, Stacy asks if there is something that she can discuss. "My husband and I have been trying to get pregnant for several months now. It's not happening." Her voice begins to shake. "My ex-husband and I tried to have a baby for years and it never came to be, even though the doctors couldn't find anything wrong. It's one of the reasons my first marriage did not work out. I am so afraid the same thing will happen again."

Nurses working with such clients need to understand the material in this chapter to manage care effectively and address each issue appropriately. Before beginning this chapter, consider the following points related to the above scenarios.

- What additional information does the nurse require from each client?
- How would you suggest the nurse balance the physical needs of each client with the emotional, psychosocial, and spiritual challenges that infertility may impose?
- What measures can the nurse consider for involving the male partners in these scenarios?
- What next steps would you expect for Ted and Joan? For Stacy?

*Contributor to first U.S. edition.

KEY TERMS

assisted hatching
assisted human reproduction (AHR)
cervical stenosis
endometriosis
gamete intrafallopian transfer (GIFT)
impaired fecundity
infertility

intracytoplasmic sperm injection (ICSI)
in vitro fertilization (IVF)
polycystic ovarian syndrome
premature ovarian failure
primary infertility
secondary infertility
zygote intrafallopian transfer (ZIFT)

Infertility, a medical diagnosis of the reproductive system, is defined as the inability to achieve pregnancy after 1 year of frequent, unprotected intercourse (American Society for Reproductive Medicine [ASRM], 2013). Women older than 35 years and having difficulty conceiving may receive a diagnosis of infertility before a full 12 months. **Primary infertility** applies to a man or woman who has never been able to conceive. **Secondary infertility** applies to an inability to conceive after one or both partners have conceived previously. **Impaired fecundity** is the term used when a couple can achieve pregnancy, but the woman cannot carry the pregnancy to a viable birth. A diagnosis of impaired fecundity is usually given after a woman has had two miscarriages.

Health Canada (2013) reports infertility affects about one in eight couples. Recent estimates of the prevalence of current infertility in Canada range from 11.5% to 15.7% (Bushnik et al., 2012). Both women and men may experience conditions that contribute to infertility. Although many people tend to think of infertility as a problem affecting heterosexual couples desiring to have children, infertility may be a problem for single women, single men, and gay and lesbian couples. People in many kinds of situations may seek services to treat infertility.

For most women, family planning involves taking measures to ensure that they can avoid unintended pregnancy, and then taking steps to conceive a child when they are ready to have children. These women have

control of their fertility. These choices and control over human reproduction are not available to women with infertility. Loss of these alternatives can be devastating, placing stress on relationships and self-identity, and leading to decreased self-esteem and depression (Brucker & McKenry, 2004; McCarthy, 2008; Spector, 2004).

HISTORICAL PERSPECTIVES

Infertility has likely existed as long as humans have. Historical accounts of kings disposing off wives because of their inability to bear children are numerous. It seems that, because the woman bore the pregnancy, the inability to achieve the pregnancy was always thought to be her fault. In many parts of the world, this myth still persists.

RELIGIOUS AND CULTURAL PERSPECTIVES

Most religions and cultures view children as a blessing. Some cultures place a value on children of a specific gender. For example, couples whose ancestry can be traced to India or China often express a strong preference for male children (Fuse & Crenshaw, 2006; Jha et al., 2006). In many developing countries, infertility is associated with adverse psychosocial outcomes such as loss of social status, social isolation, marital instability, fear, guilt, and stress (Ombelet et al., 2008).

Jewish Perspectives

Dorff (1998) notes that Judaism considers childbearing to be both an obligation and a commandment (*mitzvah*). Thus, observant Jews highly desire the ability to procreate, and the Jewish faith considers it acceptable to seek medical intervention to treat infertility. Lewis (2003), however, notes that because people cannot be commanded to do something of which they are incapable, the commandment to reproduce would not be an obligation for the infertile couple. Although sexual relations within marriage are seen as a part of fulfilling the commandment of procreation, Judaism has no requirement that the sole purpose of intercourse is the creation of offspring. Sex that is not for the purpose of procreation is acceptable. The *ketubah,* or marriage contract, obligates the man to provide for the woman in all matters, including physical intimacy.

There are a few situations in which sex is prohibited in Judaism, such as on the Day of Atonement (Yom Kippur) and during the immediate mourning period for a parent, sibling, or child. Orthodox Jewish families may follow the rules of *niddah,* or family purity, which considers women ritually impure during and immediately following menstruation. At this time, these women must refrain from any physical contact with men, including sexual intercourse, until they visit the *mikveh,* or ritual bath for immersion after 7 days with no vaginal bleeding have passed. These proscriptions may affect the timing of diagnostic and therapeutic interventions. Health care providers should encourage couples with these dilemmas to confer with their Rabbi.

Because sex outside heterosexual marriage is not in keeping with religious traditions, Judaism does not deal with issues of infertility among single women or lesbians.

Muslim Perspectives

Muslims look to the Qur'an for guidance regarding infertility. They generally accept assistive reproductive techniques when the husband's sperm and wife's eggs are used. Self-masturbation generally is forbidden, but it is acceptable for the wife to help with the collection of sperm. Use of donor gametes or surrogates is thought to produce an illegitimate child and is discouraged. In Islamic countries, polygamy (multiple wives) is an acceptable practice that allows a man to take a second wife if the first cannot bear children. Having a strong belief in the sovereignty of God encourages couples to look to Allah for guidance before making any reproductive decisions (Dutney, 2007).

Catholic Perspectives

Observant Catholics rely on rulings from the Vatican to determine permissible sexual activities. Catholic doctrine prohibits sexual activity outside of marriage, frowns upon masturbation, and permits no form of artificial contraception. Couples may find that the only acceptable way of collecting a semen specimen is through the use of a condom with a hole in it, so that the act of sex still carries the possibility of conception. Many assisted reproductive technologies may be unacceptable to Catholic women and men. Again, clients should seek specific guidance from the Church and the parish priest.

MYTHS, FACTS, AND RESOURCES

As discussed previously, the belief that the female partner is primarily responsible for unwanted infertility is but one common myth associated with infertility. Table 10.1 lists other myths as well as facts that refute them. Perhaps the most pervasive myth suggests that if couples adopt, they will become pregnant. Although pregnancy has followed an adoption in some cases, the thousands of couples who adopt and do not have a subsequent pregnancy are ignored. Although infertile women benefit from correct information, well-meaning but ill-informed advice from friends and colleagues can be more hurtful than helpful.

Reliable and accurate sources of information can be difficult for infertile men and women to access. While many turn to the internet, the sheer amount of information can be overwhelming. For example, a search using the word "infertility" on www.google.com yielded 21.5 million hits. Not all of these sources contain accurate information; some are vague and misleading, or contain biases related to commercial sponsorship. Others focus on personal stories with suggestions that do not apply to all women. Because of the intensely personal nature of infertility, many women are incredibly vulnerable. Nurses can assist women to critically analyze information from the internet so that they do not become victims of unscrupulous people and practices. Some Canadian and US web resources are listed in Box 10.1.

For health care providers, the Nursing Special Interest Group (NSIG) of the Canadian Fertility and Andrology Society (CFAS) (www.cfas.ca) provides information, educational workshops, and teleconferences, as well as connections to other nurses working in the field.

 Remember Stacy, the 42-year-old woman undergoing a routine examination who voices concerns about her ability to get pregnant. What if Stacy states, "Maybe this is God's way of telling me I wasn't supposed to be a mother." What nursing responses would be most appropriate?

(text continues on page 322)

● TABLE 10.1 **Infertility Myths and Facts**

Myth	Fact
Infertility is a woman's problem.	Male factors account for 30% of cases of infertility. Of the remainder, female factors account for 40%, combined factors account for 20%, and unexplained factors are responsible for 10% (Government of Canada, 2013a).
Infertility is rare.	Estimates are that one in six people experience infertility at some point. Approximately one in eight couples experience infertility each year. Fewer than two million infertile couples actually seek medical help. It is a common health problem.
Infertility is all in your head. If you relax and stop thinking about it, you will get pregnant.	Infertility causes stress; stress doesn't cause infertility. Infertility is a medical problem and disorder of the reproductive system.
If you adopt a baby, you will get pregnant.	The pregnancy rate after adopting is the same as for those who do not adopt.
People who can't have babies do not know proper sex techniques.	Infertility is not a sexual disorder. It is a medical condition.
Sex every day will increase your chances of getting pregnant.	Sex every 36–48 hr around the time of ovulation optimizes sperm concentration and increases the chances of conception.
For some couples, getting pregnant just takes time.	Couples in which the female partner trying to achieve pregnancy is younger than 35 yr should seek consultation after 12 mos of unprotected intercourse and no conception. Couples in which the female partner trying to achieve pregnancy is 35 yr or older should seek consultation after 6 mos of unprotected intercourse without conception.
Infertility happens only to couples who have never had a child before.	Secondary infertility (infertility after successful past pregnancies) is possible.
Maybe this is God's way of telling you that you aren't meant to be parents.	Such a statement is painful for anyone to hear and can be very discouraging. Infertility is a medical condition.
My spouse or partner might leave me if we can't conceive a child.	Although infertility can put stress on any relationship, most couples survive infertility crises with their relationship intact. Many couples find that the process of learning new ways of relating to each other during the experience of infertility brings them closer together.
Painful menstruation causes infertility.	Painful menstruation alone does not affect fertility. Progressively worsening menstrual pain may indicate endometriosis, a condition that may affect fertility. The pain escalates with each menstrual cycle and over time as scarring and adhesions form.
Blood group "incompatibility" between husband and wife can cause infertility.	There is no relationship between blood groups and fertility.
I'm not getting pregnant because most of the sperm leaks out after intercourse.	Loss of seminal fluid after intercourse is perfectly normal, and most women notice some discharge immediately after sex. This discharge is not a cause of infertility.
If you work at it and want it enough, you'll get pregnant.	Unlike many aspects of life, infertility may be beyond your control.
A man can judge his fertility by the thickness and volume of his semen.	Semen consists mainly of seminal fluid, secreted by the seminal vesicles and prostate. Volume and consistency of semen are not related to potential for fertility, which depends on sperm count. Microscopic examination is necessary for assessment of sperm count.
Infertility is hereditary.	If your mother, grandmother, or sister had difficulty becoming pregnant, this does not mean you will have the same problem. Most infertility problems are not hereditary. The exception is if a family had a genetic problem that interfered with fertility.
A retroverted (tipped) uterus causes infertility because the semen cannot swim into the cervix.	Approximately 20% of women have a retroverted uterus. If the retroverted uterus is freely mobile, this normal physiologic variation will not cause infertility.
A woman ovulates from the left ovary 1 mo and the right ovary the next month.	It is true that only one ovary ovulates each month. The pattern, however, is not necessarily regular from side to side.
Placing pillows under the woman's hips during and after intercourse enhances fertility.	Sperm are already swimming in cervical mucus as sexual intercourse is completed. They will continue to travel up the cervix to the fallopian tube for the next 48–72 hr. Hip position really does not matter.
Menstrual cycles shorter or longer than every 28 d are irregular.	The length of a woman's menstrual cycle often varies. As long as a woman can count on having her period at a regular interval each month, the number of days in her particular cycle is normal.

(continued)

● TABLE 10.1   **Infertility Myths and Facts** (continued)

Myth	Fact
A man's sperm count will be the same each time it is examined.	Sperm counts vary, based on the time between ejaculations, illness, and medications.
I have no problems having sex. Because I am virile, my sperm count must be normal.	There is no correlation between male fertility and virility. Men with totally normal sex drives may have no sperm at all.
Azoospermia (no sperm) results from excessive masturbation in childhood.	Masturbation is normal, and most boys and men indulge in it. It does not affect sperm count. Men do not "run out" of sperm because the testes constantly produce sperm.
Women who have had voluntary abortions are at risk for infertility when they want to become pregnant.	A woman's subsequent fertility is not adversely affected by abortion (Rowlands, 2011). Precautions are taken with elective abortions to prevent subsequent infertility. Antibiotics are given both during and after the procedure to prevent infection and possible scarring and adhesions. The risk for perforation of the uterus or its arteries is minimal.

From American Society of Reproductive Medicine. (2006). *Frequently asked questions about infertility.* Retrieved from http://www.asrm.org/Patients/faqs.html

● **BOX 10.1**   **Internet Resources for Infertility**

General Information Sites

www.ihr.com/infertility. The site for Internet Health Resources (IHR) provides extensive information about IVF, ICSI, infertility clinics, donor egg and surrogacy services (eg, surrogate mothers), natural infertility treatment, male infertility services, sperm banks, pharmacies, infertility books and videotapes, sperm testing, infertility support, and drugs and medications (eg, Metrodin, Pergonal, Clomid).

www.inciid.org. The InterNational Council on Infertility Information Dissemination, Inc. website includes comprehensive, consumer-targeted coverage of cutting-edge technologies and treatments. It has a good glossary, basic and advanced articles about specific topics, and excellent bulletin boards.

www.iaac.ca. This site provides educational material, support, and assistance to individuals and couples who are experiencing the anguish of infertility, a reproductive health disease which affects over half a million Canadian men and women.

www.infertilitynetwork.org. Infertility Network is a registered Canadian charity providing information and support to those who have difficulty conceiving or carrying a pregnancy to term, to help them make informed choices.

www.resolve.org. The National Infertility Association, Resolve's Helpline, Medical Call-In Hour, Physician Referral Services, Member-to-Member Contact System, and Family Building Magazine focus on supporting couples navigating the maze of infertility.

www.integramedfertility.com. IntegraMed America is a national network of fertility centers dedicated to helping women achieve pregnancy. Their website allows users to contact fertility centers, apply for loans online, and more.

Sites for Particular Medical Conditions

http://endo-online.org. The Endometriosis Association is a nonprofit, self-help organization dedicated to providing information and support, educating the public and medical community, and conducting and promoting research about endometriosis.

www.pcosupport.org. The Polycystic Ovarian Syndrome Association is a voluntary organization dedicated to promoting research and understanding of PCOS.

Sites for Support in Pregnancy Loss

www.growthhouse.org/natal.html. Growth House, Inc. provides end-of-life support, including for grief related to pregnancy and infant death.

www.hannah.org. Hannah's prayer is a Christian infertility and pregnancy loss support network.

www.fertilityplus.org/faq/miscarriage/resources.html. This site provides linkages to miscarriage and perinatal loss resources and support groups.

www.sandsvic.org.au. SANDS is a support group for parents who experience miscarriage, stillbirth, or neonatal death.

Sites for Medical Specialists and Clinical Research

www.cfas.ca/. The CFAS provides leadership in reproductive health for women and men through research, education, and advocacy and continuing educational opportunities for health care professionals.

www.asrm.com. The American Society of Reproductive Medicine is committed to supporting and

(box continues on page 322)

● **BOX 10.1** **Internet Resources for Infertility** (continued)

sponsoring educational activities for the lay public and continuing medical education activities for professionals engaged in the practice and research of reproductive medicine.

www.smru.org. This site for the Society for Male Reproduction and Urology (SMRU) contains information about male reproduction and urology physicians.

www.socrei.org. This professional website for the Society for Reproductive Endocrinology and Infertility (SREI) contains a search function for finding Reproductive Endocrinologists.

www.reprodsurgery.org. This site for the Society of Reproductive Surgeons (SRS) contains information about reproductive surgeons.

Surrogacy Sites

www.opts.com. The Organization of Parents Through Surrogacy (OPTS) website provides mutual support and surrogate parenting information.

www.surromomsonline.com. Surrogate Mothers Online provides information, support, and friendship to actual and potential surrogate mothers as well as parents and prospective parents.

Sites About Adoption

www.adoption.ca. The Adoption Council of Canada is the umbrella organization for adoption in Canada to help raise public awareness of adoption, promote placement of waiting children, and offers linkages to various resources.

www.Adoption.com. This site contains extensive adoption information, including Usenet Newsgroups, Mailing Lists, E-mail help, and search capabilities.

www.adoptionstogether.org. Adoptions Together, Inc is an adoption agency.

www.Adopting.org. This site contains extensive adoption information.

CAUSES OF INFERTILITY

Box 10.2 categorizes the major causes of infertility. Generally, causes tend to be biologic, environmental, related to lifestyle, or physical in nature. The physical factors can be grouped further as female factor, male factor, or combined.

Biologic Factors

Chief among biologic factors in infertility is age. In general, a woman's fertility begins at menarche, peaks during her 20s, and then declines gradually until age 35. Beyond age 35, the decline is more precipitous until menopause, when it ends. Because women are increasingly electing to become established in their careers

● **BOX 10.2** **Causes of Infertility**

Biologic

Age
Genetics
STIs

Environmental/Occupational

Heat
Chemicals
Radiation
Environmental toxins

Lifestyle

Smoking
Alcohol use
Substance/drug use
Delaying pregnancy
Decreased frequency of coitus
Obesity

Physical

Female Factors

Cervical factors

Uterine factors
Tubal factors
Hormonal factors
Ovulatory factors
Coital factors
Endometriosis

Male Factors

Sperm production
Sperm transport
Ejaculatory problems
Coital factors
Genetic factors

Combined Factors

Sperm antibodies
Coital difficulties

Unknown Cause

before they have children, they often delay attempting pregnancy until after their peak years of fertility. Women who delay pregnancy until later in life may find that their biologic clock has moved more quickly than anticipated. The quality and number of ova, as well as the quality of sperm, decline with age (Lane, 2006; Swanton & Child, 2005). The timing of the hormonal changes associated with menopause varies in women, which may pose challenges for some older women who have delayed pregnancy to a point at which they are perimenopausal.

Sexually Transmitted Infections

Women who have multiple sexual partners, have sex with partners who have had multiple partners, or have unprotected sex, are at increased risk for acquiring sexually transmitted infections (STIs) (Anonymous, 2004; Niccolai et al., 2004). Some infections, such as chlamydia, are associated closely with decreased fertility (Idahl et al., 2004). Women with untreated or chronic pelvic infections are at risk for having narrowed or blocked fallopian tubes, which decreases the possibility of fertilization, increases the risk for ectopic pregnancy, or both (Mardh, 2004).

Genetic Conditions

The cause of infertility may be genetic. For example, Turner syndrome is a condition in which one of the two sex chromosomes is completely or partially absent, resulting in a phenotypic female with gonadal dysgenesis in 90% of cases (Powell-Hamilton, 2012). Those with Turner syndrome have markedly compromised or completely absent fertility. Men with cystic fibrosis, another genetic condition, are almost always infertile because of a congenital bilateral absence of the vas deferens (Cystic Fibrosis Medicine, 2008). Many men with mild cystic fibrosis are diagnosed with the condition only when they seek counselling and treatment for infertility (Kolettis & Sandlow, 2002; Sharlip et al., 2002). Clients with infertility related to genetic conditions require counselling about their chances of passing the same conditions to offspring, should they be able to achieve pregnancy and carry a fetus to viability.

Environmental Factors

Many environmental toxins can affect fertility. As women gain increasing access to employment opportunities, they become exposed to workplace hazards from which they were once shielded. Environmental hazards include toxic chemicals, excessive heat, air pollution, and noise. For example, until gas scavenging systems were required in operating rooms, women working in operating rooms were at increased risk for spontaneous abortions (Panni & Corn, 2002).

Lifestyle Factors

Many lifestyle choices can affect fertility adversely. Cigarette smoking negatively affects both male and female fertility (Akushevich et al., 2007; Practice Committee of the ASRM, 2012; Windham et al., 2005). Heavy alcohol consumption negatively influences fertility and has adverse effects on the developing fetus (Klonoff-Cohen et al., 2003). Use of illegal substances can interfere with the hypothalamic–pituitary feedback loop and the production of gonadotropins (Langford et al., 2011). Dual-career couples with heavy job demands may find themselves with decreased opportunities for sexual activity at the optimal time for conception.

Obesity can affect fertility (Pasquali et al., 2007). Fat cells convert adrenal hormones into estrogens. A steady supply of estrogen from this peripheral source will ultimately interfere with the ovarian production of estrogen, disrupting ovulation and causing infertility.

Several of the lifestyle factors affecting fertility are modifiable. Nurses should encourage clients to decrease behaviours that may compromise their fertility. They should promote healthy lifestyles that include abstention from cigarettes, recreational drugs, and excessive alcohol consumption. Exercise, healthy diet, and stress management are essential (see Chapter 2). Clients should also be counselled on safe sexual practices and be made aware of potential environmental hazards that may affect fertility. See Teaching Tips 10.1 for more information.

Physical Factors and Classification

Approximately one third of infertility problems are attributable to female factor infertility; slightly less than one third are tied to male factor infertility (ASRM, 2013). Approximately one third of problems result from combined male and female factors (ASRM, 2013). In approximately 20% of cases, infertility cannot be classified as attributable to any one party or cause (ASRM, 2013).

Female Factor Infertility

Hormonal Problems. In women, infertility can result from alterations in hormonal activity of the hypothalamus, pituitary gland, thyroid gland, adrenal glands, or ovaries. Each organ has an important role in secreting hormones necessary for a normal menstrual cycle (Fig. 10.1).

Hypothalamus. Alterations in the hypothalamus cause changes in levels of estrogen and gonadotropin-releasing hormone (GnRH). Such alterations may result from stress, eating disorders, or intensive exercise (eg, gymnastics). Conditions in which body fat and total body weight are decreased markedly may lead to anovulation. If a cause for the hypothalamic disturbance can be identified, the condition may be easily reversible.

● **TEACHING TIPS 10.1** **Methods to Enhance Fertility**

The nurse counsels the client or couple as follows:

- Reduce stress, particularly stress related to the issue of becoming pregnant. Discuss your desires and frustrations with your partner, particularly if sex starts to become a "chore."
- Avoid use of douches and lubricants before, during, and after intercourse. These substances can interfere with sperm motility and alter the chemical balance of cervical mucus.
- After engaging in intercourse, the woman trying to become pregnant should remain flat in bed. This

position can help sperm flow more steadily to the cervix. The woman should not rise from this position for 20 to 30 minutes.
- The best timing for sexual intercourse is every 36 to 48 hours while the woman is ovulating. Discuss methods for predicting ovulation and planning intercourse to achieve pregnancy directly with your health care provider.
- Maintain good nutrition.
- Get regular exercise.
- Avoid tobacco, alcohol, and recreational drugs.

Treatment is more difficult if the etiology of the disturbance is unknown (Star et al., 2004).

Pituitary Gland. The pituitary gland secretes follicle-stimulating hormone (FSH) and luteinizing hormone (LH), both of which are key regulators of ovulation.

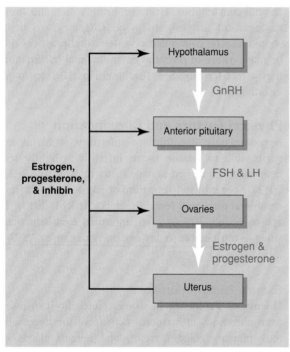

FIGURE 10.1 Role of hormones in fertility. Gonadotropin-releasing hormone (*GnRH*) released from the hypothalamus regulates production of luteinizing hormone (*LH*) and follicle-stimulating hormone (*FSH*) in the anterior pituitary. *LH* stimulates the release of estrogen and progesterone from the ovaries. *FSH* stimulates maturation of the ovarian follicle. Estrogen, a hormone produced by the ovaries, is responsible for secondary sex characteristics and cyclic changes in the lining of the uterus and vagina. Progesterone, another hormone produced by the ovaries, prepares the uterus for the development of the fertilized ovum and maintains the uterus throughout pregnancy.

FSH is responsible for the events that trigger the development of the ovarian follicle, and LH level surges with ovulation. The pituitary gland is also responsible for the production of prolactin, which normally emerges after childbirth to promote lactation. Elevated prolactin levels in the non–breastfeeding woman can cause anovulatory cycles and resultant infertility. Although a common cause of elevated prolactin levels is a tumour called pituitary adenoma, certain medications can lead to this problem, as can hypothyroidism (Star et al., 2004).

Thyroid Gland. Alterations in thyroid hormones also may be related to infertility. In the hypothyroid state, a woman may experience increased frequency of menstruation. The unopposed thyroid-releasing hormone (because the thyroid is not producing enough thyroid hormones) from the hypothalamus stimulates the pituitary gland to make excess prolactin. In turn, this situation interferes with the pituitary feedback cycle and may affect production of LH and FSH.

In the hyperthyroid state, the woman may experience decreased or absent menses. Hyperthyroid conditions are often autoimmune in nature and coexist with autoimmune ovarian problems, in which antibodies are targeted at the ovaries and prevent them from participating in menses (Thyroid Foundation of Canada, 2013).

Hyperthyroidism and hypothyroidism in men can alter spermatogenesis by interfering with the hypothalamic–pituitary feedback loop (Shaban, 2007).

Adrenal Gland. Adrenal dysfunction can lead to male and female infertility. The adrenal glands produce androgens in men and women (in women, estrogen and progesterone usually counter these androgens). In some conditions, such as adrenal hyperplasia and adrenal tumours, excess androgen is produced. Secondary to this excess steroid production, women may experience ovulatory failure; men may experience compromised spermatogenesis (Rebar, 2013a).

Ovaries. The ovaries also secrete hormones, and alterations in ovarian function may be related to infertility. **Polycystic ovarian syndrome** (PCOS) is a common cause of ovarian dysfunction (Lane, 2006). Manifestations of PCOS include the following symptoms in any combination: obesity, hirsutism, amenorrhea or irregular menses, and subsequent infertility. The condition is associated with a hypothalamic–pituitary–ovarian imbalance that results in elevated levels of estrogen, testosterone, and LH. There is also associated hyperinsulinemia and impaired glucose tolerance. The condition is also linked with the adverse health outcomes of cardiovascular disease glucose intolerance and type 2 diabetes mellitus (Randeva et al., 2012). (See Chapter 4 for more information.)

Treatment of PCOS depends on the symptoms most bothersome to the client. The health care provider may prescribe oral contraceptives to regulate menstruation and decrease the levels of LH and testosterone (decreasing hirsutism). If the client desires pregnancy, the health care provider may prescribe clomiphene (Clomid) to correct the hormone imbalance and induce ovulation. He or she also may prescribe metformin to treat impaired glucose tolerance. Metformin reduces glucose produced in the liver and increases the cellular uptake of glucose. Another drug class that may be prescribed is the glitazones to increase insulin sensitivity in the muscles and adipose tissue and to inhibit hepatic glucose production.

Another common condition is **premature ovarian failure**. All the eggs that a woman will ever produce develop in a rudimentary fashion while she is still in utero (see Chapter 11). Her number of eggs decreases steadily until menopause (Swanton & Child, 2005). In some women, however, this process is accelerated, so that they begin to experience symptoms of menopause 10 or more years earlier than would normally be expected (Swanton & Child, 2005). Causes include genetic conditions with chromosomal abnormalities, autoimmune disease, surgical removal of the ovaries, or damage to the ovaries by a virus, chemotherapy, or radiation. Women with premature ovarian failure may not be able to become pregnant with their own eggs. Symptoms of menopause (eg, hot flashes, vaginal dryness, decreased libido) can be treated with hormone replacement. Clients with this condition need to take preventive measures against osteoporosis and heart disease (see Chapter 2).

Tubal Problems. In some women, the cause of infertility is tubal. Fallopian tubes can become narrowed or scarred from ascending pelvic infection, inflammation from an intrauterine device (IUD), surgical adhesions, or previous ectopic pregnancy. Pelvic adhesions from conditions such as endometriosis (see later discussion) can prevent free movement of the fallopian tubes, making them less able to capture extruded eggs. Tubal problems can result in the inability of egg and sperm to meet or of the fertilized ovum to reach the uterus. Some women may be able to achieve fertility after reversal of previous sterilization surgery. Other women, even though their tubes were successfully reanastomosed, may be unable to become pregnant.

Cervical Problems. The reason for infertility may be a problem in the uterine cervix. Examples include cervical stenosis and suboptimal cervical mucus.

Cervical stenosis is the narrowing or closing of the cervical os. It may be congenital or the result of improper healing or scarring from previous surgery. This closing of the cervical opening can impair the ability of sperm to enter the uterus for fertilization of an egg.

Cervical mucus provides nutrients for sperm as they move toward the egg. This mucus can either facilitate or prevent the passage of sperm into the uterus. The structure of cervical mucus acts as a filter for abnormally formed sperm and sperm with antibodies attached. Cyclic influences of hormones on mucus also make it more or less navigable by sperm. Near ovulation, estrogens cause the mucus to become watery and penetrable by sperm so that the sperm can swim easily toward the egg awaiting fertilization. Progesterone causes the mucus to become viscous and impenetrable by sperm.

Uterine Problems. Some women have anatomic alterations of the uterus that compromise fertility. For example, fibroid tumours can mechanically obstruct the cervix, endometrial cavity, or fallopian tubes, preventing the union of egg and sperm. They can also distort the endometrial cavity and interfere with proper implantation of a fertilized egg. A tumour may impede blood flow to the developing embryo because the tumour requires vasculature to support it. This is frequently found to be the cause of infertility in women who have had multiple miscarriages (Marchionni et al., 2004).

Diethylstilbestrol (DES) is a synthetic estrogen that was used from the 1950s to the 1970s to reduce the incidence of early pregnancy loss, intrauterine fetal demise, and preterm delivery. It was later determined that DES actually may have increased the rates of spontaneous abortion, preterm delivery, and perinatal death; its use was banned in Canada and the United States over 30 years ago (Health Canada, 2003). Unfortunately, the effects of DES were not limited to the women who took it themselves. Recent research concludes that DES crosses the placenta and acts as a carcinogen causing reproductive cancer in offspring (Newbold, 2008). Women whose mothers took DES during their pregnancies may have congenital abnormalities that compromise fertility. DES is believed to interfere in müllerian duct development, with subsequent reproductive structure abnormalities.

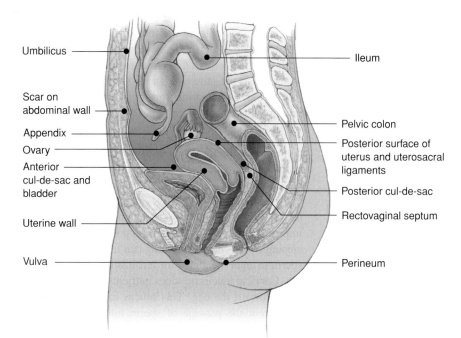

FIGURE 10.2 Common sites of endometriosis.

A "DES-exposed daughter" may have vaginal abnormalities (eg, adenosis), cervical abnormalities (eg, collars, hoods, septae), and uterine malformations (eg, T-shaped uterus, constriction bands) (Rubin, 2007). In addition to structural reproductive abnormalities, DES also may cause poor cervical mucus, endometriosis, and irregular menses, which can all contribute to infertility (Rubin, 2007). Men with in utero exposure to DES may have sperm and semen abnormalities that do not affect their fertility (Schrager & Potter, 2004).

Endometrial Problems. Endometriosis is a condition in which bits of the endometrial lining, normally attached to the inner lining of the uterus, become part of the abdominal cavity (Fig. 10.2). This displaced endometrial tissue undergoes the same cyclic changes as intrauterine endometrium. Resulting cyclic stimulation and bleeding of the endometrial tissue cause local inflammation, scarring, and adhesions. These problems, in turn, can lead to anatomic distortions that preclude normal functioning and, subsequently, to infertility. In addition, the woman with endometriosis can experience dyspareunia (severe discomfort with intercourse), which may cause her to avoid or to limit coitus.

Male Factor Infertility

Sperm Problems. Male infertility can result from problems with sperm production or transport (Table 10.2). Normal semen contains at least 20 million sperm per millilitre, of which at least 50% demonstrate normal forward progression and 35% or more have normal morphology (Taylor et al., 2012). The normal ejaculate is at least 2 mL in volume (Taylor et al., 2012). Decreased volume may result from retrograde ejaculation, a condition in which the sphincter between the urethra and bladder relaxes. As a result, some ejaculate enters the bladder rather than being expelled through the penis into the vagina of the female partner. A low sperm count may result from increased scrotal temperature, infection, or chronic illness. Trauma or infection may lead to decreased sperm motility. High number of sperm with abnormal morphology may result from environmental toxins or testicular cancer (Star et al., 2004).

Sperm transport problems are often anatomic in nature. Hydroceles, spermatoceles, or varicoceles are abnormalities that cause increased vascularity, raising the temperature in the scrotum and diminishing the viability of sperm (Saner-Amigh & Halvorson, 2011). Congenital bilateral absence of the vas deferens causes total obstruction of the transport system. In this condition, sperm are manufactured in normal quantities and of normal quality, but their ability to traverse the tubules is impaired. Men with cystic fibrosis almost always

● TABLE 10.2 **Normal Values for Semen Analysis**

Volume	2–5 mL
Liquefaction	Complete in 20–30 min
Count	>20 million per mL
Motility	>60% mobile after 1 hr
	>50% mobile after 2 hr
Morphology	>30% have normal morphology
White blood cells	None
Bacteria	None too few

have congenital bilateral absence of the vas deferens, causing absolute infertility.

Erectile and Ejaculatory Problems. The penis must introduce sperm into the vagina for successful transfer of sperm through the cervix and into the uterus and fallopian tubes. Some men have difficulty achieving and maintaining an erection, making successful completion of intercourse impossible. Other men can achieve an erection, but suffer from premature ejaculation, in which they ejaculate before sperm are introduced into the vagina, thereby eliminating the chance for fertilization of an egg. Men with spinal cord injury or neuropathies may fail to ejaculate or have retrograde ejaculation, in which case semen is delivered to the man's bladder instead of to the woman's vagina.

Hypospadias. Still other men have hypospadias, a condition in which the urethral opening is on the underside of the penis rather than at its tip (Fig. 10.3). In some cases, the urethral opening is at the juncture of the penis and the scrotum. A man with hypospadias may be able to have sexual intercourse, but the ejaculate is not delivered deep into the vagina, making it less likely that sperm will reach the outer third of the fallopian tube. A man with severe hypospadias may deliver his ejaculate totally on his partner's external genitalia.

Other Causes of Infertility

Some couples have *combined factor infertility,* in which the woman makes antibodies to her partner's sperm. These people may not have impaired fertility alone; however, as a couple, the antisperm antibodies in the female's cervical mucus cause the sperm to become immobile before they can traverse the cervix.

Other couples have difficulty with sexual intercourse because of anatomic factors. Examples include obesity and confusion or limited knowledge about coi-

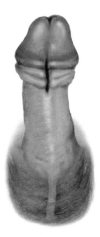

FIGURE 10.3 Hypospadias may be a male physical factor contributing to infertility.

tal technique. Environmental factors such as inadequate privacy may lead to hasty coital episodes that end prematurely.

Infertility of Unknown Cause
QUOTE 10-1

"The most difficult parts of dealing with infertility for us have been the uncertainty and the lack of closure. No one has been able to explain why we can't get pregnant. Every time we make love, I wonder if maybe this time we'll be lucky. The ongoing disappointments are sometimes unbearable."

A man who has been trying with his wife for pregnancy for more than 3 years

Infertility for which a definitive cause cannot be identified accounts for 20% of all cases (Government of Canada, 2013a). This situation can be especially frustrating for clients, particularly because they never know whether their situation is modifiable or unchangeable. They may feel guilty if they decide to give up trying; alternatively, they may feel increasing frustration for continuing their quest to have a biologic child without results. These clients may need additional counselling and resources to handle the especially challenging physical and psychological effects of this situation.

 Ted and Joan, the couple described at the beginning of the chapter, have decided to pursue further testing for infertility. During a visit, Ted states, "What if they can't find anything wrong?" How should the nurse respond?

COLLABORATIVE CARE: INFERTILITY
The realization that a couple has a problem with infertility can generate stress and negative emotions. Societal and cultural messages exalt sexual prowess and performance. Couples who cannot successfully achieve pregnancy may feel isolated, inadequate, and that they do not measure up to societal standards (Brucker & McKenry, 2004; Cousineau & Domar, 2007).

Couples who seek fertility treatment find themselves talking about the most intimate details and activities with complete strangers. Some couples disagree about the acceptability of doing so, thereby placing stress on a relationship that already may be strained. Sometimes women seek consultation during their annual gynecologic examinations and wish to have diagnostic assessment alone because their male partners are unwilling to discuss the issue.

Assessment

For some couples, the assessment process can present significant challenges. While primary care physicians and specialists such as gynecologists or urologists can perform some of the diagnostic workup and testing, access to a fertility clinic or reproductive endocrinologist may be more difficult, given that most clinics tend to be located in large urban areas. Costs are a further barrier to accessing care. Although the public health care system may cover the costs of routine diagnostic tests, specialized tests and most treatments are increasingly provided by the private health care sector. Couples might delay assessment and diagnosis because of the difficulty in accessing a specialist and concerns about the anticipated costs. Diagnostic tests often require several visits, may be scheduled at specific times during a woman's cycle, and often necessitate that she miss work. These absences can lead to further loss of income at a time when the cost of the infertility evaluation is increasing expenses.

Nurses caring for those experiencing infertility should be aware of the emotional stress that this condition can place on individuals, couples, and those who care for them (Assessment Tool 10.1). Sensitivity and support from nurses may make a difference in the ability of clients to maintain self-esteem and control during a difficult time. Nurses can remind couples that other options, such as adoption and child-free living, exist. If clients or couples express interest in such alternatives, nurses can act as advocates and supply resources and information. In all cases, the nurse works to ensure that clients understand that they themselves maintain control over options they wish to pursue and when they want to cease treatment (Fig. 10.4).

Assessment of the Man

Assessment of the male partner should be completed early in the diagnostic process because it involves fewer invasive procedures and is less costly than is the process for women. Although some reproductive endocrinologists evaluate both men and women, a urologist usually completes the workup of the male partner.

Health History

The first step is gathering a complete health history, which should include the following information:

- Whether the man has ever achieved pregnancy with this or any other partner
- Exposure to environmental agents, such as chemicals or other toxins
- Exposure to heat, including the use of steam baths or wearing tight underwear or trousers
- Smoking, alcohol, or recreational drug use

- History of STIs
- History of postpubertal mumps or orchitis (which cause testicular atrophy), or genital trauma
- Family history, including whether his mother took DES during her pregnancy with him
- Family history of cystic fibrosis (congenital absence of vas deferens)
- Use of prescription or over-the-counter medications, or use of chemotherapeutic drugs
- Dietary adequacy

Assessment Tool 10.2 provides a sample history form to evaluate for male factor infertility.

Physical Examination

The physical examination focuses on secondary sex characteristics as well as the structure and function of the male reproductive organs.

Laboratory and Diagnostic Testing

Laboratory testing is done to ensure general well-being and may include assessment of serum FSH and testosterone levels (Sharlip et al., 2002). Depending on the results of these tests, LH, free testosterone, and prolactin levels may be tested (Fritz & Speroff, 2011). See Table 10.3 for a complete summary of male hormone levels that may be examined.

Conditions such as diabetes should be ruled out first. Diabetes in men can cause bladder neck dysfunction and result in retrograde ejaculation. A complete semen analysis should be performed on a specimen collected after 2 to 3 days of abstinence from intercourse. During a semen analysis, the examiner evaluates the volume of ejaculate, the percentage of motile sperm, the percentage of sperm with normal morphology, the total sperm count, liquefaction (semen should become liquefied within 60 minutes), and the number of white blood cells (indicates possible inflammation). The specimen is usually collected by masturbation. It is acceptable for the man to collect the specimen at home or in another private setting and deliver it to the laboratory within a specified period. If the specimen requires transport to the laboratory, the man should carry the specimen in an inner pocket so that it remains at body temperature until it can be analyzed.

Some men cannot produce a specimen by masturbating or have religious or other personal reservations about masturbating. Collecting the specimen in an unlubricated condom that does not contain any spermicides and is used during intercourse is possible. For the couple whose religion prohibits both masturbation and the use of condoms, poking a small hole in the condom before applying it may satisfy those concerns.

● **ASSESSMENT TOOL 10.1**   **Infertility Questionnaire**

FertiQoL International
Fertility Quality of Life Questionnaire (2008)
For each question, kindly check (tick the box) for the response that most closely reflects how you think and feel. Relate your answers to your current thoughts and feelings. Some questions may relate to your private life, but they are necessary to adequately measure all aspects of your life.

Please complete the items marked with an asterisk (*) only if you have a partner.

	For each question, check the response that is closest to your current thoughts and feelings	Very Poor	Poor	Nor good nor poor	Good	Very Good
A	How would you rate your health?	☐	☐	☐	☐	☐

	For each question, check the response that is closest to your current thoughts and feelings	Very Dissatisfied	Dissatisfied	Neither Satisfied Nor Dissatisfied	Satisfied	Very Satisfied
B	Are you satisfied with your quality of life?	☐	☐	☐	☐	☐

	For each question, check the response that is closest to your current thoughts and feelings	Completely	A Great Deal	Moderately	Not Much	Not At All
Q1	Are your attention and concentration impaired by thoughts of infertility?	☐	☐	☐	☐	☐
Q2	Do you think you cannot move ahead with other life goals and plans because of fertility problems?	☐	☐	☐	☐	☐
Q3	Do you feel drained or worn out because of fertility problems?	☐	☐	☐	☐	☐
Q4	Do you feel able to cope with your fertility problems?	☐	☐	☐	☐	☐

	For each question, check the response that is closest to your current thoughts and feelings	Very Dissatisfied	Dissatisfied	Neither Satisfied Nor Dissatisfied	Satisfied	Very Satisfied
Q5	Are you satisfied with the support you receive from friends with regard to your fertility problems?	☐	☐	☐	☐	☐
*Q6	Are you satisfied with your sexual relationship even though you have fertility problems?	☐	☐	☐	☐	☐

	For each question, check the response that is closest to your current thoughts and feelings	Always	Very Often	Quite Often	Seldom	Never
Q7	Do your fertility problems cause feelings of jealousy and resentment?	☐	☐	☐	☐	☐
Q8	Do you experience grief and/or feelings of loss about not being able to have a child (or more children)?	☐	☐	☐	☐	☐
Q9	Do you fluctuate between hope and despair because of fertility problems?	☐	☐	☐	☐	☐
Q10	Are you socially isolated because of fertility problems?	☐	☐	☐	☐	☐
*Q11	Are you and your partner affectionate with each other even though you have fertility problems?	☐	☐	☐	☐	☐
Q12	Do your fertility problems interfere with your day-to-day work or obligations?	☐	☐	☐	☐	☐
Q13	Do you feel uncomfortable attending social situations like holidays and celebrations because of your fertility problems?	☐	☐	☐	☐	☐
Q14	Do you feel your family can understand what you are going through?	☐	☐	☐	☐	☐

	For each question, check the response that is closest to your current thoughts and feelings	An Extreme Amount	Very Much	A Moderate Amount	A Little	Not At All
*Q15	Have fertility problems strengthened your commitment to your partner?	☐	☐	☐	☐	☐
Q16	Do you feel sad and depressed about your fertility problems?	☐	☐	☐	☐	☐
Q17	Do your fertility problems make you inferior to people with children?	☐	☐	☐	☐	☐
Q18	Are you bothered by fatigue because of fertility problems?	☐	☐	☐	☐	☐
*Q19	Have fertility problems had a negative impact on your relationship with your partner?	☐	☐	☐	☐	☐
*Q20	Do you find it difficult to talk to your partner about your feelings related to infertility?	☐	☐	☐	☐	☐
*Q21	Are you content with your relationship even though you have fertility problems?	☐	☐	☐	☐	☐
Q22	Do you feel social pressure on you to have (or have more) children?	☐	☐	☐	☐	☐
Q23	Do your fertility problems make you angry?	☐	☐	☐	☐	☐
Q24	Do you feel pain and physical discomfort because of your fertility problems?	☐	☐	☐	☐	☐

(continued)

● ASSESSMENT TOOL 10.1   Infertility Questionnaire *(Continued)*

FertiQoL International
Optional Treatment Module

Have you started fertility treatment (this includes any medical consultation or intervention)? If Yes, then please respond to the following questions. For each question, kindly check (tick the box) for the response that most closely reflects how you think and feel. Relate your answers to your current thoughts and feelings. Some questions may relate to your private life, but they are necessary to adequately measure all aspects of your life.

	For each question, check the response that is closest to your current thoughts and feelings	Always	Very Often	Quite often	Seldom	Never
T1	Does infertility treatment negatively affect your mood?	☐	☐	☐	☐	☐
T2	Are the fertility medical services you would like available to you?	☐	☐	☐	☐	☐

	For each question, check the response that is closest to your current thoughts and feelings	An Extreme Amount	Very Much	A Moderate Amount	A Little	Not At All
T3	How complicated is dealing with the procedure and/ or administration of medication for your infertility treatment(s)?	☐	☐	☐	☐	☐
T4	Are you bothered by the effect of treatment on your daily or work-related activities?	☐	☐	☐	☐	☐
T5	Do you feel the fertility staff understand what you are going through?	☐	☐	☐	☐	☐
T6	Are you bothered by the physical side effects of fertility medications and treatment?	☐	☐	☐	☐	☐

	For each question, check the response that is closest to your current thoughts and feelings	Very Dissatisfied	Dissatisfied	Neither Satisifed nor Dissatisfied	Satisfied	Very Satisfied
T7	Are you satisfied with the quality of services available to you to address your emotional needs?	☐	☐	☐	☐	☐
T8	How would you rate the surgery and/or medical treatment(s) you have received?	☐	☐	☐	☐	☐
T9	How would you rate the quality of information you received about medication, surgery and/or medical treatment?	☐	☐	☐	☐	☐
T10	Are you satisfied with your interactions with fertility medical staff?	☐	☐	☐	☐	☐

Source: Boivin, J., Takefman, J., & Braverman, A. (2011). Development and preliminary validation of the fertility quality of life (FertiQoL) tool. *Human Reproduction, 26*(8), 2084–2091.

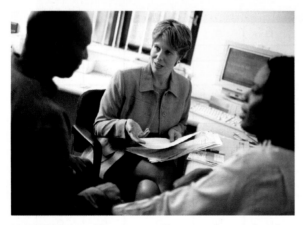

FIGURE 10.4 The nurse works as an advocate for clients and ensures that all decisions related to fertility rest with the woman or the woman and her partner.

Stacy, the 42-year-old woman from the beginning of the chapter, reports that in her previous marriage, the health care providers couldn't find anything wrong. What questions would be important for the nurse to ask when assessing Stacy's situation?

Assessment of the Woman
Health History

Assessment of the woman includes a detailed health history. The health care provider asks about genetic conditions like sickle cell anemia, β-thalassemia, or Tay–Sachs disease; a history of DES use by the woman's mother; previous pregnancies with this or another partner; surgery or trauma; infectious diseases;

● **ASSESSMENT TOOL 10.2** **Infertility History Form for Men**

Name:	Date:
Address:	Tel.:
Occupation:	Age: Religion:
Employer:	Name Rel./Friend:
Bus. Tel.:	Address:
Referred by:	
Birth Place:	
Birth Date:	

All previous occupations: | List all provinces or countries in which you have lived:

Education: Please encircle the last   Grade 5   High School 1 2 3 4   Post Grad. _____ yrs.
Grade you completed   6 7 8   College 1 2 3 4   Degrees

CHIEF COMPLAINTS
Please list all symptoms you have NOW.
1. _____
2. _____
3. _____
Routine checkup—no symptoms [ ]

P.I. Please do not write in this space.

Family History	Age	If Living Health	Age at Death	If Deceased Cause	Please Encircle Has any blood relative had		Who
Father					Cancer	no yes	
Mother					Tuberculosis	no yes	
Brother or sister 1.					Diabetes	no yes	
2.					Heart trouble	no yes	
3.					High blood pressure	no yes	
4.					Stroke	no yes	
5.					Epilepsy	no yes	
Husband or wife					Mental illness	no yes	
Son or daughter 1.					Suicide	no yes	
2.					Congenital deformities	no yes	
3.							
4.							
5.							
6.							
7.							

NOTE:
This is a confidential record of your medical history and will be kept in this office. Information contained here will not be released to any person except when you have authorized us to do so.

PERSONAL HISTORY
ILLNESS: Have you had
(Please Encircle all Answers no or yes)

Measles or German measles	no yes
Chickenpox or mumps	no yes
Whooping cough	no yes
Scarlet fever or scarlatina	no yes
Pneumonia or pleurisy	no yes
Diphtheria or smallpox	no yes
Influenza	no yes
Rheumatic fever or heart disease	no yes
Arthritis or rheumatism	no yes
Any bone or joint disease	no yes
Neuritis or neuralgia	no yes
Bursitis, sciatica or lumbago	no yes
Polio or meningitis	no yes
Bright's disease or kidney infection	no yes

Gonorrhea or syphilis	no yes
Anemia or jaundice	no yes
Epilepsy	no yes
Migraine headaches	no yes
Tuberculosis	no yes
Diabetes or cancer	no yes
High or low blood pressure	no yes
Nervous breakdown	no yes
Food, chemical or drug poisoning	no yes
Hay fever or asthma	no yes
Hives or eczema	no yes
Frequent colds or sore throat	no yes
Frequent infections or boils	no yes
Any other disease	no yes
ALLERGIES: Are you allergic to	
Penicillin or sulfa	no yes
Aspirin, codeine or morphine	no yes

Mycins or other antibiotics	no yes
Merthiolate or mercurochrome	no yes
Any other drug	no yes
Any foods	no yes
Adhesive tape	no yes
Nail polish or other cosmetics	no yes
Tetanus antitoxin or serums	no yes
INJURIES: Have you had any	
Broken bones	no yes
Sprains or dislocations	no yes
Lacerations (extensive)	no yes
Concussion or head injury	no yes
Ever been knocked out	no yes
TRANSFUSIONS: Have you ever had	
Blood or plasma transfusion	no yes
Weight: now _____ one year ago _____
Max _____ when _____ Height _____

Please review the section you have just completed and wherever you answered "yes" fill in the year (guess if necessary) and also where there is more than one illness to a line encircle the ones you have had. Example: Chickenpox or mumps............1961 .... no (yes)

(continued)

● **ASSESSMENT TOOL 10.2** **Infertility History Form for Men** *(Continued)*

SURGERY: Have you had

Tonsillectomy .... no   yes
Appendectomy .... no   yes
Any other operation (give details)... no   yes

Give DETAILS below of all hospitalizations for surgery or illness including name and address of Doctor and Hospital ....

Have you ever been advised to have any surgical operation which has not been done? [1] no [2] yes what.....................

Systems: Please check those you have had.
Eye disease [ ], Eye injury [ ], Impaired sight [ ], Ear disease [ ], Ear injury [ ], Impaired hearing [ ],
Trouble with: Nose [ ], Sinuses [ ], Mouth [ ], Throat [ ], Have you checked any in this group?.......................... no   yes
Fainting spells [ ], Loss of consciousness [ ], Convulsions [ ], Paralysis [ ], Frequent or severe headaches [ ],
    Dizziness [ ], Depression or anxiety [ ], Hallucinations [ ], Have you checked any in this group? .... no   yes
Enlarged glands [ ], Goiter or enlarged thyroid [ ], Skin disease [ ], Have you checked any in this group? .... no   yes
Chronic or frequent cough [ ], Chest pain or angina pectoris [ ], Spitting up of blood [ ], Night sweats [ ],
    Shortness of breath [ ], Palpitation or fluttering heart [ ], Swelling of hands, feet, or ankles [ ],
    Varicose veins [ ], Extreme tiredness or weakness [ ], Have you checked any in this group?.......................... no   yes
Kidney disease or stones [ ], Bladder disease [ ], Albumin, sugar, pus, etc. in urine [ ],
    Difficulty in urinating [ ], Awake to urinate nightly [ ], Have you checked any in this group?.......................... no   yes
Stomach trouble or ulcers [ ], Indigestion [ ], Liver or gallbladder disease [ ], Colitis or other bowel disease [ ]
    Appendicitis [ ], Hemorrhoids or rectal bleeding [ ], Constipation or diarrhea [ ], Recent change in bowel
    action or stools [ ], Recent change in appetite or eating habits [ ], Have you checked any in this group?....... no   yes

HABITS: Do you

Sleep well?............................. no   yes
Use alcoholic beverages .... no   yes
    Every day?....................... no   yes
Smoke?................................ no   yes
    How much? ....
Exercise enough.................. no   yes
Is your diet well balanced?.... no   yes

List any drugs or medications you take regularly or frequently:

_____

_____

_____

_____

_____

_____

_____

MARITAL HISTORY

Prior marriage? ....
Was pregnancy achieved?...

When? (Dates) ....
Any other proof of fertility?.......................................
....
....

Is sex entirely satisfactory?.......................................
Reaction of wife:..

Estimated frequency of coitus (intercourse) per month: ......
Remarks:...
....
....
....

INFERTILITY STUDIES

	Result	Date	Where Done
Semen analysis:....................................			
Thyroid tests:......................................			
Hormone tests:....................................			
Medicines given:..................................			
Other tests:			

....
....

Source: Boivin, J., Takefman, J., & Braverman, A. (2011). Development and preliminary validation of the fertility quality of life (FertiQoL) tool. *Human Reproduction, 26*(8), 2084–2091.

● TABLE 10.3   **Male Hormone Levels**

Hormone to Test	Normal Values	What Value Means
Testosterone	270–1,100 ng/dL	Testosterone production is stimulated by Leydig cells in the testicles. Low levels of testosterone combined with low FSH and LH are diagnostic of hypogonadotropic hypogonadism.
Free testosterone	0.3–2 pg/mL	
% free testosterone	0.3–5%	A normal male has about 2% free, unbound testosterone.
Follicle-stimulating hormone (FSH)	5–15 IU/L	Basic hormone testing for males often only includes FSH and testosterone.
Prolactin	<20 µg/L	A level two or three times that of normal may indicate a pituitary tumour, such as a prolactinoma, which may lead to decreased sperm production. Elevations can be treated with bromocriptine.
Luteinizing hormone (LH)	1–9 IU/L	LH stimulates Leydig cells and production of testosterone. A problem with LH levels alone is rarely seen, so testing is only needed if testosterone level is abnormal.
Estradiol (E2)	10–60 pg/mL	
Progesterone (P4)	0.3–1.2 ng/mL	

Adapted from: http://www.fertilityplus.org/faq/hormonelevels.html and Healthwise. (2012). BCHealthGuide: Fertility problems. Accessed from http://www.healthlinkbc.ca/kb/content/special/aa39523.html#hw214498

substance use; chronic illness; and dietary adequacy. He or she also elicits use of drugs, cigarettes, and alcohol; and family history of unexplained mental retardation, birth defects, perinatal or neonatal deaths, and chronic or early-onset health problems (ACOG, 2012). Assessment Tool 10.3 provides a sample form used to evaluate for female factor infertility.

Physical Examination

The physical examination focuses on secondary sex characteristics, structure and function of the reproductive organs, and general well-being.

Laboratory and Diagnostic Testing

Laboratory tests to evaluate for infertility in the woman include routine analyses, evaluation of hormonal levels (serum progesterone, FSH, LH, and prolactin), Pap testing, and testing for chlamydia. See Table 10.4 for a complete summary of female hormone levels that may be examined.

Early in the workup, the health care team must document the status of the woman's immunity to rubella, so that those clients without an appropriate titer can receive immunization in a timely fashion. Also, the health care provider should ensure that the woman is taking a folic acid supplement, as is recommended for all women of childbearing age, to reduce the risk for having a pregnancy in which the fetus has a neural tube defect.

Monitoring of Basal Body Temperature

This technique is used to predict the time of ovulation based on the thermogenic properties of serum progesterone. Body temperature should increase by 0.2°C to 0.4°C when progesterone levels are highest, just after ovulation (Fritz & Speroff, 2011). The health care provider will ask the woman to keep a chart for several months monitoring her basal body temperature. Each morning, the client records her temperature immediately upon awakening (at rest) using the same thermometer. She plots the temperatures on a chart so that a pattern develops; subsequently, she can establish the time of ovulation, which precedes the increase in temperature. The woman also records her menses, any events that would alter her temperature (eg, infections, insomnia), and when she has intercourse. She can also record any symptoms such as twinges during ovulation and the nature and character of her cervical mucus.

The nurse evaluates the chart with the couple, helping to determine whether ovulation is occurring (just before the increase in body temperature) and, if cycles are regular, when to time intercourse to maximize chances of conception. A sample temperature chart is provided in Figure 10.5.

Postcoital Testing

Another test performed early in the workup is a *postcoital test*. It may be scheduled on or just before the expected date of ovulation, if a recurrent pattern can be determined from the basal body temperature chart. The health care provider instructs the woman to have intercourse 6 to 8 hours before her scheduled appointment and to avoid showering or douching between having sexual relations and arriving for the test. After a pelvic examination, the clinician removes and microscopically

(text continues on page 338)

● **ASSESSMENT TOOL 10.3**   **Infertility History Form for Women**

Name: Date: Unit No.:
(Nee):   Tel.:   Husb.:
Address: Age: Name Rel./Friend: Occupation: Age:
Occupation: Address: Employer
Employer: Bus. Address:
Bus. Tel.:   Bus. Tel.:
Referred by: Religion: Hus-   Wife:
                                                               band:

Birth Place: [ ] Single   [ ] Divorced
Birth Date: [ ] Married   [ ] Widow

All previous occupations:	List all provinces or countries in which you have lived:

| Education: | Please encircle the last | Grade | 5 | High School | 1 | 2 | 3 | 4 | Post Grad. _____ yrs. |
| | Grade you completed | 6 | 7 | 8 | College | 1 | 2 | 3 | 4 | Degrees |

Date of last physical exam.   P.I. Please do not write in this space.

Chief Complaints: Please list all symptoms you
have NOW.

1. _____

2. _____

3. _____

Routine checkup—no symptoms [ ]

Family History	Age	If Living Health	Age at Death	If Deceased Cause	Please Encircle Has any blood relative had			Who
Father					Cancer	no	yes	
Mother					Tuberculosis	no	yes	
Brother or sister 1.					Diabetes	no	yes	
2.					Heart trouble	no	yes	
3.					High blood pressure	no	yes	
4.					Stroke	no	yes	
5.					Epilepsy	no	yes	
Husband or wife					Mental illness	no	yes	
Son or daughter 1.					Suicide	no	yes	
2.					Congenital deformities	no	yes	
3.					NOTE: This is a confidential record of your medical			
4.					history and will be kept in this office. Information			
5.					contained here will not be released to any person			
6.					except when you have authorized us to do so.			

PERSONAL HISTORY
ILLNESS: Have you had
(Please Encircle all Answers no or yes)

Measles or German measles	no	yes	Gonorrhea or syphilis	no	yes
Chickenpox or mumps	no	yes	Anemia or jaundice	no	yes
Whooping cough	no	yes	Epilepsy	no	yes
Scarlet fever or scarlatina	no	yes	Migraine headaches	no	yes
Pneumonia or pleurisy	no	yes	Tuberculosis	no	yes
Diphtheria or smallpox	no	yes	Diabetes or cancer	no	yes
Influenza	no	yes	High or low blood pressure	no	yes
Rheumatic fever or heart disease	no	yes	Nervous breakdown	no	yes
Arthritis or rheumatism	no	yes	Food, chemical or drug poisoning	no	yes
Any bone or joint disease	no	yes	Hay fever or asthma	no	yes
Neuritis or neuralgia	no	yes	Hives or eczema	no	yes
Bursitis, sciatica or lumbago	no	yes	Frequent colds or sore throat	no	yes
Polio or meningitis	no	yes	Frequent infections or boils	no	yes
Bright's disease or kidney infection	no	yes	Any other disease	no	yes
			ALLERGIES: Are you allergic to		
			Penicillin or sulfa	no	yes
			Aspirin, codeine or morphine	no	yes

Mycins or other antibiotics	no	yes
Merthiolate or mercurochrome	no	yes
Any other drug	no	yes
Any foods	no	yes
Adhesive tape	no	yes
Nail polish or other cosmetics	no	yes
Tetanus antitoxin or serums	no	yes
INJURIES: Have you had any		
Broken bones	no	yes
Sprains or dislocations	no	yes
Lacerations (extensive)	no	yes
Concussion or head injury	no	yes
Ever been knocked out	no	yes
TRANSFUSIONS: Have you ever had		
Blood or plasma transfusion	no	yes
Weight: now _____ one year ago _____		
Max _____ when _____ Height _____		

Please review the section you have just completed and wherever you answered "yes" fill in the year (guess if necessary) and also where there is more than one illness
to a line encircle the ones you have had. Example: Chickenpox or mumps.............................1961 ....no   (yes)

(continued)

● **ASSESSMENT TOOL 10.3** **Infertility History Form for Women** *(Continued)*

SURGERY: Have you had

Tonsillectomy .... no   yes

Appendectomy .... no   yes

Any other operation (give details)................ no   yes

Give DETAILS below of all hospitalizations for surgery or illness including name and address of Doctor and Hospital....

Have you ever been advised to have any surgical operation which has not been done? [1] no   [2] yes   what..................

Systems: Please check those you have had.

Eye disease [ ], Eye injury [ ], Impaired sight [ ], Ear disease [ ], Ear injury [ ], Impaired hearing [ ],..

Trouble with: Nose [ ], Sinuses [ ], Mouth [ ], Throat [ ], Have you checked any in this group?.. no   yes

Fainting spells [ ], Loss of consciousness [ ], Convulsions [ ], Paralysis [ ], Frequent or severe headaches [ ],

    Dizziness [ ], Depression or anxiety [ ], Hallucinations [ ], Have you checked any in this group?.......................... no   yes

Enlarged glands [ ], Goiter or enlarged thyroid [ ], Skin disease [ ], Have you checked any in this group? .... no   yes

Chronic or frequent cough [ ], Chest pain or angina pectoris [ ], Spitting up of blood [ ], Night sweats [ ],

    Shortness of breath [ ], Palpitation or fluttering heart [ ], Swelling of hands, feet, or ankles [ ], Varicose veins [ ],

    Extreme tiredness or weakness [ ], Have you checked any in this group? .... no   yes

Kidney disease or stones [ ], Bladder disease [ ], Albumin, sugar, pus, etc. in urine [ ], Difficulty in urinating [ ],

    Awake to urinate nightly [ ], Have you checked any in this group?.. no   yes

Stomach trouble or ulcers [ ], Indigestion [ ], Liver or gallbladder disease [ ], Colitis or other bowel disease [ ]

    Appendicitis [ ], Hemorrhoids or rectal bleeding [ ], Constipation or diarrhea [ ],

    Recent change in bowel action or stools [ ], Recent change in appetite or eating habits [ ],

    Have you checked any in this group? .... no   yes

HABITS: Do you

Sleep well?.................................. no   yes

Use alcoholic beverages .... no   yes

    Every day?.............................. no   yes

Smoke?.. no   yes

    How much? ....

Exercise enough .... no   yes

Is your diet well balanced?........... no   yes

List any drugs or medications you take regularly or frequently:

_____

_____

_____

_____

_____

_____

OBSTETRICAL–GYNECOLOGICAL REVIEW

Age at first menstruation _____ Age at first coital experience __ Number of living children (at present) _____

Number of pregnancies _____

Number of live births _____ Number of multiple pregnancies _____ Number of stillbirths (more than 20 weeks) _____ Number of abortions, miscarriages (20 weeks or less) _____ Number of children dead _____ Age of oldest child _____ Number of births with deformities _____

GYNECOLOGICAL HISTORY

Are menstrual cycles regular?...................... Are your periods similar? ....

Interval between periods...

Length of flow .... Date of last menstrual cycle ....

Amount of flow .... [1] Light   [2] Moderate   [3] Heavy

Was the quality, quantity, and duration of flow for this last cycle similar in comparison with previous cycles?...

    [1] No (specify how it differed) ....

    .... [2] Yes

Has there been any bleeding in between periods? ....

    [1] No   [2] Yes (specify) ....

Were any medications taken during cycle?...

    [1] No   [2] Yes (specify)

Dysmenorrhea (menstrual discomfort) ....

    [1] None   [2] Intermittent   [3] Constant

Type of menstrual discomfort experienced

    [1] None   [3] Dull   [5] Cramp

    [2] Sharp   [4] Ache   [6] Backache

PREMENSTRUAL SYMPTOMS

Bloating .... no   yes

Breast tenderness .... no   yes

Pelvic pain... no   yes

Backache.. no   yes

Headache.. no   yes

Irritability .... no   yes

Edema... no   yes

Acne .... no   yes

INTERMENSTRUAL DISCHARGE

Type   [1] None   [3] Yellow   [5] White

          [2] Tan   [4] Bloody   [6] Other (specify)

Amount .... Scant   Heavy

Itching .... no   yes

Odourless .... no   yes

Frequent .... no   yes

Regular pattern .... no   yes

(continued)

● **ASSESSMENT TOOL 10.3** **Infertility History Form for Women** *(Continued)*

MARITAL HISTORY

Prior marriage? .... When? (Dates) .... Was pregnancy achieved?..

Is sex entirely satisfactory? .... Dyspareunia (discomfort during coitus): no ....yes ....

Estimated frequency of coitus .... Does coitus occur during menses? Yes......................................No

(sexual intercourse) per month:..

Reaction of husband: .... On which days of flow? ....

Remarks:...Is this consistent? ....

....

....

INDICATE THE INFORMATION FOR ANY OF THE FOLLOWING STUDIES WHICH YOU HAVE HAD

	Date	Result	Doctor

Basal body temperature record:..

Biopsy test:...

Thyroid test:..

Gas (Rubin) test:..

X-ray of uterus and tubes:..

Postcoital test: (survival of seed in your secretions) ....

Cautery of cervix:...

Hormone test: ....

Inseminations:..

Medicines given:..

Other: ....

(Source: Boivin, J., Takefman, J., & Braverman, A. (2011). Development and preliminary validation of the fertility quality of life (FertiQoL) tool. *Human Reproduction, 26*(8), 2084–2091.

● TABLE 10.4 **Female Hormone Levels**

Hormone to Test	Time to Test	Normal Values	What Value Means
Anti-müllerian Hormone (AMH)	Anytime	Medium reserve: 16–29 pmol/L High reserve: 29–49 pmol/L	AMH is a newer test used in complement with FSH and day 3 antral follicle count as a measurement of ovarian reserve. This hormone has little fluctuation during the menstrual cycle and can therefore be measured at any time. Levels greater than 49 pmol/L may be indicative of PCOS. Levels less than 16 may indicate declining ovarian reserve or premature ovarian failure.
Follicle-stimulating hormone (FSH)	Day 3	5–20 IU/L	FSH is often used as a gauge of ovarian reserve. In general, under 6 is excellent, 6–9 is good, 9–10 fair, 10–13 diminished reserve, 13+ very hard to stimulate. In PCOS testing, the LH : FSH ratio may be used in the diagnosis. The ratio is usually close to 1:1, but if the LH is higher, it is one possible indication of PCOS.
Estradiol (E2)	Day 3	25–75 pg/mL	Levels on the lower end tend to be better for stimulating. Abnormally high levels on day 3 may indicate existence of a functional cyst or diminished ovarian reserve.
Estradiol (E2)	Day 4–5 of meds	100+ pg/mL or 2 × day 3	There are no charts showing E2 levels stimulation because there is a wide variation depending on how many follicles are being produced and their size. Most doctors will consider any increase in E2 a positive sign, but others use a formula of either 100 pg/mL after 4 d of stims, or a doubling in E2 from the level taken on cycle day 3.

(continued)

● TABLE 10.4 **Environmental Risks and Protective Measures** (continued)

Hormone to Test	Time to Test	Normal Values	What Value Means
Estradiol (E2)	Surge/hCG day	200+ pg/mL	The levels should be 200–600 per mature (18 mm) follicle. These levels are sometimes lower in overweight women.
Luteinizing hormone (LH)	Day 3	1–18 IU/L	A normal LH level is similar to FSH. An LH that is higher than FSH is one indication of PCOS.
Luteinizing hormone (LH)	Surge day	8.7–80 IU/L	The LH surge leads to ovulation within 48 hr.
Prolactin	Day 3	<25 µg/L	Increased prolactin levels can interfere with ovulation. They may also indicate further testing (MRI) should be done to check for a pituitary tumour. Some women with PCOS also have hyperprolactinemia.
Progesterone (P4)	Day 3	<50 ng/dL or <1 ng/mL	Often called the follicular phase level. An elevated level may indicate a lower pregnancy rate.
Progesterone (P4)	Days 15–28	300–1,500 ng/dL or 3–25 ng/mL	A progesterone test is done to confirm ovulation. When a follicle releases its egg, it becomes what is called a corpus luteum and produces progesterone. A level over 5 probably indicates some form of ovulation, but most doctors want to see a level over 10 on a natural cycle, and a level over 15 on a medicated cycle. There is no midluteal level that predicts pregnancy. Some say the test may be more accurate if done first thing in the morning after fasting.
Thyroid-stimulating hormone (TSH)	Day 3	2–10 mU/L	Midrange normal in most laboratories is about 1.7. A high level of TSH combined with a low or normal T_4 level generally indicates hypothyroidism, which can have an effect on fertility.
Free triiodothyronine (T_3)	Day 3	1.4–4.4 pg/mL	Sometimes the diseased thyroid gland will start producing very high levels of T_3 but still produce normal levels of T_4. Therefore, measurement of both hormones provides an even more accurate evaluation of thyroid function.
Free thyroxine (T_4)	Day 3	0.8–2 ng/dL	A low level may indicate a diseased thyroid gland or may indicate a nonfunctioning pituitary gland that is not stimulating the thyroid to produce T_4. If the T_4 is low and the TSH is normal, that is more likely to indicate a problem with the pituitary.
Total testosterone	Day 3	<70 ng/dL	Testosterone is secreted from the adrenal gland and the ovaries. Most would consider a level above 50 to be somewhat elevated.
Free testosterone	Day 3	0.3–2 pg/mL	
Dehydroepiandrosterone sulfate (DHEAS)	Day 3	35–430 µg/dL	An elevated DHEAS level may be improved through use of dexamethasone, prednisone, or insulin-sensitizing medications.
Androstenedione	Day 3	0.7–3.1 ng/mL	
Sex hormone-binding globulin (SHBG)	Day 3	18–114 nmol/L	Increased androgen production often leads to lower SHBG
17-Hydroxyprogesterone	Day 3	20–100 ng/dL	Midcycle peak would be 100–250 ng/dL; luteal phase, 100–500 ng/dL
Fasting insulin	8–16 hr fasting	<30 mIU/mL	The normal range here doesn't give all the information. A fasting insulin of 10–13 generally indicates some insulin resistance, and levels above 13 indicate greater insulin resistance.

MRI, magnetic resonance imaging; PCOS, polycystic ovary syndrome.

Adapted from: http://www.fertilityplus.org/faq/hormonelevels.html and Healthwise. (2012). *BCHealthGuide: Fertility problems.* Accessed July 2, 2013, from http://www.healthlinkbc.ca/kb/content/special/aa39523.html#hw214498 and ReproMed. (2009). *Anti-müllerian hormone (AMH) blood test information sheet.* Retrieved July 2, 2013, from http://www.repromed.com.au/custom/files/AMH%20Information%20 Sheet%20for%20Doctors%203.4.09.pdf

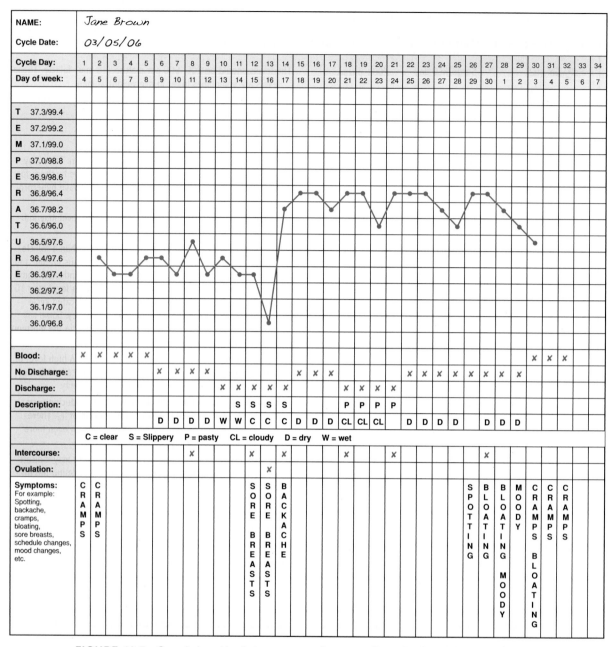

| NAME: | Jane Brown |
| CycleDate: | 03/05/06 |

Cycle Day:	1	2	3	4	5	6	7	8	9	10	11	12	13	14	15	16	17	18	19	20	21	22	23	24	25	26	27	28	29	30	31	32	33	34
Day of week:	4	5	6	7	8	9	10	11	12	13	14	15	16	17	18	19	20	21	22	23	24	25	26	27	28	29	30	1	2	3	4	5	6	7

Temperature scale (reading down): T 37.3/99.4, E 37.2/99.2, M 37.1/99.0, P 37.0/98.8, E 36.9/98.6, R 36.8/96.4, A 36.7/98.2, T 36.6/96.0, U 36.5/97.6, R 36.4/97.6, E 36.3/97.4, 36.2/97.2, 36.1/97.0, 36.0/96.8

Blood:	×	×	×	×	×																									×	×	×		
No Discharge:						×	×	×	×						×	×	×				×	×	×	×	×	×	×	×	×					
Discharge:								×	×	×	×	×				×	×	×	×														
Description:								S	S	S	S					P	P	P	P														
					D	D	D	D	W	W	C	C		C	D	D	D	CL	CL	CL		D	D	D	D		D	D	D					

C = clear   S = Slippery   P = pasty   CL = cloudy   D = dry   W = wet

| Intercourse: | | | | | | | | × | | | × | | × | | | | × | | × | | | | | | × | | | | | | | | |
| Ovulation: | | | | | | | | | | | | × | | | | | | | | | | | | | | | | | | | | | | |

| Symptoms: For example: Spotting, backache, cramps, bloating, sore breasts, schedule changes, mood changes, etc. | CRAMPS | CRAMPS | | | | | | SORE BREASTS | SORE BREASTS | BACKACHE | | | | | | | | | | | | | | | SPOTTING | BLOATING | BLOATING MOODY | MOODY | CRAMPS BLOATING | CRAMPS | CRAMPS | | | | |

FIGURE 10.5   Sample basal body temperature chart recordings. Retrieved July 31, 2013, from http://baby2see.com/preconception/basal_body_temperature.html

examines the woman's cervical mucus to determine its quality and character, as well as the number and motility of sperm (Fig. 10.6).

Many couples find this test stressful, viewing it as a quantitative assessment of sexual functioning. Because of this pressure, they often cannot complete intercourse at the prescribed time. Providers should warn them of this development ahead of time and reassure them that it is common. Some health care facilities do not schedule the appointment ahead of time but have a clinician available for walk-in appointments, so that the woman can

call to schedule the appointment after completing intercourse. Other couples agree for the woman to not let her partner know which specific day the test is scheduled, thus decreasing performance anxiety that may affect the male partner.

Endometrial Biopsy

An *endometrial biopsy*, performed during the second phase of a woman's menstrual cycle, provides information about hormonal influences on the adequacy of the endometrial lining and its ability to support a fertilized

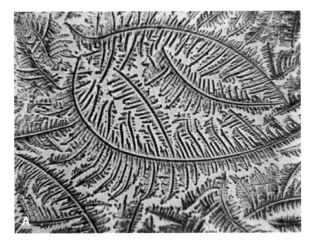

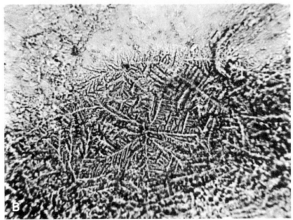

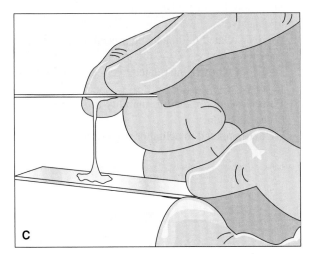

FIGURE 10.6 During assessment of cervical mucus, examiners will look for a ferning pattern to the mucus under the microscope. **A:** shows ferning; **B:** shows incomplete ferning. Another quality they will evaluate for is spinnbarkeit (the ability to stretch a distance before breaking), shown in part (**C**).

egg (Fig. 10.7). It is relatively noninvasive but gives basically the same information as serum progesterone levels or the basal body temperature (ie, that the client is ovulating). For this reason, it is not used unless the

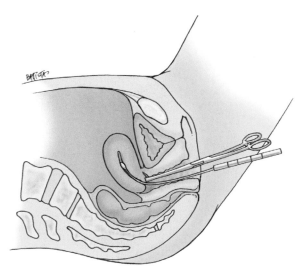

FIGURE 10.7 During endometrial biopsy, the examiner takes samples from the uterine lining to assess the hormonal levels of the endometrial tissue.

diagnostician also wishes to rule in or out endometrial hypertrophy.

Hysteroscopy and Hysterosalpingography

A *hysteroscopy* or *hysterosalpingography* may be performed to view the uterine cavity and determine tubal patency. These tests are often performed immediately after menses, when the woman is unlikely to be pregnant and the chance of disrupting a spontaneous pregnancy is minimal. Dye may be injected through the cervix under fluoroscopy (Fig. 10.8). The examiner then notes whether the dye traverses the uterus and fallopian tubes into the abdominal cavity. This test also can help determine the shape of the uterine cavity. Congenital defects of the uterine cavity (eg, septate uterus) or endometrial polyps or fibroids may be interfering with implantation or embryonic development. The hysterosalpingogram will show uterine or fallopian abnormalities but will not differentiate the cause. Laparoscopy is used to pinpoint the cause.

Laparoscopy

The most invasive test, usually saved for last, is *laparoscopy*, which is performed under general anaesthesia. The surgeon makes a small incision and inserts an instrument into the woman's abdominal cavity to introduce gas, which is used to extend the abdominal cavity. The surgeon then inserts the laparoscope. He or she can then view the woman's internal organs, looking for causes of infertility such as adhesions, structural abnormalities, or endometrial implants (Fig. 10.9). He or she also may perform some minor ablation of endometrial implants.

Some physicians forego the hysterosalpingography and insert dye through the cervix, looking for spillage

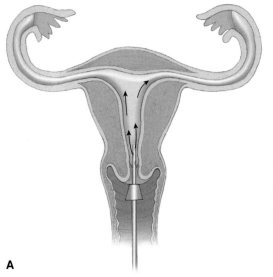

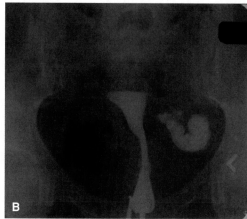

FIGURE 10.8 A: During a hysterosalpingography, examiners inject a dye into the woman's uterus. The dye outlines the uterus and fallopian tubes during radiography for evaluation of patency. **B:** This image shows blockage of the right fallopian tube (left on image). The area remains dark and difficult to discern, indicating the inability of contrast medium to pass through.

into the abdominal cavity under direct vision during the laparoscopy. In rare occasions, complications arise during the procedure, necessitating a laparotomy. Such complications include bleeding and inadvertent injury to internal structures, which may include scarring and adhesions of the ovaries and fallopian tubes, potentially further compromising a woman's fertility.

 Joan, described at the beginning of the chapter, is scheduled to undergo a laparoscopy. She asks, "How will this test help us?" What teaching should the nurse provide?

Select Potential Nursing Diagnoses

Many nursing diagnoses can apply to the client or couple experiencing infertility. Some common examples include the following:

- **Ineffective Coping**
- **Situational Low Self-Esteem** related to the inability to conceive
- **Anxiety** related to diagnostic procedures, treatments, and outcomes
- **Deficient Knowledge** related to effects of lifestyle on fertility
- **Powerlessness** related to inability to control aspects of the situation
- **Grieving** related to actual or perceived losses

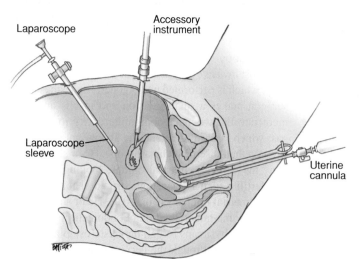

FIGURE 10.9 Diagnostic laparoscopy, the most invasive test for infertility, is used to visualize the internal pelvic organs directly, as well as to check for tubal patency.

Planning and Intervention

Expected outcomes are individualized based on the client's particular circumstances (Nursing Care Plans 10.1 and 10.2). Some expected outcomes common to most clients might be as follows:

- The client (couple) will verbalize a realistic understanding of their circumstances and knowledge about any identified causes, as well as possible options.
- The client (couple) will discuss emotions related to the situation. *(text continues on page 345)*

NURSING CARE PLAN 10.1

●

The Couple Undergoing Examination of Infertility

 Recall Ted and Joan from the beginning of this chapter. Health history taking indicates that Joan's menstrual cycle is regular. Baseline vital signs and laboratory test results are normal. While discussing their situation, Joan says, "I know that Ted and I have to have some tests, but it sounds like there are so many. What are all these tests? This whole situation is so overwhelming. And, forget privacy. That's a thing of the past."

NURSING DIAGNOSIS

Deficient Knowledge related to infertility testing procedures and their indications.

EXPECTED OUTCOMES

1. The client will identify the reasons for different testing procedures.
2. The client will state the implications of the results of testing.

INTERVENTIONS	RATIONALES
Assess the client's level of understanding about infertility testing.	Assessment provides a baseline to identify specific client needs and to develop an individualized teaching plan.
Explore the client's exposure to previous infertility testing; correct any misconceptions or myths related to these methods; allow time for questions.	Information about exposure provides additional foundation for teaching and provides opportunities to clarify or correct misinformation and teach new information.
Explain the different tests available and the information that each can reveal. Describe the various methods used for testing and indications for each; include the client's husband in the discussion.	This information will help alleviate anxiety about unknown aspects of the process. Infertility testing involves testing of the male and female client. Involving the client's husband aids in preparing him for the tests.
Obtain a health history and physical examination of client and her husband.	Health history and physical examination aid in revealing possible factors contributing to infertility.
Inform the client's husband about blood tests and semen analysis; instruct the husband how to collect semen sample and transport it to the laboratory properly.	Blood testing reveals information about hormonal levels; semen analysis provides information about the adequacy of the husband's sperm. Proper timely transport to the laboratory of the semen specimen is necessary for accurate results.

(continued)

NURSING CARE PLAN 10.1 ● The Couple Undergoing Examination of Infertility *(Continued)*

INTERVENTIONS	RATIONALES
Instruct the client how to monitor basal body temperature, explaining that ovulation usually precedes the increase in temperature. Also encourage the woman to record additional information such as menses, times of intercourse, and events such as insomnia or infection.	Basal body temperature is used as a measure to determine ovulation. Documentation of additional information provides data about possible factors affecting temperature readings.
Teach client about postcoital testing, endometrial biopsy, hysteroscopy and hysterosalpingogram, and laparoscopy as appropriate.	Additional testing with these procedures may be indicated to determine possible causes of infertility.
Review the results of testing, explaining the findings in terms the couple can understand.	Knowledge of test results aids in couple's understanding of the underlying cause of infertility and proposed methods for treatment.
Offer support and guidance throughout the testing period.	Infertility testing can be a source of anxiety and frustration.

EVALUATION

1. The client explains the rationale for specific testing procedures.
2. The couple demonstrates understanding of the tests and results.

NURSING DIAGNOSIS

Powerlessness related to lack of privacy involving sexual activity secondary to infertility testing.

EXPECTED OUTCOMES

1. The couple will state that they feel some control over their sexual activity.
2. The couple will verbalize feelings of being less overwhelmed with testing.

INTERVENTIONS	RATIONALES
Assess the couple's concerns and feelings related to testing.	Assessment provides a baseline from which to develop an individualized plan of care.
Allow the couple to verbalize their feelings related to lack of privacy and feelings of sexual functioning on demand; encourage couple to role-play situations.	Verbalization of feelings allows for sharing and offering of support; role-playing provides an outlet for concerns and provides opportunities for teaching and support.
Reassure couple that their feelings are common; encourage them to participate in support groups.	Reassurance that feelings are common reduces anxiety and fear; participation in support groups promotes sharing of feelings with others who have similar experiences.

(continued)

NURSING CARE PLAN 10.1 ● The Couple Undergoing Examination of Infertility *(Continued)*

INTERVENTIONS	RATIONALES
Encourage couple to actively participate in decision making related to testing as appropriate, such as which tests to complete first; advise the couple to focus on one aspect of testing at a time.	Active participation promotes feelings of control; focusing on one aspect minimizes feelings of being overwhelmed.
Remind couple about their reason for undergoing infertility testing, the ultimate outcome of having a child.	Reminding the couple helps to reinforce their commitment and desire for the outcome.

EVALUATION

1. The couple states they feel some control over their current situation.
2. The couple participates in infertility testing with minimal anxiety.

NURSING CARE PLAN 10.2

●

The Client Contemplating Fertility Testing

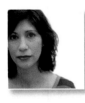

Remember Stacy, the 42-year-old woman from the beginning of the chapter. During her visit she openly talks about her situation. "As much as I want to know if we can hold out hope for having a baby, I'm afraid to learn the results. What if I am the one with the problem? I don't want to rob my husband of his chance to have a family."

NURSING DIAGNOSES

- **Situational Low Self-Esteem** related to feelings of failure secondary to concerns about inability to conceive a child
- **Anxiety** related to uncertainty of fertility status

EXPECTED OUTCOMES

1. The client will verbalize positive feelings about self and her relationship with her husband.
2. The client will state reduced anxiety about her fertility status.
3. The client and husband will verbalize feelings about their relationship and effect of infertility and its treatments on their relationship.

(continued)

NURSING CARE PLAN 10.2 ● The Client Contemplating Fertility Testing (Continued)

INTERVENTIONS	RATIONALES
Assess the client's beliefs about her reproductive function, self-esteem, and body image. Explore her current understanding about fertility and its effect on her self-esteem and body image.	Assessment provides a baseline from which to develop appropriate strategies for teaching and care.
Communicate accurate facts and answer questions; clarify any misconceptions or misinformation.	Clear communication helps to provide accurate information to aid in alleviating fears and clarifying misinformation.
Explain the different tests available and the information that each can reveal.	This information will help alleviate anxiety about unknown aspects of the process.
Ask the client about measures used to cope with previous stressful situations; determine which measures were successful.	Identifying previous coping strategies helps to determine effective strategies for use in this situation.
Encourage client to include husband in visits.	Participation of client and husband promotes sharing.
Provide the couple with a chance to discuss any concerns, fears, or worries about their situation; encourage client and husband to share feelings.	Communication can reveal sources of stress and any problematic areas that need to be addressed; sharing of feelings aids in promoting positive coping.
Ask the couple about available support systems (eg, family, friends).	Identifying available support systems helps to establish sources of assistance when one or both partners need help from other people.
Provide the couple with information about support groups, websites, and other avenues for education and assistance.	Shared experiences and knowledge of similar situations for others can help the couple prepare for what to expect and to realize that they are not alone.
Work with the client and her husband to establish measures to deal with infertility testing; role-play situations involving possible outcomes.	Establishing measures and role-playing helps clients be prepared for situations to promote adequate coping.
Assess client and partner for behaviours indicative of maladaptation or difficulty coping.	Early identification of problems fosters prompt treatment and can help prevent a crisis from escalating.

EVALUATION

1. The client demonstrates positive coping strategies related to infertility status.
2. The client and her husband identify helpful supports to deal with stresses related to infertility and its treatment.
3. The couple verbalize support and a firm commitment to each other regardless of the outcome.
4. The couple verbalize a realistic plan to handle their feelings about the situation and to address matters appropriately once they know more information.

Treatment options depend on the diagnosis. For some couples, financial concerns contribute to choices about which treatment options to pursue and how long to continue them. All options require strict adherence to complex regimens that involve expensive medications, scheduled sex, and repeated visits to the health care facility to monitor the woman's cycle and to plan treatment. The stress of the process can strain the couple's relationship and finances (Schneider & Forthofer, 2005). When working with clients considering treatments, the nurse emphasizes that the decision on whether to have treatment, which options to try, and when to say "enough" are theirs and theirs alone.

Many couples spend thousands of dollars pursuing the dream of having a biologic child. Because of the emotional and financial investments involved, the nurse should counsel clients to ensure that they are accurately informed about success rates and the modality of treatment most appropriate for the particular fertility problem. Most Canadian clinics voluntarily report their success rates to the Canadian Assisted Reproductive Technologies Register (CARTR), an initiative of the CFAS, although the information is released in aggregate form and is not clinic-specific (CFAS, 2007). This may change under new rules associated with the Assisted Human Reproduction Act (Government of Canada, 2013b). The legislation allows for the Assisted Human Reproduction Agency to inspect and license clinics, to monitor aspects that pertain to health and safety, and to help facilitate informed choices by patients about treatment options. Costs and success rates for various treatments vary. Some women have insurance coverage for fertility drugs, but it is less common for insurance to cover the costs of actual treatment procedures. Health care providers may advise some couples to try options for different durations depending on their diagnosis, age, and personal preferences. See Box 10.3 for a summary of progressive treatment options for infertility.

Assisted Human Reproduction (AHR)

Health Canada defines any activity undertaken for the purpose of facilitating human reproduction as "**Assisted Human Reproduction**" (Health Canada, 2013). This includes procedures such as in vitro fertilization (IVF), donor insemination, and intracytoplasmic sperm injection, all of which are referred to as "controlled activities" under the Assisted Human Reproduction Act (Government of Canada, 2013b).

Artificial Insemination

Artificial insemination involves the use of a thin, flexible catheter to insert sperm directly into the vagina or directly into the uterus (Fig. 10.10). This procedure reduces the distance that sperm have to travel and can

● **BOX 10.3   Progressive Treatment Options for Infertility**

Male Infertility

Intrauterine insemination
Therapeutic donor insemination

Female Infertility

Ovulation induction
Assisted reproductive therapy
    IVF
    GIFT or ZIFT
    IVF with donor oocytes
Intracytoplasmic sperm injection
Gestational carrier

be effective in maximizing the chances of conception if the male partner's sperm count is relatively low. The semen sample is obtained by masturbation. After liquefaction, the specimen is centrifuged to separate the sperm from the seminal fluid. The sperm pellet is then resuspended in a nutritive medium and inserted into the uterus through a thin flexible catheter. The seminal fluid is removed because prostaglandins in the fluid could cause a painful anaphylactic reaction if delivered directly into the uterus. This procedure can be effective if the woman's cervical mucus contains antisperm antibodies by bypassing the vagina and cervix and delivering the sperm directly into the uterus. It also might be inserted into the vagina (unwashed sperm). The male partner who has a neurologic deficit rendering him incapable of erection and ejaculation can undergo electrical stimulation for ejaculation and delivery of the sperm into the vagina.

Donor Sperm

In cases in which the male partner has a genetic condition that the couple does not want to risk transmitting, there is a serious sperm quality problem, or there is no male partner, a frozen specimen from an anonymous donor can be used. In Canada, health screening standards for donor sperm are prescribed by Health Canada regulations (Health Canada, 1996), although in the United States (US), sperm banks are self-regulated (Fritz & Speroff, 2011). Canadian fertility clinics have increasingly relied on US commercial sperm banks in recent years, importing samples of donor sperm from banks that comply with Canadian standards for screening. This practice meets the standards of the Assisted Human Reproduction Act, which prohibits commercialism and payment to donors, other than expenses (Government of Canada, 2013b). In terms of health and safety, sperm donors should be screened for any transmittable

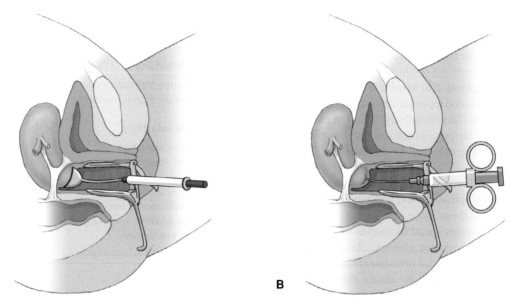

FIGURE 10.10 Procedure for artificial insemination. **A:** A cervical capping device is used to place semen directly in contact with the cervix. **B:** Semen is injected directly into the uterine cavity.

problematic conditions before they donate. Processing and distribution of semen for assisted conception regulations (Health Canada, 1996) require that there be repeat screenings (at each donation) for syphilis, gonorrhea, chlamydia, hepatitis B and C, cytomegalovirus, and HIV. The specimens must be frozen and quarantined for 6 months, at which time the donor should return for additional HIV testing. If the donor is found to be HIV negative, then the sample (whose sperm must be viable and motile after freezing) is released for use. Genetic screening should be included to determine carrier status of conditions like cystic fibrosis. Family and personal history and physical examination are conducted to ensure the donor's general health.

Couples requiring donor sperm can usually access profiles of donors' physical characteristics, family background, and personal profiles. In most cases donors are anonymous, but some sperm banks offer the option of selecting "open identity" donors who are willing to later release identifying information to offspring. Lesbians and single women who desire pregnancy are increasingly seeking donor insemination as an option. Some may prefer to use a personal or "known" donor as opposed to an anonymous one, although the same Health Canada Standards for screening apply, thus requiring testing, cryopreservation, and quarantine before the insemination can be carried out by a physician.

Ovarian Induction (Fertility Drugs)

Women who have alterations in ovulation may be treated with ovulation-inducing drugs (eg, clomiphene citrate [Clomid]) (Table 10.5). Medication regimens may take several months to achieve a satisfactory response, and the medications may have significant side effects. The risk for ovarian hyperstimulation is significant. In this condition, because of high levels of circulating hormones (serum estradiol and exogenous gonadotropins), the ovaries become enlarged. In extreme cases, intravascular fluid volume can shift into the peritoneal space, with resultant hypovolemia, oliguria, hemoconcentration, and massive ascites, which can result in death (Rebar, 2013b). Thus, health care providers must monitor the woman's cycles to prevent this condition. If hyperstimulation does occur, the provider should instruct the woman to stop medication, avoid intercourse, and reduce the level of medication during a subsequent cycle.

Use of fertility drugs increases the chance of multiple gestation, which poses several risks to the mother and fetus (see Chapter 13). Parents may face the prospect of reducing the number of fetuses for the safety of the mother and other fetuses. Often, one medication is used to mature and develop several follicles at once, and another is used to suppress the release of the follicles. With some medications, especially in combination, titrating the dose to provide the desired response and minimize untoward responses can be difficult. The level of risk depends on the medications and should be considered when planning treatment.

Women undergoing ovulation induction may engage in sexual intercourse or artificial insemination,

● TABLE 10.5 **Commonly Used Fertility Drugs**

Category	Action	Dose	Example
Selective estrogen receptor modulator (SERM)	Stimulates ovulation by causing the hypothalamus to produce GnRH, which causes the pituitary to produce more FSH and LH, which stimulates the ovary to release an egg	Tablets, start with 50 mg/d for 5 d; may increase to 200 mg/d	Clomid or Serophene (clomiphene citrate)
Follitropins (gonadotropins)	Similar to body's FSH; stimulates growth and maturation of ovarian follicle	75 IU/d	Fertinex or Braville (urofollitropin)
Menotropins (gonadotropins)	Promotes growth and maturation of ovarian follicle	Intramuscular regimens vary	Pergonal or Menopur (FSH and LH from urine)
Human chorionic gonadotropin (hCG)	Induces ovulation by stimulating release of egg from mature follicle	2,000–10,000 units IM	Pregnyl (hCG extracted from urine)
GnRH agonists	Suppress production of LH and FSH, preventing premature LH surge and development of only one dominant follicle	Lupron Depot—375 mg every 28 d for 6 mos; Synarel—200 µg intranasally twice daily for 6 mos	Lupron (leuprolide acetate) Synarel (nafarelin acetate)
GnRH antagonists	Inhibits release of LH from pituitary to prevent premature LH surge	250 µg/d injected under the skin	Antagon or Orgalutran (ganirelix acetate)
Progesterone	Prepares uterus for implantation of fertilized egg and maintain pregnancy	Vaginal suppositories, 25–50 mg twice daily or 50 mg each night; rectal suppositories, 12.25 mg every 12 hr; capsule, 100 mg orally 3 times a day	Progesterone suppository, troche, or gel
Ergot alkaloid	Interrupts prolactin feedback to pituitary, allows for release of LH and FSH	Oral dose of 5–7.5 mg/d	Bromocriptine (Parlodel)

FSH, follicle-stimulating hormone; GnRH, gonadotropin-releasing hormone; LH, luteinizing hormone.

depending on the availability of a male partner and the presence of male factor infertility.

In Vitro Fertilization (IVF)

For some couples, artificial insemination, use of donor sperm, and administration of fertility drugs do not result in pregnancy. They then must decide whether to pursue more advanced treatment options such as IVF, a procedure that involves surgically removing eggs from a woman's ovaries, combining them with sperm in the laboratory, and returning them to the woman's body or donating them to another woman. This procedure is expensive and considerably invasive. Success rates vary widely and depend on the specific procedure, the experience of the clinician, the age of the woman, the quality of the sperm, and the quality of the eggs. Many of the procedures involve similar steps, but some techniques may be more acceptable to couples than others, based on religious and personal beliefs.

The **IVF** process (Fig. 10.11) involves the woman taking ovulation-inducing medications so that multiple follicles develop and mature. Serial ultrasounds are used to monitor the follicles. When the lead follicle reaches the appropriate size, the woman or her partner administers an intramuscular injection of a drug such as human chorionic gonadotropin. The purpose of the injection is to determine the timing of ovulation accurately, so that an egg retrieval procedure can be scheduled just before the expected ovulation. The retrieval is done under conscious sedation and with ultrasound guidance.

After the eggs are retrieved, they are fertilized with sperm from the male partner or a donor. An endocrinologist or laboratory technician performs the fertilization in the laboratory. Several days later, the woman returns to the physician's office for transfer of a set number of embryos into her uterus through the cervix. Any excess embryos can be cryopreserved for future use or destroyed. In some cases, a fourth option may be to donate them to another couple.

Gamete Intrafallopian Transfer

Another AHR is called **gamete intrafallopian transfer (GIFT)**. In this procedure, the eggs are retrieved as described previously, but then the eggs and sperm are deposited directly into the woman's fallopian tube. Fertilization takes place *in vivo*. For some couples, this procedure satisfies religious prohibitions against artificial

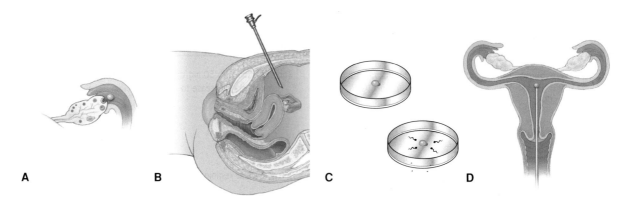

FIGURE 10.11 In vitro fertilization. **A:** Follicular release of the mature oocyte from the ovary in ovulation. **B:** Clinicians remove ova (here, through an intra-abdominal procedure). **C:** The ova are fertilized with sperm and are left to grow in a culture medium. **D:** The fertilized ova are inserted into the woman's uterus for potential implantation.

fertilization because any fertilization takes place within the woman and no embryos are left for cryopreservation.

Zygote Intrafallopian Transfer

Zygote intrafallopian transfer (ZIFT) involves egg retrieval, fertilization in the laboratory, and transfer of the zygotes directly to the fallopian tube. This is done at an earlier stage of development than the embryos inserted into the uterus in an IVF.

In Vitro Fertilization With Donor Eggs

Women who do not ovulate or who are of advanced age (ie, older than 35 years) may wish to use donor eggs. These may come from family members, friends, or anonymous donors. With donor eggs, ovulation-inducing medications are used to synchronize the cycles of the egg donor and the recipient. Eggs are then retrieved and fertilized with sperm obtained from the male partner or a donor. The embryos are then transferred to the recipient as in IVF. The use of donor eggs is a relatively new development and, with the passage of the Assisted Human Reproduction Act, it is illegal in Canada for donors to be paid a fee other than legitimate expenses associated with the donation (eg, the medical costs of the procedure). In the United States, where there is no such prohibition on payment, donor egg agencies are found throughout the country. These agencies are self-regulated and should be researched carefully. Because of the necessity for synchronization of the cycles of both the egg donor and egg recipient, and because preservation of unfertilized eggs is still considered experimental, women wishing to undergo IVF with donor eggs must travel to the location of the participating clinic, often staying there for several weeks until transfer can be accomplished and appropriate diagnostic tests can be conducted to determine success. In addition, because of the invasive nature of the procedure for the egg donor,

the use of donor eggs is more expensive than the use of donor sperm. Furthermore, in the absence of legislation in most provinces and territories relating to the rights, obligations, and status of the parties involved in egg donation, legal consultation is usually recommended. Legal contracts should relinquish parental rights by the egg donor, require parties to agree that any child born as a result of egg donation is indisputably considered the child of the recipient, and clarify that the egg donor has no responsibility for rearing and caring for the child. The legal contract should also establish who has the rights to any unused embryos, or whether they are to be destroyed or donated to other infertile couples.

Intracytoplasmic Sperm Injection

If the male partner's sperm count is very low, chances of success may increase with direct injection of a single sperm into the egg, a process called **intracytoplasmic sperm injection (ICSI)**. The procedure is similar to IVF, except that the sperm are introduced directly into the cytoplasm of the egg. If the eggs are from a woman of advanced maternal age, microscopic holes may be drilled in the zona pellucida, a procedure referred to as **assisted hatching**.

 Ted and Joan, from the beginning of the chapter, have undergone fertility testing and decide to pursue AHR. Their religious beliefs, however, forbid artificial fertilization. Which method would be most appropriate for them to choose?

Surrogate or Gestational Carriers

Some women cannot carry a pregnancy to term because of an absent or malformed uterus. In such cases, the client may choose to employ a surrogate or gestational carrier to produce a baby genetically related to the mother, father, or both. In this case, a procedure similar to IVF is performed, and then the resultant embryos are placed in the surrogate's uterus. After the child's birth, the surrogate surrenders him or her to the party or parties who legally adopt the child.

There have been several highly publicized cases in which, after birth, the surrogate declines to relinquish the child. For this reason, this procedure involves extensive preconception contracts to protect against future legal problems. In such contracts, the surrogate, who often is a married woman who has completed her family, agrees to certain conditions, including refraining from sexual activity with her own partner, so that there is no possibility of spontaneous conception. She also agrees to abstain from activities that may put the fetus at risk (eg, smoking, alcohol, or illegal drug consumption) and agrees to comply with the obstetrician's instructions. Most important, the contract should cover such issues as parental obligations of the infertile couple regardless of the child's mental and physical condition, and release of all parental obligations and rights of the surrogate and her partner. In Canada, surrogacy is covered under the provisions of the Assisted Human Reproduction Act (Government of Canada, 2013b). It is illegal to pay a woman to be a surrogate, although certain expenses are permitted under the Act. Receiving payment for brokering a surrogacy contract is also prohibited, and women under the age of 21 may not be surrogates.

Multifetal Reduction

In recent years, the incidence of multiple pregnancy in Canada has risen sharply, as a result of the increased use of fertility treatments (CFAS, 2007). Reports indicate that the births of 30% to 50% of twins, and more than 75% of higher order multiples (3+ infants) result from fertility treatments, and over 25% of these are born preterm and with a low birth weight (Fauser et al., 2005; Medical Advisory Secretariat, 2006). The associated risks of multiple birth and premature birth are well known. Babies are at increased risk for respiratory distress syndrome, intracranial hemorrhage, cerebral palsy, blindness, low birth weight, and neonatal morbidity and mortality (see Chap. 22). Mothers also experience increased risk for gestational hypertension/preeclampsia, gestational diabetes, anemia, and polyhydramnios with multiple gestations (Fauser et al., 2005). If more than one or two embryos implant and begin development by use of fertility medication alone or by other forms of assisted reproduction, reduction of the number of viable fetuses may be suggested. The Society of Obstetricians and Gynaecologists of Canada (SOGC) has developed recommendations for the number of embryos that should be transferred, in an effort to proactively deal with the issue of multiple pregnancy (Min et al., 2008). The possibility should be discussed and a plan decided before treatment begins. Nurses can facilitate this conversation and help the client or couple to develop a plan before they are faced with the decision to reduce the number of fetuses.

Evaluation

The couple should have a reasonable expectation of the probability of success of any treatment. Infertility practices vary widely in the experience of the clinicians and the success rates of their protocols. Statistics can be difficult to interpret because "success" rates may be reported in terms that are not comparable. For example, definitions of what is considered a pregnancy, demographics and risk factors of the client populations served, and variability among clinicians are all variables that may change across practice settings.

Although women undergo infertility treatment in hopes of achieving a pregnancy, those who do become pregnant face additional challenges. Although the woman may have achieved a pregnancy, the pregnancy has not "cured" the infertility. The infertility diagnosis remains and, for the woman, seems like a chronic condition. There is some speculation that women who have infertility may have differences in how they act as parents. There is concern that parents may treat these highly desired, long-hoped-for children differently by being more intense or overprotective as a consequence of the incredible risks and investments involved in conceiving. Evidence suggests that infertility treatment might be associated with idealized parenthood, which could negatively affect adjustment and the development of a confident parental identity (Hammarberg et al., 2008). A recent systematic review examining quality of life and infertility (Rigol-Chachamovich et al., 2010) found that individuals with a history of infertility, particularly women, experience some degree of health-related quality of life impairment.

Women dealing with secondary infertility also may not receive the support they need. Because they have successfully had at least one child, others may dismiss their feelings of loss and desperation. Nurses sensitive to the issues raised by infertility and its related emotional costs can better support parents and help them cope effectively with the normal stresses of parenthood.

SUMMARY

- Infertility, or the inability to achieve pregnancy after 1 year of regular, unprotected intercourse, affects approximately one in eight Canadian couples.
- Causes of infertility include biologic, chemical, environmental, and lifestyle factors. Male and female

factors, as well as combined factors, account for most cases. For some couples, no identifiable cause can be ascertained.

- Diagnostic assessment includes evaluating both partners. Assessment of the male partner should be completed early in the diagnostic process.
- Treatment options depend on the diagnosis and can cause significant financial and practical burdens. Nurses can help couples understand the reasonable expectation of the probability of success and refer clients to sources for support.
- Religious, ethnic, cultural, and personal values may play important roles in couples' responses to diagnosis and may influence their acceptance of various options.

Questions to Ponder

1. A woman whose husband has azoospermia tells the nurse that she plans to become pregnant using donor sperm without her husband's knowledge. She is afraid that he will not approve of this, but is confident that once she gives birth, he will love the child on first sight.
   - What are your personal feelings about her decision?
   - What obligations do you have to share her plans with her husband?
   - What resources are available to you?
2. A couple who is attempting pregnancy through the use of AHR is debating whether they will tell friends, relatives, or the resultant offspring about circumstances surrounding the conception.
   - What are the benefits and risks of secrecy?
   - What resources are available to the couple?

REVIEW QUESTIONS

1. The nurse is providing anticipatory guidance to a couple about to undergo an infertility workup. Of the following components for the male partner, the nurse should explain which one will be evaluated initially:
   A. Ejaculatory response
   B. Serum prolactin levels
   C. Serum testosterone level
   D. History and physical examination

2. A nurse is reviewing the potential findings that fertility testing may reveal. One partner says, "It will be such a relief to find out what the problem is so we can fix it." Which of the following responses from the nurse would be most appropriate?
   A. "I'm sure it will be a great relief, but testing can be very stressful, so be prepared."
   B. "Because of the time involved in testing, you may feel discouraged and want to give up. Don't."

   C. "It is important for you to review each test carefully before we start so you know exactly what to expect."
   D. "Although testing often identifies the cause of infertility, some cases of infertility remain unexplained even after testing."

3. A nurse is reviewing the laboratory test results of a client's cervical mucus. Which of these findings indicates that the client's cervical mucus is conducive to conception?
   A. pH of 5
   B. Ferning
   C. No spinnbarkeit
   D. Rectal temperature of 36.3°C

4. The nurse instructs a male client about the proper technique for collecting a semen specimen for analysis. Which of these statements, if made by the client, would indicate that he understands the instructions?
   A. "I will ejaculate into a sterile container."
   B. "I will deliver the ejaculate to the laboratory within 30 minutes."
   C. "I will place ice around the container in which I am transporting the ejaculate."
   D. "I will not ejaculate for 3 days before providing you with the specimen."

5. The nurse should include which of the following statements when teaching a woman about monitoring her basal body temperature?
   A. "Look for an increase in body temperature of approximately 3 degrees."
   B. "Look for a decrease in your temperature followed by a sharp increase."
   C. "Look for periodic dips in your temperature over 24 hours about 1 week before your period is due."
   D. "Look for an increase in your temperature for 2 days, followed by a return to your baseline temperature."

6. A client who is experiencing difficulty becoming pregnant asks the nurse if her infertility is the result of an induced abortion she had several years ago. The nurse's response should be based on the understanding that
   A. spontaneous abortions are related to infertility.
   B. infertility is generally independent of a history of induced abortions.
   C. there is a direct relationship between induced abortions and subsequent infertility.
   D. infertility may be related to guilt and remorse women feel following abortions.

7. The 40-year-old male partner of an infertile couple shares all the following information with the nurse during his health history. Which piece of data indicates the need for health education to improve the chances of achieving a pregnancy?

A. The man is moderately obese.

B. The man is a writer who works out of his home.

C. The man smokes one-half a pack of cigarettes per day.

D. The man drinks 1 to 2 alcoholic beverages per day.

8. The nurse is reviewing the chart of a 32-year-old client who has been diagnosed with impaired fecundity. Which of these data support the diagnosis?

A. The woman has a history of first-trimester spontaneous abortion.

B. The woman's sexual partner's semen analysis revealed a low sperm count.

C. The woman has not become pregnant after 1 year of unprotected intercourse.

D. The woman had two induced abortions during her late teens and early twenties.

9. The 34-year-old female in an infertile couple shares all the following information with the nurse during the health history. Which piece of data indicates the need for health education to improve the chances of achieving a pregnancy?

A. The woman is moderately obese.

B. The woman works as a massage therapist in a health spa.

C. The woman drinks approximately three alcoholic beverages per week.

D. The couple have had unprotected intercourse every other day during the middle of her menstrual cycle for 6 months.

10. The nurse is discussing the use of infertility medications with an infertile couple. Which of these statements, if made by one or the other of the partners, would suggest that additional information is needed?

A. "A number of different medications may be needed during each cycle."

B. "We will both take medication at different times of my wife's menstrual cycle."

C. "Depending on the medication, you will be teaching my husband how to give me a daily injection."

D. "The risk of having a multiple gestation is related to the length of time that we will be needing the medication."

REFERENCES

Akushevich, I., Kravchenko, J., & Manton, K. (2007). Health-based population forecasting: Effects of smoking on mortality and fertility. *Risk Analysis, 27*(2), 467–482.

American College of Obstetricians and Gynecologists. (2012). Evaluating infertility. Retrieved from https://www.acog.org/~/media/For%20Patients/faq136.pdf?dmc=1&ts=20140514T1103535430

American Society for Reproductive Medicine. (2013). *Frequently asked questions about infertility.* Retrieved July 2, 2013, from http://www.asrm.org/awards/index.aspx?id=3012

Anonymous. (2004). Infectious diseases. *Canadian Journal of Public Health, 95*(Suppl.), S30–S36.

Brucker, P. S., & McKenry, P. C. (2004). Support from health care providers and the psychological adjustment of individuals experiencing infertility. *Journal of Obstetric, Gynecologic, and Neonatal Nursing, 33*(5), 597–603.

Bushnik, T., Cook, J., Yuzpe, A., Tough, S., & Collins, J. (2012). Estimating the prevalence of infertility in Canada. *Human Reproduction, 27*(3), 738–746.

Canadian Fertility and Andrology Society. (2007). Incidence and complications of multiple gestation in Canada: Proceedings of an expert meeting. *Reproductive BioMedicine Online, 14*(6), 773–790.

Cousineau, M., & Domar, A. (2007). Psychological impact of infertility. *Best Practice & Research. Clinical Obstetrics & Gynaecology, 21*(2), 293–308.

Cystic Fibrosis Medicine. (2008). Fertility and cystic fibrosis. Retrieved from http://www.cfmedicine.com/cfdocs/cftext/fertility.htm

Dorff, E. N. (1998). *Matters of life and death: A Jewish approach to modern medical ethics.* Philadelphia: Jewish Publication Society.

Dutney, A. (2007). Religion, infertility and assisted reproductive technology. *Best Practice & Research. Clinical Obstetrics & Gynaecology, 21*(1), 169–180.

Fauser, B. C. J., Devroey, P., & Macklon, N. S. (2005). Multiple birth resulting from ovarian stimulation for subfertility treatment. *Lancet, 365*(9473), 1807–1816.

Fritz, M., & Speroff, L. (2011). *Clinical gynecologic endocrinology and infertility* (8th ed.). Philadelphia: Lippincott Williams & Williams.

Fuse, K., & Crenshaw, E. (2006). Gender imbalance in infant mortality: A cross-national study of social structure and female infanticide. *Social Science & Medicine, 62*(2), 360–374.

Government of Canada. (2013a). *Fertility.* Retrieved July 31, 2013, from http://healthycanadians.gc.ca/health-sante/pregnancy-grossesse/fert-eng.php

Government of Canada. (2013b). *Assisted human reproduction act.* Ottawa, ON: Canadian Government Publishing. Retrieved July 2, 2013, from http://laws-lois.justice.gc.ca/eng/acts/A-13.4/FullText.html

Hammarberg, K., Fisher, J., & Wynter, K. (2008). Psychological and social aspects of pregnancy, childbirth and early parenting after assisted conception: A systematic review. *Human Reproduction Update, 14*(5), 395–414.

Health Canada. (1996). *Processing and distribution of semen for assisted conception regulations.* Retrieved from http://laws.justice.gc.ca/en/F-27/SOR-96-254/index.html

Health Canada. (2003). *Advisory on diethylstilbestrol (DES) and the risk of genital and obstetrical complications-Health professional advisory.* Retrieved July 3, 2013, from http://www.healthy canadians.gc.ca/recall-alert-rappel-avis/hc-sc/2003/14738 a-eng.php

Health Canada. (2013). *Assisted human reproduction.* Retrieved July 3, 2013, from http://www.hc-sc.gc.ca/dhp-mps/brgtherap/legislation/reprod/index-eng.php

Idahl, A., Boman, J., Kumlin, U., & Olofsson, J. (2004). Demonstration of *Chlamydia trachomatis* IgG antibodies in the male partner of the infertile couple is correlated with a reduced likelihood of achieving pregnancy. *Human Reproduction, 19*(5), 1121–1126.

Jha, P., Kumar, R., Vasa, P., Dhingra, N., Thiruchelvam, D., & Moineddin, R. (2006). Low female[corrected]-to-male [corrected] sex ratio of children born in India: national survey of 1.1 million households. *Lancet, 367*(9524), 211–218.

Klonoff-Cohen, H., Lam-Kruglick, P., & Gonzalez, C. (2003). Effects of maternal and paternal alcohol consumption on the success rates of in vitro fertilization and gamete intrafallopian transfer. *Fertility and Sterility, 79*(2), 330–339.

Kolettis, P., & Sandlow, J. (2002). Clinical and genetic features of patients with unilateral absence of the vas deferens. *Urology, 60,* 1073–1076.

Lane, D. E. (2006). Polycystic ovary syndrome and its differential diagnosis. *Obstetrical & Gynecological Survey, 61*(2), 125–135.

Langford, D., Baron, D., Joy, J., Del Valle, L., & Shack, J. (2011). Contributions of HIV infection in the hypothalamus and substance abuse/use to HPT dysregulation. *Psychoneuroendocrinology, 36*(5), 710–719.

Lewis, J. A. (2003). Jewish perspectives on pregnancy and childbearing. *MCN—The American Journal of Maternal Child Nursing, 28*(5), 306–312.

Marchionni, M., Fambrini, M., Zambelli, V., Scarselli, G., & Susini, T. (2004). Reproductive performance before and after abdominal myomectomy: A retrospective analysis. *Fertility and Sterility, 82*(1), 154–159.

Mardh, P. (2004). Tubal factor infertility, with special regard to chlamydial salpingitis. *Current Opinion in Infectious Diseases, 17*, 49–52.

McCarthy, M. (2008). Women's lived experience of infertility after unsuccessful medical intervention. *Journal of Midwifery & Women's Health, 53*(4), 319–324.

Medical Advisory Secretariat. (2006). In vitro fertilization and multiple pregnancies: An evidence-based analysis. *Ontario Health Technology Assessment Series, 6*(18), 1–63.

Min, J. K., Claman, P., & Hughes, E. (2008). Joint SOGC-CFAS Guideline: Guidelines for the number of embryos to transfer following in vitro fertilization. *Journal of Obstetrics & Gynaecology Canada, 102*(2), 203–216.

Newbold, R. (2008). Prenatal exposure to diethylstilbestrol (DES). *Fertility & Sterility, 89*(2 Suppl.), 55–56.

Niccolai, L., Ethier, K., Kershaw, T., Lewis, J., Meade, C., & Ickovics, J. (2004). New sex partner acquisition and sexually transmitted disease risk among adolescent females. *Journal of Adolescent Health, 34*, 216–223.

Ombelet, W., Cooke, I., Dyer, S., Serour, G., & Devroey, P. (2008). Infertility and the provision of infertility medical services in developing countries. *Human Reproduction Update, 14*(6), 605–621.

Panni, M., & Corn, S. (2002). The use of a uniquely designed anesthetic scavenging hood to reduce operating room anesthetic gas contamination during general anesthesia. *Anesthesia & Analgesia, 95*(3), 656–660.

Pasquali, R., Patton, L., & Gambineri, A. (2007). Obesity and infertility. *Current Opinion in Endocrinology, Diabetes & Obesity, 14*(6), 482–487.

Practice Committee of the ASRM. (2012). Smoking and infertility: A committee opinion. *Fertility and Sterility, 98*(6), 1400–1406.

Powell-Hamilton, N. N. (2012). *Sex chromosome anomalies.* Retrieved July 2, 2013, from http://www.merckmanuals.com/professional/index.html

Randeva, H., Tan, B., Weickart, M., Lois, K., Nestler, J., Sattar, N. et al. (2012). Cardiometabolic aspects of the polycystic ovary syndrome. *Endocrine Review, 33*(5), 812–841.

Rebar, R. W. (2013a). *Sperm disorders.* Retrieved July 2, 2013, from http://www.merckmanuals.com/professional/index.html

Rebar, R. W. (2013b). *Ovulatory dysfunction.* Retrieved July 2, 2013, from http://www.merckmanuals.com/professional/index.html

Rigol-Chachamovich, J., Chachamovich, E., Ezer, H., Fleck, M., Knauth, D., & Passos, E. (2010). Investigating quality of life and health related quality of life in infertility: A systematic review. *Journal of Psychosomatic Obstetrics & Gynecology, 31*(2), 101–110.

Rowlands, R. (2011). Misinformation on abortion. *The European Journal of Contraception and Reproductive Health Care, 16*(4), 233–240.

Rubin, M. (2007). Structural variations in DES daughters. *Obstetrical & Gynecological Survey, 62*(8), 548–555.

Saner-Amigh, K., & Halvorson, L. (2011). Andrology and fertility assessment. *LabMedicine, 42*, 41–50.

Schneider, M. G., & Forthofer, M. S. (2005). Associations of psychosocial factors with the stress of infertility treatment. *Health Social Work, 30*(3), 183–191.

Schrager, S., & Potter, B. (2004). Diethylstilbestrol exposure. *American Family Physician, 69*(10), 2395–2400.

Shaban, S. (2007). *Male infertility overview: Assessment, diagnosis, and treatment.* Retrieved from http://www.ivf.com/shaban.html

Sharlip, I., Jarow, J., Belker, A., Lipshultz, L., Sigman, M., Thomas, A. et al. (2002). Best practice policies for male infertility. *Fertility and Sterility, 77*(5), 873–882.

Spector, A. (2004). Psychological issues and interventions with infertile patients. *Women & Therapy, 23*(3/4), 91–105.

Star, W. L., Lommel, L. L., & Shannon, M. T. (2004). *Women's primary health care: Protocols for practice* (2nd ed.). San Francisco: UCSF Nursing Press.

Swanton, A., & Child, T. (2005). Reproduction and ovarian ageing. *Journal of the British Menopause Society, 11*(4), 126–131.

Taylor, H. S., Aldad, T. S., McVeight, E., Homburg, R., & Guillebaud, J. (2012). *Oxford American handbook of reproductive medicine.* New York, NY: Oxford University Press.

Thyroid Foundation of Canada. (2013). *Thyroid disease, pregnancy and fertility.* Retrieved from http://www.thyroid.ca/pregnancy_fertility.php

Windham, G. C., Mitchell, P., Anderson, M., & Lasley, B. L. (2005). Cigarette smoking and effects on hormone function in premenopausal women. *Environmental Health Perspectives, 113*(10), 1285–1290.

Genetics, Embryology, and Preconceptual/ Prenatal Assessment and Screening

Luisa Ciofani, Robin J. Evans, Taranum Sultana, and Shirley Jones*

Carmen, 22 years old and recently married, comes to the health care facility to discuss preconception health screening. During her interview, Carmen states, "My spouse and I would like to start trying for a baby right away. But my mother mentioned a genetic problem a distant cousin had years ago. Several of my relatives have diabetes, heart disease, and other chronic conditions. I'm afraid that if my baby had a problem, it would be my fault."

April, 36 years old, and her husband Alex, 37 years old, come to the prenatal clinic. April is at 13 weeks' gestation. She gave birth to their first child, a healthy daughter, 4 years ago. With this pregnancy, the couple attempted to conceive for 2 years. During this appointment, April states, "According to the Internet, I'm now considered of 'advanced maternal age.' The risk of having a child with genetic problems has increased so much! Should I be worried about Down syndrome?"

Nurses working with such clients need to understand the material in this chapter to manage care and address issues appropriately. You will read more about these clients later. Before beginning, consider the following points:

- How should the nurse tailor care to best suit the needs of these clients and their families?
- What aspects of teaching do these clients require?

---

*Contributor to first U.S. edition.

- What issues are similar for the women? What issues are different?
- What factors might affect April's pregnancy adversely?
- Which types of screening and diagnostic testing would the nurse expect April to undergo? Carmen?
- How would the nurse intervene to enhance each client's health, well-being, and comfort?

LEARNING OBJECTIVES

On completion of this chapter, the reader should be able to:
- Summarize gametogenesis, embryogenesis, and fetal growth and development.
- Identify the etiology of risk factors that can adversely affect conception, gestation, and embryonic/fetal growth and development.
- Discuss preconception health risk assessment and counselling from the view of health care providers, clients and families, and sociocultural communities seeking these services.
- Describe the effect of advances in human genetics on informed decision making and consent.
- Discuss strategies to enhance the health, well-being, and comfort of clients and partners seeking preconception or prenatal health risk assessment and counselling.
- Describe the scope of preconception, prenatal, and postnatal screening and diagnostic procedures available to clients and families.

KEY TERMS

allele	meiosis
aneuploidy	mitosis
association	monozygotic twins
blastomere	morula
chromosome	multifactorial disorder
chronic sorrow	mutations
deformation	nucleotide
disruption	oocyte
dizygotic twins	phenotype
dominant	recessive
dysmorphology	sequence
gametogenesis	sex linked
genes	spermatid
genetic counselling	syndrome
genetics	teratogen
genotype	variation
informed decision making and consent	zygote
malformation	

Major congenital anomalies are detected in 2% to 3% of births every year (Public Health Agency of Canada, 2013). The risk for conceiving a child with a birth defect is increased for some people with medical, genetic, or parental age factors. In this chapter, we provide the reader with awareness and understanding of the many preconception and prenatal development issues that await clients in their journey to have a healthy biologic child. The material found here serves to provide health care professionals with the knowledge and resources needed to identify reproductive risks and to present information about alternatives to clients. The foundation for this knowledge is built through a review of basic genetics, embryology, and fetal development. We continue with discussions of appropriate preconception screening and assessment techniques. We also explore in detail prenatal screening and evaluation techniques and associated collaborative care interventions.

GENETICS AND CELL BIOLOGY

Variation is the life cycle outcome of each person's unique response to nature (genetic code) and nurture (environment), beginning before conception and ending with death. It is ever changing and ever present throughout a person's biopsychosocial growth and development. **Genetics** is the field of study that investigates variations within the human genome.

The breadth and diversity of genetic characteristics are remarkable, given that each person is 99.69% the same as any other human being (Feero et al., 2010). The Human Genome Project, completed in 2003, led to an ever-accelerating period of biomedical discovery, with significant health benefits and new approaches to common conditions, as well as controversy over the cost–benefit ratio of introducing costly medical technologies (Feero et al., 2010). The importance and potential influence of the seemingly small level of variation becomes self-evident when one considers that the human genome consists of 6 billion base pairs, each solely or jointly responsible for the myriad of human characteristics, and the difference between any two people is about 24 billion base pairs (Feero et al., 2010).

Chromosomes, Genes, and DNA

Somatic cells are the basic biologic foundation of every human organ and system. They help maintain the growth, development, and well-being of each person. *Germ cells* are the reproductive cells located in the *gonads* (ovaries, testes). The sole function of germ cells is to preserve the human species through replication. Both somatic and germ cells consist of a nucleus surrounded by cytoplasm (Fig. 11.1). The nucleus contains 46 chromosomes (two copies of each of 23 different chromosomes) that together compose the entire human genome. **Chromosomes** are thread-like strands that carry genes and transmit hereditary information. Within the cytoplasm are multiple organelles, including ribosomes and mitochondria.

Each chromosome consists of deoxyribonucleic acid (DNA), proteins, and a small amount of ribonucleic acid (RNA). DNA is made up of sugar (deoxyribose), a phosphate group, and a nitrogenous base (purine or pyri-

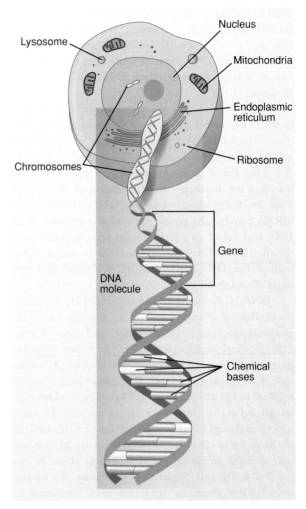

FIGURE 11.1 Schematic drawing of the contents of a cell and the physical structure of DNA. Note that each chemical base only pairs with its reciprocal chemical base.

midine). The purine bases are *adenine (A) and guanine (G)*—and pyrimidines are *cytosine (C) and thymine (T)*. Together, these substances form a **nucleotide** that joins with other nucleotides to create a strand-like chain. DNA is responsible for the genetic code required for the synthesis of all amino acids. First described by Watson and Crick (1953), the double helix structure of DNA is the product of two strands of DNA held together by hydrogen bonds formed from the complementary pairing of nitrogen bases: adenine with thymine and cytosine with guanine. The molecular structure is similar to a ladder twisted into a spiral staircase, with the strands of DNA forming the sides and the base pairs forming the rungs. The specific one-to-one pairing of the nitrogenous bases is the foundation of DNA's ability to perfectly and intrinsically replicate itself. During the process of DNA replication, the two complementary strands are separated and each serves as a template for a new DNA molecule. When mistakes in this process occur, the cell attempts to mediate and repair these errors (Friedberg, 2003). Not all **mutations** are repaired, however, and those that remain become part of the new DNA molecule and all future replications of that DNA strand. These errors are manifested as birth defects or increased susceptibility to cancer (Pfau & Amon, 2012).

RNA is also composed of a sugar (ribose), a phosphate group, and a nitrogenous base (purine or pyrimidine). Unlike DNA, however, RNA is single-stranded and uses the pyrimidine uracil (U) instead of thymine. All three types of RNA (messenger, ribosomal, and transfer) are necessary for translation of the genetic code into the synthesis of polypeptides (Allison, 2012). mRNA conveys the genetic information encoded in the DNA and serves as a template for protein synthesis in the ribosomes. The unidirectional flow of genetic information from DNA to RNA to protein is the central principle of molecular genetics.

DNA is organized into genes, which are defined as the fundamental units of genetic information. Each gene is a unique sequence (both number and order) formed from the nucleotides along the DNA strands. The four nitrogenous bases (A = adenine, T = thymine, C = cytosine, G = guanine) of DNA form three-letter "words" referred to as *codons*. From the 64 possible codons (four unique letters in three-letter combinations), 20 major amino acids are formed. Multiple codons can indicate the same amino acid, but each codon will code for only one specific amino acid. These amino acids in turn are the multiword "sentences" providing the instructions for the generation of all proteins. Thus, genes are the "recipe book" for the functional products that the human body requires.

Errors (mutations, duplications, or deletions of a gene) may affect the body's ability to maintain health and well-being. Such changes in a person's genetic code (**genotype**) may or may not alter the product coded for by that gene. Any alterations will be expressed as an observable change in the person's growth, development, or wellness (**phenotype**).

The *autosomes* are the 22 chromosomes not involved in the determination of gender. They are generally numbered from largest to smallest beginning with 1 and ending with 22. (Note, however, that chromosome 21 is actually the smallest autosome.) The *sex chromosomes,* identified as "X" and "Y," are the alternative forms of chromosome 23 and are responsible for gender. Germ cells have one set of the 23 chromosomes (one each of the 22 autosomes and one of the two sex chromosomes). Somatic cells have 46 chromosomes, two each of the 22 autosomes and two sex chromosomes (Fig. 11.2). The 46 chromosomes result from the fusion of an **oocyte** (one set of 23 chromosomes) and a sperm (one set of 23 chromosomes) to form a **zygote** (fertilized oocyte). During this fusion, those who receive two X chromosomes are female (46, XX), whereas those who receive one X and one Y chromosome are male (46, XY). Because females may give only an X to their children but males may give either an X or a Y, the chromosome complement of each sperm determines the zygote's gender.

Mitosis and Meiosis

All cells (somatic and germ) undergo a life cycle of birth, maturation, replication, and death. The process undertaken by somatic cells is called **mitosis** (Fig. 11.3). The process used by germ cells is called **meiosis;** it leads to the formation of gametes (Fig. 11.4). The similarities and differences between the two processes may be summarized as replication *with* (meiosis) or *without* (mitosis) a reduction in total chromosome count (diploid cell = 2*n,* or $2 \times 23 = 46$ chromosomes). Both mitosis and meiosis are critical to the accurate and consistent transmission of genetic information from parent to all descendant cells.

Mitosis

Mitosis is the cellular process that enables duplication of a cell into two genetically identical daughter cells. It is the body's natural process of growth and development performed in association with cellular repair and replacement.

The five phases of mitosis are interphase, prophase, metaphase, anaphase, and telophase.

- During *interphase,* the cell "rests" from mitotic division but performs metabolic functions, depending

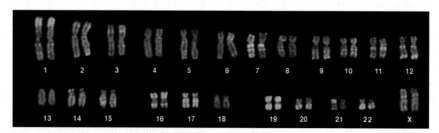

FIGURE 11.2 Normal female karyotype (46, XX). (From: Bolzer, A., Kreth, G., Solovei, I., Koehler, D., Saracoglu, K., Speicher, M. R. (2005). Three-dimensional maps of all chromosomes in human male fibroblast nuclei and prometaphase rosettes. *PLOS Biology, 3*(5), e157. doi:10.1371/journal.pbio.0030157

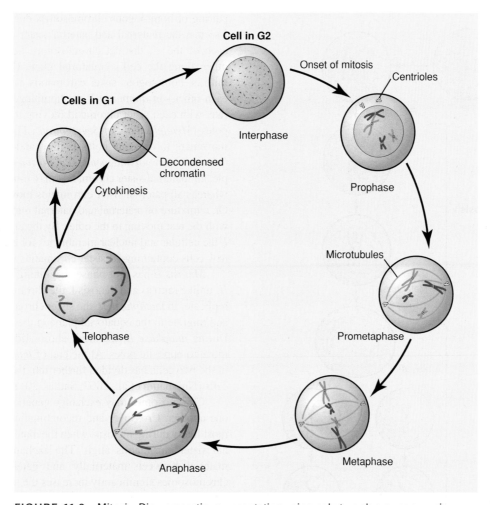

FIGURE 11.3 Mitosis. Diagrammatic representation using only two chromosome pairs. *Purple* represents maternal chromosomes; *coral* represents the paternal chromosomes. During metaphase, each chromosome lines up along the equatorial plane. In total, 46 chromosomes compose each cell.

on the type of cell (e.g., nerve, skin, muscle, brain, blood). The cell also prepares for mitotic replication and division by gathering the additional RNA, amino acids, and nucleotides it will need at the end of this phase. The replicated sides of each chromosome (*sister chromatids*) are joined together at the *centromere.*

- *Prophase* is the beginning of cellular division. This phase is identified microscopically by visualization of the condensed chromosomes and migration of the duplicated centrioles to opposite poles of the cytoplasm. Once the chromosomes have reached their highest density, they begin to migrate to the cell's equatorial plane. The spindle fibres also form.
- The key aspects of *metaphase* are complete migration of the chromosomes and linkage by the spindle fibres of the centrioles to the centromeres of each chromosome. At this point, the chromosome appears microscopically in the traditional notation of either an "X" or inverted "U."

- *Anaphase* is marked by splitting of the centromeres as the two sets of spindle fibres pull them to opposite cellular poles. The result is separation of the sister chromatids and formation of new daughter chromosomes. As the daughter chromosomes reach their respective poles, an indentation begins to form in the cell membrane.
- During the last stage of *telophase,* two new cellular membranes form through the furrowed region of the original cell, and two new daughter cells appear. The chromosomes within each uncoil and become less dense. The nuclear membrane surrounding the chromosomes re-forms in each daughter cell (Fig. 11.3) (Lashley, 2007; Nussbaum et al., 2007).

Meiosis

The process of meiosis enables the diploid germ cells to divide and produce haploid gamete cells ($n = 23$ chromosomes). Meiosis is marked by two separate

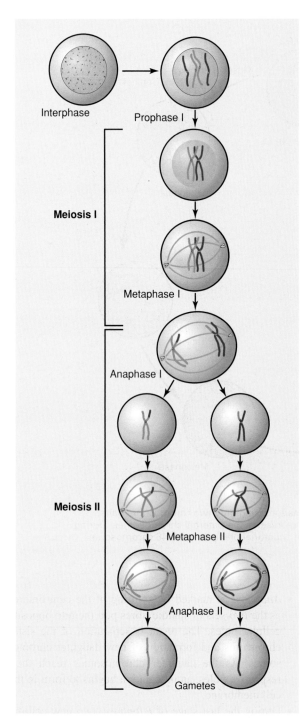

FIGURE 11.4 Meiosis. Diagrammatic representation using two homologous pairs of chromosomes. The 23 homologous pairs line up along the equatorial plane during metaphase I. This permits the potential for exchange of pieces of sister chromatids during metaphase I pairing.

reductions in the number of chromosomes after completion of their initial replication during interphase. The outcome of meiosis is four new haploid cells rather than two diploid cells.

Meiosis I includes prophase I, metaphase I, anaphase I, and telophase I. The hallmark of meiosis I is the pairing of homologous chromosomes during *metaphase I* so that the maternal and paternal sister chromatids for each of the 23 distinct chromosomes lie next to each other along the cell's equatorial plane (Fig. 11.4). (In mitosis, homologous sister chromatids do not pair with each other.) In *anaphase I,* the homologous pairs separate, with each sister chromatid moving toward opposite poles (*Mendel's Law of Segregation*). Furthermore, the movement to opposite poles is in a random assortment (*Mendel's Law of Independent Assortment*). For example, all maternal sister chromatids may move to one pole, whereas all paternal sister chromatids move to the other. Or, a mixture of maternal and paternal may move to one, with the rest moving to the other. By the end of *telophase I,* the cellular and nuclear membranes for each of the two new cells containing 23 sister chromatids have formed.

Meiosis II has four phases beginning with *prophase II;* unlike mitosis and meiosis I, the chromosomes do not replicate. In *metaphase II,* the sister chromatids elongate and migrate to the equatorial plane in the two new cells. During *anaphase II,* the sister chromatids separate and move to opposite poles. At the end of *telophase II,* each of the two cells has divided further into two new haploid cells (Nussbaum et al., 2007; Sadler, 2011).

Chromosomes may exchange genetic material with one another. Crossover and recombination of DNA are most likely during meiosis, when the maternal and paternal sister chromatids align. The exchange of genetic material between maternally and paternally derived chromosomes significantly increases the number of genotypes a man or woman may generate in gamete cells. To underscore the magnitude of possible variations, more than 30,000 known genes across 46 chromosomes can be recombined into any number of outcomes. Genetic exchange also can occur during mitosis and may result in adverse effects on metabolism and chromosomal defects (Alberts, 2003; Webster & De Wreede, 2012).

Gametogenesis

Gametogenesis is the process by which primordial germ cells yield gametes (oocytes and **spermatids**) to help maintain continuity of the human species. The cells that give rise to gametes are formed by the 3rd week of gestation and join with somatic cells to form primitive gonads by the 5th week of gestation (Sadler, 2011). Male primordial germ cells remain dormant in the testes until puberty. Female primordial germ cells, however, begin to differentiate after formation of the primitive ovary in the embryo. Development of germ cells is by mitotic division. Mature oocytes and spermatids form through meiosis.

Spermatogenesis and Spermiogenesis

Each testis is composed of tightly coiled seminiferous tubules, in which *spermatogenesis* occurs, and the

Leydig cells, residing in the interstitial space, are the source of testosterone (Kobayashi et al., 2013). At puberty, the male germ cells form two types of cells: spermatogonia A and spermatogonia B. The ongoing mitotic division of spermatogonia A ensures a constant supply of sperm stem cells critical for spermatogenesis. These stem cells have been shown to have therapeutic potential to restore fertility in infertile males (Kobayashi et al., 2013). Throughout the adult male's reproductive life, selected spermatogonia A cells go on to form spermatogonia B cells. Spermatogonia B cells in turn give rise to primary spermatocytes, which in turn produce spermatids through meiotic division.

The final maturation of spermatids is called *spermiogenesis* and consists of four critical components that provide sperm with progressive motility and the ability to fertilize oocytes (Hess & de Franca, 2008; Sofikitis et al., 2008). Step 1 is condensation of the spermatid nucleus. Step 2 is shedding of most of the spermatid cytoplasm. Step 3 is formation of the acrosome cap, which covers the nuclear surface of the spermatid and contains the enzymes necessary to penetrate the outer layers of the oocyte. This penetration permits transfer of the sperm nucleus with its chromosomes into the cytoplasm of the oocyte. Step 4, the final step, is formation of the neck, midpiece, and tail of the sperm, which facilitates its movement through the female cervix and uterus to the fallopian tubes in preparation for fertilization of the oocyte (Fig. 11.5). The seminiferous tubules transport sperm to the epididymis, where full motility is reached in preparation for ejaculation through the vas

deferens and movement through the female reproductive tract. The process of spermatogenesis takes approximately 70 days to complete (Hess & de Franca, 2008).

Oogenesis

After fertilization, the primitive gonads complete differentiation and become the testes or ovaries. In the female embryo, oogenesis begins at this point, as opposed to initiation of spermatogenesis at the onset of puberty in the male.

The genetic female's primordial germ cells become oogonia. Each oogonium replicates many times through mitotic division to increase in overall number and form clusters surrounded by epithelial (somatic) cells from the ovarian surface. From 3 to 5 months' gestation, the oogonia begin to differentiate into primary oocytes. Epithelial cells from the ovarian cortex encase each oocyte and eventually form the primordial follicle. Once a primary oocyte forms, DNA replication is complete, and the cell enters meiosis I. It remains suspended in this phase throughout childhood. Starting with menarche and continuing with each subsequent menstrual cycle over the next 35 to 40 years of a woman's reproductive life, one or more oocytes "awaken" and continue maturation by completing meiosis II (Nussbaum et al., 2007; Sadler, 2011; Fritz & Speroff, 2011).

By the 5th month of gestation, the number of oogonia reaches a lifetime maximum of approximately 6 to 7 million. Over the next 4 months, that number decreases to 1 to 2 million. This magnitude of rapid depletion, however, slows. By puberty, the number of primary oocytes has diminished to between 300,000 and 500,000 (Fritz & Speroff, 2011). Given that the reproductive female will have approximately 500 menstrual cycles in her lifetime, the surviving primary oocytes provide ample potential for conception.

With each menstrual cycle, 15 to 20 primordial follicles begin to mature in response to follicle-stimulating hormone (FSH) (Sadler, 2011). (See Chapter 6 for discussion of the endometrial cycle.) The primary oocyte within the primordial follicle also responds and begins to complete meiosis I. Usually one primordial follicle matures faster than the others and becomes the primary or "lead" follicle. In response to luteinizing hormone (LH), the primary oocyte completes meiosis I and forms a secondary oocyte and first polar body. During meiosis, the oocyte replicates its DNA and transfers 23 sister chromatids to each new daughter cell, but it does not equally divide the cell's cytoplasm between the two new cells. The primary oocyte receives nearly all the cytoplasm. This process repeats when the secondary oocyte and second polar body are formed. Each receives 23 chromatids, but the secondary oocyte receives the largest portion of the cytoplasm. Therefore, oogenesis results in one mature secondary oocyte from a single

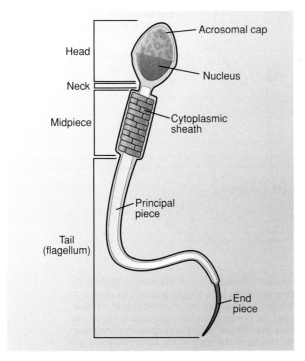

FIGURE 11.5 Normal sperm morphology.

oogonium, whereas spermatogenesis results in four secondary spermatocytes from a single spermatogonium.

With the formation of the secondary oocyte, the graafian (mature) follicle releases the developing oocyte from the ovary (ovulation), and the fimbriae brush the oocyte into the fallopian tube. The oocyte enters meiosis II as it travels down the fallopian tube. Fertilization of the oocyte by a sperm occurs in the fallopian tube. If fertilization does not occur, the oocyte dies and is reabsorbed. The secondary oocyte completes meiosis II only if a sperm fertilizes it. At completion of meiosis II, a zygote (fertilized oocyte) and second polar body have formed.

Fertilization and Implantation

Each menstrual cycle provides a narrow window of opportunity for fertilization. The ovulated oocyte remains capable of fusing with a sperm for only 24 hours. Sperm survive in the female reproductive tract for no more than 72 hours. In addition to these short lifespans, multiple sperm must encounter the secondary oocyte and use the cumulative enzymes within their acrosome caps to assist a single sperm to penetrate and fuse with the secondary oocyte. Although the normal ejaculate has 200,000,000 to 300,000,000 sperm, only a few hundred actually reach the oocyte, further decreasing the odds of conception (Fritz & Speroff, 2011).

Before sperm encounter the secondary oocyte, they must undergo capacitation in the female reproductive tract. This process lasts approximately 7 hours and results in the removal of the protective protein covering the acrosome cap. It must happen for sperm to penetrate the cells (corona radiata) that surround the oocyte (Fig. 11.6).

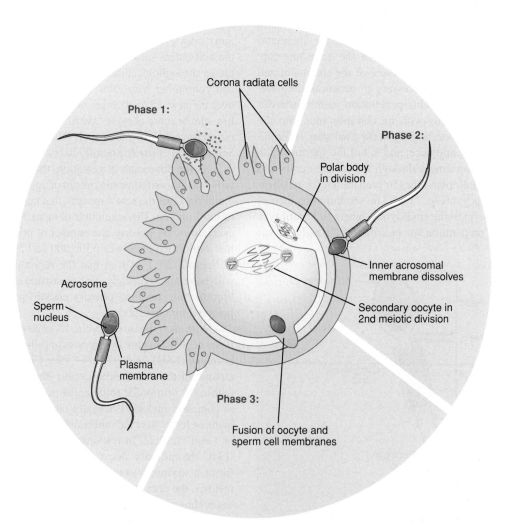

FIGURE 11.6 The three phases of fertilization. Phase 1: Penetration of the corona radiata by several sperm cells. Phase 2: Penetration of the zona pellucida by a single sperm. The proteins on the zona pellucida bind sperm to its surface. This binding causes capacitated sperm to lose the plasma membrane and release enzymes required for penetration. This process is known as the *acrosome reaction.* Phase 3: Fusion of the oocyte membrane with the posterior membrane of the sperm head. Upon fusion of the membranes, chemical changes in the zona pellucida prevent any other sperm from entering the oocyte's cytoplasm. (Adapted from Sadler, T. W. [2011]. *Langman's medical embryology* [12th ed.]. Philadelphia, PA: Lippincott Williams & Wilkins.)

After entry of the sperm, the oocyte continues with the final steps of meiosis II, forming the second polar body and the mature oocyte with its pronucleus containing 23 chromosomes. The head of the sperm contains its pronucleus with 23 chromosomes; the sperm sheds its neck and tail. The two pronuclei come to lie next to each other and begin to replicate their DNA. At the conclusion of fertilization, the normal diploid number is returned to the developing cell, the gender is determined, and cleavage of the zygote by mitotic division is initiated (Sadler, 2011).

As the developing zygote travels down the fallopian tubes to the uterine cavity, it repeats mitotic cell division, forming new cells (**blastomeres**) enclosed within the zona pellucida of the former oocyte. Each new blastomere is smaller than the parent cells. Approximately 5 days after fertilization, the **morula** (dividing embryo that contains 16 or more blastomeres) enters the uterine cavity. Fluid enters the intercellular spaces, and the blastomeres differentiate. Some blastomeres flatten along the circumference of the former oocyte to form the trophoblast, whereas others migrate to one pole to form the embryoblast. The space left by this segregation of the two cell masses is the blastocele. At this point, the zona pellucida is dissolved and lost, allowing the cells of the developing embryoblast to embed into the uterine mucosa. Full implantation is completed approximately 7 days after fertilization if the endometrium has responded appropriately to the proliferative and secretory phases of the menstrual cycle (Sadler, 2011).

EMBRYOLOGY AND DEVELOPMENT

Human gestation lasts 40 weeks (10 lunar months). The first 2 weeks correlate with development of the oocyte and endometrial lining. The field of embryology uses 38 weeks as the total length of gestation, beginning from the day of oocyte fertilization and zygote formation rather than from the first day of the last menstrual period (LMP) (Sadler, 2011). *The following discussion of embryology uses the standard of 38 weeks' gestation. Unless otherwise stated, all other references to gestation in the rest of this chapter use the obstetrical standard of 40 weeks.*

The 1st and 2nd weeks of gestation are known as the *pre-embryonic period,* which begins with fertilization and ends with the appearance of the fetal pole within the blastocyst. The *embryonic period* extends from the 3rd to the 8th week of gestation and is marked by differentiation of the embryonic tissue into the multiple and specialized tissue cells of the human body. The *fetal period* lasts from the 9th to the 38th week of gestation, and is characterized by the growth and development of fetal organs and tissues. See Table 11.1 for a summary of embryonic and fetal development.

Pre-embryonic Development

As described earlier, the zygote has the normal diploid number of 46 chromosomes. This single cell enters into a series of rapid mitotic divisions, which continue as the zygote travels down the fallopian tube to the uterine cavity. Once the zygote begins mitotic cellular division, it is referred to as an embryo. The number of cells visible on microscopic examination is used to describe the stage of embryo development (e.g., 2-cell embryo, 5-cell embryo, 10-cell embryo).

By the beginning of the 2nd week, the blastocyst has embedded partially into the endometrium. At this time, it consists of the outer cells (trophoblast), the inner cell mass (embryoblast), and the blastocele cavity. The embryoblast appears flat and is known as the bilaminar germ disk with two layers: hypoblast and epiblast. The amniotic cavity and membrane (amnion) begin to form within the epiblast. Growth of the germ disk is slow during this period. Endometrial changes as a result of implantation lead to a decidual reaction that appears as a halo around the gestational sac (Fig. 11.7).

Normally, the blastocyst implants in the main uterine body on either the anterior or posterior wall. This permits the placenta to develop embedded within the tissue prepared for the invasive fusion of the trophoblast. If the blastocyst implants near or over the internal os, a partial or complete placenta previa occurs (see Chapter 13). With careful monitoring, this abnormality of implantation can result in a vaginal birth. Implantation can also occur outside the uterus (extrauterine or ectopic pregnancy) (Cunningham et al., 2010). It may occur in the ampullary (90%) or isthmic (8%) portion of the fallopian tube (Fig. 11.8). The remaining 2% of ectopic pregnancies develop in the interstitial tissue of the abdominal cavity, the narrow portion of the fallopian tube, or on the ovary.

Membranes and Placenta

Structural Development. Differentiation of the trophoblast during the pre-embryonic phase begins the formation of the placenta and fetal membranes (chorion and amnion) (Figs. 11.9A–C). Vacuoles appear in the syncytiotrophoblast (syncytium) and form lacunae (Fig. 11.9A). The lacunar (intervillous) spaces form an intercommunicating network; the expanding syncytiotrophoblast carries these spaces into the endometrial lining. This expansion causes erosion of maternal capillaries, which become distended with increased maternal blood to the endometrium. The lacunae merge with the capillaries to establish the flow of maternal blood to the trophoblast layer of the blastocyst (Fig. 11.9B). By the end of the 2nd week, the cytotrophoblast

● TABLE 11.1 **Embryonic and Fetal Development**

Week 3

Beginning development of brain, spinal cord, and heart
Beginning development of the gastrointestinal tract
Neural tube forms, which later becomes the spinal cord
Leg and arm buds appear and grow out from body

Week 4

Brain differentiates
Limb buds grow and develop further

4 weeks

Week 5

Heart now beats at a regular rhythm
Beginning structures of eyes and ears
Some cranial nerves are visible
Muscles innervated

Week 6

Beginning formation of lungs
Fetal circulation established
Further development of the brain
Primitive skeleton forms
Central nervous system forms
Brain waves detectable

Week 7

Straightening of trunk
Nipples and hair follicles form
Elbows and toes visible
Arms and legs move
Diaphragm formed
Mouth with lips and early tooth buds

Week 8

Rotation of intestines
Facial features continue to develop
Heart development complete
Resembles a human being

8 weeks

Weeks 9–12

Embryo now known as a fetus
Sexual differentiation continues
Buds for all 20 temporary teeth laid down

Digestive system shows activity
Head comprises nearly half the fetus size
Face and neck are well formed
Urogenital tract completes development
Urine begins to be produced and excreted
Fetal gender can be determined by week 12
Limbs are long and thin; digits are well formed

12 weeks

Weeks 13–16

A fine hair develops on the body of the fetus called *lanugo*
Fetal skin is almost transparent
Bones become denser
Fetus makes active movement
Sucking motions are made with the mouth
Amniotic fluid is swallowed
Weight quadruples

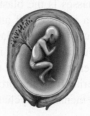

16 weeks

Weeks 17–20

Rapid brain growth occurs
Fetal heart tones can be heard with stethoscope
Kidneys continue to secrete urine into amniotic fluid
Vernix caseosa, a white greasy film, covers the fetus
Eyebrows and head hair appear
Brown fat deposited to help maintain temperature
Nails are present on both fingers and toes
Muscles are well developed
Fetal movement (also known as *quickening*) detected by
    mother

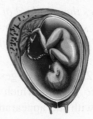

20 weeks

(continued)

● TABLE 11.1 **Embryonic and Fetal Development** (continued)

Weeks 21–24

Eyebrows and eyelashes are well formed
Fetus has a hand grasp and a startle reflex
Alveoli forming in lungs
Skin is translucent and red
Lungs begin to produce *surfactant*

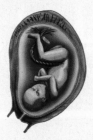

25 weeks

Weeks 25–28

Fetus reaches a length of 38 cm
Rapid brain development
Eyelids open and close
Nervous system controls some functions
Fingerprints are set
Blood formation shifts from spleen to bone marrow
Fetus usually assumes head-down position (cephalic
  presentation)

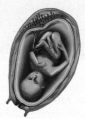

28 weeks

Weeks 29–32

Rapid increase in the amount of body fat
Increased central nervous system control over body functions
Rhythmic breathing movements occur
Lungs are developed but immature
Fetus stores iron, calcium, and phosphorus

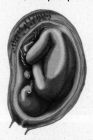

32 weeks

Weeks 33–38

Testes are in scrotum of male fetus
Lanugo begins to disappear
Increase in body fat
Fingernails reach the end of fingertips
Small breast buds are present on both sexes
Mother supplies fetus with antibodies against disease
Fetus is considered full term at 37 completed weeks
Fetus fills uterus

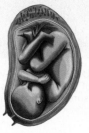

37 weeks

develops villous structures that penetrate the syncytiotrophoblast. The syncytium surrounds the cytotrophoblast columns, but the two tissues do not fuse. This side-by-side interstitial proximity of the lacunae and primary villi is the beginning of uteroplacental circulation. During the 3rd week of development, the villi at the embryonic pole further differentiate into two types of structures used to (1) anchor the chorionic plate to the maternal decidua and (2) exchange nutrients and other products with the mother (Fig. 11.9C).

Concurrent with development of the villi, cells from the hypoblast form the cavity at the pole opposite the embryoblast. (*Note: Embryologists use spherical geography to describe the location of structures within an embryo, e.g., pole, equator, or circumference.*) This cavity is the primitive yolk sac. Cells from the primitive yolk sac begin to form the extraembryonic mesoderm, a connective tissue that fills the space between the trophoblast and amnion. This mesoderm gives rise to the extraembryonic coelom (chorionic cavity) that surrounds the yolk sac and amniotic cavity.

About day 13, cells from the hypoblast form the secondary yolk sac, which nourishes the developing embryo until the placenta fully forms. The connecting stalk attaches the embryoblast within the amniotic cavity to the trophoblast; the amniotic membrane does not cross this stalk (Fig. 11.9C). The stalk develops blood vessels and surrounds the allantois by the 5th week of development. It fuses with the elongating secondary yolk sac (vitelline duct) and vitelline vessels to become the primitive umbilical cord by 10 weeks' gestation. By 12 weeks, the allantois, vitelline duct, and vitelline vessels regress, leaving the umbilical vessels (two arteries and one vein) encased within the Wharton jelly. The Wharton jelly serves as a protective surface barrier for the otherwise exposed umbilical vessels. At term, the

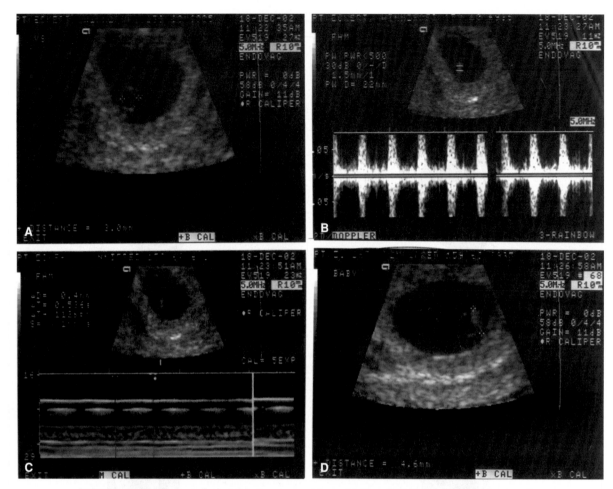

FIGURE 11.7 Five-week obstetrical sonographic evaluation. **A:** Yolk sac. **B:** Doppler recording of fetal heart tones. **C:** Measurement of fetal heart rate of 112 beats/min. **D:** Crown–rump measurement of fetal pole. (Courtesy of M. Munch, The Fertility Center, York, PA.)

umbilical cord is approximately 50 to 60 cm long and 2 cm in diameter.

By the 8th week of development, the small villous projections cover the entire surface of the gestational sac. Initially, these villi are attached loosely to the trophoblast and are easily aspirated during chorionic villus sampling (CVS) (discussed later in this chapter). Over the next 4 weeks, the villi over the embryonic pole continue to grow (forming the bushy chorion frondosum), while the villi at the abembryonic pole degenerate, creating the smooth chorion laeve. Similarly, the uterine decidua in proximity to the abembryonic pole thins and disintegrates as the gestational sac increases. The exposed chorion laeve expands with growth of the sac and fuses with the surfaces of the uterine cavity opposite the embryonic pole. This fusion creates a temporary closure of the uterine opening, which remains in place until gestation ends. Conversely, the decidual plate proliferates over the surface of the chorionic plate of the chorion frondosum. Within the gestational sac, the amnion also expands and obliterates the chorionic

cavity. With this loss of space between the amnion and chorion, the two membranes fuse to form the "amniotic sac," the amniochorionic membrane (bag) that surrounds the developing fetus.

The area between the chorionic and decidual plates contains the intervillous spaces (lakes) filled with maternal blood. It is into these intervillous lakes that the villi grow. By the 4th month, the chorion frondosum has developed 15 to 20 large villus trunks. The decidua basalis forms septa that grow between each villus trunk and surrounds the free villi branches. The septa do not descend to the chorionic plate, permitting the villus trees to remain connected to each other and the chorionic plate. Importantly, syncytial cells cover the outer layer of the septa, which together create the critical placental membrane barrier between the maternal blood in the intervillous spaces and the vessels of the embryonic villi. Growth of the septa segregates the villus trunks into compartmental structures known as *cotyledons*. These structures are visible on the maternal side of the placenta and appear as rugated liver. The fetal side of

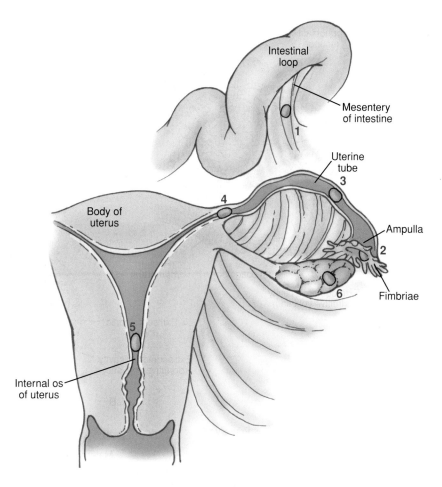

FIGURE 11.8 Diagrammatic representation of abnormal implantation sites: (*1*) abdominal cavity, most frequently in retro-uterine cavity; (*2*) ampulla region of fallopian tube; (*3*) within the fallopian tube itself; (*4*) within the narrow portion of the fallopian tube; (*5*) in the region of the internal uterine os; or (*6*) on the ovary. (Adapted from Sadler, T. W. [2011]. *Langman's medical embryology* [12th ed.]. Philadelphia, PA: Lippincott Williams & Wilkins.)

the placenta is smooth with evidence of large arteries and veins that converge toward the insertion site of the umbilical cord (Fig. 11.10). At the end of 38 weeks' gestation, the placenta covers approximately 15% to 30% of the internal uterine surface. It is approximately 15 to 20 cm in diameter, 3 cm deep, and weighs 500 to 600 g. This growth is the result of the continued proliferation of the existing villus trunks (Sadler, 2011).

Spiral arteries (80 to 100) traverse the decidual plate to enter the intervillous lakes and provide maternal blood to the cotyledons. Endometrial veins return the blood to the maternal circulation. The differences in the pressure gradients between the maternal and fetal circulations force maternal blood into and out of the intervillous lakes in cycle with maternal blood pressure changes. The spiral arteries have a pressure of 70 mm Hg, the intervillous spaces have a pressure of 10 mm Hg, and the closed vascular system of the fetus maintains a fairly constant pressure of 30 mm Hg (Tuchmann-Duplessis et al., 1975). Placental circulation of 150 mL of blood occurs three to four times per minute. Further differentiation of the tissues between the chorionic and decidual plates during the 4th and 5th months of development enhance this process, bringing the syncytial membrane of the intervillous lakes into close proximity with the endothelial lining of the fetal vessels. Given the approximate 4 to 14 m^2 of villi surface area, this rate of exchange is achieved easily. Monitoring the pregnancy for placental function is necessary, however, given that the placenta begins to undergo changes suggesting a diminishing exchange between maternal and fetal circulations. Possible changes in the villi and fetal capillaries may reduce their permeability. Occasionally, these changes result in the infarction of an intervillous lake or an entire cotyledon. If changes are substantial, they affect the exchange of metabolic and gaseous products, potentially harming the unborn fetus.

Function of the Placenta. The placenta serves two primary functions: exchange of metabolic and gaseous products between the fetal and maternal circulatory systems (Table 11.2) and production of hormones necessary for fetal development and continuation of the pregnancy. The exchange of metabolic and gaseous products across the placental membrane occurs by three mechanisms.

- *Simple diffusion:* the passive movement of molecules from a higher concentration to a lower concentration. Substances exchanged across the placenta by simple diffusion include oxygen, carbon dioxide, water, hormones, electrolytes, and many drugs.

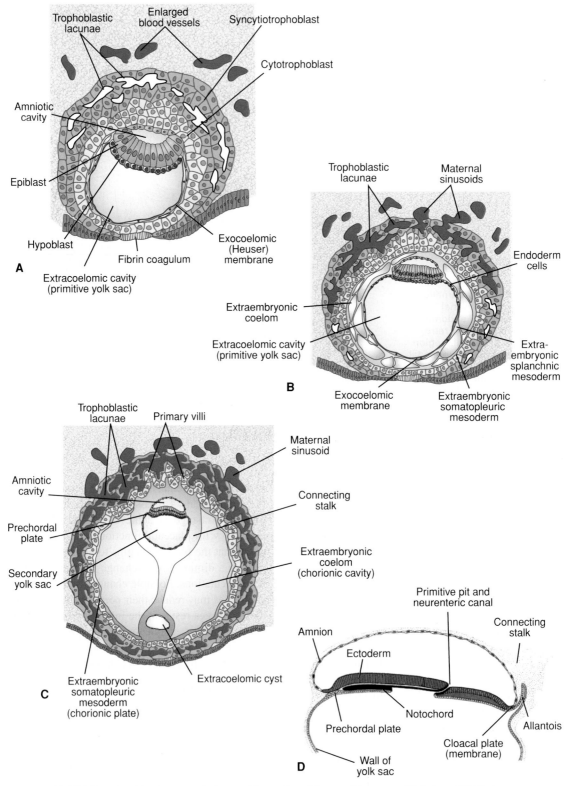

FIGURE 11.9 Membrane and placental formation. A human blastocyst **(A)** 9 days, **(B)** 12 days, **(C)** 13 days after fertilization, and **(D)** trilaminar germ disc forms during 3rd week after fertilization. (Adapted from Sadler, T. W. [2011]. *Langman's medical embryology* [12th ed.]. Philadelphia, PA: Lippincott Williams & Wilkins.)

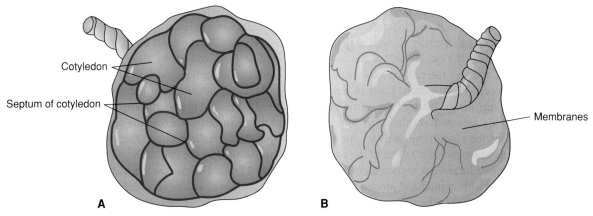

FIGURE 11.10 Placenta. **A:** Maternal side. **B:** Fetal side.

- *Facilitated or active transport:* the energy-consuming movement of molecules against an electrochemical gradient. Amino acids, free fatty acids, carbohydrates, and vitamins pass through the placenta by active transport.
- *Pinocytosis:* protrusion of the cell surface membrane to engulf a molecule. Albumin and maternal antibodies require pinocytosis for placental transport.

Transfer of maternal antibodies to the fetus confers acquired passive immunity on the newborn for several months after birth. The placenta produces the hormones progesterone, estriol, human chorionic gonadotropin (hCG), and human placental lactogen (hpL) (also sometimes referred to as chorionic somatomammotropin). Progesterone helps maintain the pregnancy. Estriol (estrogen) stimulates uterine growth and development of the maternal mammary glands. The hCG indicates the presence and health of a gestation. hpL, a polypeptide placental hormone, has an anti-insulin or "diabetogenic" action and plays a role in maternal lipolysis, thus providing the fetus with a source of energy for fetal nutrition (Cunningham et al., 2010).

Function of the Amniotic Fluid. Amniotic fluid fills the amniotic cavity and protects the developing fetus. This clear fluid increases from 30 mL at 10 weeks' gestation to approximately 900 mL by 37 weeks. It is produced primarily by substances from the maternal blood supply and cells of the amniotic cavity. The fetus begins to swallow amniotic fluid and void at approximately 5 months' gestation. Fetal urine, however, consists largely of water, given that the placenta, not the fetal kidneys, filters fetal waste products to the maternal circulation.

The amniotic fluid is replaced every 3 hours and serves several key functions (Cunningham et al., 2010).

- Prevents injury to the fetus by providing a shock-absorbing cushion.
- Provides for movement early and throughout gestation, which is critical to fetal growth and musculoskeletal development.

Without an adequate volume of amniotic fluid, fetal malformations develop.

Circulation

The cardiovascular system begins to develop midway through the 3rd week of gestation (Sadler, 2011). The heart, blood vessels, and blood cells form from the mesoderm layer of the trilaminar embryo. In response to embryologic changes in the endoderm, the splanchnic mesoderm produces angioblasts that form clusters of angiocysts on the lateral sides of the disk-shaped embryo. These clusters migrate toward the cephalic pole, where they merge and form a horseshoe-shaped structure of small blood vessels. The anterior central segment of this structure becomes the cardiogenic area and, later, part of the heart tube. A second set of angiogenic cells appears on each side of the cardiogenic area. These bilateral cell

● TABLE 11.2 **Substances that Traverse the Placental Membrane**

Substances	Substances
Leaving Maternal Circulation	Leaving Fetal Circulation
Oxygen	Carbon dioxide
Water	Water
Electrolytes	Urea
Carbohydrates	Waste products
Lipids	Hormones
Proteins	
Hormones	
Antibodies	
Viruses[a]	
Drugs[a]	

[a]Most viruses and many drugs (prescribed, over-the-counter, and recreational) cross the placenta from the maternal to fetal circulation and may adversely affect the fetus.

clusters form the two dorsal aortae. Closure of the neural tube, followed by rapid brain development, causes the germ disk to fold cephalocaudally as well as laterally. This dual folding brings the caudal ends of the two dorsal aortae together, and they merge. The very distal ends of each tube, however, remain open. Later in development, these openings merge through the aortic arches with the cardiogenic area to form the heart tube. This folding also causes the cardiogenic area to move caudally from the cervical to thoracic region of the embryo. Simultaneously, the endocardium, myocardium, and epicardium of the heart form within and around the primitive heart tube. In response to the embryo's diminishing ability to receive all necessary nutrients by simple diffu-

sion, the developing heart begins to receive blood from the embryonic veins.

By day 28, the heart tube elongates and creates the cardiac loop, caused by the caudal and ventral movement of the cephalic portion of the tube and the dorsal and cranial movement of the caudal portion. Thus, the atrial portion of the heart forms from the caudal section of the heart tube, whereas the ventricular portion forms from the cephalic portion. The major septa of the heart have formed by the end of the 5th week of development (Fig. 11.11). Differentiation of the four-chamber heart and associated valves is complete by the 8th week.

Pharyngeal arches appear in the primitive gastrointestinal tract of the endoderm layer during the 4th

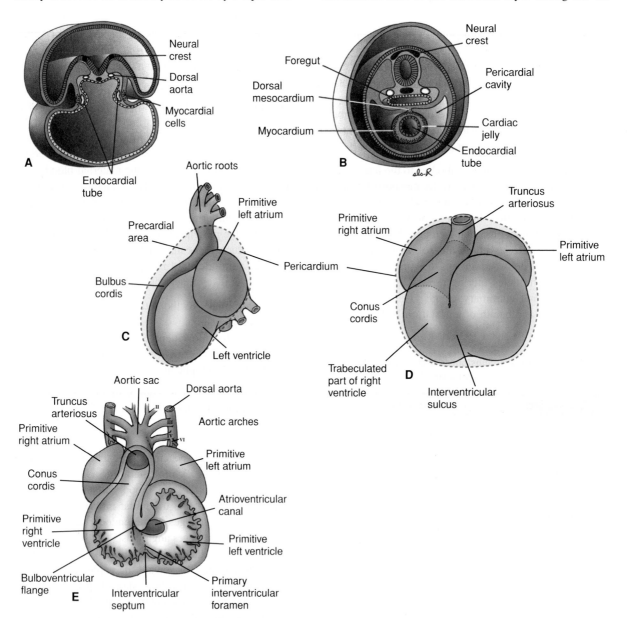

FIGURE 11.11 Embryonic development of the heart. **A, B:** 21 to 27 days. **C:** Left-side view at 28 days. **D:** Frontal view at 28 days. **E:** Frontal view at 30 days. (Adapted from Sadler, T. W. [2006]. *Langman's medical embryology* [10th ed.]. Philadelphia, PA: Lippincott Williams & Wilkins.)

and 5th weeks of development. A cranial nerve and an artery innervate each arch. These six arteries are known as the aortic arches and arise from the distal portion of the truncus arteriosus. The first, second, and fifth aortic arches disappear by the 29th day of development. The third, fourth, and sixth continue to grow and form the common carotid artery, medial portion of the internal carotid artery, part of the aortic arch, left subclavian arteries, proximal segment of the right subclavian artery, proximal portion of the right pulmonary artery, and ductus arteriosus. During this time, the vitelline and umbilical arteries form. The vitelline arteries initially supply the yolk sac; in the infant, they fuse to form the celiac, superior mesenteric, and inferior mesenteric arteries that nourish the gastrointestinal tract. The umbilical arteries form as paired branches of the dorsal aorta, travel alongside the allantois, and fuse with the connecting stalk to become the umbilical cord. The proximal portions of these arteries form the internal iliac and superior vesical arteries, whereas the distal segments form the medial umbilical ligaments after birth.

Concurrent with the development of the fetal arterial system, the venous system is established with the appearance of the vitelline, umbilical, and cardinal veins by the end of the 5th week of development. In later embryonic development, the vitelline veins give rise to the portal system (hepatocardiac portion of the inferior vena cava, portal vein, and superior mesenteric vein). The main drainage system of the early embryo consists of the cardinal veins. Later, these veins will form the caval system. Only one of the umbilical veins is sustained beyond the early embryonic period. As placental circulation increases, the left umbilical vein enlarges to form a primary communication with the ductus venosus and secondary branches with the hepatic sinusoids. At birth, the umbilical vein and ductus venosus lose their lumens and, respectively, become the ligamentum teres and ligamentum venosum.

The placenta is the main source of fetal nourishment and oxygen–carbon dioxide balance. The fetal respiratory and gastrointestinal systems do not have primary responsibility for these functions until after birth. The umbilical vein captures the maternal oxygen (80% saturation) crossing the placenta and transports it to the ductus venosus, where it continues through the inferior vena cava to the right and left atria. From there, the increasingly desaturated blood empties into the descending aorta and travels back to the placenta through the two umbilical arteries (58% saturation upon return to the placental membrane) (Sadler, 2011; Tuchmann-Duplessis et al., 1975).

With cessation of placental blood at birth and pressure changes in the heart and lungs that accompany postnatal circulation and spontaneous respiration, four major changes occur in the infant vascular system (Sadler, 2011). The closure of the umbilical vein, umbilical arteries, and ductus venosus are the result of the constriction caused by the umbilical cord clamp. The increased pressure in the right atrium closes the oval foramen (foramen ovale) between the left and right atria. Spontaneous respiration results in the release of bradykinin, which signals the smooth muscle surrounding the ductus arteriosus to contract and force closure of this structure (Sadler, 2011). Figure 11.12 compares human circulation before and after birth. Chapter 20 discusses fetal-to-newborn transitions in more detail.

Embryonic Development

As mentioned earlier, the embryonic phase lasts from the 3rd to 8th week of development (Table 11.1). The 3rd week is critical to further development because it is when *gastrulation* occurs. Gastrulation is the process by which the primitive streak begins to form on the surface of the epiblast and in turn initiates formation of the trilaminar germ disk composed of ectoderm, mesoderm, and endoderm. By day 15 or 16, the primitive streak that begins at the caudal pole of the germ disk migrates toward the prechordal plate at the cephalic pole. The primitive node is a raised area encompassing the cephalic end of the pit that forms within the primitive streak. Through the process of invagination, epiblast cells selectively journey to the primitive streak, separate from the epiblast, and then migrate beneath it to lie between the epiblast and hypoblast layers. These cells differentiate into the endoderm and mesoderm. The remaining epiblast becomes the ectoderm. This migration continues until the cells move beyond the boundaries of the germ disk to join with the yolk sac and amnion; they travel bilaterally around the prechordal plate to meet, fuse, and form the cardiogenic plate (Sadler, 2011).

Through the same process of invagination, prenotochordal cells punctuate the hypoblast to create two layers along the midline of the embryo from the primitive pit to the prechordal plate. The notochord forms when cells of the notochordal plate propagate and detach in response to the developing endoderm around the primitive streak. The notochord develops cranially to caudally as the primitive streak moves toward the caudal pole. It lies beneath the neural tube and becomes the source of the axial skeleton. Throughout these two processes of invagination, the germ disk changes shape from nearly round to an elongated teardrop, with the cephalic end broader than the caudal pole. This change results from the significant migration of cells to the cephalic region, which continues through the 4th week. The primitive streak begins to disappear at the cephalic pole by the end of the 4th week, while it remains functional at the caudal pole through the 5th week before disappearing entirely. This process of cephalic (first) to caudal (last)

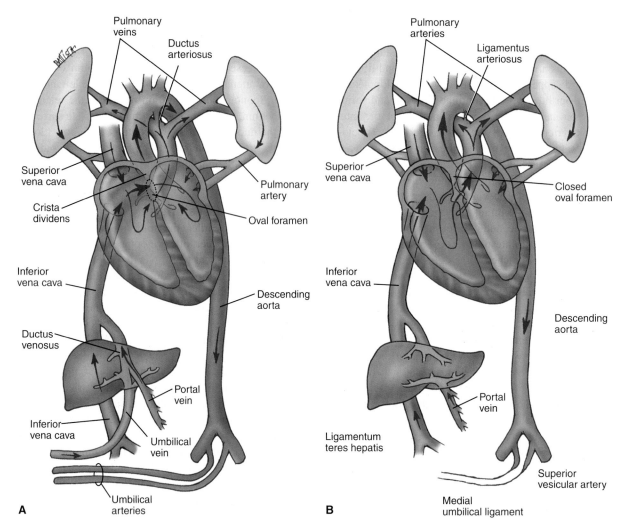

FIGURE 11.12 Human circulation **(A)** before birth and **(B)** after birth. (Adapted from Sadler, T. W. [2006]. *Langman's medical embryology* [10th ed.]. Philadelphia, PA: Lippincott Williams & Wilkins.)

development is constant throughout the embryonic phase (Fig. 11.13) (Sadler, 2011).

Organogenesis

Organogenesis begins on day 19 with the formation of the neural plate, the foundation of the central nervous system (Table 11.3). The neural plate develops from the thickening of the ectoderm lying atop the notochord. It grows toward the primitive streak while the bilateral edges become more prominent and form the neural folds. These folds proliferate until they join and fuse medially in the midsection to form the beginning of the neural tube. The neural folds of the cephalic pole close by day 25 and grow rapidly to form the vesicles of the brain. The caudal neural folds seal to form the spinal cord by day 27. Over the next 5 weeks, the ectoderm gives rise to the peripheral nervous system; sensory epithelium of the nose, eye, and ear; epidermis; subcutaneous, mammary, and pituitary glands; and tooth enamel.

The mesoderm further differentiates into three layers: paraxial, intermediate, and lateral (parietal and visceral). The paraxial mesoderm gives rise to somites, which develop cephalocaudally from days 20 to 35, creating a maximum 42 to 44 pairs. Six to eight of these pairs are lost, leaving 3 occipital, 7 cervical, 12 thoracic, 5 lumbar, 5 sacral, and 3 to 5 coccygeal pairs. Each somite produces sclerotome (cartilage and bone surrounding the notochord and spinal cord), myotome (striated and smooth muscle), and dermatome (skin) cells. The nephrogenic cord is formed by intermediate mesoderm and gives rise to the excretory components of the urinary and reproductive systems. Parietal mesoderm and ectoderm adhere to form the lateral and ventral body wall. The serous membranes of the peritoneal, parietal, and pericardial cavities and the spleen, blood vessels, and blood are all derivatives of visceral mesoderm (Sadler, 2011).

The rapid growth of the central nervous system and somites precipitates cephalocaudal and lateral folding

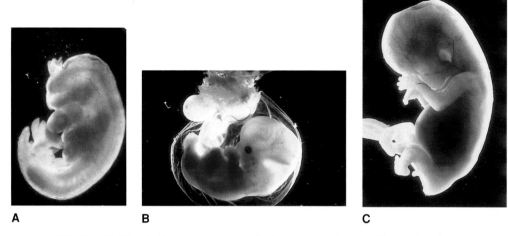

FIGURE 11.13 A: Four-week embryo. **B:** Five-week embryo. **C:** Six-week embryo.

of the embryo, respectively. This positional change profoundly affects development of the gastrointestinal tract, the primary organ system formed by endoderm. As the embryo becomes crescent shaped, the layer of endoderm forms a continuous tube from the cephalic to caudal ends of the embryo and passively changes its orientation in response to cephalocaudal bending. As a result, the yolk sac is pulled inside the body of the embryo and is constricted to form the vitelline duct. The endoderm also generates the parenchyma of the thyroid, parathyroid glands, liver, and pancreas; the epithelial lining of the respiratory tract, urinary bladder, urethra, tympanic cavity, and auditory tube; the tonsils; and the thymus gland (Sadler, 2011).

Appearance

The appearance of the embryo changes significantly from the 3rd to the 8th week. Initially, the embryo looks like a flattened spherical disk. By the end of this phase, eyes, ears, fingers, and toes are readily identifiable. Embryo size during this period is determined by measuring the distance from the vertex of the cranium to the midpoint between the apices of the buttocks (crown–rump length) (Table 11.4) (Sadler, 2011).

Recall April, described at the beginning of the chapter. Her pregnancy is of 13 weeks' gestation. Suppose April asks, "How much does my baby weigh now?" How would the nurse respond?

Teratology

The embryonic phase consists of 6 weeks of rapid growth and development. Alterations may develop from the genotype determined at conception, a spontaneous change in maturation, or an adverse gestational environment. These changes are referred to as *congenital malformations, congenital anomalies,* or *birth defects.* Once the oocyte has been fertilized, the alterations related to the genotype or to maturation are unchangeable. Alterations related to an adverse gestational environment are preventable. Nurses should remember, however, that most women are not aware they are pregnant until they are of 6 to 8 weeks' obstetrical age, which correlates with the 4th to 6th week of embryonic development. This period is significant in its level of organogenesis (Table 11.3). Thus, the effects of an adverse gestational environment may already be present before confirmation of pregnancy and initiation of prenatal care.

Teratology is the field of study that investigates and evaluates the causes of structural or functional damage to the developing embryo or fetus. The outcome for the embryo or fetus exposed to a **teratogen** may include any of the following (Lashley, 2007; Wilson, 2007):

- No apparent effect
- Congenital anomalies
- Prenatal or perinatal death
- Altered fetal growth
- Postnatal functional or behavioural deficits or aberrations
- Carcinogenesis

The principles of teratology describe the factors considered when evaluating the probable cause for any alteration in normal embryonic and fetal development. Fundamental to these principles is the gestational age when intrauterine exposure occurs, dose and length of contact with the suspected teratogen, and genotype of the fetus (Lashley, 2007; Sadler, 2011). Table 11.5 presents agents associated with human malformations.

Congenital anomalies are the second leading cause of death in Canada for children aged 1 to 4 (Public Health Agency of Canada, 2013). Approximately 1 in 25 infants

(text continues on page 374)

● TABLE 11.3 **Timing of Organogenesis by Embryonic Layer**

Layer	Tissue Formed	Embryonic Week Development Begins	Associated Developmental Defects
Ectoderm	Central nervous system	3	Encephalocele Exencephaly Holoprosencephaly Hydrocephalus Neural tube defects
	Eye	4	Coloboma iridis Congenital cataracts Cyclopia Microphthalmia
	Peripheral nervous system	4	Meningomyelocele Myeloschisis
	Tooth enamel	6	Natal teeth
	Mammary and sweat glands	7	Polymastia Polythelia
	Ear (external)	8	Preauricular appendages Preauricular pits
	Pituitary	8	Pharyngeal hypophysis
	Skin and nails	8	Ichthyosis Nail hypoplasia
	Hair	12	Hypertrichosis
Mesoderm			
Parietal (somatic)	Parietal layer of serous membranes of peritoneal, pleural, and pericardial cavities	3–4	Cleft sternum Diaphragmatic hernia Gastroschisis
Visceral (splanchnic)	Cardiac muscle (myocardium)	3	Atrial and ventricular septal defects Tetralogy of Fallot Transposition of the great vessels
	Visceral layer of serous membranes covering abdominal organs, lungs, and heart	3–4	
	Smooth muscle of arteries, veins, lymph vessels, and blood and lymph cells	4–5	Coarctation of the aorta Cystic hygroma Patent ductus arteriosus
	Stromal and muscular wall of gastrointestinal tract	4–5	Congenital hiatal hernia Duodenal atresia Esophageal stenosis Extrahepatic biliary atresia Imperforate anus Omphalocele Pyloric stenosis Rectoanal atresia
Paraxial → somitomeres and somites	Cartilage, bone	4	Achondroplasia Amelia Cleft palate Clubfoot Cranioschisis → anencephaly Craniosynostosis Mandibulofacial dysostosis Osteogenesis imperfecta Polydactyly
	Subcutaneous tissue	4	No pectoralis major muscle
	Skeletal muscle	4–5	Prune belly syndrome

(continued)

● TABLE 11.3   **Timing of Organogenesis by Embryonic Layer** (continued)

Layer	Tissue Formed	Embryonic Week Development Begins	Associated Developmental Defects
Intermediate	Kidneys, ducts, cortex of adrenal glands	4	Congenital adrenal hyperplasia Horseshoe kidney Pelvic kidney Polycystic kidney disease Renal agenesis → oligohydramnios
	Gonads, ducts, uterus	6–7	Cryptorchism Gonadal dysgenesis Hydrocele Hypospadias Inguinal hernia Testicular feminization Uterine bicornis Uterine didelphys
Endoderm	Respiratory tract epithelium	4	Esophageal atresia → polyhydramnios Tracheoesophageal fistula
	Gastrointestinal tract epithelium, including stomach, liver, gallbladder, and pancreas	4–5	Hirschsprung's disease Meckel's diverticulum Meconium ileus
	Urinary bladder epithelium	6	Exstrophy of the bladder
	Parenchyma of thyroid, parathyroids, liver, and pancreas	6–7	Hepatic tumor Thyroglossal cyst
	Tympanic cavity and eustachian tube	6–7	Deafness

Data from Sadler, T. W. (2011). *Langman's medical embryology* (12th ed.). Philadelphia, PA: Lippincott Williams & Wilkins; Sanders, R. C. (2002). *Structural fetal abnormalities: The total picture.* St. Louis, MO: Mosby.

● TABLE 11.4   **Embryo and Fetal Size by Gestational Age**

Gestational Age (wks)	CRL Length	Weight (gm)	Biparietal Diameter[a] (cm)	Femur Length[a] (cm)
4	0.2 mm			
5	2–3 mm			
6	4–6 mm			
7	5–8 mm			
8	10–14 mm			
9	17–22 mm			
10	28–30 mm			
11–14	5–8 cm	10–45	2.5–3	1–1.7
15–18	9–14 cm	60–200	3.1–4.5	1.8–2.7
19–22	15–19 cm	250–450	4.6–5.5	2.8–3.8
23–26	20–23 cm	500–820	5.6–6.6	3.9–4.8
27–30	24–27 cm	900–1,300	6.7–7.4	4.9–5.7
31–33	28–30 cm	1,400–2,100	7.5–8.4	5.8–6.6
35–38	31–34 cm	2,200–2,900	8.5–9.2	6.7–7.4
39–40	35–36 cm	3,000–3,400	9.2–9.7	7.5–7.9

[a]BPD and femur are typically not measured until 12 weeks' gestation.

Data from Sadler, T. W. (2011). *Langman's medical embryology* (12th ed.). Philadelphia, PA: Lippincott Williams & Wilkins; Sadler (2007). *Ultrasonography in obstetrics and gynecology* (5th ed.). Philadelphia, PA: W. B. Saunders.

● TABLE 11.5 **Selected Agents Associated with Human Malformations**

Category	Agent	Congenital Malformation
Chemical	ACE inhibitors	Growth restriction, pulmonary hypoplasia, renal failure, fetal death
	Alcohol	Fetal alcohol spectrum disorder characterized by short palpebral fissures, maxillary hypoplasia, heart defects, intellectual challenges
	Amphetamines	Cleft lip, cleft palate, heart defects
	Aminopterin	Anencephaly, hydrocephaly, cleft lip, cleft palate
	Cocaine	Growth restriction, microcephaly, behavioral abnormalities, gastroschisis
	Diphenylhydantoin	Fetal hydantoin syndrome characterized by facial defects, intellectual challenges
	Formaldehyde	Growth restriction
	Iodine	Hypothyroidism, goiter
	Isotretinoin	Vitamin A embryopathy characterized by small, abnormally shaped ears, mandibular hypoplasia, cleft palate, heart defects
	Lead	Growth restriction, neurologic disorders
	Lithium	Heart malformations
	LSD	Limb defects, central nervous system defects
	Methotrexate	Limb defects, central nervous system defects
	Organic mercury	Multiple neurologic symptoms similar to cerebral palsy
	PCB	Growth restriction, gum hyperplasia, skull anomalies, developmental delays
	Quinine	Deafness, limb anomalies, visceral defects, visual problems
	Streptomycin	Eighth cranial nerve damage (ear)
	Tetracycline	Discoloration and hypoplasia of tooth enamel
	Thalidomide	Limb defects, heart malformations
	Trimethadione	Cleft palate, heart defects, urogenital and skeletal abnormalities
	Valproic acid	Neural tube defects, heart, craniofacial, and limb anomalies
	Warfarin	Chondrodysplasia, microcephaly
Hormonal	Androgens	Masculinization of female genitalia
	Diethylstilbestrol (DES)	Malformations of the uterus, fallopian tubes, upper vagina, uterine cancer, malformed testes
	Maternal diabetes	Heart and neural tube defects
Infectious	Cytomegalovirus	Microcephaly, blindness, intellectual challenges
	Hepatitis virus	Biliary atresia, hepatic damage
	Herpes simplex virus	Microphthalmia, microcephaly, retinal dysplasia
	HIV	Microcephaly, growth restriction, HIV/AIDS
	Parvovirus B19	Growth restriction
	Rubella virus	Cataracts, glaucoma, heart defects, deafness
	Syphilis	Intellectual challenges, deafness
	Toxoplasmosis	Hydrocephalus, cerebral calcifications, microphthalmia
	Varicella virus	Limb hypoplasia, intellectual challenges, muscle atrophy
Physical	Radiation (x-ray)	Microcephaly, spina bifida, cleft palate, limb defects
	Smelter emissions	Growth restriction, Wilms tumor, multiple system anomalies
	Hyperthermia	Anencephaly

Note: This is a selected list of teratogenic agents. Absence of an agent from this list does not imply safe use during pregnancy. Not all fetuses will develop the congenital malformations described above.

ACE, angiotensin-converting enzyme; LSD, lysergic acid diethylamide; PCB, polychlorinated biphenyls.

Data from Lashley, F. R. (2007). *Essentials of clinical genetics in nursing practice.* New York: Springer; Sadler, T. W. (2011). *Langman's medical embryology* (12th ed.). Philadelphia: Lippincott Williams & Wilkins.

are diagnosed yearly with one or more congenital anomalies (Public Health Agency of Canada, 2013). Minor congenital anomalies may be benign or associated with other birth defects that together significantly affect the newborn's health or well-being. The probability of an associated major defect increases with the number of minor anomalies. There is a 3% chance of a major defect with one minor anomaly, a 10% chance with two minor anomalies, and a 20% chance with three or more (Sadler, 2011).

Anomalies are classified as malformations, disruptions, or deformations and may occur as part of a syndrome, association, or sequence event.

- A **malformation** is the complete or partial absence of a fetal structure.
- A **disruption** is a change in the morphology of a structure after its formation (e.g., bowel atresia, amniotic bands).

- A **deformation** is the result of a mechanical event that abnormally moulds an otherwise healthy tissue; it is often reversible after birth (e.g., clubfeet).
- A **syndrome** is a clustering of multiple anomalies known to be primary outcomes of a single event.
- A **sequence** is a number of secondary alterations that develop from a major defect.
- An **association** is the presentation of a cluster of anomalies known not to be associated with either a syndrome or sequence event (Sadler, 2011).

Multiple Gestations

The number of multiple gestations has risen sharply over the past two decades. The incidence of multiple births in Canada (excluding Ontario) rose from 2.2 per 100 births in 1995 to 3 per 100 births in 2004 (Public Health Agency of Canada, 2008). The most common form of multiple gestation is twins (Centers for Disease Control and Prevention, 2014). The two types of twins are monozygotic and dizygotic. Traditionally, **monozygotic twins** are called "identical," and **dizygotic twins** are called "fraternal." Triplets and all other high-order multiple gestations may be monozygotic, dizygotic, or both.

Monozygotic twins share the same genotype, although exposure to different environmental factors throughout their individual lives may result in the expression of different **phenotypes**. The natural incidence of monozygotic twins is 3 to 4 per 1,000 births (Sadler, 2011). These gestations result from an alteration in zygote development. Early in this process, the single cell mass becomes two or more independent structures, each capable of developing into a normal fetus (Fig. 11.14). The timing of the separation determines whether monozygotic babies share the same chorion, placenta, amnion, or all these. If the early embryo divides into two separate and distinct structures before the trophoblast has formed, they will not share the same chorion, placenta, or amnion. These monozygotic twins are noted to be dichorionic–diamniotic and may be identified initially as dizygotic. Their relationship requires genetic studies to determine that they are monozygotic infants. The most common incidence of monozygotic twins occurs 5 to 7 days after fertilization and results from the splitting of the inner cell mass of the blastocyst before formation of the amnion. These monozygotic twins have one placenta and one chorion, but two amnions (monochorionic–diamniotic). A rare

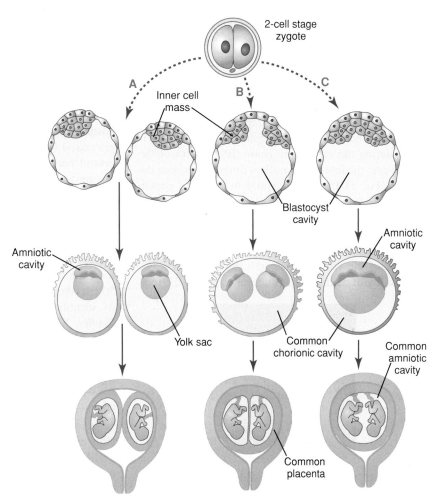

FIGURE 11.14 Diagrammatic representation of three types of monozygotic twins. **A:** Separation occurs at the two-cell stage; twins are dichorionic–diamniotic. **B:** Complete separation of the inner cell mass; twins are monochorionic–diamniotic. **C:** Late separation of the inner cell mass; twins are monochorionic–monoamniotic. (Adapted from Sadler, T. W. [2006]. *Langman's medical embryology* [10th ed.]. Philadelphia: Lippincott Williams & Wilkins.)

form of monozygotic twinning is division of the bilaminar germ disk just before the primitive streak develops approximately 8 to 10 days after fertilization. This type creates a monochorionic–monoamniotic gestation. Conjoined (Siamese) twins are the result of the incomplete separation of the bilaminar germ disk. These twins may be joined at the chest–abdomen (thoracopagus), spine (pygopagus), or cranium (craniopagus). Some conjoined twins have been successfully separated (Sadler, 2011).

Dizygotic twins represent more than two thirds of twin births and are reported to have a natural incidence of 7 to 11 per 1,000 births (Sadler, 2011). Their occurrence is known to be influenced by the mother's age, parity, nutrition, family history, and use of fertility treatments and assisted conception. Incidence increases with advancing maternal age and parity, good nutrition, and the presence of twins in the maternal family history. Dizygotic or multizygotic gestations result when separate sperm independently fertilize two or more oocytes within a single menstrual cycle. The placenta and chorion of each gestation may fuse together if the implantation sites for each embryo are in close proximity. This may result in the identification of a dizygotic twin gestation as monozygotic. Dizygotic and multizygotic siblings share the same genetic relationship as any siblings born to the same genetic mother and father, whether birth occurs on the same day or years apart.

Fetal Development

The 9th to 38th weeks of development are called the fetal phase and are characterized by the exponential growth and maturation of the organs and systems developed during the embryonic phase. By the end of the 12th week, the fetus is 2.5 million times bigger than the zygote (Fig. 11.15). The exception to this rapid growth is the fetal head, which at 12 weeks makes up 50% of the crown-rump length and by 20 weeks represents only 35% of the total crown-heel length. This ratio further decreases over the next 20 weeks; at birth, the head is 25% of the crown-heel length (Sadler, 2011). The probability of malformations decreases during the fetal

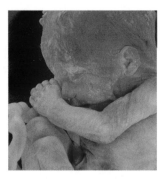

FIGURE 11.15 A fetus at approximately 14 weeks' gestation.

phase, although the central nervous system remains sensitive to teratogens. The risk of malformations may also continue if the uterus, volume of amniotic fluid, and fetus do not develop in synchrony.

 Think back to April, the 36 year old who is pregnant for the second time. In which period of gestational development is her pregnancy, according to the embryologic standard?

At the end of the 12th week, the eyes are in their medial location, the ears are rotated upward and outward, the limbs are proportional to the fetal trunk, the external sex is differentiated, and primary ossification centers are evident in the skull and long bones. Fetal movement is visible on ultrasound, but the mother typically is not aware of this activity.

At the end of the 20th week, the fetus has grown to 50% of its expected crown-heel length at birth; however, fetal weight increases minimally from weeks 9 to 20 (Table 11.4). Fine hair called *lanugo* covers the fetus; scalp hair and eyebrows are evident by the end of the 5th month. The mother begins to experience fetal movement between the 16th and 20th weeks.

Between 29 and 36 weeks, the fetus gains 50% of its birth weight. Deposits of subcutaneous tissue are laid down during this period in preparation for newborn metabolic functions and fluctuations in temperature in the postnatal environment. Chances of extrauterine survival prior to 34 weeks are much lower than after, because the central nervous and respiratory systems undergo vast maturation during these last months of gestation. Critical physiologic processes associated with these systems must be completed during the last 2 months to enhance the neonate's survival (see Chapter 22).

By 38 weeks, the normally developed fetus has the anatomic structures and physiologic maturity necessary for extrauterine life. The crown-heel length is about 50 cm. Weight is 3,000 to 3,400 g, and gender is readily identifiable by the well-defined external genitalia (Sadler, 2011).

PRECONCEPTION HEALTH ASSESSMENT AND SCREENING

Health assessment, screening, and counselling are vital behaviours for clients (see Chapter 2). Throughout the 20th century, scientific evidence mounted supporting health promotion and risk assessment to enhance the odds of the conception, gestation, and birth of a healthy child. The advent of modern medical genetics in the

1950s and the initiation of the Human Genome Project in 1990 further supported the important role of health promotion and risk screening for positive reproductive outcomes.

Despite many years of public education by the Public Health Agency of Canada, and other groups about the importance of preconception health, preparation for and timing of most conceptions remain unplanned (Moos, 2004). Lack of reproductive planning can postpone health promotion behaviours until after the first prenatal appointment, ideally within the first 12 weeks of the last menstrual period. The significance of this delay becomes clear when one remembers that the embryonic development of most organs and body systems is nearly complete by 9 to 10 weeks' gestation. The scope of preconception health assessment, screening, and counselling continues to advance with knowledge identified through the ongoing Human Genome Project. Health care is moving broadly from an orientation of disease management to one of risk identification and prevention to promote lifelong health and wellness (Collins et al., 2003). This paradigm shift is especially important for clients who wish to optimize not only their own health, but also the long-term well-being of their children.

Many clients who seek preconception health assessment are aware of a positive history for a risk factor. Examples include prior spontaneous loss of one or more pregnancies, inability to conceive, prior fetal anomaly, or a known genetic disorder within the reproductive family. Among women who seek preconception counselling because they will be 35 years or older when they give birth, many are identified to have risk factors that are not age-related. These risk factors would not have been addressed had they not sought counselling because of their age. Such risk factors are not exclusive to clients of advanced maternal age and may encompass chronic conditions (e.g., hypertension, diabetes, cardiovascular disease, renal disease) and adult genetic disorders (e.g., cystic fibrosis, sickle cell anemia) (see Chapter 4).

To eliminate gaps in service, many programs and agencies attempt to increase public awareness of preconception health assessment. Examples include Health Canada's Folic Acid Campaign; initiatives of provincial governments through Public Health Departments; the March of Dimes through national, regional, and local educational programs; and the media through public service campaigns. In order to assess the efficacy of such efforts, a formal network for congenital anomalies surveillance was created in 2002 by Health Canada, which includes participants from the provinces and territories. The 2013 Canadian Congenital Anomalies Surveillance Network report provides a concise overview of six important categories of congenital anomalies, preventive measures, and recommendations for early diagnosis and management (Public Health Agency of Canada, 2013).

All nurses need to be knowledgeable about the "basics of genetics and genomics and their applications to clinical care so that they can provide quality healthcare that is appropriate to their setting, population, geographical location, access, and coverage" (Lea et al., 2011, p. 5). Nurses can provide information about or support during preconception screening and counselling. One opportunity to disseminate such information is during annual gynecologic examinations; however, many women of childbearing age fail to seek this service. Examples of other settings in which nurses may share preconceptual health information are Planned Parenthood, pediatric offices, employee health services, school health services, and any health care encounter that includes a discussion of implications for reproduction (i.e., diagnosis of a chronic disease).

Genetic Services

People who seek genetic services may be concerned about their own risk for a genetic disorder, a genetic disorder in their child, the risk for transmission of a genetic disorder to their child, or the effects of adverse environmental exposure on their health or that of their child. Most clients do not express concern for possible genetic risk until they approach conception and birth. Other people seek genetic services only when they or their child are suspected to have a genetic disorder, and further evaluation is recommended (Lashley, 2007).

Providing Genetic Counselling

Genetic counselling is the framework that guides the performance of genetic screening, diagnosis, evaluation, and intervention (Fig. 11.16). It is a process of information gathering, clinical and laboratory evaluation, and information sharing about the occurrence of or risk for a genetic disorder within a family. The goal is to provide appropriate and accurate information in a nondirective manner so that the client can make an informed decision about personal or family health and health care (Gaff & Bylund, 2010).

Nurses routinely provide counselling to clients about genetic concerns. Health professionals, including genetics nurses, genetic counsellors, medical geneticists, clinical geneticists, and other health professionals with advanced training in human genetics provide genetic counselling, evaluation, diagnosis, therapy, and services to individuals, families, and communities (International Society of Nurses in Genetics, 2010b). Collaboration between the nurse, the genetics specialist, and other members of the health care team is integral to the provision of preconception and prenatal health assessment and care. The nurse should integrate knowledge of genetics and associated health care implications to engage in the dialogue inherent within this collaborative relationship (International Society of

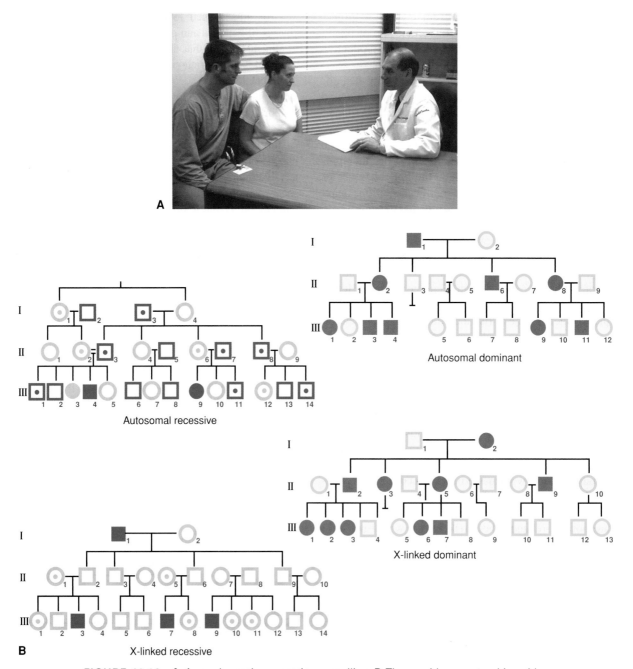

FIGURE 11.16 **A:** A couple receives genetic counselling. **B:** The provider uses teaching aids to assist the couple to understand genetic principles. (Courtesy of Main Line Perinatology, Wynnewood, Pennsylvania.)

Nurses in Genetics, 2011). Importantly, the nurse needs to assimilate and synthesize this knowledge to provide comprehensive and appropriate care to each client (International Society of Nurses in Genetics, 2011).

Understanding Basic Genetic Principles

To provide appropriate client care and give accurate information, nurses need to be aware of genetic evaluation, research, and treatment developments. Nurses work in partnership with other health care providers and

clients to ensure the rights of all: to participate in the process of informed decision making, ensure confidentiality and privacy are maintained, and ensure equitable access to services (International Society of Nurses in Genetics, 2010a).

Mendelian Patterns of Inheritance. Mendelian patterns of inheritance are based on the fundamental biologic principle that each human gene has two copies: one on the maternal chromosome and one on the paternal chromosome. Genes are categorized based on their location on a specific chromosome (loci). They are described as autosomal (chromosomes 1 to 22) or **sex linked** (X or Y chromosome). As a result of human genetic evolution, many genes have one or more alternative forms, known as **alleles**. If both the maternal and paternal alleles for a specific locus are the same, then the person is said to be *homozygous* for that gene. Conversely, if the maternal and paternal alleles for a specific locus are different, then the person is said to be *heterozygous*. Because more than 30,000 genes are in the human genome, all humans are heterogenic as a result of genetic evolution. In addition, some genetic traits require only one copy of an allele to be expressed (**dominant** trait), whereas others require two copies of the same allele to be expressed (**recessive** trait). If a trait is caused by an autosomal dominant, autosomal recessive, X-linked dominant, or X-linked recessive gene, a specific pattern of inheritance is found within families, which is identified easily with the construction of a genogram. See Table 11.6 for more information.

People with one dominant allele and one recessive allele for a given loci that requires two recessive alleles for expression are considered "carriers" of the recessive allele. Because they are not homozygous for the recessive allele, they do not express the associated phenotype; however, they can pass the recessive allele to any children. If the child subsequently receives two copies of the recessive allele (one from each parent), he or she will be homozygous for the recessive trait and will express its effects. For example, let's say a father has brown eyes and a mother has blue eyes. The expression of brown eyes requires only one copy of the dominant allele (brown) for eye colour. The expression of blue eyes requires two copies of the recessive form (blue). If the brown-eyed parent is homozygous, then all children of this couple will have brown eyes because the father can transmit only the dominant allele. If, however, he is heterozygous with one dominant allele (brown) and one recessive allele (blue), then each child has a 50% chance to be a brown-eyed heterozygote like the father and a 50% chance to be a homozygous blue-eyed child like the mother.

An inheritable permanent change in the DNA of a gene is known as a *mutation*. Some mutations have a benign or no effect; others result in an adverse alteration. Typically, such changes affect growth, development, and wellness. As with all other human traits, disorders caused by a single copy of an altered gene follow dominant patterns of inheritance, whereas disorders that require two copies of the altered gene follow recessive patterns of inheritance. Approximately 20,000 autosomal disorders, 1,200 X-linked, 59 Y-linked, and 65 mitochondrial disorders, have been identified (Online Mendelian Inheritance in Man, 2014).

Some dominant disorders (e.g., Huntington disease) do not appear until adulthood and are referred to as *adult-onset disorders*. In some cases, an altered dominant gene confers a 100% chance of expression, but clinical features have not yet developed; this is considered a *presymptomatic disorder.*

Several recessive disorders have increased frequencies among specific ethnic groups, for instance, Tay–Sachs disease in individuals of Ashkenazi descent (see Chapter 4). This may be the result of generations of people consistently establishing reproductive relationships within and among the same ethnic group, causing repeated transmission of carrier status from parent to child.

Penetrance and Expression. Some variations that occur between genotype and phenotype are explained through the principles of *penetrance* (the percentage of people with a certain mutant gene who actually show the associated characteristics, at least to some extent) and *expressivity* (the degree to which the characteristics of a disease are manifest among individuals with the same disease-causing genotype). These differences in expression account for the difficulty in the past in classifying some congenital disorders according to Mendelian principles. Such conditions did not appear to follow any of the four standard patterns of inheritance, although they consistently recurred within extended families (Lashley, 2007; Nussbaum et al., 2007). The relationship between

● TABLE 11.6   **Characteristics of Single-Gene Disorders**

Characteristic	Autosomal Recessive	Autosomal Dominant	Sex-Linked Recessive	Sex-Linked Dominant
Gender bias	None	None	Males only	Higher percentage in females
Transmission	Horizontal	Vertical	Vertical	Sporadic
Risk for occurrence	25% affected; 50% carriers	50% affected	50% affected males; 50% carrier females	50% children of affected females; 100% daughters of affected males
Unique characteristics	Consanguinity	Male-to-male transmission	Unequal X-inactivation results in affected daughters	X-inactivation modifies effect on daughters

penetrance and expressivity for those at risk for transmission of an adverse genetic trait is profound. For example, some people with the autosomal dominant form of osteogenesis imperfecta express the disorder by having blue sclera and no other problems; others experience recurrent skeletal fractures even with mild trauma. In addition, within the same family, parent and child may express the disorder to different degrees. An example is seen in families with a history of tuberous sclerosis, a disorder characterized by epilepsy, learning difficulties, behavioural problems, and skin lesions. Some individuals in these families have no disorder-related problems, even though they have both a parent and a child with clinical manifestations (tuberous sclerosis is due to a highly penetrant gene). These individuals, however, would still be assumed to have the gene (Lashley, 2007; OMIM, 2014).

Imprinting and Anticipation. Imprinting and anticipation further explain the variability in findings among people with Mendelian single-gene disorders. *Imprinting* means that an allele demonstrates a different phenotypic effect depending on whether the child received the allele from mother or father (Lashley, 2007; Nussbaum et al., 2007). It affects the expression of a gene, but not its primary sequence. An example involves Prader–Willi and Angelman syndromes. Prader–Willi syndrome is characterized by obesity, muscular hypotonia, intellectual challenges, short stature, and hypogonadotropic hypogonadism. Angelman syndrome is characterized by severe intellectual challenges, ataxia, hypotonia, epilepsy, absence of speech, and unusual facies. It is now understood that the same gene on chromosome 15 causes both Prader–Willi syndrome and Angelman syndrome, but expression depends on the parent of origin. Prader–Willi syndrome is the outcome of maternal transmission, whereas Angelman syndrome is the outcome of paternal transmission (Kubota et al., 2013; OMIM, 2014).

In most cases, the amount of DNA within a gene is stable and does not change from one generation to the next. Nevertheless, primarily among certain autosomal dominant disorders, this biologic principle may be false, and the genetic disease increases in severity and appears at an earlier age with subsequent generations (Aziz et al., 2011; Cunningham et al., 2010; Lashley, 2007). Examples include myotonic dystrophy, fragile X syndrome, and Huntington Disease. The cause is an expansion in the number of trinucleotides within the gene. This increased repetition of trinucleotides occurs during meiotic division and does not follow any established pattern; that is, a change may or may not occur in any or all subsequent generations of successive meioses. This is the biologic principle of *anticipation*.

Multifactorial Inheritance. *Multifactorial inheritance* means that multiple genes and their interactions

● **BOX 11.1** **Common Multifactorial Disorders**

Congenital Anomalies

Anencephaly
Cleft lip with/without cleft palate
Cleft palate
Clubfoot
Dislocation of the hip
Heart defects
Hypospadias
Pyloric stenosis
Spina bifida

Childhood and Adult Disorders

Asthma
Cancers
Crohn disease
Diabetes (type 1)
Hypertension
Multiple sclerosis
Peptic ulcer
Psoriasis
Systematic lupus erythematosus

with environmental factors regulate the expression of a phenotypic trait. It is the most common form of inheritance in the general population (Box 11.1). The presence or absence of a critical mass of interacting factors mediates expression of the disorder. Using the threshold model (Fig. 11.17), if the threshold is exceeded, then the person manifests signs of the disorder. Unlike Mendelian inheritance, the risk for a **multifactorial disorder** in a first-degree relative is disorder specific and depends on *heritability* (historical frequency of the disorder when manifested within an extended family) and incidence within the overall population. Generally, the frequency of the defect in first-degree relatives is equal to the square root of the general population incidence (Lashley, 2007). Thus, if a couple has given birth to one child with spina bifida (general population frequency 1:1,000), the specific risk for recurrence in a subsequent pregnancy is approximately 1:32. The risk for occurrence within a nuclear family increases if the woman and her reproductive partner are related genetically (Lashley, 2007). The likelihood of transmission of a Mendelian or multifactorial disorder is thus increased to a child conceived with their gametes.

In addition to the genes contained on the chromosomes within the nucleus of every cell, the mitochondria found in the cytoplasm of the cell contain at least 60 unique genes (OMIM, 2014). The mutation rate among mitochondrial genes is higher than for the genes found on the chromosomes (Lashley, 2007). Mitochondrial disorders typically affect the brain and the skeletal

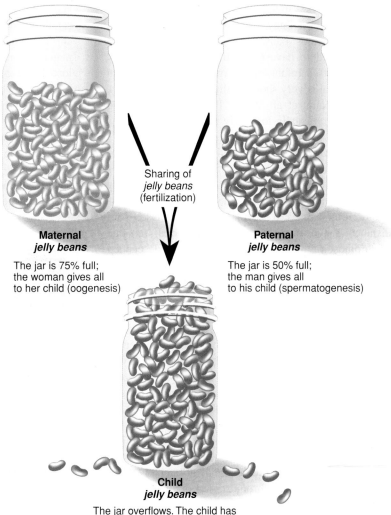

Sharing of
jelly beans
(fertilization)

Maternal
jelly beans

The jar is 75% full;
the woman gives all
to her child (oogenesis)

Paternal
jelly beans

The jar is 50% full;
the man gives all
to his child (spermatogenesis)

Child
jelly beans

The jar overflows. The child has
enough jelly beans for one and one
half jars. Also, the jar should be shrunk
a bit from environmental wear and tear.

FIGURE 11.17 Jelly bean jar
threshold model.

and heart muscles (Lashley, 2007). Importantly, these disorders are transmitted maternally. Sons and daughters are affected equally, but if paternal mitochondrial transmission occurs, it is lost very early in embryogenesis (Lashley, 2007).

Duplications, Deletions, and Translocations. Structural changes in chromosomes result from deletions, duplications, or translocations.

A *deletion* is the breakage and removal of a portion of a chromosome. It may occur on either distal end or within the chromosome itself (broken middle sections reattach to form a single structure). The best known deletion syndrome is *cri-du-chat,* which results from the absence of the "p" arm of chromosome 5. Infants with cri-du-chat have an abnormal cry that sounds like a cat's. DiGeorge syndrome results from the absence of a small portion of the "q" arm of chromosome 22 (McDonald-McGinn & Sullivan, 2011).

A *duplication* is an insertion of additional DNA within a chromosome, which may or may not have adverse phenotypic effects. Charcot–Marie–Tooth syndrome, a peripheral neuropathy, results from a replicated segment on the "p" arm of chromosome 17.

Disorders may also result from deletions or duplications of one or more entire chromosomes. Such changes either increase or decrease the amount of genetic material found in that person's genome. They are categorized as alterations in either number or structure. *Euploidy* is the correct complement of 46 chromosomes (diploid, $2n = 46$ chromosomes). *Polyploidy* is a change in the total number of chromosomes. Examples include multiple haploid sets ($n = 23$ chromosomes) such as triploidy ($3n = 69$ chromosomes) and tetraploidy ($4n = 92$ chromosomes). Triploidy most frequently results from the simultaneous fertilization of the oocyte by two separate sperm. A failure in meiotic division of the diploid oocyte or sperm also can produce a triploid zygote.

Failure of the first mitotic division of the zygote most often causes tetraploidy. Approximately 25% of spontaneous abortions caused by chromosomal anomalies are found to have either triploidy or tetraploidy (Lashley, 2007). Infants with triploidy are rarely born alive; survival is very short for those who are (Lashley, 2007; Nussbaum et al., 2007). Pregnancies involving tetraploids are usually lost early in gestation (Lashley, 2007).

Aneuploidy is characterized by the addition or deletion of one or more but fewer than 23 chromosomes ($2n \pm 1$ or two or three chromosomes). Aneuploidy results from *nondisjunction,* or the failure of two homologous chromosomes to separate during anaphase. Nondisjunction may occur during meiosis I or II (change in chromosome number appears in all cells descended from the zygote) or mitosis (change appears in some, but not all, somatic cells; referred to as mosaicism). The two most common forms of aneuploidy are *monosomy* (45 chromosomes; $2n - 1$) and *trisomy* (47 chromosomes; $2n + 1$). Turner syndrome (45, X) is the only monosomy that is not lethal. The most common trisomies observed in live-born infants include Down syndrome (47, XX or XY + 21: also known as trisomy 21), Edwards syndrome (47, XX or XY + 18; also known as trisomy 18), and Patau syndrome (47, XX or XY + 13; also known as trisomy 13) (Nussbaum et al., 2007) (Fig. 11.18).

If nondisjunction occurred during mitosis, clinical findings depend on which and how many cell lines were affected. People with chromosomal mosaicism (when two or more different chromosome complements are present) tend to have fewer and milder clinical findings than those with other aneuploidies (Nussbaum et al., 2007). Each mosaicism mentioned previously is compatible with life beyond the neonatal period, but each is associated with significant phenotypic findings. However, the majority of these fetuses are lost prior to term (Cunningham et al., 2010).

A *translocation* is the transfer of a segment of one chromosome to another. The three types of translocations are reciprocal, nonreciprocal, and Robertsonian.

- Reciprocal translocation is the breakage and exchange of segments between two chromosomes; usually, no genetic material is lost.
- Nonreciprocal translocation is the breakage of a single segment from one chromosome with attachment to another. Each translocation may be balanced (all genetic material is retained) or unbalanced (genetic material increases or decreases). The incidence of balanced translocations in the general population is 1 in 625; affected individuals generally have a normal phenotypic appearance.
- Robertsonian translocations involve only chromosomes 13, 14, 15, 21, and 22. They are referred to as

acrocentric because the "p" arm is replaced by short satellite projections. The long arms of two of these chromosomes fuse at the centromere, and the genetic material contained within the satellite projections is lost. This rearrangement is found in approximately 1 in 1,000 newborns (Cunningham et al., 2010).

- Importantly, all translocations profoundly affect gametogenesis. It is necessary for the gametes of a balanced or Robertsonian translocation carrier to segregate and divide during meiosis to maintain the integrity of the proper genetic complement. If not, a zygote is produced without the correct amount of genetic material, which may be the basis for recurrent loss of pregnancy.

April mentioned concern over an increased risk for Down syndrome during her recent examination with the nurse. How does this type of genetic disorder occur?

Health History Assessment

A health history can identify reproductive and perinatal risk factors. This assessment includes information about the medical, social, environmental, nutritional, gynecologic, and reproductive history of the woman desiring pregnancy, as well as assessment of the history of her reproductive partner. A health history also contains the medical and reproductive history of the parents, siblings, nieces, nephews, aunts, uncles, cousins, and grandparents of the woman and her partner, which the health care provider assesses for risk factors.

Health care providers use the information obtained to provide appropriate preconception or prenatal health counselling. They also use the assessment findings to identify risk factors that require further investigation and follow-up. Nurses may initiate a referral for genetic counselling if findings indicate that the client, reproductive partner, or both are at risk for having a child with a birth defect or genetic disorder.

A preconception health assessment may reveal information that clients perceive as sensitive, private, and highly confidential. Such assessment has the profound potential to alter a client's self-image and relationships. Many clients fear that insurers, employers, and social communities will use genetic information to discriminate against them and their family. In many Western countries, there appears to be little legislation dealing specifically with genetic privacy and discrimination. However, the list of laws and proposed laws applying specifically to genetics is growing, primarily in three areas—insurance, employment, and criminal forensics. In Canada, apart from legislation dealing

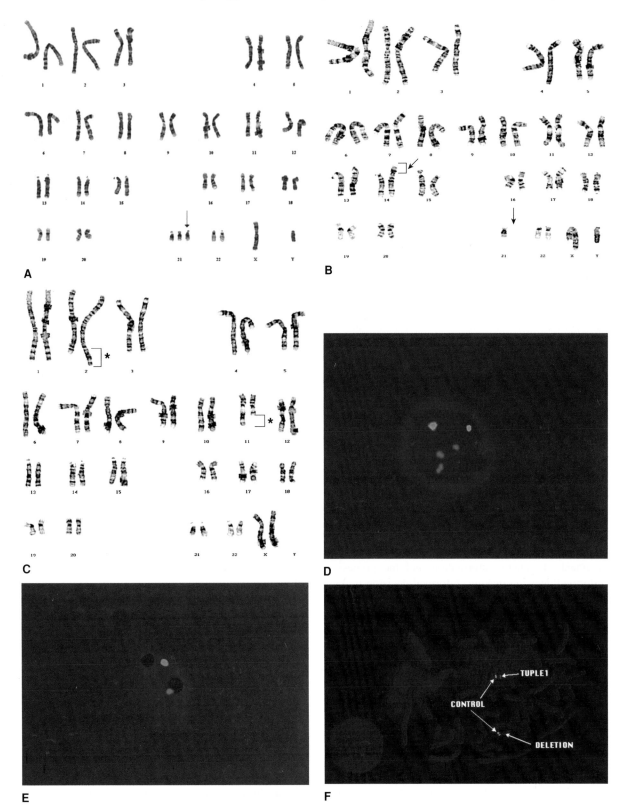

FIGURE 11.18 Karyotypes of abnormal and normal chromosome complements. **A:** Male with trisomy 21. **B:** Robertsonian translocation of chromosomes 14 and 21. Note that missing chromosome 21 is attached to chromosome 14. **C:** Translocation of distal portion of chromosome 11 to chromosome 2. **D:** Female with trisomy 21. **E:** Normal male. **F:** Normal for DiGeorge syndrome probe. (Courtesy of A. Donnenfeld, Main Line Perinatology, Wynnewood, Pennsylvania.)

with the use of DNA in criminal investigations, most provisions relevant to genetic privacy and discrimination are not found in laws dealing specifically with genetics issues. Instead, they appear in more general legislation—constitutional law, laws governing professional confidentiality, data protection (privacy), and human rights laws among them (Oscapella, 2012).

Legislation in the United States was passed in 2008 to protect genetic information against insurance or employment discrimination. In Canada, although there has been significant consideration of the issue in multiple forums, there are currently no laws that address the use of this information by insurance companies (Office of the Privacy Commissioner of Canada, 2012). Some portions of the Canadian Human Rights Act and provincial human rights codes, which prohibit discriminatory practices on the basis of a number of factors, may be relevant to this issue (Office of the Privacy Commissioner of Canada, 2012). Therefore, nurses in health care settings consider and address the following questions carefully (International Society of Nurses in Genetics, 2010b):

- Where is the appropriate place to record genetic information?
- What constitutes appropriate informed consent for genetic testing and evaluation?
- What is the nurse's responsibility to provide genetic information to clients?
- What is the nurse's responsibility to the client and family confronted with genetic information?
- Is the level of confidentiality required by genetic information different from other medical information?

These questions are critical for appropriate management of genetic information and the process of informed decision making. Informed decision making, which integrates the ethical principles of autonomy, justice, and beneficence (Harper, 2010; Nussbaum et al., 2007), is the hallmark of preconception health assessment. Its goals are as follows:

1. Methodical, organized, and complete identification of personal risk factors
2. Provision of individualized, nondirective, nonjudgemental education and counselling
3. Timely access to complementary services, such as genetic and nutritional counselling and behavioural modification programs (Moos, 2010).

If these goals are met, then the client can approach reproductive issues with the knowledge necessary to make informed choices.

Screening Process

Preconception health assessment provides the opportunity for clients and partners/families to initiate health behaviours known to be beneficial to the conception, development, and birth of children. Initiating this process tends to engender positive feelings among those who do so, because they feel empowered to optimize the health and well-being of future children. Conversely, this process also may cause feelings of anger, guilt, and anxiety as clients learn and share information. Therefore, nurses protect the right of clients *to choose* or *to choose not* to seek preconception health screening and counselling (i.e., "right to know" vs. "right not to know"). To that end, nurses precede each step of the health assessment with (1) an explanation of the process, information that may or may not be learned, and possible implications of that knowledge; and (2) an opportunity for dialogue. This is the foundation of the process of informed decision making (Box 11.2) and is part of the informed consent process (the process of assessing and documenting consent after informed decision making).

Using Standardized Risk Assessment Forms

To ensure *methodical, organized, and complete identification of personal risk factors,* the woman and her reproductive partner may complete a standardized health risk assessment form. However, research shows that few

● **BOX 11.2**   **Components of Informed Decision Making and Consent for Genetic Testing or Evaluation**

The process of informed decision making and consent includes, but is not limited to, the presentation of the following information before the performance of a genetic test or evaluation:

- The purpose of the screening or diagnostic test
- The nature of the disorder in question
- Reasons for completing the testing or evaluation
- Benefits of the testing or evaluation
- Risks of the testing or evaluation, including physical, psychological, social
- Alternative procedures
- Available interventions or treatments, including the lack of such interventions
- Subsequent decisions that will be likely after results are disclosed
- Available counselling services
- Implications of results for family members
- Institutional confidentiality standards
- Sensitivity and specificity of the test
- Unexpected results

Adapted from Rantenen, E., Hietala, J., Kristoffersson, U., Irmgard, N., Schmidtke, J., Sequeiros, J., et al. (2008). What is ideal genetic counseling? A survey of current international guidelines. *European Journal of Human Genetics, 16,* 445–452. doi:10.1038/sj.ejhg.5201983

family health questionnaires have been formally evaluated; few if any have been validated against a reference standard. This brings into question the accuracy of these assessment tools (Reid et al., 2009). They may have some positive impact on screening for cancer. They have not been shown to cause any harm (Reid et al., 2009).

In some cases, the woman's partner is not involved in this process, either by choice or by circumstance. Although the full complement of risks will not be available in such cases, it is still helpful for the woman to go through this screening to identify potential maternal risk factors.

Examples of other areas appropriate to address are as follows:

- Social history—exposure to or use of alcohol, cigarettes, drugs, radiation, or toxic chemicals
- Nutrition history—required or chosen dietary restrictions, any eating disorders, use of dietary supplements
- Medical history—any systemic condition (e.g., thyroid, kidney, cardiovascular disease)
- Infectious disease history—occurrence of or exposure to any infectious disease or blood-borne pathogen such as herpes simplex, hepatitis, or HIV
- Reproductive history—any male or female reproductive organ anomalies such as congenital bilateral absence of the vas deferens, gonadal dysgenesis, or bicornuate uterus
- Ethnic background—family history as well as the exploration of any disorder known to occur more frequently in a specific population

Common Areas of Concern

Parental Age. As maternal age advances, so does the rate of aneuploidy (Chitayat et al., 2011; Langlois & Brock, 2013). The result is increased rates of pregnancy loss and birth of infants with chromosomal anomalies. Most women and men are aware that advanced maternal age may affect a pregnancy adversely. This awareness is the direct outcome of (1) the adoption of practice standards that obligate obstetricians, gynaecologists, midwives, nurse practitioners, and women's health nurses to appropriately disseminate this information; and (2) the considerable media exposure about this issue through public service campaigns, news programs, and storylines in popular entertainment. However, the Society of Obstetricians and Gynaecologists of Canada (Chitayat et al., 2011) recommends that maternal age, as the sole factor for invasive testing below age 40 at the estimated date of delivery, should be reconsidered because of the improved use of biochemical markers.

The general public and some health care providers are less aware that advanced paternal age (older than 45 years at conception) affects the risk of miscarriage and issues with fetal development, including increased

risk of schizophrenia and autism (Bhandari et al., 2013; Hultman et al., 2011; Sartorius & Nieschlag, 2010). As discussed earlier, spermatogenesis begins at puberty and continues throughout the rest of the man's life. Estimates are that one new gene mutates each time spermatogonia replicate before spermatocyte meiosis. Most of these mutations are benign or nonlethal to embryo development; however, the incidence of new autosomal dominant mutations in newborns whose fathers are 40 years of age is approximately 0.3% (Cunningham et al., 2010). Natural selection through programmed cell death (apoptosis) eliminates many of these anomalous spermatocytes from the pool of viable sperm. Apoptosis declines as paternal age advances, however, and correlates with decreased male fertility and increased incidence of fetuses with single gene disorders of paternal origin (Sartorius & Nieschlag, 2010).

Many clients seeking preconception counselling because one or both partners are of advanced reproductive age have limited knowledge of the biologic mechanisms that adversely alter their probability of giving birth to a healthy child. The nurse identifies their level of knowledge and preconception counselling expectations. Collection of the health screening information facilitates recognition by clients of the importance of preconception health risk assessment and counselling.

Presentation and discussion of reproductive alternatives assist clients to make an informed choice as to which reproductive option aligns best with their beliefs and values. Social communities (family, friends, work, and culture) and religious doctrines often influence or dictate viable and nonviable reproductive services to consider. Some people choose to realize their goal (addition of a child to the family unit) by pursuing alternatives that violate the beliefs of their community. Assistance may be required from health care providers to access specialized services confidentially and privately to minimize the risk for social discrimination.

Reproductive History. The reproductive history of both the woman and her partner can identify potential risk factors as they pursue the desire for a biologic child. If both have previously achieved the birth of a child (together or with different partners), it is highly probable that this couple will conceive and give birth. Absence of a prior conception and birth alone is not sufficient evidence to warrant a reproductive evaluation, but additional questioning can help eliminate or identify potential risks that together indicate potential reproductive failure.

To ensure a comprehensive review, the nurse identifies and assesses reproductive history for potential risk factors and provides education about the implications of findings. Congenital or acquired reproductive malformations (e.g., congenital absence of the vas deferens, septate uterus); loss of ovarian or testicular reserve (i.e., decreased numbers of oocytes or spermatocytes); irregular menstrual cycles (e.g., premature ovarian failure); infections; autoimmune disorders; and hormonal imbalances (e.g., hyperprolactinemia, thyroid disorders, insulin resistance) may lead to an inability to conceive or carry a pregnancy to term (see Chapter 10).

Chromosomal rearrangements in the fetus from an inherited unbalanced translocation or microdeletion may result in spontaneous pregnancy loss during the first trimester. *Recurrent miscarriage,* also called *recurrent pregnancy loss,* is the loss of three or more pregnancies before 20 weeks' gestation (Cunningham et al., 2010; Puscheck & Jeyendran, 2007). Analyses performed on the products of conception from sporadic miscarriages suggest a strong correlation between chromosomal anomalies and pregnancy loss (more than half of cases show chromosomal rearrangements). Most of these losses result from nondisjunctions rather than from parental transmissions of unbalanced translocations. Among those couples experiencing recurrent pregnancy loss, approximately 1% to 4% have a parental chromosomal rearrangement (Puscheck & Jeyendran, 2007).

The complexity of establishing the probable cause of a suspected conception failure or history of recurrent pregnancy loss is increased by the potential need for the client to be evaluated by both reproductive endocrinology (infertility) and genetics specialists. A history of recurrent pregnancy loss or a fetal demise in the second or third trimester may be an indication for thrombophilia testing. Sotiriadis et al., (2007) suggest that more research is indicated before routine testing is implemented; the research of Ebrahim et al. (2010) suggests that screening should be offered to women with a personal or family history of thrombosis, as well as those with a history of recurrent adverse pregnancy outcomes. Many of the diagnostic tests required for these specialty evaluations may be completed within the primary care setting. The health care provider coordinates the completion of requisite tests (serum hormone levels, physical examinations, chromosome analysis) and reviews results before referral of the client to one or more specialists. The results of the initial evaluation may lead to elimination or redirection of a planned referral. The health care provider counsels the client about the importance of and the method for obtaining a fetal karyotype if pregnancy loss recurs.

If an irreversible cause (e.g., parental chromosomal anomaly, malformation of reproductive organs, sterility) of reproductive failure is identified, the health care provider teaches the client about the scope of reproductive options available. The nurse also encourages and assists clients as they evaluate and reflect on their feelings and beliefs about these alternatives; referral for counselling may be appropriate.

Family History and Ethnicity. Screening and diagnostic tests within the preconception health risk assessment process can identify and eliminate potential concerns for clients proactively seeking a healthy pregnancy outcome. Allele form analysis for a single gene may be indicated. This type of screening test is used in preconception and prenatal settings to identify healthy people at risk for transmitting an altered allele to their child. Its use is indicated when there is a family history of an adult-onset disorder not yet apparent in the at-risk reproductive partner. Depending on the disorder, this form of testing is known as presymptomatic (e.g., Huntington disease) or predisposition (e.g., breast cancer). Carrier screening is also appropriate if the family history or ethnic group of either reproductive partner suggests the potential transmission of a single copy of an altered recessive allele.

If both the woman *and* her partner have the same altered recessive allele, then each pregnancy has a 25% chance of resulting in the birth of a child with a genetic disorder. Likewise, each pregnancy has a 25% chance of the birth of a healthy child without an altered allele. There is a 50% chance that each pregnancy produces a child who is a healthy carrier of one copy of the altered allele just like the parents.

If a woman *or* her partner is at risk for transmitting a dominant altered allele to the fetus, then each pregnancy has a 50% chance of resulting in the birth of a child with the same presymptomatic or predisposition risk as the at-risk parent. Similarly, each pregnancy has a 50% chance of ending with a child without the altered allele and its associated phenotypic risk.

A basic preconception screening tool is the question, "What is your ethnic group?" This information initiates and directs one aspect of assessment of risk factors for a specific client. For example, if a woman is Caucasian and of French Canadian ancestry, her carrier risk is increased for cystic fibrosis and Tay–Sachs disease. Likewise, if her reproductive partner is Caucasian and of Icelandic ancestry, his carrier risk is increased for cystic fibrosis and phenylketonuria.

Completion of a genogram assists with identification of family members who have or are at risk for other single-gene disorders not necessarily specific to any ethnic or population group. Advances in molecular, biochemical, and cytogenetic testing permit determination of individual risk (present, absent, probable) for many known genetic disorders. Professional practice standards form the basis of protocols for recommended genetic screening tests (Chitayat et al., 2011; Johnson & Tough, 2012; Langlois & Brock, 2013). Current clinical protocols include a basic scope of preconception or prenatal tests.

The nurse is prepared that inquiry into a client's ethnic or population background may elicit fears of racial bias or other discrimination, resulting in the client's conscious decision not to provide requested data. Although a clinical protocol may dictate performance of one or more genetic screening tests, the principles of **informed decision making and consent** require the nurse to educate and counsel before doing so. Typically, an explanation of the science and basis of the protocol assists the client with decision making. The nurse works with clients to ensure that they understand the rationale for testing. He or she is obligated to (1) assist with the process of informed decision making, (2) document that process, and (3) support the decision, whether the client elects to pursue or not to pursue genetic testing.

If a family history of a dominant or recessive genetic disorder is suspected or positive, the nurse, based on his or her own knowledge and scope of practice, provides education and counselling, or referral for genetic counselling specific to that disorder. The need for dissemination of information and dialogue about common genetic disorders (e.g., cystic fibrosis, sickle cell anemia) in primary care settings is growing. Multiple resources are available to learn about and prepare materials for use when discussing such disorders with clients (Amos et al., 2011; Canadian Cystic Fibrosis Foundation, nd; Sickle Cell Disease Association of Canada, 2013). The nurse coordinates all referral services and provides supportive counselling throughout the process.

Environmental Influences. A preconception screening assessment can identify environmental influences that may affect pregnancy outcome. Health care providers assess paternal health during a cycle of spermatogenesis, maternal health before conception as well as throughout gestation, and the ecologic environment in which the woman and partner reside and work. Men exposed to toxic substances such as heat, radiation, viruses, bacteria, alcohol, and prescription and recreational drugs are more likely to have decreased morphologically and genetically normal sperm in a single ejaculate. This results in reproductive failure preconception and postfertilization (Fritz & Speroff, 2011). Women exposed to similar toxic agents experience diminished ovarian reserve, poor endometrial lining development, and abnormal fetal development (Table 11.5). Likewise, chronic and acute diseases decrease fecundity (fertility) (Jameson et al., 2010).

Men and women alike require proper nutrition and normal endocrine function to sustain gametogenesis and, for the woman, gestation and normal fetal development. Abnormal levels of prolactin, thyroid-stimulating hormone, gonadotropin-releasing hormone, FSH, testosterone, estrogen, and progesterone interfere with normal gametogenesis and embryo implantation (see Chapter 10). Women require additional vitamins and minerals to support fetal growth and development (see Chapter 3). Especially important is additional folic acid

to reduce the risk for neural tube defects (Public Health Agency of Canada, 2012).

The nurse evaluates the client and her partner's health and exposure to toxic substances. Ideally, each reproductive partner completes a medical health history and preconception screening questionnaire. The nurse reviews the responses and clarifies any ambiguities. This aspect of preconception health risk assessment addresses the following areas of concern (Lashley, 2007; Ward, 2008).

1. Lack of natural or acquired immunity to common infectious diseases: rubella, rubeola, hepatitis B, varicella, mumps, toxoplasmosis.
2. Any chronic or uncontrolled disorders: diabetes, hypertension, thyroid disorders, systemic lupus erythematosus, kidney disease, epilepsy.
3. Use of or exposure to radiation or hormonal, chemical, or biologic agents detrimental to fetal development: alcohol, radioactive materials, oral contraceptives, prescribed or recreational drugs.
4. Any maternal genetic disorder that affects normal fetal development (e.g., phenylketonuria, factor V Leiden).
5. Maternal nutrition assessment to address an improper diet or a lack of supplemental vitamins and minerals sufficient to assist with proper fetal development.

Many environmental factors that adversely affect conception, fetal growth, and fetal development are reversible, controllable, or both. The nurse identifies reversible health risks and educates clients about actions required to confirm and subsequently eliminate those risks. Recommended standards for some risk factors are available from professional organizations; the nurse uses them during discussion. For example, all women who could become pregnant should begin taking a multivitamin containing 0.4 mg of folic acid daily (Public Health Agency of Canada, 2012). Since 1998, the Government of Canada has required folic acid to be added to all white flour, enriched pasta, and cornmeal products sold in Canada (Public Health Agency of Canada, 2012).

The nurse assesses immune levels for diseases known to have available vaccines. He or she coordinates appropriate laboratory testing and subsequent recommendations for vaccination. Internists, endocrinologists, or nephrologists refer women with chronic or uncontrolled diseases for evaluation based on the specific diagnosis. The nurse coordinates the referral services and gathers summary reports for each completed referral.

The nurse educates and counsels clients about social or work environment activities that affect fetal development. He or she provides support for people who require assistance to eliminate a risk factor from the environment or refers them to the appropriate non–health care agency. Examples include Human Resources at their employment site, the Canadian Centre for Occupational Health and Safety, or Alcoholics Anonymous.

Women with a chronic disease (e.g., diabetes) or genetic disorder (e.g., phenylketonuria) can take steps to control glucose and insulin levels or reduce circulating phenylalanine. However, they cannot reduce the risk to a level similar to those without diabetes or phenylketonuria. The nurse provides education and counselling about alternative reproductive options when desired (see Chapter 10).

Constructing Genograms

To assist with mapping family patterns, understanding repetitive patterns of behavior, and recognizing hereditary tendencies, the health care provider may construct a genogram (pedigree) (Bokhare et al., 2014). The genogram typically contains general information such as the name, gender, and relationship of individuals, etc.; some also contain information on illnesses and addictions that run in families (Bokhare et al., 2014). Figure 11.19 presents standard symbols used in the construction of the genogram (Bokhare et al., 2014). After drawing the genogram, the health care provider reviews it with the client for accuracy and completeness. It is not unusual for this review to elicit additional and important information that the client forgot when responding to questions "about the family" rather than "about the individual family member." This careful review of individual family members helps to identify whether there are any areas that need further investigation before the information is compiled.

 Remember Carmen, the recently married client who wants to begin having children. Carmen is concerned about the possibility of disease transmission to her fetus. Would completing a genogram be helpful in this situation? Why or why not?

Care of the client who is intending to become, or is, pregnant requires that healthcare providers be knowledgeable and comfortable with discussing teratogens and their effects (Table 11.5), as well as with mitochondrial and chromosomal disorders. See Nursing Care Plan 11.1.

Information Sharing

After carefully reviewing the available results, the health care provider drafts a summary of the findings in preparation for the provision of individualized, nondirective, nonjudgemental education and counselling with the client and her partner. This initial analysis may highlight the need for additional information or referral

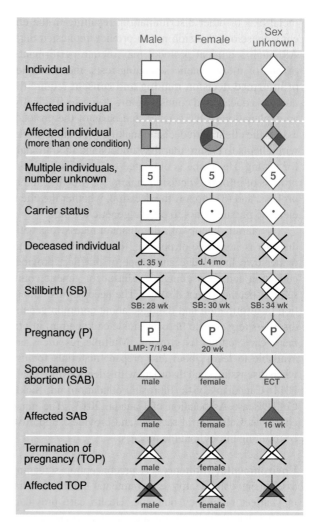

FIGURE 11.19 Common symbols used in the construction of a genogram.

to a specialist, such as a geneticist, neurologist, endocrinologist, or cardiologist. The necessity to evaluate one or more family members with a developmental delay, intellectual challenges, musculoskeletal anomaly, suspected metabolic disorder, congenital malformation, or progressive neurologic disorder to establish a definitive diagnosis is the basis of such a referral. This process element is critical to the accurate delineation of preconception risk for some clients.

The setting chosen for preconception health counselling should be quiet, private, and free of frequent interruption. The nurse allows sufficient time to disseminate information and assess the client's understanding of preconception risk, recommended health promotion behaviours, and available reproductive options. The nurse identifies and corrects misinterpretations and misunderstandings through the iterative process of reflective questioning (Lashley, 2007). In addition, he or she prepares and shares information in

NURSING CARE PLAN 11.1

●

The Client Seeking Preconception Health Screening

 Remember Carmen, the 22-year-old who desires pregnancy but is concerned about transmitting genetic or other disorders to her baby. Further assessment of Carmen reveals the following: history of seasonal allergies with use of over-the-counter decongestants, weight appropriate for height, and vital signs within acceptable parameters.

Further discussion of family history reveals that twins run in Carmen's family. "What if I have twins?" she says. "I'm not sure I could handle that!"

NURSING DIAGNOSIS

Anxiety related to uncertainty about fetal health secondary to family history

EXPECTED OUTCOMES

1. The client will identify specific areas causing her concern.
2. The client will state measures to minimize anxiety.
3. The client will report a decrease in anxiety levels.

INTERVENTIONS	RATIONALES
Assess the client's level of understanding about pregnancy and fetal health.	Assessment provides a baseline to identify specific client needs and develop an individualized plan.
Discuss with the client her concerns, feelings, and perceptions related to pregnancy and fetal health and possible effects on current family situation.	Discussion provides opportunities to emphasize positive aspects; verbalization of concerns aids in establishing sources of stress and problem areas to address.
Communicate accurate facts and answer questions honestly. Reinforce facts. Encourage the client not to blame herself if problems are found.	Open and honest communication promotes trust and helps to correct misperceptions or misinformation. Facts help dispel unfounded fears, myths, and guilt.
Evaluate which past coping strategies have been most effective.	Use of appropriate coping strategies aids in reducing anxiety.
Emphasize that the client can use this time to make health or lifestyle changes.	Health promotion behaviors can help reduce risks in pregnancy.
Obtain an assessment risk and complete a client genogram.	Assessment risk and genogram aid in determining possible areas that may pose threats to fetal health.
Review with the client measures used throughout pregnancy to monitor fetal well-being; include appropriate screening and diagnostic testing that may be done.	Knowledge of ongoing surveillance techniques aids in alleviating stress related to the unknown.
Encourage the client to include her partner in follow-up visits.	Participation of the client's partner promotes sharing, provides support, and enhances the chances for success.
Question the client about available support systems, such as family, friends, and community.	Additional sources of support are helpful in alleviating anxiety.
Provide client with information about support groups, websites, and other sources of information related to pregnancy and fetal health.	These resources can help the client to prepare for what to expect.

(continued)

NURSING CARE PLAN 11.1 ● The Client Seeking Preconception Health Screening *(Continued)*

EVALUATION

1. The client openly verbalizes concerns about potential pregnancy and fetal health.
2. The client demonstrates positive methods of coping.
3. The client reports that her anxiety level has diminished.

NURSING DIAGNOSIS

Deficient Knowledge related to pregnancy and factors affecting fetal health

EXPECTED OUTCOMES

1. The client will verbalize accurate information about pregnancy and ways to optimize fetal health.
2. The client will identify possible screening and diagnostic tests needed to optimize fetal health.

INTERVENTIONS	RATIONALES
Assess the client's knowledge about her body and typical changes in pregnancy.	This information establishes a baseline from which to develop appropriate teaching strategies.
Describe fetal growth and development and factors that may affect fetal health, including exposure to teratogens.	An accurate description of fetal growth and development is essential to understanding risk factors.
Encourage the client to avoid exposure to possible teratogens; urge her to contact her primary health care provider about the use of an over-the-counter decongestant during pregnancy.	Exposure to teratogens can result in fetal malformations, disruptions, and deformations.
Explain the basic principles of genetics, including inheritance of disorders; review the client's genogram and correlate information with explanation.	Information about genetics provides an understanding about the need for possible screening and testing.
Discuss multiple gestation, including factors that increase the risk; review the client's genogram for possible risks associated with twin births.	A maternal family history of twin births increases the client's risk for twins.
Instruct the client about possible screening and testing based on history, risk assessment, and genogram.	Information about possible upcoming testing helps to prepare the client and minimize anxiety and fear of the unknown.
Provide the client with written material about healthy behaviors and testing.	Written material provides additional means of teaching and provides opportunities for review and reinforcement.

EVALUATION

1. The client demonstrates healthy behaviors during the preconception period so that pregnancy and fetal health are optimized.
2. The client verbalizes an understanding of the rationale for screening and diagnostic testing.

a way that aligns with and accommodates the client's culture, language, education level, and prior knowledge (Uhlmann et al., 2011).

To ensure the appropriate provision of information, nurses identify the full scope of reproductive options available to the client based on specific preconception risk. Concurrently, nurses carefully identify and seek to understand their own values and beliefs as well as their accompanying inherent biases. This self-assessment is critical to providing individualized, nondirective, nonjudgemental education and counselling.

The client's reaction to the information identified through a preconception health risk assessment may be positive or negative. When an unexpected or anticipated risk is presented, the client may express anger and hostility toward the "bearer of bad news." Health care providers develop the skills necessary to assist clients to understand the basis of such a response and are prepared to transfer care to another provider if a therapeutic relationship cannot be re-established. This is essential for clients and families to achieve increased knowledge and understanding about the importance of (1) good maternal health and health care before and during pregnancy; (2) implementation of health promotion behaviours; (3) identification and reduction of perinatal risk factors; (4) elimination of toxic exposures; (5) stabilization of maternal disorders; and (6) informed dialogue and shared decision making.

Anticipatory Care

The results of preconception health risk assessment may reveal the need for multiple health care providers, community, or family services. Clients may be unaware of the breadth, availability, and accessibility of such services. The nurse's knowledge and skills align well with the role of care coordinator; he or she may help clients to identify and navigate diverse forms of assistance they seek or identify as a need (Lea et al., 2011). A key aspect of anticipatory care *is timely access to complementary services such as genetic and nutritional counselling and behavioural modification programs.*

Through anticipatory care, nurses assist clients to respond to the recommendations from the preconception health risk assessment. Nursing interventions include the following:

- Establishment of institutional protocols and policies for the completion of a referral
- Timely initiation of appropriate referrals
- Reduction or elimination of barriers to services (Guttmacher et al., 2007), such as geographic location (use of teleconferencing), knowledge (education of professional and administrative staff), or time (coordination of services to limit total number of visits required)
- Management of genetic information
- Protection of confidentiality and privacy

- Written summary of the findings and recommendations appropriate for the client's knowledge level
- Development of materials sensitive to the client's culture whether defined as geographic, ethnic, sexual orientation, social, disability, or language (Uhlmann et al., 2011)
- Dissemination of information to other individuals, family members, or health care providers (as requested by the client)

The nurse uses the skills, knowledge, and interventions integral to the completion of a comprehensive preconception health risk assessment after a pregnancy is established or a child with a suspected or known genetic disorder is born. The information gleaned can help clients anticipate concerns for the current situation as well as anticipate future pregnancy considerations. As the Human Genome Project further advances knowledge of human genome variation and the molecular basis of disease, such knowledge and skills will be requisite for nurses in all health care settings.

PRENATAL SCREENING AND DIAGNOSTIC PROCEDURES

The goal of prenatal screening is to offer a noninvasive test to all pregnant women to determine whether or not invasive prenatal diagnostic tests are necessary (Chitayat et al., 2011). These noninvasive prenatal screening tests are offered both for couples at risk or in couples with no identified risk factors (Chitayat et al., 2011). However, the Society of Obstetricians and Gynaecologists of Canada (SOGC) recommends that screening should only be undertaken when "the disorder is considered to be serious enough to warrant intervention" (Chitayat et al., 2011, p. 738). Informed decision making and consent direct this aspect of prenatal care. Clients and partners should be informed that prenatal screening does not usually result in identification, treatment, or cure. Rather, the process leads to identification of the risk of a fetus having an anomaly requiring the client to decide, after counselling, whether or not to choose to have invasive prenatal testing done (Chitayat et al., 2011; Langlois & Brock, 2013).

Before clients give procedural consent, health care providers apprise clients and families of the benefits and limitations of prenatal screening or invasive prenatal diagnosis. This includes discussion of the following key points in language that is understandable for the client and family (Nussbaum et al., 2007; Langlois & Brock, 2013).

- What is the risk the fetus will be affected?
- What are the nature and probable consequences of the disorder of concern?

- Are appropriate postnatal treatments available for the disorder of concern?
- What are the risks, benefits, and limitations of the available and disorder-appropriate procedures?
- How long will it take to receive the results of the screening or diagnostic procedures?
- What is the frequency and possible need for a repeat procedure?
- Is the risk of the procedure perceived outweighed by the information to be learned?

This dialogue may lead to the discovery of sensitive information (e.g., nonpaternity) with social implications and subsequent worry resulting from the information learned. Importantly, most couples who seek prenatal screening and diagnosis receive reassuring information after the performance of one or more such procedures. All couples should understand that seeking this service does not imply an obligation to terminate a pregnancy found to have a fetus with an anomaly. The primary goal of prenatal diagnosis is to identify whether a fetus has an anomaly. It is the sole decision of the woman and her reproductive partner to determine how to use that information, including termination of the pregnancy or preparation through knowledge acquisition for the birth and parenting of a child with a specific disorder.

Prenatal Screening

Screening is a process that uses specific marker(s) and defined cut-off points when surveying a population (e.g., the Canadian prenatal population). It "identif[ies] the individuals in the population at higher risk for a particular disorder. Screening is applicable to a population; diagnosis is applied at the individual level" (Chitayat et al., 2011, p. 738). In the mid-1960s, maternal age >35 at estimated date of delivery was the only screening criterion that was used to identify a pregnancy at risk of fetal aneuploidy. Maternal serum marker screening later became available in prenatal care settings as an adjunct to maternal age. Maternal serum alpha fetoprotein (MSAFP) was the first biochemical marker to be analyzed. In the 1970s it was identified as a second trimester marker for open neural tube defects (Fig. 11.20), gastroschisis, and omphalocele. In the 1980s, low MSAFP levels were found to be present in cases of trisomy 18 and Down syndrome.

Screening for genetic disorders has now evolved to the point where it should be a program rather than just a test (Chitayat et al., 2011). Important aspects of a comprehensive program include information that is understandable to the client and family, timely access to screening tests, a system of notification of results, referral for follow-up testing, access to interventions, regular clinical audits to evaluate local performance, and flexibility to include new technologies (Chitayat et al., 2011).

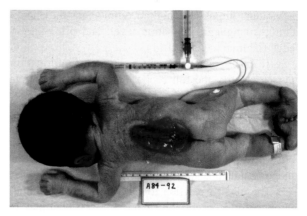

FIGURE 11.20 Stillborn infant with neural tube defect. (Courtesy of A. Donnenfeld, Main Line Perinatology, Wynnewood, Pennsylvania.)

"Counselling must be non-directive and must respect a woman's right to accept or decline any or all of the testing or options offered at any point in the process" (Chitayat et al., 2011, p. 740).

A combination of maternal age and two or more biochemical tests, with or without an ultrasound, produces a single value for the risk of Down syndrome, trisomy 18, and open neural tube defects (Chitayat et al., 2011) (Table 11.7). A screening test is considered positive when "the risk of one or more of the screened disorders falls above a designated risk cut-off" (Chitayat et al., 2011, p. 738). False positive rate and detection rate are terms that are commonly used when discussing prenatal screening. "As screening performance improves, the false positive rate decreases and/or the detection rate increases…. A risk cut-off is expressed as the risk or likelihood of the condition being present in the fetus at term or at midtrimester" (Chitayat et al., 2011, p. 738). Approximately 23% of pregnancies with fetuses with Down syndrome are lost between midtrimester and term; therefore, the risk of the condition being present at midtrimester will be higher than at term (Chitayat et al., 2011).

Nursing Care Plan 11.2 describes a scenario in which a couple faces decision making related to prenatal screening and diagnostic procedures. It describes the difficulties that clients and partners can face when trying to determine how much information they want to know in the early stages of pregnancy.

Screening programs may vary across provinces and territories, creating a responsibility for health care practitioners to be aware of the program in their jurisdiction. A number of factors need to be considered when determining the appropriateness of including (a) specific test(s) in a screening program. The screening test(s) selected should have the highest detection rate with the lowest false positive rate. Cost and logistics need to be considered; a comprehensive cost comparison for many screening options is still incomplete. Because of the

● TABLE 11.7   Current Available Screening Options and Their Screening Performance[a]

Screening Option	Markers	1st/2nd Trimester	Term Risk Cut-Off	DR (%)	FPR (%)	OAPR
Options that meet the minimum standard						
FTS	NT, free β-hCG, PAPP-A, MA	1st	1 in 325	83	5	1:27
Quad screening	AFP, uE3, free β-hCG, inhibin A, MA	2nd	1 in 385	77	5.2	1:50
IPS	NT, PAPP-A, AFP, uE3, free β-hCG/total hCG, inhibin A, MA	1st & 2nd	1 in 200	87	1.9	1:10
IPS without inhibin A	NT, PAPP-A, AFP, uE3, total hCG, MA	1st & 2nd	1 in 200	88	3	1:20
Serum IPS	PAPP-A, AFP, uE3, free β-hCG/total hCG, inhibin A	1st & 2nd	1 in 200	85	4.4	1:26
Options that do not meet the minimum standard						
Maternal age	MA	1st & 2nd	1 in 385	44	16	1:218
Triple screening	AFP, uE3, total hCG, MA	2nd	1 in 385	71	7.2	1:59

DR, detection rate; FPR, false positive rate; OAPR, odds of being affected given a positive result; FTS, first trimester combined screening; NT, nuchal translucency; PAPP-A, pregnancy-associated plasma protein-A; MA, maternal age; AFP, serum Alpha fetoprotein; uE3, unconjugated estriol; IPS, integrated prenatal screening.

[a]Some centres in Canada may offer variation on IPS (sequential screening or contingent screening) with cut-offs set that achieve at least the minimum standard.

Reprinted with permission of the Society of Obstetricians and Gynaecologists of Canada from SOGC Clinical Practice Guideline. (2001). *Prenatal Screening for Fetal Aneuploidy* (p. 741).

variations in resource availability and geographic limitations, SOGC guidelines refer to performance characteristics rather than specific tests.

SOGC (Chitayat et al., 2011) recommends that all pregnant women in Canada, regardless of age, should be offered noninvasive prenatal screening for the most common clinically significant fetal aneuploidies in addition to second trimester ultrasound for dating, growth, and anomalies. Options for this noninvasive prenatal screening include maternal age *combined* with first trimester screening, second trimester serum screening, and two-step integrated screening (Chitayat et al., 2011).

First Trimester Screening

First trimester programs should offer screens that, at a minimum, provide a 75% detection rate with no more than a 3% false positive rate (Chitayat et al., 2011). Using maternal age and maternal serum markers alone has a detection rate of 61% with a false positive rate of 5%. Thus, these screening tools alone do not fulfil guideline requirements and are less efficacious than second trimester screening (Chitayat et al., 2011). However, when these first trimester maternal serum markers are combined with nuchal translucency, the detection rate increases to 83% detection, with a 5% false positive rate (Chitayat et al., 2011).

First trimester maternal serum biochemical markers are pregnancy-associated plasma protein-A (PAPP-A) and free β-hCG. In pregnancies with Down syndrome, PAPP-A is decreased while free β-hCG is increased

(Chitayat et al., 2011). Nuchal translucency is the subcutaneous layer of fluid behind the fetal neck and lower cranium, which can be seen on ultrasound. On an ultrasound done at 12 to 15 weeks' gestation, an increased size of this fluid is associated with an increased risk of fetal Down syndrome (Chitayat et al., 2011). Nuchal translucency is also associated with other chromosome abnormalities, cardiac defects, diaphragmatic hernia, and a number of single-gene disorders—especially those associated with decreased fetal movement (Chitayat et al., 2011). PAPP-A is decreased and nuchal translucency is increased in pregnancies with trisomy 18 and trisomy 13.

The use of first trimester screening is limited by the need for high-quality equipment and appropriately trained sonographers available to perform nuchal translucency. The availability of chorionic villi sampling as a diagnostic testing option for those who have a positive screening result also places limitations on the use of first trimester screening. Because a program of quality control that includes audit by an external body is necessary to meet the SOGC guidelines, this may also contribute to these limitations. Women who have undergone first trimester screening should also have a second trimester serum alpha fetoprotein screening and/or an ultrasound to screen for open neural tube defect (Chitayat et al., 2011).

Second Trimester Screening

Screening programs offered in the second trimester should offer screens that provide a minimum 75%

NURSING CARE PLAN 11.2

●

The Client Facing Prenatal Diagnosis Options

 As discussed at the beginning of the chapter, April and Alex have conceived after 2 years. During the interview, the nurse notes that April is concerned about her increased risk for chromosomal anomalies, given her "advanced maternal age." April states, "I read that our chance of having a child with Down syndrome has risen to the point that invasive testing is the lesser of the two risks. If we have such testing, what if I am one of the women who miscarries a healthy fetus after an amniocentesis? I could never forgive myself. But if I give birth to a child with Down syndrome, I just don't know how I'll handle it...."

NURSING DIAGNOSES

- **Decisional Conflict** related to personal values and beliefs secondary to lack of knowledge
- **Anxiety** related to increased risks for genetic abnormalities and potential complications associated with prenatal screening and testing

EXPECTED OUTCOMES

1. The couple will identify the advantages and disadvantages of the prenatal diagnosis options.
2. The couple will express concerns about age-related risk and the scope of prenatal testing options.
3. The couple will describe the resources and support needed to make an informed decision.
4. The couple will make a timely and informed decision.

INTERVENTIONS	RATIONALES
Take measures to protect privacy and to facilitate a relaxed atmosphere of trust.	Clients who feel comfortable and accepted and understand that the nurse is maintaining privacy are more likely to be frank about concerns related to prenatal screening and testing.
Include both partners in the discussion; encourage them to work together in the informed decision-making process.	Disturbances in self-esteem, body image, and personal relationships are more likely if clients do not support each other.
Provide education and counselling about the identified risk factors and available diagnostic options.	Lack of information causes stress; in turn, stress fosters the inability to make an informed decision.
Explore the couple's exposure to prenatal screening and testing; assist them to identify and list their fears and concerns; correct any misunderstandings related to these methods; allow time for questions.	Such information provides an additional foundation for teaching and opportunities to clarify or correct misinformation. Unrecognized fears can lead to indecision from not understanding fully the basis of the anxiety.
Review possible options for screening and testing, including risks and benefits of each; provide the couple with written information about the various methods; suggest other sources of information, such as couples who have undergone testing and local community agencies.	Increased knowledge promotes informed decision making. Use of written material allows opportunities for review and discussion. Talking with others who have had similar experiences allows the couple to share feelings and to feel that they are not alone.

(continued)

NURSING CARE PLAN 11.2 ● The Client Facing Prenatal Diagnosis Options (Continued)

INTERVENTIONS	RATIONALES
Encourage the couple to discuss concerns, fears, and beliefs with each other.	Sharing of feelings promotes mutual decision making.
Explore the risks of not deciding.	Prenatal diagnosis has a limited window of opportunity. It requires a timely decision before options become unavailable.
Assure the couple that it is solely their choice about whether to undergo prenatal diagnosis.	The client needs support in a potential decision to *not* pursue prenatal diagnosis.
Explore the couple's ethical and spiritual beliefs; arrange for a possible referral to a spiritual leader or encourage them to speak with a spiritual leader of their choice.	Prenatal diagnosis may include voluntary interruption of pregnancy as one potential outcome. Ethics and values affect the decision whether to terminate a pregnancy. A spiritual leader may assist the couple to understand personal ethics and values in the context of prenatal choice.
Arrange for a follow-up visit with the client and her partner in 2 to 3 weeks.	Follow-up is necessary to determine the couple's progress to a decision and provides opportunities for additional teaching, support, and guidance.

EVALUATION

1. The couple states appropriate information related to prenatal testing and diagnosis.
2. The couple identifies the risks and benefits of prenatal testing.
3. The couple makes an informed choice to participate or not participate in prenatal counselling and diagnosis by the mid second trimester.
4. The couple states that they are comfortable with their decision.

---

detection rate with no more than a 5% false positive rate (Chitayat et al., 2011). Triple screening between 15 and 20 weeks' gestation began in 1991 in Canada, combining maternal age, MSAFP, unconjugated estriol (uE3), and hCG (Chitayat et al., 2011). Triple screening is able to detect 72% of fetuses with Down syndrome with a false positive rate of 7% and also screens for open neural tube defects, other open defects (gastroschisis, oomphalocele), placental dysfunction, Smith–Lemli–Opitz syndrome, and trisomy 18 (Chitayat et al., 2011). Triple screening, however, no longer meets the SOGC guideline of a 75% detection rate for Down syndrome with no more than a 3% false positive rate (Chitayat et al., 2011). When inhibin-A is added, creating a quad screen, the detection rate is increased to 75% to 80% with a false positive rate of 3%, thus meeting the SOGC minimum standard (Chitayat et al., 2011).

Two-Step Integrated Screening

The integrated prenatal screen combines the use of PAPP-A and nuchal translucency in the first trimester and the quad screen in the second trimester to achieve a detection rate of 85% to 87% with a false positive rate of 0.8% to 1.5% (Chitayat et al., 2011). First trimester measurements are usually done between 11 and 14 weeks, as this is the most favourable time for the tests to be done. This narrow time window requires that the pregnancy be accurately dated.

Serum integrated prenatal screening is done when nuchal translucency is not available. It includes PAPP-A tests done in the first trimester and either the triple screen or quad screen in the second trimester. This combination of tests results in a detection rate of 83% with a false positive rate of 4%. Virtually the same performance is achieved with PAPP-A and free β-hCG done in the first trimester and AFP and uE3 in the second trimester (Chitayat et al., 2011).

Cell-Free Fetal DNA

Intact fetal cells and cell-free fetal DNA (cffDNA) have been found in maternal serum, leading to the development of noninvasive prenatal diagnosis of certain conditions (Langlois & Brock, 2013). Fragments of cffDNA, obtained through sampling of maternal serum, have been amplified and sequenced, then mapped to the human genome and analyzed for the frequency and density along each chromosome (Langlois & Brock, 2013). The presence of an overrepresentation of chromosome 21 is highly accurate in detecting fetal Down syndrome (Langlois & Brock, 2013). The detection rate for Down syndrome, in studies conducted and reviewed so far, is very close to 100% with a false positive rate of less than 1%. The same approach has been used to detect other chromosomal abnormalities, specifically trisomy 13 or 18, with less success to date (Langlois & Brock, 2013). While the evidence to date suggests another way to conduct prenatal screening, studies have focused on women in a high-risk category; validation studies of the use of the test in average risk pregnancies are warranted (Langlois & Brock, 2013). Thus, although the development of this screening method is positive in avoiding risks associated with invasive testing, the method should not be considered equivalent to conventional amniocentesis or CVS, which detects 100% of cases of Down Syndrome, trisomy 18, and trisomy 13 (Langlois & Brock, 2013). Since the test currently screens only for Down syndrome, trisomy 13, and trisomy 18, it is not useful for detection of other abnormalities. SOGC recommends that cffDNA should be an option to test for trisomies 21, 13, and 18 and available to women who are at increased risk in lieu of amniocentesis; pretest counselling should include a discussion of the limitations of the testing (Langlois & Brock, 2013). Because there is a risk of a false positive result, SOGC further recommends that "no irrevocable obstetrical decision should be made in pregnancies with a positive noninvasive prenatal testing result without confirmatory invasive diagnostic testing" (Langlois & Brock, 2013, p. 180).

Ultrasound Evaluation

Introduced in the 1970s, ultrasound is a valuable resource for dating a pregnancy and assessing fetal health, appropriate growth, and fetal development (Salem et al., 2014). As a result of advances in this technology, the general public may expect a child's first picture to be an ultrasound snapshot taken during the second trimester. This parental expectation may be the result of news and marketing campaigns that demonstrate the clear depiction of the fetus' individual physical features through the use of three-dimensional

sonographic imaging. However, SOGC and the Canadian Association of Radiologists (CAR) recommend prudent use of the technology with only minimal, medically necessary exposure and "strongly oppose the nonmedical use of fetal ultrasound" (Sierra & Okun, 2014, p. 185). Ultrasound is performed with a transabdominal or transvaginal handheld device called a *transducer.* Sound waves pass through the transducer and abdominal or vaginal wall to bounce off the fetus. The transducer captures a moving ("real-time") or still image of the fetus and sends it back to the ultrasound machine. The image appears as a two- or three-dimensional volume snapshot of the fetus. Three-dimensional imaging transforms sound waves into sculpture-like fetal images that can provide a realistic view of the fetal face (Tache et al., 2008).

Ultrasound is a safe, noninvasive tool with no known teratogenic risks to the mother or fetus. The perceived lack of harm and the availability of routine visualization of the fetus increase the likelihood that a prenatal ultrasound scan will be performed. Nevertheless, the general public often neglects to understand the limitations of ultrasound and the potential for limited diagnostic information if an anomaly is identified. This may lead to parental worry and possible interruption in prenatal parent–fetus bonding. Ultrasound requires the dissemination of information about the potential for unanticipated findings and associated consequences (Research Highlight 11.1).

SOGC recommends that all women should be offered an ultrasound at 18 to 20 weeks' gestation, which should detect most major fetal anatomic anomalies, including open neural tube defects (Chitayat et al., 2011). This ultrasound also detects "soft markers," features that increase the risk of fetal aneuploidy but that can also be variations of normal. Soft markers by themselves do not provide effective discrimination between unaffected fetuses and those with Down syndrome. However, results can be used to modify risks established by age or prior screening when the ultrasound has been done in an established centre that performs tertiary level ultrasound (Chitayat et al., 2011). If ultrasound services are unable to provide comprehensive screening for open neural tube defects, women should be offered MSAFP in the second trimester to provide the screen.

COLLABORATIVE CARE: ULTRASOUND
Assessment

Informed decision making and consent have *not* been traditional components of the performance of ultrasound for screening or diagnosis. The nurse assesses the

● RESEARCH HIGHLIGHT 11.1   A Randomized Trial of a Prenatal Genetic Testing

Interactive Computerized Information Aid

OBJECTIVE

To determine whether an interactive computer program could improve pregnant women's knowledge regarding genetic screening.

DESIGN

150 women who were at 6 to 26 weeks' gestation were randomly assigned to two groups. Women in the two groups were similar in demographic characteristics.

One group received provider-based counselling and the other group received augmented counselling with an interactive computer program that provided information about genetic testing options. Women were tested for content knowledge immediately after the counselling session and again at 2 to 4 weeks.

RESULTS

Women in the computer group correctly answered a significantly greater number of questions than the women in the standard counselling group, both immediately following the session and in the follow-up test.

CONCLUSIONS

A patient-directed interactive computer program may provide a useful tool for provision of relevant information about genetic screening and diagnosis.

From Yee, L. M., Wolf, M., Mullen, R., Bergeron, A. R., Bailey, S. C., Levine, R. et al. (2014). A randomized trial of a prenatal genetic testing interactive computerized information aid. *Prenatal Diagnosis*, Wiley Online Library. doi:10.1002/pd.4347

client's understanding of the scope of potential benefits, risks, and limitations of sonographic imaging before performance of the procedure. Informed consent before screening or diagnostic ultrasound is highly desirable and assists with preparation for any subsequent need to disclose unexpected findings. In addition, real-time two- and three-dimensional volume imaging allows the client to visualize fetal movement before she may experience physical perception.

Early gestation (less than 12 weeks) is visualized using a transvaginal approach (provider preferred for best visualization) or transabdominal approach (requires the woman's bladder to be full to assist with transmission of the sound waves to the fetus). Some clients may not agree to the use of a transvaginal probe for social or cultural reasons. The nurse informs the person performing the scan of the client's preference.

Ultrasound imaging of the second- and third-trimester fetus is generally accomplished using transabdominal ultrasound. The available volume of amniotic fluid precludes the need for a full bladder during these scans.

Select Potential Nursing Diagnoses

The following are examples of potentially applicable diagnoses:

- **Risk for Impaired Parent/Fetal Attachment** related to identification of fetal anomalies

- **Risk for Powerlessness** related to parental perception of inability to alter fetal outcome
- **Deficient Knowledge** related to advantages and disadvantages of fetal sonographic evaluation

Planning/Intervention

Screening during the first trimester includes assessment of gestational age, viability (cardiac activity), number of embryos, size of gestational and yolk sacs, and growth (Fig. 11.7). In addition to these components, trained and accredited sonographers can evaluate nuchal translucency. This structure lies between the skin and soft tissue atop the cervical spine and is evident during 10 to 14 weeks' gestation. An increased nuchal translucency measurement between 11 and 14 weeks correlates highly with an increased risk for fetal chromosome aneuploidy (Nicolaides, 2011). Except in the case of multiple gestation, nuchal translucency should not be offered as a screen without biochemical markers (Chitayat et al., 2011).

Assessment of the fetal nasal bone through ultrasound may be done in the first or second trimester (Chitayat et al., 2011; Nicolaides, 2011). Delayed ossification of the nasal bone has been found to be indicative of Down syndrome in fetuses, with a higher detection rate in the first trimester than in the second trimester (Chitayat et al., 2011; Nicolaides, 2011). Because evaluation of the fetal nasal bone is difficult in the first trimester, SOGC recommends that it should not be incorporated as a screen at this time (Chitayat et al., 2011).

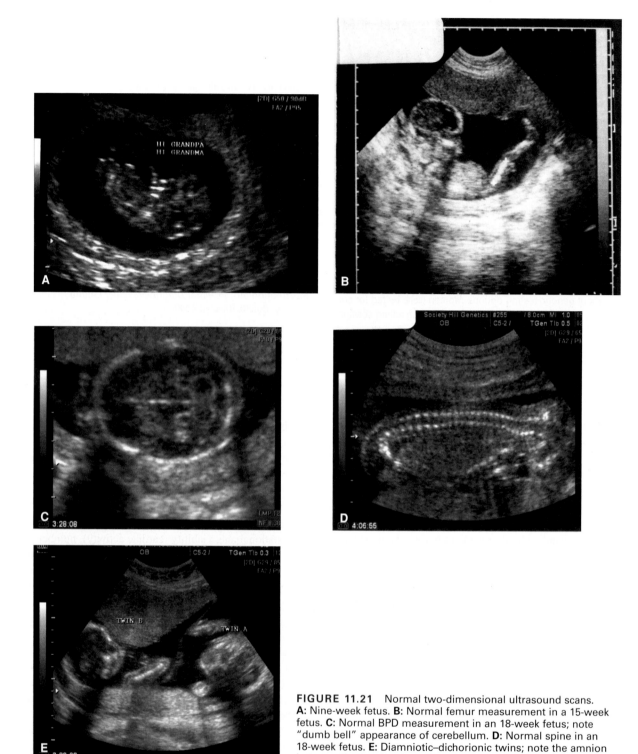

FIGURE 11.21 Normal two-dimensional ultrasound scans.
A: Nine-week fetus. B: Normal femur measurement in a 15-week fetus. C: Normal BPD measurement in an 18-week fetus; note "dumb bell" appearance of cerebellum. D: Normal spine in an 18-week fetus. E: Diamniotic–dichorionic twins; note the amnion between the two heads and arms.

Throughout gestation, ultrasound is used to screen for and diagnose fetal structural anomalies (Box 11.3, Figs. 11.21 and 11.22). The health care practitioner educates and counsels the woman about this technology. It is especially important for the client to understand that the presence of a structural anomaly is a confirmatory diagnosis. The absence of a structural anomaly, however, is not absolute. The procedure may fail to reveal an anomaly as a result of fetal position or limited skill of the person performing the ultrasound scan. The sensitivity and specificity of diagnostic ultrasound continue to advance with ongoing improvement of three-dimensional volume imaging (Fig. 11.23) and yield a declining incidence of false-negative scans.

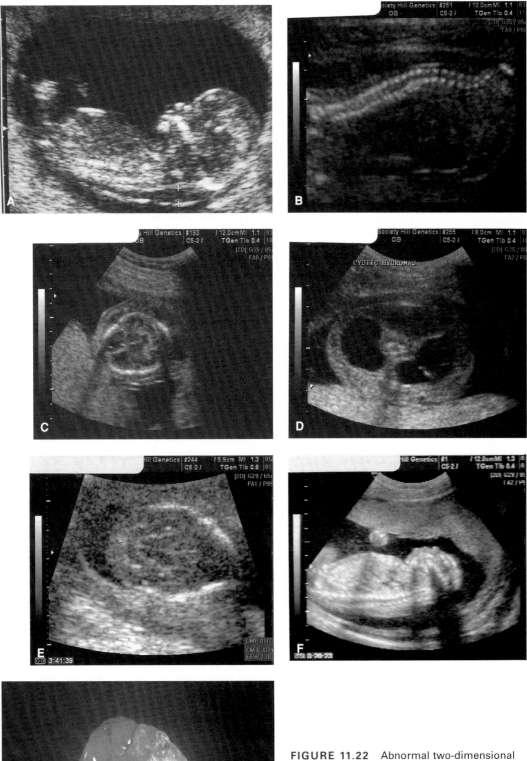

FIGURE 11.22 Abnormal two-dimensional ultrasound scans. **A:** Nuchal fold of 4 mm in a 12-week fetus. **B–D:** Abnormal spine, skull, and cystic hygromas in a 17-week fetus with normal chromosomes. **E:** Abnormal BPD with "banana sign" of the cerebellum and "lemon sign" of the pointed frontal skull in a 16-week fetus. **F:** Anencephalic 21.5-week fetus with normal spine. **G:** Anencephalic abortus. (Courtesy of S. Majewski and A. Donnenfeld.)

● BOX 11.3   Selected Examples of Structural Defects that Ultrasound Imaging can Confirm

Agenesis of the corpus callosum
Anencephaly
Cardiac malformations
Cerebellar hypoplasia
Cleft lip
Cleft palate
Clubfoot
Conjoined twins
Cystic hygroma
Diaphragmatic hernia
Duodenal atresia
Encephalocele
Exomphalos
Genital anomalies
Holoprosencephaly
Hydrocephalus
Neural tube defects
Nuchal edema
Nonimmune hydrops
Obstructive uropathy
Omphalocele
Polycystic kidney disease
Polydactyly
Radial ray defects

Evaluation

Evaluation of the knowledge and expectations of the couple who seeks or is referred for gestation ultrasound are of significant importance to the process of informed decision making, the client's comfort and well-being, and the undisrupted preservation of the growing bond between the parent and fetus. Evaluation of the couple's knowledge and understanding of possible follow-up interventions are also required.

Invasive Diagnostic Tests

In the past, invasive testing was recommended to women in Canada when the risk of having a pregnancy with a chromosomal anomaly was greater than the risk associated with the invasive testing procedure (Wilson et al., 2007). However, the advent of improved noninvasive serum and ultrasound screening facilitates identification of pregnancies at a high enough risk to warrant invasive testing, even with a risk of pregnancy loss (Chitayat et al., 2011). Invasive diagnostic tests are used to confirm or to eliminate suspected anomalies among those women who have a positive screening test. The most common invasive prenatal tests available to evaluate fetal chromosomes or genes include CVS and amniocentesis. Each is performed to obtain a specimen for analysis and evaluation. Given their invasive nature, neither is performed

unless there are multiple marker screening results above the designated cut-off point or unless the woman is over the age of 40 (Wilson, 2007) (Table 11.7).

Ultrasound is the method of choice for detection of anatomical problems but provides no information on genetic issues (Alfirevic et al., 2009). However, physicians use ultrasound to assist with the safe performance of amniocentesis and CVS. The health care practitioner educates and counsels the client about each procedure, the benefit of adjunct sonography in the reduction of fetal risk, and the risk associated with both the potential "background" risk that is inherent with the stage of pregnancy and the additional risk associated with the procedure (Wilson, 2007). He or she shares with the client the importance of understanding the scope of identifiable findings in this nondiagnostic use of sonography to ensure informed decision making and consent.

Amniocentesis. *Amniocentesis* (often referred to simply as "amnio") became available in the clinical setting in the 1960s, following closely behind the confirmation of the correct number of chromosomes in the human genome. The establishment of the positive correlation between advanced maternal age and increased risk for birth of a child with a chromosomal anomaly provided further impetus for the adoption and integration of this technology as a standard of care within the prenatal setting (Nussbaum et al., 2007). Amniocentesis done in the second trimester is safer than amniocentesis done in the first trimester, which poses a higher risk of spontaneous abortion and deformed or club foot. Transcervical CVS increases the risk of pregnancy loss compared with the risk of second trimester amniocentesis (Alfirevic et al., 2009; Cunningham et al., 2010; Dugoff, 2008).

Ultrasound is performed before the amniocentesis to determine fetal viability, gestational age, location of the placenta, number of fetuses, and fetal anatomy (Dugoff, 2008). During amniocentesis, a needle is inserted through the maternal abdominal and uterine walls to place the needle tip within the amniotic sac in a space filled with amniotic fluid and free of fetal parts (Fig. 11.24). Concurrent ultrasound is used to identify an appropriate site and to guide the needle to that area safely. Approximately 1 mL for each week of gestation up to a maximum of 20 mL of amniotic fluid is withdrawn (the initial 1 to 2 mL is discarded to prevent contamination with maternal cells) (Cunningham et al., 2010). The developing skin of the fetus sheds cells into the amniotic fluid. These cells are separated from the amniotic fluid, grown in laboratory culture dishes, and analyzed for chromosomal (method: cytogenetic analysis) or single gene (method: molecular genetic analysis) disorders. The amniotic fluid is used to determine the level of MSAFP. A third-trimester amniocentesis can be performed to assess the lecithin-to-sphingomyelin (L/S)

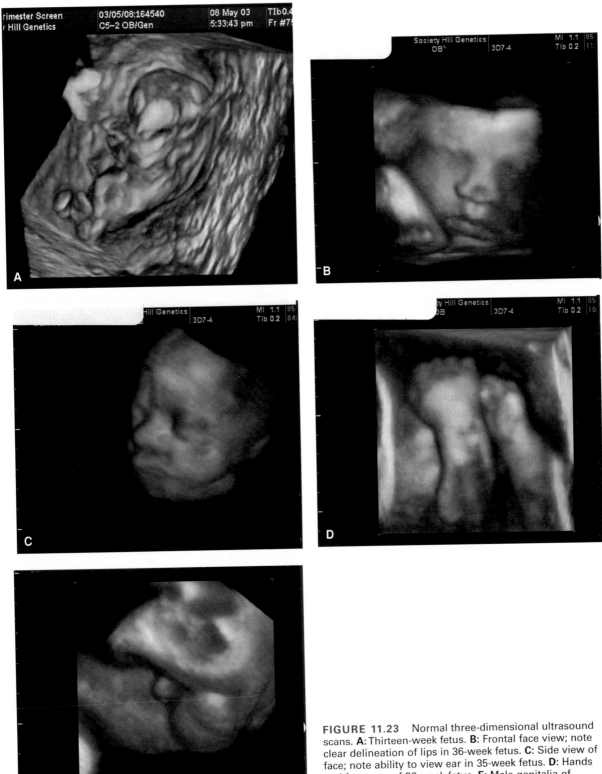

FIGURE 11.23 Normal three-dimensional ultrasound scans. **A:** Thirteen-week fetus. **B:** Frontal face view; note clear delineation of lips in 36-week fetus. **C:** Side view of face; note ability to view ear in 35-week fetus. **D:** Hands and forearms of 36-week fetus. **E:** Male genitalia of 29-week fetus. (Courtesy of S. Majewski.)

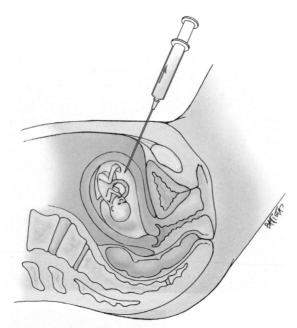

FIGURE 11.24 Amniocentesis.

ratio or the TDx-FLM II, which assesses the surfactant (mg) to albumin (g) ratio to evaluate fetal lung maturity in the gestation at risk for preterm delivery.

Following amniocentesis, the client may experience some vaginal spotting and leakage of amniotic fluid (Cunningham et al., 2010). Complications can include amnionitis and needle puncture of the fetus (Dugoff, 2008).

Chorionic Villus Sampling. CVS is another test used in the first trimester to evaluate fetal karyotype and

molecular and biochemical abnormalities. It is typically performed between 10 and 13 weeks' gestation (Cunningham et al., 2010; Dugoff, 2008). It may be done transvaginally or transabdominally (Cunningham et al., 2010). Contraindications include vaginal bleeding or spotting, active genital tract infection, or any structural anomalies that may preclude easy access or visualization of the uterus or its contents (Cunningham et al., 2010).

As with amniocentesis, an ultrasound is initially done to assess fetal viability, gestational age, and placental position (Dugoff, 2008). While using ultrasound concurrently for continuous observation, performance of CVS is completed by applying gentle syringe suction through a needle (transabdominal approach) or catheter (transvaginal approach) to detach chorionic villi tissue from the site of the developing placenta (Fig. 11.25). Similar to amniocentesis, cytogenetic and molecular genetic testing is performed on the tissue. Because CVS is done at an earlier gestational age than amniocentesis and different techniques allow for more rapid analysis, earlier results can be obtained. This decreases parental concern and anxiety when results are normal (Cunningham et al., 2010). If the results indicate a chromosomal or DNA abnormality that results in a parental request for termination of the pregnancy, some of the complications and stresses associated with termination at a later gestational age may be lessened (Cunningham et al., 2010; Dugoff, 2008).

Following CVS, the client may experience some postprocedure spotting or bleeding (more common with the transvaginal technique), or increased uterine

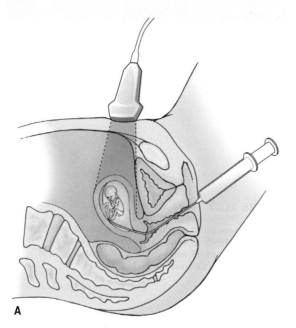

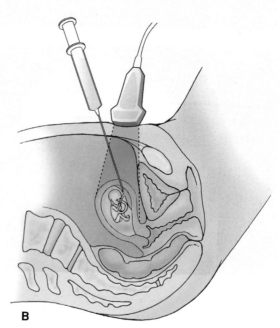

FIGURE 11.25 Chorionic villus sampling. **A:** Transvaginal sampling. **B:** Transabdominal sampling.

discomfort and cramping (more common with the transabdominal technique). There is an increased risk for pregnancy loss with CVS, slightly higher than with amniocentesis (Dugoff, 2008).

COLLABORATIVE CARE: INVASIVE DIAGNOSTIC TESTS

Assessment

Positive prenatal screening may be an indication for invasive prenatal diagnosis. CVS at 10 to 14 weeks is offered with a positive first trimester screen; amniocentesis is offered after 15 weeks for a positive first or second trimester screen. Before performance of or referral for invasive prenatal diagnostic services, the health care practitioner assesses the client's knowledge and understanding of each procedure. Informed decision making and consent are an integral component of this process and direct the type and level of assessment performed and should be nondirective. It is the responsibility of the health care practitioner to respect a woman's choice to accept or to refuse any or all testing or options offered at any point (Chitayat et al., 2011).

Select Potential Nursing Diagnoses

The following are examples of potentially applicable diagnoses:

- **Decisional Conflict** related to scope of treatment options
- **Risk for Infection** related to performance of invasive procedures
- **Anticipatory Grieving** related to identification of a fetal anomaly and "loss" of expected healthy child

Planning/Intervention

As knowledge of genetics advances, the ability to provide appropriate and disorder-specific prenatal genetic counselling and diagnosis increases. It is incumbent on nurses to integrate this developing body of clinical genetics knowledge and associated nursing care implications into professional practice. A limited number of centres throughout Canada perform CVS; however, amniocentesis is usually available in primary obstetrical settings. The nurse assisting with these procedures ensures sterile technique to minimize the potential for a maternal or fetal infection following amniocentesis or CVS.

Most people do not perceive the field of clinical genetics, and specifically, prenatal genetics, as eugenic. Clients opposed to prenatal genetic diagnosis may assume that they are required to terminate a pregnancy if a genetic anomaly is identified (Harper, 2010). Sometimes, family, social, cultural, or religious communities impose such perceptions. The nurse provides supportive counselling and teaching to assist clients to make an informed decision about services they wish to pursue. Although the prognosis for most genetic disorders or congenital anomalies cannot be altered, many people desire prenatal genetic counselling and diagnosis to prepare for the birth of a child with special needs. This includes learning about specialized care, programs available to assist with care, and determination of the best location and method for delivery of the child (i.e., choosing a hospital with an established neonatal intensive care unit versus a hospital with a level I newborn nursery, or consideration of cesarean versus vaginal birth).

A limited number of identified disorders are amenable to prenatal treatment and therapy. The health care provider assists clients to assess the risk and burden of the prenatally untreated disorder in comparison to the risk and benefit of prenatal treatment. If clients and health care providers perceive the long-term benefit to the fetus who is a candidate for prenatal treatment to outweigh the immediate risk, then the nurse assists by coordinating referral services for this highly specialized prenatal health care. An example is the fetus identified with urinary bladder outlet obstruction. It is critical for the fetus to void in utero to ensure the necessary volume of amniotic fluid for proper musculoskeletal development, as well as reduction of kidney damage subsequent to the blockage of urinary explosion. Prenatal treatment may include the placement of a vesicoamniotic shunt performed under ultrasound guidance; this treatment is currently being re-evaluated for effectiveness (Farrugia & Woolf, 2010).

Nurses expect that clients who seek prenatal genetic counselling and diagnosis desire the birth of a child without genetic disorders or congenital anomalies. The nurse assesses expectations to ensure a collective understanding of viewpoints by client and partner, as well as health care providers. For example, researchers describe the preferential desire of some people within the deaf community to have children with hearing impairment (Martini et al., 2007). The nurse carefully evaluates his or her own values and beliefs to ensure the provision of nondirective, nonjudgemental care to clients who desire an alternative outcome for their child.

Evaluation

The focal point for evaluation of the interventions associated with prenatal invasive procedures is the assessment of the informed decision making and consent processes requisite to the education, counselling, or performance of these tests. The nurse evaluates all interventions initiated for completion and success in the establishment or maintenance of the comfort and well-being perceived by the client.

Preimplantation Genetic Diagnosis and Related Technologies

Multiple marker screening, ultrasound, CVS, and amniocentesis are recognized and readily available methods of prenatal screening and diagnosis. All these procedures share one common disadvantage: each is performed after the fetus is well established within the uterus. If prenatal screening and diagnosis identifies a fetal anomaly, options available to the client are limited. Historically, clients known to be at risk for transmission of a genetic disorder to their child before conception have had five reproductive options: adopting, choosing to have no children, using donor gametes, chancing the conception and birth of a child free of the genetic disorder, and undergoing prenatal diagnosis with prenatal choice about whether to continue or to terminate a pregnancy found to have a genetic disorder. For some people, none of these reproductive alternatives is acceptable within the context of their social, cultural, or religious community. For others, selective termination is the least harmful choice in a set of emotional land mines.

Together, the development of in vitro fertilization (IVF) (see Chapter 10) and advances in molecular genetics provide a sixth reproductive alternative. *Preimplantation genetic diagnosis* is the genetic evaluation of the early, cleavage-stage embryo created through IVF for chromosomal aneuploidy and genetic defects (Sierra & Okun, 2014). First described in 1990, preimplantation genetic diagnosis may be performed on the third day of early embryonic development, although some centres routinely perform it on day 5 (Sierra & Okun, 2014).

COLLABORATIVE CARE: PREIMPLANTATION GENETIC DIAGNOSIS

Assessment

Preimplantation genetic diagnosis provides a reproductive alternative for those opposed to clinical interruption of a pregnancy. Clients identified through preconception assessment to be at risk for transmission of a genetic disorder are referred to a specialist in genetics who should offer nondirective genetic counselling (Sierra & Okun, 2014). The genetics specialist assists the client and her reproductive partner to make an informed decision about reproductive options and alternatives to preimplantation genetic diagnosis (Sierra & Okun, 2014) by providing information and counselling, including information about the reliability, significance, and limitations of this testing.

Select Potential Nursing Diagnoses

The following are examples of potentially applicable diagnoses:

- **Spiritual Distress** related to perceived status of the human embryo
- **Dysfunctional Grieving** related to desire for a "healthy" child
- **Ineffective Sexuality Patterns** related to fear of conception and transmission of genetic risk to a biologic child

Planning/Intervention

Dissemination of information and discussion about preimplantation genetic diagnosis occurs prior to conception so that it can be considered a reproductive option. Once a pregnancy is confirmed, preimplantation genetic diagnosis is no longer a viable alternative. The health care provider in the preconception setting provides this information to the family. If a client presents after conceiving, the health care provider identifies an appropriate time to apprise her of this reproductive alternative for consideration before any future conception.

Evaluation

Evaluation varies according to the individualized plan of care and related interventions. The nurse assesses the client's response to the information and interventions and provides additional education, counselling, support, and referral, as indicated.

POSTNATAL SCREENING AND DIAGNOSTIC PROCEDURES

For most clients, the birth of a child is a special and memorable event. They anxiously await confirmation from their obstetric and pediatric care providers of the child's gender and health. The obstetric care providers initially assess newborns in the delivery room; other health care providers complete more comprehensive evaluations after transfer of the baby to the newborn nursery or, if necessary, the neonatal intensive care unit (see Chapters 20 and 22). Initial assessment focuses on clinical markers included in the Apgar score (colour, respiratory effort, muscle tone, heart rate, and reflex irritability) and physical appearance. Comprehensive evaluation includes a head-to-toe assessment of all body systems.

Two facets of newborn assessment require knowledge of genetic principles and their associated clinical implications: newborn screening for inherited metabolic and hearing disorders, and evaluation of the newborn with one or more dysmorphic features. If an abnormality is identified, the family unit typically is referred for follow-up with a genetics specialist.

Newborn Screening Programs

The original and primary purpose of a newborn screening program is to identify genetic disorders (typically resulting in altered biochemical function) and to institute treatment before the onset of clinical symptoms (Grosse et al., 2010). Universal newborn screening in Canada is under provincial and territorial jurisdiction; the number of diseases screened for varies among them. There are also variations in the ability of jurisdictions to provide follow-up and treatment as well as to cover the costs associated with treatments (Therrell & Adams, 2007). In addition to screening for metabolic disorders, newborn hearing screening is advocated. Most provinces and territories have screening programs offered to select populations. All jurisdictions screen for congenital hypothyroidism and phenylketonuria; Saskatchewan is the only one where this is a legal requirement (Morrison & Dowler, 2011). British Columbia, Alberta, Saskatchewan, Ontario, Yukon, and the Kitikmeot region of Nunavut screen for cystic fibrosis (Morrison & Dowler, 2011).

Since newborn screening programs are regulated and managed at the provincial level, national consistency is limited in relation to the disorders included in individual screening programs, the delivery of services, and the retention period for samples (Morrison & Dowler, 2011). Testing methods are similar among programs. In contrast, the principles that guide the development, establishment, and continuation of a newborn screening program are universal and well established (Box 11.4). Chapter 20 discusses newborn screening in more detail.

Dysmorphology Assessment

Dysmorphology, the branch of clinical genetics that specializes in birth defects, diagnoses a child with a birth defect, suggests further diagnostic evaluations, gives

prognostic information about the range of outcomes that could be expected, develops a plan to manage the expected complications, provides the family with an understanding of the causation of the malformation, and gives recurrence risks to the parents and other relatives (Nussbaum et al., 2007). It is the most rapidly growing area within clinical genetics as a result of advances in molecular DNA analysis that permit identification of the genotypes of many disorders previously categorized solely according to phenotype expression. A dysmorphologic assessment is used to evaluate stillborn infants, newborns, children, and adults with disorders thought to result from a malformation, deformation, or disruption in development caused by altered genes, chromosomal rearrangements, or in utero teratogen exposure.

COLLABORATIVE CARE: DYSMORPHOLOGY ASSESSMENT

A dysmorphic feature is an abnormality of shape, size, or structure. Each finding is traditionally classified as minor or major. If an infant is found to have two minor dysmorphic features, the health care provider carefully assesses for one or more major anomalies that may not be readily apparent. This is especially important if three or more minor anomalies are identified. A cluster of dysmorphologic features may be categorized as a syndrome, sequence, or association (see Embryonic Development).

Assessment

The nurse determines whether a comprehensive family, medical, and reproductive history was completed in the preconception or prenatal setting. If the parent acknowledges this assessment and evaluation, the nurse assists in procuring this information. If it does not exist, then the nurse requests that the woman and her reproductive partner complete a health assessment questionnaire. The construction and review of a three- or four-generation genogram is especially important.

A careful review of the pregnancy history specific to the conception and birth of the person under evaluation is critical to the differential diagnosis in cases of a suspected genetic or environmental cause for dysmorphic findings. For example, infants with fetal alcohol spectrum disorder can have cardiac malformations (e.g., ventricular septal defect), central nervous system anomalies (e.g., microcephaly), facial abnormalities (e.g., micrognathia), truncal and skeletal anomalies (e.g., diaphragmatic hernia), and genitourinary malformations (e.g., hypoplastic external genitalia). Similarly, DiGeorge syndrome (velocardiofacial syndrome) is characterized by conotruncal abnormalities (e.g., tetralogy of Fallot), facial abnormalities (e.g., micrognathia), renal obstruction, thymic disorders (absent), and diaphragmatic hernia. Fetal alcohol

● **BOX 11.4** **Key Elements of a Newborn Screening Program**

1. Treatment is available.
2. Early intervention prevents morbidity and mortality.
3. A test is required to identify the disorder in a timely manner.
4. The test is highly sensitive (no false-negative results) and reasonably specific (limited false-positive results).
5. Frequency and severity of the disorder warrant identification.
6. Available infrastructure includes:
   a. Parental education (and consent if required)
   b. Timing screening
   c. Follow-up programs
   d. Referral resources
   e. Accurate data collection systems
   f. Access to interventions and treatment
   g. Policies to protect confidentiality and privacy

spectrum disorder results from the ingestion of alcohol by the woman during her pregnancy and has a 0% recurrence risk if the same woman does not consume alcohol in any future pregnancy. DiGeorge syndrome results from a microdeletion of the "q" arm of chromosome 22, and has a 50% recurrence if the microdeletion also is identified in the parents (McDonald-McGinn & Sullivan, 2011).

Physical examination is the primary tool of a dysmorphologic evaluation. The nurse precisely measures height, weight, head, neck, face, eyes, limbs, hands, feet, and trunk. He or she records information about the appearance of the skin, nails, teeth, genitalia, and cry. This permits accurate analysis of serial observations of these findings. Photography in conjunction with precise measurements provides the most accurate documentation of the findings. The nurse educates, counsels, and reassures the woman, child, or man of the importance of this method of documentation, although highly sensitive and personal. In addition, radiography is used to assess bone density and structure to rule out disorders such as lethal bone dysplasias and osteogenesis imperfecta. Cytogenetic, biochemical, and DNA analyses are also performed as part of the dysmorphologic assessment to confirm or rule out a genetic basis. It is particularly important to perform an autopsy on a stillborn infant to evaluate the structure and formation of internal organs, the site of many major malformations.

Select Potential Nursing Diagnoses

The following are examples of potentially applicable diagnoses:

- **Chronic Sorrow** related to recurring feelings of loss of a healthy child
- **Caregiver Role Strain** related to overwhelming daily needs of infant
- **Social Isolation** related to uncertainty that others will accept the infant

Planning/Intervention

Some obstetric and pediatric providers believe that the completion of a dysmorphologic evaluation does not contribute to the child's welfare and provides only an academic research opportunity for the dysmorphologist. In fact, dysmorphologic evaluations are important to provide if multiple minor or major anomalies are identified, including for deceased or stillborn infants. The correct diagnosis permits dissemination of appropriate and accurate information about recurrence risk for a future pregnancy. It also reduces the likelihood of a child being labelled with an incorrect diagnosis, leading to potential life-threatening or life-restricting events. For example, the person diagnosed with fetal alcohol spectrum disorder has cognitive challenges, whereas the person with DiGeorge syndrome does not. A reversal of these diagnoses can profoundly affect long-term well-being.

The parents of children diagnosed with genetic or congenital disorders may experience **chronic sorrow**. The nurse assists these clients to identify community resources to assist with daily care, health requirements, and educational needs. He or she provides information about parent support groups, respite care, school programs, and public health services. Given that the resources provided or mandated vary widely among provinces, the nurse becomes familiar with his or her provincial or territorial program to assist the family with the identification of, navigation through, and coordination of services. The nurse also assists the family by aligning services with the language, social, cultural, and religious beliefs of the identified community.

Evaluation

Evaluation is based on the individualized plan of care for each woman, man, or child. Evaluation of the perceived success of the available resources and programs within the community is essential. Ongoing evaluation of the family unit is central to this process to ensure that members are accessing the appropriate services.

SUMMARY

- Variation is the life-cycle outcome of each person's unique response to nature and nurture beginning before conception and ending with death.
- *Somatic cells* make up every organ and system and maintain growth, development, and well-being. *Germ cells* are the reproductive cells of the ovary and testis; their function is preservation through replication of the human species.
- Each chromosome consists of DNA, proteins, and a small amount of RNA. Genes, the basic units of heredity, are located along the DNA of each chromosome. Each gene is a unique sequence formed from the nucleotides along the DNA strands.
- A change in the genetic code may or may not alter the product coded for by that gene. An alteration will be expressed as a change in growth, development, wellness, life expectancy, or all these factors.
- *Mitosis* is the body's natural process of growth and development performed in association with cellular repair and replacement. *Meiosis* is the unique cell division that occurs in the diploid germ cells to produce gamete cells containing only 23 chromosomes.
- Male germ cells remain dormant in the testes until puberty. Then, the life cycle of each sperm is approximately 75 to 90 days. Female embryos begin differentiation of the germ cells after the primitive ovary

forms. Oogonia remain suspended until puberty; over the next 40 years, oocytes develop as part of the menstrual cycle.

- The oocyte can fuse with sperm for only 24 hours after ovulation. Sperm survive no more than 72 hours after they are deposited in the female reproductive tract.

- Once the zygote begins to cleave (mitotic cellular division), it is referred to as an embryo. The number of cells visible microscopically is used to describe the stage of embryo development.

- Before formation of the blastocyst (5 to 7 days after fertilization), each blastomere can differentiate into any type of tissue (totipotency). With differentiation, totipotency is lost.

- Normally, the blastocyst implants on either the anterior or posterior wall of the main uterine body. The placenta thus develops embedded within tissue prepared for the invasive fusion of the trophoblast and fetal growth to full term.

- The two primary functions of the placenta are exchange of metabolic and gaseous products between the fetal and maternal circulatory systems, and production of hormones necessary for fetal development and continuation of gestation.

- Amniotic fluid surrounds and protects the developing fetus. It separates the fetus from other placental membranes, providing for the movement critical to normal fetal growth and development. Without adequate amniotic fluid, fetal malformations occur.

- Differentiation of the four-chamber heart and associated valves is complete by the 8th embryologic week.

- The *ectoderm* gives rise to the peripheral nervous system; sensory epithelium of the nose, eye, and ear; epidermis; subcutaneous, mammary, and pituitary glands; and tooth enamel. The *mesoderm* gives rise to cartilage and bone; striated and smooth muscles; skin cells; excretory components of the urinary and reproductive systems; serous membranes of the peritoneal, parietal, and pericardial cavities; spleen; blood vessels; and blood. The *endoderm* gives rise to the gastrointestinal tract; parenchyma of the thyroid, parathyroids, liver, and pancreas; epithelial lining of the respiratory tract, urinary bladder, urethra, tympanic cavity, and auditory tube; tonsils; and thymus gland.

- The incidence of major structural congenital anomalies at birth is 2% to 3% and rises to 4% to 6% by 5 years of age, when additional findings are identified upon admittance to school. Anomalies are classified as malformations, disruptions, or deformations and may be part of a syndrome, association, or sequence event.

- Multiple gestations have risen sharply over the past 2 decades. Monozygotic gestations result from altered zygote development. They share the same genotype, although exposure to different environmental factors throughout their lives may result in different phenotypes. Dizygotic gestations share the same genetic relationship as any siblings born to the same genetic mother and father.

- The goal of genetic counselling is to provide appropriate, accurate, and nondirective information so that clients can make informed decisions about their own and their children's health and health care.

- Preconception health assessment may elicit sensitive, private, and highly confidential information. It has the profound potential to alter a client's self-image and relationships.

- Informed decision making links the goals of preconception screening and counselling with the principles of autonomy, justice, and beneficence to ensure appropriate management of genetic information.

- Each step of the health assessment should be preceded by an explanation of the process, information that may be learned, and possible implications of that knowledge; and the opportunity for dialogue between the client, the reproductive care partner, and the health care provider.

- Multifactorial inheritance is the expression of a phenotypic trait regulated by multiple genes and their interaction with environmental factors. It is the most common form of inheritance in the general population.

- Chromosomal rearrangements are categorized as alterations in either number or structure.

- Aneuploidy increases as maternal age advances. This results in a higher rate of pregnancy loss and birth of infants with chromosome anomalies.

- Advanced paternal age is associated with increased incidence of spontaneous new mutations in the fetus.

- Congenital or acquired malformations of the reproductive organs, loss of ovarian or testicular reserve, irregular menstrual cycle, infections, autoimmune disorders, and hormonal imbalances may result in the inability to conceive, carry a pregnancy to term, or both.

- Recurrent miscarriage is the loss of three or more pregnancies before 20 weeks' gestation.

- *Screening* typically is used to assess large populations to identify individuals in the population at higher risk for a particular disorder, using (a) specific marker(s) and a defined screening cut-off level. *Invasive diagnostic tests* generally are used to confirm or eliminate suspected anomalies among clients who have screened positive for a particular disorder.

- Invasive diagnostic tests available to evaluate fetal chromosomes, genes, or blood chemistry are CVS and amniocentesis.

- The primary purpose of newborn screening is to identify genetic disorders and institute treatment in the newborn before the onset of clinical symptoms.
- A dysmorphologic assessment can evaluate stillborns, infants, children, and adults with disorders thought to result from a malformation, deformation, or disruption in development from altered genes, chromosomal rearrangements, or in utero teratogen exposure.

Questions to Ponder

1. A woman and her reproductive partner come for preconception counselling. The nurse performs a preconception health risk assessment and evaluation. The results show that both carry the ΔF508 mutation of the *CFTR* gene associated with CF. The couple does not wish to have a child with CF. They request information about the scope of available reproductive options, but are concerned that their family and religious community will not support any choice they make.
   - What information should the nurse be aware of before responding to the couple about their reproductive options?
   - What support might help the couple as they process the information and choose an appropriate reproductive alternative?
   - What are your personal feelings about prenatal diagnosis and choice (therapeutic termination of a pregnancy)?
2. A young couple, both 28 years old, reports a paternal family history of Huntington disease. The mother of the young man, diagnosed with Huntington disease at 45 years old, is now in an assisted living facility because of the severity of her neuromuscular degeneration. The young man's two older siblings had DNA analysis performed, and both have received the Huntington disease gene, although neither is currently symptomatic. This couple very much wants to have a child without the Huntington disease gene and prefers that they both are the genetic parents of the child. The young man does not want to know his Huntington disease status; he currently has no manifestations of Huntington disease. They have heard about nondisclosure of preimplantation genetic diagnosis as a way to achieve these dual goals. They state that they want preliminary information from a primary care provider before seeking out a preimplantation genetic diagnosis program.
   - What are your personal feelings about facilitating someone to have preimplantation genetic diagnosis when there is a reasonable likelihood that embryos found to have the Huntington disease gene will be disposed of and not transferred to the woman's uterus?
   - Do you believe that someone can make an informed choice not to be informed?
   - What information do you need to know before responding to the couple?
   - What are your views about effectively communicating the current state of knowledge about the risk factors and lack of long-term knowledge associated with preimplantation genetics?

REVIEW QUESTIONS

1. A client presents with a clinical diagnosis of tuberous sclerosis. To determine his or her phenotype, which method of assessment would the nurse expect to be used?
   A. Construction and review of a genogram
   B. Chromosome analysis
   C. Direct DNA analysis
   D. Physical examination and evaluation
2. A woman gives birth to twins. The provider informs the woman that the children are likely dizygotic. This information is best determined by
   A. identification of one distinct placenta and one bag of water.
   B. identification of one distinct placenta and two separate bags of water.
   C. identification of two distinct placentas and two separate bags of water.
   D. same gender for both infants.
3. Parents of monozygotic twins ask if the children will experience identical growth and development. To best answer the parents, the nurse should explain
   A. each infant shares the same genotype and phenotype; thus, growth and development can be expected to be identical.
   B. each infant shares the same genotype, but the environment will alter phenotype; thus, growth and development may vary.
   C. each infant has a different genotype, but the same phenotype; thus, growth and development will not vary.
   D. each infant is the same as any other two siblings and will have variable growth and development.
4. The placenta functions to
   A. prevent passage of antibodies from mother to child.
   B. provide a direct exchange of blood between mother and child.
   C. provide an exchange of metabolic and gaseous products between mother and child.
   D. prevent passage of teratogenic agents from mother to child.

5. A 32-year-old woman comes to the clinic and reports a history of three pregnancy losses before 12 weeks' gestation. She would like to become pregnant again, but is anxious that she may spontaneously abort. To determine an appropriate plan for this woman, the nurse should next
   A. ask whether chromosome analysis was performed on any of the abortuses.
   B. construct a family genogram.
   C. obtain a peripheral blood sample for chromosome analysis.
   D. obtain a peripheral blood sample for serum hormone analysis.

6. A 28-year-old woman comes for counselling after receiving abnormal results on her quad screen at 15 weeks' gestation. To determine an appropriate plan for this woman, the nurse should next
   A. confirm gestational age and viability.
   B. refer the woman for genetic counselling.
   C. refer the woman for amniocentesis.
   D. obtain a new specimen and repeat the analysis.

7. A Caucasian woman comes for prenatal care. Her family history is negative for any known incidence of a genetic disorder. Her immediate plan of care should include
   A. collection of a blood sample for cystic fibrosis mutation screening.
   B. construction of a genogram.
   C. education about her risk to be a carrier for CF and the availability of a screening test.
   D. no further education about genetic risk factors.

8. A 37-year-old woman presents for prenatal care at 7 weeks' gestation. She requests information about CVS and wants to know when this procedure is best performed. The nurse correctly shares that CVS is performed at
   A. 6 to 8 weeks of gestation.
   B. 8 to 9 weeks of gestation.
   C. 10 to 12 weeks of gestation.
   D. 15 to 16 weeks of gestation.

9. A client arrives for an amniocentesis following a positive quad screening at 17 weeks' gestation. Which of the following would be appropriate to include in teaching associated with the amniocentesis?
   A. There is no pain associated with the test during or following.
   B. She will need to have a full bladder for the test.
   C. Although small, there is a risk of pregnancy loss associated with the test.
   D. An ultrasound will be done following the test.

10. A nurse is performing a home visit for a new mother and baby. After assessing health and breastfeeding ability, the most important inquiry the nurse should make is

   A. how much support the woman is receiving from family and friends.
   B. if a blood sample was obtained from the infant for newborn screening.
   C. if the infant is being supplemented with formula.
   D. if the mother can sleep when the infant sleeps.

REFERENCES

Alberts, B. (2003). DNA replication and recombination. *Nature, 421*(6921), 431–435.

Alfirevic, Z., Mujezinovic, R., & Sundberg, K. (2009). Amniocentesis and chorionic villus sampling for prenatal diagnosis. *Cochrane Database of Systematic Reviews, 2003*(3), CD003252. doi:10.1002/14651858.CD003252.

Allison, L. A. (2012). *Fundamental molecular biology* (2nd ed.). Malden, MA: Blackwell Publishing.

Amos, J., Feldman, G. L., Grody, W. W., Monaghan, K., Palomaki, G. E., Prior, T. W., et al. (2011). Standards and guidelines for clinical genetic laboratories. *American College of Medical Genetics.* Retrieved from http://res.illumina.com/documents/reimbursement/acmg-cftr-testing-standards-and-guidelines_2011.pdf

Aziz, N. A., Jurgens, C. K., Landwehrmeyer, G. B., van Roon-Mom, W. M. C., van Ommen, G. J. B., Stijnen, T., et al. (2011). Normal and mutant HTT interact to affect clinical severity and progression in Huntington disease. *Neurology, 73*, 1280–1285, Erratum: Neurology 73: 1608 only, 2009; Erratum: Neurology 76: 202 only, 2011.

Bhandari, A., Sandlow, J. I., & Brannigan, R. E. (2013). Risks to offspring associated with advanced paternal age. *Journal of Andrology, 32*(2), 121–122. doi:10.2164/jandrol.110.010595

Bokhare, S. F., Zinon, W. M. N. W., & Talib, A. Z. (2014). A study on visual representation of medical family tree using genograms. *The 2013 International conferences on computer Graphics, visualization, Computer vision, and Game Technology.* Atlantis Press.

Canadian Cystic Fibrosis Foundation. (nd). About cystic fibrosis. Retrieved from http://www.cysticfibrosis.ca/about-cf/what-is-cystic-fibrosis/?lang=en

Centers for Disease Control and Prevention. (2014). *Multiple births.* Hyattsville, MD: National Center for Health Statistics. Retrieved from http://www.cdc.gov/nchs/fastats/multiple.htm

Chitayat, D., Langlois, S., & Wilson, R. D. (2011). Society of Obstetricians and Gynaecologists of Canada (SOGC) Canadian College of Medical Geneticists (CCMG) Clinical practice guideline: Prenatal screening for fetal aneuploidy in singleton pregnancies. *Journal of Obstetrics and Gynaecology of Canada, 33*(7), 736–750.

Collins, F. S., Green, E. D., Guttmacher, A. E., & Guyer, M. S. (2003). A vision for the future of genomics research: A blueprint for the genomic era. *Nature, 422*(6934), 835–847.

Cunningham, F. G., Leveno, K. J., Bloom, S. L., Hauth, J. C., Gilstrap, L. C., & Wenstrom, K. D. (2010). *Williams obstetrics* (23rd ed.). New York: McGraw Hill.

Dugoff, L. (2008). Prenatal diagnosis. In R. S. Gibbs, B. Y. Karlan, A. F. Haney, & I. Nygaard (Eds.), *Danforth's obstetrics and gynecology* (10th ed.). Philadelphia, PA: Lippincott Williams & Wilkins.

Ebrahim, S. H., Kulkarni, R., Parker, C., & Atrash, H. K. (2010). Blood disorders among women: Implications for preconception care. *American Journal of Preventive Medicine, 38*(4S), S459–S467. doi:10.1016/j.amepre.2009.12.018

Farrugia, M. K., & Woolf, A. S. (2010). Congenital urinary bladder outlet obstruction. *Fetal and Maternal Medicine Review, 21*(1), 55–73. doi:10.1017/S0965539509990192

Feero, W., Guttmacher, A., & Collins, S. (2010). Genomic medicine—an updated primer. *New England Journal of Medicine, 362*(21), 2001–2011.

Friedberg, E. C. (2003). DNA damage and repair. *Nature, 421*(6921), 436–440.

Fritz, M., & Speroff, L. (2011). *Clinical gynecologic endocrinology and infertility* (8th ed.). Philadelphia, PA: Lippincott Williams & Wilkins.

Gaff, C. L., & Bylund, C. L. (2010). *Family communication about genetics: Theory and practice.* USA: Oxford Univ. Press.

Grosse,S. D., Rogowski,W. H., Ross, L. F., Cornel, M. C., Dondorp,W. J., & Khoury, M. J.(2010) Population screening for genetic disorders in the 21st century: Evidence, economics, and ethics. *Public Health Genomics, 13,* 106–115. doi:10.1159/000226594

Guttmacher, A. E., Porteous, M. E., & McInerney, J. D. (2007) Educating health-care professionals about genetics and genomics. *Nature Reviews Genetics, 8,* 151–157.

Harper, P. S. (2010). Special issues in genetic counselling. In P. S. Harper *Practical genetic counselling* (7th ed., pp. 135–144). London: Hodder Arnold.

Hess, R. A., & de Franca, L. R. (2008). Spermatogensis and cycle of the seminiferous epithelium. In C. Y. Cheng (Ed.), *Molecular mechanisms in spermatogenesis.* Austin, TX: Springer Science + Business Media.

Hultman, C. M., Sandin, S., Levine, S. Z., Lichtenstein, P., & Reichenberg, A. (2011). Advancing paternal age and risk of autism: New evidence from a population-based study and a meta-analysis of epidemiological studies. *Molecular Psychiatry, 16,* 1203–1212. doi:10.1038/mp.2010.121

International Society of Nurses in Genetics. (2010a). *Position Statement: Access to genomic healthcare: The role of the nurse.* Retrieved from http://www.isong.org/ISONG_position_statements.php

International Society of Nurses in Genetics. (2010b). *Position statement: Privacy and confidentiality of genetic information: The role of the nurse.* Retrieved from http://www.isong.org/ISONG_position_statements.php

International Society of Nurses in Genetics. (2011). *Position Statement: Informed decision making and consent: The role of nursing.* Retrieved from http://www.isong.org/ISONG_position_statements.php

Jameson, J. L., De Groot, L. J., de Kretser, D., Grossman, A., Marshall, J. C., Melmed, S., et al. (2010). *Endocrinology: Adult and pediatric* (6th ed.). Elsevier Inc.

Johnson, J., & Tough, S., (2012). Society of Obstetricians and Gynaecologists of Canada (SOGC) Committee Opinion: Delayed childbearing. *Journal of Obstetrics and Gynaecology of Canada, 34*(1), 80–93.

Kobayashi, H., Nagao, K., & Nakajima, K.(2013). Human testis–derived pluripotent cells and induced pluripotent stem cells. In D. Bhartya & N. Lenka (Eds.), *Pluripotent stem cells.* InTech Open Access Company. doi:10.5772/45917. Retrieved from http://cdn.intechopen.com/pdfs/45191/InTech-Human_testis_derived_pluripotent_cells_and_induced_pluripotent_stem_cells.pdf

Kubota, T., Miyake, K., & Hirasawa, T. (2013). The mechanisms of epigenetic modifications during DNA replication. In D. Stuart (Ed.), *Mechanism of DNA replication.* InTech Open Access Company. doi:10.5772/51592. Retrieved from http://www.intechopen.com/books/the-mechanisms-of-dna-replication/the-mechanisms-of-epigenetic-modifications-during-dna-replication

Langlois, S., & Brock, J. (2013). Society of Obstetricians and Gynaecologists of Canada (SOGC) committee opinion: Current status in non-invasive prenatal detection of Down Syndrome, Trisomy 18, and Trisomy 13 using cell-free DNA in maternal plasma. *Journal of Obstetrics and Gynaecology of Canada, 35*(2), 177–181.

Lashley, F. R. (2007). *Essentials of clinical genetics in nursing practice.* New York: Springer.

Lea, D. H., Skirton, H., Read, C. Y., & Williams, J. K. (2011). Implications for educating the next generation of nurses on genetics and genomics in the 21st century. *Journal of Nursing Scholarship, 43,* 3–12.

Martini, A., Stephens, D., & Read, A. P. (2007). *Genes, Hearing, and Deafness: From molecular biology to clinical practice.* Informa Healthcare.

McDonald-McGinn, D. M., & Sullivan, K. E. (2011). Chromosome 22q11.2 deletion syndrome (DiGeorge syndrome/velocardiofacial syndrome). *Medicine, 90*(1), 1–18. doi:10.1097/MD.0b013e3182060469

Moos, M. K. (2004). Preconceptional health promotion: Progress in changing a prevention paradigm. *Journal of Perinatal & Neonatal Nursing, 18*(1), 2–13.

Moos, M. K. (2010). From concept to practice: Reflections on the preconception health agenda. *Journal of Women's Health, 19*(3), 561–567.

Morrison, A., & Dowler, J. (2011). *Newborn screening for disorders and abnormalities in Canada.* [Environmental Scan issue 26]. Ottawa, ON: Canadian Agency for Drugs and Technologies in Health. Retrieved from http://www.cadth.ca/products/environmental-scanning/environmental-scans/newborn-screening

Nicolaides, K. H. (2011). Screening for fetal aneuploidies at 11 to 13 weeks. *Prenatal Diagnosis, 31,* 7–15. doi:10.1002/pd

Nussbaum, R. I., McInnes, R. R., & Willard, H. F. (2007). *Thompson and Thompson genetics in medicine* (7th ed.). Philadelphia, PA: W. B. Saunders.

Office of the Privacy Commissioner of Canada. (2012). Genetic information, the life and health insurance industry and the protection of personal information: Framing the debate. Retrieved from http://www.priv.gc.ca/information/research-recherche/2012/gi_intro_e.asp

Online Mendelian Inheritance in Man (OMIM). (2014). Baltimore, MD: McKusick-Nathans Institute of Genetic Medicine, Johns Hopkins University. Retrieved from http://omim.org/

Oscapella, E. (2012). *Genetics, privacy and discrimination: An overview of selected major issues.* Vancouver, BC: British Columbia Civil Liberties Association.

Pfau, S. J, & Amon, A. (2012). Chromosomal instability and aneuploidy in cancer: From yeast to man. *EMBO Reports, 13*(6), 515–527. doi:10.1038/embor.2012.65

Public Health Agency of Canada. (2008). *Canadian perinatal health report 2008 edition.* Ottawa, ON: Author. Retrieved from http://www.phac-aspc.gc.ca/publicat/2008/cphr-rspc/index-eng.php

Public Health Agency of Canada. (2012). Folic acid and prevention of neural tube defects. Retrieved from http://www.phac-aspc.gc.ca/fa-af/fa-af08-eng.php

Public Health Agency of Canada. (2013). Congenital anomalies in Canada 2013: A perinatal health surveillance report. Ottawa, ON: Minister of Public Works and Government Services. Retrieved from http://www.phac-aspc.gc.ca/ccasn-rcsac/cac-acc-2013-eng.php

Puscheck, E. E., & Jeyendran, R. S. (2007). The impact of male factor on recurrent pregnancy loss. *Current Opinion in Obstetrics & Gynecology, 19*(3), 222–228.

Reid, G. T., Walter, F. M., Brisbane, J. M., & Emery, J. D. (2009). Family history questionnaires designed for clinical use: A systematic review. *Public Health Genomics, 12,* 73–83. doi:10.1159/000160667

Sadler, T. W. (2011). *Langman's medical embryology* (12th ed.). Philadelphia, PA: Lippincott Williams & Wilkins.

Salem, S., Lim, K., & Van den Hof, M. C. (2014). Joint Society of Obstetricians and Gynaecologists of Canada (SOGC)/Canadian Association of Radiologists (CAR) policy statement on non-medical use of fetal ultrasound. *Journal of Obstetrics and Gynaecology Canada, 36*(2), 184–185.

Sartorius, G. A., & Nieschlag, E. (2010). Paternal age and reproduction. *Human Reproduction Update, 16*(1), 65–79. doi:10.1093/humupd/dmp027

Sickle Cell Disease Association of Canada. (2013). Retrieved from http://www.sicklecelldisease.ca/

Sierra, S., & Okun, N. (2014). Society of Obstetricians and Gynaecologists of Canada (SOGC) Clinical practice guidelines: Pregnancy outcomes after assisted reproduction technology. *Journal of Obstetrics and Gynaecology of Canada, 36*(1), 64–83.

Sofikitis, N., Giotitsas, N., Tsounapi, P., Baltogiannis, D., Giannakis, D., & Pardalidis, N. (2008). Hormonal regulation of spermatogenesis and spermiogenesis. *Journal of Steroid Biochemistry and Molecular Biology, 109,* 323–330. doi:10.1016/j.jsbmb.2008.03.004

Sotiriadis, A., Makrigiannakis, A., Stefos, T., Paraskevaidis, E., & Kalantaridou, S. N. (2007). Fibrinolytic defects and recurrent miscarriage: A systematic review and meta-analysis. *Obstetrics & Gynecology, 109*(5), 1146–1155.

Tache, V., Tarsa, M., Romine, L., & Pretorius, D. H. (2008). Three-dimensional obstetric ultrasound. *Seminars in Ultrasound CT and MRI, 29,* 147–155. doi:10.1053/j.sult.2007.12.004

Therrell, B. L., & Adams, J. (2007). Newborn screening in North America. *Journal of Inherited Metabolic Disease, 30*(4), 447–465.

Tuchmann-Duplessis, H., David, G., & Haegel, P. (1975). *Illustrated human embryology,* (Vol. 1). New York: Springer Verlag.

Uhlmann, W. R., Schuette, J. L., & Beverly, Y. (Eds.) (2011). *A guide to genetic counseling* John Wiley & Sons.

Ward, K. (2008). Genetics in obstetrics and gynecology. In R. S. Gibbs, B. Y. Karlan, A. F. Haney, & I. Nygaard (Eds.), *Danforth's obstetrics and gynecology* (10th ed., pp. 88–110). Philadelphia, PA: Lippincott Williams & Wilkins.

Watson, J. D., & Crick, F. H. C. (1953). Molecular structure of nucleic acids. *Nature, 171*(4356), 737–738.

Webster, S., & De Wreede, R. (2012). *Embryology at a glance.* Chichester, West Sussex: Wiley-Blackwell.

Wilson, R. (2007). Principles of human teratology: Drug, chemical, and infectious exposure. SOGC clinical practice guideline no. 199. *Journal of Obstetrics and Gynaecology of Canada, 29*(11), 911–917.

Wilson, R. D., Langlois, S., & Johnson, J. (2007). Mid-trimester amniocentesis fetal loss rate. SOGC clinical practice guideline No. 194. *Journal of Obstetrics and Gynaecology of Canada, 29*(7), 586–595.

WEB RESOURCES

American Society of Human Genetics (ASHG). Professional society for genetics healthcare specialists. http://www.ashg.org

Association of Women's Health, Obstetric and Neonatal Nurses (AWHONN). Develops resources and the education for nurses. https://www.awhonn.org/awhonn/

Canadian Association of Perinatal and Women's Health Nurses (CAPWHN). http://www.capwhn.ca/en/capwhn/index.php?page=4086

Canadian Organization for Rare Disorders (CORD). http://www.raredisorders.ca/

Centers for Disease Control and Prevention (CDC): Updates and publishes aggregate incidence of birth defects. http://www.cdc.gov/

Cystic Fibrosis Canada. http://www.cysticfibrosis.ca/

Gene Tests. Catalog and description of genetic tests currently available. http://www.genetests.orghttp://www.genetests.org

Genetic Alliance. http://www.geneticalliance.org/

International Society of Nurses in Genetics (ISONG). http://www.isong.org

March of Dimes. Prevention of birth defects through education and research. http://www.marchofdimes.com

National Human Genome Research Institute (NHGRI). Management and coordination of the national Human Genome Project. http://www.genome.gov

Online Mendelian Inheritance in Man, OMIM. http://omim.org/

Sickle Cell Disease Association of Canada. http://www.sicklecelldisease.ca/about.php

PREGNANCY

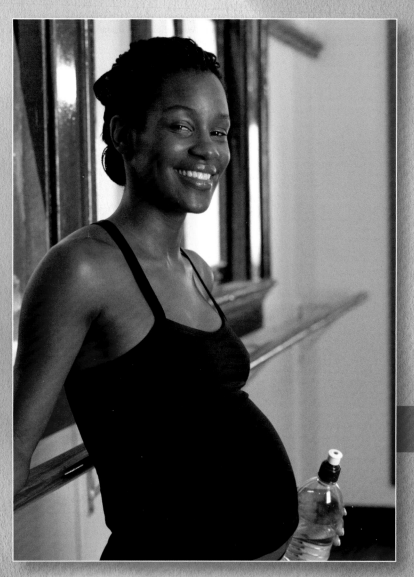

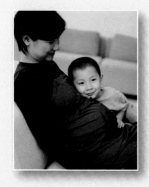 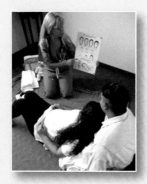 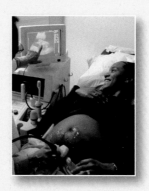 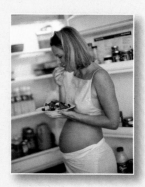

Few life events are as wonderful, ambivalent, memorable, and defining as pregnancy. While the process of gestation has many common threads and themes for all women, each mother's experience is unique. Furthermore, the same woman may experience pregnancy differently each time that she goes through it. The changes that the expectant woman undergoes involve her physical, psychological, spiritual, emotional, interpersonal, and social dimensions. Providing appropriate support for the pregnant client, as well as her partner, significant others, and extended family and friends, is one of the most important aspects of quality collaborative health care.

In this unit we describe the process of normal pregnancy, expected changes in each trimester, and associated management approaches for the normal discomforts and adjustments that accompany this life event. We also discuss those conditions and circumstances that render a pregnancy at high risk, with measures that health care providers should take to protect the health of mother and fetus. We explore different methods of preparing for pregnancy, childbirth, and parenthood, emphasizing the role that educational programs can play in improving outcomes not only for individual clients, but also for families and the overall public.

CHAPTER 12

Process of Pregnancy

Robin J. Evans and Jodie Bigalky

Millie, 38 years old, GTPAL 3-2-0-0-2, has just learned that she is at 12 weeks' gestation with an unplanned pregnancy. Although she expresses excitement, Millie also verbalizes apprehension. "I thought I was done forever with diapers and night feedings. I also forgot how tired and nauseous you feel during the first trimester." She says she is concerned about fetal well-being, because she is older than when she went through her previous pregnancies. She also wonders how she'll have enough time for the rest of her family once the new baby arrives.

Kathy, 26 years old, GTPAL 1-0-0-0-0, comes to the prenatal clinic for a regular visit at 32 weeks' gestation. While the nurse is collecting assessment data, Kathy relates that her feet have been swollen and that she has been constipated. She states, "I never expected pregnancy to have so many physical effects. I'm worried about my feet. Do you think something is wrong with the pregnancy?"

You will learn more about Millie's and Kathy's stories later in this chapter. Nurses working with these clients and others like them need to understand the material in this chapter to manage care and address issues appropriately. Before beginning, consider the following points related to the above scenarios:

- How can the nurse reassure both clients, while appropriately addressing any problems for each that might exist?
- What differences might these clients experience based on their ages, previous pregnancy histories, and other circumstances?
- What topics and assessment questions might the nurse focus on next for each woman?
- How can the nurse effectively integrate each client's physical, psychological, and sociocultural pregnancy-related concerns?

On completion of this chapter, the reader should be able to:
- Discuss variations in pregnancy.
- Describe common physical and psychological changes in pregnancy.
- Identify the presumptive, probable, and positive signs of pregnancy.
- Summarize the components of an assessment for pregnant women, focused on appropriate history taking, physical examination, and laboratory evaluation.
- Summarize the components of the assessment of fetal activity and well-being.
- Discuss strategies to enhance women's health and comfort during pregnancy.
- Discuss substances that may have teratogenic effects on the fetus.

amenorrhea	lordosis
Braxton-Hicks contractions	Montgomery tubercles
cephalopelvic disproportion	morning sickness
Chadwick's sign	multigravida
chloasma	Naegele's rule
diastasis	nulligravida
fundus	oligohydramnios
Goodell's sign	operculum
Hegar's sign	primigravida
Leopold manoeuvres	quickening
leukorrhea	striae gravidarum
lightening	supine postural hypotension syndrome
linea nigra	teratogen

Pregnancy is one of life's most profound experiences. During the early part of the 20th century, women spent a considerable portion of their reproductive years pregnant, producing large families. The advent of birth control provided options previously not available to limit family size (see Chapter 8). In the latter part of the 20th century, some countries actually began to limit the number of children people could have, enforcing deterrents to producing more than one child.

In this chapter we address the components of appropriate care of pregnant women, examining the process of pregnancy from several perspectives. A common and incorrect assumption is that all women experience pregnancy the same way. Many factors, however, contribute to women's varied responses. Knowledge and understanding of these variations allow nurses to give anticipatory health education, as well as to provide care specific to the client's and family's actual needs. Physical and psychological changes during pregnancy are explored, including the associated etiology. Appropriate assessments necessary to identify any potential or actual challenges to the well-being of the woman, the fetus, or both are described. Maintenance of maternal and fetal well-being contributes to a positive outcome of the pregnancy. Strategies that may enhance the health and comfort of pregnant clients are discussed. This knowledge provides nurses an opportunity to assist clients to improve self-image and self-care.

VARIATIONS IN RESPONSES TO PREGNANCY

The way the client and family experience pregnancy is influenced by such factors as age, sociological and cultural background, and religion. Differences are often ignored as if they do not exist; however professionals must aim to provide care that meets the needs of each woman. Viewing all women of the same age, ethnic origin, race, culture, sexual orientation, economic status, or religious beliefs as of a single type will not lead to provision of sensitive and appropriate health care. The nurse needs to see each individual as just that—an individual who may or may not subscribe to stereotypes or generalizations. For example, although women may be of a particular culture or ethnic origin, the extent to which they follow traditional customs varies. The nurse views each woman within the context of her environment, including cultural, historical, political, and economic factors, while remembering that the client is unique and requires individualized, pertinent, and specific care (Callister, 2005, 2014).

Age-Related Variations

A woman's potential to become pregnant may cover a span from early adolescence to her late 40s. The average age of mothers in Canada has been steadily increasing. In 1975, the average age of Canadian mothers began to rise; by 2009 half of all women giving birth were 30 years of age or over, 2.5 times the percentage in 1974 (Human Resources and Skills Development Canada [HRSDC], 2013). The average age of mothers who gave birth in Canada during 2011 was 29.7 years (Statistics Canada, 2013b), increased from 26.7 years in 1975 (HRSDC, 2013). Mothers giving birth to their first baby have also become progressively older over the past decade (Statistics Canada, 2013a). During the 1960s the average age of a first-time mother was 23.5 years; by 2008 this number was 28.1 (Statistics Canada, 2011a).

Pregnancy in Adolescence

The rate of teen pregnancy in Canada declined substantially during the last quarter of the 20th century. Between 2006 and 2010, adolescent pregnancy decreased by more than 20% (McKay, 2012). In 2009, just over 4% of all live births were to women aged 15 to 19 years (Statistics Canada, 2013a). Canada's rate of live births to young women aged 15 to 19 years in 2009 was 14.2 per 1,000 women, down from 24.6 in 1989 (Statistics Canada, 2013a). While the abortion rate itself has remained relatively stable, the decline in the birth rate has resulted in about half of these pregnancies ending in abortion (McKay, 2012).

Teen mothers bring unique perspectives to pregnancy that may not always be consistent with how society views them (Fig. 12.1). Teen pregnancy is often considered a social problem with significant economic impact (McKay & Barrett, 2010). Because teen mothers often have not completed schooling, their ability to provide adequate support for themselves and their children is viewed as compro-

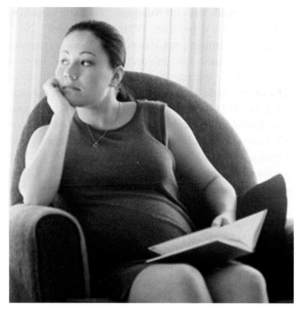

FIGURE 12.1 Although pregnancy in adolescence poses unique challenges, expectant teens may see parenthood as a demonstration of responsibility, a transformative experience, a source of stability, and a life turning point.

mised. The developmental time of adolescence often presents challenges that can be further complicated by pregnancy. Generally, teen mothers are seen as a problem attributed either to individuals making poor decisions or to a symptom of a failing society (Breheny & Stephens, 2010). Attitudes have begun to shift during the past decades. Researchers are attempting to understand from various perspectives the choices and experiences of these young women (Hanna, 2001; Seamark & Lings, 2004; SmithBattle, 2007), rather than only focusing on the more traditional view of teen mothers as immature, inexperienced, irresponsible "children raising children" (SmithBattle, 2000b), whose lack of parenting skills may put children at risk. For example, Hanna (2001) and SmithBattle (2000a) showed that teen mothers viewed raising a child as a way to demonstrate responsibility, in contrast to the more common public discourse. A metasynthesis by Clemmens (2003) revealed that although parenthood was challenging for them, teen mothers also saw motherhood as a positively transforming and stabilizing influence, as well as a turning point for the future.

Nevertheless, teen mothers do have challenges. Many teen pregnancies are unintended (Clear et al., 2012; Phipps & Nunes, 2012). When a pregnancy is unintended, the mother may not be emotionally ready for the pregnancy or parenting. The lack of emotional readiness may lead to delayed or inadequate prenatal care, delayed use of vitamins, cigarette smoking, drinking, and depression (Phipps & Nunes, 2012). Adolescent mothers are more likely than average-age mothers to have low socioeconomic status, have no partner, have experienced physical or sexual abuse, and often would have preferred to have been pregnant later in life (Al-Sahab et al., 2012). Research suggests that becoming an adolescent mother does not necessarily lead to low socioeconomic status but, rather, young women of low socioeconomic status are more likely to become teen mothers (Kearney & Levine, 2012; Luong, 2009). Teen mothers are less likely to complete high school or postsecondary education, making them less likely to get good paying jobs, further perpetuating the poverty (Luong, 2009). They may have differing levels of support from family or partners, a concept that may be somewhat culturally determined. For the families of teen mothers, the transition to parenthood and grandparenthood can be abrupt and complicated (Dallas, 2004). Teens themselves tend to emphasize the need for support and knowledge to be successful in their new role of parenting (Stiles, 2005), influenced in part by their interactions with health care providers (Peterson et al., 2007). Nurses also have identified the need for support in development of skills in their care for adolescent mothers (Peterson et al., 2012) (See Research Highlight 12.1).

Remember Kathy, the 26-year-old at the beginning of the chapter who is in her 32nd week of gestation. Imagine that Kathy were 16 years old and single. What areas would be especially important for the nurse to assess?

Pregnancy After 35

The birth rate for women over the age of 35 has increased by 2.5 times over the past 20 years (Statistics Canada, 2013a). Mothers aged 40 to 44 have had the highest increase, from 8.4 births to 9.2 births per 1,000 (Statistics Canada, 2013a). Women between the ages of 35 and 39 account for about 15% of the live births in Canada (Statistics Canada, 2011a).

Delayed childbearing has been defined as pregnancy at or after the age of 35 (Johnson & Tough, 2012). With advances in safe contraception, women have been able to delay pregnancy in order to complete postsecondary education, obtain a career, and assume financial security. However, women who choose to delay childbearing face significant risks. Women older than 35 years have an increased risk of infertility and require a longer time to conceive (see Chapter 10) (Johnson &

● RESEARCH HIGHLIGHT 12.1 Hospital-Based Perinatal Nurses Identify the Need to Improve Nursing Care of Adolescent Mothers

OBJECTIVE

To determine whether hospital-based nurses identified a need to improve in-patient experiences for adolescent mothers and their perceptions of how well perinatal units supported nurses to provide care that was friendly to adolescent mothers.

DESIGN

This descriptive quantitative study used a key informant survey approach.

PARTICIPANTS AND SETTING

Twenty-seven key informants, identified by managers and colleagues and perinatal clinical educators, from eight perinatal units at three hospitals (four separate sites) in a Canadian city completed the survey.

RESULTS

Respondents rated their own skill in caring for adolescent mothers higher than that of other nurses on their units.

The lower rankings were related to a number of factors; nurses' judgmental manner in dealing with adolescent mothers; a lack of knowledge of community-based resources; insufficient education programs on adolescent mother-friendly care; and a lack of availability, or knowledge of, policies that could inform the nursing care of adolescent mothers.

CONCLUSIONS

The findings indicate that a minority of nurses have expertise in mother-friendly nursing care of adolescents. There is an opportunity for nursing units to develop strategies and interventions that would support perinatal nurses in developing these skills. Strategies that may be identified include peer mentoring and self-reflective practices.

Source: Peterson, W. E., Davies, B., Rashotte, J., Slavador, A., & Trépanier, M. J. (2012). Hospital-based perinatal nurses identify the need to improve nursing care of adolescent mothers. *Journal of Obstetric, Gynecologic and Neonatal Nurses, 41*, 358–368.

Tough, 2012; Liu & Case, 2011). They are more likely to be obese or to have underlying medical conditions such as endometriosis, fibroids, and polyps, which may also affect fertility (Johnson & Tough, 2012). The incidence of genetic conditions and congenital anomalies is increased in babies born to older mothers; for this reason, pregnant women older than 35 years should be offered screening for fetal anomalies and should have a detailed second trimester ultrasound (Johnson & Tough, 2012).

Other complications associated with delayed childbearing include increased risk for spontaneous abortion, ectopic pregnancy, diabetes, hypertension, placental abnormalities, perinatal morbidity related to preterm birth, multiple pregnancy, caesarean section, and maternal morbidity (Johnson & Tough, 2012). Women may experience increased anxiety as concern about potential outcomes for both self and baby become more prominent, although little evidence indicates that such worry has a detrimental effect on pregnancy outcome.

Although there are many risks associated with delaying childbearing, there are also many benefits. Older parents are more mature and are more likely to be financially secure and to cope with the stresses that come with being parents (Johnson & Tough, 2012). Fortunately, many pregnancies to older parents do end with healthy maternal and neonatal outcomes; however parents should be informed about the risks associated with delayed childbearing (See Nursing Care Plan 12.1.).

Pregnancy from 20 to 35 Years

Traditionally, the age span of 20 to 35 years has been considered the most opportune time for pregnancy. Women in this age group have fewer risk factors associated with pregnancy and birth, although socioeconomic factors unrelated to age may play a role in the outcome of the pregnancy. They may be at increased risk for preterm labour related to their occupation if it requires long periods of standing or heavy work.

Sociocultural Variations

Many nurses and health care professionals assume that all women and their significant others experience pregnancy and its associated rites of passage similarly. Pregnancy and parenthood, however, have different meanings and rituals for each woman. These experiences are influenced by language and cultural differences, ethnicity, sexual orientation, and socioeconomic status.

Cultural, Racial, and Ethnic Influences

The population of Canada is truly multicultural, made up of individuals who self-identify as belonging to many different ethnic and cultural groups (Statistics Canada, 2011b). Between 1991 and 2006, the average number of immigrants to Canada was 229,000 annually (Statistics Canada, 2011b). The proportion of Canada's society that is multicultural will continue to grow with ongoing immigration and as children and grandchildren of immigrants add to Canada's diversity (Statistics Canada, 2011b). It is estimated that, if current trends continue, by 2031 about 30% of Canada's population will belong to a visible minority (Statistics Canada, 2011b). Canadian births are reflective of this ethnic and cultural diversity. Women of visible minority in Canada are younger than the overall female population. The median age for women who are of visible minority was 33.3 years in 2006, compared with 41.5 years for nonvisible minority women and 40 years for the total female population (Chui & Maheux, 2011). These demographics can influence the care provided during the antepartum and perinatal periods.

Variations among people within a culture may influence how much an individual follows culturally related beliefs (Callister, 2014; Lauderdale, 2011). For example, 616 different First Nations have been identified in Canada as well as a diverse population of Inuit and Métis communities (Wilson et al., 2013). Although they are often grouped together under the umbrella term "Aboriginal," "each First Nations, Inuit, and Métis community has its own traditions, values, and communication practices" (Wilson et al., 2013, p. S3) that have an impact on health and health care experiences.

Some women may have no affiliation with the associated culture, while others may continue to have strong affiliations. Brathwaite and Williams (2004) found that recent immigrants may follow fewer traditional practices than women who have been in Canada for many years; in contrast, Grewal et al. (2008) found that recent immigrants continue to follow traditional beliefs and practices. An important part of cultural assessment and sensitivity, therefore, is learning the client's degree of affiliation with her cultural group; the cultural beliefs and practices that she follows; her patterns of decision making, language, and communication; the family's parenting style and roles; dietary practices; and culturally influenced expectations of the health care system (Callister, 2014).

Sociocultural beliefs can influence a woman's experience of pregnancy and her beliefs about and practices during gestation. For example, people in some cultures believe that the personality is formed before birth and is affected by the mother's emotions (Callister, 2014). Other beliefs may include those related to fertility rites or what determines the gender of the fetus (Callister, 2014). Some may see cultural traditions and beliefs about childbirth as "old wives tales" (Lauderdale, 2011). Pregnancy and birth will vary for each woman based on the extent

NURSING CARE PLAN 12.1

●

The Client in Early Pregnancy

Recall Millie from the beginning of this chapter. Review of her pregnancy history reveals that both previous pregnancies were normal and resulted in vaginal births at 38 and 39 weeks, respectively. Her oldest child weighed 3,265 g at birth; her second child weighed 3,084 g. In addition to problems with "morning sickness," Millie also reports constipation and hemorrhoids. She states, "My children are very active in after-school activities and sports. And I'm the one who drives them back and forth. Sometimes I feel like a chauffeur. My husband helps when he can, but he usually has to go out of town for a few days each month for business. I'm just worried that I won't be able to keep up with everything."

NURSING DIAGNOSIS

Anxiety related to client's age and the increased physical and psychological demands associated with current pregnancy and current family lifestyle

EXPECTED OUTCOMES

1. The client will verbalize concerns related to pregnancy.
2. The client will identify areas in which she needs assistance.

INTERVENTIONS	RATIONALES
Assess the client's level of understanding about age and pregnancy	This information serves as a baseline for specific client needs and an individualized plan
Discuss with the client her concerns, feelings, and perceptions related to pregnancy and age and possible effects on current family situation.	Discussion provides opportunities to emphasize positive aspects; verbalization of concerns helps establish sources of stress and areas that need to be addressed
Communicate accurate facts and answer questions honestly	Open, honest communication promotes trust and helps correct any misinformation
Review the client's previous pregnancy history	This information gives clues to potential problems and aids in identifying the client's reactions and coping abilities
Discuss possible effects of increased age on pregnancy and measures to reduce risks	Adequate knowledge of possible effects and risk-reduction measures helps alleviate concerns related to the unknown
Ask the client to describe her typical daily schedule and activities; review with her areas that might be problematic	Knowledge of a typical routine offers a baseline; identifying potential problem areas facilitates teaching and anticipatory guidance
Investigate sources of available support, such as family, friends, and community; encourage the client to use them	Additional sources of support are helpful in alleviating anxiety and stress
Encourage the client to obtain adequate rest and nutrition; discuss ways to accomplish them within her current situation	Adequate rest and nutrition are essential to promote a positive pregnancy outcome

(continued)

NURSING CARE PLAN 12.1 • The Client in Early Pregnancy (Continued)

INTERVENTIONS	RATIONALES
Include the client, partner, and children in discussion about the pregnancy, client needs, and necessary adaptations	Client and family participation increases feelings of control over the situation and promotes support and sharing
Provide the family with information about support groups, websites, and other sources of appropriate information	Shared experiences and knowledge of similar situations can aid in preparing the client and family for what to expect
Continue to assess the family's adaptation and functioning at subsequent visits	Continued assessment aids in monitoring progress of the situation and provides opportunities to address concerns that may arise as the pregnancy progresses

EVALUATION

1. The client identifies realistic measures to cope with the demands of pregnancy and family.
2. The client and family develop a workable schedule that promotes maternal, fetal, and family health.
3. The client demonstrates use of appropriate support services.
4. The client reports a decrease in anxiety at next visit.

to which she practices cultural beliefs. The amount of support and involvement from extended family during pregnancy, birth, and childrearing is another area with cultural, ethnic, and racial determinants (Callister, 2014). For example, some cultural groups may consider it inappropriate for men to be present at birth (Callister, 2014). In such cases, it would be most appropriate for a woman's health care providers to be female. As part of delivering culturally sensitive care, respect is a primary responsibility for nurses working with pregnant women. However, respect may be understood differently in different cultures. For example, a nurse who includes the consequences of not adhering to specific instructions in his/her teaching may be perceived by a woman of Aboriginal descent, who adheres to the cultural ethic of non-interference, as disrespectful (Smylie, 2001). Traditional First Nations culture is built on a strong spiritual foundation with an orientation focused on the circular medicine wheel. Living in complete harmony with nature is important. People who follow this culture value listening and the role of elders. They may avoid eye contact, viewing it as disrespectful.

The growing immigrant population may present additional challenges in providing obstetrical care to women from diverse backgrounds. Recent immigrants may be separated from supports. Language may present challenges that may be only partially met by the use of interpreters. Hospitals often use nonprofessional employees who are not familiar with medical terminology to act as interpreters, which can lead to inaccurate translations (Callister, 2014). The results of cultural rituals such as female circumcision may lead to severe pain and birth complications (Callister, 2014). Culture may affect diet. For example, the concepts of "hot" and "cold" are common to several cultures. Asian and Hispanic women (Callister, 2014) may believe that balance should be maintained between hot and cold; during pregnancy (considered to be a hot condition), women eat cold foods; following birth (believed to deplete the woman's body of the hot element) they eat hot foods to balance the cold state. The designation of foods as hot or cold is unrelated to the temperature of the food; rather, it refers to the effect that the food has on the body.

Lesbian Pregnancy

Artificial insemination, in vitro fertilization, surrogacy, and adoption have enabled people who have struggled with fertility issues to achieve pregnancy and childbirth (see Chapter 10); these methods also have facilitated parenthood for gay and lesbian parents

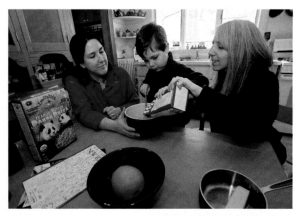

FIGURE 12.2 Families with lesbian parents are increasing in Canadian societies. These families benefit from health care provision that is sensitive, respectful, and supportive.

(Chapman et al., 2012; Lauderdale, 2011) (Fig. 12.2). Easier access to fertility treatment has contributed to the increasing number of lesbian women who choose to start a family; however gay and lesbian families seeking pregnancy often encounter hostile societal attitudes and negative experiences with health care professionals. Their most common fear is unsafe and inadequate care (Chapman et al., 2012; Lauderdale, 2011; Lee et al., 2011). Nevertheless, pregnancies are more likely to be planned, and lesbian families generally have a more equitable distribution of child care, which may provide some protective effects on mental health (Chapman et al., 2012; Ross, 2005). Studies have shown that an attitude of respect for and understanding of their choices is of primary importance (Chapman et al., 2012; Lauderdale, 2011). Lesbian couples who successfully conceive need to be supported by family, friends, and health care professionals (Chapman et al., 2012).

Influence of Income Distribution

Poverty creates problems for pregnant women, regardless of age, race, ethnicity, or sexual orientation. Limited resources compromise the ability of poor women to provide adequate housing and food for themselves and their children. Lack of money leads to problems accessing reliable transportation and child care, both of which frequently lead to inadequate prenatal care. Women enrolled in a program that provides extra food may share the food with other impoverished family members. Attitudes of health care workers may influence the mother's perceptions of herself and her environment. For example, community workers who visit the mother in her home can contribute to decreased self-respect by unconsciously making inconsiderate remarks about the home environment (Allender & Spradley, 2005).

Religious Variations

Religion may be a factor in the pregnant woman's life and response to pregnancy. Just as with culture, assessing each client and family individually is essential, because the degree to which they adhere to religious beliefs and teachings may vary. As well, some religions are divided into orthodox and nonorthodox sects, with even more variation in the views and laws to which members adhere.

As with culture, women of the same religious background may have varying degrees of affiliation with their associated religion. In some situations, other factors may override religious beliefs and must be taken into consideration when providing care. Thus, it is important to assess each woman individually to determine what aspects of care may be affected by those religious practices to which she and her significant others adhere.

PHYSIOLOGIC CHANGES IN PREGNANCY

During pregnancy, several changes occur within the body (Table 12.1). Some are obvious, whereas others are less noticeable.

Weight

Average weight gain during a singleton pregnancy is approximately 11.5 to 16 kg for women with a normal prepregnancy body mass index (BMI) (Barron, 2014; Cunningham et al., 2010). Women who gain more than the recommended amount of weight are at increased risk for macrosomia, augmented labour, gestational hypertension, and neonatal metabolic abnormalities, while those women with appropriate weight gain demonstrate fewer adverse outcomes (Davies et al., 2010). During the first several days following birth, the woman excretes the additional fluid that is gained during pregnancy in urine once she loses the placenta's fluid-retaining hormones. See Chapter 3 for more detailed discussion of recommendations for weight gain depending on the woman's prepregnancy weight and BMI.

Cardiovascular System

Major changes occur within the woman's cardiovascular system during pregnancy. These changes are necessary for adequate placental and fetal circulation.

Because of increasing uterine size, the maternal heart shifts upward and to a more transverse position, causing it to appear enlarged on radiographic examination. Blood pressure remains relatively unchanged despite the increased blood volume; it actually decreases slightly during the second trimester (approximately 5–10 mm Hg for both systolic and diastolic pressures), returning to prepregnancy values by the third trimester. These changes to

● TABLE 12.1 **Physiologic Changes in Pregnancy and Expected Time Frames**

Trimester	Week	Physiologic Changes
First	1–2	Implantation of blastocyst Human chorionic gonadotropin secreted
	6	Nausea and vomiting
	8	Fetal outline visible on ultrasound
	10–12	Fetal heart audible by Doppler
	16	Changes in skin pigmentation Possible expression of colostrum
Second	18–20	Quickening Fetal heart audible on fetoscope
	20	Fetal outline palpable through abdominal wall Human placental lactogen secreted
Third	27	Increased blood volume, cardiac output, and pulse Uterine enlargement, leading to supine postural hypotension, shortness of breath, edema, hemorrhoids, and lordosis
	38	Lightening

blood pressure may result from increased production of prostaglandins or altered vascular resistance (Blackburn, 2014; Cunningham et al., 2010).

Maternal blood volume begins to rise in the first trimester, increases most significantly during the second trimester, and then increases at a slower rate in the third trimester, eventually stabilizing in the last weeks of pregnancy. In the late stages of pregnancy, approximately 500 mL of blood flows through the maternal circulation to the placenta each minute, and blood volume at birth is increased approximately 45% above prepregnancy values to approximately 1,500 mL (Cunningham et al., 2010). Increased levels of aldosterone and renin are primarily responsible; these hormones cause the kidneys to retain more fluid. The increased blood volume provides adequate circulation to the placenta to ensure appropriate oxygen and nutrients for the developing fetus. It also helps to compensate for the blood loss experienced during childbirth, which usually ranges from 500 to 600 mL with a vaginal birth, and up to 1,000 mL with a caesarean birth (Blackburn, 2014).

Because of the increased blood volume and stroke volume, maternal cardiac output increases 30% to 50%; the largest increase occurs as early as 6 weeks' gestation, peaks in the second trimester, and then plateaus until term (Blackburn, 2014). Stroke volume increases as early as 8 weeks, peaks at 16 to 24 weeks, and declines until term (Blackburn, 2014). The woman's pulse increases approximately 10 to 20 bpm, peaking at 32 weeks' gestation (Hegewald & Crapo, 2011). The increase in cardiac output is greater in multiple gestations (Blackburn, 2014).

Cardiac output is influenced by maternal position. It is optimized in the lateral position and markedly decreased in the supine position (Blackburn, 2014). When the pregnant woman lies supine, especially in the third trimester when the fetus experiences its greatest growth spurt, she may experience what is referred to as **supine postural hypotension syndrome**. Characteristics of this syndrome include light-headedness, faintness, and palpitations. This syndrome develops from the pressure of the gravid uterus pushing the inferior vena cava against the vertebrae. Occlusion of the inferior vena cava decreases blood flow from the extremities, causing decreased cardiac output and hypotension. Maternal hypotension is potentially dangerous, because it leads to decreased placental circulation and subsequent decreased oxygen to the fetus. A preventive measure for supine postural hypotension is to tell the woman early in pregnancy to refrain from lying on her back and instead to lie on her side or to sit upright. A corrective measure is for the woman to lie laterally, preferably on the left side, or to put a wedge under her right hip (Fig. 12.3).

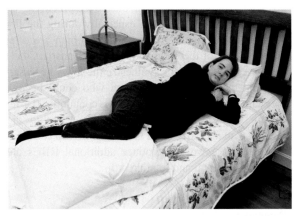

FIGURE 12.3 To avoid supine hypotension syndrome and to provide relief to her back, the client should lie on her side.

Edema in the lower extremities may result from impeded venous return caused by pressure of the growing fetus on the pelvic and femoral areas (Cunningham et al., 2010). Edema worsens with dependency, especially prolonged standing or sitting. Decreased venous return also predisposes the woman to varicosities, including hemorrhoids, which are exacerbated by the vascular relaxation resulting from circulating progesterone.

Hematologic System

Plasma volume increases approximately 40% to 60% by term to 1,200 to 1,600 mL. Erythropoiesis results from increased estrogen and progesterone and accompanies this increased fluid, resulting in an increased red blood cell (RBC) mass as the RBC volume increases 20% to 30% to 250 to 450 mL (Blackburn, 2014). As the increase in RBC volume is relatively less than the increase in plasma, hemodilution results, which is often referred to as *physiologic anemia of pregnancy* (Blackburn, 2014; Cunningham et al., 2010). This occurs most frequently during the second trimester; in the third trimester, plasma volume decreases, while the RBC mass continues to increase (Cunningham et al., 2010). For this reason, anemia is defined as less than 110 g/L in the first and third trimesters and less than 100 g/L during the second.

Most pregnant women require some iron supplementation. Women may enter pregnancy with relatively low iron stores because of the depletion that occurs during monthly menses. A daily supplement of 16 to 20 mg of iron is recommended for healthy pregnant women and is effective in reducing iron deficiency anemia that results from the increased circulating RBC mass (Health Canada, 2009). When an iron supplement is added to a healthy diet, pregnant women should have all the iron they need for pregnancy (Health Canada, 2009).

The need for folic acid also increases during pregnancy to prevent maternal megaloblastic anemia (large nonfunctioning RBCs), which has been linked to an increased risk for neural tube defects (Health Canada, 2013). Folate is essential in the development of the spine and brain of the fetus, especially during the first 4 weeks of pregnancy, a time when women are often not yet aware of the pregnancy (Health Canada, 2013). Because folic acid helps synthesize the DNA necessary for rapid cell growth, all women who could become pregnant should take a multivitamin containing 0.4 mg of folic acid daily, in addition to eating a healthy diet (Health Canada, 2013) (see Chapter 3). Extra folic acid also helps the woman produce additional RBCs and supports placental and fetal growth.

Respiratory System

Pregnancy affects the respiratory system, most notably in the later stages. As a result of increased oxygen demands of the fetal and maternal tissues, the amount of oxygen the woman uses increases throughout pregnancy (Blackburn, 2014). A corresponding amount of carbon dioxide also forms. The effect of these changes, thought to be caused by progesterone, is increased respiratory effort, occasional dyspnea, and $PaCO_2$ decreased to slightly below normal (Blackburn, 2014; Cunningham et al., 2010).

The growing fetus puts pressure on and displaces the diaphragm upward (Fig. 12.4). This crowding causes a distinct feeling of shortness of breath, especially during the late stages. Once **lightening** (movement of the presenting part into the pelvis) occurs, the woman experiences relief from dyspnea and again can breathe easily.

Gastrointestinal System

In early pregnancy, many women experience nausea and vomiting. Although researchers have hypothesized that the cause may be increased levels of human chorionic gonadotropin (hCG) and estrogen, they have not established a clear etiology. Nausea and vomiting are commonly referred to as "morning sickness" because many women experience it when first rising in the morning. Morning sickness is actually a misnomer, however, because it can occur any time of day. It usually subsides by the third month of pregnancy.

Hyperemesis gravidarum, a more severe form of nausea and vomiting, may be diagnosed in women with nausea and vomiting that lasts beyond 3 months

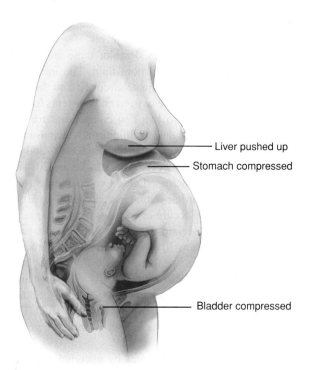

Liver pushed up
Stomach compressed

Bladder compressed

FIGURE 12.4 The growing uterus and fetus push up the liver, compress the stomach and bladder, and displace the diaphragm upward.

or that imposes dangerous health effects. Examples of such effects include weight loss, dehydration, electrolyte imbalance, ketonuria, and ketonemia. Clients with this condition may require hospitalization with fluid and electrolyte replacement. Any underlying pathophysiology must be ruled out. See Chapter 13 for more discussion.

Many gastrointestinal system changes occur predominantly in the second and third trimesters. Women may experience heartburn as the growing fetus displaces the stomach. A decrease in gastric smooth muscle tone and motility, resulting from effects of progesterone, also may cause reflux of gastric contents into the esophagus, adding to heartburn (Blackburn, 2014). Decreased intestinal motility results from pressure of the growing fetus on the intestine and the effects of progesterone, leading to constipation. The function of the gallbladder is also altered during pregnancy. Increased progesterone levels cause a hypotonic condition which may lead to slow emptying time. Subsequent stasis of bile and the increased cholesterol levels in pregnancy may predispose women to gallstones (Blackburn, 2014).

Integumentary System

Extra pigmentation often appears, caused by increased melanocyte-stimulating hormone secreted by the pituitary and the melanocyte-stimulating effects of estrogen and progesterone (Blackburn, 2014; Cunningham et al., 2010). A dark line (**linea nigra**) may be visible from just under the sternum to the pubis, separating the abdomen vertically into two hemispheres (Fig. 12.5). Darkened areas also may appear on the face, primarily over the nose and cheeks (**chloasma**). Chloasma is also referred to as the "mask of pregnancy." Once melanocyte-stimulating hormones decrease in the

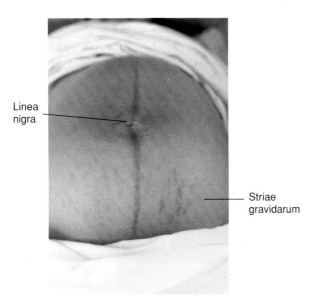

FIGURE 12.5 Skin changes in pregnancy include linea nigra and striae gravidarum.

postpartum period, the increased pigmentation usually disappears (Cunningham et al., 2010). Pigmentation may again appear with exposure to sun or oral contraceptive use (Blackburn, 2014).

As pregnancy advances, the abdominal skin becomes stretched. This results in small ruptures in the connective layer of the skin, leading to what are commonly referred to as "stretch marks" or **striae gravidarum**. These marks tend to fade following the birth of the baby, becoming more silver or white, although they never completely disappear (see Fig. 12.5). Striae also may appear on the breasts as they enlarge and on any other body parts with large weight gain. Some women use moisturizers, including cocoa butter, in an attempt to prevent or decrease these body changes, although there is no scientific basis for this practice (Buchanan et al., 2010). Some women also believe that the massage that accompanies application of these products is beneficial in preventing or decreasing skin changes.

With the progression of pregnancy, the rectus muscle may stretch to the point that it actually separates. This is known as **diastasis**. If it occurs, a pyramid shape may appear in the lower abdomen when the woman raises her head from a flat surface, as the underlying muscles protrude through the separation. If a diastasis does occur, the client should refrain from doing sit-ups until the gap reduces and should avoid lifting anything heavy, both of which may exacerbate the separation or lead to development of a hernia.

 Remember Millie, the 38-year-old woman from the beginning of the chapter who just found out that she was pregnant with her third child. When performing her physical assessment, would you expect to find striae gravidarum? Why or why not?

Endocrine System

The biggest change to the endocrine system is caused by the placenta, which produces several hormones, including estrogen, progesterone, hCG, human chorionic somatomammotropin or human placental lactogen (hPL), and relaxin (Silverthorn, 2013). The following are the bodily changes caused by these hormones:

- Estrogen causes breast and uterine enlargement.
- Progesterone helps maintain the endometrium, inhibits uterine contractility, and aids in breast development.
- The trophoblast cells of the placenta secrete hCG early in pregnancy; hCG stimulates progesterone and estrogen, which help maintain the pregnancy until the placenta can assume this function at approximately 7 weeks' gestation.

- The placenta secretes hPL at approximately 20 weeks' gestation; hPL acts as an insulin antagonist, freeing up fatty acids for energy so that glucose is available for fetal growth.
- Relaxin is responsible for softening the collagen in joints and the cervix; it also plays a role in inhibition of uterine contractions.
- The thyroid gland grows up to 50% during pregnancy, causing increased release of thyroxin. Increased secretion of adrenocortical hormones, together with increased thyroxin, leads to an increased BMR (Hall, 2011). Consequently, the pregnant woman frequently has sensations of overheating, which is also related to increased blood volume. The parathyroid gland also enlarges slightly, causing increased use of calcium and vitamin D.

Reproductive System

Pregnancy-related changes affect the uterus, cervix, ovaries, vagina, and breasts. The most obvious change is in the uterus, which gradually enlarges to encompass the growing fetus.

Uterus

The uterus grows constantly and predictably throughout pregnancy. It increases in weight from 70 to 1,100 g, and in capacity from 10 to 5,000 mL. The uterine wall thickens from 1 to 2 cm, although by the end of pregnancy the wall thins, so that it is supple and only approximately 1.5 cm thick (Cunningham et al., 2010).

At approximately 6 weeks' gestation, the lower uterine segment just above the cervix becomes extremely soft. The provider can assess for this finding by performing bimanual examination, in which he or she puts one finger of one hand in the vagina while using the other hand to palpate the abdomen. The examiner will barely be able to feel the lower uterine segment, or it will feel extremely thin. The uterus flexes easily over the cervix. This softening is referred to as **Hegar's sign** (Fig. 12.6).

Uterine contractions begin at approximately 12 weeks' gestation and last for the duration of gestation; they become stronger as pregnancy advances. The woman may begin to feel these **Braxton-Hicks contractions**, which contribute to increased placental perfusion, as waves across the uterus in the early part of the third trimester. They can be palpable and visible on monitor strips. During the last month of pregnancy, Braxton-Hicks contractions may be strong enough to make the client mistake them for labour contractions. Most clients are taught about Braxton-Hicks contractions, with the expectation that they will be able to distinguish between them and true labour contractions. Whenever the woman learns about Braxton-Hicks contractions, it is essential for nurses to provide

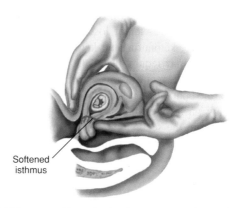

FIGURE 12.6 Hegar's sign in pregnancy is a softening of the lower uterine segment just above the cervix. Upon palpation, the area becomes difficult to feel or feels extremely thin; in addition, the uterus flexes easily over the cervix.

comprehensive education about the signs of premature labour (see Chapter 16).

By 20 to 24 weeks, the uterine wall becomes thin enough to allow a skilled examiner to palpate the fetal outline. This palpation, termed **Leopold manoeuvres**, assists providers to determine the position of the fetus. It also facilitates auscultation of the fetal heart. Both of these assessments are presented later in this chapter.

The height of the **fundus** (the top of the uterus) should correspond with the week of gestation in a singleton pregnancy (Fig. 12.7). For example, at 28 weeks' gestation, the distance from the pubis to the fundus should be approximately 28 cm. At 34 weeks' gestation, it should be 34 cm. At approximately 38 weeks in the primigravida, uterine height decreases to the level of its height at 36 weeks. This phenomenon, termed *lightening*, occurs as the presenting part settles into the pelvis in preparation for birth.

Health care providers can measure symphysis–fundal height in one of the two ways (Fig. 12.8). In the

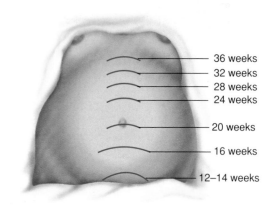

FIGURE 12.7 Fundal height corresponds to the week of gestation.

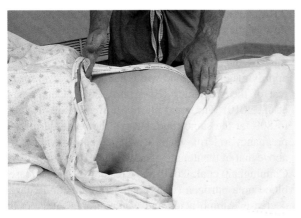

FIGURE 12.8 The nurse assesses symphysis–fundal height with a tape measure.

first method, the nurse places one end of a tape measure at the client's symphysis pubis and extends the tape up to and over the curve of the fundus. In the second method, the nurse places one end of the tape measure at the symphysis pubis of the woman. He or she then extends the tape up to the curve of the fundus, but stops before going over the curve. Either method is acceptable; however, all practitioners should consistently use the same method to prevent discrepancies in measurements. Evidence suggests that the measurement of symphysis–fundal height is less diagnostic of fetal weight abnormalities than ultrasound measurement of fetal abdominal circumference (Kayem et al., 2009).

Cervix

The cervix becomes more vascular and edematous in response to increased circulating estrogen from the placenta (Cunningham et al., 2010). Increased vascularity causes the cervix to become dark violet rather than pale pink. Increased fluid between the cells causes the cervix to soften; this softening, called **Goodell's sign**, is significant. The consistency of the nonpregnant cervix is similar to the tip of the nose, whereas the consistency of the pregnant cervix is like that of the ear lobe. Just before labour, the cervix further softens until it can be compared to the consistency of butter. This finding is a characteristic of being "ripe" for birth.

Ovaries

Ovulation ceases because of the feedback of estrogen and progesterone produced by the corpus luteum in early pregnancy and the placenta later. This feedback causes cessation of secretion of follicle-stimulating hormone (FSH), which leads to **amenorrhea**.

Vagina

The vaginal epithelium undergoes changes as a result of circulating estrogen. Increased vascularity changes the colour of the vaginal wall from the prepregnant pink to deep violet (**Chadwick's sign**). Increased estrogen also affects the vaginal epithelium and underlying tissue, causing them to become hypertrophic and enriched with glycogen. As the endocervical glands hypertrophy and increase, they form a tenacious coating of mucus, or **operculum**. This mucus plug serves as a barrier to prevent bacteria from entering the vagina, thus preventing infection in the fetus and membranes.

The pH of vaginal secretions changes from an alkaline value above 7 to an acidic value of 4 or 5. The primary cause is the bacteria *Lactobacillus acidophilus*, which grows in the glycogen-enriched environment (Cunningham et al., 2010). This pH change has favourable effects, because it helps prevent bacterial invasion of the vagina during pregnancy. However, it also has unfavourable effects, because it provides an environment that encourages the growth of *Candida albicans*, a yeast infection that causes itching, burning, and a white, cheesy discharge. Although treatment of *C. albicans* primarily aims to promote comfort, it also is necessary to prevent transmission to the newborn as he or she passes through the vaginal canal at birth.

Breasts

Breast changes result from high levels of circulating estrogen and progesterone and increased blood flow (Chow et al., 2013). During the first trimester, women may report symptoms such as tingling, fullness, or tenderness. As pregnancy progresses, the weight and size of the breasts increase (Fig. 12.9). Women require a larger bra to accommodate this increased size.

The areola darken and increase in size. The sebaceous glands of the areola (**Montgomery tubercles**) become enlarged and may be protuberant. Secretions from these glands help keep the nipples supple and prevent drying and cracking during lactation. Blue veins may become prominent over the breasts as vascularity to the area increases. By 16 weeks, the nipples may begin to express colostrum, the thin, watery, high-protein fluid that is the precursor to breast milk (see Chapter 21).

Urinary System

During the first trimester, the pregnant woman may experience urinary frequency until the uterus rises out of the pelvis and relieves pressure on the bladder. Such frequency returns in the later stages of pregnancy as lightening occurs and the fetal head again puts pressure on the bladder (Fig. 12.10).

Total body water increases by approximately 6.5 L by the end of pregnancy (Cunningham et al., 2010). During pregnancy, the woman's kidneys must filter both maternal and fetal waste products. The kidneys also must be able to handle the increased renal blood flow. Kidney size increases approximately 1 cm (Blackburn,

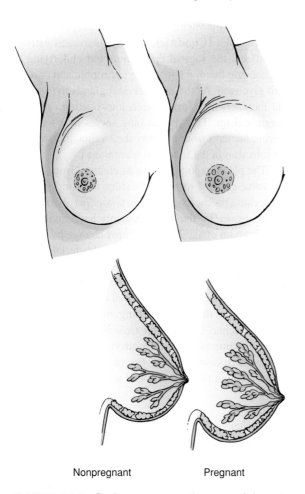

FIGURE 12.9 During pregnancy, the woman's breasts grow. The areolae darken and increase, and the sebaceous glands become enlarged and may be protuberant.

Nonpregnant   Pregnant

2014). Glomerular filtration rate (GFR) and renal plasma flow begin to increase in early pregnancy to meet the increased need of the circulatory system. By the beginning of the second trimester, the GFR has increased approximately 50% and will remain at this level for the rest of the pregnancy (Blackburn, 2014; Cunningham et al., 2010). The renal plasma flow increases by 50% to 80% at the same time, but will decrease during late pregnancy to term, where it will be approximately 50% above that of the nonpregnant woman (Blackburn, 2014; Cunningham et al., 2010). As a result of these increases, blood urea nitrogen (BUN) and serum creatinine levels decrease. Amino acids and water-soluble vitamins are lost in greater amounts in the urine.

The increased GFR, antidiuretic hormone (ADH), prostaglandins, and progesterone, as well as the decreased vascular resistance cause the woman to excrete sodium. The body increases its sodium reabsorption in the tubules to aid in maintenance of osmolarity. Progesterone causes an increased response of the renin–angiotensin–aldosterone system, leading to increased aldosterone production, which promotes sodium reabsorption. Estrogen, aldosterone, and cortisol also have an effect on increasing sodium absorption (Blackburn, 2014; Cunningham et al., 2010).

The higher GFR leads to increased filtration of glucose into the renal tubules. Because glucose is reabsorbed by the tubule cells at a fixed rate, some glucose will spill into the urine during pregnancy. Glucose is also spilled into the urine at lower levels of serum glucose.

The ureters increase in diameter because of the increased progesterone level. Ureteral compression

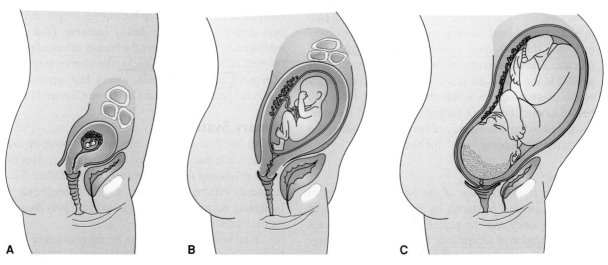

FIGURE 12.10 Urinary frequency in pregnancy is related to the changing position of the uterus as the fetus grows. **A.** In early pregnancy, pressure of the uterus against the bladder leads to increased urinary frequency. **B.** In the second trimester, the uterine position changes so that bladder pressure is relieved. **C.** Toward the end of pregnancy, the uterus once again is pressing on the bladder, leading to increased frequency.

A   B   C

from the enlarging uterus and ovarian vein plexus and pressure of the ureters against the pelvic brim may lead to hydronephrosis and hydroureter (Cunningham et al., 2010). Pressure on the urethra may lead to poor bladder emptying and subsequent bladder infection. During later gestation, the enlarging uterus may cause pressure on the bladder that may lead to urinary stasis and pyelonephritis, if not relieved. These infections are significant, because each increases the risk for preterm labour (Cunningham et al., 2010).

Musculoskeletal System

Calcium and magnesium needs increase because the fetal bones are forming and plasma levels are low. Calcium intake should be between 1,000 and 1,300 mg/day, depending on age (Health Canada, 2012). Vitamin D intake should be 15 µg/day or 600 IU/day (Health Canada, 2012). There may be an association between calcium intake and preeclampsia. The Society of Obstetricians and Gynaecologists of Canada (SOGC) recommends calcium supplementation of 1,000 mg/day for women with low dietary intake to decrease the incidence of preeclampsia (Magee et al., 2008).

As pregnancy progresses, the pelvic joints become more pliable under the influence of relaxin. This increased flexibility facilitates delivery of the fetus, but may also cause discomfort to the woman. Sometimes the symphysis pubis separates up to 3 to 4 mm, leading to difficulty walking.

The increasing weight of the fetus and protrusion of the belly cause **lordosis,** an abnormal forward curvature of the spine in the lumbar region, as the woman attempts to maintain a centre of gravity (Fig. 12.11). She may subsequently experience a chronic backache.

Physiologic Differences Related to Age and Race/Ethnicity

Many physiologic changes during pregnancy are common to all women regardless of age, race, or ethnicity. Some differences, however, are unique to certain age groups or to people of specific race or ethnicity.

Adolescent mothers who have not yet completed their own growth may be at increased risk for related complications, including **cephalopelvic disproportion (CPD),** which increases the risk for caesarean birth. They are at increased risk for low-birth-weight babies, preterm labour, and gestational hypertension, although some studies suggest that the risk for gestational hypertension is more related to parity than age (Al-Sahab et al., 2012; Ozalp et al., 2003; Stevens-Simon et al., 2002). These risks are increased with younger adolescents, especially those who conceive within 2 years of menarche (Stevens-Simon et al., 2002). Risks such as inadequate nutrition, poor health, and those related

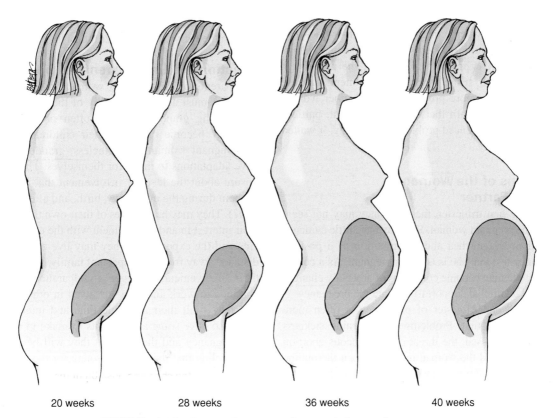

20 weeks   28 weeks   36 weeks   40 weeks

FIGURE 12.11 Progressive maternal postural changes in pregnancy.

to poverty may have negative effects on a pregnancy (Al-Sahab et al., 2012; Stevens-Simon et al., 2002).

Women older than 35 years have higher incidences of pre-existing conditions, such as diabetes and hypertension (Johnson & Tough, 2012; Ozalp et al., 2003). Hypertension increases the risk for developing abruptio placentae and preeclampsia (Magee et al., 2008; Poole, 2014). The risk for caesarean birth is increased for women who delay childbearing (Johnson & Tough, 2012). Questions have been raised about whether the increased rate of preterm and caesarean births is related to a higher incidence of maternal complications or simply age (Johnson & Tough, 2012; Kozinsky et al., 2002).

Several diseases or alterations that may affect pregnancy seem to be prevalent in women of childbearing age from different ethnic or racial backgrounds. For example, the incidence of sickle cell anemia is increased in African American women and Tay–Sachs disease is more common in the Ashkenazi Jewish population (Callister, 2014). See Chapter 4 for more discussion.

PSYCHOLOGICAL AND EMOTIONAL CHANGES IN PREGNANCY

Many psychological changes for the woman and her significant others are common throughout pregnancy. Even if a pregnancy is planned, many women are surprised to find they are actually pregnant. They may feel somewhat ambivalent, questioning whether the timing is right or how they should modify career plans. A woman may experience fears about the pregnancy, labour, and birth. If the pregnancy is unintended, these feelings may be more pronounced. Still other women are overjoyed to learn that they are pregnant, particularly if they experienced problems conceiving or waited a long time to try.

Reactions of the Woman and Her Partner

During the first trimester, the pregnancy may not seem real to the pregnant woman. She may have little evidence other than amenorrhea and confirmation of a positive pregnancy test that she is actually pregnant. As a consequence, she may become conscious of any body changes that lend additional support to validate the pregnancy.

The second trimester of pregnancy is often more idyllic than the first. Problems with morning sickness have usually passed, the threat of spontaneous abortion is decreased, and the woman may have seen the outline of the fetus on an ultrasound to confirm that there actually is a pregnancy. Women, particularly primigravidas, may choose to wear maternity clothes before truly needing them as outward confirmation of the pregnancy.

Alternatively, some women experience feelings of grief at the loss of usual body shape and size. One highlight of the second trimester is quickening, which usually occurs at approximately 20 weeks' gestation. The nurse needs to be sure that he or she is not projecting onto the woman and her significant others how they should feel. Sometimes, ambivalence remains, or expected feelings do not occur. This is also a time when the partner can be more involved in the pregnancy. Feeling the baby's movements and hearing the fetal heart during visits to the care provider help to increase the partner's involvement.

The woman often experiences mounting apprehension about what is to come as the pregnancy progresses. She may fear pain, losing control, or the responsibilities of parenthood that will come after birth (Perry et al., 2013). Physical discomforts return as the baby grows. The mother begins to prepare for the birth of the baby. Both parents are more involved in planning for labour and birth. This may be when they attend prenatal classes together. The partner may feel increased concern for the woman as she becomes more uncomfortable and the end of the pregnancy nears. Near the end of the pregnancy, the woman often experiences a surge of energy (Pillitteri, 2007). She may use this increased energy to clean and organize the home. The nurse informs the mother about this phenomenon and encourages her to resist the temptation to work, resting instead to save her energy for the stress of the labour ahead. In the weeks leading up to her due date, she may want to consider preparing meals ahead of time and freezing them to be used in the early days after her return home postpartum.

Reactions of Grandparents-to-be

The parents of the pregnant woman (and of her partner) also must accept the reality of the pregnancy and the coming grandchild. They often provide support and may become closer to their children, especially the pregnant woman. Nevertheless, grandparents also have adaptations to make for themselves. They may be unsure about the level of involvement that is expected of them during the pregnancy, birth, and after (Pillitteri, 2007). They may have issues of their own that influence their interest in and involvement with the expectant parents and the experience. They may live a considerable distance away from the expectant family, which curtails their involvement. Younger grandparents-to-be often continue to work and to be involved in other activities that may limit their available time and interest. They may also have some adjustments to make in accepting the pregnancy and the fact that they will be grandparents, feeling that they are too young for the role. Other issues such as retirement, death of friends, or menopause of the grandmother may influence reactions and subsequent involvement with the pregnancy and child. Nurses remain sensitive to any cultural patterns of communication or interaction that may influence the plan of care.

Reactions of Other Children

The idea of a younger sibling coming into the family may present challenges for other children. There is no "best" time to accomplish this; however, the introduction of the coming addition of the sibling should be based on the age, developmental level, and experience of the other children. Parents should tell the child about the coming baby before or when they tell other family members, to decrease any risk that they will hear the news accidentally or from someone else. Depending on the child's age, it may be most appropriate to begin actions to minimize potential sibling rivalry early in the pregnancy. Children who are very young may experience anxiety and frustration when the expectant mother is more fatigued. The child may feel deprived of attention. Young children need consistency. They need to know that familiar places, people, and things will continue once the new baby arrives. If planning for the new arrival involves moving children from a crib to another bed, parents should do so at a minimum of several weeks before the baby's birth.

Young toddlers frequently show regressive behaviour, reverting to thumb sucking, wanting to drink from a bottle, or wetting or soiling after having been toilet trained. One possible reason is that the toddler sees the new baby getting attention for doing these things (Pillitteri, 2007). If the new parents are aware of this possibility, they are much less frustrated if it occurs.

Families should include school-aged children as the pregnancy progresses. Information should be provided in a quantity and at a level appropriate for the child's developmental stage and interest. Feeling fetal movements, listening to the fetal heart, and attending sibling preparation classes help children to feel that they are part of the pregnancy (Fig. 12.12).

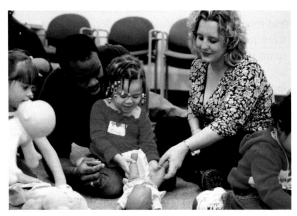

FIGURE 12.12 Sibling preparation classes can help children adjust to the changes in their family and make them feel like they are part of the experience.

Older children and adolescents may appear to be knowledgeable, but have many misconceptions. They may feel uncomfortable with the evidence of their parents' sexuality or may worry about changes to the family structure. They may be concerned that they will be expected to shoulder additional responsibilities. Parents should provide the older child or adolescent the opportunity to voice any concerns. Opportunities can be created for them to be involved in the preparation for the new child.

Changing attitudes and facility policies frequently allow children to be present at the child's birth. This changing practice facilitates involvement of siblings in the birth and feeling a part of the process. Children often attend classes that prepare them to be present at the birth. In addition to the positive aspects of involving the children, however, negative aspects also may arise. Children may become frightened or upset at seeing their mother in pain. A specific person should be designated to provide support to the children during the labour and birth. If the children cannot continue to be present, this person will provide support and care to them. Following the birth, parents need to continue to focus on assisting children to feel that they are part of the family.

SIGNS OF PREGNANCY

Several changes that women experience are used to diagnose pregnancy. These include *presumptive* or subjective signs, *probable* or objective signs, and *positive* or diagnostic signs.

Presumptive Signs

Presumptive signs of pregnancy are those subjective changes the woman herself experiences. They do not confirm a pregnancy, because other factors also may cause the same changes. In conjunction with other signs, however, they can be diagnostic.

The first sign that women generally experience is amenorrhea. In a woman with regular cycles, one or two missed menstrual periods suggest pregnancy. Another presumptive sign is "**morning sickness**"—nausea and vomiting that often occurs in the morning and fades during the day. Women may experience variations in nausea and vomiting, however, which range from distaste for certain foods or odours, vomiting throughout the day, and/or vomiting at night. Nausea and vomiting usually appear 6 weeks after the first day of the last menstrual period and last for approximately 6 to 12 weeks, ending with the beginning of the second trimester. Occasionally, nausea and vomiting are prolonged beyond this time frame.

Excessive fatigue may begin within a few weeks after the first day of the last menstrual period and may be present during the entire first trimester. Women in the first trimester may experience urinary frequency, which develops as the enlarging uterus exerts pressure on the bladder. This will diminish as the uterus rises in the abdomen, returning again near the end of pregnancy.

The woman may notice breast changes, including enlargement, tingling sensations, and tenderness, during the first few weeks of pregnancy. Pigmentation of the nipples and areolae may change, along with increased visibility of the veins, especially in those women with fair skin, occurring after the second month.

The woman may experience **quickening**, the first perception of fetal movement. Women often describe quickening as a fluttering in the abdomen that increases in frequency and duration until the movements become perceptible as distinct fetal movements that will continue throughout the pregnancy. Quickening usually occurs between 16 and 20 weeks' gestation (Cunningham et al., 2010).

Probable Signs

Probable signs of pregnancy are those objective changes assessed by the examiner. Even though they are more diagnostic than presumptive signs, they are not a definitive diagnosis—again, probable signs may result from other factors.

Changes to the uterus and vagina are the only probable signs detectable in the first trimester. They include softening of the cervix (Goodell's sign); the dark violet colouration of the cervix, vagina, and vulva (Chadwick's sign); and the softening of the lower part of the uterus between the cervix and the body (Hegar's sign). Increased circulation to the area and circulating estrogen cause these changes, which are usually evident by 6 to 8 weeks' gestation.

Progressive uterine enlargement, especially accompanied by continuing amenorrhea, is usually evidence of pregnancy. This enlargement may be more pronounced in multigravidas, whose abdominal musculature has lost some tone from previous pregnancies. The fundus of the uterus is palpable just above the symphysis pubis at 10 to 12 weeks' gestation, and at the level of the umbilicus at 20 to 22 weeks. The examiner may use Leopold manoeuvres to feel the fetal outline, beginning at approximately 24 weeks' gestation. Abdominal palpation may reveal Braxton-Hicks contractions at approximately the 28th week.

Human chorionic gonadotropin (hCG) is the chemical detected by pregnancy tests (Silverthorn, 2013). It appears in the serum early in pregnancy after implantation of the fertilized oocyte (Silverthorn, 2013). The hCG level peaks between 60 and 70 days' gestation, and then declines until about 100 to 130 days, when the level reaches its lowest point (Cunningham et al., 2010). Pregnancy tests are based on maternal blood or urine tests assessing for hCG. Blood serum tests are used more frequently than urine tests, because hCG is detected earlier in serum and therefore results can be obtained earlier. Findings are considered probable rather than positive, because luteinizing hormone, secreted by the pituitary, is similar to hCG and can sometimes cause a false-positive result. As well, conditions other than pregnancy can cause increased hCG.

Several different over-the-counter home pregnancy kits are available that manufacturers indicate are up to 99% accurate if used exactly according to directions (U.S. Department of Health and Human Services, 2009). These tests are based on recognition of hCG in the urine (U.S. Department of Health and Human Services, 2009). The woman dips the reagent strip into her urine stream or into a container containing her urine. If she detects a colour change on the strip or a line appears, the result is positive. The indicated time frame of the test is 3 to 5 minutes.

Most manufacturers suggest the woman wait until the day of her missed menstrual period to test; if done too early, results are unreliable. Some pregnancy tests on the market suggest that they can detect hCG at lower levels and thus test for pregnancy as early as 7 to 10 days after ovulation (see http://www.early-pregnancy-tests.com/pregnancytests.html). However, it may be difficult to accurately predict when conception has actually occurred. Implantation does not always occur before the expected onset of menses, nor is the hCG level produced this early in sufficient amounts for home pregnancy kits to detect.

Millie has just found out that she is 12 weeks pregnant. What probable signs would you expect Millie to have exhibited that suggest pregnancy?

Before the advent of home pregnancy kits, women had to visit their health care provider to find out if they were pregnant. Because it is now possible for women to do pregnancy tests at home, they may delay accessing prenatal care. The nurse can encourage early and regular prenatal care once a client has identified probable signs of pregnancy. He or she can instruct the client that a positive pregnancy test result confirms only that trophoblastic tissue has secreted hCG. The test does not provide positive confirmation of either pregnancy or its location. For example, gestational trophoblastic neoplasia (an uncommon but serious cancer that secretes hCG) results in a positive pregnancy test with no accompanying pregnancy. An ectopic pregnancy also may produce a positive result and may be missed if the woman does not seek early prenatal care. The client should discontinue use of oral contraceptives at least 5 days before the test to prevent false-positive results.

Because of the possibility of false-negative results with home pregnancy tests, a provider must further evaluate any negative test result when the woman continues to show other signs of pregnancy.

Evaluation focuses on the response of the client and her significant others. The nurse recognizes that a range of responses is possible. Whether the pregnancy is intended or not, reactions vary widely. Clients may experience joy, excitement, ambivalence, apprehension, or fear, even if a pregnancy was intended. Reactions may depend on past experiences with pregnancy, stories relayed by others, and anticipation. The nurse and client will plan further care based on this evaluation.

If a pregnancy is unintended or unwanted, the woman may consider abortion as an option in the early months (see Chapter 9). If the pregnancy is unwanted and therapeutic abortion is not an option, the woman may consider adoption as an alternative. The nurse provides consultations with other health care workers, including social workers, to enable the woman to obtain additional information about the options available and to make preliminary plans.

Positive Signs

Positive signs are those signs that absolutely confirm pregnancy: a fetal heart, fetal movements that the examiner can feel, and visualization of the fetus on ultrasound. Positive signs are completely objective and cannot result from any other cause or pathology. They are usually undetectable until the third month.

An examiner may hear the fetal heart or see it on ultrasound (Fig. 12.13). The fetal heart is detectable by ultrasound Doppler as early as 10 weeks' gestation (Cunningham et al., 2010). It can be detected by 16 to 19 weeks on auscultation with a stethoscope or fetoscope (Cunningham et al., 2010). Normal at a rate of 110 to 160 bpm, it is best heard over the fetal back. Movement of the fetal heart first occurs at approximately the fourth week and can be detected by echocardiography as early as 48 days after the first day of the last normal menses or by transvaginal sonography (see Chapter 11) by the fifth week (Cunningham et al., 2010).

Auscultation of the abdomen over the uterus may reveal the uterine souffle. This soft swooshing sound results from the flow of the increased blood volume and vascularity of the uterus and placenta. Because the rate of the uterine souffle matches the maternal pulse, the examiner palpates the radial pulse of the mother simultaneously with auscultation of the abdomen. If it is the uterine souffle that is heard, the beats of the souffle will match the palpated maternal pulse beats. If the beats that are heard do not match the palpated maternal pulse beats, the examiner can be confident that he or she is hearing the fetal heart tones. This assessment is essential because the fetal heart rate (FHR) may be decreased in some instances.

An examiner can usually feel fetal movements after 20 weeks' gestation (Cunningham et al., 2010), although maternal obesity may interfere until later in the pregnancy when the fetus is larger. If ultrasound is done at 4 to 6 weeks, a gestational sac may be seen, which confirms the pregnancy.

ANTEPARTAL HEALTH ASSESSMENT

Health care providers offer information about assessment findings and their meanings to the pregnant client and her designated significant others. They use information gathered during assessments to plan individualized care throughout the pregnancy and for labour and birth. Nurses also provide information about anticipated changes to assist the client and family to plan interventions related to such changes.

Assessment of maternal health is an extremely important part of care, both at the initial prenatal visit

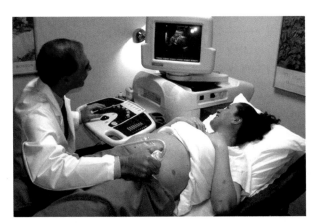
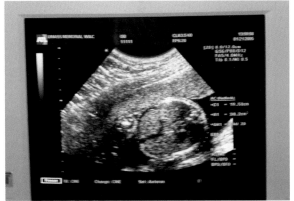

FIGURE 12.13 The appearance of the fetal heart on ultrasound is a positive sign of pregnancy.

and throughout pregnancy. Any alterations in maternal health pose concerns for the woman's well-being and can potentially hinder fetal growth, development, and well-being, thus requiring close monitoring. Nurses and other health care providers can identify risk factors that may pose problems for the woman, fetus, or both during pregnancy, labour, and birth. They can then plan care to decrease such risks. Continuing prenatal care can identify additional risk factors that may not exist or manifest themselves at the first visit and assist the health care team to ensure healthy pregnancy outcomes.

Initial Prenatal Maternal Health Assessment

Once a client identifies herself to a health care practitioner as believing she is pregnant, the provider performs an assessment to confirm the pregnancy. Nurses and other health care providers conduct a thorough assessment (history taking and physical examination) of the pregnant client at the first prenatal visit. The health history should cover a complete menstrual, sexual, and pregnancy history; family history of the woman to determine whether any familial or genetic disorders may affect maternal or fetal health (see Chapter 11); history of any previous pregnancies and births; and past illnesses. The physical examination should be comprehensive, with accompanying laboratory and diagnostic evaluations.

If pregnancy is not confirmed, the provider assesses for alternative causes of the identified symptoms (Table 12.2). The nurse can educate the pregnant client about relief measures for symptoms to promote comfort as much as possible.

● TABLE 12.2   Signs of Pregnancy and Possible Alternative Explanations

Signs of Pregnancy	Possible Alternative Explanations
Presumptive Signs	
Amenorrhea	Endocrine disorder
	Lactation
	Malnutrition, including anorexia nervosa or bulimia
	Excessive exercise
	Emotional stress
	Early menopause
Nausea and vomiting	Gastrointestinal disorders
	Emotional stress
	Acute infection
Fatigue	Lack of sleep
	Overexertion
	Anemia
	Other illnesses
Urinary frequency	Urinary tract infection
	Cystocele
	Emotional stress
Breast changes	Premenstrual changes
	Chronic cystic mastitis
	Breast cysts
Quickening	Increased peristalsis
	Flatus
	Abdominal muscle contractions
Probable Signs	
Goodell's sign	Estrogen–progesterone contraceptive pill
Chadwick's sign	Increased vascular congestion
Hegar's sign	Other hormonal influences
	Anatomically soft walls of nonpregnant uterus
Enlarged uterus	Uterine tumour
	Uterine fibroids
Braxton-Hicks contractions	Hematomas
	Soft myoma
Changes in pigmentation	Contraceptives
Positive pregnancy test results	Luteinizing hormone secreted by pituitary
	Gestational trophoblastic neoplasia
	Ectopic pregnancy

Health History

During the first prenatal visit, a comprehensive health history provides a wealth of information that nurses and other health care providers use to assess risks associated with the pregnancy, plan appropriate care, and help ensure positive outcomes. The woman's physical and emotional health before pregnancy is as important as her physical and emotional health during gestation. Assessment Tool 12.1 provides a suggested organization for a thorough health history, along with rationales and recommended questions.

Menstrual History. The nurse obtains the client's menstrual history, which includes age at onset of menarche; frequency, regularity, duration, and amount of blood loss with normal menstrual periods; any history of dysmenorrhea; and date of the first day of the last normal menstrual period. This portion of the history helps identify any irregularities in the client's normal menses that may affect calculation of the estimated date of delivery (EDD). Irregular menstrual periods often correspond with irregular ovulation; in such cases, the EDD may be less reliable. It is also important to identify that the last menstrual period was normal. Some clients experience bleeding with implantation and may misinterpret this event as a menstrual period.

Sexual and Sexually Transmitted Infection (STI) History. An appropriate sexual history includes type of birth control used and when the woman discontinued it. Recent use of hormonal contraception (eg, oral contraceptives) may delay ovulation, which may affect calculation of the EDD. Use of an intrauterine device (IUD), if still in place, may threaten the integrity of the pregnancy, and increases the risk for spontaneous abortion, sepsis, or preterm birth (Cunningham et al., 2010). Failure to use a latex condom may, depending on the situation, increase risks for HIV and other STIs. A pregnancy that occurs despite use of contraception may necessitate discussion of the desirability of the pregnancy.

The nurse identifies any history of STIs, which may be transmitted through sexual intercourse or sexual contact with the genitals, rectum, or mouth. STIs also may be transmitted in other ways. These STIs include gonorrhea; syphilis; HIV; human papillomavirus (HPV), which commonly manifests as genital warts; herpes simplex virus (HSV), which causes genital herpes; chlamydia; hepatitis B and C; and vaginitis, which may be caused by organisms such as trichomonas and *C. albicans*. Identification of a history of STIs is important, because it may affect care planned during pregnancy and delivery (See Chapter 4 for further discussion of STIs).

Along with the risks for cervical and other cancers, chronic hepatitis, cirrhosis, and other complications common for all women, pregnant women have additional consequences that may arise from STIs, which may be apparent at birth or appear at a later date. Pregnancies complicated by STIs have an increased risk for stillbirth, preterm labour, low birth weight, conjunctivitis, pneumonia, neonatal sepsis, neurologic damage, congenital abnormalities, and meningitis (Centers for Disease Control and Prevention [CDC], 2012; Cunningham et al., 2010). Congenital abnormalities may include blindness, deafness, or other organ damage.

Mothers can transmit STIs to newborns before, during, or after birth. For example, syphilis can cross the placenta and infect the fetus, causing congenital syphilis (Perry et al., 2013). Gonorrhea and chlamydia are transmitted as the infant passes through the birth canal during delivery and can cause neonatal conjunctivitis (Dapaah & Dapaah, 2009; Perry et al., 2013).

The number of women who are HIV positive in Canada is on the rise (Loutfy et al., 2012). Between 1984 and 2012, there were 3,805 infants identified as exposed to HIV perinatally, with the number increasing significantly between 2005 and 2008 (from 191 to 241); the number has fluctuated since (Public Health Agency of Canada, 2013b). HIV can cross the placental barrier and infect the fetus. Medication is available to help decrease fetal susceptibility to HIV; it is often initiated in the preconceptual period or early in the pregnancy and continued until birth under the guidance of an HIV specialist (Loutfy et al., 2012). HIV can be transmitted during birth and through breast milk (Dapaah & Dapaah, 2009). Delivery via caesarean section when indicated and abstinence from breastfeeding have helped to decrease vertical transmission from the mother to the newborn to less than 1% (Loutfy et al., 2012).

Past Pregnancies. The nurse obtains a history of past pregnancies, including whether they were planned. Complications arising in previous pregnancies may predispose the woman to a higher risk for the same complications in the present pregnancy. Information about the course of past labours and births may be useful in planning the course of this pregnancy.

A woman who has never been pregnant is called a **nulligravida**. If this is the client's first pregnancy, she is referred to as a **primigravida**. If this is a second or subsequent pregnancy, the term **multigravida** is used. The term *para* was previously used to denote the number of births after the 20th week of gestation. Because this term provides less clarity and health care providers sometimes interpreted it inconsistently, a system that provides more comprehensive data about the status of past pregnancies and births is now used. Providers use the acronym GTPAL to obtain a comprehensive pregnancy history:

- G—the total number of pregnancies that the woman has had, including the current one

(text continues on page 438)

● **ASSESSMENT TOOL 12.1** **Prenatal Health Assessment Form**

MENSTRUAL HISTORY

RATIONALE: *Identify irregularities in normal menstrual cycle that may affect the calculation of estimated date of delivery (EDD).*

Suggested questions:

- Tell me about your normal menstrual cycle.
- Tell me about your last menstrual period. When did it occur? Was it the same as or different from your normal periods?
- When did you begin to menstruate?
- How frequently do you get your menstrual period?
- Do your cycles stay the same or change from month to month? Is there any variation between cycles?
- How many days does your period normally last?
- How many pads/tampons do you saturate each day?

SEXUAL HISTORY

RATIONALE: *Recent use of birth control pills may delay ovulation. An IUD in place increases risk for spontaneous abortion or ectopic pregnancy. Early identification of sexually transmitted infections will prevent prolonged fetal exposure to effects of infection and will facilitate planning of appropriate care.*

Suggested questions:

- Tell me about what type of birth control you have been using.
- When did you discontinue using it?
- Tell me about any sexually transmitted infections you may have had.
- Have you ever had gonorrhea (clap), syphilis, HIV, genital warts, genital herpes, chlamydia, or hepatitis? If you have, describe when and how you were treated.
- Has your partner ever had any of these infections? If so, describe when and how your partner was treated.
- Have you ever had a vaginal infection? If you have, tell me about what it was like and how it was treated.
- How many sexual partners have you had?
- Have you ever had unprotected sex? If you have, tell me when this happened.

PAST PREGNANCY HISTORY

RATIONALE: *A history of past pregnancies helps identify potential complications in the current pregnancy. A history of past labours and births will assist in planning for the current pregnancy.*

Suggested questions:

- Tell me about any other pregnancies you have had.
- How many other pregnancies have you had?

- What dates were your children born?
- Have you had any babies that were premature or born earlier than they were supposed to be?
- How early were they born?
- Have you had any miscarriages or abortions? If you had a therapeutic abortion, how was it done and were there any complications?
- How far along were you in your pregnancy when you had any miscarriage or abortion?
- How is the current health of your other children?
- Did you have any problems with any of your other pregnancies such as bleeding, high blood pressure, headaches, blurring of your vision or spots before your eyes, pain, or diabetes? If you have, describe when the problems occurred and how they were treated.
- How much did each of your children weigh at birth?
- What gender was each of your children?
- What type of birth did you have with each of your children?
- Did you have any problems with other births? If you did, can you describe what happened?
- Did you have any babies that were born other than head first?
- Were you given any medicine to start your labour?
- Did you have any complications from your other births?
- Was the placenta delivered on its own?
- Did you have anything to help with pain during your previous labour(s)?

CURRENT PREGNANCY HISTORY

RATIONALE: *A history of the current pregnancy will provide baseline information that will guide planning for future evaluation and health promotion activities.*

Suggested questions:

- Was this pregnancy planned or unplanned?
- Did you become pregnant on your own or did you use some intervention? If so, what intervention did you use?
- Have you had any problems with this pregnancy such as nausea or vomiting, bleeding, pain, or headache? If so, please elaborate.

PAST MEDICAL AND SURGICAL HISTORY

RATIONALE: *Some illnesses or conditions may predispose the woman to increased risk during the pregnancy.*

Suggested questions:

- Tell me about any past illnesses or surgeries.
- Have you had any problems with your heart such as rheumatic fever or hypertension?

(continued)

● ASSESSMENT TOOL 12.1   **Prenatal Health Assessment Form** *(Continued)*

- Has anyone ever told you that you had diabetes?
- Have you had any lung problems such as difficulty breathing, asthma, or tuberculosis?
- Have you ever had seizures or been told you have epilepsy?
- Have you ever had problems with your kidneys or urinary infections?
- Have you ever had surgery before? If so, why did you have surgery?
- What kind of anaesthetic did you have? Did you have any problems with the anaesthetic?
- Have you ever had a blood transfusion? If so, why did you have it and when? Did you have any problems with it?
- What kinds of illnesses did you have when you were a child?
- What kinds of vaccinations have you had?
- Have you ever had any problems with feelings of anxiety, sadness, depression, fatigue, or had difficulty getting up?
- Have you experienced any major changes such as moving, a change in or loss of a relationship, job (your or family member)? What happens when such things occur? How do you react?

FAMILY HISTORY

RATIONALE: *Some conditions may be hereditary or familial.*

Suggested questions:

- Tell me about any illnesses in your family or the baby's father's family.
- Has anyone in your family had heart trouble, lung problems, diabetes, tuberculosis, or asthma?
- Has anyone in the baby's father's family had any of these problems?
- Has anyone in either family been diagnosed with cancer? If so, what kind?
- Has anyone in either family been born with any birth defects?
- Has anyone in either family been born with any inherited disease, blood disorders, mental retardation, or any other problems?
- Have there been twins or triplets born in either family?
- Has anyone in your family delivered a baby before the ninth month of pregnancy?

SOCIAL/CULTURAL HISTORY

RATIONALE: *Information may increase knowledge about potential risks to mother or fetus. Information about cultural history may influence plan of care.*

Suggested questions:

- Tell me about your habits and anything that I should know to assist you to incorporate your culture into your pregnancy experience.
- Tell me about anything that I should know to assist you to incorporate your religious beliefs into your pregnancy experience.
- Do you smoke cigarettes? If so, how much do you smoke?
- Do you drink alcohol? How much alcohol do you drink each day? What kind of alcohol do you drink?
- Do you use any street drugs such as cocaine, speed, marijuana, or anything else? If you do, what kind of drugs do you use and how often do you use them?
- Do you use any prescription or over-the-counter drugs?
- Do you use any herbal or natural preparations or treatments?
- Does any of your family or friends consider your habits to be a problem?
- Do any of your habits interfere with your daily living?
- Are there any special practices that you or your partner want to incorporate from your culture into your plan for this pregnancy? Is there anything that we can assist you with to accomplish this?
- If you needed help (such as someone to babysit, lend you money, listen when you are upset), whom would you ask?

HISTORY OF INTIMATE-PARTNER VIOLENCE

RATIONALE: *Intimate-partner violence affects a significant number of women and frequently escalates during pregnancy. Physical, emotional, and sexual violence crosses race, culture, ethnicity, social class, and gender. Therefore, all women may be at potential risk. Violence may have serious consequences for both the mother and fetus.*

Suggested questions:

- Have you been hit, slapped, kicked, or otherwise physically hurt by someone within the last year?
- If yes, by whom and how many times?
- Have you been hit, slapped, kicked, or otherwise physically hurt by someone since you have been pregnant?
- If yes, by whom and how many times?
- Has anyone forced you to have sexual activities within the last year?
- If yes, by whom and how many times?
- Are you afraid of your partner or anyone else?
- Have you had negative comments made about you or your sexual performance within the last year?
- If yes, by whom and how many times?
- Can you freely access your family's money?

- T—the number of term births (at 37 or more weeks' gestation)
- P—the number of preterm births (after 20 weeks' gestation but before 37 weeks' gestation)
- A—the number of pregnancies that ended in either therapeutic or spontaneous abortion (before 20 weeks' gestation)
- L—the number of children currently alive to whom the woman has given birth

Thus, a woman currently pregnant for the fifth time, with three children currently alive (delivered at 38, 40, and 32 weeks), and who had a spontaneous abortion at 14 weeks will have a GTPAL recorded as 5-2-1-1-3. In the case of multiple gestation, such as twin and triplet pregnancies, the birth is counted only once regardless of how many babies are born. For example, a woman currently pregnant for the third time who gave birth to twins at 35 weeks and a single baby at 42 weeks, all of whom are currently alive, will have a GTPAL of 3-1-1-0-3. After delivering her baby at 39 weeks, her GTPAL will change to 3-2-1-0-4.

The nurse assesses past pregnancies for their duration. If a woman has had multiple pregnancy losses before 20 weeks, it may suggest cervical insufficiency (see Chapter 13). The nurse also assesses for complications in previous pregnancies that may have significance or implications for this pregnancy. Examples include bleeding, hypertension, headaches, blurred vision, pain, and gestational diabetes. Bleeding in a past pregnancy may have implications for the current pregnancy, based on the cause and outcome. For example, if the bleeding resulted in a spontaneous abortion, the risk for recurrence may be increased (Cunningham et al., 2010). Hypertension, headaches, blurred vision, or pain may have been indicative of a hypertensive disorder of pregnancy. If a hypertensive disorder of pregnancy or gestational diabetes complicated a previous pregnancy, risk for recurrence in this pregnancy will be increased (Daley, 2014; Poole, 2014).

The nurse identifies the birth weight of previous children. If any were classified as small for gestational age (SGA), intrauterine growth restriction (IUGR) may have complicated the pregnancies. If so, risk for recurrence in the current pregnancy may be increased. The risk for an infant who is large for gestational age (LGA) in the current pregnancy is increased if a previous pregnancy produced an LGA infant (Cunningham et al., 2010). Women whose infants are LGA are at increased risk for CPD or shoulder dystocia (Cunningham et al., 2010; Daley, 2014). Regardless of whether a previous pregnancy resulted in an SGA or LGA infant, the nurse should always closely monitor the rate of fetal growth in the current pregnancy.

The nurse identifies the types of previous births, including any that were through caesarean section, required instruments such as forceps or vacuum extractors, or were complicated by a presentation other than vertex (head first). He or she identifies the reasons for any previous caesarean births. Indications may have no influence on this birth or may continue to be significant. For example, caesarean birth because of breech presentation will have fewer implications unless it recurs in this pregnancy (Cunningham et al., 2010). If caesarean birth occurred because of dystocia (failure to progress), chances are increased that this will continue to present indications for caesarean birth in this pregnancy.

Assessment includes a review of any complications of previous pregnancies, including postpartum hemorrhage. The risk for this recurring increases in subsequent pregnancies (James, 2014), so it is useful to have this information to monitor the birth and postpartum period more closely.

The nurse documents any labour analgesia or anaesthesia used during previous births. This information will be useful in assessing the woman's tolerance for pain and planning care for labour and childbirth.

Consider Millie, described at the beginning of the chapter and in Nursing Care Plan 12.1. Based on the information provided, how would you document her history of past pregnancies using the GTPAL method? Imagine that Millie had also had a spontaneous abortion at age 22 and that her 11-year-old was born at 34 weeks' gestation instead of 39 weeks. What would her GTPAL be now?

Past Medical and Surgical History. The nurse can elicit information about the woman's past medical and surgical history. He or she reviews cardiovascular or bleeding disorders; respiratory illnesses, including asthma and tuberculosis; renal illnesses, including urinary tract infections (UTIs); hypertension; diabetes; epilepsy; past surgeries; anaesthetic problems; transfusions; allergies; childhood illnesses; and mental health concerns.

Cardiovascular disorders may predispose the client to increased risk, because pregnancy generates increased blood volume and BMR and subsequent increased cardiac output (see Chapter 13). Bleeding disorders may predispose the woman to thrombophlebitis, episodes of bleeding, and postpartum hemorrhage.

Respiratory illnesses have implications for both maternal and fetal well-being. Women with asthma may have decreased respiratory capacity, which may be further compromised by fetal growth and subsequent pressure on the diaphragm. This decreased respiratory capacity also may affect the fetus, because decreased oxygen in the maternal circulation decreases oxygen to the placenta and subsequent diffusion to the fetus. Although not prevalent in Canada, active tuberculosis may spread from mother to newborn, following birth (Chow et al., 2013).

Women who have had a previous UTI may be at increased risk for developing subsequent infections. A UTI in pregnancy can lead to increased risk for preterm labour (Reedy, 2014).

Women with a history of hypertension are at increased risk for developing preeclampsia (Cunningham et al., 2010; Magee et al., 2008). Knowledge of pre-existing hypertension, then, should lead to increased surveillance during pregnancy. Women with pre-existing diabetes are at increased risk during pregnancy. See Chapter 13 for further information on these conditions.

Women with epilepsy often have little or no difficulty during pregnancy; however, in some instances, seizure activity may be exacerbated (Cunningham et al., 2010). The plan of care for these women includes close follow-up to ensure maintenance of appropriate medication. Medication must be balanced to provide the antiseizure characteristics the mother requires without posing a risk for congenital anomalies to the fetus, which may be caused by some anticonvulsants (Cunningham et al., 2010).

The nurse uses information about past surgeries and anaesthesia to anticipate care that may be needed should caesarean birth be required. In addition, past surgery, depending on its nature, may have implications for the plan of care during pregnancy. The nurse can use information about past transfusions to plan further assessment that may be needed to determine the woman's hepatitis B and C status.

Information about childhood illnesses is a valuable resource about immunity that the client probably has acquired, although occasionally immunity is not achieved after exposure to an illness. The nurse obtains the mother's vaccination history, if known. Live-attenuated virus vaccines such as MMR or varicella are contraindicated in pregnancy related to a theoretical risk to the fetus, associated with administration of live vaccines (Public Health Agency of Canada, 2013a). Because research studies have shown no evidence of congenital rubella syndrome, pregnancy termination should not be recommended for women who have been inadvertently vaccinated during pregnancy or within 3 months prior to conception (Public Health Agency of Canada, 2013a). Other live-attenuated vaccines should be evaluated according to an individual risk/benefit analysis (Public Health Agency of Canada, 2013a). There is no evidence to suggest that maternal administration of inactivated viral and bacterial vaccines, toxoids, or immune globulin for passive immunization pose any risk to the fetus or pregnancy (Public Health Agency of Canada, 2013a).

Using both information about childhood illnesses and the vaccination history to ascertain the client's immunity status, the nurse may provide information about appropriate avoidance of exposure to others who may be ill. Exposure to rubella and chickenpox in the nonimmune woman can result in miscarriage, stillbirth, or congenital anomalies, including congenital heart disease, cataracts, and deafness (Public Health Agency of Canada, 2013a).

Family History. The nurse assesses the family background of the mother and, if known, the father for any known conditions or alterations relating to the cardiovascular and respiratory systems, kidney disease, and bleeding disorders. He or she identifies any history of diabetes, congenital or fetal anomalies, epilepsy or seizures, emotional problems, cancer, HIV, or hepatitis. A history of any of these variations from normal may provide important information in identifying potential risks to the pregnant woman or unborn child. Identification of multiple births, especially fraternal, in the family may indicate ovulation twice in 1 month, which may predispose the woman to multiple births.

History of Substance Use. Assessment includes the use of cigarettes; alcohol; illicit, prescribed, and over-the-counter drugs; and any herbal remedies, including amounts and types consumed. Smoking increases the risk for problems related to spontaneous abortion, birth weight, placental abnormalities, preterm birth, and sudden infant death syndrome (Anderson et al., 2005; Keegan et al., 2010; Magee et al., 2004; Zdravkovic et al., 2005). Alcohol increases the risk for fetal alcohol spectrum disorders (FASD) (Floyd et al., 2005; Stade et al., 2009). The use of drugs like cocaine and narcotics during pregnancy is associated with congenital anomalies, SGA, risk for placental abruption, and neonatal abstinence syndrome (Cunningham et al., 2010; Fraser, 2014; Irner et al., 2012). In their clinical practice guideline, the SOGC recommends that health care providers are flexible in their approach with pregnant women who use substances and that all women are counselled about the risks of drug use during pregnancy (Wong et al., 2011).

Nutrition History. A review of the pregnant woman's dietary habits, preferences, and knowledge is critical. Chapter 3 discusses nutritional assessment and pregnancy-related needs and adjustments in detail.

History of Violence. The incidence of physical and sexual violence has been found to be as high as 10.9% in childbearing women (Daoud et al., 2012). See Research Highlight 12.2 Intimate-partner violence has remained stable at 6% since 2004 (Statistics Canada, 2011c). Acts of violence frequently escalate during pregnancy (Anderson, 2002; Cherniak et al., 2005), although in

● RESEARCH HIGHLIGHT 12.2 Prevalence of Abuse and Violence Before, During, and After Pregnancy in a National Sample of Canadian Women

OBJECTIVE

To describe the prevalence of abuse and violence before, during, and after pregnancy in a national sample of Canadian new mothers.

DESIGN

The prevalence, frequency, timing, and types of physical and sexual abuse before, during, and after pregnancy was estimated. The category of perpetrator was identified. The onset and cessation of abuse around pregnancy was examined, using a weighted sample from the Maternity Experiences Survey (2006–2007).

PARTICIPANTS AND SETTING

The Maternity Experiences Survey collected information from a stratified random sample of mothers in Canadian provinces and territories, using recent births from the 2006 Canadian Census of Population. This study used the data collected from this survey.

RESULTS

The prevalence of any abuse in the 2 years prior to the interviews was 10.9%. The prevalence was higher among low-income, lone, and Aboriginal mothers. In the majority of cases, the perpetrator was an intimate partner. Sixty one percent of the abused mothers identified that they had received information on what to do.

CONCLUSION

The results from this large population-based sample were consistent with other studies that identified lone women and those with low socioeconomic position as at high risk for abuse. The findings suggest that women should be monitored for abuse before and after, as well as during, pregnancy. Emphasis should be put on ensuring that women have information on what to do if they experience abuse.

Source: Daoud, N., Urquia, M. L., O'Campo, P., Heaman, M., Janssen, P. A., Smylie, J. et al. (2012). Prevalence of abuse and violence before, during, and after pregnancy in a national sample of Canadian women. *American Journal of Public Health*, *102*(10), 1893–1901.

---

some studies the incidence has been found to decrease (Brownridge et al., 2011; Scribano et al., 2013). Factors that may be associated with an increased risk for violence include young age, geographical isolation, poverty, substance use by the woman and/or her partner, and unintended pregnancy (Bhandari et al., 2011; Cherniak et al., 2005; Daoud et al., 2012; Hellmuth et al., 2012). Women who have experienced violence tend to have more episodes of depression and anxiety and fewer sources of support; they also tend to begin prenatal care later (Cherniak et al., 2005; Espinosa & Osborne, 2002). Serious consequences of violence during pregnancy include placental abruption, premature rupture of the membranes, low birth weight, and death of the mother, fetus, or both (Brownridge et al., 2011; Cherniak et al., 2005; Kramer et al., 2012; Scribano et al., 2013; Shah & Shah, 2010).

Violence may be physical, emotional, or sexual; pregnant women are significantly more likely to report experiencing all forms of violence (Brownridge et al., 2011). Women may experience violence differently and understandings of violence may be framed by cultural understandings of "normal" relations between intimate partners and gender inequality (Bhandari et al., 2011; Cherniak et al., 2005). This may also be true of women who are lesbian or who have physical disabilities. These differences may also impact barriers to reporting (Cherniak et al., 2005).

Because the woman may have had only one prenatal visit or be afraid to disclose violence until a trusting relationship is established, health care providers should ask direct questions at every visit (Anderson, 2002; Cherniak et al., 2005). Because violence crosses race, culture, religion, social status, and gender, they do this assessment with all pregnant women. Women who are not in violent situations generally do not express offence at being asked such questions, perhaps because intimate-partner violence is so prevalent that many women know someone who has been in that situation (Renker & Tonkin, 2006). The nurse asks questions in privacy, away from the partner, other family members, or significant others (Chow et al., 2013; Stenson et al., 2005). Because she may be slow to respond, the woman needs adequate time to answer. Although there has been increased emphasis on the importance of screening and improved detection rates, Shah and Shah (2010) found that there has not been consistent impact in improvement in the outcomes for these women.

Assessment findings that may suggest violence include infrequent prenatal visits that begin late in the pregnancy, poor weight gain, signs of possessiveness or jealousy in the woman's partner, apparent fear of her partner, or lack of eye contact or conversation (Anderson, 2002; Cherniak et al., 2005). Although the nurse may believe that the woman should leave the situation, he or she must understand that the woman may

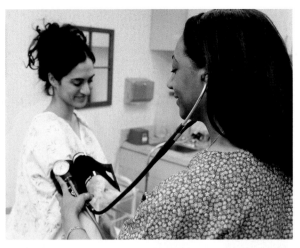

FIGURE 12.14 The nurse takes the client's blood pressure during the first prenatal visit and at all subsequent appointments.

not be at a stage where this is seen as a viable option (Chow et al., 2013; Lutz, 2005).

Physical Examination

A complete physical examination should be performed. Vital signs and an initial weight need to be established as baseline data (Fig. 12.14). If the prepregnancy weight is known, the nurse includes it. Nurses and other providers can then use these baseline data to compare with changes that occur throughout pregnancy and to identify potential problems identified.

Estimated Date of Delivery. Providers calculate the EDD. This date was formerly known as expected date of confinement (EDC). Because childbirth is no longer seen as a "confinement," the terminology has changed to estimated date of delivery (EDD), or estimated date of birth (EDB).

The most common way to calculate the EDD is to use **Naegele's rule**. The woman identifies the first day of her last normal menstrual period; Naegele's rule subtracts 3 months and adds 7 days to this date to give an EDD. For example, the first day of a client's last normal menstrual period was May 6. Subtracting 3 months would be February; adding 7 days would be 13. Therefore, the EDD is February 13 of the following year. Providers also can use an EDD wheel to calculate the EDD (Fig. 12.15). To do so, providers match the line indicating the day of the last period with the appropriate date. The date on the outside wheel that falls on the line indicating 40 weeks is the EDD. Alternatively, websites frequently provide simple

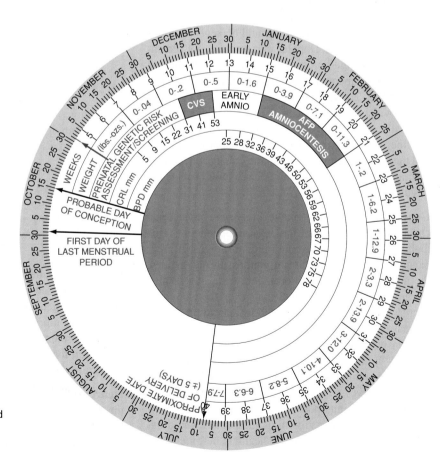

FIGURE 12.15 The EDD wheel helps health care providers estimate a client's due date. This client's last menstrual period (LMP) was October 1. Her due date according to the wheel is July 8 of the following year.

calculators to determine EDD (http://www.marchofdimes.com/pregnancy/calculating-your-due-date.aspx).

Some women have irregular periods or bleed throughout their cycle, which makes the use of Naegele's rule or the EDD wheel less reliable. As well, some women are simply not sure of the date of their last menstrual period, especially in the case of an unplanned pregnancy or when the woman pays little attention to the frequency of her periods. In these cases, providers use alternative methods to determine EDD. One such method to date pregnancy is ultrasound to visualize the gestational sac and regular measurements of the embryo/fetus (see Chapter 11). The most common measurements include biparietal diameter (distance from side to side) of the fetal head, head circumference, crown–rump length, abdominal circumference, and femoral length. Standard measurements have been established at different gestations, facilitating estimation of the pregnancy (Cunningham et al., 2010).

To date, there have been no adverse biological effects proven to be associated with obstetric diagnostic ultrasound (Bly & Van den Hof, 2005). However, because of the potential for an unidentified risk, the SOGC recommends that ultrasound should not be used for nonmedical reasons and should only be used when the "potential medical benefit outweighs any theoretical or potential risk" (Bly & Van den Hof, 2005, p. 575). In addition, ultrasound exposure should be kept to a minimum. The use of the Doppler ultrasound is not recommended during the first trimester of pregnancy because of the high temperatures that may be produced (Bly & Van den Hof, 2005).

Providers can also use the EDD wheel to determine the weeks of gestation of the pregnancy. They match up the line indicating the EDD with the appropriate date and then find the current date on the outside wheel. Following that line toward the inner circle will provide the gestation in weeks and days.

General Survey. The nurse assesses physiologic changes that the woman has been experiencing. This includes both presumptive and probable signs of pregnancy. Although these do not confirm the pregnancy, the nurse also uses the information to develop a plan of care to identify anticipated changes to the woman to decrease anxiety and to assist the woman to prevent or decrease the symptoms.

An organized approach, often according to body systems, is usually easiest to follow to complete the physical examination. The initial assessment includes a general survey of the woman and her state of nourishment, grooming, posture, mood, affect, and general appearance. Poor grooming and posture and a flat affect may suggest some mental health issues, including

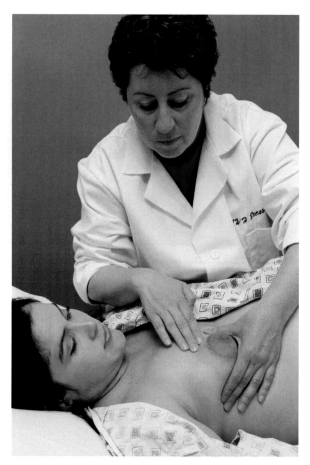

FIGURE 12.16 The nurse examines the pregnant client's breasts.

depression. A woman appearing poorly nourished with poor grooming may have decreased resources and may benefit from a social services consultation.

Skin. Assessment of the skin includes evaluation of any scars. These may be from a previous caesarean section or tracks caused by intravenous drug use. In combination with bruising, scars may suggest physical violence. Skin variations may include chloasma, linea nigra, and striae.

Breasts. The client is assessed with a clinical breast examination (see Chapter 2). The pregnant breasts may appear enlarged, perhaps with striae (Fig. 12.16). The areolae and nipples may also appear enlarged and with darker pigmentation. Montgomery tubercles may be visible on the areola; the nipples may begin to express colostrum during the last trimester.

Heart and Lungs. When assessing the heart and lungs, the nurse may hear a functional, soft, blowing systolic murmur from the increased cardiac volume (Fig. 12.17). The nurse notes any other murmur and refers

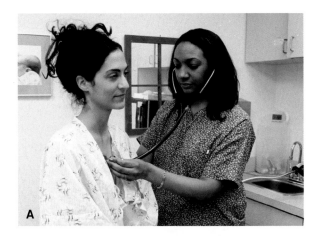

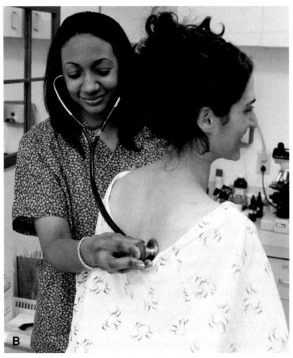

FIGURE 12.17 The nurse assesses the client's (**A**) heart and (**B**) lungs. A soft, blowing systolic murmur from the increased cardiac volume is a normal finding.

the finding to appropriate health care team members. The increased blood volume and resulting increased cardiac output add significantly to the workload of the heart.

Abdomen. The nurse palpates and inspects the abdomen. Striae and linea nigra may be present. Depending on the gestation of the pregnancy, the nurse may assess symphysis–fundal height.

Genitalia. The examination includes assessment for cervical and vaginal changes as part of assessment of the probable signs of pregnancy, including Chadwick's, Hegar's, and Goodell's signs. A Pap smear and vaginal cultures will provide baseline data.

Pelvimetry. Assessment includes the pubic arch, inclination, and curve of the side walls; the prominence of the ischial spines; and the shape of the sacrum.

The pelvic bones are assessed for size and shape to determine the adequacy of the pelvis for vaginal birth. The two most important measurements are the *diagonal conjugate* and the *biischial diameter*. The diagonal conjugate indicates the anterioposterior diameter of the pelvic inlet. It is measured by pointing the second and third fingers, when placed within the vagina, toward the sacral promontory (Fig. 12.18A). The distance of the fingers is then measured to estimate the diagonal conjugate. The measurement ideally is at least 11.5 cm.

To measure the biischial diameter, the examiner forms his or her hand into a closed fist, which he or she then places across the woman's perineum between the ischial tuberosities (Fig. 12.18B). This measurement ideally is at least 8 cm.

Laboratory Evaluation and Disease Screening

Laboratory evaluation will identify the mother's ABO blood type and Rh, as well as any antibodies. If the mother's Rh is negative, the father's blood type should be identified, if possible. This is useful in determining any potential for Rh incompatibility (see Chapter 16). Ideally, a woman would have received necessary immunizations prior to conception. However, this is often not possible, because many pregnancies are not planned. Immunization status is therefore often assessed during pregnancy. Because of the potential risk to the fetus, women should not receive any vaccines that contain a live virus (eg, varicella, measles–mumps–rubella) during pregnancy and should avoid pregnancy for a minimum of 28 days following immunization.

Pregnant woman are in the high priority category for receiving inactivated (not live) influenza vaccine, which has been shown to be safe during pregnancy. Influenza vaccination during pregnancy has been shown to decrease maternal morbidity, prematurity, low birth weight, and influenza in the neonate (Public Health Agency of Canada, 2013). Pregnant women should be tested for hepatitis B surface antigen (HBsAG). The woman who tests negative and is at high risk for hepatitis B infection should be offered the hepatitis B vaccine series (Public Health Agency of Canada, 2013). Other immunizations that may be indicated include hepatitis A, tetanus toxoid, reduced diphtheria toxoid-containing vaccine, acellular pertussis-containing vaccine (Tdap), poliomyelitis, pneumococcal, meningococcal, and rabies vaccines (Public Health Agency of Canada, 2013). HPV vaccine is not recommended.

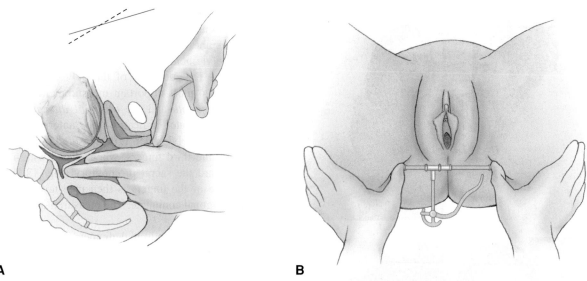

A

B

FIGURE 12.18   **A.** Diagonal conjugate (*solid line*). **B.** Ischial diameter.

A rubella titer is done to identify immunity. The nurse needs to be aware of the specific value for immunity in his/her setting, as these values are dependent on the type of test used by the laboratory that performs the test. If the pregnant woman is nonimmune, she should avoid exposure to rubella during her pregnancy, because of the associated risk for spontaneous abortion and congenital anomalies. Once she has delivered the baby, she should be offered an MMR (measles, mumps, rubella) vaccination to increase her immunity. She should not become pregnant within 4 weeks of receiving the vaccine (Public Health Agency of Canada, 2013). Breastfeeding is not a contraindication (Public Health Agency of Canada, 2013).

The woman will also have a baseline hemoglobin and urinalysis. The urinalysis will indicate any asymptomatic bacteriuria, which is common in pregnancy. If this is not treated, it may lead to acute symptomatic UTI. Bacteria in the urine, combined with urinary stasis that occurs in pregnancy, put the woman at increased risk for pyelonephritis. Bacteriuria or pyelonephritis increases the risk for preterm labour (Cunningham et al., 2010).

The hemoglobin is done as a baseline on which to evaluate future values. Hemoglobin normally decreases during pregnancy, because iron is actively transferred to the fetus and the RBC mass of the mother increases. Continued evaluation is essential to ensure that hemoglobin values are maintained within safe ranges. Abnormal values, especially in late pregnancy (considered to be less than 110 g/L), are usually the result of iron deficiency and indicate the need for additional exogenous iron (Cunningham et al., 2010).

All women should be offered HIV testing at the first prenatal visit. Repeat testing in the third trimester before 36 weeks' gestation is recommended for women at high risk for acquiring HIV, including those who have multiple sex partners, use illicit drugs, or have a partner infected with HIV. A Venereal disease research laboratory (VDRL) test for syphilis is recommended for all women at the first prenatal visit and for anyone who has a stillbirth. Serological testing for HbsAG is advised at the first visit for all women and repeated during the third trimester for those at risk for hepatitis B, including those who use injection drugs or who have other STIs. Those at high risk for contracting hepatitis C, including those who use injection drugs or have repeated exposure to blood products, prior blood transfusion, or organ transplantation, are tested at the first prenatal visit. Testing for chlamydia is offered at the first visit and repeated in the third trimester for women who have new or multiple sex partners.

All pregnant women can be offered a prenatal screening test, following informed consent, for fetal aneuploidies (including Down syndrome and trisomy 18), in addition to a detailed second trimester ultrasound regardless of age (Chitayat et al., 2011). See Chapter 11 for a discussion of these screening tests.

The SOGC (Money & Dobson, 2004) recommends that all pregnant women be offered screening for group B streptococci (GBS) at 35 to 37 weeks' gestation. GBS are among the normal vaginal flora, although colonization can be transient and variable. It is common for pregnant women to be asymptomatic carriers; 20% to 30% of pregnant women will have a positive culture (Cunningham et al., 2010). Mothers who are carriers

● TABLE 12.3   **Frequency of Prenatal Visits**

Weeks of Gestation	Frequency of Visits	Special Investigations
Up to 28	Every 4 wk	If opt for first trimester screening for aneuploidy, should have second trimester screen and/or ultrasound for alpha fetoprotein If opt for integrated screening for aneuploidy, PAPP-A and NT at 9–10 wk, Quad screening in second trimester 16–20 wk: ultrasound 24–28 wk: Gestational diabetes
28–36	Every 2–3 wk	28 wk: Anti-D antibodies if mother is Rh negative. If none present, give anti-D immune globulin 35–37 wk: culture for Group B streptococcus
36+	Every week	

of GBS are more prone to preterm labour, premature rupture of membranes, chorioamnionitis, and puerperal infections (Cunningham et al., 2010).

Mothers can pass GBS to babies during pregnancy, labour, or delivery; 50% of infants born to colonized women will be colonized themselves at birth (Money & Dobson, 2004). This bacterium is a leading cause of fetal infections and neonatal sepsis (Cunningham et al., 2010). Antibiotic treatment with penicillin G at the time of rupture of membranes or during labour is recommended for women who test positive for GBS at 35 to 37 weeks' gestation, who have had an infant previously infected with GBS, or who have had previously documented bacteriuria in the current pregnancy (Money & Dobson, 2004). If penicillin G is unavailable, ampicillin may be used. For women with penicillin allergies, cefazolin, clindamycin, or erythromycin are the alternative drugs of choice (Cunningham et al., 2010).

Follow-Up Maternal Assessments

Once a pregnancy is confirmed, regular follow-up visits are planned. See Table 12.3 for a sample of a normal prenatal visit schedule. During the prenatal and subsequent visits, as well as during phone calls and other interactions that may occur with the client, the nurse provides anticipatory guidance to assist the woman to understand expected changes, their timelines, and potential comfort measures.

Continuing prenatal assessments during each subsequent visit include vital signs and weight, FHR when audible, symphysis–fundal height, position of the fetus when palpable, edema, discomforts of pregnancy, any risk factors, and any concerns that the woman may have. The examiner may palpate the fetal outline using Leopold manoeuvres and auscultate and assess the fetal heart. See Nursing Procedures 12.1 and 12.2.

Continued regular prenatal care is essential for the remainder of the pregnancy to monitor maternal well-being and fetal growth and well-being. Once the pregnancy is confirmed positively and the client can see or hear evidence of the fetus, it may be the first time she realizes that she is truly pregnant. It provides positive proof to her that a baby really is growing inside her. This may be the first time that she feels confident enough to begin to plan for the arrival. The nurse continues to provide support and anticipatory guidance to the pregnant woman and her significant others in continuing prenatal care. He or she can give information about prenatal classes as well as other support services that may be available in the woman's community.

Assessment of Fetal Activity and Well-Being

Assessment of fetal activity and well-being throughout the pregnancy is vital to ensuring a favourable outcome. Health care providers use several methods and tools to accomplish this assessment, including fetal movement counting, nonstress test (NST), contraction stress test (CST), sonographic assessment of fetal behaviour and/or amniotic fluid volume, uterine artery Doppler, and umbilical artery Doppler (Liston et al., 2007). They may be used simultaneously or hierarchically, but are tailored to the underlying etiology and perceived risk (Liston et al., 2007). Maternal awareness of fetal activity is the only assessment recommended for all pregnant women, regardless of whether or not any risk factors are present (Liston et al., 2007). Routine antenatal testing for pregnant women who are less than 41 weeks' gestation with an uncomplicated pregnancy is not supported (Liston et al., 2007).

Fetal Movement Counting

All pregnant women can be encouraged to be aware of fetal movements during the third trimester and to perform a fetal movement count if they perceive a decrease in fetal movement (Liston et al., 2007). The woman

NURSING PROCEDURE 12.1
Performing Leopold's Maneuvers

PURPOSE

To determine fetal presentation, position, and attitude

ASSESSMENT AND PLANNING

- Assess the client's knowledge of and previous experience with the procedure.
- Review the client's medical record to determine estimated date of delivery (EDD) and week of gestation.
- Gather necessary equipment
- Warmed, clean hands

IMPLEMENTATION

1. Explain the procedure to the client *to help alleviate anxiety*.
2. Have the client empty her bladder *to promote client comfort and minimize uterine distention from interfering with palpation*.
3. Perform hand hygiene.
4. Assist the client to the supine position with her knees slightly flexed *to help relax abdominal muscles*; place a small pillow under one side *to prevent supine hypotension syndrome*.
5. Expose the abdominal area and inspect the abdomen *to identify any bulging prominences, asymmetry, and indentations*.
6. Position yourself at the side of the bed, facing the client. Place both hands on the uterine fundus and palpate for its contents *to identify the fetal body part occupying the fundus*. Identify the fetal body part palpated by consistency, shape, and mobility. *A soft irregular object that does not move freely suggests the buttocks; a smooth, firm, regular object that moves independently suggests the head (breech presentation)*.
7. Then move your hands to the sides of the maternal abdomen, placing the palmar surface one hand on each side of the abdomen. Gently palpate one side of the abdomen while using the opposite hand to support the abdomen and uterus *to locate the fetal back and extremities*. Repeat using the opposite action. *The fetal back will feel hard and smooth; the extremities will feel irregular and nodular.*

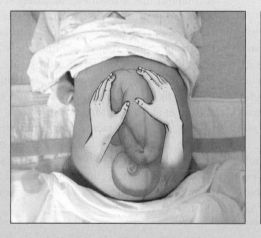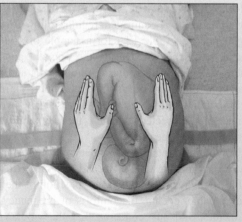

(continued)

NURSING PROCEDURE 12.1 (CONTINUED)
Performing Leopold's Maneuvers

8. Place one hand just above the symphysis pubis and, using your thumb and fingers, attempt to grasp the presenting part of the fetus. Feel for a hard, round object *to identify the head as the presenting part* or a soft irregularly shaped object *to identify breech presentation.* While palpating, attempt to move the object *to determine possible engagement of the head. Free movement denotes that the presenting part is not engaged.*

9. Turn and face the client's feet. Using the first three fingers of each hand, begin to palpate in a downward fashion moving toward the symphysis pubis, along both sides of the abdomen, *to identify the degree of fetal flexion.* Feel for a hard bony area. If this area is on the opposite side of where the fetal back was palpated, then the fetus is in an attitude of flexion; if the area is on the same side as the fetal back, the fetus is in an attitude of extension.

10. Assist the woman to a comfortable position.

11. Document the findings in the client's medical record.

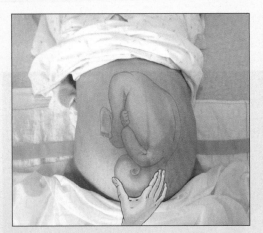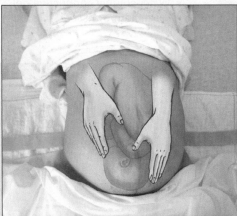

EVALUATION

* The client tolerated the procedure without difficulty.
* The fetal position, presentation, and attitude were within normal parameters.

AREAS FOR CONSIDERATION AND ADAPTATION

Perinatal Considerations

* Remember that Leopold's maneuvers can be performed throughout a woman's pregnancy.
* Use Leopold's maneuvers to assist in determining where best to auscultate fetal heart tones.
* If the woman is in labour, perform these maneuvers in between contractions.
* Place a pillow under the client's shoulders if necessary to promote comfort.
* Do not perform the fourth maneuver (palpating for fetal attitude) if the fetus is in the breech position.

---

with risk factors for adverse perinatal outcomes monitors fetal movements daily (Cunningham et al., 2010). While there are a number of methods available for counting fetal movements, the SOGC recommends that women count six distinctive fetal movements; if there are less than 6 movements in 2 hours, further antenatal testing is indicated (Liston et al., 2007). It is best if the count is performed in the early evening when in a reclined (not supine) position.

(text continues on page 450)

NURSING PROCEDURE 12.2
Assessing Fetal Heart Rate

PURPOSE

To evaluate fetal well-being

ASSESSMENT AND PLANNING

- Assess the client's knowledge of and previous experience with the procedure.
- Determine the client's estimated date of delivery (EDD) and number of weeks' gestation.
- Check the client's medical record for baseline information related to fetal heart rates.
- Review the client's medical record for information related to any previous pregnancies and outcomes.
- Gather equipment
  - Ultrasonic Doppler device
  - Water-soluble conductive gel
  - Washcloth or tissue

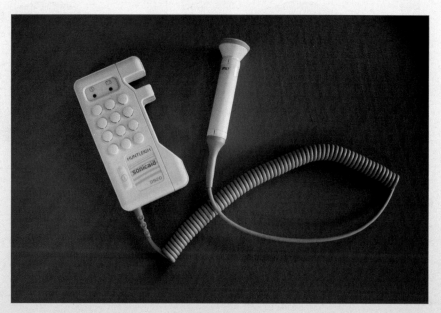

Ultrasound doppler.

IMPLEMENTATION

1. Explain the procedure to the client and answer any questions that she may have *to help allay any fears and anxieties.*
2. Assist the woman to the supine position *to allow for easy access to the abdominal area.* Provide privacy.
3. Perform hand hygiene.
4. Expose the client's abdomen and perform Leopold's maneuvers *to identify fetal back and best location to hear fetal heart tones.* (See Nursing Procedure 12.1.)
5. Apply water-soluble gel to client's abdomen in the area of the fetal back or to the device *to ensure adequate contact of the device to the client's skin and enhance sound transmission.*
6. If the ultrasonic device has ear pieces, place them into the ears; then turn on the device.

(continued)

NURSING PROCEDURE 12.2 (CONTINUED)
Assessing Fetal Heart Rate

7. Position the device on the client's abdomen at the location of the fetal back *to hear the heart sounds*; alternatively, place the device beginning at the midline, midway between the umbilicus and symphysis pubis, and apply slight pressure; if necessary, slowly move the device laterally *to hear the heart sounds*; move the device slowly and slightly until you hear the sounds the loudest.

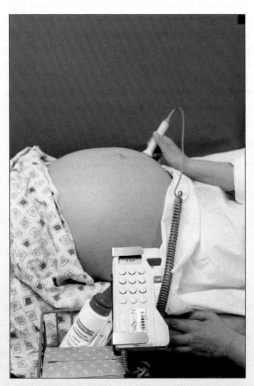

Step 7. The examiner applies the ultrasound Doppler device.

8. Count the client's pulse rate *to determine that what is heard is the fetal heart rate and not the maternal heart rate*. If the rates are the same, reposition the device and count again.
9. Once you have confirmed the fetal heart rate, count it for one full minute; also note the rhythm and presence of any accelerations or decelerations.
10. Remove the device and wipe the client's abdomen with a washcloth or tissue *to remove water-soluble gel*; provide the client with information about fetal well-being based on fetal heart rate.
11. Wipe the device *to remove the gel*; perform hand hygiene.
12. Document the fetal heart rate, rhythm, presence of any accelerations or decelerations, and location of fetal heart sounds.

EVALUATION

* The fetal heart rate was within the normal range of 110 to 160 bpm. The fetal heart rate was regular, with accelerations present.
* The client tolerated the procedure without difficulty.

(continued)

NURSING PROCEDURE 12.2 (CONTINUED)
Assessing Fetal Heart Rate

AREAS FOR CONSIDERATION AND ADAPTATION

Perinatal Considerations

- If this is the client's first prenatal visit, assess the client for presumptive, probable, and positive signs of pregnancy.
- Keep in mind that fetal heart rate assessment is performed at every prenatal visit.
- During labour, monitor fetal heart rate immediately after a contraction for one full minute. Monitoring of the fetal heart rate may be done intermittently or continuously, as per the facility's policy, using ultrasonic Doppler device, or external or internal electronic fetal monitoring. The Society of Obstetricians and Gynaecologists of Canada recommends the use of intermittent auscultation as the preferred method of intrapartum fetal surveillance in low-risk women in the active phase of labour (Liston et al., 2007).
- When using electronic fetal monitoring during labour, evaluate fetal heart rate and rhythm in light of uterine contractions. (See Chapter 15 for more information.)

COMMUNITY-BASED CONSIDERATIONS

- Expect to assess fetal heart rate at every home visit.
- Notify the client's primary care provider about changes in fetal heart rate outside the normal range of 110 to 160 bpm.

Nonstress Test

While a NST may be performed in clinical practice, there is poor evidence that it reduces perinatal morbidity or mortality. Therefore, SOGC recommends that it be used only in women with risk factors for adverse perinatal outcomes (Liston et al., 2007). During a NST, an electronic fetal monitor provides a tracing of the FHR and accelerations of the FHR with movement during the period when the uterus is relaxed and no contractions are present. It is relatively simple, quick, and noninvasive. It can be done on an outpatient basis and interpreted with relative ease.

The woman should have voided and be in bed or on a recliner in the left lateral recumbent position. Each of the two transducers is held in place with soft fabric belts snugly fastened. The tocodynamometer transducer (which measures uterine activity) is placed over the fundus of the uterus. The Doppler FHR transducer (which measures FHR) is covered with transducer gel and placed over the position where the FHR is most readily heard (usually over the fetal back, ascertained by using Leopold manoeuvres). The tracing should last a minimum of 20 minutes.

Nonstress tests are classified as normal, atypical, or abnormal (Liston et al., 2007). In a normal tracing, the baseline FHR should be between 110 and 160 bpm,

variability between 6 and 25 bpm, and the tracing should show two or more accelerations that reach a peak of at least 15 bpm above baseline FHR, and that last at least 15 seconds from onset to return to baseline (Cunningham et al., 2010; Liston et al., 2007). The two accelerations must occur within 20 minutes. A tracing that does not meet the heart rate acceleration criteria is continued for another 20 minutes. This takes into consideration the average period of sleep when fetal movement and subsequent heart rate variability are reduced (Cunningham et al., 2010; Liston et al., 2007). If accelerations are not present after 40 minutes, the primary care provider should be notified and the electronic monitoring continued (Liston et al., 2007). Evidence has shown that the administration of glucose and manual stimulation do not increase the incidence of normal tests (Liston et al., 2007). In addition, the predictive reliability and safety of vibroacoustic stimulation is not known; therefore, none of these interventions are recommended to stimulate FHR accelerations (Liston et al., 2007).

In most cases, a normal tracing is predictive of good perinatal outcome for 1 week, provided the maternal–fetal condition remains stable (Liston et al., 2007). Repeat testing is recommended at least twice a week in women with insulin-dependent diabetes or with a postdate pregnancy (Liston et al., 2007).

Because of the relative immaturity of fetal sympathetic innervation, criteria used to determine a normal tracing need to be adapted early in pregnancy. Accelerations of 10 bpm that last 10 seconds are considered normal at less than 32 weeks' gestation (Liston et al., 2007).

A nonstress test is classified as atypical if the baseline FHR is 100 to 110, or greater than 160, for up to 30 minutes; a rising baseline is present; there is absent or minimal (<6 bpm) variability for 40 to 80 minutes; variable decelerations (see Chapter 15) lasting 30 to 60 seconds are present; or if the two accelerations occur in 40 to 80 minutes (Liston et al., 2007). Atypical tracings require further evaluation of the total clinical picture and fetal status, which may include further assessment (Liston et al., 2007).

An abnormal tracing is characterized by a persistent lack of accelerations after 80 minutes; a significant abnormality of the baseline FHR or variability; and/or evidence of significant deceleration (Liston et al., 2007). An abnormal NST should lead to further investigation and may potentially result in delivery.

Contraction Stress Test

A CST is rarely used in Canada anymore, although it may be used in pregnancies complicated with diabetes, hypertension, growth restriction, or postdates, or as an alternative in centres that do not have access to biophysical profiles (BPPs) (Liston et al., 2007). Because it most closely resembles intrapartum surveillance of the fetus at risk, it may still be used when a client might be a candidate for a vaginal delivery if the contractions are tolerated (Liston et al., 2007). It indicates response of the FHR to uterine contractions and is designed to indicate poor placental function. Because the uteroplacental circulation is compromised during a contraction (as a result of decreased blood flow to the intervillous space by the contracting uterus), there is transient decreased oxygen exchange during the contraction (Cunningham et al., 2010). A deceleration in the FHR that begins at the peak of the contraction and ends after the completion of the contraction (late deceleration) will occur if the fetus experiences hypoxia (Chow et al., 2013) (see Chapter 15). Recurrent late decelerations indicate fetal hypoxemia. Variable decelerations may be seen in response to contractions as a result of fetal umbilical cord compression, which may be associated with oligohydramnios (Cunningham et al., 2010).

The CST should only be performed in a facility where there is access to emergency caesarean delivery (Liston et al., 2007). It should not be used when uterine activity is contraindicated, such as with placenta previa or a previous vertical uterine scar (Liston et al.,

2007). It should not be used when the gestation is so early that interventions would not be implemented if the results of the CST were abnormal (Liston et al., 2007).

An initial 20-minute NST provides a baseline recording. In 10% to 15% of the time, spontaneous uterine activity seen during the NST is adequate and further stimulation of contractions is not needed (Cunningham et al., 2010). Adequate uterine activity for a CST is defined as three uterine contractions, each lasting 1 minute, during a 10-minute period (Liston et al., 2007). If spontaneous uterine activity is not adequate but late decelerations occur, further stimulation of uterine activity is contraindicated. See Fig 12.19 for examples of tracings.

If there is no, or inadequate, spontaneous uterine activity and no late decelerations have occurred, contractions are stimulated using either nipple self-stimulation or, an exogenous oxytocin infusion. Nipple stimulation is used most frequently, since the risk of hyperstimulation is no greater than with oxytocin and there is a shorter average testing time (Liston et al., 2007). With nipple self-stimulation, the woman rapidly but gently rubs one nipple through light clothing with the palm of her hand for 2 minutes and then stops for 5 minutes (Liston et al., 2007). During this time, uterine activity continues to be monitored. If adequate contractions do not result, the woman further stimulates her nipple for an additional 2 minutes (Liston et al., 2007). If this is unsuccessful, then bilateral stimulation is used. Once adequate contractions occur, stimulation is stopped. If adequate contractions do not result from nipple stimulation, exogenous dilute oxytocin may be administered to stimulate contractions (Liston et al., 2007). It is delivered as a low-dose infusion piggyback by pump at an initial rate of 0.5 to 1 mU/min (Liston et al., 2007). The rate is increased by 1 mU/min every 15 to 30 minutes until three uterine contractions lasting 1 minute each are achieved in a 10-minute period (Liston et al., 2007). Because hyperstimulation has been found to occur in up to 10% of tests when the oxytocin increases occur every 15 minutes, SOGC suggests it may be more appropriate to increase the rate every 30 minutes (Liston et al., 2007).

The CST is said to be negative if a normal baseline FHR tracing is obtained with no late decelerations seen with any contraction (Liston et al., 2007). It is considered positive if late decelerations accompany 50% or more of the induced contractions, regardless of whether or not the criterion for adequate contractions is reached (Liston et al., 2007). The test is considered equivocal if there are repetitive decelerations that are not late in either timing or pattern (Liston et al., 2007). If there are fewer than three contractions that last

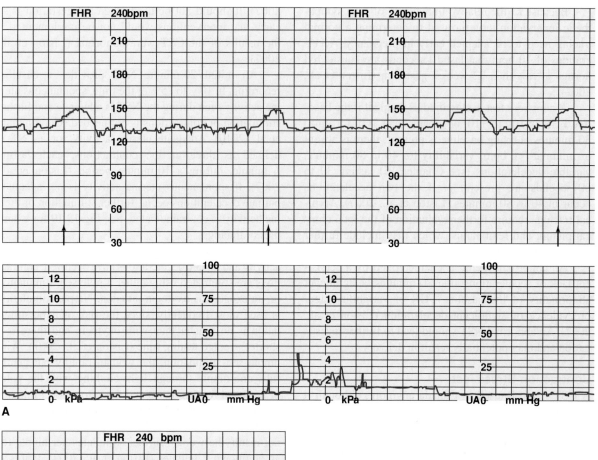

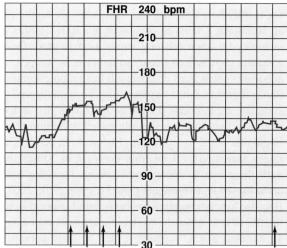

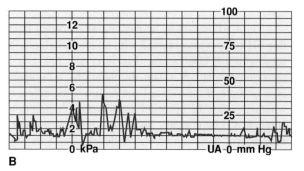

FIGURE 12.19 **A.** A rhythm strip. The upper portion is the fetal heart rate (FHR), and the lower portion is uterine activity. Arrows represent fetal movement. **B.** Baseline FHR is 130 to 131 bpm. The strip shows FHR accelerations in response to fetal movement (*arrows*).

1 minute in 10 minutes, or the tracing is not interpretable, the test is considered unsatisfactory (Cunningham et al., 2010; Liston et al., 2007). The CST has a high negative predictive value, but is poor in predicting perinatal morbidity. As a result, a CST alone is not recommended to guide clinical action (Liston et al., 2007).

Sonographic Assessment of Fetal Behaviour and/or Amniotic Fluid Volume

A number of fetal behavioural and physiologic characteristics can be assessed simultaneously with the use of sonography. The BPP is used to evaluate current fetal well-being. The BPP assesses fetal breathing movements, body movements, tone, and amniotic fluid volume over a 30-minute period (Liston et al., 2007). It may be done in conjunction with a NST, usually when one of the ultrasound components is absent (Liston et al., 2007). Because the BPP provides a more comprehensive examination of fetal well-being than does evaluation of FHR alone, the false-negative rate is often superior to any single test (CST or NST) used to predict the fetus at risk for poor outcome (Cunningham et al., 2010; Sprong, 2008). Examples may include pregnancies complicated by maternal hypertension, diabetes, premature rupture of the membranes, postmaturity, history of previous fetal death, or maternal reports of decreased fetal movements. Although the information provided by the BPP may be useful in identifying a fetus in jeopardy at a specific point and the fetal condition over the last several weeks (Chow et al., 2013; Manning, 2002), it cannot be used as a definitive predictor of future well-being.

One component of the BPP is fetal breathing movements that are visible on ultrasound. These movements differ from those in neonates (Cunningham et al., 2010). In the fetus, the chest wall collapses paradoxically during inspiration and the abdomen protrudes; in the neonate, the opposite occurs. Gasps, sighs, and rapid irregular bursts of breathing have been identified in the fetus (Cunningham et al., 2010). At least one episode of breathing movements that lasts at least 30 seconds over 30 minutes is considered normal for the BPP (Liston et al., 2007).

Fetal body movements comprising at least three separate and distinct episodes of body or limb movements in 30 minutes are considered normal (Cunningham et al., 2010; Liston et al., 2007). Simultaneous movements of the limbs or trunk are counted as one movement. Periods of rest in the fetus must be distinguished from a lack of activity because of a compromised uterine environment.

The fetus begins to flex and stretch its arms and legs by about 13 weeks' gestation (Cunningham et al., 2010). At least one episode of both extension and flexion of fetal extremities or trunk or the opening or closing of a hand within 30 minutes indicates normal body tone (Cunningham et al., 2010; Liston et al., 2007).

Amniotic fluid volume is an important component of the BPP. The kidneys and lungs are the principal sources of amniotic fluid. When placental function is compromised, perfusion to organs such as the kidneys is decreased and can lead to decreased amniotic fluid (Chow et al., 2013). When the membranes are intact, fetal kidneys are functioning, and the urinary tract is unobstructed, decreased amniotic fluid volume is a reflection of decreased glomerular filtration as cardiac output is shunted away from the fetal kidneys in response to chronic hypoxia (Liston et al., 2007). It takes approximately 15 days for amniotic fluid to progress from a normal volume to a barely abnormal volume, and approximately 23 days to reach severe oligohydramnios (Manning, 2002). Therefore, amniotic fluid volume may be the most obvious sign of chronic fetal hypoxemia or acidemia. Abnormal amniotic fluid volumes also may indicate congenital anatomic anomalies or fetal growth restrictions (Perry et al., 2013; Schrimmer & Moore, 2002).

A pocket of amniotic fluid that measures less than 2 cm by 2 cm is considered **oligohydramnios** (Liston et al., 2007; Moise, 2013). In the maximum vertical pocket (MVP) depth technique, a pocket depth of 2 to 8 cm is normal in the latter part of the second or third trimesters, 1 to 2 cm is marginal, <1 cm is decreased, and >8 cm is increased (Liston et al., 2007; Moise, 2013). Amniotic fluid index, another technique, sums the deepest vertical pocket of fluid in the four quadrants of the uterus (the umbilicus being the centre point) to quantify the total amount of amniotic fluid (Liston et al., 2007). A range of 5 to 24 cm in the late second and third trimesters is considered normal (Moise, 2013). Nabhan and Abdelmoula (2008) concluded, in a Cochrane review, that the MVP technique seemed to be a better choice in assessment of amniotic fluid volume for fetal surveillance, since the use of the amniotic index has been associated with increased frequency of interventions with no improvement in outcomes.

Table 12.4 indicates the interpretation of the variables, each of which is assigned a score of 2 or 0. A score of 1 is not an option. The maximum score is 8, when only the BPP is done; 10, when it is done in conjunction with a NST (Liston et al., 2007). The score result informs the management of the pregnancy. A score of 10/10, 8/8, and 8/10, with a normal amount of amniotic fluid, indicates a normal fetus with an extremely rare risk of asphyxia (Cunningham et al., 2010; Liston

● TABLE 12.4   **Biophysical Profile**

Variable	Normal (Score = 2)	Abnormal (Score = 0)
Fetal breathing movements	At least one episode of breathing movements lasting at least 30 s in a 30-min period	Absent respirations or no episode of breathing movements lasting at least 30 s in a 30-min period
Gross body movements	At least three separate and distinct episodes of body or limb movements in 30 min	Two or fewer episodes of body or limb movements in 30 min
Fetal tone	At least one episode of extension and flexion of fetal extremities or the spine	Slow extension with return to partial flexion or movement of limb in full extension only or no movement
Amniotic fluid volume	At least one pocket of amniotic fluid measuring at least 2 cm in vertical diameter	Either pocket of fluid is less than 2 cm in vertical diameter or no pocket
Fetal heart reactivity	Two or more accelerations of the fetal heart of at least 15 bpm above baseline and lasting at least 15 s associated with fetal movement within 20 min	Less than two accelerations or acceleration less than 15 bpm in a 20-min period

et al., 2007). A score of 8/10 with abnormal fluid suggests that there is a probability of chronic fetal asphyxia and the term fetus should be delivered (Cunningham et al., 2010; Liston et al., 2007). A score of 6 is considered equivocal and indicative of possible fetal asphyxia. If the amniotic fluid volume is abnormal, fetal asphyxia is probable and the term fetus should be delivered (Cunningham et al., 2010; Liston et al., 2007). When the score is 6/10 or 8/10, with abnormal fluid, and the preterm fetus is less than 34 weeks, intensive surveillance may be instituted to maximize fetal maturity. If the amniotic fluid volume is normal with a score of 6/10, the BPP should be repeated within 24 hours. This reassessment will be reassuring in 75% of cases; in those cases where an equivocal result persists, the fetus should be delivered (Liston et al., 2007). A score of 4 or less is considered to be a high to certain risk of fetal asphyxia, and the fetus should be delivered (Cunningham et al., 2010; Liston et al., 2007).

Uterine Artery Doppler

Impaired trophoblastic implantation of the placenta is associated with pre-existing hypertension and subsequent development of hypertensive disorders of pregnancy, IUGR, abruptio placentae, and intrauterine fetal demise (Liston et al., 2007). The resistance of vessels that supply the placenta can be assessed by Doppler ultrasound of the uterine arteries (Liston et al., 2007). In the normal pregnancy, there is increased blood flow velocity and decreased resistance to flow (Liston et al., 2007). In pregnancies complicated by hypertensive disorders, there is increased resistance to flow, early diastolic notching, and decreased diastolic flow (Liston et al., 2007).

Umbilical Artery Doppler

Umbilical artery Doppler is based on the belief that the shape of uterine artery velocity waveform is unique and differs in the fetus with normal growth and the fetus with growth restriction. In a normal pregnancy, continuous forward flow to the placenta increases as the pregnancy progresses and the branching of the villus vasculature develops, resulting in decreased resistance to forward flow (Liston et al., 2007). Increased resistance to forward flow in the umbilical circulation implies that there is a problem with the vasculature within the placenta (Liston et al., 2007). When end-diastolic flow is decreased, IUGR occurs (Berkley et al., 2012; Cunningham et al., 2010). This is thought to result in part from the poorly vascularized placenta villi (Berkley et al., 2012; Cunningham, 2010). With extreme cases of placental dysfunction, the end-diastolic flow may be absent or reversed (Berkley et al., 2012; Cunningham et al., 2010). Absent or reversed end-diastolic flow is considered an ominous sign indicating fetal compromise that may precede fetal death (Berkley et al., 2012; Cunningham et al., 2010). Perinatal mortality in reversed end-diastolic flow has been reported to be approximately 33%, while mortality in absent end-diastolic flow is 10% (Cunningham et al., 2010).

Although abnormal Doppler studies have been associated with lower arterial and venous pH values, increased intrapartum nonreassuring FHR patterns, and a higher incidence of neonatal respiratory distress syndrome (Berkley et al., 2012; Cunningham et al., 2010; Sprong, 2008), it is currently recommended for assessment of the fetal placental circulation in women with suspected placental insufficiency (Liston et al., 2007).

Umbilical artery Doppler is the only form of fetal surveillance that research has shown to improve perinatal mortality (Liston et al., 2007).

Collaborative Management

The nurse examines the findings from any assessment of fetal well-being to anticipate the appropriate plan of care. Although antenatal fetal surveillance implemented across Canada may include a variety of methods, there is limited Level 1 evidence (obtained from at least one properly randomized controlled trial) to support this practice. Level 1 evidence is only available for umbilical artery Doppler for fetuses with growth restriction (Liston et al., 2007). It is therefore suggested that antenatal testing for women with risk factors should only take place when the results will guide decisions about future care (Liston et al., 2007). It is important for nurses to remember that the mother and significant others will be concerned about the tests and the results and possible implications for the fetus and pregnancy. A major component of the nurse's care includes emotional support for the woman and her significant others.

ANTICIPATORY GUIDANCE RELATED TO PREGNANCY

During pregnancy, women experience many changes. Several physical discomforts are common; however, each client will have a unique experience. Therefore, not everyone will experience all discomforts, or have them to the same degree. Physical discomforts occur at different times during pregnancy. See Table 12.5 for a summary of common discomforts, their etiologies, and suggested relief measures.

After providing anticipatory guidance, the nurse should remember to evaluate the effectiveness of interventions used to assist with the discomforts of pregnancy. If implemented measures have been ineffective, the nurse may need to investigate further to ensure that there is no alternative reason for the problems. Symptoms that continue to increase with associated metabolic or psychological complications may need treatment. For example, the client with uncontrolled nausea and vomiting that leads to dehydration and significant weight loss may need intravenous fluids for hydration and nourishment. See Nursing Care Plan 12.2.

Urinary Frequency

Early in pregnancy, women experience urinary frequency from the growing uterus compressing the bladder. Although little can be done to solve this problem, the nurse can advise women who experience it to consider decreasing fluid intake in the evening before going to bed. Doing so assists in decreasing urine production, which may limit the number of times a woman has to get up during the night to void. The nurse advises women not to reduce their fluid intake during the day, because appropriate fluids are important to maintain hydration and to increase blood volume. The nurse can counsel women to void whenever they feel the urge. Urine that stays in the bladder for an extended time increases the risk for UTI (Blackburn, 2014). The nurse also teaches that urinary frequency will be alleviated when the uterus rises into the abdominal cavity, although it will return with lightening in the third trimester.

Fatigue and Sleep Problems

Pregnant women often are fatigued because of nocturia and increased metabolic requirements. They experience frequent sleep difficulties related to other signs and symptoms, such as palpitations. Suggestions to manage fatigue and sleep difficulties include taking more frequent rest periods, going to bed earlier, and resting in a modified Sims position to reposition some fetal weight onto the bed. The nurse also may advise the client to use pillows under the abdomen and between the legs for support.

Breast Sensitivity and Other Discomforts

The breasts enlarge and become more sensitive from the effects of circulating hormones, especially estrogen and progesterone. The nurse may recommend wearing a supportive bra with wide shoulder straps that decrease pressure on the shoulders, and avoiding any stimulus that tends to exacerbate breast sensitivity.

Increased estrogen levels may cause nasal stuffiness and epistaxis (nosebleeds). Suggestions to manage nasal stuffiness include humidification of the room air, and saline drops or spray. These suggestions also may help control epistaxis. Additional suggestions for epistaxis include local application of a moisturizer such as petroleum jelly, avoidance of forceful blowing of the nose, and avoidance of excessive overexertion or heating that may exacerbate epistaxis.

Ptyalism (excessive salivation) may occur for unknown reasons. Frequent mouth care and chewing gum or sucking hard candy may assist with ptyalism (Cunningham et al., 2010).

Gastrointestinal Problems

One of the most frequent discomforts of early pregnancy is nausea and vomiting, the cause of which is unknown. Hormonal and emotional factors have been investigated with inconsistent results. Because clients with nausea and vomiting often experience it as morning sickness, the nurse may recommend that they eat

● TABLE 12.5   **Common Discomforts of Pregnancy, Etiology, and Relief Measures**

Discomfort	Etiology	Relief Measures
First Trimester		
Urinary frequency	Pressure of growing uterus on bladder	Decrease fluid intake at night Maintain fluid intake during day Void when feeling the urge
Fatigue	Possibly increased metabolic requirements or nocturia	Rest frequently Go to bed earlier
Sleep difficulties	Often related to other signs and symptoms (eg, nocturia, palpitations)	Rest frequently Decrease fluid intake at night
Breast enlargement and sensitivity	Effect of hormones, especially estrogen and progesterone	Wear a good supporting bra with wide shoulder straps Assess for other conditions
Nasal stuffiness and epistaxis	Elevated estrogen levels	Avoid decongestants Use humidifiers, cool mist vaporizers, and normal saline drops
Ptyalism (excessive salivation)	Unknown	Perform frequent mouth care Chew gum or suck hard candies
Nausea and vomiting	Unknown	Avoid food or smells that exacerbate condition Eat dry crackers or toast before rising in morning Eat small, frequent meals
Second and Third Trimesters		
Urinary frequency	After lightening, pressure of fetal head on bladder	Void when feeling the urge Decrease fluid intake at night Maintain fluid intake during day
Shortness of breath	Growing fetus, which puts pressure on diaphragm	Use extra pillows at night to keep more upright Limit activity during day
Heartburn	Displacement of stomach by growing fetus Relaxation of cardioesophageal sphincter	Eat small, more frequent meals Use antacids Avoid overeating and spicy foods
Dependent edema	Impeded venous return from pressure of fetus on pelvic area	Avoid standing for long periods Elevate legs when laying or sitting Avoid tight stockings
Varicosities	Weight of uterus, which causes pooling and engorgement of veins in lower extremities Heredity, age, obesity	Rest in Sims' position Elevate legs regularly Avoid crossing legs Avoid tight stockings Avoid long periods of standing
Hemorrhoids	Constipation Pressure of enlarging uterus on pelvic and rectal veins	Maintain regular bowel habits Use prescribed stool softeners Apply witch hazel compresses and topical or anaesthetic ointments to area
Constipation	Pressure of growing fetus on intestine, causing decreased peristalsis Possibly, ingestion of iron	Maintain regular bowel habits Increase roughage in diet Increase fluids Find iron preparation that is least constipating
Leukorrhea	Response to increased estrogen levels	Take a daily bath or shower. Do not douche or use tampons Wear cotton underwear
Backache	Lumbar lordosis that develops to maintain balance in later pregnancy	Wear shoes with low heels. Walk with pelvis tilted forward Use firmer mattress Perform pelvic rocking or tilting
Leg cramps	Decreased serum calcium level Increased serum phosphorus level Interference with circulation	Extend affected leg and dorsiflex the foot Elevate lower legs frequently Apply heat to muscles Evaluate diet

(continued)

● TABLE 12.5   **Common Discomforts of Pregnancy, Etiology, and Relief Measures** (continued)

Discomfort	Etiology	Relief Measures
Balance alterations	Growing uterus, which throws off the woman's centre of gravity	Wear shoes with low heels Walk with pelvis tilted forward
Round ligament pain	Tension on round ligament from enlarging uterus	Rise slowly from sitting to standing or lying to sitting Apply a warm heating pad to abdomen or take a warm (not hot) bath Bring knees up toward abdomen
Flatulence	Decreased gastric motility Pressure of growing uterus on large intestine	Avoid gas-forming foods Chew food thoroughly Engage in regular daily exercise Maintain regular bowel routine
Carpal tunnel syndrome	Compression of medial nerve in carpal tunnel of wrist; weight gain and edema may contribute	Avoid aggravating hand movements Elevate affected arm Wear splint
Faintness	Pooling of blood in lower extremities Anemia	Rise slowly from sitting to standing Evaluate hemoglobin and hematocrit Avoid hot stuffy environments
Mood swings	Hormonal influences	The woman and her partner need information about these mood swings to understand that they are normal. This assists them to cope with them

dry crackers or toast before rising. The nurse can counsel clients to avoid foods or smells that exacerbate nausea. Small, frequent meals also may assist to control nausea. Alternative and complementary therapies that have been suggested for nausea include acupressure bracelets, acupuncture, ginger, peppermint, chamomile or lemon balm tea, reflexology, and hypnosis (BabyCentre Canada, 2012; Mayo Clinic, 2011). There is little evidence to support these options, although some women do find them effective in the relief of nausea. The woman should check with her health care provider prior to using herbal or alternative treatments (Mayo Clinic, 2011).

During the second and third trimesters, pregnant women may experience heartburn as the cardioesophageal sphincter relaxes and the growing fetus displaces the stomach upward, leading to gastroesophageal reflux. Small, frequent meals may assist with heartburn, along with avoiding overeating and spicy foods. Limiting food and fluids before bed and sleeping in a semi-Fowler's position may help. Antacids also may be useful. The most consistent relief is provided by the use of liquid forms of antacids and histamine-2 receptor inhibitors (Katz, 2008). Women are advised that antacids containing aluminum may cause constipation; those containing magnesium may cause diarrhea. The woman can discuss antacids with her primary care provider before using them. Complementary and alternative therapies that may be effective in the reduction of heartburn include ginger, chamomile and dandelion root tea, acupressure, yoga,

tai chi, acupuncture, or shiatsu (BabyCenter Canada, 2012).

The pressure of the enlarging uterus on the pelvic and rectal veins may lead to hemorrhoids. Adding to the development of hemorrhoids and the resulting discomfort, pregnant women are prone to constipation, as the pressure of the growing fetus on the intestine decreases peristalsis. The use of iron supplements may exacerbate constipation. Women may experience flatulence from decreased gastric motility and the pressure of the growing uterus on the large intestine.

The nurse can encourage regular bowel habits to decrease constipation, hemorrhoids, and flatulence. Increasing roughage and fluids in the diet, avoiding or reducing constipating foods such as cheese, and increasing fluid intake may all assist with constipation. After consultation with her primary care provider to ensure that there are no contraindications, the client may find a regular program of mild exercise helpful. Stool softeners may assist with constipation and hemorrhoids. Witch hazel compresses, topical analgesics, or anaesthetic ointments also may help if hemorrhoids accompany constipation. The woman can decrease flatulence by avoiding gas-forming foods and chewing food thoroughly.

Vascular Problems

Dependent edema, especially of the ankles and feet, results from the impeded venous return caused by the pressure of the growing fetus on the pelvic area. The pooling and engorgement of the veins in the lower

NURSING CARE PLAN 12.2

●

A Client With Common Discomforts of Pregnancy

Consider Kathy from the beginning of the chapter. Assessment of her feet reveals pitting edema. On further questioning, Kathy says that she is employed as a cashier at the local supermarket. Once she finishes work for the day, she usually goes home, makes supper, and does some housework. She goes to bed about 10 PM, having gotten up at 6:30 AM. She has been decreasing her fluid intake in the evening because she occasionally still has urinary frequency. She does not like to eat vegetables.

NURSING DIAGNOSIS

Constipation related to decreased peristalsis secondary to pregnancy

EXPECTED OUTCOMES

1. The client will verbalize the underlying etiology of constipation.
2. The client will identify two strategies to decrease constipation.

INTERVENTIONS	RATIONALES
Use both oral and written materials to teach the client about the pressure that the growing fetus places on the intestine, which causes decreased peristalsis	Assisting the client to understand the reasons for constipation will help her choose effective strategies to decrease the problem. Understanding the etiology will help decrease anxiety
Assist the client to choose vegetables and fruit that she likes in her diet	Dietary roughage helps the stool retain fluid and decreases constipation
Assist the client to plan increased fluid intake throughout the day	Doing so will facilitate softer stool. Planning the increase during the day will assist the client with the urinary frequency she experiences at night
At her next visit to the prenatal clinic, ask the client if she has experienced any changes in her stools. Assess for any further discomforts	Doing so will reveal if the actions have been successful or if further planning is needed. The client will be less anxious if she has achieved success

EVALUATION

1. The client verbalizes understanding of the reasons for constipation.
2. The client reports improvements in her stool pattern.
3. The client lists specific vegetables and fruit that she now includes in her diet.
4. The client reports that increased fluid has been successful in treating her constipation and avoiding urinary frequency at night.

NURSING DIAGNOSIS

Health-Seeking Behaviours related to discomforts of pregnancy

(continued)

NURSING CARE PLAN 12.2 ● A Client With Common Discomforts of Pregnancy *(Continued)*

EXPECTED OUTCOMES

1. The client will verbalize the underlying etiology of dependent edema.
2. The client will take measures to control swelling and to avoid overexertion.

INTERVENTIONS	RATIONALES
Using oral and written material, instruct the client about the impeded venous return from the fetal pressure on the pelvic area	Assisting the client to understand the reasons for the edema will assist her to choose effective strategies to decrease the problem. Understanding the etiology will help decrease her anxiety
Assist the client to identify ways by which she can decrease the time that she stands	Doing so will assist with venous return and should decrease the edema. Having the client identify the strategies assists both client and nurse to plan realistic interventions. The client will be more likely to continue to use suggestions if she has had more control
Assist the client to identify appropriate clothing that will prevent further occlusion of the venous return	Avoiding tight stockings will assist with prevention
At the client's next visit to the clinic, assess the edema	Doing so facilitates further planning and interventions if these are not successful

EVALUATION

1. The client identifies two strategies to decrease dependent edema.
2. The client verbalizes understanding of the causes of edema and repeats material taught.
3. The client reports more frequent rest periods and going into work 30 minutes later each day.

extremities also leads to varicose veins, which can be exacerbated by heredity, age, or obesity. Leg cramps may develop from decreased serum calcium level, increased serum phosphorus level, and interference with circulation of the extremities.

The nurse can advise the client to avoid long periods of standing and to elevate the legs while sitting, which may help decrease dependent edema, varicosities, and leg cramps (Fig. 12.20). If the woman develops a leg cramp, she should extend the affected leg and dorsiflex the foot. Application of heat to the muscle also may be helpful. Women should avoid crossing their legs and wearing tight stockings to prevent varicosities. They also should avoid massaging the calf muscle.

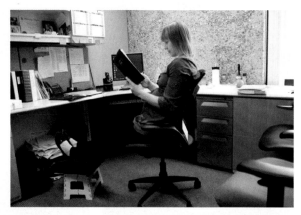

FIGURE 12.20 Leg elevation can prevent or decrease edema, varicosities, and leg cramps during pregnancy. (Used with permission from Robin J. Evans.)

Dyspnea

Dyspnea arises from the crowding caused by the growing fetus on the diaphragm, the increased oxygen the client uses, and the resulting carbon dioxide that forms. Use of extra pillows at night to prop the client in bed into a more semisitting position may assist with shortness of breath. If shortness of breath occurs during the day as well, the client may need to limit her activities.

Leukorrhea

Leukorrhea (increased vaginal secretions) often results in response to increased estrogen levels. A daily bath or shower, along with the use of cotton underwear and panty liners, will increase comfort and decrease risk of infection. The woman is advised to avoid douching because of the risk of vaginal infection.

Round Ligament Pain

As the uterus enlarges, tension is put on the round ligament, often resulting in pain. Rising slowly from a sitting to standing position, or from a lying to sitting position may decrease this pain. Bringing the knees up to the abdomen also may help decrease some of the pain. Assuming a position on the hands and knees and lowering the head to the floor while keeping the buttocks in the air, may alleviate unremitting ligament pain.

Carpal Tunnel Syndrome

Weight gain, edema, and traction on the median nerve from postural changes resulting in median nerve compression, may contribute to the development of carpal tunnel syndrome, a condition that causes tingling, numbness, and burning in the fingers and hands (Bahrami et al., 2005). The nurse can advise the woman that gentle range of motion of the affected hand every 4 hours may assist with mild symptoms. If symptoms are more severe, the woman may need a soft wrist splint to avoid pressure on the median nerve in the mid-palm area. The nurse may counsel the woman to avoid repetitive wrist motion, flexion, or extension and encourage her to alternate and take frequent breaks from activities.

Supine Hypotension Syndrome

Women in the later stages of pregnancy may be at increased risk for faintness as blood pools in the lower extremities. If the woman lies on her back, pressure from the gravid uterus compresses the vena cava, causing supine hypotensive syndrome. This results in hypotension with diaphoresis and possible syncope. The woman can avoid supine hypotensive syndrome by maintaining a side-lying position during pregnancy, especially resting on the left side, which increases placental circulation and oxygenation. Slowly rising from sitting to standing and avoiding hot, humid environments also will help prevent postural hypotension.

Backache

The growing uterus disrupts the pregnant woman's centre of gravity, compromising her balance (Fig. 12.21). Backache and lordosis may develop in late pregnancy, as she tries to maintain her balance. The woman can relieve backache by wearing shoes with lower heels, performing pelvic rocking or tilting exercises, and walking with the pelvis tilted backward. Warm (not hot)

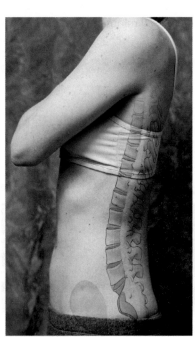

A. Early pregnancy

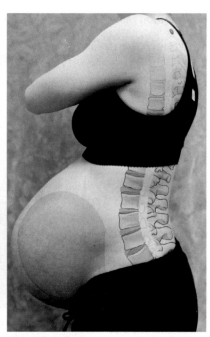

B. Late pregnancy

FIGURE 12.21 The postural changes from the first trimester (**A**) to the third trimester (**B**) disrupt the pregnant client's centre of gravity and sense of balance.

baths that do not exceed 30 minutes may be helpful. Use of a firmer mattress also may provide relief. The woman should also practice good body mechanics by bending both knees when lifting, holding objects close to her body, lifting with her leg muscles, and avoiding heavy lifting. Regular exercise (after consultation with the primary care provider) may assist with strengthening the back and abdominal muscles and thus decreasing backache.

Bathing

Tub bathing is acceptable during pregnancy as long as the woman's membranes are intact. Bathing with ruptured membranes is contraindicated because of the risk for infection. Because of the problems with balance in the last trimester, showers at the end of pregnancy may be preferable. The temperature of the water should not exceed 39°C to avoid raising the core body temperature, which may lead to postural hypotension. The use of saunas and whirlpool baths is not recommended because of the intense heat.

Working

Working during pregnancy generally is not contraindicated, although there may be particular instances in which it is not recommended. If the woman works in a high-risk area (ie, an occupation that is physically or emotionally hazardous), additional precautions may be necessary, or she may need to transfer to another area. Pregnant women who continue to work should take the opportunity to rest periodically throughout the day whenever possible. Those whose work requires prolonged standing should be especially conscious of sitting frequently; prolonged standing has been found to increase the risk of preterm labour (Cunningham et al., 2010).

Travel

There is no contraindication to travel for pregnant women, unless they have medical or obstetrical complications. Travel may be contraindicated for women with cardiovascular conditions complicated by pregnancy, congenital or acquired heart disease, multiple gestations after 22 weeks, or cervical insufficiency. Long-distance travel may not be advisable when pregnancy is complicated by threatened abortion, vaginal bleeding, history of preterm labour, or other obstetrical complications.

Travel by car is often tiring, especially late in pregnancy. Frequent rest stops are necessary to assist with maintenance of circulation to extremities. The woman should wear lap and shoulder seatbelts throughout her pregnancy to decrease risk for maternal injury (Motozawa et al., 2010; Transport Canada, 2007). For correct use, the woman places the lap portion of the seatbelt over the upper portion of her thighs, under her abdomen. She then positions the shoulder harness

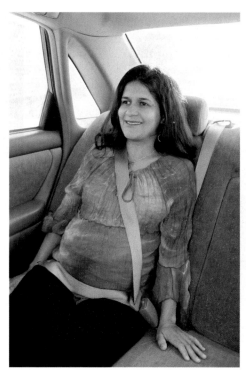

FIGURE 12.22 The pregnant client should wear a seatbelt as shown.

between the breasts. Both belts should be snugly applied. Seatbelts also will decrease exaggerated flexion of the woman's torso, which may lessen the risk for placental separation (Fig. 12.22).

Pregnant women may choose to travel by air during pregnancy, although most airlines restrict travel in later pregnancy (Government of Canada, 2014). Flying is permitted for women with singleton pregnancies up to the end of the 36th week of pregnancy (Government of Canada, 2014). During flights, they are advised to wear support hose and periodically exercise the legs and ankles, walking in the aisles if possible, to decrease the risk of thrombophlebitis (Government of Canada, 2014).

Exercise

In uncomplicated pregnancies, women are encouraged to participate in aerobic and strength conditioning exercises regardless of whether their previous lifestyle has been sedentary or active (Davies et al., 2003) (Fig. 12.23). Absolute and relative contraindications to exercise in pregnancy are listed in Table 12.6. The woman makes the decision about whether to be active or not in collaboration with her health care provider. The Canadian Society for Exercise Physiology has developed a tool called the PARmed-X for pregnancy, available at www.csep.ca/cmfiles/publications/parq/parmed-xpreg.pdf. This tool, endorsed by the Society of Obstetricians and Gynaecologists of Canada, can be

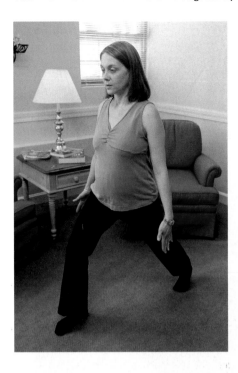

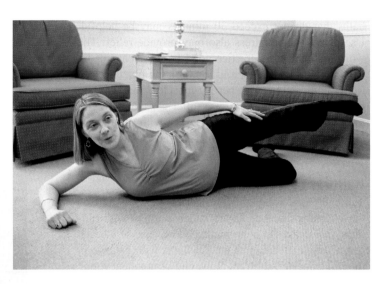

FIGURE 12.23 The client with an uncomplicated pregnancy can participate in aerobic and strength conditioning exercises, which may strengthen the abdominal and back muscles. The decision to be active or not should be made with her health care provider.

used for screening women interested in exercise during pregnancy.

Most women find that the second trimester is the best time to initiate an exercise program. The nausea, vomiting, and fatigue of the first trimester have usually passed and the physical limitations associated with the third trimester have not yet begun. Women who have been exercising prior to pregnancy can continue their exercise regimen, without trying to reach peak fitness or train for an athletic competition. Women who have been previously sedentary can begin with 15 minutes of continuous exercise 3 times a week, increasing gradually to 30-minute sessions 4 times a week (Davies et al., 2003).

All pregnant women are advised to modify exercises so that they do not spend time in the supine position after 16 weeks' gestation. They may choose activities that minimize the risk of loss of balance and fetal trauma, avoiding such activities as horseback riding, ice hockey, gymnastics, downhill skiing, cycling, or hiking where they might fall (Davies et al., 2003). Women should not scuba dive during pregnancy; the fetus is not protected from decompression sickness or gas embolism (Davies et al., 2003). Exercise should be stopped and medical attention sought if the woman has excessive shortness of breath, chest pain, painful uterine contractions, leakage of amniotic fluid, vaginal bleeding, or presyncope (Davies et al., 2003).

● TABLE 12.6   **Contraindications to Exercise in Pregnancy**

Absolute Contraindications	Relative Contraindications
● Ruptured membranes ● Preterm labour ● Hypertensive disorders of pregnancy ● Incompetent cervix ● Growth-restricted fetus ● High-order multiple gestation (≥ triplets) ● Placenta previa after 28th week ● Persistent second or third trimester bleeding ● Uncontrolled type 1 diabetes, thyroid disease, or other serious cardiovascular, respiratory, or systemic disorder	● Previous spontaneous abortion ● Previous preterm birth ● Mild/moderate cardiovascular disorder ● Mild/moderate respiratory disorder ● Anemia (Hb <100 g/L) ● Malnutrition or eating disorder ● Twin pregnancy after 28th week ● Other significant medical conditions

Reprinted with permission of the Society of Obstetricians and Gynaecologists of Canada from Davies, G. A., Wolfe, L. A., Mottola, M. F., & MacKinnon, C. (2003). Joint SOGC/CSEP clinical practice guideline: Exercise in pregnancy and the postpartum period. *Canadian Journal of Applied Physiology, 28*(3), 3.

Dental Care

Good dental care during pregnancy is important. Studies have suggested that active periodontal disease increases the woman's risk for preterm birth, low birth weight, and preeclampsia (Cockney, 2003; Contreras et al., 2006; George et al., 2011). The woman is advised to schedule a dental checkup in early pregnancy, and inform the dentist about her pregnancy to assist in avoiding teratogenic substances. Dental x-rays may be taken if a lead apron fully covers the abdomen (Katz, 2008). There is no evidence that suggests that pregnancy aggravates dental caries (Cunningham et al., 2010).

Sexual Concerns

Sexual intercourse is safe in an uncomplicated pregnancy (Society of Obstetricians and Gynaecologists of Canada [SOGC], 2012b). Both the woman and her partner may express concerns about sexuality and intercourse during pregnancy. Although there is no reason why the healthy woman needs to abstain from intercourse or orgasm during pregnancy, some sources suggest that women should avoid coitus and orgasm in the last 4 weeks of pregnancy (Cunningham et al., 2010). Clients may engage in intercourse less frequently because of decreased desire or fear of causing harm in the pregnancy.

Intercourse or orgasm is contraindicated in cases of known placenta previa or ruptured membranes (Cunningham et al., 2010; Perry et al., 2013; SOGC, 2012a). The amniotic sac provides protection from infection; once it has ruptured, the risk of infection increases. Nipple stimulation, vaginal penetration, or orgasm may cause uterine contractions secondary to the release of prostaglandins and oxytocin (Katz, 2008; Perry et al., 2013). Therefore, women who are predisposed to preterm labour or threatened abortion may choose to avoid intercourse (Katz, 2008; Perry et al., 2013).

It is normal for desire for sexual intercourse to either decrease or increase during pregnancy (SOGC, 2012a). Sometimes, the cause is discomforts of pregnancy, such as nausea or vomiting. Discussing these changes with the woman's partner helps decrease misunderstandings and feelings of inadequacy in either partner. Other changes that may influence sexual desire or activity include the normally increased amount and odour of vaginal secretions and increased breast sensitivity, especially in the first trimester, that may be exacerbated by touching of breasts or positions that increase the pressure put on them.

In later stages, once the abdomen is significantly enlarged, alternate positions may be more comfortable for some women. Examples of positions that may increase comfort include the woman in the superior position or a side-by-side position. If the woman experiences discomfort from vaginal penetration, the couple may find alternative methods of sexual expression, such as cuddling, masturbation, or oral sex.

Some women report increased sexual desire during pregnancy. Possible reasons for this increase include not having to worry about birth control, as well as the increased blood flow to the pelvic region that increases libido and sexual satisfaction. Decreased desire may result from those times when the woman is not feeling well. Occasionally, concerns may develop about potential changes in the woman's body and the couple's relationship. The nurse provides the opportunity for each to verbalize their concerns and correct any misinformation or myths. The nurse also encourages the couple to initiate and maintain an open dialogue.

Clothing

As the client's abdomen enlarges, the need for different clothing becomes apparent. Clothing that fits more loosely or stretches easily promotes comfort and accommodates the growing abdomen. Because new clothing can be expensive and is worn for a relatively short time, women may choose to economize by sharing clothes with friends and family, sewing one's own clothing, purchasing clothing on-line, and buying used clothing. Stores that sell slightly used clothing at reduced prices may be an option.

As the woman's breasts enlarge, she will require a larger bra and will benefit from bras that provide maximum support. Although some recommend purchasing nursing bras during the last trimester of pregnancy, the breasts will change in size once lactation has been established. Thus, purchasing nursing bras while pregnant may not be helpful.

Nutrition

Nutrition is important because the client must ensure that both she and the fetus receive the calories and nutrients they require. Chapter 3 provides a discussion of nutritional needs and adaptations required during pregnancy.

Pets

Pets provide companionship, especially to women who may be home more than usual during pregnancy. They may present additional challenges, however, to expectant mothers and their significant others. Pets may demonstrate jealousy of the new baby, similar to sibling rivalry, when they have held a central position in the family. It might be helpful for the expectant woman to pretend to carry a baby around the house. In addition, many pregnant women give additional time and affection to their pets, in anticipation of their having less time to do so once the baby is born. Rather than helping the pet, however, this may increase the animal's feelings of jealousy, because it emphasizes the differences in attention that they are receiving once the baby is part of the family. Books and other resources are available that will provide assistance to the family in dealing with this.

The protozoan *Toxoplasma gondii* causes toxoplasmosis, an illness that presents few problems to adults but can produce profound effects on the fetus, including spontaneous abortion and congenital toxoplasmosis, if contracted during pregnancy. The likelihood of fetal infection increases with gestation (Cunningham et al., 2010). Eating undercooked meat, drinking unpasteurized milk, or having contact with the feces of infected cats facilitates contact with *T. gondii* (Cunningham et al., 2010). Fecal oocytes are spread through the air and can cause infection through inhalation. The nurse counsels the pregnant woman to avoid contact with the cat litter box or areas of the garden frequented by cats. Otherwise, contact with cats is safe.

Teratogens

Substances that women come into contact with during pregnancy may affect fetal growth and development adversely. Such substances are called **teratogens** (see Chapter 11). Some teratogens are legal, whereas others are illegal. Some effects of teratogens are evident at birth, whereas others are not detected until years later. For example, female children of women who took the drug diethylstilbestrol (DES) during pregnancy did not show any adverse effects until years later, when those who had been exposed in utero developed vaginal and cervical cancer in adolescence. Structural abnormalities of the reproductive tract in female children led to infertility and increased risk for ectopic pregnancy, spontaneous abortions, and preterm labour (Cunningham et al., 2010). Exposed male children had increased risk for epididymal cysts, microphallus, cryptorchidism, and testicular hypoplasia (Cunningham et al., 2010). On the other hand, babies demonstrated the adverse effects of thalidomide (shortened limbs) as soon as they were born.

Many substances can be teratogens or have teratogenic effects, including x-rays and pesticides. Medications are the most frequently recognized and researched teratogens. Other examples include rubella, alcohol, syphilis, and toxoplasmosis.

Complementary and Alternative Medicine

The term *complementary and alternative medicine* (CAM) encompasses treatments that are not considered to be part of conventional medicine. Complementary treatments are additional to, and alternative treatments are replacements for standard or established practices in Western medicine (Gossler, 2010; Hall et al., 2010). There appears to be relatively widespread use of complementary or alternative therapies by pregnant women (Hall et al., 2010). Those most commonly used include massage, vitamin and mineral supplements, relaxation techniques, and aromatherapy (Hall et al., 2010).

COLLABORATIVE CARE: TERATOGENS

Assessment

Maternal use of teratogenic substances may be known or unknown during pregnancy, either to the woman herself or to health care providers. Assessment focuses primarily on determining any substances that the woman may come into contact with. The health care provider also can discuss with the client the frequencies and amounts of such contact (eg, how often and the amount of alcohol ingested).

Select Potential Nursing Diagnoses

The following are examples of commonly applicable nursing diagnoses:

- **Risk for Fetal Injury** related to prenatal exposure to drugs
- **Deficient Knowledge** related to substances that adversely affect fetal development

Planning/Intervention

During pregnancy, the woman needs information about substances that may have teratogenic effects on the fetus and what those effects may be. The health care provider can engage in such discussion and answer questions as needed.

Medications, including both over-the-counter and prescription drugs, are the most well-documented teratogens. Although women may be aware of the hazards of prescription drugs during pregnancy, such awareness does not always extend to over-the-counter medications (Mitchell et al., 2011; Werler et al., 2005). Over the last 30 years, the use of prescription medication in the first trimester has increased by more than 60%, suggesting that its use in pregnancy is growing (Mitchell et al., 2011). The greatest danger to the fetus is during the organogenesis of the first trimester (see Chapter 11). Maternal exposure to medications may occur before a woman knows that she is pregnant. Therefore, if possible, the nurse can suggest that the woman begin avoiding medications once she makes the decision to become pregnant.

Caffeine has not been directly implicated as a teratogen; however, excessive intake may be implicated in spontaneous abortion (Cunningham et al., 2010; Katz, 2008). Caffeine also interferes with the absorption of iron (Lloyd, 2009). The commonly accepted recommendation is for women to try to limit their intake of caffeine during pregnancy.

Nicotine has been demonstrated to cause decreased birth weight in neonates (Bernstein et al.,

2005; Keegan et al., 2010). It also has been associated with an increased risk for abruptio placentae, preterm birth, and perinatal death (Amasha & Jaradeh, 2012; Cunningham et al., 2010). Babies born to mothers who smoke during pregnancy, or are exposed to second hand smoke have an increased incidence of lower Apgar scores, sudden infant death syndrome and lower respiratory tract infections (Amasha & Jaradeh, 2012; Lannero et al., 2006; Viccars, 2009). The nurse can provide information to women about the risks. If it is difficult for a woman to quit smoking, the nurse informs her that any decrease is beneficial. If significant others around the client smoke, rather than the woman herself, the nurse can suggest that they smoke in places other than around the woman.

Infants of mothers who ingest alcohol are at increased risk for FASD, including fetal alcohol syndrome (FAS) and fetal alcohol effects (FAE) (see Chapter 22). No level of alcohol has been determined safe during pregnancy, so the nurse cautions women to avoid all alcohol during pregnancy. Alcohol can pass through the placental barrier, resulting in an alcohol content in the fetal blood equivalent to the maternal alcohol content.

The use of cocaine during pregnancy increases the risk for abruptio placentae, stillbirth, low birth weight, neonatal addiction and subsequent withdrawal, and some birth defects (Cunningham et al., 2010; Fraser, 2014; Irner et al., 2012). Marijuana has not proven to be a teratogen (Chow et al., 2013; Yankowitz, 2008); however, it may be used in combination with other drugs that may be teratogens (Pillitteri, 2007). Therefore, the health care provider assesses the woman for use of marijuana. Because the use of marijuana is more acceptable in society today, women may admit to using it while denying other drug use. Other licit and illicit substance use may also impact pregnancy. Collaborative care involving nurses, physicians, midwives, nurse practitioners, social workers, and others focuses on harm-reduction strategies for pregnant women. Pollution also may be a teratogen. The nurse can caution pregnant women to limit their exposure outside on days when pollution levels are significant. Other environmental teratogens include mercury, found in certain fish, and lead, which may be found in paint in older buildings.

Evaluation

Health care providers continue to evaluate the client's behaviours. They may determine that additional teaching and support are necessary. Referral to support groups may be appropriate. Providers should closely monitor newborns exposed to teratogenic substances in utero.

COMMUNITY AND HOME CONCERNS

The role of the community in a client's pregnancy varies, often depending on cultural practices of the woman and her partner. For example, women and families from some cultures may be more likely to have significant support from the community and extended family. Other women may have little knowledge of community programs and resources. Many women, however, are interested in prenatal classes and may access these from public health offices, private groups, or other organizations. The nurse needs to be aware of the availability of these classes within the community and provide accurate information to women and support people. See Chapter 14 for further information.

Many families today face difficult issues, such as poverty, homelessness, unemployment, chemical dependency, family and neighbourhood violence, and lack of support systems. Early recognition of any of these problems may assist the nurse to provide referrals to appropriate resources. Examples include social workers, food and nutrition supplement programs, and social services.

SUMMARY

- Women experience pregnancy in various ways. In addition to age, ethnicity, race, culture, sexual orientation, economic status, and religion also have effects. Each woman is unique. Nurses should not make assumptions that a particular client fits into any one stereotype. For example, although a woman may be from a particular culture, the extent to which she follows traditional customs may vary. The nurse must view each woman within the context of her environment.

- Women who present with pregnancy may range in age from younger than 15 to older than 45 years. Each age group faces unique challenges with pregnancy.

- Blood volume at delivery increases approximately 45%. Cardiac output increases by 30% to 50%. Pulse increases by approximately 10 to 20 bpm.

- Supine hypotension syndrome may present problems of light-headedness and faintness as the pressure of the gravid uterus compresses the vena cava if the woman lies on her back.

- Impeded venous return to the legs and pelvis may result in edema of the lower extremities, varicosities, and hemorrhoids.

- As the fetus grows, it pushes the diaphragm up so that the woman experiences shortness of breath in the latter stages of pregnancy. As it exerts pressure on other abdominal organs, it causes constipation, flatus, and heartburn.

- Changes to the integumentary system include pigmentation changes of the face and abdomen and the development of striae.
- Hormones that are increased in pregnancy, including estrogen, progesterone, hCG, hPL, and relaxin, cause breast enlargement and tingling, leukorrhea, and mood swings.
- The glomerular filtration rate and the renal plasma flow increase in the kidneys.
- As the woman's abdomen grows, she develops a lordosis in an attempt to maintain her balance with her shifting centre of gravity. This may lead to chronic backache.
- Women may experience a number of psychological changes as they move through pregnancy, including surprise, fear, excitement, and apprehension. Changes also are experienced by partners, grandparents, and siblings.
- Presumptive signs are the subjective signs that the mother experiences. They include amenorrhea, morning sickness, excessive fatigue, urinary frequency, changes in the breasts, and quickening. Probable signs are those objective signs that the examiner assesses. They include Goodell's sign, Chadwick's sign, Hegar's sign, enlargement of the uterus, Braxton-Hicks contractions, skin pigmentation changes, and pregnancy tests. Positive signs absolutely confirm pregnancy. They include the presence of a fetal heart, fetal movements that can be felt by the examiner, and visualization of the fetus on ultrasound.
- The health history of the pregnant woman includes a menstrual history, sexual history, history of STIs, history of past pregnancies, past medical and surgical history, history of intimate-partner violence, childhood illnesses, family background of the mother and father, and the use of drugs, alcohol, and tobacco.
- Physical examination of the pregnant woman includes the EDD, physiologic changes the woman has been experiencing, and a complete physical examination of all body systems. A pelvic examination includes assessment of the pelvis. The mother's ABO and Rh, rubella titer, hemoglobin, and urinalysis are also assessed.
- Fetal well-being can be evaluated through maternal assessment of fetal activity, the NST, the CST, sonographic assessment of fetal behaviour and/or amniotic fluid volume, and the umbilical artery Doppler velocimetry. Each of these alone provides relatively limited information; in combination, however, greater confidence in care decisions will be achieved.
- Women may not be able to solve the common problems associated with pregnancy, but they may be able to manage the symptoms sufficiently to be comfortable for most of the pregnancy. Strategies include decreasing fluid intake in the evening, taking frequent rest periods, wearing a supportive bra, avoiding foods that are bothersome, eating small and frequent meals, elevating legs regularly, increasing roughage in the diet, and rising slowly from sitting to standing.
- Several substances are teratogenic to the developing fetus. Examples include prescription and over-the-counter medications, nicotine, alcohol, cocaine, and pollution.

Questions to Ponder

During an appointment with the prenatal clinic, a woman's partner tells the nurse that the woman has been using cocaine throughout her pregnancy and continues to do so. He says that he is concerned about the health of the fetus and wants something done to prevent her from continuing to use drugs.

1. Discuss your personal feelings about a pregnant woman who knowingly continues to use drugs that she has been repeatedly told will cause serious harm to the baby.
2. Explore your personal feelings about the partner wanting to have something done to prevent her from continuing to use drugs.
3. Identify the additional information that might be helpful for the nurse to have before responding.
4. Clarify the legal and ethical considerations that need to be considered.

REVIEW QUESTIONS

1. During a prenatal visit, a 38-year-old primigravida, who is at 28 weeks' gestation, expresses increased concerns about the pregnancy. Which of the following would the nurse recognize as the most likely potential cause for anxiety?
   A. Fear of the unknown
   B. Fear of losing the pregnancy
   C. Ambivalence about the pregnancy
   D. Changes in the woman's mental health
2. A woman calls the Labour & Birth unit needing to come to have a nonstress test done. She is new to the area, having recently arrived from Bangladesh. She identifies herself as a Muslim. Which intervention would be most important to consider when scheduling her request?
   A. Ensure an interpreter is available.
   B. Ask her about what traditions of the Muslim faith she follows.
   C. Ensure the appointment is not scheduled on a Friday.
   D. Assign her to a provider with a small workload so that more time can be spent with her.

3. A woman who is at 26 weeks' gestation calls the office nurse and shares that she has been experiencing all the following symptoms. Which symptom would suggest to the nurse that additional information is needed?
   A. Nasal stuffiness
   B. Urinary frequency
   C. Tingling in the breasts
   D. Darkened spots on the nose and cheeks

4. A woman, GTPAL 2-0-0-1-0, who is at 14 weeks' gestation, says that she is not sure she is pregnant. She believes that her symptoms may indicate something is wrong with her. Which of these statements would it be most appropriate for the nurse to use to reassure the woman?
   A. "Once you feel the baby move you will feel better about being pregnant."
   B. "Many women feel this way early in pregnancy, so you are not alone."
   C. "Your pregnancy test came back positive, so you don't need to worry."
   D. "An ultrasound will provide the best assurance that you are pregnant."

5. During a health assessment of a woman who is in labour, she indicates that she has 5-year-old twin boys who were born at 32 weeks and a 3-year-old daughter born at 41 weeks. She relates that she miscarried last year. All her children are currently healthy. What is the appropriate way to record her GTPAL status?
   A. 4-2-1-1-3
   B. 4-1-2-1-3
   C. 4-1-1-1-3
   D. 3-1-1-1-3

6. A young woman comes to the emergency unit. She indicates that the first day of her last normal menstrual period was December 2. Using Naegele's rule, her estimated date of delivery (EDD) is September
   A. 2
   B. 5
   C. 9
   D. 12

7. The nurse is preparing a teaching plan in anticipation of meeting with a client who is at 34 weeks' gestation, GTPAL 3-2-0-0-2, and is concerned about the development of varicose veins in both legs. Which of the following should the nurse include in the teaching plan?
   A. Shoes should have flat or minimal heels
   B. Massage both legs daily
   C. Plan exercise focusing on the lower extremities
   D. Reassure the client that they will disappear after birth

8. A client, G2TPAL 2-1-0-0-1, who is 33 weeks pregnant, comes to the nurse–midwifery office for a routine visit. She shares with the nurse that she has been experiencing difficulty getting to sleep, backaches, swelling of her ankles, and shortness of breath. Which of these statements would it be best for the nurse to make?
   A. "Tell me more about each of these."
   B. "These are normal changes of pregnancy."
   C. "They will go away in another few weeks."
   D. "These are normal, you don't need to worry about them."

9. During a prenatal assessment, a woman indicates that she has several cats and dogs at home. Which of the following information should the nurse share with the woman?
   A. No changes are necessary to the woman's routines.
   B. The client should avoid emptying the cats' litter box.
   C. Someone else should feed the animals.
   D. The client should avoid cleaning up the dog's waste.

10. A woman, G4TPAL 4-2-1-0-3, who is at 38 weeks' gestation, has had a NST and ultrasound. Results show a pocket of amniotic fluid measuring 2 cm in vertical diameter and that the fetus is stretching and flexing its arms and legs and has moved discretely 3 times in 30 minutes. The FHR is 132 bpm, with three increases to 160 bpm accompanying movements. The ultrasound showed breathing movements lasting 45 seconds. Based on these findings, the nurse should conclude that the fetus is
    A. Healthy
    B. Sleeping
    C. In need of immediate birth
    D. In need of repeat testing in 4 to 6 hours

REFERENCES

Allender, J. A., & Spradley, B. W. (2005). *Community health nursing concepts and practices* (6th ed.). Philadelphia, PA: Lippincott Williams & Wilkins.

Al-Sahab, B., Heifets, M., Tamim, H., Bohr, Y., & Connolly, J. (2012). Prevalence and characteristics of teen motherhood in Canada. *Maternal and Child Health Journal, 16*, 228–234.

Amasha, H. A., & Jaradeh, M. S. (2012). Effect of active and passive smoking during pregnancy on its outcomes. *Health Science Journal, 6*(2), 335–352.

Anderson, C. (2002). Battered and pregnant: A nursing challenge. *AWHONN Lifelines, 6*, 95–99.

Anderson, M. E., Johnson, D. C., & Batal, H. A. (2005). Sudden infant death syndrome and prenatal maternal smoking: Rising attributed risk in the Back to Sleep era. *BMC Medicine, 3*(1), 4.

BabyCenter Canada. (2012). *Natural remedies for pregnancy ailments*. Retrieved from http://www.babycenter.ca/c1003018/natural-remedies-for-pregnancy-ailments

Bahrami, M. H., Rayegani, S. M., Fereidouni, M., & Baghbani, M. (2005). Prevalence and severity of carpal tunnel syndrome (CTS) during pregnancy. *Electromyography and Clinical Neurophysiology, 45*(2), 123–125.

Barron, M. L. (2014). Antenatal care. In K. R. Simpson & P. A. Creehan (Eds.), *AWHONN's perinatal nursing* (4th ed., pp. 89–121). Philadelphia, PA: Lippincott Williams & Wilkins.

Berkley, E., Chauhan, S. P., & Abuhamad, A. (2012). Doppler assessment of the fetus with intrauterine growth restriction. *American Journal of Obstetrics and Gynecology, 206*(4), 300–308.

Bernstein, I. M., Mongeon, J. A., Badger, G. J., Solomon, L., Heil, S. H., & Higgins, S. T. (2005). Maternal smoking and its association with birth weight. *Obstetrics and Gynecology, 106*(5 Pt. 1), 986–991.

Bhandari, S., Bullock, L. F. C., Anderson, K. M., Danis, F. S., & Sharps, P. W. (2011). Pregnancy and intimate partner violence: How do rural, low-income women cope? *Health Care for Women International, 32,* 833–854.

Blackburn, S. T. (2014). Physiologic changes of pregnancy. In K. R. Simpson & P. A. Creehan (Eds.), *AWHONN's perinatal nursing* (4th ed., pp. 71–88). Philadelphia, PA: Lippincott Williams & Wilkins.

Bly, S., & Van den Hof, M. C. (2005). SOGC clinical practice guidelines: Obstetric ultrasound biological effects and safety. *Journal of Obstetrics and Gynaecology Canada, 160,* 572–575. Retrieved from http://www.sogc.org/jogc/pdf/abstracts/200506-senikas_e.pdf

Brathwaite, A. C., & Williams, C. C. (2004). Childbirth experiences of professional Chinese Canadian women. *Journal of Obstetric, Gynecologic, & Neonatal Nursing, 33*(6), 748–755.

Breheny, M., & Stephens, C. (2010). Youth or disadvantage? The construction of teenage mothers in medical journals. *Culture, Health and Sexuality, 12*(3), 307–322.

Brownridge, D. A., Taillieu, T. L., Tyler, K. A., Tiwari, A., Chan, K. L., & Santos, S. C. (2011). Pregnancy and intimate partner violence: Risk factors, severity, and health effects. *Violence Against Women, 17*(7), 858–881, doi:10.1177/1077801211412547

Buchanan, K., Fletcher, H. M., & Reid, M. (2010). Prevention of striae gravidarum with cocoa butter cream. *International Journal of Gynecology & Obstetrics, 108*(1), 65–68.

Callister, L. C. (2005). What has the literature taught us about culturally competent care of women and children? *MCN. The American Journal of Maternal Child Nursing, 30*(6), 380–388.

Callister, L. C. (2014). Integrating cultural beliefs and practices when caring for childbearing women and families. In K. R. Simpson & P. A. Creehan (Eds.), *AWHONN's perinatal nursing* (4th ed., pp. 41–70). Philadelphia, PA: Lippincott Williams & Wilkins.

Centers for Disease Control and Prevention [CDC]. (2012). *STDs and pregnancy – CDC fact sheet.* Retrieved from http://www.cdc.gov/std/pregnancy/STDFact-Pregnancy.htm

Chapman, R., Wardrop, J., Zappia, T., Watkins, R., & Shields, L. (2012). The experiences of Australian lesbian couples becoming parents: Deciding, searching, and birthing. *Journal of Clinical Nursing, 21,* 1878–1885.

Cherniak, D. Grant, L., Mason, R., Moore, B., & Pellizzari, R. (2005). Intimate partner violence consensus statement. *Journal of Obstetrics and Gynaecology Canada, 157,* 365–387. Retrieved from http://www.sogc.org/jogc/pdf/abstracts/200504-ipv.pdf

Chitayat, D., Langlois, S., & Wilson, R. D. (2011). SOGC clinical practice guideline: Prenatal screening for fetal aneuploidy in singleton pregnancies. *Journal of Obstetrics and Gynecology Canada, (261),* 736–750. Retrieved from http://sogc.org/wp-content/uploads/2013/01/gui261CPG1107E.pdf

Chow, J., Ateah, C. A., Scott, S. D., Ricci, S. S., & Kyle, T. (2013). *Canadian maternity and pediatric nursing.* Philadelphia, PA: Lippincott Williams & Wilkins.

Chui, T., & Maheux, H. (2011). *Visible minority women. Women in Canada.* Ottawa, ON: Statistics Canada. Retrieved from http://www.statcan.gc.ca/pub/89-503-x/2010001/article/11527-eng.pdf

Clear, E. R., Williams, C. M., & Crosby, R. (2012). Female perceptions of male versus female intendedness at the time of teenage pregnancy. *Maternal Child Health Journal, 16,* 1862–1869.

Clemmens, D. (2003). Adolescent motherhood: A meta-synthesis of qualitative studies. *MCN. The American Journal of Maternal Child Nursing, 28*(2), 93–99.

Cockney, C. D. (2003). On the edge: Periodontal disease linked to preeclampsia risk. *AWHONN Lifelines, 7,* 211.

Contreras, A., Herrera, J. A., Soto, J. E., Arce, R. M., Jaramillo, A., & Botero, J. E. (2006). Periodontitis is associated with preeclampsia in pregnant women. *Journal of Periodontology, 77*(2), 182–188.

Cunningham, F. G., Leveno, K. J., Bloom, S. L., Hauth, J. C., Rouse, D. J., & Sprong, C. Y. (2010). *Williams obstetrics* (23rd ed.). New York: McGraw-Hill.

Daley, J. M. (2014). Diabetes in pregnancy. In K. R. Simpson & P. A. Creehan (Eds.), *AWHONN's perinatal nursing* (4th ed., pp. 203–223). Philadelphia, PA: Lippincott Williams & Wilkins.

Dallas, C. (2004). Family matters: How mothers of adolescent parents experience adolescent pregnancy and parenting. *Public Health Nursing, 21*(4), 347–353.

Daoud, N., Urquia, M., O'Campo, P., Heaman, M., Janssen, P., Smylie, J. et al. (2012). Prevalence of abuse and violence before, during, and after pregnancy in a national sample of Canadian women. *American Journal of Public Health, 102*(10), 1893–1901.

Dapaah, S., & Dapaah, V. E. (2009). Sexually transmissible and reproductive tract infections in pregnancy. In E. M. Fraser & M. A. Cooper (Eds.), *Myles textbook for midwives* (15th ed., pp. 415–431). Philadelphia, PA: Elsevier Science.

Davies, G. L., Maxwell, C., & McLeod, L. (2010). SOGC clinical practice guideline: Obesity in pregnancy. *Journal of Obstetrics and Gynaecology Canada, 239,* 165–173. Retrieved from http://sogc.org/wp-content/uploads/2013/01/gui239ECPG1002.pdf

Davies, G. A. L., Wolfe, L. A., Mottola, M. F., & MacKinnon, C. (2003). Joint SOGC/CSEP clinical practice guideline: Exercise in pregnancy and the postpartum period. *Journal of Obstetrics and Gynaecology Canada, 25*(6), 516–522. Retrieved from http://sogc.org/guidelines/exercise-in-pregnancy-and-the-postpartum-period/

Espinosa, L., & Osborne, K. (2002). Domestic violence during pregnancy: Implications for practice. *Journal of Midwifery & Women's Health, 47,* 305–317.

Floyd, R. L., O'Connor, M. J., Sokol, R. J., Bertrand, J., & Cordero, J. F. (2005). Recognition and prevention of fetal alcohol syndrome. *Obstetrics & Gynecology, 106*(5 Pt 1), 1059–1064.

Fraser, D. F. (2014). Newborn adaptation to extrauterine life. In K. R. Simpson & P. A. Creehan (Eds.), *AWHONN's perinatal nursing* (4th ed., pp. 581–596). Philadelphia, PA: Lippincott Williams & Wilkins.

George, A., Shamim, S., Johnson, M., Ajwani, S., Bhole, S., Blinkhorn, A. et al. (2011). Periodontal treatment during pregnancy and birth outcomes: A meta-analysis of randomized trials. *International Journal of Evidenced-Based Healthcare, 9,* 122–147.

Gossler, S. M. (2010). Use of complementary and alternative therapies during pregnancy, postpartum, and lactation. *Journal of Psychosocial Nursing & Mental Health Services, 48*(11), 30–36.

Government of Canada. (2014). Travelling while pregnant. Retrieved from http://travel.gc.ca/travelling/health-safety/travelling-pregnant

Grewal, S. K., Bhagat, R., & Balneaves, L. G. (2008). Perinatal beliefs and practices of immigrant Punjabi women living in Canada. *Journal of Obstetric, Gynecologic, and Neonatal Nursing, 37,* 290–300.

Hall, H. G., McKenna, L. G., Griffiths, D. L. (2010). Complementary and alternative medicine: Where's the evidence. *British Journal of Midwifery, 18*(7), 436–440.

Hall, J. E. (2011). *Guyton and Hall textbook of medical physiology* (12th ed.). Philadelphia, PA: W.B. Saunders.

Hanna, B. (2001). Negotiating motherhood: The struggles of teenage mothers. *Journal of Advanced Nursing, 34,* 456–464.

Health Canada. (2009). *Prenatal nutrition guidelines for health professionals – iron contributes to a healthy pregnancy.* Retrieved from http://www.hc-sc.gc.ca/fn-an/pubs/nutrition/iron-fer-eng.php

Health Canada. (2012). *Vitamin D and calcium: Updated dietary reference intakes.* Retrieved from http://www.hc-sc.gc.ca/fn-an/nutrition/vitamin/vita-d-eng.php

Health Canada. (2013). *Prenatal nutrition guidelines for health professionals – folate contributes to a healthy pregnancy.* Retrieved from http://www.hc-sc.gc.ca/fn-an/pubs/nutrition/folate-eng.php

Hegewald, M., & Crapo, R. (2011). Respiratory physiology in pregnancy. *Clinics in Chest Medicine, 32*(1), 1–13.

Hellmuth, J. C., Gordon, K. C., Stuart, G. L., & Moore, T. M. (2012). Risk factors for intimate partner violence during pregnancy and postpartum. *Archives of Women's Mental Health, 16,* 19–27.

Human Resources and Skills Development Canada. (2013). *Family life – age of mother at childbirth.* Retrieved from www4.hrsdc.gc.ca/.3ndic.1t.4r@-eng.jsp?iid=75

Irner, T. B., Teasdale, T. W., Nielsen, T., Vedal, S., & Olofsson, M. (2012). Substance use during pregnancy and postnatal outcomes. *Journal of Addictive Diseases, 31*, 19–28.

James, D. C. (2014). Postpartum care. In K. R. Simpson & P. A. Creehan (Eds.), *AWHONN's perinatal nursing* (4th ed., pp. 530–558). Philadelphia, PA: Lippincott Williams & Wilkins.

Johnson, J., & Tough, S. (2012). SOGC committee opinion: Delayed child-bearing. *Journal of Obstetrics and Gynaecology Canada, 34*(1), 80–93. Retrieved from http://sogc.org/wp-content/uploads/2013/01/gui271CO1201E.pdf

Katz, V. L. (2008). Prenatal care. In R. S. Gibbs, B. Y. Karlan, A. F. Haney, & I. E. Nygaard (Eds.), *Danforth's obstetrics and gynecology* (10th ed., pp. 1–21). Philadelphia, PA: Lippincott Williams & Wilkins.

Kayem, G., Grange, G., Breart, G., & Goffinet, F. (2009). Comparison of fundal height measurement and sonographically measured fetal abdominal circumference in the prediction of high and low birth weight at term. *Ultrasound in Obstetrics & Gynecology, 34*(5), 566–571.

Kearney, M. S., & Levine, P. B. (2012). Why is the teen birth rate in the United States so high and why does it matter? *Journal of Economic Perspectives, 26*, 141–166.

Keegan, J., Parva, M., Finnegan, M., Gerson, A., & Belden, M. (2010). Addiction in pregnancy. *Journal of Addictive Diseases, 29*, 175–191.

Kozinsky, Z., Orvos, H., Zoboki, T., Katona, M., Wayda, K., Pal, A. et al. (2002). Risk factors for cesarean section of primiparous women aged over 35 years. *Acta Obstetricia et Gynecologica Scandinavica, 81*, 313–316.

Kramer, A., Nosbusch, J. M., & Rice, J. (2012). Safe mom, safe baby: A collaborative model of care for pregnant women experiencing intimate partner violence. *The Journal of Perinatal and Neonatal Nursing, 26*(4), 307–316.

Lannero, E., Wickman, M., Pershagen, G., & Nordvall, L. (2006). Maternal smoking during pregnancy increases the risk of recurrent wheezing during the first years of life (BAMSE). *Respiratory Research, 5*(7), 3.

Lauderdale, J. (2011). Transcultural perspectives in childbearing. In M. M. Andrews & J. S. Boyle (Eds.), *Transcultural concepts in nursing care* (6th ed., pp. 91–122). Philadelphia, PA: Lippincott Williams & Wilkins.

Lee, E., Taylor, J., & Raitt, F. (2011). "It's not me, it's them": How lesbian women make sense of negative experiences of maternity care: A hermeneutic study. *Journal of Advanced Nursing, 67*(5), 982–990.

Liston, R., Sawchuck, D., & Young, D. (2007). SOGC clinical practice guideline: Fetal health surveillance: Antepartum and intrapartum consensus guideline. *Journal of Obstetrics and Gynaecology Canada, 29*(9), S3–S56.

Liu, K., & Case, A. (2011). SOGC clinical practice guideline: Advanced reproductive age and fertility. *Journal of Obstetrics and Gynaecology Canada, 269*, 1165–1175. Retrieved from http://sogc.org/wp-content/uploads/2013/01/gui269CPG1111E_000.pdf

Lloyd, C. (2009). Medical disorders associated with pregnancy. In D. M. Fraser & M. S. Cooper (Eds.), *Myles textbook for midwives* (15th ed., pp. 361–396). Philadelphia, PA: Elsevier Science.

Loutfy, M., Margolese, S., Money, D., Gysler, M., Hamilton, S., & Yudin, M. (2012). SOGC clinical practice guideline: Canadian HIV pregnancy planning guidelines. *Journal of Obstetrics and Gynaecology Canada, 278*, 575–590. Retrieved from http://sogc.org/wp-content/uploads/2012/09/gui278CPG1206E1.pdf

Luong, M. (2009). Life after teenage motherhood. *Perspectives on Labour and Income, 9*(5). Retrieved from http://www.statcan.gc.ca/pub/75-001-x/2008105/article/10577-eng.htm

Lutz, K. F. (2005). Abused pregnant women's interactions with health care providers during the childbearing year. *Journal of Obstetric, Gynecologic, and Neonatal Nursing, 34*(2), 151–162.

Magee, B. D., Hattis, D., & Kivel, N. M. (2004). Role of smoking in low birth weight. *Journal of Reproductive Medicine, 49*(1), 23–27.

Magee, L. A., Helewa, M., Moutquin, J. M., & von Dadelszen, P. (2008). SOGC clinical practice guideline: Diagnosis, evaluation, and management of the hypertensive disorders of pregnancy. *Journal of Obstetrics and Gynaecology Canada, 30*(3), S1–S48.

Retrieved from http://sogc.org/wp-content/uploads/2013/01/gui206CPG0803hypertensioncorrection.pdf

Manning, F. A. (2002). Fetal biophysical profile: A critical appraisal. *Clinical Obstetrics and Gynecology, 43*(4), 975–985.

Mayo Clinic. (2011). *Morning sickness*. Retrieved from http://www.mayoclinic.com/health/morning sickness/DS01150/DSECTION=alternative-medicine

McKay, A. (2012). Trends in Canadian national and provincial/territorial teen pregnancy rates: 2001–2010. *The Canadian Journal of Human Sexuality, 21*(3–4), 161–175.

McKay, A., & Barrett, M. (2010). Trends in teen pregnancy rates from 1996 to 2006: A comparison of Canada, Sweden, U.S.A., and England/Wales. *Canadian Journal of Human Sexuality, 19*(1/2), 43–52.

Mitchell, A. A., Gilboa, S. M., Werler, M. M., Kelley, K. E., Louik, C., & Hernandez-Diaz, S. (2011). Medication use during pregnancy, with particular focus on prescription drugs: 1976–2008. *American Journal of Obstetrics and Gynecology, 205*(1), 51.e1–51.e8.

Moise, K. J. (2013). Toward consistent terminology: Assessment and reporting of amniotic fluid volume. *Seminars in Perinatology, 37*(5), 370–374.

Money, D. M., & Dobson, S. (2004). SOGC clinical practice guideline: The prevention of early-onset neonatal Group B streptococcal disease. *Journal of Obstetrics and Gynaecology Canada, 26*(9), 826–832. Retrieved from http://sogc.org/wp-content/uploads/2013/01/149E-CPG-September2004.pdf

Motozawa, Y., Hitosugi, M., Abe, T., & Tokudome, S. (2010). Effects of seat belts worn by pregnant drivers during low-impact collisions. *American Journal of Obstetrics and Gynecology, 203*(1), 62.e1–62.e8.

Nabhan, A. F., & Abdelmoula, Y. A. (2008). Amniotic fluid index versus single deepest vertical pocket as a screening test for preventing adverse pregnancy outcome. *Cochrane Database of Systematic Reviews, (3)*, Art. No. CD006593. doi:10.1002/14651858.CD006593.pub2

Ozalp, S., Tanir, H. M., Sener, T., Yazan, S., & Keskin, A. E. (2003). Health risks for early (or = 35) childbearing. *Archives of Gynecology and Obstetrics, 268*(3), 172–174.

Perry, S. E., Hockenberry, M. J., Lowdermilk, D. L., Wilson, D., Sams, C., & Keenan-Lindsay, L. (2013). *Maternal child nursing care in Canada*. Toronto, ON: Elsevier Canada.

Peterson, W. E., Davies, B., Rashotte, J. Salvador, A., & Trepanier, M. J. (2012). Hospital-based perinatal nurses identify the need to improve nursing care of adolescent mothers. *Journal of Obstetric, Gynecologic, and Neonatal Nursing, 41*, 358–368.

Peterson, W. E., Sword, W., Charles, C., & DiCenso, A. (2007). Adolescents' perceptions of inpatient postpartum nursing care. *Qualitative Health Research, 17*(2), 201–212.

Phipps, M. G., & Nunes, A. P. (2012). Assessing pregnancy intention and associated risks in pregnant adolescents. *Maternal and Child Health Journal, 16*, 1820–1827.

Pillitteri, A. (2007). *Maternal & child health nursing* (5th ed.). Philadelphia, PA: Lippincott Williams & Wilkins.

Poole, J. H. (2014). Hypertensive disorders of pregnancy. In K. R. Simpson & P. A. Creehan (Eds.), *AWHONN's perinatal nursing* (4th ed., pp. 89–121). Philadelphia, PA: Lippincott Williams & Wilkins.

Public Health Agency of Canada. (2013a). *Canadian immunization guide: Part 3*. Retrieved from www.phac-aspc.gc.ca/publicat/cig-gci/p03-04-eng.php

Public Health Agency of Canada. (2013b). At a glance – HIV and AIDS in Canada: Surveillance report to December 31, 2012. Retrieved from http://www.phac-aspc.gc.ca/aids-sida/publication/survreport/2012/dec/index-eng.php

Reedy, N. J. (2014). Preterm labor and birth. In K. R. Simpson & P. A. Creehan (Eds.), *AWHONN's perinatal nursing* (4th ed., pp. 166–202). Philadelphia, PA: Lippincott Williams & Wilkins.

Renker, P. R., & Tonkin, P. (2006). Women's views of prenatal violence screening: Acceptability and confidentiality issues. *Obstetrics & Gynecology, 107*(2 Pt 1), 348–354.

Ross, L. E. (2005). Perinatal mental health in lesbian mothers: A review of potential risk and protective factors. *Women's Health, 41*(3), 113–128.

Schrimmer, D. B., & Moore, T. R. (2002). Sonographic evaluation of amniotic fluid volume. *Clinical Obstetrics and Gynecology, 45*, 1026–1038.

Scribano, P., Stevens, J., & Kaizar, E. (2013). The effects of intimate partner violence before, during, and after pregnancy in nurse visited first time mothers. *Maternal & Child Health Journal, 17*(20), 307–318.

Seamark, C. J., & Lings, P. (2004). Positive experiences of teenage motherhood: A qualitative study. *British Journal of General Practice, 54*(508), 813–818.

Shah, P. S., & Shah, J. (2010). Maternal exposure to domestic violence and pregnancy and birth outcomes: A systematic review and meta-analysis *Journal of Women's Health, 19*(11), 2017–2029.

Silverthorn, D. U. (2013). *Human physiology: An integrated approach* (6th ed.). Boston, MA: Pearson.

SmithBattle, L. (2000a). Developing a caregiving tradition in opposition to one's past: Lessons from a longitudinal study of teenage mothers. *Public Health Nursing, 17*, 85–93.

SmithBattle, L. (2000b). The vulnerabilities of teenage mothers: Challenging prevailing assumptions. *Advances in Nursing Science, 23*, 29–40.

SmithBattle, L. (2007). Learning the baby: An interpretive study of teen mothers. *Journal of Pediatric Nursing, 22*(4), 261–271.

Smylie, J. (2001). SOGC policy statement: A guide for health professionals working with Aboriginal peoples: Cross cultural understanding. *Journal SOGC, 23*(2), 157–167.

Society of Obstetricians and Gynaecologists of Canada. (2012a). *Sexual health: Sex during pregnancy*. Retrieved from http://www.sexualityandu.ca/sexual-health/sex-during-pregnancy

Society of Obstetricians and Gynaecologists of Canada. (2012b). *SexualityandU.ca Frequently asked questions*. Retrieved from http://www.sexualityandu.ca/faqs/single/is-it-safe-to-have-sex-when-you-are-pregnant

Sprong, C. Y. (2008). Assessment of fetal well-being. In R. S. Gibbs, B. Y. Karlan, A. F. Haney, & I. E. Nygaard (Eds.), *Danforth's obstetrics and gynecology* (10th ed., pp. 152–164). Philadelphia, PA: Lippincott Williams & Wilkins.

Stade, B., Ali, A., Bennett, D., Campbell, D., Johnston, M., Lens, C. et al. (2009). The burden of prenatal exposure to alcohol: Revised measurement of cost. *Canadian Journal of Clinical Pharmacology, 16*(1), e91–e102.

Statistics Canada. (2011a). *Births 2008*. Retrieved from http://www.statcan.gc.ca/daily-quotidien/110427/dq110427a-eng.htm

Statistics Canada. (2011b). *Ethnic diversity and immigration. Canada Year Book*. Retrieved from http://www.statcan.gc.ca/pub/11-402-x/2011000/chap/imm/imm-eng.htm

Statistics Canada. (2011c). *Family violence in Canada: A statistical profile*. Ottawa, ON: Author. Retrieved from http://www.statcan.gc.ca/pub/85-224-x/85-224-x2010000-eng.pdf

Statistics Canada. (2013a). Live births, by age of mother, Canada, provinces and territories. Retrieved from http://www5.statcan.gc.ca/cansim/pick-choisir?lang=eng&p2=33&id=1024503

Statistics Canada. (2013b). *Mean age of mother at time of delivery (live births), Canada, provinces and territories*. Retrieved from http://www5.statcan.gc.ca/cansim/a26;jsessionid=9CFAF88A93A22ED0D31FDA38F62C9680?lang=eng&retrLang=eng&id=1024504&pattern=102-4501..102-4516&tabMode=dataTable&srchLan=-1&p1=-1&p2=31

Stenson, K., Sidenvall, B., & Heimer, G. (2005). Midwives' experiences of routine antenatal questioning relating to men's violence against women. *Midwifery, 21*(4), 311–321.

Stevens-Simon, C., Beach, R. K., & McGregor, J. A. (2002). Does incomplete growth and development predispose teenagers to preterm delivery? A template for research. *Journal of Perinatology, 22*, 315–323.

Stiles, A. S. (2005). Parenting needs, goals, and strategies of adolescent mothers. *MCN. The American Journal of Maternal Child Nursing, 30*(5), 327–333.

Transport Canada. (2007). *Seat belt sense*. Ottawa, ON: Author. Retrieved from http://www.tc.gc.ca/media/documents/roadsafety/TP14646e.pdf

US Department of Health and Human Services, Office on Women's Health. (2009). *Pregnancy Tests*. Retrieved from http://womenshealth.gov/publications/our-publications/fact-sheet/pregnancy-tests.pdf

Viccars, A. (2009). Antenatal care. In D. M. Fraser & M. S. Cooper (Eds.), *Myles textbook for midwives* (15th ed., pp. 263–287). Philadelphia, PA: Elsevier Science.

Werler, M. M., Mitchell, A. A., Hernandez-Diaz, S., & Honein, M. A. (2005). Use of over-the-counter medications during pregnancy. *American Journal of Obstetrics and Gynecology, 193*(3 Pt 1), 771–777.

Wilson, D., de la Ronde, S., Brascoupe, S., Apale, A. N., Barney, L., Guthrie, B. et al. (2013). SOGC clinical practice guideline: Health professionals working with First Nations, Inuit, and Métis consensus guideline. *Journal of Obstetrics and Gynaecology Canada, 293*, S1–S52. Retrieved from http://sogc.org/wp content/uploads/2013/06/gui293CPG1306ErevC.pdf

Wong, S., Ordean, A., & Kahan, M. (2011). SOGC clinical practice guideline: Substance use in pregnancy. *Journal of Obstetrics and Gynaecology Canada, 256*, 367–384.

Yankowitz, J. (2008). Drugs in pregnancy. In R. S. Gibbs, B. Y. Karlan, A. F. Haney, & I. E. Nygaard (Eds.), *Danforth's obstetrics and gynecology* (10th ed., pp. 122–136). Philadelphia, PA: Lippincott Williams & Wilkins.

Zdravkovic, T., Genbacev, O., McMaster, M. T., & Fisher, S. J. (2005). The adverse effects of maternal smoking on the human placenta: A review. *Placenta, 26*(Suppl. A), S81–S86.

WEB RESOURCES

British Columbia Centre of Excellence for Women's Health
http://bccewh.bc.ca/
Canadian Harm Reduction Network
http://www.canadianharmreduction.com/taxonomy/term/673
March of Dimes
http://www.marchofdimes.com/
Public Health Agency of Canada
http://www.phac-aspc.gc.ca/hp-gs/index-eng.php
South Riverdale Community Health Centre Women's Harm Reduction
http://www.srchc.ca/program/womens-harm-reduction
The Sensible Guide to a Healthy Pregnancy
http://www.phac-aspc.gc.ca/hp-gs/guide-eng.php

CHAPTER 13

High-Risk Pregnancy

Nancy Watts

Keyla, a 23-year-old Aboriginal Canadian woman, comes to the clinic at 27 weeks' gestation with her first pregnancy. During this routine prenatal visit, she will undergo screening for diabetes. Keyla states, "My mother found out 2 years ago that she has diabetes and my sister was diagnosed with diabetes during her first pregnancy. Am I now at risk?"

Lindsey, a 33-year-old client at 28 weeks' gestation with her second pregnancy, is being evaluated in the health care provider's office. During her first pregnancy, Lindsey developed gestational hypertension managed with bed rest at home for several weeks. Her obstetrical history (GTPAL) is documented as 20101. "My first baby was born at 34 weeks because of my blood pressure problems," she reports. Her child is 2 years old.

You will learn more about Keyla's and Lindsey's stories later. Nurses working with these and similar clients need to understand this chapter's content to manage care and address issues appropriately. Before beginning, consider the following points:

- Does anything about either scenario above present issues of immediate concern? Explain.
- Would you consider each client's pregnancy to be high risk? Why or why not?
- How are Keyla and Lindsey similar? How are they different?
- What details does the nurse need to investigate with Keyla? What about Lindsey?
- What areas of concern and teaching would the nurse need to address with each client?

LEARNING OBJECTIVES

On completion of this chapter, the reader should be able to:

- Explain what is meant by the term *high-risk pregnancy*.
- Identify the role of risk assessment in pregnancy, as well as areas of focus in performing such evaluation.
- Outline a comprehensive approach to the care of the pregnant woman with asthma.
- Describe factors that may contribute to pregnancy outcomes in pregnant women with cardiovascular disease and appropriate management strategies for various types of clients.
- Discuss common signs and symptoms associated with anemia during pregnancy and their management.
- Identify the major problem related to concurrent pregnancy and systemic lupus erythematosus.
- Describe appropriate screening and treatment measures for various infections that pose dangerous risks to mother, fetus, or both during pregnancy.
- Compare several renal and urinary problems that can develop in the expectant woman and associated levels of care.
- Outline key interventions for the pregnant woman with diabetes.
- Discuss why psychosocial disorders may be more prevalent in pregnant women and the appropriateness of management strategies within the context of gestational and fetal growth.
- Understand reasons for universal screening of all pregnant women for intimate-partner violence.
- Identify potential indicators that suggest intimate-partner violence in a pregnant client.
- Explain why screening for smoking, alcohol use, and other substance use in pregnancy is essential.
- Define the criteria for a diagnosis of hyperemesis gravidarum.
- List the various classifications of hypertension in pregnancy.
- Outline general treatment strategies and interventions for women with hypertension in pregnancy.
- Describe what is meant by acute HELLP syndrome and measures for evaluating successful treatment.
- Explain the usual management of pPROM.
- Identify complications associated with neurologic disease, specifically epilepsy.
- Identify why pregnant women are at increased risk for disseminated intravascular coagulation.
- Compare and contrast various placental problems in pregnancy that can pose risks to maternal and fetal health.
- Name complications commonly associated with pregnancy in adolescence.
- List ideal outcomes in cases of multiple gestation.
- Explain the difference between miscarriage and stillbirth.
- Compare and contrast ectopic pregnancy with gestational trophoblastic disease.

KEY TERMS

cerclage	ectopic pregnancy
cervical insufficiency	gestational diabetes mellitus (GDM)
disseminated intravascular coagulopathy (DIC)	gestational trophoblastic disease
	high-risk pregnancy
eclampsia	hyperemesis gravidarum

hypertension
miscarriage
multiple pregnancy
obesity
peripartum cardiomyopathy

placenta previa
placental abruption
preeclampsia
stillbirth

A high-risk pregnancy may be defined as one "in which there is a maternal or fetal factor that may adversely affect the outcome" (Queenan et al., 2007). Approximately 25% of pregnancies are considered high risk based on this definition (Youngkin et al., 2013). Health problems that predispose the mother, fetus, or both to complications frequently exist before conception, although sometimes they develop or show manifestations for the first time during pregnancy. Examples of common health problems in pregnancy include obesity, cardiac disease, autoimmune disorders, and diabetes. Obstetric complications involve those conditions directly related to gestation itself (Gilbert, 2011). Examples include placental abnormalities and preterm premature rupture of membranes (pPROM). In addition, some pregnancies are considered high risk because of specific circumstances related to the mother's age, lifestyle, environment, or situation. Examples include adolescent pregnancy and/or pregnancy complicated by violence, poverty, mental illness, problematic substance use, lack of access to prenatal care, and trauma.

This chapter reviews medical, obstetric, and other factors that may compromise pregnancy and general measures taken to monitor and manage gestational complications. Discussions of conditions that pose special or increased risks in labour and birth and their management are found in Chapter 16.

PREGNANCY RISK ASSESSMENT

Many pregnant clients with chronic pre-existing health conditions can anticipate close monitoring of their gestation and may not associate a need for hospitalization or home care as a crisis or emergency. Differences in risk perception between pregnant women at high risk and health professionals have implications of care and pregnancy outcomes (Lee et al., 2012). A client who develops unexpected complications, however, may experience great stress, anger, and anxiety and feel unprepared to deal with the threat to herself and to her fetus. She may need more time to adjust to the situation and to express feelings to supportive others (Gilbert, 2011).

Regardless of when a pregnancy risk develops, high-risk pregnancy is stressful for any family anticipating a baby's birth. The major reason for risk assessment is to guide rational planning for appropriate care, including the need for ongoing consultation and site of birth. Such planning is especially important in geographic areas lacking intensive or special care facilities. In such cases, special modifications may be necessary, such as increased prenatal visits to a family physician, nurse practitioner or midwife, more intensive involvement from an obstetrician, ongoing home care, monitoring in an acute care setting, or admission to a tertiary-level facility in advance of labour and birth. For First Nations, Metis, or Inuit women it may mean leaving their families and traveling distances to be monitored in facilities where there is appropriate care (Society of Obstetricians and Gynecologists of Canada [SOGC], 2013a).

Variables such as anxiety, stress, social support, and self-esteem influence a client's risk status. Women may view their risk status differently than the health care provider does. The client's personal perceptions and understandings are important to consider when care providers assess pregnancy and plan care (Gupton et al., 2001). Assessment Tool 13.1 gives guidelines for areas of the health history and physical examination to focus on when evaluating a pregnancy's risk.

Psychosocial Risk Factors

For some clients, pregnancy is unplanned, unwanted, or both. At times, women also face other challenges during pregnancy, such as job changes, unemployment, relocation, unstable relationships, death of a significant person, or onset or worsening of a medical condition. Stress related to these developments may intensify or be the risk factor leading to psychological problems. Hormonal changes associated with reproduction also increase the possibility of mental health diagnoses.

Psychosocial stressors associated with high-risk pregnancy include the following:

- Lack of control
- Concern or anxiety over fetal well-being
- Boredom
- Feelings of helplessness and powerlessness
- Sense of isolation and confinement
- Missing out on normal activities
- Separation from home and family
- Physical discomforts
- Medication side effects

● ASSESSMENT TOOL 13.1   **Common Risk Factors in Pregnancy**

BIOPHYSICAL FACTORS	PSYCHOSOCIAL FACTORS
● Genetic disease ● Cardiovascular disease ● Hypertension ● Diabetes ● Autoimmune disorder ● Adolescent pregnancy ● Late-life pregnancy ● Uterine, cervical, or placental abnormalities ● Infections (including sexually transmitted infections) ● Asthma ● Poor nutrition ● Underweight or overweight ● Multiple gestation	● Mood disorders ● Anxiety disorders ● Eating disorders ● Stress ● Substance use ● Intimate-partner violence **SOCIAL FACTORS** ● Poverty ● Lack of social support ● Decreased or absent access to health care ● Family problems (eg, divorce, illness, relocation) ● Geographical location

- Changing self-image
- Sick role
- Concerns about other children
- Role reversal
- Difficulties in relationship with partner
- Lack of privacy (if hospitalized)
- Incompatible roommates (if hospitalized)

Antenatal psychosocial health assessment is a critical component of prenatal care. Completion of the Antenatal Psychosocial Health Assessment (ALPHA) document (Assessment Tool 13.2) at 20 weeks' gestation can assist care providers to screen for the above problems, in addition to poor parenting skills, substance use, and mood disorders (Austin et al., 2009; SOGC, 2005).

Economic Risk Factors

Low-income women may struggle to gain access to health care. Lack of prenatal care is associated with adverse perinatal outcomes (Cannon et al., 2000). Many women with low-paying jobs are not educated for other positions, or must take whatever work they can

find because of family responsibilities. Over the past two decades, the number of women in the workforce has increased significantly, with 58% of all Canadian women 15 years old and older currently employed, 66.8% of whom are single female parents with children 5 years of age or younger (Statistics Canada, 2011). As a result, more Canadian women hold part-time positions, and women continue to be paid less than their male counterparts for the same job (Statistics Canada, 2011). In 2008, 43% of all children in a low-income family were living with a single female parent, whereas these families accounted for only 13% of all children aged 17 and under.

In 2008, 21% of families headed by lone-parent mothers had incomes that fell below the definition for low-income cut-off in Canada. Butterworth (2004) describes an association between single-parent status and increased risk for mental illness. Single mothers report sexual abuse in childhood, anxiety, and depression (Butterworth, 2004). In the midst of poverty and inadequate resources, these women must juggle work and responsibility for their family's well-being. The health status of those with high poverty rates is compromised,

● ASSESSMENT TOOL 13.2   **Antenatal Psychosocial Health Assessment (ALPHA)**

● How do you and your partner solve arguments? ● Do you ever feel frightened by what your partner says or does? ● Have you ever been hit, pushed, shoved, or slapped by your partner?	● Has your partner ever humiliated or psychologically abused you? ● Have you ever been forced to have sex against your will?

as this group consists largely of single women and their families (Keating-Lefler & Wilson, 2004). Single mothers also experience great stress from physical, emotional, and psychological challenges. They are at risk for significant losses in pregnancy, because they may be isolated from friends, male partners, family, themselves (their "old self"), and their dreams (Keating-Lefler & Wilson, 2004).

Statistics Canada (2011) reports that 16.4% of Canadian women are members of a visible minority. Of this group, 33% had a university degree, so on average were better educated than the majority of women; however, they were less likely to be employed and earned less at their jobs (Statistics Canada, 2011). In our multicultural world, particularly in Canada, cultural diversity challenges health care providers and organizations to consider cultural diversity as a priority in health care delivery (Campinha-Bacote, 2003). For perinatal nurses, a critical element of care is understanding the lifeworlds of women from different cultural backgrounds who will be represented in their patient populations, namely, their beliefs about health, pregnancy, labour, birth, and newborns.

Most clients who develop a high-risk pregnancy and can no longer work experience economic stress; such problems are compounded when a woman is single and must provide economically for herself and others. Nurses working in occupational health or in an ambulatory clinic setting are in a strategic position to assist such women to continue to support themselves and their dependents. Advocacy for childbearing women to have flexible work hours, to coordinate prenatal visits within working hours, to obtain information on various health and wellness topics associated with pregnancy, and to facilitate rest periods throughout the day can enable them to continue working. Working women may also be older, having chosen to wait for childbirth until their careers were advanced. Advanced maternal age, defined as age greater than 35 years, is a risk factor for Caesarean birth, preterm birth, stillbirth and chromosomal abnormalities (Bayrampour & Heaman, 2010). Assessment for occupational teratogens is also important. Substances to look for include lead, mercury, medications, and extremely high temperatures (Cannon et al., 2000).

Nurses working with single women need to help identify potential sources of support (including forming new groups of pregnant single women), encourage dreams and visions for the future, and assist with practical financial assistance. Strategies that also enhance personal capacity and resources may have the most potential for success (Fig. 13.1).

Nutrition-Related Risk Factors

Overall, poor nutrition can compromise maternal weight gain, resulting in a low–birth-weight infant. In

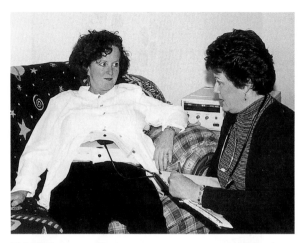

FIGURE 13.1 Single pregnant women, especially those with other risk factors in pregnancy, need additional systems of support and help with obtaining resources. (Photo by Melissa Olson, with permission of Health Home Coming, Inc., Bensalem, PA.)

Canada, the small-for-gestational-age rate is defined as the number of live births whose birth weight is below the standard 10th percentile of birth weight for gestational age; in 2006/7, this rate was 8.3% of all infants born (Canadian Institute for Health Information, 2009) (see Chapter 22). Deficiencies in iron, iodine, and calcium affect a woman's ability to maintain a healthy pregnancy. One significant nutritional risk to fetal development is deficiency of folic acid, specifically in the first trimester. At least 50% of neural tube defects can be prevented with folic acid supplementation that begins before conception and continues into the first trimester (Comley & Mousmanis, 2003) (see Chapters 3, 11, and 22).

Poor nutrition can result from inadequate financial resources to obtain food, poor appetite, lifestyle choices such as smoking or alcohol use, or ongoing nausea and vomiting associated with pregnancy (Luke, 2005b). Slowed fetal weight gain has been linked to preterm labour (Luke, 2005b). This risk is increased if the mother herself was born with low birth weight (twofold increase in giving birth to a low–birth-weight infant and doing so prematurely) (Luke, 2005b).

Counselling with a dietician and referral to appropriate community resources may help ensure maternal and fetal health. Pattern of weight gain is more important than total number of pounds in ensuring optimal birth outcomes (Fowles, 2002). Adequate intake of both water and milk is critical. Women taking prenatal vitamins within the first 3 gestational months are significantly less likely to have low–birth-weight babies as women who do not use such supplements (Fowles, 2002). Approximately 25% to 50% of women do not take prenatal vitamins consistently (Gennaro et al., 2011). The nurse should offer nutritional information

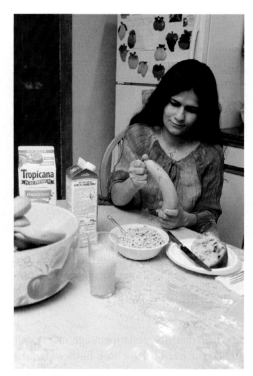

FIGURE 13.2 Ensuring adequate and appropriate nutritional choices in pregnancy is a significant area of nursing focus in all clients and one area requiring ongoing monitoring for risk.

throughout the pregnancy, assessing types of foods as well as numbers of servings and emphasizing the importance of higher intake of fruits and vegetables and importance of taking prenatal vitamins (Fig. 13.2). If the client and nurse have a cultural or language barrier, an interpreter can assist as necessary to ensure that the client understands nutritional needs and practices and to offer culturally integrated suggestions (Fowles, 2002).

Family-Related Considerations

Researchers and theorists have described pregnancy and childbirth as a crucial period in which the steady state of the family is disrupted, requiring its members to use coping mechanisms for adaptation. When coping skills are strong, growth or change results (Zwelling & Phillips, 2001). If coping abilities are insufficient to meet the challenges, crisis occurs (see Chapter 7). High-risk pregnancy poses even greater challenges than usual. The ABCX model of family response to stress illustrates this adaptation and the potential for crisis (Fig. 13.3). Support for the entire family unit as well as each person within it is a critical enhancement to inherent coping abilities and strategies.

Family-centred care, with its emphasis on the family unit and collaboration, can promote positive coping with high-risk pregnancy. Knowledge can empower families; information about specific conditions, treatments, and overall plans of care can help them deal with expected and unexpected developments. Sensitivity and integration of unique customs is respectful and fosters collaboration (Zwelling & Phillips, 2001).

A high-risk pregnancy carries the potential for separation of the client from her newborn, other family members, or both. This threat increases the chance for family crisis and the need for support from health care providers. Encouragement of family-centred practices,

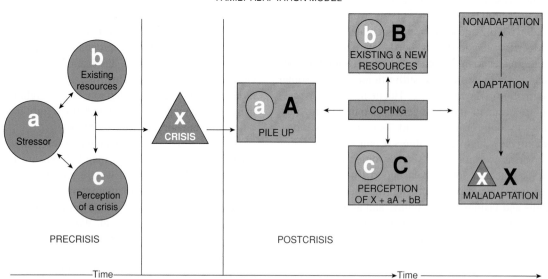

FIGURE 13.3 The ABCX model for assessing family dynamics. (From McCubbin, H. I., Thompson, E. A., Thompson, A. L., & Futrell, J. A. (2000). *The dynamics of resilient families.* Thousand Oaks, CA: Sage Publications.)

policies, and collaboration in health care facilities can strengthen the family unit and prepare relatives for this transitional period.

Consider Lindsey, the 33-year-old woman pregnant with her second child described at the beginning of the chapter. During her previous pregnancy, she was placed on bed rest at home. If bed rest is necessary with this pregnancy, how might this affect the family unit?

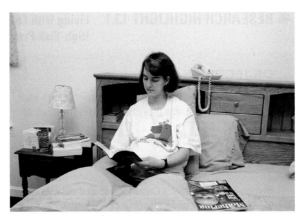

FIGURE 13.4 Bed rest may be used in high-risk pregnancies. Sources of activity (eg, reading) and interaction (eg, telephone) are important for women requiring bed rest to help prevent loneliness, isolation, and depression.

COMMON INTERVENTIONS IN HIGH-RISK PREGNANCY

Certain interventions are common in high-risk pregnancy, regardless of the presenting problem. This section focuses on some common methods of monitoring and preserving maternal and fetal health in cases of high-risk pregnancy.

Fetal Health Surveillance

Fetal surveillance is critical to the management of high-risk pregnancy. Involving women in their care, including fetal surveillance, by teaching them about fetal movements, providing written instructions, and reviewing what to do if they are concerned helps to prevent stillbirth and fosters maternal attachment (Berndl et al., 2013). Regular monitoring of fetal well-being allows health care providers to assess perfusion and oxygenation, as well as the potential for hypoxia or acidosis (Armour, 2004). As discussed in detail in Chapter 12, fetal surveillance methods include fetal movement counting, nonstress testing (NST), contraction stress testing, sonographic assessment of fetal behaviour and/or amniotic fluid volume, uterine artery Doppler, and umbilical artery Doppler. Together, these methods can minimize the chances of fetal morbidity and mortality (Malcus, 2004). Evaluations of fetal circulation, neurology, and heart rate also can give crucial information throughout the antenatal period (Malcus, 2004).

Bed Rest

Bed rest for the mother, whether in a health care facility or at home, may be prescribed in cases of high-risk pregnancy (Fig. 13.4). However, two systematic reviews reveal inconclusive evidence for the use of bed rest in preventing miscarriage in high-risk pregnancies or preterm births (Aleman et al., 2005; Sosa et al., 2004). Bed rest restricts movement and can isolate the woman from family and friends. Hospitalization usually is necessary if the client lives far from family or other support people, or if she, the fetus, or both require increased medical attention. This treatment carries its own risks, such as decreased muscle tone and atrophy, constipation, sleep disturbance, fatigue, fear, and depression (Rubarth et al., 2012). Weight loss during bed rest has been linked to decreased muscle mass, intracellular and extracellular fluid loss, bone loss, cardiovascular or physical deconditioning, and psychological distress (Rubarth et al., 2012). Regardless of the setting for bed rest, clients may experience negative emotions. Social isolation can have a negative effect, because contact with family and friends may be vital to maternal psychosocial well-being (MacDonald & Jonas-Simpson, 2009). Increased anxiety and emotional lability over weeks or months of bed rest can strain relationships and alter family dynamics. Absence from the home or decreased involvement in daily routines also can be hard on children or those caring for them (Maloni et al., 2001). Financial costs can be extensive. The woman may be required to leave her job, other children may need care from paid providers, or the family may need to pay for transportation back and forth to the facility giving care.

Women asked about bed-rest therapy in the hospital described their experience as "feeling like a prisoner" but as "something that needed to be done for the baby" (Rubarth et al., 2012). Stress-related symptoms included mood swings, boredom, isolation, grief over the loss of a normal pregnancy, and loneliness. Some women, however, described feeling safer as a result of the reassurance provided by frequent fetal assessments, and the ability to have health care providers see them more often for assessment (Simmons & Goldberg, 2011). See Research Highlight 13.1.

● **RESEARCH HIGHLIGHT 13.1**   Living With Changing Expectations for Women With
High-Risk Pregnancies: A Parse Method Study

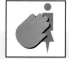

OBJECTIVES

To understand from women how their expectations and understanding of pregnancy changed with the label of "high risk."

SAMPLE

Women hospitalized at a Canadian hospital were asked to talk about their understanding of "high risk" and then comments were analyzed based on the parse method.

METHOD

Multiple interviews were held with women on their experience of being "high risk" and on how this affected their views of their pregnancies.

RESULTS

A sample of three was described, using the parse method to view their stories.

CONCLUSIONS

It is important for nurses to be able to spend time listening to women and understanding their paradoxical feelings of wanting to be safe in the hospital and at home with their families at the same time. Women have voiced their concerns about enforced restrictions while in hospital, and, for those providing care, it is important to genuinely work with women to understand how they can live within those limits.

From MacDonald, C., & Jonas-Simpson, C. (2009). Living with changing expectations for women living with high-risk pregnancies: A Parse method study. *Nursing Science Quarterly, 22*(1), 74–82.

HEALTH COMPLICATIONS IN PREGNANCY

Health complications in pregnancy can pose significant challenges for the woman, fetus, family, and health care team. Ideally, clients whose problem existed before gestation were prepared for the pregnancy and received appropriate preconception counselling and care (see Chapter 11). Referral to an obstetrician specializing in maternal and fetal medicine or a medical specialist, genetic counsellor, or both may have been completed before pregnancy. Beginning this care and continuing to assess this woman and family up through the postpartum period is extremely important for healthy outcomes and is best done with an interprofessional team that includes nurses, social workers, physiotherapists, and pharmacists as well as physicians.

Some conditions (eg, asthma) may improve during pregnancy; others (eg, diabetes) may shift continually with other physiologic adjustments that naturally accompany the various stages of gestation. Part of admission for a woman in labour includes review of significant components of her health history, such as current conditions, previous surgeries, psychiatric disorders, problematic substance use, and medications taken during pregnancy.

ASTHMA

Asthma, the most common obstructive pulmonary disorder in pregnant women, is a concurrent factor in 4% to 8% of pregnancies (Blaiss, 2004; Frye et al., 2011;

Kwon et al., 2004). Morbidity and mortality from asthma during pregnancy are increasing. The most common exacerbation period is from 24 to 36 weeks' gestation, with the most infrequent and usually mildest incidents in the last month (Blaiss, 2004). Risk for prenatal asthma exacerbation is related directly to asthma severity, which increases in approximately 30% of pregnant women, decreases in 30%, and stays stable in the remaining 40% (Schatz et al., 2003). Asthma is more common and severe in women of all races with lower socioeconomic status. Beckmann (2002) describes the physical effects of asthma in pregnancy as decreased exercise, walking outside, climbing stairs, and even performing housework because of shortness of breath, coughing, wheezing, and increased upper respiratory infections. Low birth weight may result from ongoing chronic asthmatic changes.

Pregnant clients with asthma should receive care from a team of asthma specialists and an obstetrician, family physician, nurse, or midwife. Initial treatment should include a review of the environment and potential removal of any irritants/allergens or triggers that have been identified, if possible (Frye et al., 2011). Team members should perform frequent pulmonary function tests, because abnormalities in pulmonary gas exchange produced by worsening asthma can lead to fetal hypoxia. Pregnant clients can participate in self-care by using a peak expiratory flow (PEF) meter to determine their lung volume and capacity three times a day, particularly morning and evening, recording findings to review with health care providers (Beckmann, 2002) (Fig. 13.5). Monthly assessment of such findings

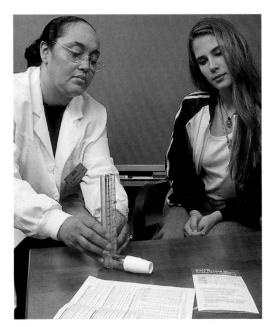

FIGURE 13.5 The nurse teaches the pregnant client with asthma how to use the peak flow monitor.

is beneficial, as is spirometry (National Institutes of Health [NIH] & National Asthma Prevention Program Working Group [NAPPWG], 2004).

Prenatal asthma treatment is based on a stepwise approach focused on maintaining adequate control (Fig. 13.6). Evidence of such control includes minimal or no chronic symptoms day or night, minimal exacerbations, no activity limitations, maintenance of pulmonary function, minimal use of short-acting inhaled β_2-agonists, and minimal or no adverse effects from medications (NIH & NAPPG, 2004). Clients may be prescribed corticosteroids, which may decrease birth weight and increase the risk for gestational hypertension. The team should review concerns regarding fetal weight gain and well-being and collaborate with the pregnant woman regarding risks and benefits in their approach to her care. They also may need to revise the plan if concerns increase over time.

During labour, initial maternal assessments focus on vital signs (especially respiratory rate and temperature), coping ability, and pain management preferences. Because stress may cause or trigger an asthma attack, continual monitoring for any signs or symptoms is essential. Positive findings include shortness of breath, increased respiratory rate (above the normal range of 12 to 24 breaths/min), and increased inspiratory or expiratory effort. An oxygen saturation monitor may be attached to the client's finger; a level less than 95% indicates a need for increased oxygenation. The health care team should assess the client's progress depending on any presenting symptoms. The labouring client may require intravenous (IV) fluids for ample hydration,

and more frequent assessments of vital signs, including oxygen saturation monitoring (Rey & Boulet, 2007). Medications taken throughout pregnancy (eg, inhalers) should remain available. The nurse should stay with the client and provide continuous support, because a consistent nursing presence can decrease anxiety and increase security.

The team should avoid administering pain medications such as meperidine (Demerol) or morphine, because of their associated histamine release. Prostaglandin E preparations should not be used in clients with asthma undergoing labour augmentation or induction, because they may contribute to bronchospasm. In such cases, oxytocin (Syntocinon) is the medication of choice. The team must review the risks and benefits of any procedure or test before beginning.

Assessment of fetal health during pregnancy varies according to the severity of maternal asthma, maternal respiratory rate, fetal growth measurements, and other individual circumstances. If no fetal risk factors exist when a client is in labour, fetal health may be evaluated by auscultation as long as the fetal heart rate remains within the normal range. If any change in fetal heart rate causes concern (eg, decelerations), or if the maternal asthma worsens, electronic fetal monitoring may be required. Normal findings include variability of 6 to 25 beats per minute (bpm), with a baseline rate of 110 to 160 bpm and no abnormal decelerations (SOGC, 2007a).

Adequate respiratory function, ability to cope with labour and birth, presence of support person(s) as per the client's wishes, and verbalized understanding of all aspects of care and fetal well-being are desired outcomes. Documentation that demonstrates consistency of care, would include identification of all triggers, medications, appropriate therapies, and monitoring.

CYSTIC FIBROSIS

Cystic fibrosis (CF) is a genetic disorder affecting multiple organs (see Chapter 4). In the past, clients with CF often did not live to adulthood. Recently, however, advances in treatment have prolonged the life span of these clients. Some women with CF are becoming pregnant.

Normal pregnancy causes decreased residual volume. Some women with CF cannot maintain the vital capacity or increased cardiac output of pregnancy, which increases risk for premature birth (Barak et al., 2005) (see Chapter 22). In pregnant clients with CF, nurses should observe for signs of malabsorption and monitor maternal weight and pancreatic enzymes during each visit. To ensure adequate nutrition, the nurse administers oral supplements as ordered. During the intrapartal period, the nurse monitors the client's fluid and electrolyte balance and frequently assesses results of laboratory

Classify severity: clinical features before treatment or adequate control			**Medications** required to maintain long-term control
Symptoms/day **Symptoms/night**	**PEF or FEV₁** **PEF variability**		**Daily medications**
4 Severe persistent	Continual ——— Frequent	60% ——— >30%	**Preferred treatment:** • High-dose inhaled corticosteroid 　　AND • Long-acting inhaled β₂-agonist 　　AND, if needed • Corticosteroid tablets or syrup long term (2 mg/kg/day, generally not to exceed 60 mg/day). (Make repeat attempts to reduce systemic corticosteroid and maintain control with high dose.) **Alternative treatment:** • High-dose inhaled corticosteroid* 　　AND • Sustained-release theophylline to serum concentration of 5–12 μg/mL
3 Moderate persistent	Daily ——— >1 night/week	>60% – <80% ——— >30%	**Preferred treatment:** 　EITHER • Low-dose inhaled corticosteroid* and long-acting inhaled β₂-agonist 　OR • Medium-dose inhaled corticosteroid* 　　IF Needed (particularly in patients with recurring severe exacerbations): • Medium-dose inhaled corticosteroid* and long-acting inhaled β₂-agonist **Alternative treatment:** • Low-dose inhaled corticosteroid* and either theophylline or leukotriene receptor antagonist† 　　IF Needed • Medium-dose inhaled corticosteroid* and either theophylline or leukotriene receptor antagonist†
2 Mild persistent	>2 days/week but <daily ——— >2 nights/month	>80% ——— 20% – 30%	**Preferred treatment:** • Low-dose inhaled corticosteroid* **Alternative treatment** (listed alphabetically): •Cromolyn, leukotriene receptor antagonist†, OR sustained-release theophylline to serum concentration of 5–12 μg/mL
1 Mild intermittent	2 days/week ——— 2 nights/month	80% ——— <20%	• No daily medication needed • Severe exacerbations may occur, separated by long periods of normal lung function and no symptoms. A course of systemic corticosteriods is recommended.
Quick relief All patients			• Short-acting bronchodilator: 2–4 puffs short-acting inhaled beta₂-agonist‡ as needed for symptoms. • Intensity of treatment will depend on severity of exacerbation; up to 3 treatments at 20-minute intervals or a single nebulizer treatment as needed. Course of systemic corticosteroid may be needed. • Use of short-acting inhaled beta₂-agonist‡ >2 times a week in intermittent asthma (daily, or increasing use in persistent asthma) may indicate the need to initiate (increase) long-term control therapy.

Step down
Review treatment every 1–6 months; a gradual stepwise reduction in treatment may be possible.

Step up
If control is not maintained, consider step up. First, review patient medication technique, adherence, and environmental control.

Goals of therapy: asthma control

- Minimal or no chronic symptoms day or night
- Minimal or no exacerbations
- No limitations on activities; no school/work missed
- Maintain (near) normal pulmonary function

- Minimal use of short-acting inhaled beta₂-agonist‡
- Minimal or no adverse effects from medications

Notes

- The stepwise approach is meant to assist, not replace, the clinical decision making required to meet individual patient needs.
- Classify severity: assign patient to most severe step in which any feature occurs (PEF is percent of personal best; FEV₁ is percent predicted).
- Gain control as quickly as possible (consider a short course of systemic corticosteroid), then step down to the least medication necessary to maintain control.
- Minimize use of short-acting inhaled μ₂-agonist‡ (eg, use of approximately one canister a month even if not using it every day indicates inadequate control of asthma and the need to initiate or intensify long-term control therapy).
- Provide education on self-management and controlling environmental factors that make asthma worse (eg, allergens, irritants).
- Refer to an asthma specialist if there are difficulties controlling asthma or if in Step 4 care is required. Referral may be considered if Step 3 care is required.

* There are more data on using budesonide during pregnancy than on using other equal inhaled corticosteroids.
† There are minimal data on using leukotriene receptor antagonists in humans during pregnancy, although there are reassuring animal data submitted to FDA.
‡ There are more data on using albuterol during pregnancy than on using other short-acting inhaled β₂-agonists.

FIGURE 13.6 Stepwise approach to asthma management in pregnancy and lactation. (From U.S. Department of Health and Human Services. (2005). *NAEPP working group report on managing asthma during pregnancy: Recommendations for pharmacological treatment.* 2004 Update. Rockville, MD: Author.)

testing and vital signs. Adequate oxygenation is essential. The nurse monitors the results of pulse oximetry and, if problems arise, administers oxygen as ordered. Generally, local or epidural anaesthesia is preferred for clients with CF ready to give birth. Breast-feeding is permitted once sodium content has been determined; if the sodium content of the mother's milk is high, breast-feeding is contraindicated (Lawrence & Lawrence, 2005).

CARDIOVASCULAR DISEASE

Cardiovascular complications occur in approximately 1% to 3% of pregnancies (Arafeh & Baird, 2006; Davies & Herbert, 2007). Cardiac disease is responsible for 10% to 25% of maternal deaths (Dobbenga-Rhodes & Prive, 2007). The two most common categories are acquired and congenital disorders. The incidence of acquired disorders is decreasing in Western countries (largely as a result of the decline of rheumatic fever), but remain a concern in developing areas. The number of women of childbearing age with congenital heart disease is increasing because advances in both diagnosis and intervention have improved survival rates and health, facilitating the ability of these clients to achieve and to maintain pregnancy (Arafeh & Baird, 2006; Kuczkowski, 2004).

Maternal factors that determine fetal growth include nutrition, oxygenation, and cardiovascular adaptation. In the presence of maternal cardiac disease, the most frequent fetal complication is small for gestational age, in some studies as high as 60% (see Chapter 22) (Gelson et al., 2011). These women also have a high rate of preterm births, which may contribute to the difference in weight. However, the fetal birth weight is associated with maternal risk factors of reduced cardiac output or cyanosis, left heart obstruction, anticoagulation, smoking, and multiple gestation (Gelson et al., 2011).

Etiology and Pathophysiology

Physiologic adaptations in pregnancy pose significant risks for women with cardiovascular disease (Ramsey et al., 2001). Increases in blood volume and cardiac output are detectible within the first 2 months of pregnancy (Kilpatrick & Purden, 2007). With some conditions (eg, Marfan syndrome), the additional volume may increase the risk for congestive heart failure, aneurysm, or both. Toward the end of pregnancy, the increased uterine size encroaches on the inferior vena cava, decreasing venous return and lowering cardiac output when in the supine position (Ramsey et al., 2001). The uterine blood flow significantly increases from 50 mL/minute prior to pregnancy to 500 mL/minute by the third trimester (Davies & Herbert, 2007). Risks for women who have cardiovascular problems are further increased because of the hypercoagulable state normal to pregnancy. The cardiac muscle

shows a mild hypertrophy caused by an increase in cardiac valve diameters and increased blood flow to the heart (Dobbenga-Rhodes & Prive, 2007). Pregnant women with artificial valves and atrial fibrillation are at increased risk for arterial thrombosis (Arafeh & Baird, 2006). Any type of therapeutic anticoagulation increases the risk of hemorrhage. Electrocardiographic changes also are common in pregnancy, including sinus tachycardia, shift in the QRS axis, and atrial and ventricular dysrhythmias (Ramsey et al., 2001). Hypertensive disorders are the most common complication, with rates as high as 16% in certain cardiac conditions such as aortic stenosis, and aortic coarctation (Fernandes et al., 2010).

Certain risk factors can help predict which clients are at highest risk for morbidity and mortality: (1) history of a cardiac event or dysrhythmia prior to pregnancy, (2) prepregnancy heart disease class III or IV on the New York Heart Association (NYHA) system, or cyanosis and (3) left ejection fraction less than 40% and (4) left heart obstruction (Fernandes et al., 2010). Smoking, multiple gestation, and use of heparin or warfarin also are linked to a greater potential for neonatal complications (Martin & Foley, 2003). Overall, adverse fetal and neonatal outcomes complicate 15% to 39% of pregnancies with preterm birth, small for gestation age, stillbirth, and respiratory distress (Fernandes et al., 2010).

Types
Manifestations depend on the specific cardiac problem (Gilbert, 2011). Maternal functional status is based on the following Canadian Cardiovascular Society (2008) categories:

- Class I: angina only during strenuous or prolonged physical activity
- Class II: slight limitation, with angina only during vigorous physical activity
- Class III: symptoms with everyday living activities, ie, moderate limitation
- Class: IV: inability to perform any activity without angina or angina at rest, ie, severe limitation

Generally, pregnant clients with class I or II heart disease have a favourable prognosis, although their functional status may worsen (Davies & Herbert, 2007). For example, 44% of women with cardiac disease develop congestive heart failure and pulmonary edema in the third trimester (Ramsey et al., 2001).

Newborns of parents with congenital heart disease have a 2% to 5% risk for congenital heart malformations (Lupton et al., 2002; Ramsey et al., 2001), particularly on the maternal side. The health care team must review the functional status associated with the condition, together with the potential risk for congenital heart disease in the newborn. A fetal echocardiogram is important at 18 to 21 weeks' gestation (Davies & Herbert, 2007).

Mitral Stenosis

Mitral stenosis is the most common rheumatic valvular lesion in pregnant clients; approximately 25% of women become symptomatic for the first time while pregnant (Arafeh & Baird, 2006). Mitral stenosis decreases left atrial outflow as well as left ventricular diastolic filling, resulting in a fixed cardiac output. These clients need adequate diastolic filling time to complete cardiac output. Any increase in heart rate shortens the diastolic period more than the systolic, decreasing time for blood to flow across the mitral valve. The increased heart rate and blood volume inherent in pregnancy contribute to the potential for symptoms in the latter half of gestation, particularly during labour and birth. Treatment may include activity restriction to prevent tachycardia, β-blockers to control heart rate, and carefully monitored diuretic therapy to treat pulmonary edema (Martin & Foley, 2003).

Mitral Valve Prolapse

Mitral valve prolapse, the most common congenital heart lesion, occurs in 17% of women with cardiac disease in the childbearing years (Ramsey et al., 2001). It can be asymptomatic or cause palpitations, chest pain, or both. The increased blood volume and decreased systemic vascular resistance of pregnancy actually improve mitral valve function, allowing women with mitral valve prolapse to tolerate pregnancy well (Martin & Foley, 2003). Auscultation may reveal a midsystolic click and murmur, which may decrease with advancing pregnancy because of increased peripheral vasodilation.

Peripartum Cardiomyopathy

Peripartum cardiomyopathy (PPCM) is the term used for heart failure in the last month of pregnancy or within 5 months of childbirth without previous heart disease or identifiable cause (Roos-Hesselink et al., 2009). Diagnostic criteria include evidence of left ventricular dysfunction confirmed by echocardiography examination (Palmer, 2007). The underlying mechanism is largely unknown, but myocarditis has a strong association (Palmer, 2007). Approximately 1 in 3,000 to 1 in 4,000 women develops PPCM, which has a mortality rate as high as 56% (Martin & Foley, 2003). Risk factors include multiparity, multiple gestation, gestational hypertension, obesity, low socioeconomic status, Black race, and advanced maternal age (>30 years) (Roos-Hesselink et al., 2009). Signs and symptoms include nocturnal dyspnea, chest pain, cough, increasing fatigue, peripheral edema, and, on physical examination, rales and murmurs (Ramsey et al., 2001). This problem is discussed in more detail in Chapter 19.

Atrial Septal Defects

Atrial septal defects are commonly seen during pregnancy and are usually asymptomatic (Ramsey et al., 2001). The increased plasma volume of pregnancy can cause dysrhythmias as gestation progresses, but generally this condition is well tolerated.

Collaborative Management: Pregnancy and Cardiac Disease

The most important factors to consider in pregnant clients with cardiac disease are the specific cardiac lesion and whether it has been corrected surgically (Table 13.1). Preconception is the best time to provide the necessary information regarding maternal and fetal risks related to the specific problem (see Chapters 4 and 11). Once pregnancy is established, fetal echocardiography

● TABLE 13.1   **Selected Heart Conditions in Pregnancy**

Problem	Explanation	Treatment/Management
Aortic stenosis	A narrowed opening of the aortic valve results in obstructed left ventricular ejection	Confirmation of diagnosis by echocardiography Antiarrhythmic drugs, β-blockers, or both to reduce the risk for other cardiac problems Bed rest, activity restrictions, and close maternal and fetal monitoring
Atrial septal defect	Congenital opening between the atria, with left-to-right shunting of blood and greater left-sided pressure	Atrioventricular nodal–blocking agents Electrical cardioversion Rest and activity limitations
Mitral valve prolapse	Prolapse of the leaflets of the mitral valve into the left atrium during ventricular contraction	Usually no special precautions needed during pregnancy
Mitral valve stenosis	Obstructed blood flow from atria to ventricle, with possible resultant pulmonary hypertension and edema, as well as right ventricular failure	Diuretics, anticoagulants, and β-blockers to treat symptoms In severe cases, bed rest and activity restriction
Peripartum cardiomyopathy	Heart failure of unknown etiology in the last month of gestation to 5 mo postpartum in women with no pre-existing heart disease	Diuretic therapy Vasodilators Inotropic agents
Ventricular septal defect	Opening in the ventricular septum	Rest and activity limitations

is critical to prenatal diagnosis of congenital heart disease and important to include in care of women with a history of congenital cardiac disease. Generally, the management of pregnant clients with serious cardiac disease should occur in health care facilities with the capacity and resources for intensive maternal, fetal, and neonatal care (Ramsey et al., 2001).

All pregnant clients require thorough and ongoing physical examination (see Chapter 12). Early in the first trimester, it is important to determine the gestational age as this will be an important element of her later plan for labour and/or birth (Davies & Herbert, 2007). Clients should be asked about heart murmurs before pregnancy, any activity limitations, chest pain, cyanosis, shortness of breath, or previous rheumatic fever. Clients with positive responses should be suspected of having cardiac disease; appropriate classification and diagnosis are important to their ongoing care. Pregnant women with known cardiovascular problems need particular attention paid to heart sounds and pulse rate, as well as questions regarding childhood illnesses, exercise, episodes of dyspnea, and surgery. Symptoms of fatigue, difficulty breathing, palpitations, and lower-extremity edema can be attributed to pregnancy or worsening cardiac disease, so it is important to determine the cause (Martin & Foley, 2003). Women with congenital heart disease are also encouraged to supplement their diet with a multivitamin containing folic acid to reduce the risk of some types of cardiac and nervous system defects in their infants (Kilpatrick & Purden, 2007).

Antepartal blood volume progressively increases, peaking at 28 to 32 weeks' gestation. This period is a critical time to observe the status of the pregnant client with a cardiac condition (Arafeh & Baird, 2006). Anemia, which may occur as a physiologic change in pregnancy, should be prevented with nutritional counselling, iron supplementation, and testing (Davies & Herbert, 2007). Beginning at 28 weeks, her visits to the health care provider may need to occur weekly to protect the client's health during this pivotal time.

Diagnostic studies include chest x-ray, electrocardiogram, arterial blood gas analysis, and echocardiogram. Usually, consultation with a cardiologist occurs during initial diagnosis and for ongoing care and follow-up. The team providing care decides the appropriate facility for labour and birth, timing of birth, additional equipment or supplies needed (eg, hemodynamic monitoring, endocarditis prophylaxis), preferred method of anaesthesia, anticoagulant therapy, and needs for early admission (Arafeh & Baird, 2006).

General treatment measures include careful use of antepartum activity restriction, bed rest, or both, based on the specific cardiac lesion and functional class; avoidance of anemia by regular laboratory testing and iron supplementation; and intensive maternal and fetal

monitoring for potential complications (Ramsey et al., 2001). Frequent rest throughout the day is necessary to meet the increased demands that pregnancy imposes on the cardiac system. Assisting with diet counselling helps ensure appropriate weight gain based on the client's prepregnancy body mass index. A fetal echocardiogram at 18 to 22 weeks' gestation, as well as ongoing monitoring of growth and development, provides clues to fetal well-being.

Collaborative Management: Labour and Birth

Assessment during labour includes careful history taking to pinpoint medications and their dosages, explanations about the effects of cardiac disease during pregnancy and labour, and physical examination, including vital signs. The team needs to understand the client's support for labour, plan for birth, initial labour stage, cervical dilation, effacement, and fetal well-being. Signs and symptoms of complications include fatigue, difficulty breathing or shortness of breath, palpitations, and increasing edema of the feet and ankles (Martin & Foley, 2003).

During labour, demands on the cardiovascular system increase by as much as 50% (Ramsey et al., 2001). Uterine contractions cause fluctuating levels in venous return and sympathetic tone. Placental separation and uterine involution cause physiologic autotransfusion of approximately 500 mL of blood, increasing risks for pulmonary edema and cardiogenic shock (Ramsey et al., 2001). Care at this time focuses on reducing maternal cardiac workload, specifically from tachycardia. Epidural analgesia is beneficial in reducing catecholamine surges from labour pains that cause tachycardia or hypertension without compromising uterine contractions (see Chapter 17). Management of the second stage of labour often includes an assisted vaginal birth using forceps or vacuum extraction and avoidance of extended breath holding (Valsalva maneuver) (Bowers et al., 2008; SOGC, 2004a). Vaginal birth after 36 weeks' gestation is the goal of care, because it poses fewer hemodynamic changes than does cesarean birth and facilitates further fetal growth and development. Each case is considered individually, however, depending on the severity of the maternal lesion, symptoms associated with pregnancy, and results of completed tests for fetal lung maturity (Gilbert, 2011). Changes in the labour plan are based on maternal and fetal well-being. The client and her family need to be kept informed of her progress throughout pregnancy and labour and of any required changes in care.

Monitoring of a labouring woman with cardiac disease may include readings of central venous pressure, pulmonary wedge pressure, and oxygen saturation. Intake and output are monitored accurately; specific assessments for individualized care (eg, anticoagulant therapy) are necessary (Gilbert, 2011). Depending on the severity of the condition, continuous maternal ECG monitoring may be required. Vital signs are assessed every 15 to 60 minutes, with auscultation of the lung fields every 1 to 4 hours. During insertion of monitoring lines, the nurse looks for changes in waveforms or dysrhythmias, which may signify a need for repositioning. Measuring urine output to ensure at least 30 mL/hour is essential for adequate circulating volume, as is careful assessment of intake. Hypovolemia or hypervolemia would be a concern for this woman during labour (Davies & Herbert, 2007). Oxygen therapy and use of the left lateral recumbent position may help. Staff from the intensive care nursery should be at hand to ensure adequate newborn care.

Maternal cardiac disease is identified as an antenatal and intrapartum condition associated with increased risk of adverse fetal outcome, and warrants intrapartum electronic fetal surveillance (SOGC, 2007a). External monitoring may be adequate; in some cases, internal monitoring with an intrauterine pressure catheter and a fetal scalp electrode is used, so that data about contraction intensity and fetal heart rate patterns are consistent. Abnormal patterns (eg, late decelerations), together with labour progress and potentially a fetal scalp pH sample, need to be evaluated.

Balancing this client's risk and care with the anticipation of birth as a joyous occasion is important. If the mother must be separated from her newborn for any period, facilitating postpartum visitation as soon as possible is vital. Assisting with breast-feeding as per the woman's wishes should begin as soon as possible (Arafeh & Baird, 2006). Helping the mother to pump her breast milk may be indicated to build and maintain milk supply if separation of mother and infant is required.

ANEMIA

Anemia, which affects approximately 50% of pregnant clients, occurs when the quantity or quality of circulatory red blood cells (RBCs) decreases (Casanova et al., 2005). Physiologic anemia is the most common form of anemia seen in pregnancy (See Chapter 12). Problems with quantity occur when RBCs are destroyed or lost earlier than their 120-day life cycle. Problems related to quality include microcytic (too small), macrocytic (too large), hypochromic (hemoglobin concentration too low), or hyperchromic (hemoglobin concentration too high) RBCs. Regardless of type, all anemias cause similar signs and symptoms: fatigue, palpitations, chest pain, and shortness of breath with exercise.

Iron-Deficiency Anemia

The iron requirement in pregnancy is 3 to 4 mg/day and increases with gestation as the woman's body works to build the maternal RBC mass, expand plasma volume, and facilitate placental growth (Scholl, 2005). This requirement is challenging to meet with a typical Western diet (Bodnar et al., 2005), and current researchers believe that 50% of women do not have adequate iron stores for pregnancy (Scholl, 2005). Risks for iron-deficiency anemia are higher among black women, clients using antacids or tetracyclines, low-income women, adolescents, and clients with a concurrent zinc deficiency (Bodnar et al., 2005).

Signs and symptoms of iron-deficiency anemia include fatigue, decreased endurance, and compromised work efficiency. Cognitive deficits and mood swings also are possible, including problems with short-term memory, verbal learning, and depression. Accompanying reduced immune function poses additional health risks (Bodnar et al., 2005). Iron-deficiency anemia has also been associated with preterm birth and low birth weight (Briggs et al., 2007; Kirkham et al., 2005).

To assess for iron-deficiency anemia, hemoglobin and hematocrit values should be tested in all pregnant clients as part of initial prenatal care. Preferably, these studies are done in the first trimester to separate true anemia from physiologic changes associated with pregnancy. Other evaluations include serum ferritin, transferrin saturation, and free erythrocyte protoporphyrin (Bodnar et al., 2005). A dietary review, possibly with a nutritionist or dietician, may be appropriate. The client may be prescribed prenatal vitamins with supplemental iron. Discussion of finances may be appropriate to ensure that the client can afford the foods and supplements needed to provide adequate iron or to offer assistance through a social worker, nutritionist, community program, or other avenue. Client teaching focuses on the importance of iron for energy, weight gain, and fetal well-being.

Sickle Cell Anemia

Sickle cell anemia occurs predominantly in African Americans (see Chapter 4). In Canada, as the Black population grows, there is a corresponding rise in the carrier rate of this gene. Canadians of Caribbean origin have a carrier rate of 10% to 14%; those of African origin have a rate of 20% to 25% (Canadian Task Force on Preventive Health Care, 2003). This homozygous recessive illness is characterized by chronic hemolytic anemia. A woman with sickle cell anemia normally has a decreased hemoglobin level (70 to 80 g/L), as well as a decreased oxygen-carrying capability, to which she likely has adjusted (Blackburn, 2013). Pregnancy, however, may pose new or added problems, as the increased blood volume also increases her anemia. Assisting the client to achieve or maintain healthy hemoglobin levels without acute episodes of vascular occlusion is the goal. Careful monitoring involves ongoing blood work and fetal assessment.

Clients with sickle cell anemia may experience chronic hemolytic anemia, acute episodes of vascular occlusion (sickle cell crises), or both. Those with chronic anemia may appear jaundiced and suffer from gallstones, splenomegaly, and slow-healing ulcers. Pyelonephritis and pneumonia are also common. Clients with acute crises may describe pain resulting from sickled cells clustering together in the microvasculature, particularly in the bones and chest. Occlusions in the brain increase the risk for stroke. The heart, liver, and spleen may be affected. Sickle cell crises may increase in frequency and severity with gestation (Blackburn, 2013). Placental infarction and fetal hypoxia can occur during one or more episodes of acute vascular occlusion, with the potential adverse effects of preterm labour, intrauterine growth restriction (IUGR), and stillbirth.

Assessment of the pregnant woman with sickle cell anemia should include a complete health history and physical examination. Laboratory testing should include a complete blood count, differential, reticulocyte count, blood urea nitrogen, glucose, direct bilirubin, and urinalysis. Questions about previous episodes should include type, amount, and location of pain, as well as any helpful treatment. Understanding potential triggers and any precipitating factors (eg, infection) is also helpful. Hydroxyurea (Droxia, Hydrea) may be ordered to reduce acute crises. Folic acid supplements may be beneficial and are usually tolerated well. For the client with sickle cell crisis, fluids and analgesics are appropriate. See Chapter 4 as well.

AUTOIMMUNE DISEASES

Autoimmune diseases affect women of childbearing age more than any other group. Research findings suggest a link with these disorders and increased levels of estrogen and other steroids, the naturally enhanced immunity resulting from pregnancy, or a combination of these factors. Chapter 4 includes discussion of various autoimmune problems common to women; the following subsections explore two of the most significant of these illnesses in relation to pregnancy.

Systemic Lupus Erythematosus

Systemic lupus erythematosus (SLE) is a complex, chronic, inflammatory autoimmune disease that can affect numerous organs, specifically the skin, joints, serous membranes, kidneys, and central nervous system (Baer et al., 2011). Deposits of antigen–antibody complexes in capillaries and various visceral structures are characteristic (Sibai & Chames, 2003). Systematic lupus erythematosus often begins or worsens during the childbearing years (Zhang & Chen, 2003); incidence may be as high as 1% of pregnancies (Hamar & Funai,

2007). The disease is marked by intermittent remissions and exacerbations (see Chapter 4). Clients are prone to clotting problems, with increased rates of pulmonary emboli, deep vein thromboses, and cerebrovascular accidents.

Fertility in women with SLE is usually normal. Pregnancy-related risk factors include IUGR, prematurity, stillbirth, and miscarriage, in addition to maternal hypertension, proteinuria, or both. One factor cited as related to pregnancy outcomes for clients with SLE is the duration of remission of the illness before pregnancy. Women who experience a flare within 6 months of pregnancy are more likely to experience pregnancy complications while those who have been in remission for at least 1 year have milder symptoms during pregnancy (Baer et al., 2011). Extensive preconception counselling should include a discussion of risks and benefits as well as planning for the best time to conceive for both maternal and fetal health.

The major difficulty in pregnancy for women with SLE involves the placenta, which can have various abnormalities and forms of compromise. The inflammatory autoimmune response inherent with this disease leads to placental vasculopathy, with subsequent fibrin deposition and areas of infarction. As a result, placental size and circulation can be decreased, and the fetus may have IUGR (Hamar & Funai, 2007). In pregnant women with SLE, placental villi are thinner and slimmer.

Nurses, obstetricians, rheumatologists, and social workers are team members likely to have significant roles in evaluating the health of the pregnant client with SLE. Visits to the primary care provider should occur every 2 weeks during the first two trimesters and then weekly beginning at 28 weeks. Evaluations of renal function, blood pressure, and fetal growth are critical to locate any changes that might suggest maternal or fetal compromise. Neonatal lupus occurs in 3.5% to 8% of pregnancies with the most serious complication being an in utero heart block. Fetal echocardiography is recommended between 18 and 24 weeks' gestation (Baer et al., 2011). Corticosteroid therapy has been shown to improve outcomes in pregnancies in women with SLE (Zhang & Chen, 2003). Glucocorticosteroids are the drugs of choice. The smallest therapeutic dose should be prescribed, with the primary care provider increasing the amount during times of stress (eg, labour).

Preterm birth, IUGR, and gestational hypertension are potential risks. Teaching about the signs and symptoms of preterm labour, scheduling fetal monitoring, and communicating with the client about findings throughout the pregnancy are therapeutic and supportive nursing interventions (see Chapter 16). Discussing the need for close follow-up, child care, and transportation assistance may help ensure the client's compliance with appointments and interventions.

Collaborative planning for labour and birth is necessary before admission. Once the client arrives at the birthing area, she needs individualized attention to her care needs. Initial assessment includes routine blood tests, evaluation of blood pressure, monitoring for signs of edema or proteinuria, and checks of creatinine clearance and urine output. Evaluation of cardiac function by ECG and invasive monitoring may be necessary. Auscultation of breath and lung sounds helps determine pulmonary function. The team must check for signs of disseminated intravascular coagulation (DIC) by evaluating complete blood count, platelet count, prothrombin time, and International Normalized Ratio (INR); additionally, maternal blood may be needed for group and cross-match. Physical examination focuses on labour's progress; a vaginal examination is performed, unless contraindicated. The client may be administered antihypertensive drugs and high-dose prednisone. SLE is considered a chronic medical condition that can affect fetal oxygenation and warrant intrapartum fetal heart rate monitoring (SOGC, 2007a). Continuous fetal monitoring and ongoing communication can decrease the woman's anxiety about fetal well-being as her labour continues. Cesarean birth may be determined safest, depending on the specific risks and benefits to both mother and fetus. Expected outcomes include a normal fetal heart rate, normal labour progress, pain management per the woman's wishes, and birth without coagulopathy.

Antiphospholipid Syndrome

Antiphospholipid syndrome is an autoimmune disorder characterized by the presence of circulating antiphospholipids. The two most common types are lupus anticoagulants and anticardiolipin antibodies. Low levels of antiphospholipids may be found in 2% to 4% of all women; however, some women (0.2%) have levels associated with pregnancy complications. Antiphospholipid syndrome is a leading cause of pregnancy loss (Salmon & Girardi, 2008). Women with this condition may experience complications, such as severe preeclampsia, utero-placental insufficiency, HELLP syndrome, oligohydramnios, fetal distress, and iatrogenic preterm birth (DiPrima et al., 2011). Thrombosis is the most serious risk associated with antiphospholipid syndrome with occlusions occurring in various locations.

Laboratory testing for antiphospholipids should be done when the maternal health history reveals recurrent spontaneous abortions, unexplained pregnancy loss in the second or third trimester, venous thrombosis, arterial thrombosis, stroke, SLE, autoimmune thrombocytopenia, or prolonged clotting assay. The client with antiphospholipid syndrome requires treatment from a team including social workers, nurses, obstetricians, hematologists, and pharmacists. Communication among members and with the client and family ensures collaborative care and desired outcomes. Fetal growth and development should be assessed weekly from 28 weeks' gestation onward through nonstress test, biophysical profiles, Doppler studies, or all these methods. Monitoring of maternal blood pressure and renal function also is essential.

One potential treatment for the pregnant client with antiphospholipid syndrome is a combination of prednisone (40 mg/day) with low-dose aspirin (81 mg/day). Although effective, this treatment increases the risks for preterm birth and gestational hypertension. Another potential treatment is low–molecular-weight heparin; this drug poses risks for abnormal bleeding and fractures but has been successful in decreasing occlusion. Individual factors need to be considered to determine the most effective therapy.

INFECTIONS

Routine prenatal care for all pregnant clients includes obtaining a detailed medical history, testing for sexually transmitted infections (STIs), and offering laboratory testing for human immunodeficiency virus (HIV) as well as Hepatitis B and C. Intrapartum infections require knowledge and skill from health care providers to decrease the risk of vertical transmission from mother to fetus. Such transmission may occur through ascending infection in the birth canal, blood exchange, or direct contact with vaginal or cervical secretions.

HIV

As discussed in Chapter 4, clients may not develop symptoms of HIV for 10 years or longer. At the end of 2011, approximately 208 people per 100,000 in Canada were positive for the HIV virus (Public Health Agency of Canada, 2011a). Canadian rates of infection are continuing to increase as treatments have improved and more people are surviving. The rate for Canadian women is increasing, currently at 28.8% with a disproportionate number of women from First Nations, Metis, or Inuit communities (SOGC, 2013a). Some clients are choosing to become pregnant as their care improves with their quality of life.

Pediatric transmission of HIV occurs primarily during the perinatal period (Burdge et al., 2003). The transmission rate from infected mother to fetus without treatment is 25% (Gilbert, 2011). Maternal HIV status should be determined during pregnancy, with appropriate counseling, consent, and testing; maternal treatment should be initiated before birth, and subsequent infant treatment initiated at birth. Nurses should provide information to women about the benefits of consenting to an HIV test at the first prenatal visit to facilitate prompt diagnosis and treatment for the mother and the fetus or newborn. Treatment during pregnancy significantly reduces the risk of the infant acquiring the disease.

Collaborative interventions focus on teaching about the risks and benefits of all aspects of care in relation to the infection. A multidisciplinary team includes practitioners with knowledge in treating HIV-positive women, nurses, obstetricians, social workers, dieticians, and pharmacists (SOGC, 2006). All care providers should use universal precautions at all times (standard of care for all women). Confidentiality and privacy are important to this woman's care and need to be respected at all times by health care providers.

The nurse should use open-ended questions to determine the client's knowledge about her infection and plans for newborn care. Some women choose not to share information about their health with family members, partners, or both; therefore, nurses must be careful to ask initial questions about HIV status in private. Assessment also should include evaluations of the client's emotional state and coping ability. The nurse should review and document community resources the client is already using when planning care during pregnancy and after the baby's birth.

An estimated 50% to 80% of perinatal transmissions of HIV occur during labour and birth (Katz, 2004). Treatment goals during labour are to provide individualized care to the client based on the clinical and immunologic stage of her disease, and to prevent perinatal HIV transmission (Katz, 2004). Combined antiretroviral therapy may have been started during pregnancy and will be given intravenously during childbirth (Pharmacology Box 13.1). The goal is to reduce the maternal viral load, thus decreasing the chances of disease transmission. Medical interventions such as rupturing the membranes or using a fetal scalp clip (internal monitoring) are avoided. Vaginal examinations should be minimal. Prolonged ruptured membranes increase the risk of HIV transmission; thus, care should be taken to decrease exposure of the fetus or newborn to maternal body fluids (Katz, 2004). Antibiotic therapy should be considered at least 4 hours before birth to reduce the rate of vertical transmission of infectious agents during the birth process. Cesarean birth is an option being studied as a way to decrease perinatal HIV transmission with a woman whose viral load is high.

Some HIV-positive women are also injection drug users. They may be ambivalent about their pregnancies or worried about fetal health (Katz, 2004). Emotional support involves being nonjudgemental during care provision. Depression also has been associated with an HIV diagnosis; encouraging the client's resourcefulness and coping skills can contribute to increasing her health behaviours (Boonpongmanee et al., 2003).

Postpartum discussions should focus on obtaining the client's feedback about care received during labour and birth, giving her opportunities to discuss her memories and perceptions of the experience. Testing for HIV in the newborn initially and in follow-up and providing ongoing prophylaxis for him or her are extensions of the care started during pregnancy. See Chapter 22 for more information on care of the newborn with HIV.

Sexually Transmitted Infections

As of 2010, the incidence of all three of the reportable STIs—syphilis, gonorrhea, and chlamydia—is increasing. Young women, in particular, account for two

---

● PHARMACOLOGY 13.1   Zidovudine (ZVD)

ACTION

Inhibits retroviral replication, including HIV; helps block maternal–fetal transmission of HIV

PREGNANCY CATEGORY

C

DOSAGE

100 mg 5 times a day from gestational week 14 to onset of labour

POSSIBLE ADVERSE EFFECTS

Nausea and vomiting, headache, skin rash, fatigue, paresthesias

NURSING CONSIDERATIONS

- Ensure that the client schedules and attends regular appointments for monitoring of blood tests.
- Emphasize to the client that she must strictly follow the dosage and administration instructions given to her with the medication.
- Assist the client to manage any nausea that may accompany use of the drug.
- Teach the client that use of zidovudine does not protect against transmitting HIV to others through sexual contact or contaminated blood.

From Karch, A. M. (2005). *2005 Lippincott's nursing drug guide.* Philadelphia, PA: Lippincott Williams & Wilkins.

thirds of the population affected, notably for chlamydia (Public Health Agency of Canada [PHAC], 2010). As discussed in detail in Chapter 4, STIs are most common during the reproductive years. Women have more frequent and more serious complications from STIs than do men (Youngkin et al., 2013). Viral STIs are often difficult to treat; the person may have the virus for the rest of his or her life.

As part of prenatal care, nurses should ask every woman questions about sexual activity, previous STIs, and risk factors for STIs (eg, number of partners). Reviewing the sexual history of a pregnant woman with an STI also is important to help determine any requirements for reporting in her geographic area. Physical examination should include thorough assessment of the perineal area for any warts, malodorous or unusual vaginal discharge, redness, or bleeding.

Treatment of bacterial STIs is tailored to the pregnant woman's situation; follow-up should be implemented during prenatal care. Treatment of viral STIs may not remove the virus; the nurse may need to educate the woman about ongoing safety and preventive health measures.

Planning for screening, treatment, and follow-up for STIs is important during pregnancy. Collaboration with the woman is key to ensuring that she continues to complete preventive measures, treatments, or both. See Table 13.2.

Group B Streptococcus

Incidence of group B streptococcus (GBS) sepsis is 0.64 per 1,000 births (SOGC, 2004b), and GBS is a major cause of neonatal morbidity and mortality (Centers for Disease Control and Prevention, 2005a). In pregnant women, GBS is usually asymptomatic and is present in 15% to 40% of women, but can cause urinary tract infections (UTIs), amnionitis, endometritis, and wound infection (Chandran et al., 2001). Newborn infection results from vertical transmission, making maternal colonization an identifiable risk factor. Other risk factors include preterm labour, birth of a previous infant colonized with GBS, and membranes ruptured longer than 18 hours.

Current recommendations for prenatal care before labour include taking a swab at 35 to 37 weeks' gestation from the vaginal introitus and anorectum of all pregnant women so that results are available during labour (Chandran et al., 2001; SOGC, 2004b). The client who tests positive for GBS has had an infant previously infected with GBS, or who has had documented GBS bacteriuria in the current pregnancy should receive information about the need for intrapartal antibiotics at the time of labour or the rupture of membranes (SOGC, 2012). Penicillin G, 5 million units IV initially, with 2.5 million units IV every 4 hours until birth, is the pre-

ferred treatment. If no swab has been taken, or if the results of testing are unavailable, treatment is based on risk factors during labour: temperature above 37.7°C, rupture of membranes greater than 18 hours, or preterm labour (SOGC, 2004b).

Further education is necessary postpartum. Although the risk for transmission of GBS is highest in the first 24 hours, it persists for up to 7 days following birth. Thus, the nurse should review signs and symptoms of infection with the family before discharge. See Chapter 22 for care of the newborn with GBS.

Rubella

Today, rubella (German or "three-day") measles is rare in Canada; since 2002, fewer than 30 cases have been reported annually (PHAC, 2005). A population-based immunization strategy has effectively decreased the risk of rubella infection during pregnancy. The greatest risk to the developing fetus occurs in the first trimester, when congenital rubella syndrome (CRS) may result. Approximately 25% of affected newborns have tremors, increased irritability, small head size, and hypotonia at birth (Comley & Mousmanis, 2003). By the end of the first year, these children may have psychomotor delays, progressive hearing loss, or visual deficits, with new impairments emerging with development (Comley & Mousmanis, 2003).

Symptoms of rubella infection include a rash that may or may not be itchy, beginning on the face and progressing to the trunk. Transmission is by droplet and may occur up to 7 days before and 7 days after the rash (CDC, 2005b). In adults, lymph node edema, joint pain, and mild fever may accompany the rash.

Screening for rubella immunity is normally part of blood testing completed at the first antenatal visit. Evidence of immunity is determined by the amount of maternal immunoglobulin G (IgG) antibodies. A client with no, or less than adequate, evidence of immunity (based on IgG antibodies in blood) should be told about her status and offered postpartum immunization. She should also be educated about this disease and alerted to take preventive measures for the first 3 months of gestation, so that she may avoid groups of children who may not be immunized.

Toxoplasmosis

Toxoplasma gondii, a protozoan parasite, infects up to one third of the world's population through ingestion or handling undercooked meat (pork and lamb) or handling cat feces (Montoya & Liesenfeld, 2004). In clients infected for the first time while pregnant, the parasite can enter the fetal circulation through the placenta. Positive maternal status before pregnancy poses little or no fetal risks, unless the infection happens close to the time of conception. Early maternal infection tends

● TABLE 13.2 **Infections in Pregnancy and Potential Fetal Effects**

Infection	Potential Fetal Effects	Collaborative Care Considerations
Toxoplasmosis	Neurodevelopmental disabilities related to damage of the central nervous system: severe neurologic or ocular disease (blindness) or cardiac and cerebral anomalies	Assess women for risk for toxoplasmosis and screen only if at risk for *Toxoplasma gondii* infection Caution pregnant women to avoid emptying cat litter boxes or working in soil contaminated with cat feces Remind women to cook all meats thoroughly If acute infection is suspected, test again in 2–3 wk and start therapy with spiramycin immediately If fetal infection has been confirmed, a combination of pyrimethamine, sulfadiazine, and folinic acid should be prescribed (SOGC, 2013b) Monitor newborn for hyperbilirubinemia if sulfonamides are prescribed
Rubella	Teratogenic, particularly to fetal eyes, ears, heart, and brain, resulting in congenital cataracts, deafness, cardiac anomalies, mental and motor deficits, congenital cleft lip and cleft palate, intrauterine growth restriction	Remind all pregnant women to avoid contact with children who have rashes; reinfection is possible in women with rubella antibodies Review results of antepartal rubella titer; provide counselling about results and possible implications Assess fetal biophysical profile and ultrasound findings Give postpartal vaccination to women who do not demonstrate immunity to rubella with cautions to avoid conception within 1 mo of vaccination Take specimens for culture from newborn's nose and throat Isolate newborn from other newborns in the nursery Assess for evidence of congenital anomalies Provide supportive and restorative care measures Teach specialized feeding techniques for cleft lip and palate Promote attachment and bonding
Syphilis	Possible fetal demise; if infection persists beyond 18 wks' gestation, cognitive deficits and orthopedic deformities (osteochondritis) Congenital syphilis	Perform VDRL on initial antepartal visit with immediate antibiotic therapy if indicated Give instructions regarding safer sex practices Monitor newborn for rash, obstructed nasal breathing, and excessive nasal secretions Give immediate antibiotic therapy and follow-up care to newborn
Cytomegalovirus (CMV)	Severe disability; damage to cranial nerves leading to blindness; deafness and hepatic dysfunction from transplacental exposure; exposure during vaginal birth or from contaminated breast milk; serious only in very low–birth-weight newborns	Detect maternal infection (asymptomatic) with CMV-IgG and IgM by ELISA testing. Routine testing for CMV in newborns is not performed, although antibodies may be isolated in maternal or newborn serum for diagnosis Provide antepartal teaching to avoid exposure Perform meticulous handwashing before meals and avoid contact with young children in crowds such as nursery schools or daycare settings (to reduce risk for droplet transmission)
Herpes simplex virus type 2 (HSV-2)	Congenital herpes virus infection from transplacental inoculation with vesicles at birth or infection during birth when vulvar lesion present Infection leading to encephalitis, convulsions, shock, and death Neurologic damage in newborn survivors	Plan for cesarean rather than vaginal birth if woman has active herpes lesions. Assess newborn for oral ulcerations and skin lesions (pinpoint clustered vesicles surrounded by erythema). Monitor for onset of birth-acquired infection, such as poor feeding, fever, and lethargy preceding eruption of skin lesions Administer prescribed antiviral agent acyclovir (Zovirax) Restrict newborn handling or feeding if active lesions present. Restrict health care providers with fever blisters or cold sores from nursery because of the severity of infection and the high risk for neurologic sequelae in the newborn

(table continues on page 490)

● **TABLE 13.2** **Infections in Pregnancy and Potential Fetal Effects** (continued)

Infection	Potential Fetal Effects	Collaborative Care Considerations
Gonorrhea	Severe eye infection resulting from conjunctival inoculation of *Neisseria gonorrhoeae* during vaginal birth (ophthalmia neonatorum) Blindness (if untreated) from corneal damage	Ensure early antepartal diagnosis; treat with penicillin or ceftriaxone (Rocephin) Give neonatal eye prophylaxis at birth Assess newborns born outside the hospital for fiery red conjunctiva and thick yellow crusting exudate from the eyes; treat with IV antibiotics and topical antibiotic ointment. Use sterile normal saline eye irrigations for thick suppuration
Hepatitis B virus (HBV)	Hepatitis B infection with potential for becoming a chronic carrier	Promptly wipe contaminated blood and secretions from the newborn after birth. Perform gentle nasal and oropharyngeal suction to avoid a break in mucous membranes, which could provide the entry route for inoculation of the virus Give first dose of HBV vaccine within 12 h of birth to prevent future HBV infection. Ensure use of chlorhexadine to prepare injection site if giving immunization prior to bathing infant Give immune serum globulin to infants of mothers testing positive for HBV. Ensure skin is prepared with chlorhexadine swab prior to giving injection if infant has not yet been bathed
Chlamydia	Eye infection from conjunctival inoculation during vaginal birth	Administer bilateral eye prophylaxis at birth with erythromycin ophthalmic ointment Assess newborns born outside the hospital for edema and erythema of the eyelids and purulent exudates Give systemic antibiotic therapy as prescribed for the newborn, mother, and mother's sexual contacts
Candidiasis	Thrush (oral *Monilia*)	Assess newborn for white-coated tongue resembling milk curds; scrape from the tongue to reveal red, raw patches Observe for poor feeding or signs of oral pain when suckling. Give prompt and aggressive topical antifungal therapy with nystatin to prevent systemic infection; application to lesions of the oral mucosa, the buccal space, or the tongue; ensuring contact with the lesion rather than allowing the infant to suck and swallow directly from the dropper Give antifungal treatment to mother and her sexual contacts to prevent reinfection
Human immunodeficiency virus (HIV)	Possible HIV infection resulting from placental transmission, perinatal exposure, or breast milk	Give antepartal zidovudine therapy to reduce placental transfer of virus to fetus. Counsel mother not to risk exposure through breast-feeding Reassure mother that because of transfer of antibodies through the placenta, all newborns will test positive for HIV, but this does not mean that the disease is present Treat toddlers who remain positive after 18 mo old with long-term strategies to support nutrition and prevent opportunistic illness
Group B streptococcus (GBS)	Early onset (day of birth): rapidly progressing pneumonia and respiratory distress Late onset (2–4 wk): meningitis, intracranial pressure, bulging fontanels; neurologic deficits in survivors	Ensure that health care providers practice strict hand washing between caring for newborns Administer IV antibiotic therapy (penicillin) during labour 4 or more hours before birth Monitor newborn blood cultures following prolonged rupture of membranes, if no prophylaxis Give antibiotic therapy to newborns of mothers who are GBS positive, if symptomatic and no prophylaxis

to result in severe congenital toxoplasmosis, including severe neurologic or ocular disease as well as cardiac and cerebral anomalies. With late maternal exposure, the newborn appears normal but may have a subclinical infection (Montoya & Liesenfeld, 2004). The incidence of congenital toxoplasmosis ranges from 1 to 10 per 10,000 births (Montoya & Liesenfeld, 2004).

Routine universal screening is not recommended. Identification of high-risk women such as those who are immunosuppressed or HIV positive is important for inclusion of screening as part of their initial prenatal bloodwork (SOGC, 2013b). Providing instructions to all women in pregnancy about cooking meat thoroughly, avoiding the handling of cat feces, and using gloves while gardening outdoors is important health promotion (Montoya & Liesenfeld, 2004). Treatment with spiramycin should be initiated as quickly as possible if diagnosis of recently acquired maternal infection is found, together with ongoing follow-up, including ultrasound assessment of the fetus and information and education for the woman and family.

Cytomegalovirus

Cytomegalovirus (CMV) is the most common cause of congenital infection leading to neurologic impairment (Damato & Winnen, 2002). The illness acquired during gestation can result in stillbirth or spontaneous abortion, IUGR, congenital anomalies, or other infections. In some cases, affected infants appear asymptomatic at birth but develop progressive sensorineural problems, including hearing impairment. The greatest risks to the pregnant woman include contact with infected children in daycare centres or health care settings. Frequent hand washing is encouraged in these environments. No treatment exists for CMV; thus, nurses should encourage women to practice sound hygiene while pregnant. Another nursing role may be to provide supportive counselling to clients if ultrasound or other diagnostic testing reveals sequelae of congenital CMV infection.

Parvovirus

Parvovirus B19 is the smallest DNA-containing virus that infects mammalian cells (White, 2003). Infection with parvovirus B19 (fifth disease or erythema infectiosum) is common among young children, particularly from March to May (Fig. 13.7). Transmission occurs by inhaled particles, hand-to-mouth contact, contaminated blood, and transplacental transfer. Symptoms include headache, fever, malaise, gastrointestinal upset, sore throat, and cough. The distinctive rash, described as "slapped cheek," has a red appearance against relatively pale skin, usually appearing on the face before spreading to the trunk and limbs and fading in colour. Approximately 50% to 65% of women of reproductive age are immune from prior infection; therefore, incidence in

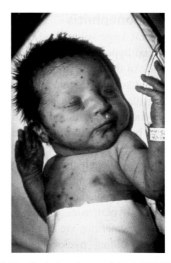

FIGURE 13.7 An infant born with congenital rubella.

pregnancy is decreased (SOGC, 2002a; White, 2003). Adults who contract the disease may describe joint pain, particularly in the hand and wrist.

Pregnant women who contract this infection transmit it to their fetuses in up to 30% of cases (Goff, 2005; White, 2003). Complications can include spontaneous abortion, fetal anemia, and fetal nonimmune hydrops (Goff, 2005; SOGC, 2002b). Clients with symptoms or history of exposure should have blood work that includes serology, IgG, and IgM (enzyme-linked immunosorbent assay [ELISA] and indirect fluorescent antibody [IFA]). Serial ultrasounds may assist in a diagnosis of hydrops; if so, the pregnant woman should be referred to an obstetrician and a tertiary care centre for management of this high-risk fetus (White, 2003).

RENAL AND URINARY PROBLEMS

During pregnancy, kidney volume, weight, and size increase, as do dilation of the ureters and renal calyces as a result of hormonal influences and obstruction by the enlarging uterus. The obstructive effect, along with urinary stasis, predisposes pregnant women to UTIs, pyelonephritis, and symptomatic infections from vesicoureteral reflux. It is also possible for bacteria from the gastrointestinal area to contaminate the perineal area.

Renal blood flow increases during gestation 70% to 85% (Thorsen & Poole, 2002). Other renal adaptations in pregnancy include changes in protein excretion, tubular function, acid–base regulation, and osmoregulation. These developments are reflected in laboratory test results; for example, protein excretion can reach an upper limit of 300 mg/day (the usual normal limit is 150 mg/day). Awareness of such pregnancy-related variations is vital to be able to quickly recognize and address abnormalities (see Chapter 12).

UTIs and Pyelonephritis

During pregnancy, large volumes of urine may remain in the ureters and hypotonic bladder. Glucose, protein, and amino acids in the urine provide an ideal environment for bacterial growth. Edema and hyperemia of the bladder mucosa also increase susceptibility to infection in pregnant women. The static column of urine in the ureters leads to bacterial migration (Blackburn, 2013). Asymptomatic bacteriuria develops in 2% to 10% of pregnant women. Although this number is similar to rates in nonpregnant women, significant complications can develop during pregnancy, such as preterm birth, low birth weight, hypertension, and maternal anemia. A further 3% of pregnancies are complicated by symptomatic UTIs, including pyelonephritis and cystitis (Thorsen & Poole, 2002).

All health care providers for pregnant women should be alert to the possibility of asymptomatic and symptomatic UTIs. Describing symptoms to be aware of (eg, urinary burning and frequency) during the first prenatal visit can help pregnant women recognize differences between UTI and normal pregnancy changes. Testing urine at every prenatal visit is crucial. The most common method of assessment is urinalysis by dipstick (Thorsen & Poole, 2002). The one exception may be the client with hypertension who should have a dipstick test, followed by 24-hour urine collection if the urinary protein level is greater than 1+. A woman with underlying renal disease should have a baseline 24-hour urine collection that may be continued with serial 24-hour tests to determine renal involvement. Diagnosis of asymptomatic bacteriuria is based on a midstream urine collection that reveals at least 100,000 colonies/mL of a single organism. The most common bacterium isolated is *Escherichia coli*.

Treatment of UTIs in pregnant women may include ampicillin if *E. coli* is identified as the causative organism. High-dose antibiotics usually are required because of the increased excretion that stems from increased renal blood flow (Gilbert, 2011). Reculturing at the end of therapy is important to ensure that the infection has cleared. If necessary, treatment can be reinitiated up to two more times. An antimicrobial agent (eg, nitrofurantoin) may be prescribed if ampicillin is ineffective. Discussion of hygiene that includes wiping from front to back after urination and sexual intercourse, extra fluid intake, and cotton underwear is important.

The most common symptoms of pyelonephritis include costovertebral angle tenderness, high fever, chills, myalgia, nausea, and vomiting. Maternal temperature typically "spikes" and then falls to normal or even hypothermic levels. These symptoms should prompt a urinalysis that typically shows numerous leukocytes and bacteria. A complete blood count usually shows a significantly increased leukocyte count with a left shift. Treatment includes admitting the client to the health care facility and beginning generalized IV antibiotic therapy until results from culture and sensitivity are available. Once results are known, drug therapy is individualized to the client's illness. If there is no response within 24 hours of therapy, blood cultures should be drawn to ensure that sepsis has not developed. IV therapy should continue until 24 to 48 hours after temperature is normal and right-sided tenderness has resolved. Oral antibiotics can then continue for 10 to 14 days as ordered (Thorsen & Poole, 2002). Ongoing assessment of urine by urinalysis, dipstick, or both throughout the rest of pregnancy is essential to prevent recurrences.

Acute Renal Failure

The rate of live births to women with a history of renal disease ranges between 64% and 98%, depending on the severity (Ramin et al., 2006). Acute renal failure may occur in clients with a prepregnancy diagnosis of renal disease, from a pregnancy-associated event such as gestational hypertension or preeclampsia, or from a nonpregnancy-associated problem such as trauma (Thorsen & Poole, 2002). Clients who experience acute renal failure have a sudden decrease in renal function, with an increased serum creatinine level and oliguria.

Management of the pregnant client with acute renal failure requires a collaborative approach to protect maternal health and fetal well-being. Determining the ability of the health care facility to manage this woman's care and to transfer her appropriately as needed is vital. A thorough health history and physical examination are important. Decreased intake (eg, hyperemesis gravidarum, laxative use with eating disorders) or diarrhea can lead to volume depletion and increased risk for acute renal failure. Hypertension and concealed hemorrhage also are risk factors. Assessment of vital signs is critical to evaluate maternal well-being. For example, increased blood pressure readings may indicate fluid overload. Increased pulse and respiratory rate may precede pulmonary edema. Maternal pulse oximetry is appropriate, as indicated by the woman's clinical condition. Fatigue, malaise, irritation, and disorientation may be seen. Laboratory testing may include complete blood count, coagulation profile, and electrolytes. A 24-hour urine collection should be started. Evaluation of hemoglobin is necessary to ensure that the client does not develop anemia from decreased erythropoietin production. Awareness of symptoms of anemia (ie, shortness of breath, easy fatigue, impaired fetal growth) can help monitor for this condition.

Fetal monitoring through NST and fetal movement counts also is mandatory. Ultrasound imaging of the kidneys may be required to assist with a diagnosis. If diuretics are used as treatment, monitoring of electrolyte levels is extremely important (Gilbert, 2011).

DIABETES MELLITUS

As discussed in Chapter 4, various types of diabetes mellitus affect women. In type 1 (10% to 20% of cases), pancreatic β-cells are destroyed gradually or suddenly, and the client requires administration of insulin to stay alive (Kozak, 2002). In type 2 (80% to 90% of cases), the client has abnormal insulin secretion as well as insulin resistance. Hereditary and environmental factors are involved in the development of both conditions.

Women with type 1 or type 2 diabetes who become pregnant require adaptations to manage their condition and their pregnancy successfully. Ideally, these clients plan their pregnancy carefully with health care team members at a high-risk pregnancy clinic. The goal is to maintain or achieve "ideal" blood glucose control to decrease the risk for congenital anomalies, fetal macrosomia, and spontaneous abortion (see Chapters 16 and 22). A woman with type 1 or 2 diabetes will need to alter her treatment during pregnancy to reflect changes in insulin requirements, assessment for retinal and renal disease, and glucose monitoring. Careful follow-up by a multidisciplinary team throughout pregnancy in preparation for labour and birth is essential.

In **gestational diabetes mellitus (GDM)**, a woman develops or recognizes carbohydrate intolerance for the first time during pregnancy. Approximately 4% of Canadian pregnant women experience GDM, which varies in severity for each client (Canadian Diabetes Association [CDA], 2013). Risk factors include previous history of GDM, previous birth of a large-for-gestational-age infant, history of stillbirth or spontaneous abortion, family history of type 2 diabetes, obesity, age over 35 years, BMI over 30, multiple pregnancy, and hypertension. High-risk ethnic groups include Aboriginals, Hispanics, Pacific Islanders, and South or East Asian people (Kozak, 2002; SOGC, 2002b). Studies related to the prevalence of GDM among Aboriginal women in Canada have shown regional rates of 8% to 18% (excluding those with pre-existing diabetes) (CDA, 2013).

Current recommendations are for all pregnant women to undergo screening for gestational diabetes between 24 and 28 weeks' gestation and screening to be offered at any time during pregnancy to women with risk factors for GDM (CDA, 2013). This screening is done with a 1-hour plasma glucose measurement following a 50-g glucose load given at any time of the day. A result greater than 11.1 mmol/L confirms gestational diabetes. A result between 7.8 and 11.1 mmol/L is an indication for the woman to undergo a 75-g oral glucose tolerance test (Fig. 13.8).

An additional recommendation is to screen those at high risk at any stage in the pregnancy. This would include those whose maternal age is greater than 35, BMI over 30 kg/m², previous diagnosis of GDM,

previous birth of a large–for-gestational-age infant, and member of an at-risk population, for example Aboriginal (CDA, 2013).

Regardless of the type of diabetes involved, the risk for congenital anomalies in infants born to mothers with diabetes is higher than in the general population (4% to 11% vs. 2% to 3%) (Kozak, 2002). Maintaining strict glucose control throughout pregnancy decreases this risk. During labour and birth, diabetes increases both maternal and fetal risks, including gestational hypertension, shoulder dystocia, polyhydramnios, and need for cesarean or operative birth (see Chapter 16). Early childhood obesity, development of metabolic syndrome in early childhood, and type 2 diabetes are also associated with maternal GDM and there is double the risk for these children as compared with the general population (Kendrick, 2011).

Think back to Keyla, the 23-year-old client pregnant for the first time. What risk factors would the nurse identify when placing Keyla at increased risk for gestational diabetes? When during pregnancy would she be most appropriately screened?

COLLABORATIVE CARE: DIABETES IN PREGNANCY

Pregnant women with diabetes may develop complications. A team approach is necessary to involve them and their families in management of the condition, promotion of health, prevention of hospitalization, and control of any complications. Balancing pregnancy and diabetes is stressful. The woman may have financial concerns related to the supplies required for monitoring. Learning about diabetes, planning meals, and testing blood glucose levels can be emotionally and physically taxing. Risks for other problems, such as gestational hypertension, polyhydramnios, UTI, intrapartal trauma, retinopathy, and depression, are increased. Health care providers need to be aware of such complications and constantly monitor for them (Kozak, 2002). Women who maintain euglycemia during pregnancy and labour seem to be at a decreased risk for complications (SOGC, 2002b).

Treatment during pregnancy includes dietary counselling and review, glucose monitoring instruction, and insulin therapy. Normally, an endocrinologist and obstetrician are members of the client's team. Others involved may include social workers, community nutrition and diabetic clinic staff, and public health nurses. In some cases, fetal size or gestational age (38 to 39 weeks) leads to a decision to induce labour (see Chapter 16). Such a choice is based on indicators of fetal well-being as monitored through assessment of fetal lung maturity and

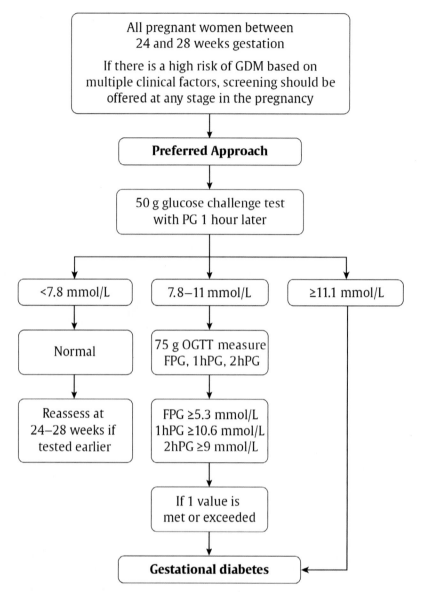

FIGURE 13.8 Screening guidelines for gestational diabetes mellitus (GDM). Canadian Diabetes Association Clinical Practice Guidelines Expert Committee. (2013). Chapter 36: Diabetes and pregnancy. Canadian Journal of Diabetes.

a nonstress test. Care in labour and birth must be ongoing; including the client and family in activities such as self-monitoring glucose during labour or consulting an endocrinologist can facilitate involvement and continuity. Level of care required during labour and birth depends on whether the client was taking insulin before labour and her blood glucose levels during labour.

Assessment

Assessment of the pregnant client with pre-existing diabetes includes type, onset, duration, and treatment. The nurse reviews a history of any complications such as retinopathy, neuropathy, or cardiovascular disease. He or she explores the client's support systems, dietary understanding, stress levels, motivation, and coping methods. The woman should undergo a glycosylated hemoglobin test (HbA1 c) to reveal her glucose control over the previous 3 months. Additional tests include serum creatinine and urinalysis for microalbumin.

The client diagnosed with gestational diabetes who is 24 to 28 weeks' pregnant requires immediate intervention from a diabetic care team. Their assessment includes reviewing support systems, nutrition and diet, coping strategies, family history, lifestyle, and genetics (CDA, 2013).

For cases of both pre-existing and gestational diabetes, careful nursing assessment on admission to the birthing unit includes review of pregnancy history, diabetes management, support systems, cultural differences (which may give clues about stress and anxiety levels), and results of screening tests (eg, urine, blood glucose levels). Recording her insulin therapy during pregnancy and last dose, if appropriate, would be important, as would her last oral intake.

Evaluation every hour for maternal hyperglycemia should be ongoing during labour and birth. The goal in labour is to prevent neonatal hypoglycemia. Insulin requirements decrease in labour while at the same time there are high maternal glucose requirements. Signs and symptoms of maternal hyperglycemia include shakiness, dizziness, sweating, clumsy or jerky movements, hunger, headache, pale skin colour, and confusion. Assessment of fetal well-being depends on institutional policy but usually includes intermittent auscultation or continuous electronic fetal monitoring, depending on the severity of the diabetes and risk to the fetus (SOGC, 2007a).

Select Potential Nursing Diagnosis

The following are examples of commonly applicable nursing diagnoses in cases of diabetes in pregnancy:

- **Anxiety** related to maternal and fetal health with diabetes and pregnancy
- **Deficient Knowledge** related to new medical diagnosis
- **Risk for Ineffective Health Maintenance** related to a new diagnosis of diabetes or previous diagnosis together with pregnancy
- **Imbalanced Nutrition: Risk for More Than Body Requirements** related to an inability to assess diet in initial stages of diet planning
- **Ineffective Coping** related to stress of managing pregnancy and diabetes

Planning/Intervention

Reviewing Blood Glucose Self-Monitoring and Urine Testing

During pregnancy, the nurse assists the client to review or to learn techniques of blood glucose monitoring (Fig. 13.9). The client needs to self-assess her blood glucose level 4 to 7 times a day (postprandial and preprandial) using an accurate monitor; she needs to record results on a written log or as electronic data that allow for easy tracking of patterns that can be reviewed by the clinic. Risk for nocturnal hypoglycemia is increased, so testing during the night may be required. The nurse should provide guidelines for findings that mandate communication with the diabetic team. Nursing Care Plan 13.1 highlights some key aspects of nursing care.

Because starvation ketosis is common in pregnancy, assessing urine regularly for presence of ketones is important (CDA, 2013).

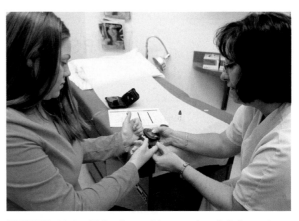

FIGURE 13.9 This client with gestational diabetes is learning techniques for self-monitoring of blood glucose levels.

Promoting Diet Management

Dietary management is extremely important when pregnancy and diabetes coexist. A dietician can assist with individualizing meals to ensure tight blood glucose control, appropriate weight gain, and adequate nutrition. Together, the nurse and dietician should consider the client's cultural and socioeconomic status when assisting her to plan meals. A diet with 2,000 to 2,500 cal/day spaced over three meals and three snacks meets the needs of most women in their second and third trimesters. The care team generally tries to structure maternal weight gain to be approximately 1 to 3 kg in the first trimester and 0.2 kg/week for the remainder of gestation (CDA, 2013; Kozak, 2002).

Encouraging Activity and Exercise

A physiotherapist may help to assess a client's history of exercise and tailor a program to meet her needs for energy balance. Walking, swimming, biking, and housecleaning should be encouraged. Good posture, positioning, and body mechanics for lifting and decreasing stress on joints (eg, the pelvic area) are important (Kozak, 2002).

Administering Insulin

Women with type 1, type 2, or gestational diabetes may require insulin during pregnancy. Some clients just starting insulin find injecting themselves difficult and require support and encouragement. The nurse reviews equipment, type of insulin, and injection tool (pen, needle) with the client and then goes over the details a second time for the client to practice.

Clients who take insulin need to be aware of their risk for hypoglycemia (abnormally low blood glucose), why it happens, when it can occur, how to prevent it, and how to treat it. They may need to have glucagon with them at all times in case of a hypoglycemic episode.

(text continues on page 499)

NURSING CARE PLAN 13.1

●

The Client With Gestational Diabetes

 The results of Keyla's screening test for gestational diabetes are positive. Her primary care provider prescribes a special diet and blood glucose self-monitoring. Keyla states, "I'm in shock. How will this affect my baby? And what if I need shots?"

NURSING DIAGNOSES

- **Deficient Knowledge** related to disease process, treatment, and effects on pregnancy and fetus
- **Anxiety** related to uncertainty about insulin therapy and possible effects on fetal outcome

EXPECTED OUTCOMES

1. The client will demonstrate an understanding of gestational diabetes and treatment.
2. The client will verbalize effects of diabetes on pregnancy and fetus.
3. The client will report less anxiety related to the condition and pregnancy.

INTERVENTIONS	RATIONALES
Assess the client's knowledge of gestational diabetes and associated risks.	Assessment provides a baseline from which to develop an individualized teaching plan.
Explore the client's exposure to diabetes, including gestational diabetes; correct any misconceptions related to experiences of family/friends; provide time for questions.	Information provides an additional foundation for teaching and opportunities to clarify misinformation.
Review the client's history for risk factors, such as previous birth of an LGA infant and family history of type 2 diabetes.	Identification provides a basis for developing appropriate measures to reduce the risk associated with these factors.
Review the physiologic mechanisms underlying gestational diabetes; teach the client about various treatment options.	Education promotes understanding and participation in care.
Work with the client to develop an appropriate plan for activity and exercise, based on her preferences and ability.	Activity and exercise assist glucose control. A client-tailored program enhances the chances for compliance. Collaboration fosters cooperation and feelings of control.
Review the client's dietary program, including the need for evenly spaced meals and snacks throughout the day. Consider ethnically appropriate nutritional intake in her dietary program. Monitor weight at each visit.	Well-timed intake of food prevents wide fluctuations in blood glucose levels. Weight monitoring provides a means for evaluating the client's adherence to the diet and fetal growth and development.

(continued)

NURSING CARE PLAN 13.1 ● The Client With Gestational Diabetes *(Continued)*

INTERVENTIONS	RATIONALES
Teach the client how to perform blood glucose self-monitoring; have her return-demonstrate the skill. Urge her to check and to record blood glucose levels as ordered. Tell the client to notify the health care provider promptly if levels are outside established parameters or if she needs help obtaining supplies.	Blood glucose self-monitoring with documentation provides objective data to evaluate glucose control. Levels outside of established parameters may indicate the need for adjustments to the regimen.
Teach the signs and symptoms of hypoglycemia to the client taking exogenous insulin, including factors contributing to its development and measures to treat it. Instruct the client to check blood glucose levels if she develops any signs and symptoms.	Early identification and prompt intervention for hypoglycemia reduce the risk for injury to the client and her fetus.
Evaluate the client's past coping strategies to determine which have been most effective.	Use of appropriate coping strategies aids in reducing anxiety.
Encourage the client to include her partner in follow-up visits.	Participation of the client's partner promotes sharing, provides support to the client, and enhances the chances for a successful experience.
Question the client about available support systems, such as family, friends, and community resources. Enlist the aid of social services as necessary to assist with possible stressors such as supplies, financial concerns, and child care.	Stress can upset blood glucose control. Additional sources of support are helpful in alleviating anxiety.
Provide information about support groups, Web sites, and other resources related to gestational diabetes, pregnancy, and fetal health.	Shared experiences and knowledge of similar situations can prepare the client for what to expect.
Discuss health promotion, such as influenzae vaccination, handwashing, and adequate rest/sleep.	Illness can increase the blood glucose levels. Regular handwashing, clean food handling, and strategies such as influenzae vaccination can help decrease the possibility of illness.

EVALUATION

1. The client describes gestational diabetes and its effect on pregnancy.
2. The client identifies the role of measures used to control gestational diabetes.
3. The client demonstrates a beginning ability to perform blood glucose self-monitoring.
4. The client shows use of positive coping measures to reduce anxiety level.

(continued)

NURSING CARE PLAN 13.1 ● The Client With Gestational Diabetes *(Continued)*

NURSING DIAGNOSIS

Risk for Injury (maternal and fetal) related to effects of diabetes on pregnancy

EXPECTED OUTCOMES

1. The client will verbalize the need for glucose control during pregnancy.
2. The client will maintain blood glucose levels within acceptable parameters.
3. The client will demonstrate progression of pregnancy with fetal growth and development appropriate for gestational age.

INTERVENTIONS	RATIONALES
Assess maternal status at each visit; monitor vital signs, including blood pressure. Reinforce the need for more frequent follow-up during pregnancy.	Ongoing assessment is essential for early identification of potential problems. Gestational diabetes increases risks for gestational hypertension. Frequent follow-up provides multiple opportunities to assess maternal and fetal well-being.
Measure fundal height at each visit; prepare the client for diagnostic and laboratory testing. Monitor fetal heart rate.	Fundal height provides an estimation of fetal growth. Diagnostic and laboratory testing provides information about maternal and fetal well-being. Fetal heart rate is an indicator of fetal well-being.
Review blood glucose levels for fluctuations. Expect to include insulin administration if blood glucose levels are outside established parameters. Instruct the client in administration and related care.	Strict blood glucose control is necessary to prevent fetal macrosomia. Insulin may be necessary to maintain blood glucose control.
Assess for signs and symptoms of hypoglycemia, if insulin is necessary. Instruct the client in measures to control hypoglycemia.	Untreated hypoglycemia poses a danger to the mother and fetus.
Prepare the client for necessary fetal surveillance, such as biophysical profiles and nonstress testing, especially during the third trimester. Teach her how to perform fetal kick counts.	Fetal surveillance provides information about fetal well-being, aids in early detection of possible complications, and promptly enables any necessary intervention.
Discuss care that may be required during labour and birth.	Discussion helps the client prepare for labour and birth and provides a baseline for additional teaching once labour starts.
Reinforce the need for client adherence to the treatment regimen and follow-up.	Adherence and follow-up enhance the chances for a successful outcome.

EVALUATION

1. The client demonstrates understanding of glucose control measures.
2. The client exhibits acceptable blood glucose levels.
3. The client progresses through pregnancy without complications.
4. The fetus demonstrates gestational age–appropriate growth and development.

Screening tests indicate that Keyla has gestational diabetes. As part of the treatment plan, she is to perform blood glucose self-monitoring 4 times a day. She says, "My mother only tests her blood twice a day. Why do I have to do it four times a day?" How should the nurse respond?

Monitoring the Fetus

Intensive fetal monitoring begins toward the end of pregnancy (third trimester) and may include fetal movement counting, ultrasound evaluation, nonstress test, and Doppler studies. These evaluations all are done to reduce the risk for trauma, stillbirth, or both.

Providing Care During Labour and Birth

The woman who comes to the birthing unit with preterm labour and receives corticosteroids to enhance fetal lung maturity (usually 12 to 24 hours between doses) requires increased insulin for 2 days. An explanation of this treatment as well as the interaction between corticosteroids and diabetes should be provided.

During labour, the goal of insulin therapy is to maintain blood glucose concentrations of 4 to 7 mmol/L (Canadian Diabetes Association, 2013) to decrease the risk for neonatal hypoglycemia (Gilbert, 2011). Insulin needs commonly decrease at the beginning of labour and fall to zero during the active phase. Maternal glucose requirements are 2.5 mg/kg/min. Her blood glucose levels should be monitored hourly. IV insulin may be administered as 50 units of regular insulin in 250 mL of NS, with the line flushed with 25 mL to decrease the insulin-binding capacity to plastic surfaces (Gilbert, 2011). The insulin solution should be maintained on an infusion pump while piggybacked to a main IV line to ensure the woman's safety.

Areas that require careful monitoring include the progress of labour (increased risk for prolonged labour from fetal macrosomia), maternal temperature every 1 to 4 hours, vital signs hourly, and continuous fetal health surveillance by electronic monitoring, depending on institutional policy. Urine should be assessed for ketones at every void or every 4 hours if the woman has an indwelling catheter. Intake and output should be evaluated hourly (Gilbert, 2011). Assessment for hypoglycemia during labour and birth should be ongoing.

Evaluation

Any type of diabetes in pregnancy increases maternal and fetal risks. Ongoing involvement from a team of specialists is essential to ensure maximum maternal and fetal health. The goals are fetal and maternal well-being throughout pregnancy, labour, and birth as evidenced by consistently normal blood glucose levels, normal fetal monitoring results, and coordinated multidisciplinary care.

PSYCHOSOCIAL DISORDERS AND PROBLEMS

Chapter 5 includes discussion of mental health and mental illness during the adolescent and adult years in detail. The following sections explore the effects of some common psychiatric problems when they develop or coincide with pregnancy. Postpartum psychiatric illnesses are explored in detail in Chapter 19.

Depression in Pregnancy

It is now known that the prevalence of depression in the antenatal period is similar to that during the first 6 months after birth (Flynn et al., 2006; Milgrom et al., 2008). However, prenatal depression is not always recognized, as many discomforts of pregnancy can be similar to depression and there is a tendency to attribute pregnancy hormones as the primary cause for any emotional changes (Brown & Solchany, 2004). As well, the stigma associated with depression and society's expectation of happiness during a pregnancy may cause a woman to underreport the symptoms of sadness and irritability she may be experiencing (Marcus, 2009). Major depression is a cluster of signs and symptoms that include at least five or more of the following that last for at least 2 weeks:

- Mood changes, usually sadness, anxiety, or irritability
- Negative changes in sleep patterns (eg, insomnia)
- Appetite changes
- Weight changes
- Change in activity levels
- Fatigue
- Decreased motivation
- Decreased interest in other things, life in general, or both
- Decreased libido
- Decreased ability to concentrate, usually with a shortened attention span
- Feelings of helplessness and worthlessness
- Thoughts of dying (American Psychiatric Association, 2000)

Depression is associated more commonly with the postpartum period (see Chapter 19); however, women can experience depression anytime in life, including pregnancy. A milder form of depression, dysthymia, is described as a loss of enthusiasm or joy and ongoing fatigue (Dietch & Bunney, 2002). See Chapter 5.

All women of childbearing age should be made aware of the signs and symptoms of depression. For pregnant women, open-ended questions to ask, particularly during the first prenatal visit, include the following:

• What changes have you noticed about how you feel lately?
• What changes have you noticed about how you have been behaving lately?
• How are these changes affecting you personally? Your family?
• How do these changes make you feel? (Dietch & Bunney, 2002)

These questions may lead to a discussion of particular signs and symptoms, especially changes in appetite, eating, sleep, and mood. Further assessment using the Edinburgh Postnatal Depression Scale (EPDS), which is specific to the perinatal period, would be appropriate as needed (Marcus, 2009).

A careful history both of the pregnancy and factors causing stress or low self-esteem is important for individualizing the care plan. Counselling, whether individual or group, is crucial to assist with review of symptoms, build on maternal strengths, and assist in developing self-esteem and interpersonal relationships (Dietch & Bunney, 2002). Behavioural therapy also may be an option; it involves completing a series of tasks to facilitate changes, enhance self-esteem, and improve problem-solving skills. Peer support groups have shown to be beneficial for women experiencing prenatal depression (Field et al., 2013).

Pharmacology may include tricyclic antidepressants, monoamine oxidase inhibitors (MAOIs), or selective serotonin reuptake inhibitors (SSRIs). Side effects include decreased appetite, nausea, decreased deep sleep, and drowsiness (Dietch & Bunney, 2002). The nurse should review these side effects during client teaching if pharmacology is part of the treatment plan. Treatment, whether counseling and/or pharmacology, is important because untreated or undertreated depression may lead to inadequate weight gain, increased substance use, and underutilization of prenatal care (Marcus, 2009). The nurse should discuss with the client and her family the risks versus benefits of using pharmacologic treatment for depression in pregnancy. The woman's support person(s) are critical to whether she identifies her symptoms as depression rather than hormonal influences of pregnancy and her decision to seek treatment and its value to her and their family. Providing information to and including support people in screening is helpful for women and their ongoing care (Henshaw et al., 2013). Collaborative approaches should explore such options as counselling and increased prenatal visits. Assisting the client to evaluate areas of stress and offering counselling to her partner and family also may be appropriate.

Bipolar Disorder

Bipolar disorder affects approximately 1% of the general population in Canada, and is characterized by cyclical patterns of depression and mania (Yatham et al., 2009). Clients usually are in their teens or early adulthood at onset of bipolar illness, putting them at risk during their reproductive years. Rapid cycling and depressive characteristics are more common in women than in men with this problem (Yonkers et al., 2004).

Review of the health history of the pregnant woman with bipolar illness should include her prior response to medications, the severity of her illness, the duration of normal mood with and without medications, the time between episodes when she has discontinued medications, and recovery with pharmacotherapy (Yonkers et al., 2004). A client with a stable condition may be able to stop taking medications for some time before conception and during the first trimester, to decrease the risk for teratogenic effects. Discontinuation of maintenance pharmacologic treatment, however, may lead to relapse, particularly if withdrawal is abrupt and not tapered (Yonkers et al., 2004). Before conception, the client and health care provider may test the stability of the woman's condition by tapering medication slowly and closely monitoring for symptoms. Should symptoms manifest, the client and provider may decide that remaining on medication during pregnancy is the best plan.

Ongoing pharmacotherapy may be necessary if the client has a tendency to self-harm, protracted recovery time, impaired insight, or lack of sufficient support systems (Yonkers et al., 2004). The risk for fetal malformations depends on the properties of the specific medication involved and when in gestation the drugs are taken. In planning treatment, it is critical to minimize risks to both mother and fetus while also limiting maternal morbidity from an active phase of bipolar disorder. An informed choice, together with prenatal care given by both an obstetrician and psychiatric specialist, is important.

For the woman who continues to take medications during pregnancy, the lowest effective dose must be used, with consideration given to those drugs that have the least teratogenic potential (Yonkers et al., 2004). Older agents with case and cohort data (research evidence for use during pregnancy) should be tried and evaluated first. Fetal screening and assessment should be part of the client's care plan. Lithium, valproate, or olanzapine may be used during pregnancy.

Intimate-Partner Violence

Intimate-partner violence is defined as "someone using power over another person to try to harm that person, or to exert control that will harm that person either immediately, or eventually if repeated over time" (Health Canada, 1999). Intimate-partner violence affecting women of childbearing age is unique among individuals experiencing violence, because outcomes are not only experienced by the woman but also affect her fetus during pregnancy and her newborn after birth (Records, 2007). Intimate-partner violence may be physical, emotional, verbal, financial, or sexual. Clients who report the highest rates of violence are typically in their childbearing years (15 to 45 years old) (Watts, 2004). Aboriginal women in Canada are at risk for violence and experience a disproportionately high rate of sexual and physical abuse (SOGC, 2013a). The ongoing pattern of control may include physical or sexual violence or threats, emotional violence, stalking, economic control, and control of social contacts.

Intimate-partner violence may begin or increase during pregnancy. Jasinski (2004) describes both maternal and fetal consequences of pregnancy-related violence. These include delayed or absent prenatal care, low birth weight, preterm labour, unhealthy maternal behaviours (eg, substance use), fetal trauma, recurrent UTIs, postpartum depression, and social isolation. In other cases, pregnancy is the woman's first entry into the health care system and her first contact with a helping profession. Those who care for pregnant women are in a unique position to screen for and to treat cases of violence. Evidence also suggests that women want health care providers to ask direct and nonthreatening questions about violence (Jasinski, 2004).

COLLABORATIVE CARE: THE PREGNANT CLIENT EXPERIENCING INTIMATE-PARTNER VIOLENCE
Assessment

All health care facilities should routinely screen all women for violence (Registered Nurses Association of Ontario [RNAO], 2012). Care providers should be alert for suggestive indicators such as chronic pain; insomnia; irritable bowel syndrome; migraines; arthritis; UTIs; injuries to the face, breasts, abdomen, and buttocks; anxiety; depression; fractures; unexplained bruises; areas of redness consistent with slaps; lacerations; and multiple injuries in various stages of healing. Any type of screening must be done with the woman privately. A nonthreatening and nonjudgemental approach may include a general statement about the prevalence of violence in society. For example:

> "Out of concern for all the women to whom I provide care, I ask whether you have ever been hit, kicked, or punched in your current intimate relationship. Also, do you feel personally safe in your home? Have you ever been hurt or frightened in your home?"

The "SOS" is a screening tool that may be used with pregnant women in a clinic setting. The letters SOS describe the process of *S*creen, *O*ffer options, and *S*afety. The nurse should first tell the woman that "We're concerned about the health effects of partner violence, so we ask a few questions of all of our clients." Then, he or she can ask the following questions:

- Do you ever feel unsafe at home?
- Has anyone at home hit you or tried to injure you in any way?
- Have you ever felt afraid of a partner? (Watts, 2004, quoting Mian, 2000, p. 232)

The woman who responds positively to experiencing violence either currently or in the past needs to know that she did not deserve this, that help can be provided, and that her situation may threaten the course of labour and birth.

For clients in labour, accurate, confidential assessment is critical. Lack of privacy has been the largest barrier to screening cited by health care providers (Furniss et al., 2007). Antenatal documentation may provide information that questions regarding violence have been asked previously. Screening for violence should take place privately in the labour assessment area, with responses documented.

Labour and birth sometimes trigger memories of childhood sexual abuse, as women experience their bodies in new and different ways. These early experiences are often formative and a survivor may not be able to recall these early adverse experiences (Haskell, 2012). Potential triggers during this time include expressions of pain, strangers in the room, vaginal examinations, pushing efforts, perineal pain, and even breast-feeding (Hobbins, 2004). Private discussion with the woman who has described past experiences of abuse would be helpful in knowing how to assist her to cope during labour and birth (Fig. 13.10).

Select Potential Nursing Diagnoses
The following are examples of commonly applicable nursing diagnoses for the client who has experienced intimate-partner violence:

- **Fear** related to possible injury or ongoing violence
- **Anxiety** related to maternal and fetal health and well-being
- **Chronic Pain** related to ongoing or beginning violence
- **Deficient Knowledge** related to safety and support
- **Pain** related to labour and birth and increased anxiety caused by violence or memories of violence
- **Impaired Parenting** related to violence or past violence

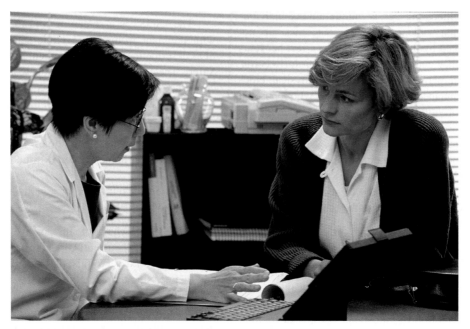

FIGURE 13.10 Well before labour begins, the nurse should try to discuss sensitive issues, such as past abuse, with the client to help prepare her for emotions and feelings she may experience during childbirth.

Planning/Intervention

If a woman responds positively about abuse during screening, nurses and other care providers must make resources available and assist her to form an emergency safety plan. Inclusion of any children in this plan is important to ensure their safety. Every effort must be made to protect this woman; therefore, charting and all information given must remain confidential. However, not all women are ready to act on the identified plan and resources at the time of disclosure; the nurse must respect the right of the woman to choose to remain in the relationship until she is ready to make a change. However, the nurse is responsible to ensure that the woman has a plan and that any children are protected. Clients entering prenatal care must be treated with respect and dignity, regardless of their stories or decisions.

Ensuring one-to-one nursing care throughout labour can facilitate the client's trust. Encouraging her choices relative to pain medications and comfort measures would be important to giving the client a feeling of control. Providing her with information regarding her care may promote her participation in and acceptance of labour and birth. Ensuring that she receives information to make a safety plan that she can implement at any time if needed would be critical to postpartum follow-up. Assisting her to verbalize concerns and questions privately also would be important. Culturally sensitive care would include the use of a translator other than a family member and asking open-ended questions.

Evaluation

The goal of care for all women is to screen for violence and, depending on answers, provide encouragement and support. For women dealing with violence issues, information about community resources and shelters is a measure by which to provide needed assistance.

Confidentiality and privacy of both the woman's records and conversations are essential. Ensuring safety and well-being is also crucial. Safety of the fetus or newborn must also be considered; measures to promote family bonding need to be enacted, even in what might be a painful and emotional atmosphere. The simple act of "screening" for intimate-partner violence as an element of care for all women is a positive outcome (Furniss et al., 2007).

Substance Use

Substance use during pregnancy in Canada is common and increasing (SOGC, 2011). Many substances can have negative consequences on maternal, fetal, and neonatal health. Antenatally, the nurse should ask all women about their use of tobacco, marijuana, cocaine, alcohol, and other recreational or prescription drugs. The use of nonjudgemental, open-ended questions is more likely to encourage disclosure (SOGC, 2011). The use of alcohol and drugs in pregnancy can cause women to decrease prenatal care attendance and have higher rates of infectious diseases (SOGC, 2011).

Alcohol use in pregnancy contributes to birth defects and developmental delays. Heavy or binge drinking has been linked to fetal alcohol syndrome/fetal alcohol effects (FAS/FAE) now known as fetal alcohol spectrum disorder. Risk factors identified for prenatal alcohol exposure include higher maternal age, social isolation, lower education level, stress, violence, smoking, drug use, lower socioeconomic status, inadequate nutrition, and limited access to prenatal and postnatal care and services (Chudley et al., 2005).

Approximately 25% of all babies born each year in Canada are exposed to some alcohol during early gestation; fetal alcohol spectrum disorder affects up to 9 out of every 1,000 babies born in the United States and Canada (Koren et al., 2003). Low levels of alcohol use may cause low birth weight (see Chapter 22). Facial anomalies as well as learning deficits have been shown to be associated with alcohol use in pregnancy. A safe level of alcohol use during pregnancy has not been determined (Comley & Mousmanis, 2003). However, the timing of exposure during pregnancy, the frequency, and the pattern of consumption are important factors associated with fetal alcohol spectrum disorder (Chudley et al., 2005).

The results of the 2011 Canadian Tobacco Use Monitoring Survey indicated that 6.9% of women between the ages of 20 and 44 reported smoking during their most recent pregnancy (PHAC, 2011b). Many of these women quit during pregnancy and others reduce their tobacco use. Women who smoke during pregnancy are at increased risk for preterm labour and low birth weight infants (SOGC, 2011). Other problems associated with maternal tobacco use include spontaneous abortion and ectopic pregnancy (Comley & Mousmanis, 2003).

Opioid addiction is increasing in Canada, particularly in Ontario, with an increased number of infants requiring care for withdrawal (neonatal abstinence syndrome) in special care nurseries. Women who report opioid use should be asked about the name of the drug, amount, frequency, duration, route(s), last use, any injection drug use, sharing of needles and other paraphernalia, or withdrawal symptoms. They should be asked about their medical history, including infectious diseases; psychiatric history, including eating disorders, abuse, mood, and anxiety disorders; and their social history, including child safety concerns, partner, and finances. Finally, an assessment is made about their stage of change; awareness of risk to the fetus with continuation of use; and need for intervention such as methadone maintenance treatment (SOGC, 2011).

Methadone is the standard of treatment in the perinatal period (RNAO, 2009). In caring for the pregnant woman, the nurse together with the rest of the health care team will:

- Reflect on his/her own values and beliefs regarding use of methadone in pregnancy

- Understand the woman's perspective by asking about "her story"
- Understand neonatal abstinence syndrome and provide information and support to the woman during pregnancy and in the postpartum period
- Support the woman in working with child protection services, if a link is there already and/or need is identified, after birth
- Understand the woman's support services, including her relationship with her partner and if he/she is continuing to use substances
- Assess for intimate-partner violence and abuse
- Provide continuous support throughout pregnancy with positive reinforcement highlighting her strengths
- Understand pain control in labour/birth and postpartum and advocate for her
- Ensure processes are in place for follow-up with community health (RNAO, 2009)

Most women who use substances in pregnancy use more than one drug (Table 13.3). It may be difficult to separate the effects of one from the other. Other factors such as poverty, lack of family support, and inadequate education may be equal risk factors in these women's pregnancies.

Effective care for women who use substances and their fetuses is multifaceted and involves cooperation and collaboration from the woman and her family, social workers, physicians, midwives, community health workers, and family and children's services. One tool that has been developed to begin the discussion about substance use is the four Ps:

- Have you ever used drugs or alcohol during this **p**regnancy?
- Have you had a problem with drugs or alcohol in the **p**ast?
- Does your **p**artner have a problem with drugs or alcohol?
- Do you consider one of your **p**arents to be an addict or an alcoholic? (Gilbert, 2011)

When a woman describes substance use during pregnancy, it is important for the health care provider to respond in relation to the effects of her behaviour on her health and on that of her fetus. Remaining nonjudgemental but assessing her motivation to taper off or quit is essential. Discussing family and social supports is important to the success of intervention. Providing smoking cessation interventions are encouraged in pregnancy, as they are effective. Counselling alone may be beneficial with use of Smoker's Helpline and other behavioural reinforcement techniques. Nicotine replacement therapy may also be offered at the lowest dose possible to be effective and potentially an intermittent therapy such as gum or lozenge rather than a continuous amount such as the patch (SOGC, 2011).

● TABLE 13.3 **Maternal Substance Use**

Substance	Effects	Management Guidelines
Alcohol	Fetal alcohol spectrum disorder Spontaneous abortion Low birth weight Low Apgar scores	Identify and confirm cases of alcohol use Educate women regarding danger to fetus: permanent cognitive impairment, facial deformity, microcephaly, growth deficiencies, and behavioural problems Refer woman to alcohol treatment facility. Use supportive network and follow-up to reduce alcohol intake
Cocaine	Congenital anomalies of the brain, kidneys, and urogenital tract Small for gestational age (SGA), intrauterine growth restriction (IUGR) Prematurity Birth asphyxia secondary to placental abruption Brain infarcts Neurobehavioural abnormalities	For newborns, perform massage therapy to soothe, calm, and reduce behavioural disorganization: stroke the prone newborn over each area of the body systematically, moving from trunk outward to extremities. Talk soothingly in low tones to calm baby. If newborn is unstable or preterm, use gentle palmar touch to head and abdomen at several intervals each day Ensure adequate nonnutritive sucking; swaddle newborn snugly. Reduce environmental stimuli. Administer sedation as ordered.
Smoking or exposure to secondhand tobacco smoke	Spontaneous abortion SGA Low birth weight Increased risk for sudden infant death syndrome (SIDS) Increased incidence of abruptio placentae and placenta previa Birth defects including congenital urinary tract anomalies	Educate women about dangers to fetus and self Evaluate woman's desire and ability to quit If woman cannot or is unwilling to quit, form a contract to ration or limit cigarettes per day Give support and positive reinforcement Provide information about alternative methods of stress relief Encourage partner/family to support client's efforts to decrease smoking.
Heroin	IUGR SGA Increased incidence of SIDS Newborn withdrawal Poor feeding in the newborn Dehydration and electrolyte imbalance related to vomiting and diarrhea	Begin maternal methadone therapy to reduce risk for spontaneous abortion or possible fetal demise (after 32–34 wks' gestation) secondary to heroin withdrawal Administer sedatives and methadone to newborn Swaddle newborn for comfort; give gentle persistence and stimulation for feeding Use soft preemie nipples to reduce energy expenditure associated with feeding Conduct massage and give gentle human touch to help decrease restlessness and improve habitation Decrease noise, noxious stimuli, and light
Marijuana	Preterm birth Decreased birth weight and length Possible delays in growth and development in preschooler	Assess for concurrent use of other harmful substances: alcohol, cocaine, methamphetamines Educate women about drug's potential long-term effects on the child's language, memory, and development. Give psychological support if drug use is a form of self-medication to avoid an unpleasant or violent home environment. Provide social service referrals as needed

Ongoing reinforcement by the nurse and/or health care provider is also beneficial in decreasing smoking during pregnancy and postpartum.

Eating Disorders

The idealization of the slender feminine body in Western culture has led to disordered eating amongst women, particularly of childbearing age (Carwell & Spatz, 2011). For some clients, the natural weight gain that accompanies pregnancy is difficult. Women may struggle with prenatal visits that require objective checks of weight.

Canadian statistics demonstrate that 0.9% to 4.5% of women have bulimia or anorexia; 90% of these women are in the childbearing years (Langlois et al., 2012). Pregnancies complicated by anorexia or bulimia are at high risk for preterm birth, gestational hypertension, gestational diabetes, intrauterine growth restriction, miscarriage, vaginal bleeding, and cesarean birth (Carwell & Spatz, 2011).

The client with an eating disorder who presents for prenatal care needs a thorough health history with questions about stress, how she feels about her body size, and what it is like for her to get on the scale while at her prenatal appointment (Zauderer, 2012). Many women attempt to deny or hide an eating disorder. If the client has been slow to gain weight or has not gained any weight for two appointments or more, seems unwilling to talk about her weight, or has a body mass index lower than 19 (prepregnant), an eating disorder should be suspected. For women who admit to having an eating disorder, important blood tests include serum electrolytes, thyroid function, blood urea nitrogen, and serum creatinine. It is important to request the client's permission before arranging a social worker visit or a referral to community services. Eating disorders frequently increase in intensity in the first postpartum year with the intent to lose the weight associated with pregnancy; some clients attempt to control the weight of their infants as well (Carwell & Spatz, 2011). Assisting women with eating disorders to find help immediately postpartum may protect not only their own health but also that of their baby. Seeking a client's consent for nutritional consultation can be beneficial and help her to establish appropriate nutritional requirements during her recovery. Involving family, with the client's permission, may assist her to achieve her goals.

OBESITY

Obesity is becoming more common in North America. Twenty-three percent of Canadian women over the age of 18 are obese, and the 25 to 34 age group has had the fastest growing obesity rate among adults over the past 25 years (PHAC, 2011a). Increased consumption of processed and fast foods, decreased exercise, and a sedentary lifestyle all increase the chances of excessive weight gain. Excess weight before pregnancy increases risks for many maternal and fetal complications (Nodine & Hastings-Tolsma, 2012). Obesity in pregnancy leads to an elevation in free fatty acids and causes a proinflammatory state that increases the risk for hypertension, vascular disease, diabetes, and the need for cesarean birth (Cesario, 2003). The fetus has an increased risk for cardiac anomalies, spinal bifida, and stillbirth (Nodine & Hastings-Tolsma, 2012). The pregnant obese woman may complain of fatigue, backache, pelvic pain, or UTI. All these common complaints in pregnancy are increased for obese women because of the additional musculoskeletal strain, cardiac workload, and chance for infection their extra weight imposes. These clients also need to be assessed regularly for any signs of labour depending on gestation because many symptoms they experience also can be indications of preterm labour. Chapter 16 discusses in detail specific issues related to obesity and the labour and birth process.

COMMON GESTATIONAL COMPLICATIONS

Major complications specifically related to gestation and pregnancy are relatively few. Nevertheless, they can pose significant risks to mother, fetus, or both. This section discusses those problems of gestation inherently related to the state of pregnancy itself. In addition, it explores two common types of special risk pregnancies: adolescent pregnancy and multiple gestation. The section concludes with those conditions leading to pregnancy loss and care for the grieving family.

HYPEREMESIS GRAVIDARUM

Most women, approximately 63% to 80%, experience mild to moderate nausea and vomiting during pregnancy, which usually begins by 4 to 6 weeks' gestation, increases in severity by 8 to 12 weeks, and improves or resolves by 20 weeks (Einarson et al., 2007; Kramer et al., 2013). Between 20% and 45% continue to have nausea and vomiting throughout pregnancy, even in the third trimester.

Less than 1% of women are diagnosed with **hyperemesis gravidarum**, which is defined as severe nausea and vomiting, a weight loss of 5% or more from their prepregnancy value, dehydration, and electrolyte imbalances (Youngkin et al., 2013). Hyperemesis gravidarum is a high-risk condition, as it increases chances for pregnancy loss, IUGR, maternal activity restriction, fatigue, and depression.

Many risk factors are associated with severe nausea and vomiting in pregnancy (NVP), including young maternal age, nulliparity, low socioeconomic status, unplanned pregnancy, previous pregnancy with NVP, increased body mass index, eating disorders, ethnicity, and fetal female gender or fetal abnormalities such as trisomy 21 (suggesting that an immune mechanism may be involved). One etiologic theory is that NVP results from an olfactory response with specific odour triggers in some women; another is that the problem stems from motion hypersensitivity. Dysregulation of gastric rhythms also has been proposed as a cause. Gestational hormones, particularly human chorionic gonadotropin (hCG), have been investigated for their role, particularly because rising levels of hCG are correlated with increased NVP in the first trimester. No etiology has yet been proven. A deficiency of vitamin B_6 is associated with NVP, but it is uncertain whether this occurs before or after NVP.

Some researchers have linked hyperemesis gravidarum to psychosocial conflicts inherent in pregnancy: fear and anxiety regarding changing or new roles, possible adverse socioeconomic repercussions of childbirth, and whether the pregnancy was planned. NVP can negatively affect family relationships and the pregnant client's ability to work: 75% of employed women with NVP reported time lost from their jobs, and 50% felt that NVP adversely compromised their relationship with their partner (Mazzotta et al., 2000). NVP has been compared with the severity of nausea experienced by clients undergoing chemotherapy (SOGC, 2002c). Hospitalized women with hyperemesis gravidarum have described social alienation and withdrawal due to the embarrassment and pervasiveness of the problem. They describe loneliness, being overwhelmed, and hopelessness, particularly when faced with little understanding from family, friends, and health care providers (O'Brien et al., 2002). See Research Highlight 13.2.

Assessment Findings

It may be a challenge for some women to find a health care provider while experiencing hyperemesis gravidarum, which usually begins during the first 10 weeks of pregnancy. Access to help may depend on whether the client already has a family doctor, has had medical confirmation of her pregnancy, and is well enough to attend appointments. Potentially, this client may present at the emergency department for assistance.

A thorough history is necessary. Frequency, severity, and duration of episodes are important to ascertain. Triggers or precipitating factors (eg, odours, times of day, specific foods) also would be helpful to know. The nurse should ask about strategies that the woman may have tried, such as dietary modifications or herbal medications such as ginger (Motherisk, 2007). Information from family and friends may provide insight about how the client is coping.

Physical examination is essential to rule out other diagnoses and to confirm the pregnancy. Routine procedures include urinalysis (protein, ketones, and glucose) as well as current weight. Blood work may include a complete blood count, electrolytes, liver enzymes, and thyroid and bilirubin levels.

Collaborative Management

Many clients with hyperemesis gravidarum have one or more admissions to a health care facility (as many as 14 per 1,000 births) (SOGC, 2002c). Hospitalization may be necessary if assessment reveals dehydration and

---

● **RESEARCH HIGHLIGHT 13.2**   Isolation From "Being Alive": Coping With Severe Nausea and Vomiting of Pregnancy

OBJECTIVE

To understand how pregnant women cope with severe nausea and vomiting.

SAMPLE

Twenty-four pregnant women admitted for nausea and vomiting to a Canadian hospital participated. They ranged in age from 18 to 41 years, came from various cultural backgrounds, and had different levels of education. Eight women were pregnant for the first time; 15 were having their second pregnancy, and 1 woman was expecting for the third time.

METHOD

This descriptive–exploratory study relied on semistructured interviews. Data analysis was concurrent with information collection. Researchers reviewed emerging results with a focus group for comment, confirmation, and clarification to ensure that participants recognized their own experience in the presented description.

RESULTS

Women identified increasing loneliness and isolation beginning early in pregnancy and continuing for the duration of their symptoms. Although the women themselves recognized that the symptoms were not minor and that strategies to deal with them were not working, their support people did not appreciate their difficulties. They also emphasized that health care professionals did not understand the extent and debilitating nature of the problem. Participants described nausea and vomiting as "taking over their lives," eventually feeling as if they had no life of their own. For many, symptoms subsided by 22 weeks' gestation. Two participants elected to have abortions, and two continued to have severe nausea and vomiting up until birth.

NURSING IMPLICATIONS

Nurses providing care to pregnant women hospitalized because of nausea and vomiting need to understand the emotional effects of this problem. Assisting clients to reduce predisposing and coexisting factors that exacerbate nausea and vomiting may help.

From O'Brien, B., Evans, M., & White-McDonald, E. (2002). *Nursing Research, 51*, 302–308.

● PHARMACOLOGY 13.2 Promethazine (Phenergan)

ACTION

Blocks cholinergic receptors in the vomiting centre of the brain, thus mediating nausea and vomiting in cases of hyperemesis gravidarum

PREGNANCY CATEGORY

C

DOSAGE

25 mg orally; repeat doses of 12.5 to 25 mg as needed every 4 to 6 hours. Drug can be given rectally if client cannot tolerate oral administration. IM dosages are 12.5 to 25 mg, not to be repeated more frequently than every 4 hours. Parenteral dosages are not given, based on potential damage to the IV site and/or circulation.

POSSIBLE ADVERSE EFFECTS

Confusion, dizziness, restlessness, epigastric distress, urinary frequency, dysuria

NURSING CONSIDERATIONS

● Implement safety precautions to protect the client against injury secondary to the drug's sedative effects.
● Emphasize to the client to try to maintain an adequate fluid intake.

From Karch, A. M. (2005). *2005 Lippincott's nursing drug guide.* Philadelphia, PA: Lippincott Williams & Wilkins.

---

a need for IV therapy to correct electrolyte imbalances. Initially, the client's status will be nothing by mouth (NPO) during IV hydration. Fluids should not be taken again until the client has gone 48 hours without vomiting.

During hospitalization, nursing care involves monitoring intake and output, including emesis; assessing urine for ketones and protein; taking daily weights; and providing nutritional counselling, as needed. Mouth care while the client is NPO, and a quiet environment with attention to minimizing odours (to try and prevent this potential cause of nausea) may decrease the severity of symptoms. Medical care may include pharmacologic therapy (Pharmacology Box 13.2).

Critical to this woman's emotional needs is support provided by health care providers combined with the recognition of her need for isolation when she is feeling nauseous. Demonstrated understanding about the severity and reality of this syndrome is essential (O'Brien et al., 2002). Women experiencing NVP have expressed concern about their inability to communicate to others the pervasiveness of their symptoms. Depression has also been found to be caused by this condition, so screening for nausea and vomiting needs to be combined with questions about mood and support for this pregnancy (Kramer et al., 2013). The nurse who provides care should assist the client and her family to discuss the experience, identify interventions that may be helpful, and communicate openly.

Depending on the severity of symptoms, total parenteral nutrition (TPN) also may be started in the hospital and continued at home. The home care nurse would focus on evaluating the results of hydration and IV therapy; he or she also would explore the client's coping strategies and support systems. Teaching parameters include eating smaller and more frequent meals (every 1 to 2 hours), taking fluids between meals, decreasing cooking odours, eating whatever the woman can tolerate, and using complementary therapies such as ginger or vitamin B_6 supplements (SOGC, 2002c). Prenatal vitamins can worsen nausea because of their size and iron content. Taking folic acid alone in the first trimester and a multivitamin without iron may help until the client is able to tolerate the prenatal vitamin in the second or third trimester. Indications of improving health include increased fluid intake, weight gain, adequate hydration, and successful employment of coping strategies (Motherisk, 2007).

HYPERTENSIVE PROBLEMS

Hypertension in pregnancy is defined as a diastolic BP value greater than or equal to 90 mm Hg, using the average of at least two measurements in the same arm. Women who present with a systolic BP value greater than or equal to 140 mm Hg should be closely monitored for development of elevated diastolic BP (SOGC, 2008).

Most pregnant women have an internal "clock" that regulates BP, showing an increase during the day, a peak during the early evening, and a decrease between midnight and 4 AM. Hypertensive disorders occur in 12% to 22% of pregnancies and are a major cause of maternal mortality (Gilbert, 2011; Jones et al., 2012). They develop most often in primiparas, particularly those who are overweight or obese (Deen et al., 2006; Samuals-Kalow et al., 2007). Multiparas are also at risk, particularly those with a new partner in the current pregnancy, pre-existing hypertension, renal disease, diabetes, or multiple gestation (SOGC, 2008).

Hypertension in pregnancy is classified into two categories: pre-existing or gestational (SOGC, 2008). Pre-existing hypertension refers to hypertension that appears before 20 weeks' gestation or prior to pregnancy. Gestational hypertension is used for hypertension first noted after 20 weeks' gestation. Both categories are divided into two subgroups: (1) with comorbid conditions (diabetes, renal disease), and (2) with preeclampsia (hypertension, proteinuria, and adverse conditions) (SOGC, 2008).

Proteinuria should be strongly suspected when urinary dipstick is 2+, and considered if greater than or equal to 0.3 g/d in a 24-hour urine collection or greater than or equal to 30 mg/mmol urinary creatinine in a randomly obtained urine sample (SOGC, 2008). Edema and weight gain are not considered part of the diagnosis for gestational or chronic hypertension.

Preeclampsia refers specifically to hypertension after 20 weeks' gestation with proteinuria. It is more common in multiparas; multiple pregnancy; women with pre-existing hypertension, diabetes mellitus, or the presence of antiphospholipid antibodies; clients with a family history of preeclampsia or who have had preeclampsia in a previous pregnancy; women with a BMI of 35 or greater; and clients with renal disease (Chobanian et al., 2003; SOGC, 2008). Preeclampsia can progress to life-threatening **eclampsia**, a medical emergency at any time in pregnancy, labour, or early postpartum. Signs of eclampsia include convulsive facial twitching and tonic–clonic contractions (Youngkin et al., 2013). These developments are usually preceded by an acute increase in BP and worsening signs of multiorgan involvement, such as increased liver enzymes, proteinuria, blurred vision, epigastric pain, and hyperreflexia.

In women who develop gestational hypertension, BP begins to increase during the second half of pregnancy; they may not experience the pregnancy-related decrease in BP at night. Normal fluctuations in BP during pregnancy are the reason for two evaluations for hypertension in pregnant women. The placental implantation or invasion into the maternal myometrium and remodeling of the uterine arteries is an important factor in the development of preeclampsia, suggesting that the condition begins with conception rather than in the second half of pregnancy (Townsend & Drummond, 2011). Narrow vessels and hypoperfusion in the circulation from the placenta into the myometrium can lead to placental hypoxia. Decreased placental perfusion occurs as the spiral uterine arteries remain thick walled with decreased capacity to accommodate the 10-fold increase in uterine blood flow necessary for fetal growth and development (Peters, 2008). This can lead to fetal

IUGR from decreased placental circulation. Vasospasm, which causes poor perfusion, is thought to be the mechanism for increased BP and total peripheral resistance throughout the maternal circulation in pregnancy. Vasospasm decreases blood flow and changes the function of many organs and systems. Intra-arterial lesions caused by vasospasm initiate the coagulation cascade, resulting in endothelial damage. As hypertension progresses, the woman may also develop an increased sensitivity to vasoactive hormones, reduced plasma volume, increased systemic vascular resistance, and activation of the coagulation cascade (Peters, 2008).

Consider Lindsey, the woman pregnant with her second child described at the beginning of the chapter. What risk factors might predispose Lindsey to preeclampsia?

COLLABORATIVE CARE: THE PREGNANT CLIENT WITH HYPERTENSION

When a client is pregnant, her health care providers need to be alert for any signs or symptoms of hypertension. Ongoing assessments of proteinuria, BP, and fetal health are critical components of each prenatal visit. Any increase in BP requires follow-up questions about headache, epigastric pain, and visual disturbance. An increase in BP may also indicate the need for a 24-hour urine collection to more accurately assess the level of protein and kidney function. Those providing care should collaborate in their assessment and planning. If hypertension is diagnosed, team members may include an obstetrician and home care nurses to provide the treatment that the woman and fetus require. Antenatal admission to the hospital may be considered based on the distance of the woman's residence from the facility; signs of increasing blood pressure, proteinuria, and/or end organ complications; and the woman's specific requirements for care.

Treatment of the client with symptoms of multiorgan involvement and hypertension during labour involves assessment of signs and symptoms, laboratory testing, monitoring of fetal well-being, and review of the prenatal history. Multiorgan involvement and subsequent symptoms can result from vascular constriction or vasospasm and movement of fluid intracellularly (Fig. 13.11). Vasospasm and endothelial damage can lead to reduced placental perfusion, which can decrease fetal development, leading to IUGR.

Severe preeclampsia is defined as preeclampsia with onset prior to 34 weeks' gestation with multiorgan

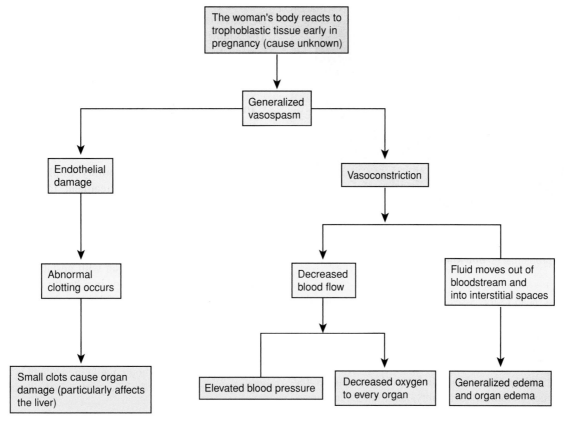

FIGURE 13.11 Gestational hypertension can cause a cascade of problems.

involvement and is considered an obstetric emergency (SOGC, 2008). This situation demands involvement from a hematologist, neonatologist, obstetrician, internal medicine specialist, neonatal nurses, maternity nurses, social workers, and pharmacists.

Assessment

Prompt recognition of hypertension in pregnancy is based on comprehensive knowledge that includes understanding of anatomy and physiology, application of clinical skills, and awareness of possible complications (eg, abruptio placenta, acute renal failure, pulmonary edema, cerebral hemorrhage, and stroke). Assessment begins with taking the woman's BP, evaluating urine for output and protein, and checking neurologic signs. Careful monitoring of vital signs, neurologic status, renal function, and hematologic values is important (Chobanian et al., 2003).

A thorough medical and family history must focus on any underlying cardiovascular disease, diabetes, pulmonary disease, migraine headaches, or seizure disorder. Preeclampsia has been associated with a first pregnancy but it is three times more common in a woman with a previous history of preeclampsia, particularly if she had signs and symptoms starting in the second trimester. Asking about her previous pregnancy or pregnancies

is critical to care planning (Townsend & Drummond, 2011). Asking about genetic history is also important, as preeclampsia in a woman's mother or sisters may increase her risk. Paternal genes are also a risk factor, as male children of preeclamptic pregnancies are twice as likely to go on to be fathers of a preeclamptic pregnancy (Townsend & Drummond, 2011). Questions about the woman's perinatal history should emphasize presence of increasing BP throughout the pregnancy, fetal demise or IUGR in a previous pregnancy, and prepregnancy BP. Other assessment parameters include amniotic fluid volume, fetal growth, and current fetal status (SOGC, 2008).

The nurse always takes BP with the client sitting and her arm at heart level (Fig. 13.12). The cuff must be of the appropriate size, with an accurate sphygmomanometer and Korotkoff phase V recorded to designate diastolic BP. The BP should not be taken within 60 minutes of smoking, caffeine ingestion, or exercise. Also if the evaluation of BP is done in a cool room or while the woman is talking, the BP can increase up to 8 to 15 mm Hg (Townsend & Drummond, 2011). The nurse takes the woman's BP in both arms initially to assess for differences that may be caused by anatomy, position, or other factors. If a difference is noted, ongoing assessment with the arm demonstrating the higher value is appropriate (Peters, 2008).

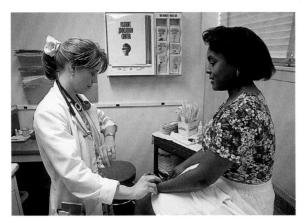

FIGURE 13.12 Although ongoing evaluations of blood pressure for all pregnant clients are essential, they are of special importance in women with a history of hypertensive problems. (© Bob Kramer.)

A head-to-toe assessment of the client with diagnosed hypertension would include taking BP with the client in the lateral position. Repeat BPs are taken in the same arm, with the client in the same position, and using the same machine for consistency. The nurse should ask the client about headaches, visual disturbances (eg, blurring, scotomata), irritability, and tremors, and investigate whether the client has experienced any bleeding, petechiae, or both. Other symptoms to investigate include any right-upper-quadrant pain, epigastric pain, nausea and vomiting, urine output and colour, and swelling. Asking about fetal activity and movements is also important.

Laboratory tests are per physician's orders. Likely studies include hemoglobin, platelet count, white blood count and differential, fibrinogen, partial thromboplastin time, prothrombin time (INR), alanine transaminase, aspartate transaminase, lactate dehydrogenase, bilirubin (liver function tests), albumin, glucose, proteinuria, creatinine, urea, and serum uric acid (SOGC, 2008).

Fetal assessment may include continuous fetal monitoring if the woman is in labour or an NST if she is not, ultrasound, umbilical artery Doppler flow studies, amniotic fluid volume assessment, and biophysical profile. IUGR is a risk in ongoing hypertension and antihypertensive medications. Ultrasound and symphysis fundal height measurements should be used to monitor fetal growth and development (Sibai & Chames, 2003; SOGC, 2003).

 Remember Lindsey, the woman at 28 weeks' gestation with a history of gestational hypertension. Imagine that she is diagnosed with gestational hypertension in this pregnancy. For what complications are she and her fetus at risk?

Select Potential Nursing Diagnoses

The following are examples of commonly applicable nursing diagnoses in a pregnant client with hypertension:

- **Anxiety** related to pregnancy and fetal growth and development with gestational hypertension
- **Ineffective Health Maintenance** related to gestational hypertension
- **Pain** related to specific symptoms of gestational hypertension
- **Risk for Compromised Family Coping** related to diagnosis of or required treatment for gestational hypertension
- **Social Isolation** related to potential bed-rest therapy

Planning/Intervention

The plan of care for a woman with gestational hypertension may occur at home or in a health care facility, depending on the distance of her residence from the institution, available resources, and her access to monitoring equipment and services (Fig. 13.13). Ongoing monitoring may include the following:

- BP readings every 4 hours while the woman is awake
- Assessments for any facial or abdominal edema
- Daily weights
- Neurologic symptoms (eg, hyperreflexia, clonus)
- Checks for any persistent occipital or frontal headaches or visual disturbances
- Monitoring for any right-upper-quadrant or epigastric pain
- Evaluation for any proteinuria by dipstick daily to be followed by a urinary creatinine in a spot random sample or 24-hour collection if greater than 1+
- Hematocrit and platelet counts twice a week
- Liver function tests one to two times per week
- Fetal movement counts twice a day

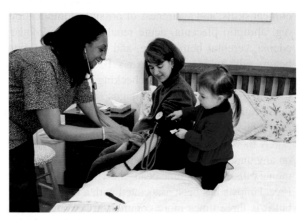

FIGURE 13.13 Depending on her condition and distance from a health care facility, the expectant client with hypertension may receive ongoing blood pressure monitoring at home.

- Nonstress test two to three times a week
- Biophysical profile once to twice a week
- Doppler studies to determine placental blood flow weekly or more often based on results and assessment of fetal growth and well-being (SOGC, 2008)

Teaching and providing information are important parts of care for any pregnant woman, especially one who is experiencing a complication like hypertension. Common concerns and questions these clients may have include the following:

- Why did this happen to me?
- Why did I not hear of this condition before I became ill?
- Why did I not feel ill?
- Will it happen again in my next pregnancy?
- Why do I feel like I have failed?
- Will this have long-term effects on my health?
- Does gestational hypertension run in families?

Pharmacologic treatments may be necessary, including those drugs that a woman with pre-existing hypertension was taking before becoming pregnant (Table 13.4). Oral β-blockers such as labetalol are the preferred medication because they minimize the severity of hypertension and the need for additional antihypertensive drugs (Montan, 2004; SOGC, 2008). Its onset is at 5 minutes with a peak effect at 10 to 20 minutes, causing a decrease in systemic vascular resistance and decreased pulse without decreasing maternal cardiac output (Townsend & Drummond, 2011). Atenolol, metoprolol, and pindolol are common agents prescribed during pregnancy. Oral nifedipine or IV hydralazine may be prescribed for severe hypertension (SOGC, 2008). Hydralazine is a peripheral arteriolar vasodilator with a gradual onset of action and a peak at 20 minutes, so care should be taken as to how frequently it is given in an acute episode (Townsend & Drummond, 2011). Side effects may include a small-for-gestational-age baby (see Chapter 22). See Nursing Care Plan 13.2 for additional information.

● TABLE 13.4 **Hypertensive Drugs Used in High-Risk Pregnancy**

Drug	Action	Dosage	Adverse Effects	Special Considerations
Furosemide (Lasix)	Inhibits resorption of sodium and chloride	Slow IV bolus of 10–40 mg over 1–2 min	Anorexia, dizziness, electrolyte imbalances, muscle cramps and spasms, orthostatic hypotension, vertigo, vomiting	Assess the client's urine output hourly
Hydralazine hydrochloride (Apresoline)	Relaxes the vascular smooth muscle, improving blood perfusion	Slow IV bolus of 5–10 mg every 20 min	Anorexia, diarrhea, headache, nausea and vomiting, tachycardia	Be sure to withdraw this drug gradually to prevent rebound hypertension
Labetalol hydrochloride (Normodyne)	α_1- and β-blockers	Bolus dose of 10–20 mg, with IV infusion of 2 mg/min until desired blood pressure is reached	Constipation, dizziness, fatigue, flatulence, gastric pain, vertigo	Regularly assess the client for development of any adverse effects; help to manage those that may arise
Magnesium sulfate	Blocks neuromuscular transmission; assists with vasodilation	IV loading dose of 4–6 g over 30 min; maintenance infusion of 2–4 g/h as ordered	Toxicity: cardiac and central nervous depression, flushing, hypotension, sweating	Be sure to monitor the client's serum magnesium levels carefully to prevent toxicity. Check deep tendon reflexes and ankle clonus. Ensure that calcium gluconate 10% is readily available as an antidote
Nifedipine (Procardia)	Calcium channel blocker	10 mg orally for three doses; then every 4–8 h	Angina, cough, diarrhea, dizziness, nasal congestion, peripheral edema	Regularly assess the client for development of any adverse effects; help to manage those that may arise. Capsule and PA tablets are appropriate
Sodium nitroprusside	Arterial and venous vasodilator	IV infusion, with dose titrated according to blood pressure values	Abdominal pain, apprehension, diaphoresis, palpitations, restlessness, retrosternal pressure	Protect medication from effects of light by wrapping drug container in foil or other opaque material

From Karch, A. M. (2005). *2005 Lippincott's nursing drug guide*. Philadelphia, PA: Lippincott Williams & Wilkins.

NURSING CARE PLAN 13.2

●

The Client With Hypertension in Pregnancy

During this prenatal visit, Lindsey's urine test for protein is 2+. Her blood pressure is 150/98 mm Hg. Lindsey is asked to return to the office the next morning to have her blood pressure checked again. On her return visit, her urine is 2+ for protein, and her blood pressure is 158/96 mm Hg. She is diagnosed with gestational hypertension with preeclampsia.

NURSING DIAGNOSIS

Risk for Injury (maternal and fetal) related to elevated blood pressure and resultant effects on maternal and fetal status

EXPECTED OUTCOMES

1. The client will demonstrate a blood pressure less than 140/90 mm Hg.
2. The client will remain free of signs and symptoms of eclampsia.
3. The fetus will demonstrate gestational age–appropriate growth and development.

INTERVENTIONS	RATIONALES
Assess the client's blood pressure at each visit; compare readings in each arm. Also assess fetal heart rate.	These assessments provide objective information about maternal and fetal status and aid in detecting trends that may signify a developing problem.
Question the client about any central nervous system complaints such as headaches, visual disturbances, irritability, or tremors.	Central nervous system disturbances may indicate possible progression to eclampsia.
Continue to assess urine by dipstick for protein or for creatinine in random urine sample; prepare client for 24-hour urine collection.	A 24-hour urine collection helps confirm proteinuria and evaluates renal function.
Administer antihypertensive agents as prescribed. Instruct the client in medication therapy.	Antihypertensive agents aid in controlling blood pressure.
Obtain fundal height measurements at each visit; assist with scheduling the client for follow-up ultrasounds.	Fundal height measurements help estimate fetal growth and development. Ultrasounds provide information about the intrauterine environment and fetal well-being.
Monitor the client's weight and assess for edema, especially of the hands and face.	Weight is a reliable indicator of fluid status. Edema of the hands and face may suggest increased edema.
Arrange for laboratory testing such as CBC, coagulation studies, renal and hepatic function tests, and serum magnesium and calcium levels.	Gestational hypertension can affect multiple organs. Laboratory testing provides a baseline for future comparison and continued monitoring. Serum calcium and magnesium levels provide a baseline should magnesium sulfate therapy be necessary.

(continued)

NURSING CARE PLAN 13.2 ● The Client With Hypertension in Pregnancy *(Continued)*

INTERVENTIONS	RATIONALES
Teach the client how to monitor fetal activity and movement.	Fetal activity and movement indicate fetal well-being.
Assist with arranging for fetal assessment studies such as nonstress test, ultrasound, Doppler flow studies, and amniotic fluid volume.	Gestational hypertension can affect placental functioning, which can interfere with fetal well-being. Fetal assessment studies aid in determining fetal status.
Teach about danger signs and symptoms to report immediately, such as severe persistent headaches or visual disturbances, right upper quadrant or epigastric pain, and change in fetal activity or movement.	These signs may indicate continued elevation of blood pressure that may progress to eclampsia. Fetal movement changes are easy for the woman to detect and count daily. A decrease or cessation would be a reason for immediate assessment.
Arrange for continued follow-up of client at home; initiate referral for home care as appropriate.	Continued follow-up provides further opportunities for assessment, teaching, and support.

EVALUATION

1. The client maintains a blood pressure below 140/90 mm Hg.
2. The client exhibits no signs and symptoms of preeclampsia progressing to eclampsia.
3. The fetus demonstrates gestational age–appropriate growth and development.
4. The client gives birth to a healthy newborn at term without complications. These assessments provide objective information about maternal and fetal status and aid in detecting trends that may signify a developing problem.

Current research is focusing on the use of calcium during pregnancy to decrease the development of hypertension. Further studies are needed, but women at high risk may benefit. Low-dose aspirin (81 mg) also may decrease gestational hypertensive effects in high-risk women (Montan, 2004).

Indications that birth should be expedited include the following:

- Persistent increase in maternal BP to severe hypertension
- Development of severe or persistent cerebral symptoms
- Persistent right-upper-quadrant or epigastric pain
- Progressive thrombocytopenia
- Abnormal liver enzymes with hemolysis
- Onset of labour, rupture of membranes, or bleeding
- Severe growth restriction shown on ultrasound or compromised placental perfusion by Doppler studies

- Abnormal NST with abnormal biophysical profile
- Decreased amniotic fluid volume (oligohydramnios)
- Gestational age of 38 to 40 weeks

A woman's BP is not a reliable indicator of her risk for seizures. The central nervous system involvement in gestational hypertension can progress to headaches and visual disturbances, decreased level of mentation, seizure, or eclampsia. Magnesium sulfate is the agent of choice in cases of hypertension and proteinuria with risk factors for eclampsia. Magnesium sulfate reduces the risk of eclampsia by 50% without significant short-term maternal or fetal adverse effects and is the drug of choice (Townsend & Drummond, 2011). The dosage initially is 4 g IV, followed by 1 to 2 g/hour IV. Side effects are weakness, paralysis, decreased respirations, and decreased urinary output. The client's reflexes are checked regularly while she is receiving magnesium sulfate and the antidote; IV calcium gluconate 10% over

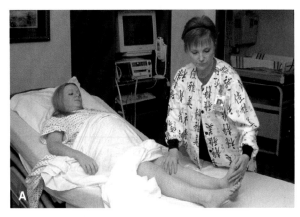
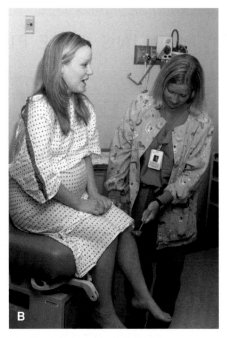

FIGURE 13.14 Monitoring for preeclampsia includes evaluations for nervous system irritability. **A:** To assess for ankle clonus, the nurse should dorsiflex and then release the woman's foot on both sides. Movements should be smooth. Jerky and rapid movements may indicate worsening hypertensive problems. **B:** The nurse can assess the client's patellar reflexes by using a reflex hammer to strike the woman's patellar tendon quickly and firmly. A patellar reflex occurs when the leg and foot move (documented as 2+). Exaggerated reflex in either leg may be a sign of developing preeclampsia.

3 minutes should be available if needed. Patellar tendon response is the most common reflex assessed because of its ease of access (Fig. 13.14). Absence of deep tendon reflex is often the first sign of magnesium toxicity. Frequent blood work to assess for the therapeutic level of magnesium is completed every 4 to 6 hours or per institutional policy. Other blood work to monitor the woman's condition, such as a complete blood count and liver function tests, would be done at the same time to minimize the number of venipunctures.

Close monitoring is required to prevent seizure activity, stroke, and intracranial pressure. Supplies kept at the client's bedside for acute episodes include diazepam, calcium gluconate 10%, ephedrine, epinephrine, hydralazine, magnesium sulfate 50%, phenytoin, and IV solutions such as sodium chloride (saline) and sterile water. Various needles, IV supplies, reflex hammer, tourniquet, blood collection tubes, and airways also are important. These could be kept together in a box taken to the bedside if a client with hypertension presents in an acute episode.

An opportunity to "debrief" after the woman has given birth would be extremely helpful in answering her questions and concerns. Reviewing information provided 1 to 2 weeks later is ideal. A public health nurse may be the best health care provider to accomplish this task.

Evaluation

Care for the woman with hypertension in pregnancy includes assessment, monitoring of both the woman and her fetus, and provision of the safest possible environment for both. Prolonging the pregnancy if the fetus is growing is preferred to a preterm birth and its associated complications. Use of low-dose aspirin and other medications may assist in avoiding the acute episodes that must be treated with advanced fetal and maternal monitoring and interventions including birth.

HELLP SYNDROME

The acronym HELLP is used to indicate a syndrome involving hemolysis (microangiopathic hemolytic anemia), elevated liver enzymes, and a low platelet count (Barton & Sibai, 2004). HELLP syndrome complicates 0.1% to 0.4% of all pregnancies (Kidner & Flanders-Stepans, 2004). It can occur independently or along with gestational hypertension (Peters, 2008). Pregnant women may develop symptoms of HELLP syndrome as early as 17 weeks' gestation or as late as 7 days postpartum. Approximately 66% of clients who develop HELLP do so antenatally, whereas 33% develop it after giving birth (Magann & Martin, 1999). Maternal hypertension can involve multiple organs and require immediate decisions about care. Complications include liver hematoma or rupture, stroke, cardiac arrest, seizure, DIC, and renal damage (Kidner & Flanders-Stepans, 2004). Obstetrical complications cause maternal mortality at rates as high as 24%, and perinatal mortality at rates of up to 70% (Mihu et al., 2007).

Endothelial dysfunction is the underlying pathology in HELLP syndrome. It begins at implantation, causing incomplete maternal spiral artery transformation and activation of intravascular coagulation. This in turn causes vascular ischemia and fibrin deposits with vasospasm and clotting cascade activation (Kidner & Flanders-Stepans, 2004).

Assessment Findings

HELLP syndrome is characterized by various vague symptoms the woman may include in the initial complaint, making it difficult to diagnose (Kidner & Flanders-Stepans, 2004). The client may describe epigastric or right-upper-quadrant pain, nonspecific virus-like symptoms, or present with nausea and vomiting (Barton & Sibai, 2004; Sibai, 2004). The pain is likely to result from obstructed blood flow in the hepatic sinusoids blocked by fibrin deposition. Any pregnant woman who presents with malaise or a viral-type illness in the third trimester needs a complete blood count and liver function testing for HELLP (Padden, 1999). Significant weight gain with generalized edema usually is associated with HELLP syndrome (Barton & Sibai, 2004).

Diagnosis is based on laboratory evidence of hemolytic anemia, hepatic dysfunction, and thrombocytopenia. A peripheral blood smear shows evidence of damaged erythrocytes (burr cells, schistocytes, and helmet cells) caused by vasoconstriction, vasospasm, and damaged endothelial cells (microvascular injury). Decreased prothrombin time and platelet count occur later because of a decreased life span of the circulating platelets (3 to 5 days rather than the normal 8 to 10 days) as well as increased platelet aggregation from decreased resistance to platelet activating factor (Magann & Martin, 1999).

Ongoing monitoring of a critically ill woman with HELLP syndrome includes visual assessments, reflexes, strict intake and output, BP, and fetal heart rate. The nurse assesses for epigastric pain or headache.

Collaborative Management

HELLP syndrome is something of a unique gestational experience, because fear of death may be prominent for the mother. Loneliness, anxiety, powerlessness, and depression are emotions commonly described by hospitalized women with high-risk pregnancies. The speed with which treatment decisions must be made when a woman has HELLP syndrome and the information provided to her, however, may heighten a sense of doom and anxiety. Some clients have described a premonition even before HELLP was diagnosed that "things were not right with this pregnancy" (Kidner & Flanders-Stepans, 2004).

A team approach is vital to providing the best care. Frequently, internists as well as obstetricians, nutritionists, physiotherapists, and pharmacists are part of treatment planning. Management approaches are based on estimated gestational age, maternal health, and fetal status (Padden, 1999). Ongoing evaluations of maternal platelet count and lactate dehydrogenase level are critical for prediction of worsening symptoms. Complaints of severe right-upper-quadrant, shoulder, or neck pain require evaluation through liver imaging to assess for subcapsular hematoma or hepatic rupture (Padden, 1999). Blood should be cross-matched continually and reserved for labour and birth. Ongoing fetal assessments include daily fetal movement counts, NSTs, biophysical profiles, and Doppler studies.

If gestational age is estimated as 32 weeks or less, therapy may include corticosteroid administration for fetal lung maturation, transfer to a tertiary care facility, bed rest, fluid replacement, and fetal assessment (Barton & Sibai, 2004). If gestation is more than 32 weeks but less than 34 weeks, corticosteroids may still be given along with conservative measures to prolong the pregnancy as long as is safe for both mother and fetus. Consultation with a health care team member can assist the family to prepare for birth regardless of gestation (Padden, 1999).

Antihypertensive therapy should be initiated if maternal BP is greater than 160/110 mm Hg. Magnesium sulfate may be used to prevent seizures. The initial bolus is 4 to 6 g followed by an infusion of 2 g/hour measured by infusion pump and assessed together with magnesium blood levels and urine output. Toxicity can be treated with 10 g of 10% IV calcium gluconate (SOGC, 2008). Hydralazine (Apresoline) or labetalol (Normodyne) may be given to decrease the risk for maternal cerebral hemorrhage and placental abruption.

Up to 25% of women with HELLP syndrome develop serious complications, such as DIC, placental abruption, adult respiratory distress syndrome, hepatorenal failure, pulmonary edema, and hepatic rupture. Many require blood products. Infant morbidity and mortality range from 10% to 60%, depending on severity of the maternal disease. These infants are at increased risk for IUGR and respiratory distress syndrome (see Chapter 22) (Padden, 1999).

Postpartum counselling should focus on the client's risk for recurrence of HELLP syndrome (19% to 27%) and hypertension (43%) in future pregnancies.

PRETERM PREMATURE RUPTURE OF MEMBRANES

Premature rupture of the fetal membranes (PROM) is a complication in approximately 8% of pregnancies

(Mercer, 2004). pPROM occurs before 37 weeks' gestation, is responsible for 30% of all cases of PROM (Mercer, 2004), and leads to 30% to 40% of all preterm births (see Chapter 22). Approximately 70% to 90% of pregnancies have up to 7 days before labour begins following pPROM.

Risk factors for pPROM include maternal nutritional deficiencies, prior pPROM, tobacco use, substance abuse, polyhydramnios, multifetal pregnancy, placental abruption, prior preterm birth, multiple gestation, and antepartal trauma (Menon & Fortunato, 2007; Mercer, 2004). Maternal connective disorders also have been linked to pPROM. Infections with trichomoniasis, chlamydia, gonorrhea, and bacterial vaginosis have been shown to lead to an inflammatory response that reduces fetal membrane strength and elasticity (Menon & Fortunato, 2007). There is also a risk for preterm labour in the current pregnancy.

Studies indicate that intrauterine infection, specifically chorioamnionitis, is strongly associated with pPROM and preterm birth particularly at 21 to 24 weeks' gestation (Goldenberg et al., 2008). Intrauterine death occurs in 1% of cases from cord accident, oligohydramnios, cord compression, or abruptio placentae. *Amniotic band syndrome,* which is the adherence of tough bands derived from the fetal membranes, may constrict fetal parts, leading to deformities and, in severe cases, potential amputation of a fetal limb. Increased incidence of neonatal morbidity is associated with pPROM (Pasquier et al., 2007). A small number of women can have spontaneous resealing of the membranes and restoration of a normal amniotic fluid volume, particularly with pPROM following amniocentesis (Mercer, 2004).

COLLABORATIVE CARE: pPROM AND PROM

During pregnancy, the nurse should be aware of a client's risk factors for pPROM, and provide counselling during routine prenatal care about smoking cessation, nutrition, and signs and symptoms of preterm labour (see Chapters 12 and 16).

Fetal fibronectin, a protein produced by the fetal membranes and normally found in the cervicovaginal fluid until approximately 20 weeks' gestation, can be tested as a predictor of pPROM, preterm labour, or both. Fetal fibronectin found between 24 and 34 weeks' gestation in the cervicovaginal fluid in a woman with intact fetal membranes may indicate an increased risk for preterm birth. Collection is done using an unlubricated speculum and placing with a specific (fetal fibronectin) swab in the posterior fornix of the external cervical os for a minimum of 10 seconds and then preserving it in a tube for analysis. The sample must be obtained before digital examination and without the use of lubricants.

Assessment

Women may describe pPROM as a "gush of fluid," a "pop," or "leaking." In such instances, the nurse discusses with the client the timing and date of the event. Questions about fluid colour, amount, and consistency are important, as are fetal movements, contractions, vaginal bleeding, and fever. Questions about frequency and burning associated with urination, as well as sexual activity and douching practices are needed to rule out a UTI and other causes of discharge.

Objective assessments include maternal vital signs, fetal heart rate, abdominal palpation for contractions, and uterine tenderness. The nurse inspects the perineal area for fluid, odour, endocervical mucus, or bloody discharge. A sterile speculum examination may be required to determine fluid leaking from the os. Such an examination also permits visualization for cord prolapse, presenting part, and any vaginal bleeding, as well as swabs for culture and sensitivity for *Chlamydia trachomatis* and *Neisseria gonorrhoeae* (Mercer, 2004). A rectal or vaginal swab for GBS is obtained at this time, if not done within the past 6 weeks (Mercer, 2004). Digital examination is avoided to decrease the immediate risk for infection (Weitz, 1999).

Nitrazine and fern tests aid in the diagnosis of pPROM. The Nitrazine test involves application of vaginal fluid secretions to sterile pH paper. Vaginal pH is normally 4.5 to 6 and does not change the yellow colour of the paper, whereas amniotic fluid is alkaline and changes the paper to dark blue. A false-positive nitrazine test can occur as a result of blood, semen, or vaginal infection (Medina & Hill, 2006). The fern test is performed by gathering vaginal secretions onto a microscopic slide (sterile swab). The fern pattern that appears microscopically is determined by the high salt content of amniotic fluid and strongly indicates pPROM.

If a client's findings indicate a need for bed rest, hospitalization, or both, individual assessment of her support systems and ability to communicate with them is vital when making plans for provision of care.

Select Potential Nursing Diagnoses

The following are examples of commonly applicable nursing diagnoses:

- **Risk for Infection** related to pPROM
- **Risk for Maternal/Fetal Injury** related to pPROM (eg, oligohydramnios causing a cord accident, maternal infection, or both)
- **Risk for Deficient Fluid Volume**
- **Constipation** related to bed rest, if indicated
- **Anxiety** related to fetal and maternal risks for injury and preterm birth
- **Fatigue** related to hospital environment for care provision

Planning/Intervention

The common treatment for pPROM is restricted activity with ongoing assessment for fever, chills, and change in amniotic fluid (colour, odour) that would indicate chorioamnionitis. Temperature assessment every 8 hours, together with a white blood cell count as part of a complete blood count every other day, assists with assessing for chorioamnionitis (Mercer, 2004). The administration of broad spectrum antibiotics following pPROM has been associated with delayed delivery and a reduction in neonatal morbidity; erythromycin is the drug of choice (Kenyon et al., 2003). Uterine tenderness and tachycardia also suggest chorioamnionitis. Uterine activity and fetal heart rate assessments should be done daily. Antenatal corticosteroids are ordered if the pregnancy is less than 34 weeks and viable (at least 23 to 24 weeks) (Mercer, 2004). If gestation is 32 to 36 weeks, amniotic fluid may be collected for fetal lung maturity testing. Amniotic fluid assessed for lecithin-to-sphingomyelin (L/S) ratio can predict fetal lung maturity if the client goes into labour.

A diagnosis of pPROM may necessitate hospitalization. Nursing interventions for the hospitalized client focus on helping her communicate with family from whom she may be separated. She also may need assistance with obtaining financial aid to help support her household while she is away. Common assistive measures include ensuring her access to a telephone, computer, and letter-writing materials; additionally, the facility should promote a liberal visiting policy. Assisting the client with passive and stretching exercises performed in bed would help to pass time. Consultation with a physiotherapist is appropriate. A nutritionist can help ensure adequate weight gain and access to preferred foods and portion sizes. Other activities are visits from the neonatal staff to assist the client in understanding care that the fetus will receive if born prematurely, show prenatal videos, and provide other educational materials focusing on preparation for labour and birth.

Evaluation

Prolonging pregnancy to allow for further fetal growth and development without maternal infection is the goal for the woman and fetus. Constant fetal and maternal assessment is required to ensure that appropriate interventions are initiated to ensure safety.

CERVICAL INSUFFICIENCY/ INCOMPETENCE

Incompetent cervix, or painless cervical dilation, can progress to pPROM and preterm birth and is the cause of 10% to 25% of second-trimester fetal losses (Terkildsen et al., 2003). The term cervical incompetence carries a negative connotation that may increase the emotions and physical burdens associated with recurrent pregnancy losses to women and families. **Cervical insufficiency** is therefore a more sensitive term, suggesting that the cervix is a dynamic structure with compliance and length unique to each woman (Williams & Iams, 2004). The sequence of events involved in insufficiency may or may not repeat itself in future pregnancies. Affected clients can therefore be placed into three groups: those with a history of three or more second-trimester pregnancy losses without labour, those with ultrasound findings during pregnancy showing a shortened cervix, and those with evidence of advanced dilation and effacement but no evidence of regular contractions (Williams & Iams, 2004). Composition of cervical tissue and maternal stress may lead to premature cervical dilation. An inverse relationship between cervical length and preterm birth is well established (Belej-Rak et al., 2003).

Risk factors for premature cervical dilation include excessive cervical dilation for curettage or biopsy, history of previous cervical lacerations during childbirth, and cervical or uterine anomalies (see Chapter 4). A history of short labours and/or losses at early gestations may also contribute.

Transvaginal ultrasound is used to assess cervical length, effacement, and dilation. Cervical length remains fairly stable throughout pregnancy until the third trimester, when it progressively shortens. The median length is 35 to 40 mm from 14 to 22 weeks, and 30 mm after 32 weeks. Effacement begins at the internal cervical os and proceeds distally through a process called *funnelling* (Williams & Iams, 2004). The discovery of cervical thinning and dilation in a woman is a stronger predictor of insufficiency in a nullipara than in a multipara.

Cerclage (suturing) early in the second trimester has the potential to decrease fetal morbidity and mortality in cases of cervical insufficiency (Williams & Iams, 2004) (Fig. 13.15). The suturing helps to prevent cervical relaxation and dilation. A cerclage may be prophylactically placed at 13 to 14 weeks' gestation for clients with a history of cervical insufficiency leading to pregnancy loss (ie, three or more second trimester losses) or who have a cervical anomaly (Abenham & Tulandi, 2009). Emergency cerclage may be performed at 20 to 23 weeks' gestation, but risks include pPROM,

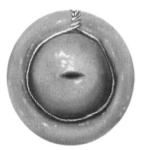

FIGURE 13.15 Cervical cerclage may be used in cases of cervical insufficiency.

chorionitis, and preterm birth. Placement at 22 weeks' gestation may help the pregnancy to proceed to at least 28 weeks, promoting the chances for a better fetal outcome. The client is advised to limit her activity (potentially bed rest at home or in the hospital) and to avoid intercourse and long periods of standing (more than 90 minutes). If cerclage successfully maintains the pregnancy, the suture is removed in the physician's office at 37 weeks' gestation (term) to encourage normal labour. If the health care team determines that an earlier cesarean birth would be best for the woman and family, the cerclage is removed at the same time.

Wherever the client is receiving care, she requires support to cope with the ongoing stress associated with her condition. Encouraging her to communicate with other mothers at home with restricted activity would be helpful, as would contact with community supports such as public health nurses, occupational therapists, and physical therapists.

Effectiveness of treatment is indicated by a pregnancy that reaches term without premature labour. Ensuring that the woman and her family have coped with decreased mobility and limitations related to avoiding labour is an integral part of successful therapy as well.

NEUROLOGIC DISEASES

Epilepsy affects almost 1% of the general population and 3 to 5 out of 1,000 women of childbearing age have been diagnosed (Harden et al., 2009). Of these women, 90% will have a healthy newborn but all of them are considered to be a high-risk pregnancy requiring increased monitoring throughout by an interdisciplinary team of health care providers (Jeha & Morris, 2005). Epilepsy is defined as the presence of recurrent, unprovoked seizures, and is usually treated with long-term antiepileptic medications (Harden et al., 2009). The major hazard to the fetus from a seizure is through direct trauma to the abdomen or through hypoxia if a seizure is prolonged (Bagshaw, 2009).

During pregnancy, it is important for the woman to review her medications with her neurologist for fetal safety and to prevent seizure activity if possible. Throughout pregnancy, it will be important to have her obstetrical specialist consult with the neurologist for any recommendations for care. Approximately one third of women will experience an increase in seizure activity related to anxiety for their fetal well-being causing a decrease in medications, nausea and vomiting related to pregnancy, or changes in the woman's metabolism. Adjusting her medications and providing encouragement about the baby's growth through serial ultrasound may be required. The risk for major congenital malformations is increased with antiepileptic medications, so an increased dose of folic acid (5 mg) is recommended (Bagshaw, 2009).

In approximately 2% to 4% of women, the stress of labour may result in a seizure during childbirth or in the first 24 hours postpartum. Having medication available to treat this is important, as well as ensuring the woman's safety with plans for one-to-one nursing care in labour, use of siderails, discussion about warning signs, having someone available to assist with baby care, and having anesthesiology nearby to assist with treatment and airway management as needed.

Counselling during pregnancy by the nurse on the multidisciplinary team is beneficial not only in coordinating specialist care but in planning for the woman's safety at home and for the future when her infant will be with her.

DISSEMINATED INTRAVASCULAR COAGULOPATHY

Disseminated intravascular coagulopathy (DIC) is a complex coagulation disorder caused by activation of both the clotting and fibrinolytic systems (Lurie et al., 2000) (Fig. 13.16). *Coagulo* refers to clotting, and *pathy* means "disease of," so DIC simply means a disorder with multiple defects in the coagulation cascade that cause inappropriate clotting throughout the vascular system (Geiter, 2003). During pregnancy, a woman's blood is hypercoagulable. Events unique to pregnancy can trigger DIC: abruptio placentae, intrauterine fetal demise, and hypertension in pregnancy. Release of placental tissue factor may activate the prothrombinase complex that causes DIC. Sepsis can also be a trigger.

The presentation of DIC can be acute, chronic, or low grade. Low-grade presentation occurs when coagulation activity increases for a short time and then is restored to normal, or if the body can compensate for a short time with the consumption of coagulation factors (Geiter, 2003). With the heightened coagulation of pregnancy, it is important to be aware of the chronic presentation of DIC and test for it, as appropriate.

Assessment Findings

Signs and symptoms of DIC can be subtle or obvious, as with hemorrhage:

- Oozing or bleeding from IV sites, previous incisions, mucous membranes, trauma from insertion of a catheter, spontaneous bleeding from the gums or nose, patchy cyanosis, gangrene
- Altered level of consciousness, subarachnoid bleeding, cerebrovascular accident
- Hemoptysis, pulmonary embolus, acute respiratory distress syndrome
- Gastrointestinal bleed, abdominal distention, bowel infarction, constipation, diarrhea
- Hematuria, oliguria, renal insufficiency or failure (Geiter, 2003)

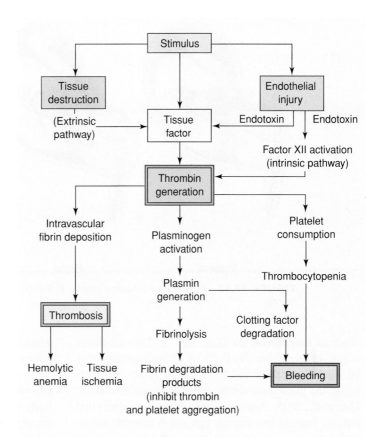

FIGURE 13.16 Pathways in normal blood coagulation and fibrinolysis versus in disseminated intravascular coagulation.

Diagnostic tests include a complete blood count (platelet count that decreases by 50% or more from baseline would be indicative), prothrombin time, activated partial thromboplastin time, fibrinogen, fibrin degradation products and D-dimer (fibrin degradation products that only increase with rapid clot dissolution).

Collaborative Management

Health care providers should be aware of potential triggers for DIC, which may develop suddenly in an obstetric client. A hematologist may be part of the multidisciplinary team. In cases of confirmed DIC, important measures include looking for the underlying cause, rapidly infusing blood and IV fluids as needed, giving continuous oxygen, and assisting with organ perfusion (Lurie et al., 2000). Once the cause has been identified, therapy specific to it (eg, antibiotics to treat gram-negative sepsis) is initiated. Adequate tissue perfusion prevents ischemia, necrosis, or both. Increasing or initiating IV therapy, as well as the delivery of packed RBCs, can be instrumental in treating hemorrhage. Closely monitoring vital signs, particularly oxygen saturation, blood pressure, and pulse, is critical to ensuring the woman's recovery (Geiter, 2003). Heparin therapy may slow coagulation, particularly in situations such as incomplete abortion. Whole blood does not contain clotting factors, so a ratio of 4 units of blood to

1 unit of fresh frozen plasma should be considered. Cryoprecipitate and platelets also may be considered. The goal is to keep the hematocrit above 100 if possible. Each unit of blood is expected to raise the hemoglobin by 15 g/L.

Communicating to the client and her family members about care, what is being done and why is essential so that they understand what is happening. Being honest while remaining supportive and competent is extremely important at this time. Ensuring that the client is receiving appropriate care in a facility that can ensure a safe birth is a primary goal. Effective treatment would be determined by a return to normal clotting time, maintenance of normal blood values, and normal level of consciousness.

PLACENTAL ALTERATIONS

When growth and development of a pregnancy are normal, the blastocyst implants in the upper uterine portion, which has the most extensive blood supply (see Chapter 11). The lower uterine segment is thinner, and placental implantations in this area put the placenta in direct contact with the myometrium.

Placenta Previa

Placenta previa is a condition in which the blastocyst implants in the lower uterine segment, over or very

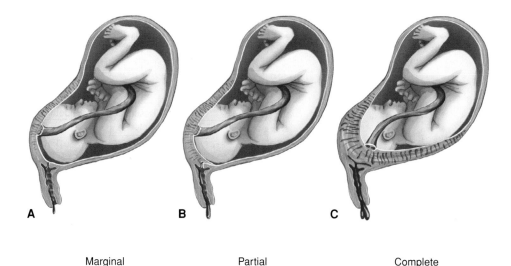

Marginal   Partial   Complete

FIGURE 13.17 **A:** Marginal placenta previa. **B:** Partial placenta previa. **C:** Complete placenta previa.

close to the internal os (Fig. 13.17). This condition occurs in approximately 0.4% of all pregnancies after 20 weeks' gestation and is the major cause of bleeding in the third trimester (Oyelese & Canterino, 2011; Usta et al., 2005). Approximately 90% of placentas that initially implant low migrate upward. A possible explanation for this migration is that as the lower uterine segment grows, the placenta moves away from the os; alternatively, chorionic villi may develop in one area but remain dormant in another (Gilbert, 2011). The degree to which the placenta covers the cervical os determines the diagnosis of total, partial, or marginal.

Placenta previa has been traditionally classified as major or minor degree and further categorized as type I, II, III, or IV. Approximately 50% of all cases are minor, and 50% are major.

Minor degree includes the following:

- Type I (lateral or low-lying) implantation: includes the lower uterine segment but not the internal os
- Type II (marginal) implantation: includes the lower edge of the placenta extending to but not covering the internal os

Major degree includes the following:

- Type III (partial): the placenta partially covers the dilated internal os
- Type IV (complete or central): the placenta completely covers the internal os, even when fully dilated (Oyelese & Smulian, 2006)

SOGC (2007b) currently suggests that when the placental edge does not reach the internal os, the distance in millimeters of the edge from the internal os should be reported; when the placental edge overlaps the internal os, the overlap in millimeters should be reported; and when the placental edge is exactly at the internal os, the distance should be reported as 0 mm.

Etiology and Pathophysiology

Early in the second trimester, the unformed lower uterine segment extends only 0.5 cm from the internal cervical os. Ultrasounds performed during this time show 5% of all placentas as low lying and close to the internal os (Baskett, 2004). As the lower uterine segment develops over the last 12 weeks, the upper uterine segment and attached placenta appear to move up and away from the cervix (placental migration). By term, only 1 in 250 placentas remain low lying (placenta previa). Transvaginal sonography is considered as the preferred method over transabdominal sonography for the accurate localization of a low-lying placenta (SOGC, 2007b). Operative interventions on the uterus that cause damage to, and scar tissue formation in, the endometrium increase the risk for low implantation. Such problems may decrease the possibility for the natural expansion that facilitates placental migration away from the cervical os.

Risk Factors

Risk factors for placenta previa include previous cesarean birth, previous placenta previa, previous pregnancy termination, prior intrauterine surgery, multiparity, maternal age older than 35 years, and use of cocaine (Usta et al., 2005). Smoking doubles the risk of placenta previa and is based on years of use rather than quantity (Oyelese & Canterino, 2011). Other possible contributing factors include uterine anomalies (eg, bicornuate or septate uterus), a short interval between pregnancies, living at a high altitude, and Asian ethnicity (an 86% higher incidence of placenta previa than in the general population).

Complications

Associated complications include coagulopathy, post-partum hemorrhage (because the lower segment contracts poorly and lacerates easily), uterine rupture, and vasa previa. Other placental abnormalities are possible because of poor development at the implantation site.

Assessment Findings

The most common signs and symptoms of placenta previa are antepartum hemorrhage and fetal malpresentation in late pregnancy because of displacement by the low-occupying placenta. Near term, the lower uterine segment is formed and stretched. The edge of a placenta implanted in this area may separate from the uterine wall, causing bleeding that is normally painless. Generally, the first bleeding episode associated with placenta previa is rarely fatal, with maternal death occurring in 0.03% of all cases (Baskett, 2004). Major degrees of placenta previa bleed earlier, more often, and more heavily than minor degrees. Bleeding is often associated with contractions; 10% of women do not begin bleeding until labour starts (Alexander & Schneider, 2000).

Other presenting symptoms include the following:

- A uterus felt to be "soft" on palpation
- Fetal heart present with a normal rate
- Shock and anemia (corresponding with the amount of blood lost)
- Increased risk for postpartum hemorrhage (lower uterine segment has less contractility)
- Abnormalities of the placenta and cord insertion (Baskett, 2004)

Any bleeding after 20 weeks' gestation warrants investigation, preferably by transvaginal or, if that is not available, transabdominal ultrasound to determine the placental location. A sterile speculum examination can help determine other causes of bleeding, such as cervicitis. An asymptomatic placenta previa identified before the last half of the third trimester has a 90% chance of moving to the normal location; therefore, an ultrasound should be performed in the third trimester to determine whether placenta previa still exists (Gilbert, 2011; SOGC, 2007b). Bleeding usually stops, but may resume at a later date.

With more women undergoing ultrasound examination early in the second trimester, more low-lying placentas are being noted and documented, with additional ultrasounds performed closer to term to monitor the condition's progress. If a woman is diagnosed with a placenta less than 20 mm from the cervical os, careful individualized plans are developed, with the expectation of a cesarean birth as close to term as possible, ensuring that blood for transfusion is available to minimize risks to the woman and fetus (SOGC, 2007b).

Collaborative Management

Antenatal admission is necessary for the client who presents with bleeding during pregnancy. At this time, nursing care focuses on the following measures:

- Clotting studies on a blood sample
- Avoidance of speculum or digital vaginal examination, if at all possible
- Establishment of a large-bore IV line (16G or 18G for blood transfusion, if needed)
- Administration of oxygen, if needed
- Monitoring of vital signs (BP, pulse, and respirations)
- Assessment of quantity, colour, and presence of clots, if bleeding
- Continuous monitoring of fetal heart rate
- Caring for the woman in a left lateral position
- Anticipation of cesarean birth and monitoring closely for postpartum hemorrhage (general anaesthesia would be considered if the woman is hypovolemic, still bleeding, or both; spinal anaesthesia would be considered if bleeding stops and volume status is within normal limits)

The nurse should speak calmly to the woman and support persons, explaining interventions and their purposes. He or she should identify the roles of various care providers and document care, teaching, and outcomes.

Signs of improved tissue perfusion include blood clotting, vital signs within normal limits, and decreased blood loss. Evidence of the woman's ability to cope with the situation includes decreased maternal tension and verbalized understanding of interventions. Signs of significant blood loss are shock (hypotension, pale, clammy skin), measured vaginal bleeding (soaked pads), and laboured breathing.

Bed rest may initially be part of the plan until bleeding has stopped and the woman's condition has stabilized for at least 24 to 48 hours, at which time the woman may be discharged to home care. Blood for transfusion must be available at all times; any anemia should be treated. The woman who is Rh negative needs to receive Rh immune globulin (see Chapter 22). Diagnostic transvaginal ultrasound is most appropriate to determine the exact placental location.

Team members collaborate with the woman regarding where she will receive ongoing care, depending on her distance from an appropriate health care facility. Options for home care depend on the degree of placenta previa, point of gestation, and safety concerns. The woman who is at less than 34 weeks' gestation needs corticosteroids, as per institutional policy, to increase fetal lung maturity. Many women with placenta previa give birth before 35 weeks' gestation. See Chapter 16 for discussions of cesarean birth and for considerations when placenta previa is first noted in a labouring client.

Invasive Placentas

Three types of invasive placentas are placenta accreta, placenta increta, and placenta percreta. *Placenta accreta* refers to abnormal development and implantation of the placenta into the myometrium. *Placenta increta* occurs when the chorionic villi invade into the myometrium. *Placenta percreta* is growth of the chorionic villi through the myometrium, into the uterine serosa and into adjacent structures such as the bladder, ureters, bowel, and omentum (Gilbert, 2011; Oyelese & Canterino, 2011).

Normally, after an infant is born, the placenta separates or shears away from the uterine surface. It is impossible for the placenta implanted into the myometrium to separate, so blood loss increases until the placenta can be removed manually. Ultrasound or magnetic resonance imaging (MRI) is necessary to determine the presence of an invasive placenta, particularly in women with a history of placenta previa or previous cesarean birth. Both these conditions significantly increase the risk for an invasive placenta (Gilbert, 2011). For example, the risk for placenta accreta is eight times greater with one cesarean birth and four times greater still with a history of two or more cesarean births (Usta et al., 2005). The woman is also at increased risk for a hysterectomy if the placenta cannot be manually removed.

Placenta accrete is a cause of significant hemorrhage. Planning for birth, including appropriate place and interdisciplinary team members, is important. An initial plan after admission of expectant management with ongoing assessment for bleeding, maternal vital signs, and fetal well-being may be appropriate. Outcomes can be optimized with a plan for cesarean birth via a vertical uterine incision in the fundus, with hysterectomy performed with the placenta still intact. Use of interventional radiologists to embolize or occlude the uterine arteries to reduce bleeding is helpful with inflation occurring after the birth of the infant and continuing until the hysterectomy is complete (Oyelese & Canterino, 2011).

If the woman suddenly begins bleeding, the cesarean birth may be done emergently for an immature fetus. Steroids may be administered to accelerate fetal lung maturation in gestations less than 34 weeks. An IV line (18G to allow for blood transfusion, as required), with blood available and/or cross-matched at all times, should be part of the nursing care of the hospitalized client. Currently, in some geographic areas, women diagnosed with placental problems are hospitalized and prescribed limited activity awaiting fetal maturation. In other areas, antenatal care is conducted at home to allow women to remain with their families while being monitored for signs of labour and/or bleeding.

Circumvallate Placenta

With a *circumvallate placenta,* the edges roll under the placenta during development, and a membrane forms around the entire outside edge (Alexander & Schneider, 2000). Causes include deep uterine implantation and bleeding early in gestation. Circumvallate placenta occurs in approximately 1% of pregnancies (Alexander & Schneider, 2000). Bleeding can occur if the membranous edge separates. If bleeding is absent or controlled, the client can receive care similar to that used for women with minor placenta previa. If bleeding persists or increases, cesarean birth is necessary (Alexander & Schneider, 2000). See Chapter 16.

Placental Abruption

Placental abruption (abruptio placentae) is the premature separation of a normally implanted placenta from the uterine wall (Fig. 13.18). This serious complication is the most common cause of intrapartal fetal death (Usta et al., 2005).

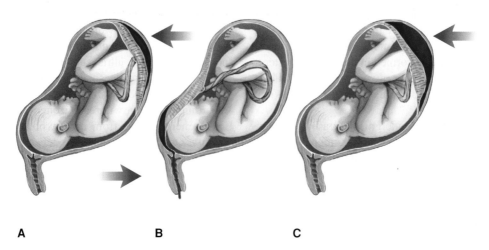

FIGURE 13.18 Types of placental abruption. **A:** Partial with concealed hemorrhage. **B:** Partial with apparent hemorrhage. **C:** Complete with concealed hemorrhage.

Etiology

The cause of placental abruption is unknown. This complication is present in approximately 0.6% to 1.2% of all pregnancies (Ananth & Kinzler, 2011). Risk factors include advanced maternal age, hypertension, cocaine, tobacco and alcohol use, unusually short cord, abdominal trauma, polyhydramnios, pPROM, intramniotic infection and diabetes. Folate deficiency, increased parity, multiple gestation, and male fetal gender also are associated. The majority of abruptions are idiopathic. Women with a history of a second trimester, third trimester, or repeated fetal loss are at high risk for placental abruption in a subsequent pregnancy. A previous abruption is the strongest predictor (Ananth & Kinzler, 2011; Lindqvist & Happach, 2006).

Placental abruption can result from bleeding followed by hematoma formation and then rebleeding. This cycle can continue, causing ongoing separation of the placenta from the uterine wall. The displaced portion of the placenta is no longer perfused, interrupting the maternal–fetal circulation. Fetal death can result, as can maternal DIC.

Classification

Placental abruption normally is classified as mild, moderate, or severe. Approximately 90% of cases are mild to moderate and do not lead to any fetal concerns, maternal hypotension, or coagulopathy (Palmer, 2002). Further classifications are as follows:

- *Marginal or apparent:* separation is near the edge of the placenta; blood can escape
- *Central or concealed:* separation is in the centre of the placenta; blood is trapped in a pocket of the placenta
- *Mixed or combined:* part of the separation is near the edge; part is concealed in the centre (Gilbert, 2011)

Assessment Findings

Presenting symptoms depend on the degree and type of detachment. Onset may be sudden. The goal of care is to recognize and to treat the cause of any visible bleeding as quickly as possible. Visible vaginal blood loss can be misleading, because the "true" maternal blood loss may be concealed behind the placenta (Palmer, 2002).

The nurse should assess for the colour and amount of vaginal bleeding, as well as for uterine tenderness and rigidity. Pain in the abdomen or back may be sudden, sharp, and severe. Concealed blood causes uterine pressure and myometrial contractions, which result in abdominal tenderness and pain. If the woman has epidural anaesthesia infusing, palpation may reveal continuous abdominal rigidity.

Because of the pregnant state, the vital signs of a woman experiencing placental abruption may not indicate accurately her degree of blood loss or shock. Symptoms of shock usually do not occur until hemorrhage is significant. They may include hypotension, tachycardia, decreased urinary output, shallow and irregular respirations, pallor, and thirst.

The fetal heart should be monitored continuously in the case of suspected placental abruption; indicators include increased or absent resting tone in the tocodynometer and repetitive late or variable decelerations.

Ongoing blood loss can result in coagulopathy and progress in a few cases to DIC. It is critical for health care providers to work together to continually evaluate through laboratory testing, physical examination, and fetal monitoring to ensure ongoing health and safety. Laboratory testing includes a complete blood count, hemoglobin and hematocrit, platelet count, fibrinogen and fibrin-split products, and type and cross-match. It also is critical to hold several units of blood in reserve.

Collaborative Management

Care depends on gestation and maternal–fetal status. The goal is stabilization. If the fetus is alive and near or at term, the team focuses on achieving cesarean birth as quickly as possible. Blood loss at birth may be substantial; medications such as oxytocin, ergometrine, and carboprost tromethamine (Hemabate) should be readily available (Palmer, 2002). Ongoing assessment of vital signs, pain, bleeding, and fetal monitoring are essential components of all plans of care. See Chapter 16.

If the fetus is immature and blood loss is slow, birth can be postponed. Discussion with the client and family is necessary to help them understand why plans might change suddenly if bleeding increases or vital signs indicate hemorrhage. Interventions must include measures for evaluating blood test results and reassessing the condition. Ultrasound to check for "concealed" bleeding may be required.

In cases of severe abruption, the fetus may die in utero. In such cases, the decision for a vaginal or cesarean delivery is based on risks for hemorrhage or other complications related to optimizing maternal health.

ADOLESCENT PREGNANCY

In recent years, the pregnancy rate among adolescents has decreased to approximately 4.1% of all live births; nevertheless, this issue continues to have serious societal implications in Canada (Fleming et al., 2013). This rate may be reflective of increased sex education in schools, increased awareness and use of contraception, and increased availability of abortion services.

In some geographical areas, the rate is higher, as Nunavut had the overall highest proportion of live births to teenage mothers in 2012 (Health Canada, 2012).

In most cases, teen pregnancy is unplanned. Developmentally, adolescents tend to be in the "concrete thinking" phase, in which use of contraception, particularly condoms, as part of future planning and avoidance of adverse consequences does not enter into decision making. The young woman (and her partner) may think that pregnancy will never happen to them and that they are somehow protected from risky behaviour (Feroli & Burstein, 2003). In some cases, teens may intentionally try to become pregnant without appreciating the responsibilities and risks inherent in assuming the parental role. Risk factors for teen pregnancy include school failures, high rates of sexual activity, sexual or physical violence at the home, and cultural values and norms that accept adolescent parenting (Anderson & McCarley, 2013; Cox, 2007).

If a pregnant teen chooses to continue with the gestation, she is at greater risk for perinatal complications than a pregnant woman between 20 and 35 years old. Some of these risks are related to aspects of her situation, such as lower rates of education and family income and higher rates of smoking and substance use. Specific perinatal concerns for expectant teens include iron-deficiency anemia, gestational hypertension, preterm birth, and low–birth-weight infant. Competition between the adolescent's own needs for growth and development and fetal demands may contribute to such problems (Youngkin et al., 2013).

COLLABORATIVE CARE: THE PREGNANT ADOLESCENT

In Canada, the pregnant adolescent is considered an independent client: it is her decision whether to inform or involve her parent(s) or other support persons in the provision of health care.

Assessment

Assessment parameters for pregnant teens are similar to those for any pregnant woman (see Chapter 12). For clients of this developmental stage, assessment of social support systems is especially critical, as these may vary between family, friends, or a partner. Encouraging teens to involve helpful family members and friends when making decisions may be beneficial because lack of support has been shown to lead to increased stress, depression, a less than positive birth experience, and risk of preterm birth (Anderson & McCarley, 2013).

Select Potential Nursing Diagnoses

The following are examples of nursing diagnoses commonly applicable to pregnant adolescents:

- **Risk for Ineffective Health Maintenance** related to inadequate prenatal care and nutrition
- **Risk for Imbalanced Nutrition: Less Than Body Requirements**
- **Risk for Delayed Growth and Development**

- **Fatigue**
- **Deficient Knowledge**
- **Risk for Situational Low Self-Esteem**

Planning/Intervention

At the first prenatal appointment, providing information about the teen's options is important. Generally, the choices are to continue with the pregnancy and raise the baby, to continue with the pregnancy and place the child with adoptive services, or to terminate the pregnancy. Educating the client about procedures, processes, and the risks and benefits involved with each choice is critical to her decision making. It is also important to ensure that the teen asks questions and verbalizes understanding of information she is given. Asking her privately if she wants someone to be present when receiving this information will help her feel supported and further develop her trust in the health care provider.

If the client decides to terminate her pregnancy, advice, instructions, or both should be given in a straightforward, nonthreatening manner (see Chapter 9). If she chooses to continue the pregnancy, scheduling follow-up appointments to review information as well as to perform the necessary examinations is important. Additional interventions may include referrals to community nursing, social services, or both for extra support (American Academy of Pediatrics and the American College of Obstetricians and Gynecologists [AAP & ACOG], 2002). Monitoring the teen's psychosocial needs throughout the gestation and attempting to find resources and ways to meet them is an integral part of client advocacy (Fig. 13.19). See Research Highlight 13.3.

Evaluation

Giving the pregnant teen a chance to collaborate with health care providers when formulating plans of care is critical. Desired outcomes are for the adolescent to

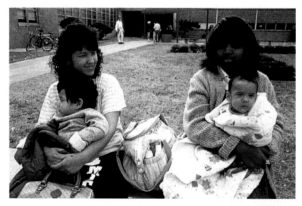

FIGURE 13.19 Adolescents may benefit socially from school-sponsored programs that continue after pregnancy to facilitate interactions with other young mothers and their children.

● **RESEARCH HIGHLIGHT 13.3** Pregnant Adolescents' Perspectives of Pregnancy

OBJECTIVE

The purpose of this qualitative study was to obtain a clearer understanding of teens' perspectives on pregnancy and parenting.

SAMPLE

Twenty unmarried teens pregnant for the first time and planning to keep the child were interviewed during the second or third trimester.

METHOD

Each teen participated in a 60- to 90-minute interview with questions such as "What was life like before you became pregnant?" and "What do you think it will be like being a mother?" The researchers grouped data into themes using grounded theory and the constant comparative method.

RESULTS

These young women described three major themes. "The Pregnant Me—Unexpected Changes" involved surprise that pregnancy-related changes included new emotions, lifestyle choices, and future plans, as well as the many unexpected physical manifestations of gestation. "Transformed Relationships" referred to responses from others including peers, partners, and significant adults. The final theme, "Envisioning Motherhood," included the responses of fear, awe, and desire to be a "good mother."

CONCLUSION

The teens in this small sample size described positive feelings about pregnancy and the hope of being good parents. They communicated a wish to protect their fetuses through lifestyle changes, such as decreasing smoking and improving eating habits.

NURSING IMPLICATIONS

Community nurses, particularly those working with teens (eg, school nurses) need to build on positive responses and give opportunities for pregnant adolescents to support one another. Assisting teens to become more aware of the process of pregnancy can help them anticipate changes, which may improve their coping. Support groups that begin during and continue after pregnancy might promote ongoing lifestyle improvements as well as enhancing parenting skills.

From Rentschler, D. (2003). Pregnant adolescents' perspectives of pregnancy. *Journal of Maternal–Child Nursing, 28*, 377–383.

understand her alternatives and to identify people she wants involved in her care. If the client elects to continue the pregnancy, desired outcomes are for care providers to develop a good working relationship with her, encourage her attendance at prenatal visits, and provide ongoing care as needed for her specific circumstances. When planning labour and birth, it is important to remember that adolescents express different needs than adults, usually with a focus on pain management, nonjudgmental nursing care, and emotional support (Anderson & McCarley, 2013). In a recent study, when asked about prenatal classes, only a small number of adolescents reported attending (Sauls, 2010). When asked about labour, adolescents indicated that they want to be treated with respect, to be advocated for in terms of pain management, to receive information on options, and to know that their support person(s) will be present and involved (Sauls, 2010). Pregnant adolescents are at a much higher risk for depression related to family history, exposure to stressful life experiences, and childhood adversity. Screening with the EDPS can be helpful pre- and postpartum with appropriate treatment and referrals.

MULTIPLE PREGNANCY

Multiple pregnancy (gestation with two or more fetuses) is considered high risk because it has an increased potential for fetal abnormalities, prematurity, discordant fetal growth, and fetal growth restriction (Malcus, 2004). Other associated risks include preeclampsia, anemia (maternal blood volume is 500 mL or more than in single pregnancy), and increased discomforts such as constipation (Watson-Blasioli, 2001). Prenatal health care providers should be alert for these complications.

Incidence of multiple pregnancy is increasing for many reasons: older maternal ages, frequent use of reproductive-assisted technology, and hereditary factors (SOGC, 2007c; Watson-Blasioli, 2001). In Canada, the rates of multiple births have increased steadily over time from 20 per 1,000 total births in 1991 to 31.4 per 1,000 total births in 2009 (Fell & Joseph, 2012). The number of twins increased by 35% and triplets by 58% (Healy & Gaddipati, 2005). See Chapter 11 for details on developmental processes that lead to multiple gestation and the different types.

Care of clients with multiple gestation is challenging throughout pregnancy, labour, and birth. Mothers are at risk for preterm labour, preeclampsia, placental dysfunction, cord abnormalities, gestational diabetes, and intrauterine fetal growth restriction (Graham & Gaddipati, 2005). Ongoing assessment of fetal well-being is important. Twin studies have shown that fetal heart rate accelerations are simultaneous 52% of the time and that both fetuses have synchronous behaviour patterns 95% of the time (sleep or awake state) (Hayward, 2003). Thus, NSTs for women with multiple gestation should be done with fetal monitors that can simultaneously record two or more fetal heart rates. Frequent review of the results is necessary to protect the health of all fetuses being assessed.

The frequency of ultrasound evaluation in multiple gestation depends on the risk factors and preferences of the primary care provider. As with singleton pregnancy, ultrasound is used to determine gestation, fetal growth, and amniotic fluid volume. In multiple gestation, ultrasound also is necessary to determine chorionicity, one of the most important determinants of outcome. This is best determined in the first trimester, as early as 10 to 14 weeks. Monochorionic twins share a placenta and vascular anastomoses in the placenta and/or growth abnormalities can put one or both twins at risk (Cleary-Goldman & D'Alton, 2008). Twin-to-twin transfusion syndrome (TTTS) complicates approximately 15% of monochorionic multiple gestations and is associated with a mortality rate of 30% to 50% (Kumar & O'Brien, 2004). Risk factors for this problem include a single monochorionic placenta, polyhydramnios, oligohydramnios, and same-sex fetuses. It is characterized by a circulation imbalance through communicating vessels across the sharing placenta, leading to an underperfusion of one twin and an overperfusion of the other (Cleary-Goldman & D'Alton, 2008). Findings may include a chronically distended bladder in one fetus, fetal growth discordance, and evidence of fetal cardiac dysfunction (Gilbert, 2011). In cases of TTTS, the family needs care from a facility that can provide individualized evaluation and counselling (Kumar & O'Brien, 2004). The other concern for monochorionic pregnancies includes the increased risk of velamentous cord insertion (13% to 21% vs. 1% to 2% of singleton pregnancies).

Monochorionic, monoamniotic placentation is a rare condition of multiple gestation associated with a mortality rate as high as 50% from cord entanglement, knots, congenital anomalies, and prematurity (SOGC, 2000). Cord entanglement occurs in almost all monoamniotic twins. Other sonographic features of a monoamniotic pregnancy include the following:

- No dividing amniotic membrane
- A single placenta
- Same-sex fetuses
- Adequate amniotic fluid surrounding each fetus
- Fetuses moving freely within the uterine cavity (SOGC, 2000)

COLLABORATIVE CARE: MULTIPLE PREGNANCIES

Care for the client with a multiple gestation mainly involves educating the client and family about their many options for care. Plans must be flexible enough to accommodate emergency interventions (eg, cesarean birth) as necessary, while facilitating the woman's participation in decision making (eg, feeding choices, support people, early comfort measures depending on gestation and fetal positions). Team members should give realistic information as pregnancy progresses to dispel myths. They should encourage the woman/family to discuss fears and worries openly. The following paragraphs focus on care during pregnancy of the woman carrying more than one fetus. Chapter 16 presents special considerations relative to labour and birth in multiple gestation.

Assessment

Ongoing prenatal assessment of cervical length may help predict the chances of preterm birth. Restricted activity may be recommended or simply initiated as a practical necessity, because of the mobility limitations imposed by the increased fetal weight. Planning for this possibility can decrease the client's social isolation and increase her ability to cope. Upper-body exercises and physiotherapy may be helpful for clients who must remain on bed rest (Mariano & Hickey, 1998). Restricted activity, bed rest, and leaving employment early in the pregnancy, however, have not been shown to decrease the likelihood of preterm birth and are therefore not routinely recommended (Crowther, 2001; SOGC, 2000).

Assessment of maternal weight gain is critical. Although specific recommendations must be tailored to each woman's prepregnant body mass index (see Chapter 12), for multiple pregnancies increased nutritional intake is especially important in the first and second trimesters (Luke, 2005a). A woman expecting twins should gain between 9.1 and 13.6 kg by 20 weeks and approximately 0.68 kg/week thereafter (Luke, 2005a). Women need to be offered nutrition counselling and dietary resources to support a pregnancy weight gain of 18 to 27 kg (SOGC, 2007c).

When discussing nutrition, the care provider emphasizes quality and variety while ensuring that the woman is eating adequate servings from all food groups (Mariano & Hickey, 1998). Other discussion topics include ways to manage constipation, consume sufficient nutrients, and deal with nausea and vomiting; problems in these areas may necessitate referral to a dietician.

Ongoing ultrasounds during pregnancy provide information on fetal growth and development and help detect any anomalies, rates of which are 40% higher in multiples (SOGC, 2000). For each fetus in a multiple pregnancy, growth is similar to that found in a single pregnancy until approximately 32 to 35 weeks' gestation, when the rate for the multiples slows.

During each prenatal visit, the primary care provider checks the lie and presentation of each fetus, which will be critical determining factors relative to the type of birth (vaginal or cesarean). Ultrasound as well as abdominal palpation should be used to confirm the fetal positions.

Select Potential Nursing Diagnoses

The following are examples of commonly applicable nursing diagnoses in cases of multiple gestation:

- **Anxiety** related to maternal and fetal health concerns
- **Fear** related to labour, birth, and the health of the mother and fetuses
- **Constipation** related to decreased gastrointestinal functioning
- **Risk for Imbalanced Nutrition** related to the demands of multiple pregnancy
- **Risk for Ineffective Health Maintenance** related to multiple pregnancy care requirements
- **Deficient Knowledge** related to specialized care for multiple pregnancy
- **Risk for Compromised Family Coping** related to the increased demands of multiple newborns

Planning/Intervention

Maternal–fetal attachment has been studied mainly in terms of single pregnancies. Damato (2000) concluded that nurses should ask nonjudgemental questions regarding a woman's emotional adjustment to a multifetal pregnancy. Differing feelings for each fetus may not be unusual, and parents should understand that such attitudes are valid. Parents may need time to process the circumstances related to their high-risk pregnancy and the potential for preterm birth. If labour happens early, interrupted antepartal attachment may compromise perinatal bonding. If the woman's partner is involved, nurses should include him or her as much as possible in prenatal care and encourage his or her support. They also should refer the client and her support people to associations or clubs that encourage the sharing of hopes and fears in cases of multiple gestation.

Multifetal pregnancies are associated with many financial, personal, and social costs for the families involved. Nurses should provide anticipatory information to these families to prepare them for the increased emotional, financial, and practical stresses they are likely to experience. Participation in organizations such as the Parents of Multiples Birth Association (POMBA) before birth helps establish a source for support and networking. Community nurses are ideally placed to visit families during the prenatal periods to prepare them. Referral to a social worker, counselling services, family support programs, or all of these may be appropriate.

Ongoing discussion with the woman and family regarding social support and preparation for infant care after birth is necessary. Parents of multiples are at increased risk for divorce, child abuse, and postpartum depression related to increased emotional and financial stress (Mariano & Hickey, 1998). Assistance in coping skills and anticipation of the need for increased social support can be extremely valuable.

Because of the risk for preterm labour associated with a multiple pregnancy, the nurse should teach the client the signs and symptoms of this problem. The mean weekly frequency of uterine contractions is higher than in a singleton pregnancy; additionally, contractions gradually increase with gestation and increased uterine size (Stock & Norman, 2010).

Evaluation

In cases of multiple pregnancy, ideal outcomes are for the woman to reach 36 to 37 weeks' gestation with all fetuses growing and developing normally, with progress toward the birth of all healthy infants while maintaining the health of the mother. Close fetal monitoring through movement counts, Doppler studies (as appropriate), biophysical profiles, and NST are measures by which to monitor progress. Verbalization from family members that they are prepared for their postpartal circumstances is equally important. See Chapter 16 for more information.

PERINATAL LOSS

From the earliest moments of learning about a pregnancy, parents envision their infant's future, with expectations and hopes for their life together (Michon et al., 2003). Regardless of the point of gestation at which it happens, a pregnancy loss can be difficult for the family involved. Parents who experience perinatal loss move through the stages of shock and numbness, searching and yearning, disorganization and depression, and reorganization. They adjust to the loss at varying paces depending on support systems, individual coping strategies, strengths, and other stressors. Generally, the bereavement process lasts 6 to 24 months. According to Michon et al. (2003), the grief experienced by mothers is usually of greater intensity than that of fathers.

Societal changes have contributed to increased parental grieving over perinatal loss. The lower infant mortality rate and scientific advances have fostered expectations for pregnancies to continue without disruption, which encourages women to bond early with their fetuses. Methods of reproductive control may increase a woman's motivation to plan pregnancy for a specific time or point in her life. When a pregnancy is lost under such conditions, sadness and mourning are likely to be greater.

Early Pregnancy Loss

Most pregnancy losses occur within the first trimester (Abboud & Liamputtong, 2003). **Miscarriage** is the lay term used for a pregnancy lost before 20 weeks' gestation. It is estimated that 25% to 50% of pregnancies result in early pregnancy loss (Callister, 2006). In Canada, the definition includes fetal weight less than 500 g. If the fetal weight is greater than 500 g, gestation is longer than 20 weeks, or both, arrangements are needed for disposition of the remains, by cremation or interment. Registration is required according to provincial Vital Statistics legislation.

The medical term for pregnancy loss before 20 weeks' gestation is *abortion,* regardless of whether the event is elective or spontaneous (Table 13.5). Nurses should be sensitive to the terminology they use when discussing a pregnancy loss with clients and their families, however, because some people may view the term "abortion" as unkind, judgemental, or inappropriate.

When a client experiences a spontaneous abortion, feelings may vary from relief (if the pregnancy was unwanted) to extreme sadness and despair (Gilbert, 2011). The woman may feel like a failure or want acknowledgement of the loss from everyone to whom she announced the pregnancy. Spontaneous abortion is unique in that the woman experiences the death of another literally inside of her and attached to her (Callister, 2006). Usually, few interventions can prevent a spontaneous abortion; however, the client may blame herself or be blamed by others (Abboud & Liamputtong, 2003). She may also have an ongoing sense of failure for being unable to maintain pregnancy. A second-trimester loss may be especially difficult, because the client and family are likely to have experienced objective validations of the pregnancy's existence, such as seeing the fetus through ultrasound, hearing the fetal heartbeat, or feeling fetal movements. Because most pregnancy losses occur before 12 weeks' gestation, a second-trimester spontaneous abortion may be more traumatic because it is less expected.

Common causes of early pregnancy loss include genetic abnormalities, uterine or cervical problems, infections, substance use, and maternal medical conditions (eg, diabetes, hypothyroidism). Two other common problems related to early pregnancy loss are ectopic pregnancy and gestational trophoblastic disease.

Ectopic Pregnancy

Ectopic pregnancy, a life-threatening condition, occurs when the products of conception implant anywhere other than the uterus (Fig. 13.20). It happens in approximately 1.5% of pregnancies (Royal College of Obstetricians and Gynaecologists [RCOG], 2002). Most ectopic implantations involve the fallopian tubes; as gestation continues, bleeding and pain develop. If untreated, the tube can rupture, causing severe hemorrhage that may lead to maternal collapse and death (Abbott, 2004).

● TABLE 13.5 **Classifications of Spontaneous Abortions**

Type	Definition	Management
Complete abortion	Passage of all products of conception, revealed by ultrasound showing an empty uterus	Follow-up care to discuss related issues, family planning needs, psychosocial concerns
Habitual abortion	Three or more consecutive spontaneous abortions	Identification and treatment of underlying cause (if possible) If related to cervical insufficiency, cerclage in future pregnancies to promote successful outcome
Incomplete abortion	Passage of some of the products of conception, revealed by ultrasound showing retained material in the uterus	Dilation and curettage (D&C) or administration of prostaglandin analog to evacuate the uterus
Inevitable abortion	Pregnancy loss that cannot be prevented	If products of conception are not passed spontaneously, vacuum curettage or administration of prostaglandin analog to evacuate the uterus
Missed abortion	Nonviable embryo retained in utero for 6 wk or more	Uterine evacuation by suction curettage or D&C, depending on the stage of the pregnancy Induction of labour as a nonsurgical option
Threatened abortion	Vaginal bleeding early in gestation, with no passage of embryonic or fetal tissue	Possibly, mild activity restriction

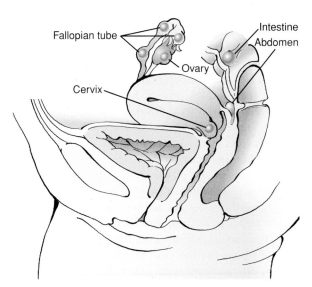

FIGURE 13.20 Sites for implantation of an ectopic pregnancy may include the fallopian tubes, ovary, intestines, abdomen, and cervix.

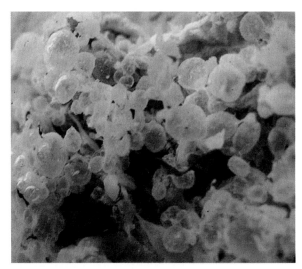

FIGURE 13.21 Complete molar pregnancy.

Causes and risk factors for ectopic pregnancy include blocked or narrowed fallopian tubes that prevent ova from reaching the uterus; previous pelvic infection; history of chlamydia infection; previous appendicitis; history of infertility or cesarean birth; age more than 35 years; and smoking (Abbott, 2004).

Presenting symptoms may include a positive pregnancy test, vaginal bleeding, and abdominal pain, which usually is one sided but not necessarily on the side of the ectopic implantation. Bleeding may range from spotting to severe hemorrhage. A classic sign of a ruptured ectopic pregnancy is shoulder tip pain caused by internal bleeding irritating the diaphragm. Bladder pain may accompany urination, and the client may feel pressure in the bowels. Dizziness, pallor, and nausea may precede collapse. Up to 75% of affected clients present with subacute symptoms (Abbott, 2004). Transvaginal ultrasound can confirm the diagnosis from 4 weeks' gestation onward.

Treatment may involve drugs (eg, c) or laparoscopic surgery. The emergency surgery and reality of the lost pregnancy can pose challenges to the client's psychological health and relationships. Women who have experienced ectopic pregnancy describe it as "a termination without consent" (Abbott, 2004, p. 33). Initial feelings may include pain, fear for personal safety, and concern for future fertility. The linkage with past STIs as a risk factor may heighten a woman's emotions over this experience. Providing supportive care and expressing sympathy are important interventions; the nurse also should give information about community resources.

Gestational Trophoblastic Disease
Gestational trophoblastic disease (molar pregnancy) is abnormal proliferation and degeneration of the tro-

phoblastic villi. When gestational trophoblastic disease occurs, gestational tissue exists, but the pregnancy is not viable. As the gestational cells degenerate, they fill with fluid (Fig. 13.21). In addition to the typical early indicators of pregnancy (ie, amenorrhea, fatigue, breast tenderness), signs and symptoms of molar pregnancy include brownish vaginal bleeding, anemia, hyperemesis gravidarum, edema, disparity between uterine size and gestational age, elevated hCG levels, absent fetal heart sounds, and a characteristic molar pattern on ultrasound.

There are two types of gestational trophoblastic disease: complete and partial hydatidiform moles. With a complete hydatidiform mole, all the villi swell and form cysts. This problem has an accompanying risk for *choriocarcinoma,* a dangerous and rapidly spreading malignancy. With a partial hydatidiform mole, some villi form normally. Partial moles rarely lead to choriocarcinoma. Regardless of type, the uterine contents must be immediately evacuated by dilation and curettage and tested for any evidence of malignancy. If no malignancy is found, the client must undergo follow-up tests of hCG levels for the next 12 months to ensure that any remaining tissue does not turn malignant. Chemotherapy may be used prophylactically or as treatment (see Chapter 4). Because of the risks for cancer, the client must be careful to avoid pregnancy for 1 year following gestational trophoblastic disease.

Late Pregnancy Loss
Stillbirth is the term used when a pregnancy of more than 20 weeks' gestation and a fetal weight of 500 grams ends in fetal death. Stillbirth is reported to have occurred at a rate of 7.1 per 1,000 births in 2009 in Canada (Joseph et al., 2013). Causes include cord accident, extreme prematurity, and congenital or chromosomal abnormalities (Gilbert, 2011). Another type of stillbirth

occurs when one fetus in a multiple gestation dies before or during labour and birth. In this event, the family may struggle with the ambivalence of celebrating the birth of the living baby or babies, while grieving for the one who has died. Another 1/4 of all stillbirths, despite extensive evaluation, have an unknown cause, which is also very difficult for families who are grieving and hoping for answers to their questions (Leduc et al., 2006).

COLLABORATIVE CARE: PREGNANCY LOSS

When a family has lost a pregnancy, health care providers must provide sensitive collaborative interventions that focus on information, understanding, and physical care. The team may involve physicians, midwives, nurses, public health nurses, and social workers. Ongoing communication about each professional's role and the care given can help ensure that the needs of the client and family are met. In some cases, families must deal with both birth and death within a short time and need extra support during this transition period (Chichester, 2005).

Assessment

Depending on when a gestation is lost, a client may come to the labour and birth area describing decreased or no fetal movements over an extended period. Fear, anxiety, and a desire for reassurance are common emotions at such times. The nurse should assess the fetal heart rate; if he or she cannot reassure the parents quickly, the nurse should notify the client's primary care provider immediately to move forward with additional evaluations. The next step may involve a biophysical profile or a real-time ultrasound scan, the results of which will indicate fetal health or confirm fetal death.

Select Potential Nursing Diagnoses

The following nursing diagnoses are commonly applicable in cases of perinatal loss:

- **Chronic Sorrow**
- **Risk for Dysfunctional Grieving**
- **Social Isolation** related to the grief process
- **Interrupted Family Processes** related to grief

Planning/Intervention

Once a gestation has been confirmed as lost, parents may feel shocked, confused, distressed, or fearful that they may have contributed to the event, or angry. Commonly, women and their partners search for an answer about what went wrong. Nurses should understand that such questioning is normal, while trying to learn whether a desire to blame someone or something for the loss is at the root of the concern (Abboud & Liamputtong, 2003). Giving short and simple explanations, allowing parents

to be together (if the woman has come alone, she should be asked about her preferences for someone to be with her), and providing a quiet place for grieving are helpful immediate interventions. Many facilities have a "quiet" room that provides privacy for families during such times. Nurses who cry at this event should feel reassured that this response is not unusual and can be a comforting expression of sympathy and empathy valued by the client and her significant others.

In cases of late pregnancy loss, the client may not experience labour immediately after fetal demise, which may be difficult for her and her family to understand. Some primary care providers encourage clients to wait for spontaneous labour rather than undergoing induction of labour. In either case, families may find it helpful if they can grieve for some time before labour begins.

Preparation of a birth plan for a family who is preparing for a stillbirth or neonatal death may include the development of a plan prior to labour. This may include asking the following questions and using the answers to develop a written plan for the health care providers, especially the nurse who will be present. Questions that might be included in such a plan are outlined in Box 13.1.

Once labour starts, care from the same supportive nurse can be comforting, especially if it helps to minimize the number of times the family needs to tell its story to health care providers. A "butterfly" or some other symbol posted on the client's door or assignment board helps to communicate the family's special circumstances so that staff members are prepared to approach them with extra sensitivity. Assisting the client to make decisions about pain relief methods and comfort measures may facilitate positive feelings about this time. Parents describe that continuing to have hope throughout this time is also helpful. This may include holding the baby, expressing love to their baby and having remembrances of the time spent together (Wool, 2013). Giving information about emotions and reactions that they may experience also can be helpful. Describing in simple terms the legal aspects necessary for an autopsy is important. An autopsy is one of the most important aspects of care for the family that wishes to seek further information. The nurse may explore with the parents options for memorial services, funeral, or other religious or ethnic traditions which deal with death and bereavement. Providing an opportunity for the health care provider to talk sensitively with the family to obtain consent as well as to follow-up with the family later with the results is important to the grieving process (Leduc et al., 2006).

Encouraging families to decide how much time to spend with their baby after birth and whether they want keepsakes such as pictures, a lock of hair, or footprints may result in better memories of the experience

● **BOX 13.1** Questions to Help Support Parents Who Experience a Stillbirth

---

- What is the name you have chosen for your baby? How would you like us to refer to your baby once she or he is born?
- Would you like help in sharing information with your other family members about your baby's problems?
- If you have children, have they ever experienced a death before? Did anything help them to cope with that experience?
- Whom would you like to be with you for your labour and birth?
- Would anything be helpful (eg, hydrotherapy, music, assistance with breathing techniques)?
- Whom would you like to be present after the baby's birth?
- Would you like your baby to be baptized or dedicated? Do you need us to call anyone?
- Would you like to assist us in dressing and bathing your baby?
- Would you like special memories of your baby (eg, lock of hair, umbilical cord clamp, ID band, footprint or mold made of hand or foot)
- Would you like photographs taken?
- Would you like help in planning your baby's memorial service? In planning for your baby's funeral?
- Do you have any special traditions that you wish us to honour?

Source: English, N., & Hessler, K. (2013). Perinatal birth planning for families of the imperiled newborn. *Journal of Obstetrical and Gynecological Nursing, 42*, 390–399.

(Gilbert, 2011). Alexander and Schneider (2000) write that respectful and compassionate pictures for parents to keep can assist in their mourning. Photos of the baby's foot or hand in a parent's or sibling's hand may be powerful and treasured remembrances. Some cultural groups, with strong religious beliefs, such as the Amish, view photographs as "graven images," however, and would not appreciate this approach.

Various cultures mourn and grieve losses differently. Most cultures highly value having children, and perinatal loss is very significant and painful. To provide culturally sensitive care, nurses must first identify their own values to facilitate respect for the wide-ranging emotions, customs, and wishes that others may bring to this experience (Chichester, 2005). Religion also may influence preferences for care. Some families may desire the presence of a support person from their faith or immediate baptism of the stillborn infant. Asking clients about such wishes helps to ensure the provision of culturally sensitive care (Chichester, 2005).

Parents who have experienced perinatal loss have described the following interventions as helpful (Gilbert, 2011):

- Support from a significant person during the experience
- Seeing the fetus
- Holding the baby
- Saving mementos
- Being given time to grieve
- Being allowed choices (decision making)
- Having sensitive caregivers
- Hearing words or phrases such as "I don't know what to say," "I am sorry, I can't imagine what this must be like for you," and "What is this like for you?" (Unhelpful statements such as "You can have another one" or "Time heals all wounds" are not comforting [Jonas-Simpson & McMahon, 2005]).

Health care providers need to acknowledge the client's physical and emotional pain (Abboud & Liamputtong, 2003). The mother requires immediate support and information to ensure that she does not blame herself for what has happened. She needs to be able to request care or counselling later if she requires it. Encouraging the partners to discuss their feelings in individual counselling and/or in support groups might be appropriate. Each member of the couple may not have legitimate means of expressing his or her own loss while supporting the other person. For the sake of their relationship, each person should be encouraged to assist the other to grieve at an individual pace and to use referrals as necessary (Abboud & Liamputtong, 2003). If the woman is stable, she will likely be discharged directly from the labour and birth area at a time when she and her partner and family are ready. If the woman needs to remain in the hospital, arrangements should be made for her to be transferred to another unit rather than remaining with other mothers and their babies, if that is her preference.

Nurses and other health care providers present for a stillbirth or an infant death describe feelings similar to those of mothers and families: anger, sadness, pain, helplessness, and isolation. Many nurses described "putting their heart" into their care and providing continuous empathetic care for the woman and her family during this time of sadness. Others report that these shared memories are among the strongest of their work life and that the emotion expressed stays with them. Nurses are encouraged to talk to one another, share their stories, and be involved in debriefing sessions if possible within 72 hours of the birth to aid in coping with these experiences (Puia et al., 2013).

Evaluation

Ensuring that family members feel that their wishes for care, privacy, comfort, and information were met is key.

Facilitating a smooth discharge from the health care facility is critical. Nurses also must do what they can to ensure that such families do not receive surveys from the facility about their experience or donation requests.

SUMMARY

- High-risk pregnancies involve conditions or complications that can endanger the safety of the mother, fetus, or both. The situation may involve the need for monitoring to prevent a maternal or fetal problem, such as with maternal obesity, substance use, or adolescent pregnancy; a significant health problem that existed before or developed during the pregnancy; or a health problem directly related to the gestation.

- A high-risk pregnancy is a stressor that requires risk assessment to guide planning for appropriate care, including the need for ongoing consultation and place of birth. Assessment of possible psychosocial, economic, nutritional, and family-related stressors is essential.

- The pregnant woman with asthma requires a step-wise approach to care to maintain adequate control of her symptoms during pregnancy. Use of corticosteroids may lead to decreased birth weight and increased risk for preeclampsia.

- The New York Heart Association's classification is used to determine the functional status of a pregnant woman with heart disease. Women with class I or II heart disease have a favourable prognosis, but their functional status may worsen with the physiologic changes of pregnancy. Gestational weeks 28 to 32 are a critical time for the pregnant woman with heart disease, because the increased blood volume peaks at this time.

- Fatigue, palpitations, and potentially chest pain or shortness of breath with exercise are common signs and symptoms associated with anemia during pregnancy. Iron-deficiency anemia is associated with preterm birth and low birth weight.

- The major problem related to pregnancy and SLE involves the placenta, with inflammatory responses that include infarctions, fibrin deposits, and small placental size. As a result, decreased placental circulation and fetal malnutrition can occur.

- Planning for screening, treatment, and follow-up for STIs is important during pregnancy. Collaboration with the woman is key to ensuring that she continues to complete preventive measures, treatments, or both. Testing for GBS (via swab obtained from the vaginal introitus and anorectum) is recommended for all pregnant women at 35 to 37 weeks' gestation.

- The most common cause of asymptomatic bacteriuria is *E. coli*. Costovertebral angle tenderness, high fever, chills, myalgia, nausea, and vomiting are common signs and symptoms of pyelonephritis. The pregnant woman with acute renal failure requires immediate therapy that includes frequent assessments of vital signs, breath sounds, fluid intake, and urine output as well as fetal monitoring such as NST and fetal movement counts.

- Key interventions for the pregnant woman with diabetes include blood glucose self-monitoring, diet management, activity and exercise, insulin administration (if required), and fetal monitoring.

- Although depression is associated more commonly with the postpartum period, women can experience depression anytime in life, including pregnancy. Women are at risk for developing bipolar disorder during their reproductive years.

- Health care providers need to be alert for indicators that may suggest that a woman is a victim of violence; these may include chronic pain and insomnia; irritable bowel syndrome; migraine headaches; arthritis; UTIs; injuries to the face, breasts, abdomen, and buttocks; anxiety; depression; fractures; unexplained bruises; areas of redness consistent with slap injuries; lacerations; and multiple injuries consistent with stages of healing.

- Alcohol use in pregnancy is a causative factor in birth defects and developmental delays; heavy or binge drinking has been linked to fetal alcohol spectrum disorder. A safe level of alcohol use during pregnancy has not been identified. Smoking during pregnancy is linked to preterm labour and intrauterine growth restriction.

- Hyperemesis gravidarum, which usually begins during the first 10 weeks of pregnancy, is manifested by nausea and vomiting, a greater than 5% weight loss, dehydration, and electrolyte imbalance.

- Hypertension in pregnancy is classified as pre-existing hypertension, pre-existing hypertension with comorbid conditions and/or with preeclampsia, gestational hypertension, and gestational hypertension with comorbid conditions and/or preeclampsia. Preeclampsia can progress to eclampsia (seizures).

- Decreased placental perfusion is a key pathophysiologic change with hypertension in pregnancy. Magnesium sulfate is the drug of choice for treating hypertension with risk factors for eclampsia. Close monitoring is necessary to prevent magnesium toxicity.

- Acute HELLP syndrome in a pregnant woman requires immediate and careful attention to both the mother and fetus. Successful treatment involves a balance between antenatal treatment and birth of a viable infant in the safest location for the family.

- A common treatment for pPROM is bed rest with ongoing assessment for fever, chills, and change in amniotic fluid (colour and odour) that would indicate chorioamnionitis.
- During pregnancy, a woman's blood is hypercoagulable, and events unique to pregnancy, such as abruptio placentae, intrauterine fetal demise, and preeclampsia, can trigger DIC.
- Placenta previa, a condition in which the placenta covers the cervical os to varying degrees, is the major cause of bleeding in the third trimester and commonly manifested by painless vaginal bleeding. Placental abruption, the premature separation of a normally implanted placenta from the abdominal wall, is manifested by vaginal bleeding, uterine tenderness, and rigidity. It is the most common cause of intrapartal fetal death.
- A pregnant adolescent is at greater risk for perinatal complications; adolescence is a risk factor for iron-deficiency anemia, preeclampsia, operative birth, preterm birth, and low–birth-weight infant.
- With a multiple pregnancy, the ideal outcomes are for the woman to reach 36 to 37 weeks' gestation with all fetuses growing and developing normally, culminating in the birth of all healthy infants and preservation of the mother's health. Close monitoring of fetal health through movement counts, Doppler studies, biophysical profiles, and NST are useful in monitoring the status of the pregnancy.
- Parents experiencing perinatal loss move through bereavement and adjust to their loss at their own pace depending on their support systems, individual coping strategies, strengths, and other stressors. This process averages about 6 to 24 months.
- Miscarriage is the term used to denote a pregnancy loss before 20 weeks' gestation. The medical term for a pregnancy loss before 20 weeks is abortion, regardless of whether it is elective or spontaneous. Stillbirth is the term used to denote a pregnancy that has lasted more than 20 weeks' gestation and ends without signs of life.
- Most ectopic pregnancies occur in the fallopian tube. The woman usually complains of pain on one side with some bleeding ranging in amount and character. Shoulder tip pain caused by irritation to the diaphragm is a classic sign of a ruptured ectopic pregnancy.
- Gestational trophoblastic disease occurs as one of the two types: complete molar pregnancy in which all the villi swell and form cysts; and partial mole in which some villi form normally. A complete molar pregnancy increases the woman's risk for developing choriocarcinoma, whereas partial moles rarely lead to this malignancy.

Questions to Ponder

1. Ms. C (GTPAL 3-1-1-0-2) has just been diagnosed with an anterior placenta previa. Her plan of care includes bed rest, biweekly biophysical and non-stress testing, vital signs every 12 hours, and fetal movement counting bid. Ms. C's two children are 5 and 3 years old, her husband is a shift worker at an automotive plant, and her parents live 300 miles away. How would you assess Ms. C's support system and teaching regarding her need for hospitalization at present?

2. Ms. C. has had no further episodes of bleeding, and the decision has been made to send her home on Home Care with weekly fetal monitoring at home, daily fetal movement counts, and instructions to return weekly for an ultrasound to monitor the baby's growth and development. Describe the teaching that you would do before Ms. C's discharge.

REVIEW QUESTIONS

1. When assessing a pregnant woman with asthma, the nurse would be most alert for exacerbation of asthmatic symptoms during which gestational weeks?
   A. 6 to 12
   B. 12 to 24
   C. 24 to 36
   D. 36 to 40

2. A pregnant woman with sickle cell anemia develops chronic hemolytic anemia. Which of the following findings would be least important for the nurse to assess?
   A. Severe bone pain
   B. Jaundice
   C. Splenomegaly
   D. Cholelithiasis

3. Which of the following should the nurse include when describing the care that will be required during labour for a pregnant client with HIV?
   A. Artificial rupture of membranes
   B. Internal electronic fetal monitoring
   C. Expected cesarean birth
   D. Antibiotic therapy before birth

4. After teaching a group of students about the effects of parvovirus infection on the fetus, which effect, if stated by the group, indicates the need for additional teaching?
   A. Fetal death
   B. Hypotonia
   C. Anemia
   D. Nonimmune hydrops

5. A pregnant woman comes to the clinic complaining of high fever, chills, and flank pain. Assessment reveals costovertebral angle tenderness. She

states, "My temperature will go up high and then go back to normal, sometimes even a little below normal." Which of the following should the nurse suspect?

A. Pyelonephritis
B. Acute renal failure
C. Gestational hypertension
D. Hypoglycemia

6. The nurse teaches a pregnant client with gestational diabetes how to perform blood glucose self-monitoring. Which statement, if made by the client, indicates effective teaching?

A. "I'll test my blood every morning before breakfast."
B. "I'll make sure to eat a light snack before testing my blood."
C. "I'll keep a log for each result with my 4-times-a-day testing."
D. "I'll give myself the insulin and then test my blood."

7. The nurse determines that a pregnant woman who has come to the clinic is a victim of intimate-partner violence. Which of the following would be least important when providing nursing care to this client at this time?

A. Maintaining confidentiality
B. Ensuring client and fetus safety
C. Making a referral to a local shelter
D. Establishing a one-to-one relationship

8. A client, admitted to the hospital with hyperemesis gravidarum resulting in dehydration and electrolyte imbalance, is NPO. When should the nurse expect that the client will be allowed to start taking oral fluids again?

A. When the client's bowel sounds return
B. After 6 hours of receiving intravenous fluids
C. When the client reports that she feels hungry
D. After the client has not vomited for 48 hours.

9. A client with preeclampsia is receiving magnesium sulfate intravenously. Which assessment finding would lead the nurse to suspect that the client is experiencing magnesium toxicity?

A. Muscle weakness
B. Absent patellar reflex
C. Seizures
D. Respiratory rate of 18 bpm

10. A client with a complete molar pregnancy comes to the clinic for follow-up after dilation and curettage. Which statement should indicate to the nurse that the client needs additional teaching about her condition?

A. "I need to make appointments to have my hormone levels checked for the next year."
B. "I know that this condition has put me at risk for a dangerous type of cancer."
C. "I hope to get pregnant again, but I know that I need to wait for at least a year."
D. "I know that the umbilical cord wrapped around my baby's neck, causing problems."

REFERENCES

Abbott, L. (2004). Ectopic pregnancy: Symptoms, diagnosis and management. *Nursing Times, 100,* 32–33.

Abboud, L. N., & Liamputtong, P. (2003). Pregnancy loss: What it means to women who miscarry and their partners. *Social Work in Health Care, 36,* 37–62.

Abenham, H., & Tulandi, T. (2009). Cervical insufficiency: Re-evaluating the prophylactic cervical cerclage. *Journal of Maternal-Fetal Medicine, 22*(6), 510–516.

Aleman, A., Althabe, F., Belizan, J., & Bergel, E. (2005). Bed rest during pregnancy for preventing miscarriage. *Cochrane Database of Systematic Reviews, 18*(2), CD003576.

Alexander, J., & Schneider, F. (2000). Vaginal bleeding associated with pregnancy. *Primary Care, 27,* 137–150.

American Academy of Pediatrics and the American College of Obstetricians and Gynecologists. (2002). *Guidelines for perinatal care* (5th ed.). Washington, DC: Authors.

American Psychiatric Association. (2000). *Diagnostic and statistical manual of mental disorders* (4th ed., text revision). Washington, DC: Author.

Ananth, C. V., & Kinzler, W. L. (2011). Placenta abruption. In E. Sheiner (Ed.), *Bleeding During Pregnancy* (pp. 121–131). New York, NY: Springer.

Anderson, C., & McCarley, M. (2013). Psychological birth trauma in adolescents experiencing an early birth. *The American Journal of Maternal/Child Nursing, 38*(3), 170–176.

Arafeh, J., & Baird, S. (2006). Cardiac disease in pregnancy. *Critical Care Nursing Quarterly, 29*(1), 32–52.

Armour, K. (2004). Antepartum maternal–fetal surveillance: Using surveillance to improve maternal and fetal outcomes. *Association of Women's Health, Obstetric, and Neonatal Nurses Lifelines, 8,* 233–240.

Austin, M. P., Priest, S. R., & Sullivan, E. A. (2009). Antenatal psychosocial assessment for reducing perinatal mental health morbidity. *The Cochrane Database of Systematic Reviews,* Issue 4. doi:10.1002/14651858.CD005124.

Baer, A. N., Witter, F. R., & Petri, M. (2011). Lupus and pregnancy. *Obstetrical and Gynecological Survey, 66*(10), 639–653.

Bagshaw, J. (2009). Women with epilepsy and pregnancy: From preconception to the postnatal period. *British Journal of Neuroscience Nursing, 4*(11), 532.

Barak, A., Dulitzki, M., Efrati, O., Augarten, A., Szeinberg, A., Reichert, N. et al. (2005). Pregnancies and outcome in women with cystic fibrosis. *Israel Medical Association Journal, 7*(2), 95–98.

Barton, J., & Sibai, B. (2004). Diagnosis and management of hemolysis, elevated liver enzymes, and low platelets syndrome. *Clinics in Perinatology, 31*(4), 807–833.

Baskett, T. (2004). *Essential management of obstetric emergencies* (4th ed.). Bristol: Clinical Press Ltd.

Bayrampour, H., & Heaman, M. (2010). Advanced maternal age and the risk of caesarean birth: A systematic review. *Birth, 37*(3), 219–226.

Beckmann, C. (2002). A descriptive study of women's perceptions of their asthma during pregnancy. *Journal of Maternal/Child Nursing, 27*(2), 98–102.

Belej-Rak, T., Okun, N., Windrim, R., Ross, S., & Hannah, M. E. (2003). Effectiveness of cervical cerclage for a sonographically shortened cervix: A systematic review and meta analysis. *American Journal of Obstetrics and Gynecology, 189*(6), 1679–1687.

Berndl, A. M., O'Connell, C. M., & McLeod, N. L. (2013). Fetal movement monitoring: How are we doing as educators? *Journal of Obstetrics and Gynaecology Canada, 35*(1), 22–28.

Blackburn, S. T. (2013). *Maternal, fetal and neonatal physiology: A clinical perspective* (4th ed.). St. Louis, MO: Saunders.

Blaiss, M. (2004). Managing asthma during pregnancy: The whys and hows of aggressive control. *Postgraduate Medicine, 115*(5), 55–65.

Bodnar, L., Cogswell, M., & McDonald, T. (2005). Have we forgotten the significance of postpartum iron deficiency? *American Journal of Obstetrics and Gynecology, 193*, 36–44.

Boonpongmanee, C., Zauszniewski, J. A., & Morris, D. L. (2003). Resourcefulness and self-care in pregnant women with HIV. *Western Journal of Nursing Research, 25*(1), 75–92.

Bowers, N. A., Curran, C. A., Freda, M. C., Krening, C. F., Poole, J. H., Slocum, J. et al. (2008). High-risk pregnancy. In K. R. Simpson & P. A. Creehan (Eds.), *AWHONN's perinatal nursing* (3rd ed., pp. 125–299). Philadelphia, PA: Lippincott Williams & Wilkins.

Briggs, M., Hopman, W., & Jamieson, M. (2007). Comparing pregnancy in adolescents and adults: Obstetric outcomes and prevalence of anemia. *Journal of Obstetrics and Gynaecology Canada, 29*(7), 546–555.

Brown, M., & Solchany, J. (2004). Two overlooked mood disorders in women: Subsyndromal depression and prenatal depression. *Nursing Clinics of North America, 39*(1), 83–95.

Burdge, D. R., Money, D. M., Forbes, J. C., Walmsley, S. L., Smaill, F. M., Boucher, M. et al. (2003). Canadian consensus guidelines for the management of pregnancy, labour and delivery and for postpartum care in HIV-positive pregnant women and their offspring (summary of 2002 guidelines). *Canadian Medical Association Journal, 168*(13), 1671–1674.

Butterworth, P. (2004). Lone mothers' experience of physical and sexual violence: Association with psychiatric disorders. *British Journal of Psychiatry, 184*, 21–27.

Callister, L. (2006). Perinatal loss: A family perspective. *Journal of Perinatal and Neonatal Nursing, 20*(3), 227–234.

Campinha-Bacote, J. (2003). Many faces: Addressing diversity in health care. *Online Journal of Issues in Nursing, 8*(1), 3. Retrieved from http://www.nursingworld.org/MainMenu Categories/ANAMarketplace/ANAPeriodicals/OJIN/Tableof Contents/Volume82003/No1Jan2003//AddressingDiversityin HealthCare.html

Canadian Cardiovascular Society. (2008). Position statement on grading of angina pectoris, 1976. Retrieved from http://www.ccs.ca/ images/Guidelines/PositionStatements/Grading_of_Angina.pdf

Canadian Diabetes Association. (2013). *Diabetes and pregnancy.* Retrieved from http://guidelines.diabetes.ca/Browse/Chapter36

Canadian Institute for Health Information. (2009). *Too early too small: A profile of small babies across Canada.* Retrieved from https://secure.cihi.ca/free_products/too_early_too_small_en.pdf

Canadian Task Force on Preventive Health Care. (2003). *Screening for hemoglobinopathies in pregnancy.* Retrieved September 7, 2008, from http://www.ctfphc.org/Abstracts_printable/Ch20abs.htm

Cannon, R., Schmidt, J., Cambardella, B., & Browne, S. (2000). High-risk pregnancy in the workplace: Influencing positive outcomes. *American Association of Occupational Health Nursing, 48*, 435–446.

Carwell, M., & Spatz, D. (2011). Eating disorders and breastfeeding. *American Journal of Maternal Child Nursing, 36*(2), 112–117.

Casanova, B., Sammel, M., & Macones, G. (2005). Development of a clinical prediction rule for iron deficiency anemia in pregnancy. *American Journal of Obstetrics and Gynecology, 193*, 460–466.

Centers for Disease Control and Prevention. (2005a). Early-onset and late-onset neonatal group B streptococcal disease–United States, 1996-2004. *MMWR: Morbidity and Mortality Weekly Report, 54*(47), 1205–1208.

Centers for Disease Control and Prevention. (2005b). *Rubella.* Retrieved September 7, 2008, from http://www.cdc.gov/rubella

Cesario, S. (2003). Obesity in pregnancy: What every nurse needs to know. *Nursing in Women's Health, 7*(2), 118–125.

Chandran, L., Navaie-Waliser, M., Zulqarni, N. J., Batra, S., Bavir, H., Shah, M. et al. (2001). Compliance with group B streptococcal disease prevention guidelines. *MCN—The American Journal of Maternal/Child Nursing, 26*(6), 313–319.

Chichester, M. (2005). Multicultural issues in perinatal loss. *Association of Women's Health, Obstetric, and Neonatal Nurses Lifelines, 9*(4), 312–320.

Chobanian, A., Bakris, G., Black, H., Cushman, W., Green, L., Izzo, J. et al. (2003). Seventh report of the Joint National Committee on prevention, evaluation and treatment of high blood pressure. *Hypertension, 42*, 1206.

Chudley, A., Conry, J., Cook, J., Loock, C., Rosales, T., & LeBlanc, N. (2005). Fetal alcohol spectrum disorder: Canadian guidelines for diagnosis. *Canadian Medical Association Journal, 172*, S1–S21.

Cleary-Goldman, J., & D'Alton, M. (2008). Growth abnormalities and multiple gestations. *Seminars in Perinatology, 32*(3), 206–212.

Comley, L., & Mousmanis, P. (2003). *Improving the odds: Healthy child development.* Toronto, ON: Ontario College of Family Physicians.

Cox, J. (2007). Teenage pregnancy. In: L. S. Neinstein, C. M. Gordon, D. K. Katzman, D. S. Rosen, & E. R. Woods (Eds.), *Adolescent health care: A practical guide* (5th ed., pp. 565–580). Philadelphia, PA: Lippincott Williams & Wilkins.

Crowther, C. A. (2001). Hospitalization and bed rest for multiple pregnancy. *Cochrane Database of Systematic Reviews,* (1):CD000110.

Damato, E. (2000). Maternal–fetal attachment in twin pregnancies. *Journal of Obstetric, Gynecologic, and Neonatal Nursing, 29*, 598–605.

Damato, E. G., & Winnen, C. W. (2002). Cytomegalovirus infection: Perinatal implications. *Journal of Obstetric, Gynecologic, and Neonatal Nursing, 31*(1), 86–92.

Davies, G., & Herbert, W. (2007). Assessment and management of cardiac disease in pregnancy. *Journal of Obstetrics and Gynaecology Canada, 29*(4), 331–336.

Deen, M., Ruurda, L., Wang, J., & Dekker, G. (2006). Risk factors for preeclampsia in multiparous women: Primipaternity versus the birth interval hypothesis. *Journal of Maternal-Fetal & Neonatal Medicine, 19*(2), 79–84.

Dietch, K., & Bunney, B. (2002). The "silent" disease: Diagnosing and treating depression in women. *Association of Women's Health, Obstetric, and Neonatal Nurses Lifelines, 6*, 140–145.

DiPrima, F., Valenti, O., Hyseni, E., Giorgio, E., Faraci, M., Redda, E. et al. (2011). Antiphospholipid syndrome during pregnancy: The state of the art. *Journal of Prenatal Medicine, 5*(2), 41–52.

Dobbenga-Rhodes, Y., & Prive, A. (2007). Assessment and evaluation of the woman with cardiac disease during pregnancy. *Journal of Perinatal and Neonatal Nursing, 20*(4), 295–302.

Einarson, A., Maltepe, C., Boskovic, R., & Koren, G. (2007). Treatment of nausea and vomiting in pregnancy: An updated algorithm. *Canadian Family Physician, 53*, 2109–2111.

Fell, D., & Joseph, K. (2012). Temporal trends in the frequency of twins and higher-order multiple births in Canada and the United States, *BMC Pregnancy and Childbirth, 12*, 103.

Fernandes, S., Arendt, K., Landzberg, M., Economy, K., & Khairy, P. (2010). Pregnancy in women with congenital heart disease: Cardiac, anesthetic and obstetrical complications. *Expert Review Cardiovascular Therapy, 8*(3), 439–448.

Feroli, K., & Burstein, G. (2003). Adolescent sexually transmitted infections: New recommendations for diagnosis, treatment and prevention. *American Journal of Maternal/Child Nursing, 28*, 113–118.

Field, T., Diego, M., Delgado, J., & Medina, L. (2013). Peer support and interpersonal psychotherapy groups experienced decreased prenatal depression, anxiety and cortisol. *Early Human Development, 89*(9), 621–624.

Fleming, N., Ng, N., Osborne, C., Biederman, S., Yasseen, A., Dy, J. et al. (2013). Adolescent pregnancy outcomes in the province of Ontario: A cohort study. *Journal of Obstetrics and Gynaecology Canada, 35*(3), 234–245.

Flynn, H., O'Mahen, H., Massey, L., & Marcus, S. (2006). The impact of a brief obstetrics clinic-based intervention on treatment use for perinatal depression. *Journal of Women's Health, 15*(10), 1195–1204.

Fowles, E. (2002). Comparing pregnant women's nutritional knowledge to their actual dietary intake. *Journal of Maternal/Child Nursing, 27*, 171–177.

Frye, D., Clark, S., Piacenza, D., & Shay-Zapien, G. (2011). Pulmonary complications in pregnancy. *Journal of Perinatal and Neonatal Nursing, 25*(3), 235–244.

Furniss, K., McCaffrey, M., Parnell, V., & Rovi, S. (2007). Challenges and barriers to screening for intimate partner violence. *The American Journal of Maternal/Child Nursing, 32*(4), 238–243.

Geiter, H. (2003). Disseminated intravascular coagulopathy. *Dimensions of Critical Care Nursing, 22*, 108–114.

Gelson, E., Curry, R., Gatzoulis, M., Swan, L., Lupton, M., Steer, P. et al. (2011). Effect of maternal heart disease on fetal growth. *Obstetrics and Gynecology, 117*(4), 886–891.

Gennaro, S., Biesecker, B., Fantasia, H., Nguyen, M., & Garry, D. (2011). Nutrition profiles of American women in the third trimester. *American Journal of Maternal/Child Nursing, 36*(2), 120–126.

Gilbert, E., (2011). *Manual of high-risk pregnancy and delivery* (5th ed.). St. Louis, MO: Mosby.

Goff, M. (2005). Parvovirus B19 in pregnancy. *Journal of Midwifery and Women's Health, 50*(6), 536–538.

Goldenberg, R., Culhane, J., Iams, J., & Romero, R. (2008). Epidemiology and causes of preterm birth. *The Lancet, 371*, 75–84.

Graham, G., & Gaddipati, S. (2005). Diagnosis and management of obstetrical complications unique to multiple gestations. *Seminars in Perinatology, 29*(5), 282–295.

Gupton, A., Heaman, M., & Cheung, L. (2001). Complicated and uncomplicated pregnancies: Women's perception of risk. *Journal of Obstetric, Gynecologic, and Neonatal Nursing, 30*, 192–201.

Hamar, B., & Funai, E. (2007) Systemic lupus erythematosus. In: J. Queenan, C. Young, & C. Lockwood (Eds.), *Management of high-risk pregnancy: An evidence-based approach* (5th ed., pp. 214–221). Oxford UK: Blackwell Publishing.

Harden, C., Hopp, J., Ting, T., Pennell, P., French, J., Hauser, W. et al. (2009). Management issues for women with epilepsy–Focus on pregnancy (an evidence-based review): I. Obstetrical complications and change in seizure frequency. *Epilepsia, 50*(5), 1229–1236.

Haskell, L. (2012). A developmental understanding of complex trauma. In: N. Poole & L. Greaves (Eds.), *Becoming trauma informed.* Toronto, ON: Centre for Addiction and Mental Health.

Hayward, K. (2003). Cobedding of twins: A natural extension of the socialization process. *Journal of Maternal/Child Nursing, 28*, 260–263.

Health Canada. (1999). *A handbook for health and social service professionals responding to abuse during pregnancy.* Retrieved September 7, 2008, from http://www.phac-aspc.gc.ca/ ncfv-cnivf/familyviolence/pdfs/pregnancy_e.pdf

Health Canada. (2012). *Canadian perinatal health report: 2012.* Ottawa, ON: Minister of Public Works and Government Services Canada.

Healy, A. J., & Gaddipati, S. (2005). Intrapartum management of twins: Truths and controversies. *Clinics in Perinatology, 32*(2), 455–473.

Henshaw, E., Sabourin, B., & Warning, M. (2013). Treatment seeking behaviours and attitudes survey among women at risk for perinatal depression or anxiety. *Journal of Obstetric and Gynecological Nurses, 42*, 168–177.

Hobbins, D. (2004). Survivors of childhood sexual abuse: Implications for perinatal nursing care. *Journal of Obstetric, Gynecologic, and Neonatal Nursing, 33*(4), 485–497.

Jasinski, J. (2004). Pregnancy and domestic violence: A review of the literature. *Trauma, Violence and Abuse, 5*, 47–64.

Jeha, L. E., & Morris, H. H. (2005). Optimizing outcomes in pregnant women with epilepsy. *Cleveland Clinic Journal of Medicine, 72*(10), 938–940.

Jonas-Simpson, C., & McMahon, E. (2005). The language of loss. When a baby dies prior to birth: Cocreating human experience. *Nursing Science Quarterly, 18*(2), 124–130.

Jones, R., Baird, S., Thurman, S., & Gaskin, I. (2012). Maternal cardiac arrest: An overview. *Journal of Perinatal & Neonatal Nursing, 26*(2), 117–123.

Joseph, K. S., Kinniburgh, B., Hutcheon, J. A., Mehrabadi, A., Basso, M., Davies, C. et al. (2013). Determinants of increases in stillbirth rates from 2000 to 2010. *Canadian Medical Association Journal, 185*(8), 345–351. Retrieved from www.cmaj.ca

Katz, A. (2004). Neonatal HIV infection. *Neonatal Network, 23*(1), 15–20.

Keating-Lefler, R., & Wilson, M. (2004). The experience of becoming a mother for single, unpartnered, medicaid-eligible, first-time mothers. *Journal of Nursing Scholarship, 36*, 23–29.

Kendrick, J. (2011). Screening and diagnosing gestational diabetes mellitus revisited: Implications from HAPO. *Journal of Perinatal and Neonatal Nursing, 25*(3), 226–232.

Kenyon, S., Boulvain, M., & Neilson, J. (2003). Antibiotics for preterm rupture of membranes. *Cochrane Database of Systematic Reviews, (2)*, CD001058. doi:10.1002/14651858.CD001058

Kidner, M. C., & Flanders-Stepans, M. B. (2004). A model for the HELLP syndrome: The maternal experience. *Journal of Obstetric, Gynecologic, and Neonatal Nursing, 33*, 44–53.

Kilpatrick, K., & Purden, M. (2007). Using reflective nursing practice to improve care. *The American Journal of Maternal/Child Nursing, 32*(3), 140–147.

Kirkham, C., Harris, S., & Grzybowski, S. (2005). Evidence-based prenatal care. I. General prenatal care and counseling. *American Family Physician, 71*(7), 1307–1316.

Koren, G., Nulman, I., Chudley, A. E., & Loocke, C. (2003). Fetal alcohol spectrum disorder [Electronic version]. *Canadian Medical Association Journal, 169*(11), 1181–1185. Retrieved September 7, 2008, from http://www.cmaj.ca/cgi/content/full/169/11/1181

Kozak, S. (2002). *Diabetes: Antepartum, intrapartum, postpartum and newborn nursing care. A self-directed learning module.* Vancouver, BC: Women's Hospital.

Kramer, J., Bowen, A., Stewart, N., & Muhajarine, N. (2013). Nausea and vomiting of pregnancy: Prevalence, severity and relation to psychosocial health. *American Journal of Maternal Child Nursing, 38*(1), 21–27.

Kuczkowski, K. M. (2004). Labor analgesia for the parturient with cardiac disease: What does the obstetrician need to know? *Acta Obstetricia et Gynecologica Scandinavica, 83*, 223–233.

Kumar, S., & O'Brien, A. (2004). Recent developments in fetal medicine. *British Medical Journal, 328*, 1002–1006.

Kwon, H., Belanger, K., & Bracken, M. (2004). Effect of pregnancy and stage of pregnancy on asthma severity: A systematic review. *American Journal of Obstetrics and Gynecology, 190*, 1201–1210.

Langlois, K. A., Samokhvalov, A. V., Rehm J., Spence S. T., Connor Gorber, S. K. (2012). *Health state descriptions for Canadians: Mental illnesses.* Statistics Canada, catalogue no. 82-619-MIE2005002. Ottawa, ON: Statistics Canada.

Lawrence, R. A., & Lawrence, R. M. (2005). *Breast-feeding: A guide for the medical profession* (6th ed.). St. Louis, MO: Mosby.

Leduc, L., Farine, D., Armson, B., Brunner, M., Crane, J., Delisle, M. et al. (2006). Stillbirth and bereavement: Guidelines for stillbirth investigation. *Journal of Obstetrics and Gynaecology Canada, 25*(6), 540–545.

Lee, S., Ayers, S., & Holden, D. (2012). Risk perception of women during high risk pregnancy: A systematic review. *Health, Risk & Society, 14*(6), 511–531.

Lindqvist, P., & Happach, C. (2006). Risk and risk estimation of placental abruption. *European Journal of Obstetrics and Gynecology, 126*(2), 160–164.

Luke, B. (2005a). Nutrition and multiple gestation. *Seminars in Perinatology, 29*(5), 349–354.

Luke, B. (2005b). The evidence linking maternal nutrition and prematurity. *Journal of Perinatal Medicine, 33*, 500–505.

Lupton, M., Oteng-Ntim, E., Ayida, G., & Steer, P. (2002). Cardiac disease in pregnancy. *Current Opinion in Obstetrics and Gynecology, 14*, 137–143.

Lurie, S., Feinstein, M., & Mamet, Y. (2000). Disseminated intravascular coagulopathy in pregnancy: Thorough comprehension of etiology and management reduces obstetricians' stress. *Archives of Gynecology and Obstetrics, 263*(3), 126–130.

MacDonald, C., & Jonas-Simpson, C. (2009). Living with changing expectations for women with high-risk pregnancies. *Nursing Science Quarterly, 22*(1), 74–82.

Magann, E., & Martin, J. (1999). Twelve steps to optimal management of HELLP syndrome. *Clinical Obstetrics and Gynecology, 42*, 532–550.

Malcus, P. (2004). Antenatal fetal surveillance. *Current Opinion in Obstetrics and Gynecology, 16*, 123–128.

Maloni, J., Brezinski-Tomasi, J., & Johnson, L. (2001). Antepartum bed rest: Effect upon the family. *Journal of Obstetric, Gynecologic, and Neonatal Nursing, 30*, 165–173.

Marcus, S. M. (2009). Depression during pregnancy: Rates, risks and consequences–Motherisk Update 2008. *Canadian Journal of Clinical Pharmacology, 16*(1), 15–22.

Mariano, C., & Hickey, R. (1998). Multiple pregnancy, multiple needs. *Canadian Nurse, 94*(9), 26–30.

Martin, S., & Foley, M. (2003). Adult-onset heart disease in pregnancy. *Patient Care for the Nurse Practitioner, 2*, 1–16.

Mazzotta, P., Magee, L., Maltepe, C., Lifshitz, A., Navioz, Y., & Koran, G. (2000). The perception of teratogenic risk by women with nausea and vomiting of pregnancy. In G. Koren & R. Bishai (Eds.), *Nausea and vomiting of pregnancy: State of the art 2000* (pp. 157–172). Toronto, ON: Motherisk, Hospital for Sick Children.

Medina, T., & Hill, D. (2006). Preterm premature rupture of membranes: Diagnosis and management. *American Family Physician, 73*(4), 659–664. Retrieved September 7, 2008, from http://www.aafp.org/afp/20060215/659.html

Menon, R., & Fortunato, S. (2007). Infection and the role of inflammation in preterm premature rupture of the membranes. *Best Practice & Research in Clinical Obstetrics & Gynaecology, 21*(3), 467–478.

Mercer, B. (2004). Preterm premature rupture of the membranes: Diagnosis and management. *Clinics in Perinatology, 31*, 765–782.

Mian, P. (2000). The role of the clinical nurse specialist in the development of a domestic violence program. *Clinical Nurse Specialist, 14*, 229–234.

Michon, B., Balkou, S., Hivon, R., & Cyr, C. (2003). Death of a child: Parental perception of grief intensity–end of life and bereavement care. *Pediatric Child Health Journal, 8*, 363–366.

Mihu, D., Costin, N., Mihu, C., Seican, A., & Ciortea, R. (2007). HELLP syndrome–a multisystemic disorder. *Journal of Gastrointestinal & Liver Diseases, 16*(4), 419–424.

Milgrom, J., Gemmill, A., Bilszta, J., Hayes, B., Brooks, J., Erickson, J. et al. (2008). Antenatal risk factors for postnatal depression: A large prospective study. *Journal of Affective Disorders, 108*(1-2), 147–157.

Montan, S. (2004). Drugs used in hypertensive diseases in pregnancy. *Current Opinion in Obstetrics and Gynecology, 16*(2), 111–115.

Montoya, J., & Liesenfeld, O. (2004). Toxoplasmosis. *The Lancet, 363*, 1965–1976.

Motherisk. (2007). *Treatment of nausea and vomiting in pregnancy.* Retrieved September 7, 2008, from http://www.motherisk.org/women/index.jsp

National Institutes of Health, & National Asthma Education and Prevention Program Working Group. (2004). *Managing asthma during pregnancy: Recommendations for pharmacologic treatment.* Retrieved from http://www.nhlbi.nih.gov/health/prof/lung/asthma/astpreg/astpreg_qr.pdf

Nodine, P. M., & Hastings-Tolsma, M. (2012). Maternal obesity: Improving pregnancy outcomes. *MCN. The American Journal of Maternal Child Nursing, 37*(2), 110–115.

O'Brien, B., Evans, M., & White-McDonald, E. (2002). Isolation from "being alive": Coping with severe nausea and vomiting of pregnancy. *Nursing Research, 51*, 302–308.

Oyelese, Y., & Canterino, J. C. (2011). Placenta previa and placenta accrete. In El. Sheiner (Ed.): *Bleeding during pregnancy: A comprehensive guide.* New York: Springer.

Oyelese, Y., & Smulian, J. (2006). Placenta previa, placenta accreta, and vasa previa. *Obstetrics and Gynecology, 107*(4), 927–941.

Padden, M. O. (1999). HELLP syndrome: Recognition and perinatal management. *American Family Physician, 60*(3), 829–836. Retrieved September 7, 2008, from http://www.aafp.org/afp/990901ap/829.html

Palmer, C. (2002). Obstetric emergencies and anesthetic management. *Current Reviews for Perianesthesia Nurses, 24*, 121–132.

Palmer, D. (2007). Peripartum cardiomyopathy. *Journal of Perinatal and Neonatal Nursing, 20*(4), 324–332.

Pasquier, J. C., Picaud, J. C., Rabilloud, M., Claris, O., Ecochard, R., Vigier, S. et al. (2007). Maternal leukocytosis after preterm premature rupture of membranes and infant neurodevelopmental outcome: A prospective, population-based study. *Journal of Obstetrics and Gynaecology Canada, 29*(1), 20–26. Retrieved September 7, 2008, from http://sogc.org/ jogc/abstracts/full/200701_Obstetrics_1.pdf

Peters, R. M. (2008). High blood pressure in pregnancy. *Nursing for Women's Health, 12*(5), 410–421.

Public Health Agency of Canada. (2005). Rubella. Retrieved September 5, 2008, from http://www.phac-aspc.gc.ca/tmp-pmv/info/rubella-eng.php

Public Health Agency of Canada. (2010). Report on sexually transmitted infections in Canada. Retrieved from http://publications.gc.ca/collections/collection_2013/aspc-phac/HP37-10-2010-eng.pdf

Public Health Agency of Canada (2011a). *Obesity in Canada.* Retrieved from http://www.phac-aspc.gc.ca/hp-ps/hl-mvs/oic-oac/assets/pdf/oic-oac-eng.pdf

Public Health Agency of Canada. (2011b). *Tobacco use.* Retrieved 2013, from http://www.hc-sc.gc.ca/hc-ps/tobac-tabac/research-recherche/stat/_ctums-esutc_2011/ann-eng.php#t7

Puia, D., Lewis, L., & Beck, C. T. (2013). Experiences of obstetric nurses who are present for a perinatal loss. *Journal of Obstetrical and Gynecological Nurses, 42*, 321–331.

Queenan, J., Spong, C., & Lockwood, C. (2007). *Management of high-risk pregnancy: An evidence-based approach* (5th ed.). Malden, MA: Blackwell.

Ramin, S., Vidaeff, A., Yeomans, E., & Gilstrap, L. (2006). Chronic renal disease in pregnancy. *Obstetrics & Gynecology, 108*(6), 1531–1539.

Ramsey, P., Kirk, D., & Ramin, S. (2001). Cardiac disease in pregnancy. *American Journal of Perinatology, 18*, 245–265.

Records, K. (2007). A critical review of maternal abuse and infant outcomes: Complications for newborn nurses. *Newborn and Infant Nursing Reviews, 7*(1), 7–13.

Registered Nurses Association of Ontario. (2009). *Best practice guidelines: Supporting clients on methadone maintenance treatment.* Toronto, ON: Author.

Registered Nurses Association of Ontario. (2012). *Best practice guidelines: Woman abuse: Screening, identification and initial response.* Toronto, ON: Author.

Rey, E., & Boulet, L. (2007). Asthma in pregnancy. *British Medical Journal, 334*, 582–585.

Roos-Hesselink, J., Duvekot, J., & Thorne, S. (2009). Pregnancy in high risk cardiac conditions. *Heart, 95*, 680–686.

Royal College of Obstetricians and Gynaecologists. (2002). *Clinical guidelines for tubal pregnancies.* London: Author.

Rubarth, L., Schoening, A., Cosimano, A., & Sandhurst, H. (2012). Women's experience of hospitalized bed rest during high-risk pregnancy. *Journal of Obstetrical, Gynecological and Neonatal Nursing, 41*(3), 398–407.

Salmon, J., & Girardi, G. (2008). Antiphospholipid antibodies and pregnancy loss: A disorder of inflammation. *Journal of Reproductive Immunology, 77*(1), 51–56.

Samuals-Kalow, M., Funai, E., Buhimschi, C., Norwitz, E., Perrin, M., Calderon-Margalit, R. et al. (2007). Prepregnancy body mass index, hypertensive disorders of pregnancy, and long term maternal mortality. *American Journal of Obstetrics and Gynecology, 199*(1), 490e1–490e6.

Sauls, D. (2010). Promoting a positive childbirth experience for adolescents. *Journal of Gynecological, Obstetrical, and Neonatal Nurses, 39*, 703–712.

Schatz, M., Dambrowski, M., Wise, R., Thom, E., Landon, M., Mabie, W. et al. (2003). Asthma morbidity during pregnancy can be predicted by severity classification. *Journal of Allergy and Clinical Immunology, 112*(2), 283–288.

Scholl, T. (2005). Iron status during pregnancy: Setting the stage for mother and infant. *American Journal of Clinical Nutrition, 8*, 1218S–1222S.

Sibai, B. (2004). Diagnosis, controversies, and management of the syndrome of hemolysis, elevated liver enzymes, and low platelet count. *Obstetrics & Gynecology, 103*(5), 981–991.

Sibai, B., & Chames, M. (2003). Hypertension in pregnancy: Tailoring treatment to risk. *OBG Management, 15*(7).

Simmons, H., & Goldberg, L. (2011). "High-risk" pregnancy after perinatal loss: Understanding the label. *Midwifery, 27,* 452–457.

Society of Obstetricians and Gynaecologists of Canada (SOGC). (2000). Management of twin pregnancies (Parts I & II). *Journal of Obstetrics and Gynaecology Canada, 91,* 519–526, 607–610.

Society of Obstetricians and Gynaecologists of Canada (SOGC). (2002a). Parvovirus B19 infection in pregnancy. *Journal of Obstetrics and Gynaecology Canada, 24*(9), 727–734.

Society of Obstetricians and Gynaecologists of Canada (SOGC). (2002b). Screening for gestational diabetes mellitus. *Journal of Obstetrics and Gynaecology Canada, 24*(11), 894–903.

Society of Obstetricians and Gynaecologists of Canada (SOGC). (2002c). The management of nausea and vomiting of pregnancy. *Journal of Obstetrics and Gynaecology Canada, 24,* 817–823.

Society of Obstetricians and Gynaecologists of Canada (SOGC). (2003). The use of fetal doppler in obstetrics. *Journal of Obstetrics and Gynaecology Canada, 25*(7), 601–607.

Society of Obstetricians and Gynaecologists of Canada (SOGC). (2004a). Guidelines for operative vaginal birth. *Journal of Obstetrics and Gynaecology Canada, 26*(8), 747–753.

Society of Obstetricians and Gynaecologists of Canada (SOGC). (2004b). The prevention of early-onset neonatal group B streptococcal disease. *Journal of Obstetrics and Gynaecology Canada, 26*(9), 826–832.

Society of Obstetricians and Gynaecologists of Canada (2005). Intimate partner violence consensus statement. *Journal of Obstetrics and Gynaecology Canada, 157,* 263–286. Retrieved from http://www.cfpc.ca/uploadedFiles/Resources/Resource_Items/Health_Professionals/Intimate_partner_violence_consensus.pdf

Society of Obstetricians and Gynaecologists of Canada (SOGC). (2006). HIV screening in pregnancy. *Journal of Obstetrics and Gynaecology Canada, 28*(12), 1103–1107.

Society of Obstetricians and Gynaecologists of Canada (SOGC). (2007a). Fetal health surveillance: Antepartum and intrapartum consensus guideline. *Journal of Obstetrics and Gynaecology Canada, 197,* S3–S56.

Society of Obstetricians and Gynaecologists of Canada (SOGC). (2007b). Diagnosis and management of placenta previa. *Journal of Obstetrics and Gynaecology Canada, 189,* 261–266.

Society of Obstetricians and Gynaecologists of Canada (SOGC). (2007c). *Women's health information: Multiple birth.* Retrieved September 7, 2008, from http://www.sogc.org/health/pregnancy-multiple_e.asp

Society of Obstetricians and Gynaecologists of Canada (SOGC). (2008). Diagnosis, evaluation, and management of the hypertensive disorders of pregnancy. *Journal of Obstetrics and Gynaecology Canada, 30*(3), S1–S48.

Society of Obstetricians and Gynecologists of Canada (SOGC). (2011). Substance use in pregnancy: Clinical practice guideline. *Journal of Obstetrics and Gynaecology Canada, 33*(4), 367–384.

Society of Obstetricians and Gynecologists of Canada (SOGC). (2012). Management of group B streptococcus bacteriuria in pregnancy: Clinical practice guideline. *Journal of Obstetrics and Gynaecology Canada, 276,* 483–486.

Society of Obstetricians and Gynecologists of Canada (SOGC). (2013a). Rowe, T. (Principal Ed.). Health professionals working with First Nations, Inuit, and Métis: Consensus guideline. *Journal of Obstetrics and Gynaecology Canada, 35*(6), S1–S52.

Society of Obstetricians and Gynecologists of Canada (SOGC). (2013b). Toxoplasmosis in pregnancy: Prevention, screening and treatment. *Journal of Obstetrics and Gynaecology Canada, 285,* 78–79.

Sosa, C., Althabe, F., Belizan, J., & Bergel, E. (2004). Bed rest in singleton pregnancies for preventing preterm birth. *Cochrane Database of Systematic Reviews,* (1), CD003581.

Statistics Canada. (2011). *Women in Canada: A gender based statistical report* (6th ed.). Retrieved from http://www.statcan.gc.ca/pub/89-503-x/89-503-x2010001-eng.htm

Stock, S., & Norman, J. (2010). Preterm and term labour in multiple pregnancies. *Seminars in Fetal and Neonatal Medicine, 15,* 336–341.

Terkildsen, M., Parilla, B., Kumar, P., & Grobman, W. (2003). Factors associated with success of emergent second-trimester cerclage. *Obstetrics and Gynecology, 101,* 565–569.

Thorsen, M., & Poole, J. (2002). Renal disease in pregnancy. *Journal of Perinatal and Neonatal Nursing, 15,* 13–29.

Townsend, N., & Drummond, S. (2011). Preeclampsia: Pathophysiology and implications for care. *Journal of Perinatal and Neonatal Nursing, 25*(3), 245–252.

Usta, I., Hobeika, E., Musa, A., Gabriel, G., & Nassar, A. (2005). Placenta previa-accreta: Risk factors and complications. *American Journal of Obstetrics and Gynecology, 193,* 1045–1049.

Watson-Blasioli, J. (2001). Double-take: Defining the need for specialized prenatal care for women expecting twins: A Canadian perspective. *Association of Women's Health, Obstetric, and Neonatal Nurses Lifelines, 5,* 34–42.

Watts, N. (2004). Screening for domestic violence: A team approach for maternal/newborn nurses. *Association of Women's Health, Obstetric, and Neonatal Nurses Lifelines, 8,* 210–219.

Weitz, B. (1999). Premature rupture of the fetal membranes: An update for advanced practice nurses. *Journal of Maternal-Child Nursing, 26,* 86–92.

White, A. (2003). Parvovirus B19 infection in pregnancy. *Perinatal Outreach Program of Southwestern Ontario, 25.*

Williams, M., & Iams, J. (2004). Cervical length measurement and cervical cerclage to prevent preterm birth. *Clinical Obstetrics and Gynecology, 47*(4), 775–783.

Wool, C. (2013). State of the science on perinatal palliative care. *Journal of Obstetrical and Gynecological Nurses, 42,* 372–382.

Yatham, L., Kennedy, S., Schaffer, A., Parikh, S., Beaulieu, S., ODonovan C. et al. (2009). Canadian Network for Mood and Anxiety Treatments (CANMAT) and International Society for Bipolar Disorders (ISBD) collaborative update of CANMAT guidelines for the management of patients with bipolar disorder: update 2009. *Bipolar Disorders, 11,* 225–255.

Yonkers, K., Wisner, K., Stowe, Z., Leibenluft, E., Cohen, L., Miller, L. et al. (2004). Management of bipolar disorder during pregnancy and the postpartum period. *American Journal of Psychiatry, 161,* 608–620.

Youngkin, E., Davis, M., Schadewald, D., & Juve, C. (2013). *Women's health: A primary care clinical guide* (4th ed.). Upper Saddle River, NJ: Pearson Education Inc.

Zauderer, C. (2012). Eating disorders and pregnancy: Supporting the anorexic or bulimic expectant mother. *American Journal of Maternal Child Nursing, 37*(1), 48–55.

Zhang, W., & Chen, S. (2003). An overview on systemic lupus erythematosus pregnancy. *Modern Rheumatology, 13,* 293–300.

Zwelling, E., & Phillips, C. (2001). Family-centered maternity care in the new millennium: Is it real or is it imagined? *Journal of Perinatal and Neonatal Nursing, 15,* 1–12.

CHAPTER 14

Educational Preparation for Pregnancy, Childbirth, and Parenthood

Karen MacKinnon, Jocelyn Churchill, and Barbara Hotelling*

Monique, 32 years old, comes to the community health centre for a prenatal visit at 14 weeks' gestation with her first pregnancy. She mentions that she and her husband have been talking about labour and birth. Monique states, "He thinks we should have 'natural childbirth,' but I might want an epidural. I don't want to be in pain. People are constantly telling me horror stories about labour."

Shelley, now at 22 weeks' gestation, comes to the clinic for a prenatal visit. Her partner of 7 years, Joel, accompanies her. During the visit, Shelley and Joel mention that their 3-year-old son has been acting out lately. "This all started right after we told him we were expecting another baby," they report.

You will learn more about these stories later in this chapter. Nurses working with women and their families during childbearing need to understand how perinatal education can promote health, prevent pregnancy risks, and address health inequities. Before beginning, consider the following points related to the above scenarios:

- What details will the nurse need to investigate with Monique? What about Shelley and Joel?
- What areas related to education need to be considered for each client?
- What educational resources or programs might be helpful for Monique? For Shelley and Joel?
- How can the nurse provide woman- and family-centred care and perinatal education in both of these situations?
- How might each client's circumstances influence the nurse's approach to care?

*Contributor to first U.S. edition.

PERINATAL EDUCATION

Perinatal education (education about childbirth) has been a consistent, powerful health promotion tool for women, children, and families since the earliest classes in maternal hygiene, nutrition, and baby care (Nichols & Humenick, 2000). Education may be provided by **perinatal educators** during pregnancy, childbirth, and postpartum. These educators may be certified by organizations such as the Childbirth and Postpartum Professional Association (CAPPA), which has a Canadian branch (www. http://www.cappa.net/canada.php). Pregnancy, for many parents, is a teachable moment. For example, as an expectant mother bonds with her fetus, she may be willing to change risky behaviours for the sake of her unborn child. She may become more careful about her diet and try harder to choose foods and beverages that optimize fetal growth and health, even if these selections are not her usual preferences (Fig. 14.1). She may consult her health care provider before taking any over-the-counter medications. She may quit or reduce her smoking. Exercise may become part of her daily routine, or she may seek information from friends, books, classes, or the internet. This information-seeking activity makes pregnancy a reachable moment as well

as a teachable one. Lifestyle changes that women and their families make may be beyond and better than what they normally would do if they were concerned only with their own welfare.

Ideally, the decision to become a parent is made consciously and within an environment that incorporates holistic, health-promoting, and empowering perinatal education. In addition, such education is rooted in collaborative communication and targeted toward relevant times during conception, pregnancy, birth, and postpartum. An example would be information about nutrition during these different stages. For the woman seeking conception, nurses and other maternity care providers would focus their teaching on ensuring that her nutrient intake optimizes fetal development and maintains or improves maternal health. They would emphasize the importance of folic acid supplementation, which can prevent fetal neural tube defects (Motherisk, 2013). During pregnancy, nutrition teaching would likely emphasize dietary measures to combat nausea, boost the immune system, and protect maternal iron stores. For women who plan to breastfeed, education would focus on measures to promote an optimal milk supply. In the postpartum period, health teaching would centre on the chosen newborn-feeding method, nutritional strategies

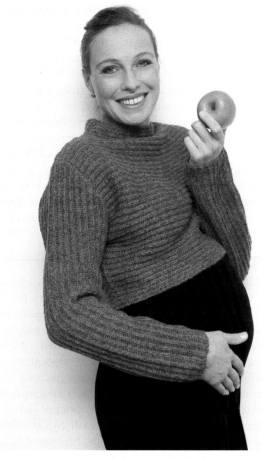

FIGURE 14.1 Pregnancy has been called a "teachable" moment. Many women are motivated to make healthier choices when they are expecting because of the direct effects of their decisions on their fetus.

to help the woman's body readjust to the nonpregnant state, and ways to obtain extra energy and nutrients needed for the demanding requirements of child rearing. At each phase, nurses and care providers need to communicate with one another to ensure that information is coordinated, accurate, and consistent. A unified approach assists clients to internalize evidence-based information and develop health-promoting behaviours that can benefit families for a lifetime.

 Recall Monique, the woman at 14 weeks' gestation described at the beginning of the chapter. What specific areas would the nurse need to address to help guide Monique and her husband in their decisions about childbirth?

Nurses and Perinatal Education

Canadian nurses have the opportunity to provide education about pregnancy, childbirth, and parenting in a variety of settings. Examples include both formal

group classes and less formal opportunities to address questions during a prenatal health visit, in community health centres or public health clinics, or over the phone. Nurse-managed health-related phone lines are increasing in popularity with today's millennial parents, along with internet-based sources of information and peer support (Agostino, 2012; Dennis & Kingston, 2008; Devolin et al., 2013).

Care providers are consistently identified by childbearing women as the "most helpful" sources of information (Public Health Agency of Canada [PHAC], 2009). Nurses need to take advantage of *all* opportunities for health promotion both before and throughout the childbearing year. Health promotion may also include referring women and their families to perinatal education classes and to reliable evidence-based sources of health information. Canadian nurses need an understanding of (1) how perinatal education has evolved over time; (2) the variety of approaches currently available for Canadian families; (3) how to work collaboratively with other health care providers and perinatal educators to promote **health literacy** (the ability to obtain, read, and understand basic healthcare information needed to make basic healthcare decisions) and provide consistent and accurate messages; (4) how to work collaboratively with childbearing women and their families in a variety of contexts and situations; and (5) how to work collaboratively with intersectoral teams to ensure that all childbearing women and their families have access to the resources needed for health (Pauly et al., 2009).

Whether a nurse or educator is facilitating learning with a home- or hospital-bound pregnant woman or with a group of women and their partners, integrating web-based resources such as videos, podcasts, and sites with interactive widgets can enhance the health literacy of participants at the same time that it makes sessions more interesting. Health literacy has been defined as "the ability of individuals to access and use health information to make appropriate health decisions and maintain basic health" (Canadian Council on Learning, 2007, p. 4).

Perinatal Education as Health Promotion

People who take prenatal classes receive extensive information about nutritional needs during pregnancy, appropriate exercise, smoking cessation, stress management, medications and street drugs that may pose dangers to the fetus or pregnancy, ways to foster healthy relationships, and the importance of avoiding alcohol. Expectant parents who receive health information before pregnancy or during the first trimester can initiate health-promoting behaviours earlier and improve their chances of giving birth to a full-term, healthy infant. Childbearing women have also been targets of social marketing health promotion campaigns (such as recent programs aimed at decreasing fetal alcohol spectrum disorder by changing women's drinking behaviours). Although many of these approaches have good intentions, they can also have negative effects on women's childbearing experiences (MacKinnon & McIntyre, 2006).

Perinatal education is an important vehicle of health promotion for women, infants, and families. We tend to think of educational preparation for pregnancy, childbirth, and parenting only as prenatal classes, but health promotion for childbearing families requires a more comprehensive, multidisciplinary, and community-based approach (see Chapter 2 for more discussion on models and theories as well as nursing approaches to health promotion.) Today the emphasis on health promotion and health education has shifted from models that emphasize healthy lifestyles and behavioural change toward more inclusive models that also consider the social, economic, and environmental conditions that determine health.

> *Health promotion is viewed as a collective, rather than individual activity, and has five key strategies: develop personal skills, create supportive environments, strengthen community action, build healthy public policy, and reorient health services (Vollman et al., 2007, p. 15)*

Nurses and perinatal educators can contribute significantly to perinatal health by helping women and family members develop healthy personal skills and by working together to create supportive environments for childbearing families. How can we promote healthy childbearing for all Canadian women and their families? Which groups of women or families are most affected by childbearing risks and by inequities in access to education and other resources needed for healthy living? What is the relationship between perinatal education and health literacy?

In this chapter we will address many of these questions as we explore educational preparation for pregnancy, childbirth, and parenting. We consider the history of childbirth education and the evolution of different approaches over time. We discuss a variety of approaches to educational preparation that promote health and health literacy. We also explore how nurses and other maternity care providers can assist women and families with health promotion, decision making, and family transitions. Finally, we discuss educational preparation as *one* important component of a more comprehensive life course approach to health promotion and risk prevention for *all* childbearing women and their families. We begin by reviewing the context for perinatal care and health promotion in Canada today.

Collaborative Approaches to Perinatal Care

Educational preparation for childbearing today takes place within the context of a collaborative and multidisciplinary approach to perinatal care. Nurses work in collaborative partnerships with childbearing women and their families (Gottlieb & Feeley, 2006). Nurses mobilize the strengths of the woman, her family, and the community (Gottlieb, 2013) to promote health, prevent known childbearing risks, and address the woman's concerns and questions. Nurses are important members of the multidisciplinary primary maternity care team and have many opportunities for offering health education. Other members of the team may include midwives, physicians, doulas, lactation consultants, and perinatal educators. Working collaboratively with physicians is common among nurses, so the contributions of some other team members are briefly explored in this introductory section.

Midwives

In Canada, a **Registered Midwife (RM)** is a person educated in midwifery who is registered with a provincial/territorial regulatory authority and is legally permitted to practice. Canadian midwives have adopted a community-based continuity-of-care model, providing care to women and their families throughout the childbearing year. Midwives use their prenatal visit time to empower women, address their concerns, and answer their questions. Time with women and their partners gives midwives the ability to discuss the difference between pain and suffering, the benefits of breath awareness and relaxation, massage techniques, and the emotional and physical transition toward parenthood. If parents are attending formal classes, midwives are available to help women and their partners understand the information they have received in class and integrate this knowledge into their plans for childbirth and early parenting. Although most midwives provide intrapartum care in birth centres, hospitals, and the home, legislation and funding models vary across the county. For current information on midwives in Canada, see the website for the Canadian Association of Midwives (www.canadian-midwives. org) or the Canadian Midwifery Regulators Consortium (http://www.cmrc-ccosf.ca/).

Doulas

Women have been helping women give birth throughout history. The term **doula** has come to mean a woman who provides continuous support to the mother before, during, and after childbirth (Fig. 14.2). Doulas of North America, formed in 1992, was the result of the effort of a small group of birth support experts to promote the importance of continuous emotional and physical support for mothers and their partners during pregnancy, childbirth, and through the early postpartum transition period. The organization was based on research that demonstrated statistically significant benefits to continuous support during labour. Benefits included decreases

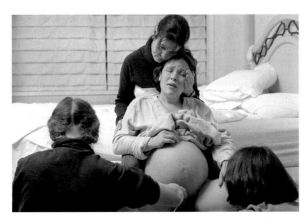

FIGURE 14.2 A woman who is having a home birth is being assisted by a doula and a midwife.

in cesarean birth, use of vacuum extractor or forceps, and requests for analgesia or anaesthesia (Hodnett et al. 2013). Some doulas are expanding their practices by also becoming certified postpartum doulas with additional knowledge about assisting families during the postpartum transition period. Although some doulas in Canada are volunteers, many charge a fee for their services. British Columbia currently has an initiative to support Aboriginal doulas for Aboriginal Women (Aboriginal Doula Advisory Committee, 2010).

Perinatal Educators

Perinatal educators (those who provide education to women and their families related to pregnancy and childbirth) have played an important role working with childbearing women and families to create supportive environments for birth and breastfeeding. Over the years, educators have also worked toward humanizing women's childbearing experiences and have significantly contributed to many current practices such as **family-centred maternity care** (an approach to birth that focuses on the needs of women and their families), mother-friendly childbirth, and baby-friendly hospitals. Perinatal educators may be nurses, many of whom obtain additional education and certification. Certification is offered for a broad approach to perinatal education through International Childbirth Education Association (ICEA), but nurses can also be certified in particular approaches, such as Lamaze and Birthing from Within. Please see the list of Web Resources at the end of this chapter for details.

Understanding health promotion and perinatal education today requires an exploration of how these complex social environments came to be. Over a period of approximately 300 years, the source of information about pregnancy, birth, parenting, and breastfeeding has changed. The pendulum has swung from information being supplied by women to other women, then by physicians to women in an authoritative, "medicalized"

fashion, and now through collaborative partnerships between women, families, and maternity care providers. A historical review of educational preparation for pregnancy, childbirth, and parenthood is a good place to begin.

HISTORICAL PERSPECTIVES: EVOLUTION OF PERINATAL EDUCATION

Throughout history women have supported other women during childbearing and have passed down their knowledge about fertility, birth control, and childbearing from woman to woman. Kitzinger (2011) describes it as "the women's network" by which women learned about birth and baby care from their mothers, sisters, and female relatives. The following paragraphs explore the evolution of perinatal education in Canada from informal women's networks to the present era of internet access to information and the use of social media.

Informal Women's Networks

First Nations' women developed rituals and taboos to keep both mother and newborn healthy and shared practical and herbal remedies for pregnancy discomforts, to promote lactation, and for postpartum recovery. Aboriginal women elders (commonly called "aunties" or "grannies") assisted during childbirth, using the knowledge they had learned over a lifetime (Benoit & Carroll, 2005). Although there is often a tendency to devalue this women's knowledge as "unscientific," women learned by carefully observing what worked and what did not.

Historically, birth was the exclusive domain of women, who aided one another during labour and throughout the postpartum *lying-in* period of 3 to 4 weeks. Female relatives and friends provided continuous emotional and physical support to mother and newborn, whereas midwives provided skilled birth care. The lying-in period gave the mother time to rest, regain strength, and successfully nurse and care for her baby without interruption. However, for many Canadian women living in rural and remote Canada, the needs of their families made a prolonged postpartum rest period impossible. Women helped each other, providing practical assistance and advice for new mothers living nearby (Biggs, 2004).

Attending births of other women and/or farm animals provided pioneer women with their education about childbirth and the stages and phases of labour. At the same time, they learned practical ways to help birthing women emotionally and physically.

The 20th Century

Although physicians provided care to childbearing women in Canada's newly forming cities, many rural and economically disadvantaged women relied on midwives or skilled neighbours for assistance during childbirth. Women continued to treat their families with home remedies, and "medical manuals" (not all written by physicians) for the home proliferated. However, "twentieth-century medicine aligned itself with science" (Mitchinson, 2002, p. 22) and the support for midwives as maternity care providers began to decline. Some physicians supported midwifery care in rural and remote communities as "better than no care at all," but also promoted the view that midwifery care was clearly inferior to medical science. In the early years of the 20th century, medical terminology developed and technology proliferated, resulting in the growth of hospitals. "Western medicine viewed the body as a machine that should run properly," which ultimately resulted in the desire to control and improve childbirth (Mitchinson, 2002, p. 23). Middle class and urban women also embraced medical science with their desire to decrease the risks of childbirth for themselves and their babies. Once maternity care moved to the hospital, women began choosing anaesthesia to deal with the painful, lonely hospital birth experience.

In 1902, a method of amnesic–analgesia which combined scopolamine and morphine delivered through the recently developed hypodermic syringe was first administered (Pitcock & Clark, 1992). Women were kept in darkened rooms with nurses quietly protecting their amnesic state. The goal was for the mother to remember nothing of labour's physical discomforts. This popular method came to be known as twilight sleep. Rallies of the Twilight Sleep Association in major cities in eastern Canada and the United States were successful in forcing physicians to provide this form of analgesia (Pitcock & Clark, 1992). Many women were eager for any modern medical method that could protect them against the pain and dangers they associated with childbirth. Use of this method began to dwindle, however, with reports of dangerous delays in newborn respirations associated with twilight sleep. The final blow came from the sudden death of one of its most visible advocates, Frances X. Carmody, in a twilight sleep birth (Pitcock & Clark, 1992). Despite the disappearance of twilight sleep, messages persisted that women did not have to suffer in childbirth and that freedom from labour pain was preferred.

In 1910 an insurance company (Metropolitan Life) set up the first visiting nurse program in Canada, which later became the Victorian Order of Nurses. These nurses urged women to seek out physician care in addition to providing "medical" surveillance, and education focused on maternal hygiene, nutrition, and baby care (Mitchinson, 2002). This service and the prenatal classes that later developed were the mainstay of perinatal education until the 1960s.

In 1926, 17.8% of births in Canada took place in hospitals; by 1940, more than 45% did (Mitchinson, 2002). By this time physicians had also assumed significant control over information about birth, and although physicians "may have disagreed with one another about what food, activities, and so on a pregnant woman should engage in" they all agreed "that the woman should have a physician and should listen to that physician and no one else" (Mitchinson, 2002, p. 299). Friends and relatives were no longer primary sources of information and were unable to regularly provide support for birthing women. Concerns about hospital-acquired infections further excluded women from supporting each other during childbirth.

By the beginning of the postwar baby boom, the shift toward hospitalized birth, for all who could afford it, was almost complete, and childbirth education had all but disappeared. It was kept alive by the relatively small number of women who could not afford birth in the hospital and were attended by other women at home. Breastfeeding had also been replaced by scientific infant "formulas" and newborns were cared for by skilled (and sterile) nurses in large nurseries.

By the 1960s, hospital rules had been liberalized to allow husbands to visit their wives on the postpartum unit and see their children through the nursery window. However, it would still be many years before siblings were allowed to visit.

Group Prenatal Classes for Childbirth Education

After World War II, women began to seek consciousness, control, dignity, and companionship in birth. Natural birth activists in England, Russia, and France were conducting research demonstrating that pain could be deconditioned and a new response to it could be created (Nichols & Humenick, 2000). Theories that began at this time are still in vogue today and form the basis of many formal education programs used internationally.

Dick-Read

In the 1940s, Grantly Dick-Read, an English obstetrician, was attending a birth and offered the mother chloroform as the fetal head began to crown. The mother rejected the medication. When Dick-Read asked her later about the refusal, she replied that it didn't hurt, nor was she expecting it to. In 1944, Dick-Read published *Childbirth Without Fear*, addressing the holistic nature of childbirth, in which the mind and body are connected. Dick-Read posited that the basic cause of labour pain was fear that produced tension. By educating pregnant women in physical exercise, relaxation, and breathing, Dick-Read believed that the fear–tension–pain cycle could be broken. Creating healthy bodies and attitudes in advance would prepare labouring women to deal with the strong physical sensations of childbirth (Nichols & Humenick, 2000).

Psychoprophylaxis
In Russia, research based loosely on Pavlov's experiments showed the mind–body connection in response to pain. Velvosky's trial-and-error experiments emphasized the prevention of pain through psychological strategies (rather than chemicals), resulting in an approach which was later named **"psychoprophylaxis"** (Ondeck, 2000). This training method emphasized controlled breathing, abdominal stroking, and applying pressure points on the hip and back to manage pain without pharmacology.

Lamaze
Fernand Lamaze brought the psychoprophylactic method of childbirth to Western Europe. It was in the Parisian Lamaze clinic that Marjorie Karmel learned about psychoprophylaxis and used it successfully with her first childbirth. When she and her husband returned to the United States, she sought a physician who would help her have the same satisfying and safe experience she had with Lamaze, and managed to have another fulfilling birth, using medication only as requested (Karmel, 1981).

In 1958, Elisabeth Bing and Marjorie Karmel began providing psychoprophylactic classes to other women. Together, they started the first education organization, the American Society for Psychoprophylaxis in Obstetrics (Lamaze International, 2013). This group sought to bring together noninterventionist obstetricians interested in reducing the use of analgesia and anaesthesia during childbirth, parents who wanted more control over labour, and educators who wanted to make psychoprophylaxis accessible. At the same time, the Maternity Center Association convened local consumer groups for the purpose of having "professionals and parents work together so that parents had knowledge of alternatives and were able to make an informed choice" (Nichols & Humenick, 2000).

Second Wave Feminism and the 1960s
Contemporary childbirth education grew out of the "self-help" movement and second wave feminism of the 1960s. By the 1980s self-help books such as *Our Bodies, Ourselves* (first printed in 1984) were available to Canadian women. This book (Boston Women's Health Book Collective, 2011) remains a valuable source of health information for women in Canada today. Perinatal education was also associated with consumer-driven efforts to humanize health care for childbearing families (such as Family Centred Maternity Care). Women, families, and childbirth educators began to advocate for changes in obstetrical practices, such as allowing partners and family members into the birthing setting.

The American Society for Psychoprophylaxis in Obstetrics (now simply Lamaze) was an organization of parents, professionals, and providers, whereas the International Childbirth Education Association began as a federation of local groups focused on creating a consumer-based organization to improve maternity services (Ondeck, 2000). Subsequent childbirth education organizations focused on reform and alternatives to medicalized practices. In the 1970s, the National Association of Parents and Professionals for Safe Alternatives in Childbirth promoted the demedicalization of childbirth. Robert Bradley, a Denver obstetrician, promoted nonmedicated birth and the need for fathers to serve as active coaches for labouring and birthing women (Ondeck, 2000).

La Leche League
Although physicians in the 1950s admitted that breastfeeding was the best for the baby, many felt that successful breastfeeding required a scientific knowledge base that few women could attain (Mitchinson, 2002). In addition, dairy producers launched an active marketing campaign for cow's milk "formulas" as the "scientific" and "modern" way to feed babies. As a result, fewer urban women were breastfeeding. In 1956 the La Leche League was founded by seven American mothers who simply wished to help each other learn to breastfeed (Ward, 2000). It is a good example of a consumer group developed to provide peer support and education. Today, La Leche League Canada gathers women together to share information and experiences about breastfeeding and offer one another support (For more information, see Web Resources.)

Learning Baby Care: The 1970s and 1980s
Until the 1980s most women learned how to care for their newborn from nurses during their postpartum hospital stay, which varied from 3 to 7 days. Women then received follow-up home visits from a Public Health Nurse (PHN) to ensure that their questions about newborn care were addressed and to promote immunization. As more was learned about how to promote successful breastfeeding, PHNs started to offer more breastfeeding assistance to women both in the home and at Breastfeeding Clinics located in public health units. Some PHNs also became certified Lactation Consultants.

Earlier, postpartum discharge required a substantial readjustment in nursing roles, as women were not ready for a lot of health teaching during the immediate postpartum rest and recovery period (first 24 to 48 hours). PHNs started visiting women in their home earlier, frequently within 24 hours of hospital discharge. However, costs and caseload considerations limited the number of home visits PHNs were able to make, with most women receiving *one* home visit so that follow-up visits could be saved for women experiencing breastfeeding difficulties or dealing with complex family and social situations (Cusack et al., 2008).

From Childbirth-Focused Education to Perinatal Education

Unlike the childbirth-focused education of the late 20th century, current perinatal education programs prepare families for the entire childbearing year. Preconception, early pregnancy, childbirth, and early parenting are all family life cycle moments when health promotion messages can invite positive lifestyle changes with long-term health benefits for the entire family (Misra et al., 2003). Perinatal education programs engage in health promotion by taking advantage of reachable and teachable moments. Women and their families are reachable because they actively seek information from books, classes, and internet sources. They are teachable because they are motivated by their pregnancy and impending transition to parenthood to learn and develop personal skills to cope with their transitions (Herrman et al., 2012).

Today, educational preparation for pregnancy, childbirth, and parenting has a health promotion focus and is offered to childbearing women and their families before conception and throughout the childbearing year. Classes are provided in community health clinics, hospitals, private clinics, community centres, or privately. In addition, there is an overwhelming amount of information available on the internet. The role of the nurse has shifted away from that of being a "giver of information" toward helping women and their family members evaluate and make sense of this information in the context of their particular lives. In the next section of this chapter, health-promoting perinatal education for the childbearing year will be discussed.

HEALTH PROMOTION FOR THE CHILDBEARING YEAR

The purposes of perinatal education include (1) health promotion throughout the childbearing year (preconception through infancy); (2) preventing known pregnancy and childbearing risks; (3) promoting informed participation in health care decision making; (4) enhancing efficacy for self-care and for adapting to the challenges of pregnancy, labour, birth, and early parenting transitions; and (5) building community support networks for new parents.

 Recall Shelley and her partner Joel from the beginning of the chapter. Shelley asks you how she can know which of the sources of information about sibling rivalry that she found on the internet are reliable and accurate. Pause here to think about how you would respond to her question.

Canadian families today want access to information that supports them throughout the childbearing year and transition to parenthood. The most useful sources of pregnancy-related information identified by Canadian women have been health care providers, books, and previous pregnancies (PHAC, 2009).

Promoting Health Before Pregnancy

Education about healthy living ideally begins early in a person's life, with emphasis on eating well, exercising, and reducing risk factors that may lead to illness. The ultimate goal is to maintain and improve health throughout life. In addition, teaching about healthy behaviours provides information for enhanced decision making. Chapter 2 presents a detailed description of major areas of health promotion for women, along with numerous suggestions for teaching and recommendations for screening.

Providing health information and educational opportunities *before* conception/pregnancy can help prevent known childbearing risks. For example, high school students can be provided opportunities to explore the realities of parenting a child and learn about how to prepare for a healthy pregnancy in the future. Preconception counselling also provides an opportunity for health promotion related to childbearing and offering information about pregnancy and ways to promote maternal and fetal well-being. See Chapter 11 for more detailed information related to preconceptual health. Areas commonly addressed during health teaching at this time are described in Table 14.1.

Pregnancy

Once a woman becomes pregnant, health teaching should include discussion about perinatal education programs available in her community. In addition, the nurse or care provider offers information about the many changes that occur in the woman's body during pregnancy and how to promote wellness during this time. The nurse may also discuss how to manage the common discomforts of pregnancy such as nausea and vomiting, breast tenderness, constipation, fatigue and muscle cramps, urinary frequency, ankle edema, and backache. In addition, he or she instructs the woman and her partner about danger signs and symptoms of pregnancy, so that they can notify a maternity care provider immediately, receive early intervention, and possibly reduce the risk for problems. See Chapter 12 for more information on these changes and appropriate interventions. Throughout pregnancy, the nurse or care provider reassesses learning needs and allows time for the client and her partner to ask questions and identify concerns and possible areas of misinformation (Fig. 14.3).

● TABLE 14.1   **Perinatal Education Classes**

Type	Attendees	Topics Covered	Timing	Purpose
Preconception	Parents planning a pregnancy	<ul><li>Assesses pregnancy readiness: emotional, financial, social, nutritional and health practices for pregnancy and parenting</li><li>Physical readiness for pregnancy: both parents play a part</li><li>Prevention of birth defects</li><li>Fertility issues</li><li>Emotional and physical changes in early pregnancy</li><li>Self-care and health care during pregnancy</li></ul>	Anytime an individual or couple is planning or considering a future pregnancy	To promote healthy lifestyles before becoming pregnant. Specific areas of focus include the following:<ul><li>Strong and safe relationships</li><li>Self-assessment of current health and lifestyle</li><li>Benefits of regular health care during pregnancy</li><li>Folic acid intake</li><li>Management of health conditions affecting pregnancy and birth</li><li>Stress reduction</li><li>Smoking cessation</li><li>Avoiding toxic substances</li><li>Environmental health and workplace safety</li></ul>
Early prenatal	Parents in the first or second trimesters whether planning birth at home, in a birth centre, or in a hospital	<ul><li>Health care during pregnancy: rights and responsibilities</li><li>Physical and emotional changes in pregnancy<ul><li>Warning signs and what to do</li><li>Coping with minor discomforts of pregnancy</li><li>Sexuality</li><li>Nutrition</li><li>Rest and sleep</li><li>Exercise</li><li>Use of drugs</li><li>Stress management</li><li>Fetal development</li><li>Finances</li></ul></li><li>Resources<ul><li>Myths</li><li>Choices in caregivers</li><li>Choices in birth sites</li><li>Practice in each class of comfort measures</li></ul></li></ul>	As early as possible in the first trimester; also valuable in the second trimester	To promote health in pregnancy, as evidenced by:<ul><li>Term birth</li><li>Adequate birth weight</li><li>Relationship maintenance</li><li>Good maternal health and energy</li><li>Good maternal mental health</li><li>Stress relief</li><li>Bonding</li><li>Financial planning</li><li>Support systems</li></ul>
Prenatal	Parents in the third trimester	All of the above, *plus:*<ul><li>Common fears and anxieties</li><li>Partner involvement in childbirth</li><li>Choice and birth preferences</li><li>Anatomy and physiology of childbirth</li><li>Comfort measures & labour support skills</li><li>Pain management strategies</li><li>Variations in birth</li><li>Hospital or birth centre routines</li></ul>	Third trimester	To promote health in the third trimester, in labour and birth, *plus:*<ul><li>Develop relaxation awareness</li><li>Plan for support during labour, birth, and postpartum</li><li>Understand hospital or birth centre culture and routines</li><li>Promote healthy lifestyles</li></ul>

(table continues on page 548)

● TABLE 14.1   **Perinatal Education Classes** (continued)

Type	Attendees	Topics Covered	Timing	Purpose
		● Obstetric interventions ● Practice in each class of comfort measures ● Informed consent/refusal ● Birth preferences		● Avoid unnecessary interventions ● Prevent complications ● Develop an understanding of the body's natural ability to give birth
Vaginal birth after cesarean (VBAC)	Parents who have had a previous cesarean	● Previous birth experience ● Reframing this labour: primipara and multipara labours ● Importance of support systems ● Benefits and risks of VBAC ● Planning for a vaginal birth ● Benefits and risks of cesarean birth ● Avoidable factors leading to cesarean ● Planning for a cesarean birth ● Variations in labour ● Comfort techniques for labour: familiar and new ● Informed consent and refusal ● Birth preferences ● Preparation of siblings ● Breastfeeding	Third trimester	To enhance the confidence of parents preparing for trial of labour after a previous cesarean birth with a goal of achieving a vaginal birth.
Refresher	Parents who have already had at least one birth	● Review of previous birth experience ● Review of comfort measures used successfully ● Comparison of primipara and multipara labours and birth ● Birth preferences	Third trimester	Parents may not have had time to focus on the new baby. Some families want to review and learn new coping skills to build their confidence for labour. Others may be having their first baby with a new partner and be learning about how they can cope and work together in labour and early parenting.
Multiple births	Parents expecting multiple births	All prenatal class topics, *plus:* ● Fetal surveillance ● Increased needs for nutrition, hydration, and rest ● Body mechanics and exercises for posture ● Relationship strengthening, and stress reduction ● Preterm labour symptoms and what to do ● Breastfeeding multiples ● Local and regional resources for parents of multiples ● Birth preferences	Late in the second trimester or early in the third trimester	Parents of multiples want information on how the birth may be different from singleton births and want to prepare for birth and postpartum.
Breastfeeding preparation	Parents at any time of pregnancy	● Breast milk production ● Benefits ● Nutrition, hydration, and relaxation for breastfeeding ● Proper latch ● Fertility ● Positions at the breast	Anytime during pregnancy	Preparation will help decrease the stress of breastfeeding for parents by providing information about the process and resources for questions after they are home.

(continued)

● TABLE 14.1   **Perinatal Education Classes** (continued)

Type	Attendees	Topics Covered	Timing	Purpose
		• Infant feeding cues and patterns • How to tell when the infant is getting enough milk • Hand expression and pumping • Storing breast milk • Complications • The partner's roles • Resources for support		
Partners in pregnancy, labour, and early parenting	Partners in the second or third trimester	• The partner's experience of pregnancy • Coping strategies for pregnancy, labour, and early parenting • Qualities and roles of a parent • Easing the transition to parenthood: the early days	Second or third trimester	Partners experience their own transitions during pregnancy. Their experience needs to be affirmed, and their roles in pregnancy, labour, and early parenting made clear. Partners need the opportunity to meet and talk about what it means to become a parent. Hearing from and talking with others can build confidence in the role.
Hospital or birth centre tour/ virtual tour	Parents giving birth in a hospital or free standing birth centre	• Facilities • Roles of members of the medical team • Hospital protocols • Comfort amenities (e.g., bath, shower, birth balls, healing touch) • Admission procedures • Creating a peaceful environment	Anytime during pregnancy	Familiarity with the hospital environment allows parents to personalize their birth space and improves relaxation. By providing access to a virtual tour families can access the resource online or in a group setting.

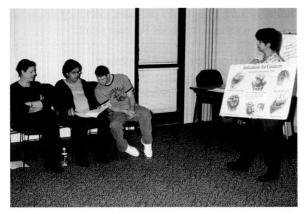

FIGURE 14.3 During individual and group teaching sessions, nurses and educators need to assess learning needs, review understanding, and answer questions.

As the woman progresses through the third trimester, teaching begins to focus more on the upcoming labour and birth. Labour support has been shown to positively influence birth outcomes and women's satisfaction with childbirth (Hodnett et al., 2013). Supportive care during childbirth is discussed in more detail in Chapter 15. The nurse or care provider explains and reviews with the woman and her partner the process of labour, expected events, procedures, and assessments so that they have a sense of what to expect. Such preparation can alleviate anxiety about the unknown and assist families to make decisions about the events surrounding birth.

To facilitate informed decision making, information about settings available for labour and birth (such as hospitals, birthing centres, and home births) may be given early in pregnancy. Later, the nurse could inquire about the decisions and choices women/families have made and address any unanswered questions. Women should be encouraged to develop a birth plan that reflects their desires and enhances communication with care providers.

Childbirth

Discussing Pain Management for Childbirth

The degree of discomfort and pain associated with labour and birth can be a major concern for the pregnant woman and her partner. Nurses are instrumental in educating the woman and her partner about the expected pain of labour and the many nonpharmacologic and pharmacologic options available to manage the pain. Once armed with this knowledge, the client and her partner can choose the methods most appropriate for their situation and beliefs.

Nonpharmacologic Methods. Women can use non-pharmacologic methods for pain relief during labour alone, in combination with other nonpharmacologic methods, or as adjuncts to pharmacologic interventions. Regardless of how such methods are used, the nurse describes and discusses the various options with the woman and her partner so that they can decide on the type(s) that would be most appropriate for them. Examples of nonpharmacologic methods can be found in Box 14.1.

The nurse may begin teaching by exploring families beliefs about pain and expected labour pain. Building on that knowledge the nurse can continue by explaining the physiology of the pain response and the factors that influence pain perception. Next, he or she may describe sources that cause pain during labour and birth (see Chapter 17). Most people are aware that uterine contractions are the major source of pain; however, they also need to understand that stretching of the cervix and perineum may contribute. An additional source

● BOX 14.1   Non-Pharmacologic Methods for Pain Relief During Labour

- Relaxation and imagery
- Mindfulness and meditation
- Music
- Breathing techniques
- Herbal preparations
- Aromatherapy
- Heat and cold applications
- Hydrotherapy
- Therapeutic touch
- Massage
- Hypnosis
- Biofeedback
- Transcutaneous electrical nerve stimulation (TENS)
- Acupressure and acupuncture

of pain can be pressure from the fetus on the surrounding structures, organs, and tissues as it moves through the birth canal (Blackburn, 2013). The nurse presents such information to the woman and partner so that they can understand the nature of the pain. As the nurse reviews the methods for pain relief, the woman and partner are better prepared to make decisions based on a fully informed understanding of what is happening to the woman's body. During such discussions, the nurse keeps in mind any sociocultural, religious, or other beliefs and concerns that may influence the reactions and choices of the woman and her partner.

The nurse explains different pain relief methods to the woman and her partner and demonstrate specific techniques or steps, such as the different types of breathing that can be used. The client and partner then can return demonstrate any steps or techniques to ensure that they are performing them properly (Fig. 14.4). Positive feedback for their performance is encouraging, along with suggestions, as necessary, to enhance their use of techniques. In addition, the nurse reminds the woman and her partner that during labour, nurses providing care will be readily available to keep them informed about the progress of labour, and provide support, suggestions, and encouragement. MacKinnon et al. (2005) have documented the importance of nursing presence during childbirth (see Research Highlight 14.1).

Pharmacologic Methods. Many different pharmacologic agents may be used during labour and birth to provide pain relief. In addition, they may be administered by different techniques. As with nonpharmacologic methods, pharmacologic methods may be used alone, in combination with other medications, or in combination with nonpharmacologic methods. Nurses ensure that clients receive adequate information about the options available related to medications. Since nurses prepare women for informed decision making, they include potential effects on the woman and her fetus as part of this teaching. Chapter 17 provides a detailed discussion of pharmacologic methods for pain relief.

Preparation for the Newborn

Preparation for baby care and infant feeding has also been an important component of group prenatal classes and popular with first time parents. An important element of educational preparation for the newborn is building parental confidence and competence (Liu et al., 2012). Group education classes also offer the opportunity to address newborn safety concerns such as the correct use of infant car restraints and preventing sudden infant death syndrome (SIDS) by positioning newborns on their back for sleeping (Ateah, 2013). In a systematic review of postnatal parental education, Bryanton and

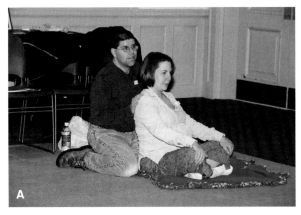 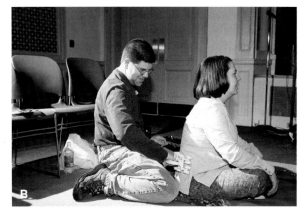

FIGURE 14.4 Ideally, during teaching sessions clients **(A)** are actively involved in learning, and **(B)** need time to practice their new skills.

Beck (2010) noted that education about infant behaviour may enhance women's knowledge and that information about ways to enhance infant sleep appears to be effective in increasing sleep duration. Connections made with other parents during group perinatal education classes can also expand the family's social support network.

Health teaching also addresses preparation for the newborn and baby care. Typically, care providers review the normal characteristics of the newborn and assist the woman to prepare for breastfeeding or bottlefeeding. They usually give information about newborn appearance, and behaviours, as well as providing assistance as the woman gets started with breastfeeding (see Chapters 20 and 21). In addition, the nurse or care provider should offer information about potential relationship changes the woman and family may expect during the postpartum period (see Chapter 18). Fathers, siblings, and grandparents also have learning needs and appreciate being included in health teaching.

● RESEARCH HIGHLIGHT 14.1 The Meaning of the Nurse's Presence During Childbirth

PURPOSE

The purpose of this exploratory study was to develop new understandings of what it means to women in labour for a nurse to be present during childbirth.

DESIGN

Hermeneutic inquiry was used to explore the phenomenon of nursing presence during childbirth. Six women from an urban centre in Canada shared their experiences through conversational, audiotaped interviews. Hermeneutic phenomenology was used to more fully explore the meaning of the women's experiences and attempt to understand what the conversations with women revealed.

RESULTS

Women attribute multiple meanings to the care provided by intrapartum nurses. What stood out in the interviews with women about their childbearing experiences was that a nurse's presence was the way that a nurse was "there" for them. Women said they valued the nurses' work of providing information about what was happening to them, suggesting strategies for working with their body, and being available to support them. Women also valued opportunities to get to know their nurse before active labour and felt that this "knowing" helped them trust their nurse in a way that they could "let go" of some of their responsibilities for "keeping their baby safe" and focus on their "labouring work." Skillful intrapartum nursing practice involves knowing about the woman, knowing how to build trusting relationships, and knowing about how to assist.

CONCLUSION

Since many things, such as triage practices, influence the birth setting, women's experiences of a nurse's presence cannot be understood apart from the institutional structures and work processes that shape the experiences of both the woman and the nurse.

Adapted from MacKinnon, K., McIntyre, M., & Quance, M. (2005). The meaning of the nurse's presence during childbirth. *Journal of Obstetric, Gynecologic & Neonatal Nursing, 34*(1), 28–36.

Preparation for Parenting and Family Transitions

The Canadian Maternity Experiences Survey asked women if they felt they had received *enough* information about a variety of topics. Women reported that they had enough information about breastfeeding, basic maternal and infant care, and community resources; they were less informed about the transition to parenthood. Gaps identified by these Canadian women included sexual changes, physical demands of newborn care, and the effects of the transition period on the relationship with their partner (PHAC, 2009).

Fox (2010) has written a book about couples' experiences of becoming parents that initially focuses on women's experiences of birthing and mothering. She also includes a relational account of parenting that addresses men and fathering. Her analysis shows how material resources and the dynamics of relationships affect the transition to parenthood. Canadian women and their family members have received variable preparation for the transition to parenting and the family adjustments required following childbirth. Learning activities related to postpartum family adjustments have been integrated into prenatal classes and some programs offer specialized classes for father, siblings, and grandparents (See Table 14.1 for details).

Resources for Fathers

Canadian fathers are becoming more engaged parents with their children, but learning to be a father takes time and practice (Best Start Resource Centre, 2012a). Since most men have little previous experience with childbearing or newborns, they need encouragement to become involved with their children during pregnancy and the postpartum period. Paternal fears related to childbirth have also been identified (Hanson et al., 2009) and should be addressed in perinatal education programs.

There is a growing body of literature about the transition to fatherhood and the roles fathers play during childbirth (Ball & Daly, 2012). The Fatherhood Involvement Research Alliance is a Pan-Canadian alliance of individuals, organizations, and institutions dedicated to the development and sharing of knowledge focusing on father involvement, and the building of a community–university research alliance supporting this work (Fatherhood Involvement Research Alliance, 2013). Their website gathers research on fathering and has a variety of resources for parents and professionals (see Web Resources).

Resources for Lesbian, Gay, Bisexual, Trans, Queer (LGBTQ) Parents

While less is written about transition to parenthood for gay and lesbian couples, it is no less significant and often requires extensive planning. Best Start has produced a useful guide for health and social care providers called "Welcoming and Celebrating Sexual Orientation and Gender Diversity in Families: From Preconception to Preschool" (Best Start Resource Centre, 2012b). The guide is intended to make it easier to welcome LGBTQ parents into childbirth and parenting programs. It includes an Organizational Checklist for LGBTQ Inclusivity and a list of useful resources including links to The Lesbian, Gay, Bisexual, Trans (LGBT) Parenting Connection (see Web Resources).

Early Child Development Programs

From conception to 5 years is an intense period of growth and development that impacts a child's future growth and development. In an effort to promote healthy families and early childhood development, prenatal and parenting programs are integrating information about this important life stage into their programming. *Prenatally*, concepts such as prenatal parenting, attachment, and brain development (Benoit, 2009; Kagan, 2012) are being included in classes and in online resources. *New parent* programming integrates or focuses on concepts such as attachment, infant and child development, and the development of positive parenting skills (Cowan & Cowan, 2009; van Ijzendoorn, 2012; Watson, 2010). Excellent resources for parents, health care providers, and program developers are available online through the Encyclopedia on Early Childhood Development (see Web Resources). The Encyclopedia is produced by the Centre of Excellence for Early Childhood Development in Montreal and the Strategic Knowledge Cluster on Early Child Development (a Canadian consortium of early childhood researchers).

Nurses can be actively involved in meeting the expressed and developmental learning needs of childbearing families. Integrating health promotion content into care will help families be better prepared and more confident for the transition to becoming a family with an infant. In the next section we will explore how women's beliefs about childbearing and childbirth pain affect their labour and birth experiences and their choice of an approach to perinatal education.

CHILDBIRTH PAIN AND PREPARATION FOR LABOUR AND BIRTH

The pendulum has swung both ways between women's desire for natural birth and anaesthetized birth. Is birth a normal physiologic process or a pathologic event? Does childbirth education provide parents with the information they need to make thoughtful and informed choices about how they give birth, or is it merely preparation for a medicalized labour? What options are available for Canadian women giving birth in a variety of settings across Canada? What influence do fear, pain, and the environment for birth have on the woman's childbirth experiences?

 Recall Monique, the woman at 14 weeks' gestation described at the beginning of the chapter. What specific areas would the nurse address to help guide Monique and her partner in their decisions about childbirth?

Women's beliefs about childbirth and childbirth pain can influence both their birth experiences and their choice of approaches for perinatal education.

Childbirth Pain

A common concern for women and their partners is how to cope with the pain of labour and birth. Childbearing women receive mixed messages about the pain of childbirth. Given the task of moving the baby from inside to outside, the physiology of pain during childbirth is normal. Pain focuses women and allows them to summon their support systems and find a safe place to give birth. Pain also facilitates endorphin release (the body's natural pain reliever) and working through pain may give the woman a tremendous sense of accomplishment (Leap & Anderson, 2004).

Most perinatal education programs include content on the development of pain-coping skills and information about medical interventions to reduce or alleviate labour pain. However, by itself, pain relief may not improve women's satisfaction with childbirth. In a classic study, Simkin (1996) found that women remember many details of their birth experiences, but their long-term satisfaction is heavily influenced by their sense of control over what happened, their participation in care-related decisions, treatment by attending professionals, and a sense of accomplishment from having given birth.

In a recent US study (the Good Birth Project), Namey and Lyerly (2010) explored the meaning of the word "control" as expressed in the birth narratives from 101 women who had given birth. For this study the investigators recruited a diverse group of participants and discovered that the concept of "control" could be understood more completely as it relates to five domains of well-being: self-determination, respect, personal safety or security, trust in oneself and others, and knowledge about the process of labour and birth. Namey and Lyerly concluded by noting that "de-emphasizing the term control may help lead the way toward a maternity care system that fosters the sort of birth—agential,

dignified, accompanied, considered—that women hope for and deserve" (p. 775).

Recent trends have documented that a move toward medicated birth and the use of epidural anaesthesia to cope with labour pain is increasing. More than half (57.3%) of the women who completed the Canadian Maternity Experiences Survey (MES) (2009) reported having epidural or spinal anesthesia for vaginal birth (PHAC, 2009, p. 16). Less than a quarter (22%) of these same women reported using "pain-killing" medications or gas, while almost another quarter (23%) reported using *only* medication-free pain relief techniques, including controlled or patterned breathing, position changes, and walking.

Women rated baths or showers the highest on the "helpfulness" scale out of all medication-free pain management techniques, second only to epidural anaesthesia for all pain management techniques. However, less than a third of the women surveyed reported using baths or showers during labour. Unfortunately, the MES did not ask about the availability of various pain management options, so some women may not have used hydrotherapy during labour because it was not available to them. Almost 70% of these Canadian women reported using *both* pharmacologic and nonpharmacologic pain management techniques during childbirth (PHAC, 2009).

While research continues into methods of pain relief with the fewest complications, other questions are rarely addressed. What effect do the values and attitudes of the caregiver have on women's perception of labour pain and the need for pharmacologic pain relief? Should labour pain be eliminated? Does it serve a useful purpose for the mother or the baby?

Recent evidence suggests that women's fears, attitudes, and beliefs about childbirth may influence their choice of approach to childbirth education *and* their birth outcomes. Researchers from Sweden (Haines et al., 2012) suggest that women's beliefs and attitudes could be clustered into three groups: "fearful" (those afraid of birth and childbirth pain); "take it as it comes" (those with no fear or strong attitudes about birth); and "self-determiners" (those who see birth as a natural process with no fear of childbirth). Women whose attitudes and beliefs were aligned with the "fearful" cluster were more likely to have reported their labour pain as very intense, to have had an epidural, and/or to have opted for an elective cesarean birth. More research may help nurses, midwives, and perinatal educators tailor their educational approaches to the particular needs of childbearing women.

Nurses providing perinatal education want to build women's confidence so they can cope with the events of labour, birth, and early parenting. A women's self-efficacy, or her confidence in her ability to cope with childbirth pain, may be enhanced by including learning activities to build maternal confidence. Efficacy is enhanced through mastery experiences (like practicing a contraction while holding ice), vicarious experience (watching videos or talking with women who have coped well with childbirth), being able to self-assess their own physiologic responses (through mindfulness or relaxation), and lastly through social or verbal persuasion, which has been shown to be the least effective over time (Salomonsson et al., 2013).

Preparation for Labour and Birth

Childbirth preparation classes today are offered by various organizations with differing views of the roles of women, partners, and health care providers during labour and birth. Table 14.2 highlights the characteristics of some common approaches to childbirth preparation. Here the following approaches will be discussed: Birthing from Within, Self-hypnosis, Bradley Method (an example of a partner-oriented approach), Caesarean

● TABLE 14.2 **Childbirth Preparation Approaches**

Type	Mission Statement or Explanation	Role of Woman	Role of Partner	Role of Provider
Birthing From Within (Birthing From Within, 2013)	To assist women to prepare for birth as a rite of passage, to honor sharing birth stories, and listening to understand the power and life-long impact of self-discovery or "birthing from within."	The purpose of childbirth preparation is to help mothers give birth-in-awareness, not to achieve a specific birth outcome.	Fathers and partners are invited to be present in a loving, gentle way, supporting the mother by sensing her needs and offering suggestions. Importance is placed not on the partner's knowledge or skill, but on the partner's presence and belief in the mother.	Parents deserve support for any birth option that might be right for them (e.g., drugs, technology, home birth, bottlefeeding). For parents, pregnancy, birth, and postpartum are continuous adjustments during which ongoing holistic support and education should be available.
Bradley Method (Bradley Method, 2013)	The Bradley Method is a system of natural labour techniques in which a woman and her coach play an active part. It emphasizes relaxed abdominal breathing and relaxation throughout labour.	Women are taught how to deal with the stress of labour by being aware of their own body.	The partner or coach is taught how to help the woman stay healthy during pregnancy, what to expect during labour & birth, how to avoid unnecessary pain during labour, and how to be an advocate and support for the mother.	Providers provide support and backup if medically necessary.
Mindfulness-Based Childbirth and Parenting Program	MBCP has been created to serve women going through childbirth transformation and for parents who nurture and care for the next generation.	Women are taught to integrate present moment awareness (mindfulness practices) such as breath awareness and meditation so they can respond to their body during labour and birth.	Focuses on learning life-long mindfulness practices for healthy living and wise parenting.	Also provides a program for care providers to learn mindfulness-based stress reduction life skills.
Lamaze (Lamaze International 2013)	To promote, protect, and support every woman's right to give birth, confident in her own ability, free to find comfort in a wide variety of ways, and supported by her family and all members of the health care team.	Women who are fully informed, confident, and supported will find comfort in a wide variety of ways.	Classes focus on partners learning how to provide quiet, gentle, encouraging support along with basic comfort measures for most women in labour. Fathers and partners learn that their presence is more important than an active coaching role.	Six "Lamaze Healthy Birth Practices help simplify the birth process with a natural approach that helps alleviate fears and manage pain. Regardless of the baby's size, labor's length and complexity, or the mother's confidence level, these care practices will help keep labor and birth as safe and healthy as possible."

Prevention, and new approaches integrating mindfulness practices.

Think back to Monique, the pregnant woman from the beginning of the chapter who wants to make decisions relative to labour pain management. How do Monique's current knowledge and her beliefs about pain reflect some of the historical influences associated with childbirth?

Birthing From Within

Pam England, midwife and artist, founded Birthing from Within to offer a soulful and holistic approach to labour. Expectant couples are invited to draw on their own knowledge to gain insight into their own meaning of labour and birth. They contribute to their own learning through interactive, creative participation using art as a way to reveal secret hopes and dark fears (England & Horowitz, 1998). Participants explore their personal and cultural beliefs about labour pain, and master a variety of powerful practices that include breath awareness, mindfulness, and visualizations. Parents are encouraged to actively practice pain-coping strategies and are believed to deserve support for any pain relief or birth option they consider right for them (see Web Resources).

Self-Hypnosis in Labour and Birth

Self-hypnosis is a pain-reduction method that empowers women and their partners during the labour and birth process. Women are educated in the techniques needed to promote a self-trance that alters their perception of reality. Methods may include a series of relaxation techniques consisting of therapeutic suggestions, visualization, and relaxation breathing. HypnoBirthing Classes (also called the Mongan method) are available to Canadian women and their families. This approach is an adaptation of the classic approach earlier developed by Grantly Dick-Read (see historical section) and is also used as the foundation for other educational approaches such as Lamaze (see Web Resources).

Bradley Method (a Partner-Oriented Approach)

Fathers and other partners have been involved in birth since the formalization of childbirth education in the early 1970s. Many of them attend prenatal classes, learn breathing techniques, and discover how to help mothers during labour (Fig. 14.5). Such partners have adopted the responsibilities of supporting or "coaching" the mother. Both Lamaze and the Bradley Method could be considered partner-oriented approaches. For additional information on Lamaze please refer to Table 14.2.

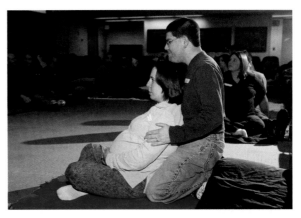

FIGURE 14.5 Many fathers and partners attend prenatal classes to learn labour support techniques and methods that will help pregnant women have a positive labour and birth experience.

Dr. Robert Bradley, a Denver obstetrician, moved the role of fathers into prominence in his book *Husband-Coached Childbirth*, first published in 1965. He developed the Bradley Method of natural childbirth classes in which mothers and fathers follow nature and give birth without the use of drugs. The Bradley Method advocates for the father's continuous presence during labour and birth. Fathers prepare so that they understand what their wives are doing, enabling them to coach, guide, and encourage women during their labour (Bradley, 1996).

Cesarean Prevention Approaches

A number of volunteer organizations have developed with a focus on education to prevent unnecessary cesarean births. The International Cesarean Awareness Network (ICAN) and the Canadian birth network, called Association for Safe Alternatives in Childbirth, are consumer movements and birth networks dedicated to educating and empowering families to make informed choices about pregnancy, birth, and parenting and to support cesarean prevention and vaginal birth after cesarean (VBAC) (See Web Resources; see also Chapter 16).

To counter a trend of interest in cesarean birth on demand, the Society of Obstetricians and Gynaecologists of Canada (SOGC), the Association of Women's Health Obstetric and Neonatal Nurses of Canada (now the Canadian Association of Perinatal and Women's Health Nurses), the Canadian Association of Midwives, the College of Family Physicians of Canada, and the Society of Rural Physicians of Canada issued a joint policy statement supporting vaginal childbirth (SOGC et al., 2008). However, ethical concerns related to not supporting the woman's informed decisions and weighing risks in a patient-centred manner make this issue more complex than it first appears (Reilly, 2009).

Integrating Mindfulness Practices

Mindfulness is development of the ability to witness changing mental and physiologic states while not working to change the states or get into another more desired state (Vieten & Astin, 2008). Mindfulness practices have been integral to how women have coped with labour over the millennia. Whether walking, swaying, chanting, or rubbing their bellies, women have sought and often found ways of being present or mindful of their experience of labour and what they need for comfort. Mindfulness practices are not identified as relaxation techniques, but they can induce a relaxed state.

Nancy Bardacke has integrated yoga, meditation, and mindfulness-based stress reduction (MBSR) into Mindfulness-Based Childbirth and Parenting classes (Bardacke, 2012). Provided as a series of classes, a retreat, and a postpartum reunion, this perinatal education approach requires a commitment on the part of families to practicing yoga and meditation 6 days a week, use CDs, a workbook and readings, while also practicing mindfulness in daily life (see Web Resources). In other health fields, MBSR has been demonstrated to "reduce anxiety and depression, improve chronic pain, quality of life and sleep" (Walker et al., 2009 p. 473).

Some women and families want to attend group perinatal education classes while others prefer to take advantage of internet sources of information and/or use social media to connect informally with other women. In the following section, a variety of approaches to perinatal education are briefly explored.

APPROACHES TO PERINATAL EDUCATION

Women and their partners who attend prenatal classes may be old or young, single or married, heterosexual or homosexual, incarcerated, or adoptive. They may have disabilities, have experienced previous pregnancy loss, or have conceived by in vitro fertilization. Their pregnancies may be planned or unplanned, desired, or unwanted. They may or may not speak the culture's predominant language. Their religious or cultural backgrounds may dictate their preferences and activities during labour and birth. They may be predominantly left- or right-brained and may be influenced by the way their families have spoken about birth. They may be limited to attending the classes available within their geographic location. They may face limitations related to cost, transportation, availability of classes, employment restrictions, and other family obligations. This amazing diversity of women and their families invites nurses to be both responsive and creative when offering any form of perinatal education.

Perinatal Education Classes

Group classes for perinatal education are offered in a variety of formats based on the unique population targeted. Many families are interested in attending a prenatal class and are able to choose between classes offered by their local health region, birth centre, hospital, or public health clinic. Although some families have the financial ability to pay fees for attending perinatal education classes, others do not (health inequities will be addressed later in the chapter). Some families seek fee-for-service private childbirth education taught from a particular perspective (eg, Birthing From Within or Lamaze).

From the Canadian Maternity Experiences Survey (PHAC, 2009) we have learned that about one third of pregnant Canadian women attend prenatal classes, two thirds are having their first baby, and only 6% are in their second or subsequent pregnancy. Women living at or below the low-income cut-off are less likely to attend classes while teens (15 to 19) are more likely to attend (PHAC, 2009). A recent Canadian study by Stoll and Hall (2012) confirmed that women who attend childbirth education classes tend to be older, more educated, and expecting their first baby (nulliparous). Families want credible, reliable, and research-based content and to access programming by making one call or contact to find it.

Perinatal education is not a standard carefully integrated into Canada's publicly funded health care system. Stoll and Hall (2012) found that higher rates of vaginal birth were associated with attending prenatal education classes. These Canadian researchers recommend that future studies explore the effects of specialized education programs on rates of interventions during labour and mode of birth. Preventing unnecessary interventions may promote better health for women and their families, reduce recovery time following childbirth, and save money for health service provision.

Other approaches to perinatal education include social marketing campaigns to raise awareness of health concerns (eg, alcohol use and preventing fetal alcohol spectrum disorder), brief educational encounters, internet sources of information, birth networks, and online perinatal education classes. The development of reliable, research-based perinatal education websites, and free written or video resources provided in languages targeting regional demographics can be considered an important strategy for health promotion. (for an online look at this type of resource see the Peel Region website listed on the *Web Resources* page).

Brief Educational Encounters

Not all families are interested in, or able to attend, prenatal classes in the formal class format offered by most health regions, hospitals, or independent providers. Families may lack finances, transportation, child care, or may not speak the language in which classes are offered. They may not know of, or have access to, subsidized, free, or language-appropriate classes. They may be located in remote rural or northern settings where classes may be less available. Some cultures do not believe that education is necessary, while other potential participants find the term "class" a barrier. These families may be contacted through brief educational encounters such as bench-style programs offered in the waiting rooms of doctor's offices or interactive learning exhibits such as Baby Care Fairs offered in accessible community sites such as malls, recreation centres, grocery stores, temples, or churches (Best Start Resource Centre, 2009).

Smoking Cessation

One place where nurses can make a difference when working with childbearing women and their families is providing brief educational interventions related to smoking cessation. The Registered Nurses Association of Ontario (RNAO) has an excellent resource designed to assist nurses to learn the skills needed for integrating smoking cessation into daily nursing practice (RNAO, 2007). This Best Practice Guideline contains evidence-based recommendations for nurses and information about the Stages of Change Model, Motivational Interviewing, the Ask, Advise, Assist, Arrange Protocol, Quit Smoking First-Line Medications, as well as a list of available resources.

Internet Resources

Access to pregnancy and early parenting information through the internet is growing as a source of information for pregnant women (Larsson, 2009). While the benefits of accessing information from the internet can be flexibility of access for families and reduction of travel and wait times often linked with accessing information from a health care provider, the most commonly used search engine does not do well at directing parents to websites with content relevant to their interests (Buultjens et al., 2012). There are also ongoing concerns that when searching for information on the internet it is difficult for families to find easy to understand information from reliable sources (Angood et al., 2010).

Having access to and being able to share unbiased, research-based information is an important skill for Canadian nurses today. The explosion of information on the internet can be overwhelming for childbearing families. Knowing and being able to direct women to current websites that provide credible, research-based, understandable, and respectful information is important. When women have accessed websites providing information that is either no longer current or provides only one view of a topic or issue, then the nurse or perinatal educator has the opportunity (some would say obligation) to promote health literacy (Tillett, 2011).

As an example, one reliable internet source on smoking cessation for pregnant women and their family members is the Health Canada (2011) website *Expecting to Quit*. This site contains helpful resources for *both* health providers (a review of Best Practices related to smoking cessation for pregnant girls and women) and for childbearing women grounded in woman-centred care and a harm reduction approach. Learning how to evaluate information available on the internet is an important skill for nurses today. A variety of tools are available, such as the link to the Georgetown University Library (2013) (see Web Resources).

Social Media and Birth Networks

Current educational trends include social media, list serves with email and RSS subscriptions, and downloadable webcasts and YouTube videos. Many of these new technologies can be accessed through portable devices such as tablets and smart phones (Jolivet & Corry, 2010). Birth networks, such as the American site "Birth Networks," are usually nonprofit advocacy groups providing information to help families find local "mother-friendly" pregnancy and childbirth care. Links to birth networks, prenatal websites, blogs, and podcasts are often posted and "liked" on social media, providing quick access to information (see Web Resources).

At the same time that social and electronic media are evolving to provide pregnant and parenting families with information, the same media may subject them to information overload (Angood et al., 2010). Families may have challenges identifying trustworthy sources of information that can help to inform their choices and decision making in pregnancy (Jolivet & Corry, 2010). Nurses can work with childbearing women and family members to help them make sense of the vast amounts of information available within the context of their particular lives.

Group Prenatal Care with an Education Component (Centering Pregnancy Models)

Rising et al. (2004) developed a model of group education and prenatal care called Centering Pregnancy in which women enter a group facilitated by their maternity care provider and a nurse or educator after their initial prenatal evaluation. At each subsequent session, women participate actively in their care by assessing and recording their own blood pressure and weight. The maternity care provider completes each woman's standard prenatal assessment within the group setting before the group discussion begins. Women meet with the same group of 8 to 12 women whose due dates are close to theirs. Discussion includes pertinent physical, emotional, social, and spiritual topics associated with childbirth (see Web Resources). This model of care has been shown to be effective in reducing preterm births and contributes to a reduction of low neonatal birth weights (Ickovics et al., 2007). Findings from recent Canadian research (Benediktsson et al., 2013; McNeil et al., 2012) suggest that this group model of care may contribute to improved mental health, social support, and health literacy. Nurses interested in learning more about group prenatal care may find Rotundo's (2011) Continuing Education article helpful.

Online Perinatal Education Programs

Online perinatal education programs are available from many different providers across North America (for an example see the *Online Birth and Babies* program listed on the Web Resources page). Some provinces and regions provide free classes online, while other online classes are fee-for-service. These interactive sites may offer information in other languages, videos, written information, handouts, and interactive "decision-points" at which time participants are invited to reflect and make decisions based on their own values and needs. Some programs offer online communities where women and families can chat, share experiences, and give or receive support. However, there is currently little published research that evaluates how frequently these sites are accessed, their impact on learning, or their impact on pregnancy, birth, or parenting outcomes.

Educational strategies are thought to improve perinatal outcomes and prevent health risks, including preterm birth, low birth weight, and congenital anomalies.

In the next section preventing childbearing risks and addressing health inequities are addressed. **Health inequities** refer to "unfair or unjust differences in health outcomes or access to care that are structurally produced, unnecessary, avoidable, and potentially remediable" (Pauly, 2013, p. 431).

PREVENTING CHILDBEARING RISKS AND ADDRESSING HEALTH INEQUITIES

Infant mortality rates are recognized as one of the best indicators of the health of populations. In Canada, rates of infant mortality are higher in Aboriginal communities, and both infant mortality and low birth weight are correlated with average neighbourhood income levels (Raphael, 2010). Nurses and perinatal educators need to be aware that *poverty* remains one of the *most* important determinants of maternal and newborn health (Raphael, 2010). How do health literacy and the social determinants of health (SDOH) relate to educational preparation for pregnancy, childbirth, and family transitions? How are pregnancy outcomes related to the social, economic, and environmental contexts of Canadian women's lives?

Health Literacy

On their website the Canadian Public Health Association defines **health literacy** simply as "the ability to access, understand and act on information for health." (Canadian Public Health Association, ND). However, in their 2008 Expert Panel Report, a more complex definition is provided: "the ability to access, understand, evaluate and communicate information as a way to promote, maintain and improve health in a variety of settings across the life-course" (Rootman & Gordon-El-Bihbety, 2008, p. 11). Raynor (2012) identified three important facets of health literacy: "the ability to read and understand health information; a wider ability to engage with the healthcare process; and the removal by healthcare systems of unnecessary complexity and barriers to patient understanding and involvement" (p. e2188).

The expert panel report from the Public Health Agency of Canada indicated that almost 12 million Canadians have inadequate health literacy skills and documented a strong relationship between health literacy and self-reported health status (Rootman & Gordon-El-Bihbety, 2008). The authors of this report noted that young working people and people with advanced levels of education have higher literacy levels, and that people who are not employed or whose first language is not French or English have lower literacy levels. Box 14.2 includes suggestions for developing health resources for childbearing families.

Although the Canadian Perinatal Surveillance System (PHAC, 2008) doesn't report directly on health literacy, it does report on low levels of maternal education as a proxy for health literacy status. Low maternal education was defined as "the number of women with

● **BOX 14.2** **Assessing Health Resources**

These simple guidelines can also be used to evaluate health-related information.

- Learn how to write in clear language.
- Keep to the point. Focus on the most important messages.
- Use short words and short sentences.
- A grade 5 to 8 reading level is appropriate for the general public.
- Test your text using readability tools on your computer.
- Choose a simple font that is easy to read.
- Use white space effectively.
- Include images that provide visual messages.
- Ask the population of interest if the literacy level is appropriate.

Adapted from Best Start Resource Centre. (2006a). *Checklist for the development of resources on preconception, prenatal and child health.* Toronto, ON.

less than a high school education who delivered a live born child, as a proportion of all women who delivered a live born child" (PHAC, 2008, p. 57). Low maternal educational levels are associated with poor perinatal health practices including maternal smoking, exposure to second-hand smoke, and alcohol use during pregnancy. Breastfeeding rates (both initiation and continuation) and folic acid supplementation increase with the level of maternal education (PHAC, 2008).

Access to Perinatal Education and Care

Although formal education programs have successfully reached many middle class, well-educated Canadian women, programs need to be tailored to the needs of particular groups (Stoll & Hall, 2012). Groups not well served by mainstream prenatal classes include adolescent women, immigrant women and those who do not speak either of Canada's two official languages, First Nations' women, homeless or migrant women, women living in remote rural and northern settings, women living in poverty, and women with disabilities. Innovative approaches to meet the needs of some of these special groups have been developed. These include pregnancy outreach programs for women living in poverty (such as the Canada Prenatal Nutrition program discussed below), and women-centred, harm-reduction programs for women who use drugs during pregnancy (Marcellus, 2007; Sword et al., 2009). Perinatal education programs across Canada also have been developed to help meet the needs of socially at-risk women and families.

Women living in rural and Aboriginal Communities (includes First Nations, Métis, and Inuit people) may also have limited access to perinatal education programs and more recently to local maternity care services, since many rural hospitals now provide limited labour and birth services (Kornelsen & Grzybowski, 2012). "Women who live more than 1 to 2 hours away from labour and delivery services have an increased risk of unplanned out-of-hospital delivery....Women who live 2 to 4 hours from services have increased rates of intervention including the highest rates of induction of labour for logistical reasons" (p. 5). Women and care providers also have different understandings and values related to childbearing risks (e.g., clinical risks vs. social risks), which sometimes results in "care providers viewing parturient women as noncompliant and women feeling abandoned" (p. 5).

Canada Prenatal Nutrition Program

The Canada Prenatal Nutrition Program is funded jointly by Federal and Provincial/Territorial governments (PHAC, 2010). This program funds community groups to develop or enhance programs for vulnerable pregnant women including pregnant women living in poverty, teens or women living in isolation, or women with poor access to services. Programs funded by the Canada Prenatal Nutrition Program use a variety of service approaches designed to feed, inform, and support women and families during the childbearing year. Positive outcomes have been demonstrated in breastfeeding initiation rates that are higher than expected for the target populations, fewer babies born with low birth weight, and impressive local community support (PHAC, 2010). These programs are designed to prevent known childbearing risks and address health inequities.

Best Start Resources

The Ontario-based organization Best Start provides information and resources for health and service providers who are "working on health promotion projects to improve the health of expectant parents and their young children. The Centre provides workshops and conferences, resources, consultations, and subject-specific information" (Best Start Resource Centre, 2013, home page). Best Start has a useful resource titled "Populations at higher risk: When mainstream approaches don't work" (Best Start Resource Centre, 2006). Best Start also has educational resources for nurses working with First Nations families (Best Start Resource Centre, 2012c) and for childbearing women and their family members available in a variety of languages. Nurses and perinatal educators might find these resources helpful (see Web Resources).

Programs for New Canadians

New Canadians, particularly those whose first language is neither English nor French, require additional health information and specialized approaches for perinatal education. Immigrant women have more difficulty understanding and using printed materials, even when available in their native language (Rootman & Gordon-El-Bihbety, 2008). An example of an integrated program developed to assist new immigrants and families living in poverty is the South Community Birth Program in Vancouver (see Web Resources). The South Community Birth Program (SCBP) includes a variety of free resources including a doula program (often with a doula who speaks the woman's native language), food and educational materials, food vouchers for fresh foods not provided by the local food banks, and access to donated infant furniture and strollers. The SCBP has adapted the Centering Pregnancy model discussed earlier and nurses provide group prenatal classes alongside midwife or physician-led prenatal care.

Programs for Aboriginal Women and their Families

Current research suggests that a complex interplay of poverty and exposure to racism, violence, trauma, and loss may result in poorer perinatal outcomes for Aboriginal

Canadian women when compared with non-Aboriginal Canadian women (Varcoe et al., 2013). "A life-long trajectory of health begins during gestation, with the health profile and social determinants affecting the health resources for pregnant women. Early child development follows, in which the circumstances of the physical and emotional environment impact not only children's current health but set the groundwork for future vulnerabilities and resiliencies" (Loppie Reading & Wien, 2009, p. 3).

Aboriginal women's childbearing experiences are influenced by rural environments for perinatal care and the effects of both historical and ongoing colonization (Varcoe et al., 2013). "Practitioners who better understand Aboriginal women's birth outcomes in context can better care in every interaction, particularly by enhancing women's power, choice and control over their experiences" (Varcoe et al., 2013, p. 1). The Aboriginal doula project mentioned earlier (Aboriginal Doulas for Aboriginal Women) is an example of one current initiative designed to enhance Aboriginal women's choices, power, and control (Aboriginal Doula Advisory Committee, 2010).

Preterm Birth Prevention Programs

Because of increasing preterm birth rates, a recommended population health strategy (Heaman et al., 2001) was implemented, as well as a number of preterm birth prevention programs across Canada. Careful analysis of the effects of these risk prevention programs on women's everyday lives illustrates the power of health education and some of the dangers of individualized risk prevention programs that only target "lifestyle behaviours" (MacKinnon & McCoy, 2006). Even though the causes of preterm labour and birth are not well understood (Centers for Disease Control and Prevention, 2013), women in one study described a profound sense of personal responsibility for preventing preterm birth (MacKinnon, 2006). Even more troubling, the women who had given birth early felt that they had failed in the work of "keeping the baby in" (MacKinnon & McIntyre, 2006). Although perinatal and parenting education provides women and their families with important health information, it is also important to carefully examine the impact of health education programs. Liaschenko (2002) warns that health promotion can result in "moral harm": "Because disease is increasingly viewed as being under individual control, people who do not engage in health promotion practices and who develop disease increasingly are reprimanded socially" (Liaschenko, 2002, p. 144). Frequently, social sanctions are directed at groups of women or families who are in some way different or "other" than the mainstream (such as teen moms, single parents, or women living in poverty). Thinking about health promotion from within a framework that includes the social, economic, and environmental determinants of health can help practitioners develop strategies where resources,

risks, and responsibility for health are shared by communities, health care providers, and individuals.

The Limits of Educational Interventions

When one considers health promotion that addresses health inequities, the limits of educational interventions are more readily apparent. Prominent discourses like "healthy lifestyles" obscure the effects of the social, economic, and environmental determinants of health. Institutional structures and a lack of the resources needed for health make healthy childbearing more difficult for some women and their families (MacKinnon & Moffitt, 2014). Health inequities in Canada are geographically distributed with people living in rural, remote, and Aboriginal communities experiencing a disproportionate burden of risk and disease (Fortier, 2012). Pauly, MacKinnon, and Varcoe note that "inequities in access to healthcare interact with inequities in access to social resources (such as housing, education, and social assistance) and with institutionalized oppression to produce inequities in health outcomes" (2009, p. 126).

Health disparities become health inequities when they are unnecessary, unfair, and preventable, resulting from social injustices that become engrained in the fabric of society through its social, economic, and political structures, laws, policies, and culture so as to become largely invisible. What become societal norms are created deliberately to advantage select members of society at the expense of others (Falk-Raphael & Betker, 2012, p. 98).

This is not to say that educational interventions are not important or even empowering, only that they are, in themselves, not sufficient for addressing health inequities.

Nurses provide leadership for and advocate *with* childbearing women and their families to reduce health inequities by removing structural and institutional barriers (MacKinnon & Moffitt, 2014; Pauly et al., 2009). Nurses are aware of the social, economic, and environmental determinants of healthy childbearing so that they can work collaboratively to ensure that *all* childbearing women have access to the resources needed for healthy living. In the next section how nurses can *both* provide and promote perinatal education will be reviewed.

COLLABORATIVE NURSING CARE

Many options are available to the woman and her family in preparation for pregnancy, childbirth, and parenting. Nurses, perinatal educators, and maternity care providers collaborate to discuss topics important to the woman and her partner, to explore their understanding of information provided, and to correct any misconceptions they might have so that the woman and her family can make the most appropriate and informed decisions. One important role for nurses today is to help women and their partners make sense of health information in the context of their lives.

Nurses maximize opportunities for health-promoting perinatal education both *before* pregnancy and *throughout* the childbearing year. Providing anticipatory guidance, referrals to local programs, and recommending reliable sources of online health information can promote health and enhance childbearing experiences. When recommending resources and programs, RNs consider the "fit" of various approaches with the woman's personal birth philosophy and goals. Nurses also help women mobilize their personal strengths and support networks to adapt to the challenges of pregnancy, childbirth, postpartum, and parenting transitions. Nurses work with others to mobilize community resources and to enhance or develop new programs. Social networks and support groups (such as mom and baby drop in groups) have been shown to both promote health and to prevent postpartum depression (Dennis, 2009). In this section, the nursing process will serve as a basis for exploring how nurses can provide health-promoting perinatal education for women and their families throughout the childbearing year.

Assessment

Assessment typically involves determining the client's knowledge about pregnancy, childbirth, and parenting. Ideally, this assessment occurs before the woman becomes pregnant to ensure that she is in the best possible health. Early assessment helps the nurse or care provider to work in partnership with women and families toward a healthy pregnancy, a positive birth experience, and a thriving baby/family.

Once a pregnancy is established, the nurse's assessment focuses on ascertaining the woman's knowledge level about the physical and psychological changes that accompany gestation, common discomforts that she may experience, and danger signs and symptoms (see Chapter 12). In addition, the client's experiences with any previous pregnancies can help provide clues about areas that need clarification or further discussion. Another key area of assessment includes the woman's knowledge level about how to promote physical and mental health in pregnancy.

As the pregnancy continues, assessment focuses on the woman's and family's ability to adapt and their preparations for labour and birth. The nurse also has an opportunity to address questions and alleviate fears about childbirth (see Chapter 15). Key areas of focus include the following:

- Understanding of normal labour and birth, including signs and symptoms of prodromal and active labour

- Goals for labour and birth, including involvement of family members (e.g., siblings)
- Preference for approach to perinatal education (e.g., group classes or online)
- Plans for birth, including birth attendant, support persons, and setting
- Labour support skills and options for pain management
- Plans for feeding the newborn and skills for getting started
- Understanding of newborn care, growth, and development
- Plans for the mother and newborn once at home
- Understanding of the transition to parenthood and plans for self/couple and family care

Nursing Care Plan 14.1 provides an example of perinatal educational interventions designed for Monique and her partner.

Assessment continues after the birth to determine the learning needs of the new parents. Common areas of focus include newborn care, infant feeding, and newborn growth and development. The nurse can also ask the woman about her childbearing experiences with the goal of promoting confidence in her abilities or identifying situations that require further assessment and/or follow-up. Assessment also addresses the woman's understanding of the events after birth, including the physical and psychological changes that aid in returning her body to its prepregnant state. These topics are discussed in detail throughout Unit 5 of this text.

Select Potential Nursing Diagnoses
Nursing diagnoses appropriate for the woman and her family related to education can be numerous, encompassing a wide range of concerns. Some of the more common nursing diagnoses may include the following:

- **Lack of Knowledge** about the events of pregnancy, childbirth, the postpartum rest and recovery phase, newborn care and infant feeding, and/or childbearing and parenting transitions
- **Lack of Knowledge** about labour support and managing labour pain
- **Health-Seeking Behaviours** related to health practices that promote optimal pregnancy health outcomes
- **Anxiety** related to lack of experience with pregnancy, childbirth fear, and lack of confidence with newborn care and breastfeeding
- **Decisional Conflict** related to lack of knowledge, misconceptions, and inaccurate information about childbearing options including labour and birth

(text continues on page 564)

NURSING CARE PLAN 14.1

●

The Couple Preparing for Labour and Birth

 Remember Monique, the 32-year-old woman at 14 weeks' gestation with her first pregnancy. Upon further assessment, Monique reveals that her partner's desire for natural childbirth results from his concern about the use of drugs during labour. Monique says, "My mom was asleep when she had me, and I was fine. I want to do what's best for my baby, but I'm afraid of the pain." Monique also shared that she has heard many "horror stories" about labour and birth.

NURSING DIAGNOSES

- **Anxiety** related to inexperience with labour, birth process, and associated pain
- **Lack of Knowledge** related to labour and birth, pain experience, and pain relief measures
- **Decisional Conflict** related to management of the labour and birth process

EXPECTED OUTCOMES

1. The woman and her partner will identify areas of concern related to the labour and birth process.
2. The woman and her partner will describe the process of labour and birth and the support available to assist both of them.
3. The woman and her partner will learn strategies for working *with* the labour and birth process.
4. The woman and her partner will describe options available for labour pain management.
5. The woman and her partner will access perinatal education resources that address their learning needs.

INTERVENTIONS	RATIONALES
Explore what Monique has heard about labour and labour pain; provide information that invites further reflection and corrects misconceptions; allow time for questions and invite her partner to participate in a future discussion.	Addressing Monique's identified concerns first provides an opening for health promoting perinatal education.
Assess Monique's level of understanding about the labour and birth process; include her partner in the assessment and discussion/teaching.	Assessment provides a baseline to identify specific client needs and to develop an individualized learning plan. Participation of the partner provides support to the client, promotes informed decision making, and enhances the chances for a positive experience for both partners.
Discuss how labour progresses and reinforce the need for adaptation during labour. Discuss the importance of supportive care stressing that nurses and other care providers will also be available during childbirth. Explore the possibility of a doula as appropriate.	Awareness of potential changes helps to prepare the couple for what to expect and work more effectively with the labour and birth process. Knowing that nurses and/or other caregivers will be available to support her may decrease her fear of labour and birth.

(continued)

NURSING CARE PLAN 14.1 ● The Couple Preparing for Labour and Birth *(Continued)*

INTERVENTIONS	RATIONALES
Explore Monique's past experiences with relaxation, stress reduction, and pain management. Discuss how different approaches to perinatal education would build on what has worked for her in the past.	Mobilizes her strengths, builds confidence, and creates receptiveness to thinking about perinatal education programs.
Discuss working with one's body during labour and birth and how childbirth pain is normal. Review nonpharmacologic comfort measures (including baths or showers) and how these techniques can be used at different phases of labour and also as an adjunct to pharmacologic approaches if desired.	Awareness of potential changes helps to prepare women for what to expect and to work more effectively with the labour and birth process. An understanding of labour pain provides a foundation for deciding on the most appropriate methods to promote comfort and control pain during childbirth.
Review pharmacologic options including epidural anaesthesia. Discuss the benefits and risks of these options and available sources of reliable evidence-based information. Review the use of close monitoring to prevent complications if pharmacologic agents are used.	Prepares the woman and her partner for informed decision making. Knowledge of measures to prevent complications can alleviate anxiety related to the effects of analgesia/anaesthesia on the fetus.
Review with Monique and her partner perinatal education classes available in the community. Describe common approaches and encourage them to investigate and enrol in classes that best meet their needs.	Perinatal education programs vary and need to fit with the woman's/couples' values, learning needs, and goals for childbirth. Enrolment fosters learning and normalizes pregnancy, childbearing, and parenting transitions. Meeting other expectant parents can also enhance the family's support network.
Encourage the couple to use reliable sources of information (including online resources) and discuss their questions and concerns with each other and their maternity care provider.	Encouraging the couple to seek out information shifts the nurse's role away from simply providing information to helping them make sense of this information in the context of their lives. Understanding evidence-based information (health literacy) is necessary for informed decision making.
Schedule a return visit for Monique and her partner to allow for follow-up discussion and teaching.	A return visit provides an opportunity to evaluate teaching as well as provides opportunities for clarification and additional instruction.

EVALUATION

1. The woman and her partner identify their learning needs.
2. The woman and her partner describe their birth preferences and realistically consider their options.
3. The woman and her partner demonstrate strategies for working with the process of labour and birth.
4. The woman and her partner choose perinatal education resources appropriate to their learning needs.

- **Lack of Resources** to support prenatal/intrapartum/ postpartum family health
- **Readiness for Enhanced Family Processes** related to seeking out information to promote a positive pregnancy and childbirth experience for the entire family

Planning/Intervention

Outcomes are highly individualized based on the client's needs. Some common outcomes may include the following.

- The woman and her partner will identify personal health practices that promote a healthy childbearing experience.
- The woman and her partner will develop an appropriate plan for labour and birth, including options for pain management.
- The woman and her partner will decide on a setting and a care provider for birth.
- The woman and her partner will seek perinatal education resources that meet their learning needs.
- The woman and her partner will state that they feel prepared for the childbirth experience.
- The woman and her partner will demonstrate newborn care measures appropriately.
- The family will demonstrate ways to support the childbearing woman and integrate the newborn into the family, such as mobilizing their support networks.

Health Promotion Goals

The ultimate goal in preparing for pregnancy, childbirth, and parenting is that the woman and her partner can make informed decisions that meet their needs and promote healthy childbearing experiences. Nurses, educators, and other care providers can collaborate with women and families for health promotion and to meet their learning needs. Individualized learning plans are based on initial assessment of the woman's knowledge, culture, and particular family situation and are adapted as needs change and pregnancy progresses.

Discussing Perinatal Education Programs

Perinatal education programs are wide ranging and vary in focus and philosophy, content, and methods of presentation (Tables 14.1 and 14.2). Some programs base information on the belief that labour is a physiologic process requiring no medical intervention unless compelling evidence supports it. Other programs present information based on the concepts of relaxation, exercise, learning, and trusting of the natural birth process. Where one program may cover pregnancy from conception through birth to early parenting, another may focus solely on labour and birth.

The nurse should be familiar with perinatal education programs offered in the community. He or she provides the woman and her partner information about the various classes and encourages them to review their goals for the pregnancy, labour, and birth. The nurse can assist parents to investigate the programs, including talking with instructors and others who have participated in them. Such information helps the couple make an informed decision based on their desires and needs.

Expectant parenting classes are also available and commonly provide information about newborn care, growth and development, and family health. Other types of programs include sibling and grandparent classes and refresher courses for parents who already have a child or children. Nursing Care Plan 14.2 provides an example of a family incorporating sibling education classes into their pregnancy preparations.

Evaluation

Working in partnership with women and families requires a shift toward collaboration for promoting health. The nurse can solicit feedback on the effectiveness of his/her teaching by asking women and family members directly. In addition, the nurse may have opportunities to evaluate health practices. Sometimes a review of the woman's nutritional patterns may be needed to show that she is drinking enough fluids and eating healthy foods that are needed for the current stage of childbearing. The nurse can also ask questions that will help identify the client's learning needs. For example, the nurse might ask questions about the preparations the expectant parents have made for labour and birth. Are they enrolled in a perinatal education program? Who will be providing supportive care during labour? Have they considered a doula? What preparations have they made for caring for mom and baby after hospital discharge? For some skills, such as massage techniques and positions for labour, birth, and breastfeeding, a demonstration followed by a return demonstration provides opportunities for the nurse to evaluate learning and give additional guidance as required.

Since childbearing families come from a variety of educational, cultural, religious, and socioeconomic backgrounds, they have different experiences with learning. Nurses and perinatal educators are involved in evaluating community resources and education programs that support childbearing women and their families. They also advocate for the development of innovative approaches to meet the special needs of *all* women and families.

NURSING CARE PLAN 14.2

●

The Expectant Family With Sibling Adjustment Difficulties

 Remember Shelley and her partner Joel from the beginning of the chapter. When questioning the couple further, they mention that their son has regressed somewhat. "He used to be able to dress himself and put on his shoes with no problem. Now he wants me to do it. And I constantly have to tell him to be careful and not jump on me. Then when I tell him to be careful, he throws a tantrum. What can we do?"

NURSING DIAGNOSES

- **Lack of Knowledge** related to growth and development and effect of pregnancy on toddler
- **Readiness for Enhanced Family Processes** related to desire for seeking help with toddler

EXPECTED OUTCOMES

1. The woman and her partner will identify and discuss the effects of current pregnancy on their son.
2. The woman and her partner will implement measures to reduce the threat of the new baby on their son.
3. The woman and her partner will state that their son is demonstrating beginning acceptance of pregnancy and birth of the new baby, including fewer regressive and acting-out behaviours.

INTERVENTIONS	RATIONALES
Assess the couple's level of understanding about growth and development of a toddler and effects of pregnancy on children.	Assessment provides a baseline for identifying specific client needs and developing an individualized teaching plan.
Review with the couple the child's struggle for developing autonomy during this period (see Chapter 5).	Knowledge of the child's need to develop independence helps foster an understanding of the child's behaviour patterns.
Explain that the child's behaviour is a reflection of feelings of jealously or fears of not being loved (e.g., not being mommy's or daddy's little boy anymore).	Children may fear the loss of parental love and experience jealousy with the prospect of the birth of a new baby.
Encourage the couple to include their son in age-appropriate activities involving the pregnancy throughout the perinatal period, such as helping to prepare the baby's room, choosing special toys, and reading stories about being a big brother.	Inclusion of the child in activities promotes feelings of security and being loved.
Urge the couple to spend time with their son in activities totally unrelated to the new baby; encourage other family members to spend individualized time with the toddler.	Individualized activities for the toddler promote a sense of security and love.

(continued)

NURSING CARE PLAN 14.2 ● The Expectant Family With Sibling Adjustment Difficulties *(Continued)*

INTERVENTIONS	RATIONALES
Suggest that the couple investigate reliable online sources of information and sibling education classes in their community.	Sibling education classes help prepare children in an age-appropriate manner for the birth of the new baby.
Have the couple observe the effects of these actions on the child's behaviour for improvement.	Improved behaviour suggests that the child is adapting to the prospect of a new sibling, although occasional setbacks might be expected.
Plan to follow up with the couple by telephone in 2 to 3 weeks.	Follow-up provides a means of evaluating the success of the plan; it also provides opportunities for additional teaching.

EVALUATION

1. The woman and her partner verbalize the effects of pregnancy on their son.
2. The woman and her partner include their son in age-appropriate preparations for the new baby (including sibling preparation classes).
3. The child demonstrates fewer regressive and acting-out behaviours.

SUMMARY

- Nurses need to take advantage of all opportunities for health-promoting perinatal education both before and throughout the childbearing year.
- Nurses and care providers need to communicate with one another to ensure that information is coordinated, accurate, and consistent.
- Education for pregnancy and childbirth has changed dramatically over the years from information about pregnancy, birth, and baby care passed woman-to-woman to information supplied by physicians in an authoritative, medicalized fashion toward collaborative partnerships between women, families, and care providers.
- Prepared childbirth methods became prominent after World War II. These included psychoprophylaxis (Lamaze), emphasizing the use of controlled breathing; abdominal stroking and pressure application on the hip and back; and the Dick-Read method, addressing the holistic nature of childbirth in which mind and body are connected. The women's movement then invited a more active and informed role for women during their childbearing experience.

- The role of the nurse has shifted away from being a "giver of information" toward helping women and their family members evaluate and make sense of health information in the context of their particular lives.
- The purpose of perinatal education includes promoting healthy lifestyles and relationships; active health care decision making; building personal skills for pregnancy, childbirth, and early parenting; and building community/social support for new parents.
- Perinatal education involves taking multiple opportunities to provide health-promoting information to childbearing women and their families in a variety of formats and settings.
- Providing health information and educational opportunities *before* conception/pregnancy can help prevent known childbearing risks.
- For the nurse attending a labouring woman, pain is a less important issue than how the woman feels she is treated by her care providers. Thus, nurses are in a position to increase or diminish a woman's feelings of self-esteem, sense of accomplishment, and overall satisfaction with birth, and to assist her in her transition to motherhood.

- Baths or showers were the medication-free pain management technique with the highest "helpfulness" rating by women, second only to epidural anaesthesia.
- Perinatal education programs/offerings are increasingly diversified in form and format to meet the needs of diverse families and communities.
- Educational strategies are thought to improve perinatal outcomes and prevent health risks including preterm birth, low birth weight, and congenital anomalies.
- Knowing and being able to direct women to current websites that provide credible, research-based, understandable, and respectful information are important.
- Nurses consider more than personal lifestyle issues and educational interventions; social factors such as the woman's employment, family situation, and available resources should also be considered.
- Nurses can work with other health care providers to address health inequities resulting from the social, economic, and environmental determinants of health.
- Nurses and other health care professionals in contact with pregnant or parenting women and men view themselves as educational resources for childbearing women and their families.
- Providing anticipatory guidance, referrals to local programs, and recommending reliable sources of health information can help promote health and enhance childbearing experiences.
- Nurses also help women mobilize their personal strengths and support networks to adapt to the challenges of pregnancy, childbirth, postpartum, and parenting transitions.

Questions to Ponder

1. How might a nurse invite further reflection for a pregnant woman who states, "I'm not using any medication for pain. I'm doing it natural all the way."
2. A pregnant client who is in a remote community in Northern Canada is inquiring about accessing an education program.
   - What considerations should the nurse make when responding to the woman?
   - What might the nurse suggest if education programs are not available locally?
3. A client in the early stages of pregnancy expresses significant anxiety about labour pain. Knowing her concern, how might the nurse invite her to prepare for labour and birth?

REVIEW QUESTIONS

1. Which of the following should the nurse identify as having a major influence on a woman's satisfaction with childbirth?
   A. Feeling respected during childbirth
   B. Use of nonpharmacologic pain relief methods
   C. The extent of education received
   D. Past experiences with pain
2. A woman interested in attending childbirth classes to prepare for labour and birth asks the nurse about what will most likely be included. Which of the following would the nurse *exclude* from her teaching?
   A. Stages of labour
   B. Breathing exercises
   C. Pain control techniques
   D. Prevention of birth defects
3. Which of the following is *correct* about the evolution of perinatal education?
   A. Historically, women knew very little about childbirth.
   B. Moving birth into hospitals improved childbirth education.
   C. The self-help movement grew out of second wave feminism.
   D. Lactation consultants became early perinatal educators.
4. Which of the following should the nurse integrate into the discussion about psychoprophylaxis for prepared childbirth?
   A. Partners can take an active role coaching the woman through childbirth.
   B. The emphasis is on psychological strategies to prevent pain.
   C. Pharmaceuticals are important in removing the pain sensation.
   D. Healthy bodies and attitudes help women cope with labour pain.
5. A woman is unable to access formal education classes for her second pregnancy due to a lack of classes in her area. Which of the following would be the *least* appropriate nursing action?
   A. Provide the information over the telephone.
   B. Take advantage of any contact for incidental teaching.
   C. Have her inform her maternity care provider during a prenatal visit.
   D. Remind her that she already knows how to give birth.
6. Which of the following *best* describes mindfulness approaches to childbirth preparation?
   A. They incorporate art to reveal fears about birth.
   B. They use deep relaxation to tune out pain.

C. They incorporate ways of being present during birth.

D. They use yoga and meditation.

7. A pregnant woman asks the nurse, "A friend of mine used a doula when she was in labour. What is this?" Which description should the nurse include in the response?

   A. A woman specially trained in the methods of breathing, relaxation techniques, and hypnosis for pain control

   B. A person who provides continuous emotional, physical, and informational support to the mother

   C. A mentor who teaches the partner about caring for the newborn and supporting the mother during the labour process

   D. A person educated in labour support who demonstrates evidence of certification and successful course completion

8. Which of the following *best* describes how nurses assist childbearing women today?

   A. Providing information about prenatal classes

   B. Demonstrating baby care techniques

   C. Recommending a doula or midwife

   D. Helping women understand available information

9. Which of the following *best* describes the purpose of perinatal education today?

   A. To ensure women avoid alcohol

   B. To promote breastfeeding

   C. To teach coping skills for labour and birth

   D. To promote health literacy for childbearing

10. Health literacy includes the ability to do all of the following except:

   A. Engage in health care decision making

   B. Understand health information

   C. Make choices about mode of delivery

   D. Navigate the health care system

REFERENCES

Aboriginal Doula Advisory Committee. (2010). *Aboriginal doulas for aboriginal women: An action plan for bringing traditional birthing support practices back into the hands of women.* Retrieved from http://www.phsa.ca/NR/rdonlyres/5B9D7E8B-F251-4EC6-B56A-A7541CC4E57F/0/AboriginalDoulaProjectReportFINALJune22010.pdf

Agostino, M. (2012). Post-discharge telephone support for the first-time, low-risk, breastfeeding mother. *Journal of Obstetric, Gynecologic, & Neonatal Nursing, 41*(1), S142–S143.

Angood, P., Armstrong, E., Ashton, D., Burstin, H., Corry, M., Delbanco, S., et al. (2010). Blueprint for action; steps toward a high quality, high-value maternity care system. *Women's Health Issues, 20*(Suppl. 1), S18–S49.

Ateah, C. (2013). Prenatal parent education for first-time expectant parents: "Making it through labor is just the beginning…" *Journal of Pediatric Healthcare, 27*(2), 91–97.

Ball, J., & Daly, K. (Eds.). (2012). *Father involvement in Canada: Diversity, renewal, and transformation.* Vancouver, WA: UBC Press.

Bardacke, N. (2012). *Mindful birthing: Training the mind, body and heart for childbirth and beyond.* New York: Harper Collins.

Benediktsson, I., McDonald, S. W., Vekved, M., McNeil, D. A., Dolan, S. M., & Tough, S. C. (2013). Comparing Centering Pregnancy to standard prenatal care plus prenatal education. *BMC Pregnancy and Childbirth, 13*(Suppl 1), S5. doi:10.1186/1471-2393-13-S1-S6. Retrieved from http://www.biomedcentral.com/1471-2393/13/S1/S6

Benoit, C., & Carroll, D. (2005). Canadian midwifery: Blending traditional and modern practices. In C. Bates, D. Dodd, & N. Rousseau (Eds.), *On all frontiers: Four centuries of Canadian nursing* (pp. 27–41). Ottawa, ON: Canadian Museum of Civilization.

Benoit, D. (2009). Efficacy of attachment-based interventions. In R. E. Tremblay, R. G. Barr, R. D. Peters, & M. Boivin (Eds.), *Encyclopedia on early childhood development [online]* (pp. 1–6). Montreal, QC: Centre of Excellence for Early Childhood Development and Strategic Knowledge Cluster on Early Child Development. Retrieved from http://www.child-encyclopedia.com/documents/BenoitANGxp_rev-Attachment.pdf

Best Start Resource Centre. (2006). *Populations at higher risk: When mainstream approaches don't work.* Toronto, ON. Retrieved from http://www.beststart.org/resources/howto/pdf/HowTOGuide_2c.pdf

Best Start Resource Centre. (2009). *Health fairs and preconception, prenatal and child health: An overview of effectiveness, strategies and examples.* Toronto, ON. Retrieved from http://www.beststart.org/resources/howto/pdf/health_fairs_manual_fnl_low%20rez.pdf

Best Start Resource Centre. (2012a). *STEP BY STEP: Engaging fathers in programs for families.* Toronto, ON. Retrieved from http://www.beststart.org/resources/howto/pdf/BSRC_Engaging_Fathers.pdf

Best Start Resource Centre. (2012b). *Welcoming and celebrating sexual orientation and gender diversity in families: From preconception to preschool.* Retrieved from http://www.beststart.org/resources/howto/pdf/LGBTQ_Resource_fnl_online.pdf

Best Start Resource Centre. (2012c). *Supporting the sacred journey: From preconception to parenting for first nations families in Ontario.* Toronto, ON. Retrieved from http://www.beststart.org/resources/rep_health/pdf/SupportingtheSacredJourney.pdf

Best Start Resource Centre. (2013). *Best start: Ontario's maternal newborn and early child development resource centre.* Retrieved from http://www.beststart.org/index_eng.html

Biggs, L. (2004). Rethinking the history of midwifery in Canada. In I. Bourgeault, C. Benoit, & R. Davis-Floyd (Eds.), *Reconceiving midwifery* (pp. 17–45). Montreal & Kingston, NY: McGill-Queen's University Press.

Birthing From Within. (2013). *Philosophy.* Retrieved from http://www.birthingfromwithin.com/philosophy

Blackburn, S. T. (2013). *Maternal, fetal, and neonatal physiology* (4th ed.). Philadelphia, PA: Elsevier.

Boston Women's Health Book Collective. (2011). *Our bodies, ourselves* (9th ed.). New York: Touchstone.

Bradley, R. A. (1996). *Husband-coached childbirth: The Bradley method of natural childbirth* (4th ed.). (Revised and edited by Marjie and Jay Hathaway). New York: Bantam Books.

Bryanton, J., & Beck, C. T. (2010). Postnatal parental education for optimizing infant general health and parent-infant relationships. *Cochrane Database of Systematic Reviews,* (1), Art. No.: CD004068. doi:10.1002/14651858.CD004068.pub3.

Buultjens, M., Robinson, P., & Milgrom, J. (2012). Online resources for new mothers: Opportunities and challenges for perinatal health professionals. *The Journal of Perinatal Education, 21*(2), 99–111.

Canadian Council on Learning. (2007). *Health Literacy in Canada: Initial results from the International Adult Literacy and Skills Survey 2007.* Retrieved from http://www.ccl-cca.ca/pdfs/HealthLiteracy/HealthLiteracyinCanada.pdf

Canadian Public Health Association. (ND). Health literacy portal. Retrieved from http://www.cpha.ca/en/portals/h-l.aspx

Centers for Disease Control and Prevention. (2013). National prematurity awareness month. Retrieved from http://www.cdc.gov/features/prematurebirth/

Cowan, P. A., & Cowan, C. P. (2009). How working with couples fosters children's development: From prevention science to public policy. In M. S. Schulz, M. K. Pruett, P. K. Kerig, & R. D. Parke (Eds.), *Strengthening couple relationships for optimal child development*. Washington, DC: APA Books.

Cusack, C., Hall, W., Scruby, L., & Wong, S. (2008). Public Health Nurses' perceptions of their role in early postpartum discharge. *Canadian Journal of Public Health, 99*(3), 206–211.

Dennis, C. (2009). Preventing and treating postnatal depression. *BMJ: British Medical Journal [Online], 338*(7689), 246–247. Retrieved from http://www.jstor.org/stable/20511904

Dennis, C., & Kingston, D. (2008). A systematic review of telephone support for women during pregnancy and the early postpartum period. *Journal of Obstetric, Gynecologic, & Neonatal Nursing, 37*(3), 301–314. doi:10.1111/j.1552-6909.2008.00235.x

Devolin, M., Phelps, D., Duhaney, T., Benzies, K., Hildebrandt, C., Rikhy, S., et al. (2013). Information and support needs among parents of young children in a region of Canada: A cross-sectional survey. *Public Health Nursing, 30*(3), 193–201. doi:10.1111/phn.12002

England, P., & Horowitz, R. (1998). *Birthing from within*. Albuquerque: Partera Press.

Falk-Raphael, A., & Betker, C. (2012). Witnessing social injustice downstream and advocating for health equity upstream: "The trombone slide" of nursing. *Advances in Nursing Science, 35*, 98–112.

Fatherhood Involvement Research Alliance. (2013). *Welcome to FIRA*. Retrieved from http://www.fira.ca/

Fortier, J. (2012). Advocacy: Inside the maze. *Canadian Nurse, 108*(3), 22–27.

Fox, B. (2010). *When couples become parents: The creation of gender in the transition to parenthood*. Toronto, ON: University of Toronto Press.

Georgetown University Library. (2013). Evaluating Internet Resources. Retrieved from http://www.library.georgetown.edu/tutorials/research-guides/evaluating-internet-content

Gottlieb, L. (2013). *Strengths-based nursing care: Health and healing for person and family*. New York: Springer.

Gottlieb, L., & Feeley, N. (2006). *The collaborative partnership approach to care: A delicate balance*. Toronto, ON: Elsevier-Mosby.

Haines, H., Rubertsson, C., Pallant, J., & Hildingsson, I. (2012). The influence of women's fear, attitudes and beliefs of childbirth on mode and experience of birth. *BMC Pregnancy and Childbirth, 12*, 55. http://www.biomedcentral.com/1471-2393/12/55

Hanson, S., Hunter, L., Bormann, J., & Sobo, E. (2009). Paternal fears of childbirth: A literature review. *The Journal of Perinatal Education, 18*(4), 12–20. doi:10.1624/105812409×474672

Health Canada. (2011). *Expecting to quit*. Retrieved from http://www.expectingtoquit.ca/

Heaman, M., Sprague, A., & Stewart, P. (2001). Reducing the preterm birth rate: A population health strategy. *Journal of Obstetric, Gynecologic & Neonatal Nursing, 30*(1), 20–29.

Herrman, J. W., Rogers, S., Ehrenthal, D. B. (2012). Women's perceptions of centering pregnancy: A focus group study. *Maternal Child Nursing, 37*, 19–28.

Hodnett, E. D., Gates, S., Hofmeyr, G. J. & Sakala, C. (2013). Continuous support for women during childbirth. *Cochrane Database Systematic Reviews*, (7), doi:10.1002/14651858.CD003766.pub5

Ickovics, J. R., Kershaw, T. S., Westdahl, C., Magriples, U., Massey, Z. Reynolds, H. et al. (2007). Group prenatal care and perinatal outcomes. *Obstetrics and Gynecology, 110*(2), 330–339.

Jolivet, R. R., Corry, M. P. (2010). Steps toward innovative childbirth education: Selected strategies from the blueprint for action. *Journal of Perinatal Education, 19*(3), 19.

Kagan, J. (2012). Temperament. In R. E. Tremblay, R. G. Barr, R. D. Peters, & M. Boivin (Eds.), *Encyclopedia on early childhood development [online]* (pp. 1–4). Montreal, QC: Centre of Excellence for Early Childhood Development and Strategic Knowledge Cluster on Early Child Development. Retrieved from http://www.child-encyclopedia.com/Pages/PDF/KaganANGxp2.pdf

Karmel, M. (1981). *Thank you, Dr. Lamaze. (A new edition of the original work.)*. New York, NY: Harper & Row Publishers.

Kitzinger, S. (2011). *Rediscovering Birth* (revised ed.). London, UK: Pinter and Martin.

Kornelson, J., & Grzybowski, S. (2012). Cultures of risk and their influence on birth in rural British Columbia. *BMC Family Practice, 13*, 108. doi:10.1186/1471-2296-13-108. Retrieved from http://www.biomedcentral.com/1471-2296/13/108

Lamaze International. (2013). *About Lamaze: History*. Retrieved from www.lamaze.org/History

Larsson, M., (2009) A descriptive study of the use of the internet by women seeking pregnancy-related information. *Midwifery, 25*(1), 14–20.

Leap, N., & Anderson, T. (2004). The role of pain in normal birth and the empowerment of women. In S. Downe (Ed.), *Normal childbirth: Evidence and debate*. London, UK: Churchill Livingstone.

Liaschenko, J. (2002). Health promotion, moral harm, and the moral aims of nursing. In L. Young & V. Hayes (Eds.), *Transforming health promotion practice* (pp. 136–147). Philadelphia, PA: F A. Davis Company.

Liu, C.-C., Chen, Y.-C., Yeh, Y.-P., & Hsieh, Y.-S. (2012). Effects of maternal confidence and competence on maternal parenting stress in newborn care. *Journal of Advanced Nursing, 68*(4), 908–918. doi:10.1111/j.1365-2648.2011.05796

Loppie Reading, C., & Wien, F. (2009). *Health Inequalities and social determinants of aboriginal peoples' health*. Retrieved from http://www.nccah-ccnsa.ca/docs/nccah%20reports/LoppieWien-2.pdf

MacKinnon, K. (2006). Living with the threat of preterm labor: Women's work of keeping the baby in. *Journal of Obstetric, Gynecologic & Neonatal Nursing, 35*(6), 700–708.

MacKinnon, K., & McCoy, L. (2006). The very loud discourses of risk in pregnancy! In P. Godin (Ed.), *Risk and nursing practice* (pp. 98–120). Basingstoke, UK: Palgrave Publishers.

MacKinnon, K., & McIntyre, M. (2006). From Braxton Hicks to preterm labour: The constitution of risk in pregnancy. *Canadian Journal of Nursing Research, 38*(2), 56–72.

MacKinnon, K., McIntyre, M., & Quance, M. (2005). The meaning of the nurse's presence during childbirth. *Journal of Obstetric, Gynecologic & Neonatal Nursing, 34*(1), 28–36.

MacKinnon, K., & Moffitt, P. (2014). Informed advocacy: Rural, remote and northern nursing praxis. *Advances in Nursing Science, 37*(2), 161–173.

Marcellus, L. (2007). Using feminist ethics to inform practice with pregnant women who use substances. In S. Boyd & L. Marcellus (Eds.), *With child: Substance use during pregnancy: A woman centred approach* (pp. 28–37). Halifax: Fernwood Publishing.

McNeil, D., Vekved, M., Dolan, S., Siever, J., Horn, S., & Tough, S. (2012). Getting more than they realized: A qualitative study of women's experience of group prenatal care. *BMC Pregnancy and Childbirth, 13*(Suppl. 1), S6. doi:10.1186/1471-2393-13-S1-S6. Retrieved from http://www.biomedcentral.com/1471-2393/13/S1/S6

Misra, D., Guyer, B., & Allston, A. (2003). Integrated perinatal health framework: A multiple determinants model with a lifespan approach. *American Journal of Preventive Medicine, 25*(1), 65–75.

Mitchinson, W. (2002). *Giving birth in Canada: 1900–1950*. Toronto, ON: University of Toronto Press.

Motherisk. (2013). *Taking folic acid before you get pregnant*. Retrieved from http://www.motherisk.org/women/folicAcid.jsp

Namey, E., & Lyerly, A. (2010). The meaning of "control" for childbearing women in the US. *Social Science & Medicine, 71*, 769–776. doi:10.1016/j.socscimed.2010.05.024

Nichols, F. H., & Humenick, S. S. (2000). Childbirth education: Practice, research and theory. (2nd ed.). Philadelphia, PA: W. B. Saunders.

Ondeck, M. (2000). Historical development. In F. H. Nichols & S. S. Humenick (Eds.), *Childbirth education: Practice, research and theory* (2nd ed.). Philadelphia, PA: W. B. Saunders.

Pauly, B. (2013). Challenging health inequities: Enacting social justice in nursing practice. In J. Storch, P. Rodney, & R. Starzomski. (Eds.), *Toward a moral horizon: Nursing ethics for leadership and practice* (2nd ed., pp. 430–447). Toronto, ON: Pearson.

Pauly, B., MacKinnon, K., & Varcoe, C. (2009). Revisiting "Who gets care?" Health equity as an arena for nursing action. *Advances in Nursing Science, 32*, 118–127.

Pitcock, C. D., & Clark, R. B. (1992). From fanny to fernand: The development of consumerism in pain control during the birth process. *American Journal of Obstetrics and Gynecology, 167,* 581–587.

Public Health Agency of Canada. (2008). Canadian perinatal health report, 2008 Edition. Ottawa, ON.

Public Health Agency of Canada. (2009). *What mothers say: The Canadian maternity experiences survey.* Retrieved from http://www.phac-aspc.gc.ca/rhs-ssg/survey-eng.php

Public Health Agency of Canada. (2010). *Summative evaluation of the Canada prenatal nutrition program 2004–2009.* Retrieved from http://www.phac-aspc.gc.ca/about_apropos/evaluation/reports-rapports/2009–2010/cpnp-pcnp/summary-resume-eng.php

Raphael, D. (2010). The health of Canada's children: Part 1: Canadian children's health in comparative perspective. *Paediatric Child Health, 15*(1), 23–29.

Raynor, T. (2012). Health literacy: Is it time to shift our focus from patient to provider? *British Medical Journal [Online], 344,* e2188. doi:10.1136/bmj.e2188 (Published 22 March 2012).

Registered Nurses Association of Ontario. (2007). *Integrating smoking cessation into daily nursing practice.* Retrieved from http://rnao.ca/bpg/guidelines/integrating-smoking-cessation-daily-nursing-practice

Reilly, D. R. (2009). Caesarean section on maternal request: How clear medical evidence fails to produce ethical consensus. *Journal of Obstetrics and Gynaecology Canada, 31*(12), 1176–1179.

Rising, S. S., Kennedy, H. P., & Klima, C. S. (2004). Redesigning prenatal care through CenteringPregnancy. *Journal of Midwifery and Women's Health, 49*(5), 398–404.

Rootman, I., & Gordon-El-Bihbety, D. (2008). *A vision for a health literate Canada: Report of the expert panel on health literacy.* Ottawa, ON: Canadian Public Health Association.

Rotundo, G. (2011). Centering Pregnancy: The benefits of group prenatal care. *Nursing for Women's Health, 15*(6), 508–517. doi:10.1111/j.1751-486X.2011.01678.x

Salomonsson, B., Berterö, C., & Alehagen, S. (2013). Self-efficacy in pregnant women with severe fear of childbirth. *Journal of Obstetric, Gynecologic, & Neonatal Nursing, 42*(2), 191–202. doi:10.1111/1552-6909.12024

Simkin, P. (1996). The experience of maternity in a woman's life. *Journal of Obstetric, Gynecologic and Neonatal Nursing, 25*(3), 247–252.

Simkin, P., & Ancheta, R. (2011). *The labor progress handbook* (3rd ed.). Malden, MA: Wiley-Blackwell.

Society of Obstetricians and Gynaecologists of Canada, the Association of Women's Health, Obstetric and Neonatal Nurses of Canada, the Canadian Association of Midwives, the College of Family Physicians of Canada, the Society of Rural Physicians of Canada. (2008). Joint policy statement on normal childbirth. SOGC Clinical Practice Guideline No. 221. *Journal of Obstetrics and Gynaecology Canada, 30,* 1163–1165. Retrieved from http://www.sogc.org/guidelines/documents/gui221PS0812.pdf

Stoll, K. H., & Hall, W. (2012). Childbirth education and obstetric interventions among low-risk Canadian Women: Is there a connection? *The Journal of Perinatal Education, 21*(4), 229–237.

Sword, W., Jack, S., Niccols, A., Milligan, K., Henderson, J., & Thabane, L. (2009). Integrated programs for women with substance use issues and their children: A qualitative meta-synthesis of processes and outcomes. *Harm Reduction Journal, 6,* 32 doi:10.1186/1477-7517-6-32. Retrieved from http://www.harmreductionjournal.com/content/6/1/32

The Bradley Method. (2013). *The Bradley method of husband coached natural childbirth.* Retrieved from http://www.bradleybirth.com

Tillett, J. (2011). The assessment of health literacy is a nursing priority. *The Journal of Perinatal & Neonatal Nursing, 25*(3), 217. doi:10.1097/JPN.0b013e318225f7b0

van Ijzendoorn, M. (2012). Attachment – synthesis. In R. E. Tremblay, R. G. Barr, R. D. Peters, & M. Boivin (Eds.), *Encyclopedia on early childhood development [online].* Montreal, QC: Centre of Excellence for Early Childhood Development and Strategic Knowledge Cluster on Early Child Development. Retrieved from http://www.child-encyclopedia.com/pages/PDF/synthesis-attachment.pdf

Varcoe, C., Brown, H., Calam, B., Harvey, T., & Tallio, M. (2013). Help bring back the celebration of life: A community-based participatory study of rural Aboriginal women's maternity experiences and outcomes. *BMC Pregnancy and Childbirth, 13,* 26. Retrieved from http://www.biomedcentral.com/content/pdf/1471-2393-13-26.pdf

Vieten, C., & Astin, J. (2008). Effects of a mindfulness-based intervention during pregnancy on prenatal stress and mood: Results of a pilot study. *Arch Women's Mental Health, 11*(1), 67–74.

Vollman, A. R., Anderson, E. T., & McFarlane, J. (2007). *Canadian community as partner* (2nd ed.). Philadelphia, PA: Lippincott Williams & Wilkins.

Walker, D., Visger, J., & Rossie, D. (2009). Contemporary childbirth education models. *Journal of Midwifery and Women's Health, 54*(6), 469–478. doi:10.1016/j.jmwh.2009.02.013

Ward, J. (2000). *La Leche League: At the crossroads of medicine, feminism, and religion.* Chapel Hill, NC: University of North Carolina Press.

Watson, C. (2010). Voices from the field – Challenges faced by parenting program designers. In R. E. Tremblay, R. G. Barr, R. D. Peters, & M. Boivin, (Eds.), (*Encyclopedia on early childhood development [online].* Montreal, QC: Centre of Excellence for Early Childhood Development and Strategic Knowledge Cluster on Early Child Development. Retrieved from http://www.child-encyclopedia.com/documents/WatsonANGps.pdf

WEB RESOURCES

Association for Safe Alternatives in Childbirth
http://www.asac.ab.ca/

Best Start Resource Centre
http://www.beststart.org/index_eng.html

Birthing from Within
http://www.birthingfromwithin.com/

Birth Network
http://www.birthnetwork.org/

Bradley Method
http://www.bradleybirth.com/Default.aspx

Canada Prenatal Nutrition Program
http://www.phac-aspc.gc.ca/hp-ps/dca-dea/prog-ini/cpnp-pcnp/

Canadian Association of Midwives
www.canadianmidwives.org

Canadian Midwifery Regulators Consortium
http://www.cmrc-ccosf.ca/

Centering® Pregnancy
http://www.centeringhealthcare.org/

Childbirth and Postpartum Professional Association (CAPPA)
www.http://www.cappa.net/canada.php

Encyclopedia on Early Childhood
www.child-encyclopedia.com

Expecting to Quit
http://www.expectingtoquit.ca/

Fatherhood Involvement Research Alliance (FIRA)
http://fira.ca/

Georgetown University Library (evaluating internet resources)
http://www.library.georgetown.edu/tutorials/research-guides/evaluating-internet-content

HypnoBirthing Canada
http://www.hypnobirthing.com/canada.htm

International Caesarean Awareness Network (ICAN)
http://www.childbirth.org/section/ICAN.html

International Childbirth Education Association
http://www.icea.org/

La Leche League Canada
http://www.lalecheleaguecanada.ca/

Lamaze International
http://www.lamazeinternational.org/

LGBT (Lesbian, Gay, Bisexual, Trans) Parenting Connection
http://www.lgbtqparentingconnection.ca/home.cfm

Mindful Birthing
http://www.mindfulbirthing.org/

Motherisk
http://www.motherisk.org/women/index.jsp

Online Birth and Babies
http://online.birthandbabies.com/

Peel Region
http://www.peelregion.ca/health/family-health/breastfeeding/.

South Community Birth Program
http://scbp.ca/

LABOUR AND CHILDBIRTH

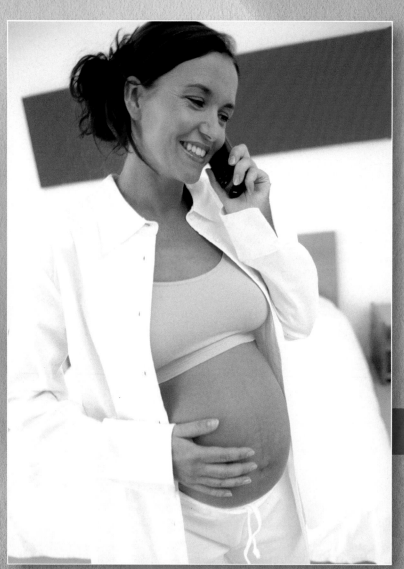

UNIT 4

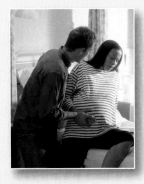 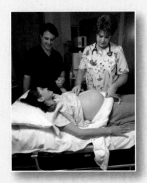 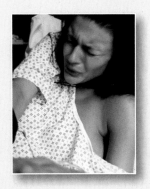 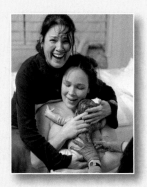

Labour and childbirth represent both an end and a beginning. The experience serves as the culmination of the approximate 9 months that the expectant family has spent preparing to welcome and to incorporate a new member. At the same time, birth represents the first separation between mother and child. As the initial step in a series of milestones, birth marks an infant's progression toward total independence from his or her parents.

Unit 4 explores the normal processes of labour and the related management to facilitate a healthy vaginal birth. It discusses conditions that pose potential risks during labour, as well as complications that arise only during the process of childbirth itself. The content also presents methods of assisted delivery, including cesarean births. This unit also examines dimensions of pain during labour and various methods that can be implemented to manage it.

CHAPTER 15

Labour and Childbirth

Erna Snelgrove-Clarke and Wendy Budin*

Tyrese, 31 years old and at 38 weeks' gestation with her first pregnancy, comes to the clinic for an appointment. During health history taking, Tyrese states, "The last few days I've been urinating more frequently than I had been. My belly doesn't seem so tight anymore. My back's been aching lately, too."

Yolanda, 29 years old and GTPAL 2-1-0-0-1, arrives at the labour and birth suite at term. Her contractions are moderate, occurring every 7 to 8 minutes and lasting approximately 30 seconds. She is accompanied by her mother. "My husband is on his way home from a business trip," Yolanda says. "I hope he gets here in time."

You will learn more about Tyrese's and Yolanda's stories later. Nurses working with these and similar clients need to understand this chapter's content to manage care and address issues appropriately. Before beginning, consider the following points related to the above scenarios:

- What are the nursing care priorities for each client? Explain your answer.
- In what stage of labour is each client? What physiologic events happen during these stages?
- How might labour and birth be similar for each woman? How might these processes be different?
- How would you expect each client's circumstances to influence the nurse's approach to assessment, teaching, and follow-up? What other factors would you want to learn?

---

*Contributor to first U.S. edition.

LEARNING OBJECTIVES

On completion of this chapter, the reader should be able to:

- Describe the signs of approaching labour.
- Differentiate prodromal labour from progressive labour.
- Recognize the influence of a client's cultural background on her choices about and responses to labour and birth.
- Discuss the current theories explaining the onset of labour.
- Describe the characteristics of the cervix and uterine contractions as labour progresses.
- Identify the landmarks of the fetal skull.
- Define the concepts used to describe fetopelvic relationships.
- Describe the mechanisms of labour when the fetus is in a cephalic presentation.
- Explain how maternal position may affect labour and birth.
- Discuss maternal system responses to labour and birth.
- Describe the monitoring techniques used to assess fetal well-being.
- Recognize various patterns in fetal heart rate and appropriate nursing implications.
- Identify the characteristics of the stages and phases of normal labour.
- Describe the emotional and social changes that women experience throughout labour and birth.
- Describe the collaborative measures to facilitate the normal course of labour and birth.

KEY TERMS

acceleration
acme
active labour
afterbirth
attitude
bradycardia
tachycardia
variability
Bishop score
bloody show
Braxton Hicks contractions
bregma
contraction
contraction duration
contraction frequency
contraction intensity
crowning
deceleration
denominator
dilation
doula
early deceleration
early labour
effacement
electronic fetal monitoring (EFM)
engagement

episiotomy
first stage of labour
fontanelles
fourth stage of labour
labour
late deceleration
lie
lightening
mechanisms of labour
moulding
occiput
pelvic inlet
pelvic outlet
position
presentation
presenting part
prodromal labour
second stage of labour
spontaneous rupture of membranes (SROM)
station
third stage of labour
transition phase
variable deceleration
vertex

"It is refreshing to know that for all the billions of times it has occurred, the birth of a child, like the wonder inspired by a sunset, can never be tarnished by repetition."

Anonymous

Childbirth is an event with meaning far beyond the actual physiologic process (Lee & Lamp, 2005). In addition to the physical sensations and work involved, labour and birth also encompass psychological, spiritual, and social dimensions. The nursing and psychosocial literature consistently describes childbirth as a life-altering experience for women and their families (Lundgren, 2004; Mercer, 2006; Vincent, 2002). It forever shapes women's thoughts of themselves and may affect their relationships, both positively and negatively, with children and other family members (Goodman et al., 2004; Lundgren, 2005; Waldenstrom, 2004). A recent Canadian study (Bryanton et al., 2008) indicates that responding to the needs of women enables care that can promote a positive experience. The care provider and place of birth can enhance or diminish a woman's confidence and ability to give birth (Matthews & Callister, 2004; Vedham et al., 2012). Nurses who provide supportive, competent care during labour can positively influence the quality of a family's childbirth experience, as well as the health and well-being of mothers and babies. Women describe having the nurse present and "there" during labour is an important part of their childbirth experience (MacKinnon et al., 2005).

To respond professionally, nurses must understand the basic physiologic and psychological aspects of childbirth. This chapter describes the process of normal labour and birth, as well as appropriate collaborative care measures for the various stages and phases of this experience. The nurse's role throughout birthing focuses on assessing maternal and fetal physical status, as well as identifying the learning and psychosocial needs of the client and her significant others. Providing care to families during labour and birth is both a privilege and an opportunity. It allows nurses to participate in a miracle, contributing to the safe arrival of a new human being and guiding the family through a multidimensional, complex, and ongoing journey.

PRELABOUR

Most women are unaware of the exact moment that labour begins. Theoretically, the process of labour starts when the cervix begins to dilate; however, this initiating event is difficult to determine (Gross et al., 2005; Ragusa et al., 2005). Therefore, health care providers typically rely on the client's report of signs and symptoms to pinpoint the time of the onset of labour.

During the last few weeks of pregnancy, several premonitory changes may indicate that the mother's body is preparing for childbirth. The cervix begins to soften, thin, and move forward; it may also begin to open. The fetus settles into the pelvis. **Contractions** (intermittent tightening of the uterine muscles) may be noticeable as achy sensations or as pressure in the lower abdomen or lower back. Such contractions are highly variable. They can be irregular—starting and stopping—or regular. Sometimes they are mild; at other times, they may be strong. These early contractions, referred to as **prodromal labour**, can last for hours to a few days.

Signs of Approaching Labour

Signs and symptoms of approaching labour may include lightening, increased Braxton Hicks contractions, backache, bloody show, spontaneous rupture of membranes (SROM), diarrhea, spurt of energy, and weight loss (Lund & McManaman, 2008). Most women experience one or more of these events in the weeks and days leading up to labour.

Lightening

Lightening is the lay term used to describe fetal engagement into the maternal pelvis. Typically, the woman's abdomen changes in shape as the uterus drops forward. Decreased fundal height measurements also indicate that the baby has "dropped" (Fig. 15.1). Lightening may happen suddenly. The woman may arise one morning entirely relieved of the abdominal tightness and diaphragmatic pressure that she experienced previously (see Chapter 12). Relief in one direction, however, is followed by greater pressure below. She may experience shooting pains down the legs from pressure on the sciatic nerves, increased vaginal discharge, and greater urinary frequency because of uterine pressure on the bladder.

In women nearing childbirth for the first time, lightening may occur approximately 10 to 14 days before

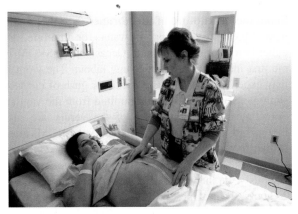

FIGURE 15.1 Decreased fundal height measurements near term indicate that the baby has "dropped" and that the woman is approaching labour.

labour. In women who have given birth before, lightening is more likely after labour already has started.

Braxton Hicks Contractions

Women may notice increased **Braxton Hicks contractions**, which are irregular, usually painless uterine contractions throughout pregnancy caused by increased estrogen levels and uterine distention (Khan & Razi, 2005). These contractions do not lead to the progressive cervical changes that indicate true labour. More frequent and intense Braxton Hicks contractions are associated with other subtle signs of approaching labour, such as a low, mild backache.

Backache

By the end of pregnancy, the woman's back may hurt persistently as a result of postural changes. Approximately two thirds of pregnant women experience low back pain (Pennick & Liddle, 2013). Such pain also may be from mild and early uterine contractions. Backache also may develop from pressure on the sacroiliac joint, which is related to the influence of relaxin hormone on the pelvic joints. A backache should be considered suggestive of labour if it fluctuates regularly, increases in intensity, or is accompanied by pelvic pressure or cramping.

Bloody Show

Another sign of impending labour is a pink or **bloody show**. This pinkish-tinged vaginal discharge, often mixed with mucus, results from dislodgment of the mucous plug that has sealed the cervical os throughout pregnancy and rupture of the cervical capillaries as effacement and dilation begin (Khan & Razi, 2005). Women may notice this discharge before recognizing any of the other preliminary signs of labour. Some women notice a bloody show following a routine vaginal examination in the last few weeks of pregnancy.

Spontaneous Rupture of Membranes

Spontaneous rupture of membranes (SROM) is the natural breaking of the bag of waters, or amniotic sac, either before or during labour. Occasionally, SROM is the first indication of approaching labour. The woman may experience SROM as a trickle or gush of clear or slightly straw-coloured amniotic fluid from the vagina. Sometimes, whitish particles of the vernix are visibly mixed with the amniotic fluid. After SROM, most women go into labour on their own within 24 hours (Gross et al., 2005, 2006). If membranes rupture spontaneously, but the woman does not go into labour within 24 hours, she is at increased risk for developing an intrauterine infection (Hannah et al., 2000; MacDonald & Saurette, 2010). In addition, any time membranes rupture there is a risk for umbilical cord prolapse (Dilbaz

et al., 2006). See Chapters 13 and 16 for more information relative to these problems, as well as a discussion of labour induction and augmentation.

Diarrhea

Some women experience increased bowel activity and mild diarrhea shortly before labour. Such developments are probably associated with the release of prostaglandin that accompanies labour. They may also be the body's attempt to empty the bowel so that the digestive system is not competing with the woman's other organs for energy during the demanding work of childbirth.

Spurt of Energy

Some women have described an unexpected spurt of physical and emotional energy, feeling better than they have in weeks, before the onset of labour. The underlying mechanism may be increased epinephrine resulting from decreased placental progesterone production (Pillitteri, 2014). Other women report a "nesting" instinct, during which they find themselves preparing their home for the newborn (e.g., organizing the nursery, cleaning) with a flurry of activity. Some health care providers advise women to ignore this feeling and to conserve energy for the approaching work of labour.

Weight Loss

After months of steady weight gain, the woman nearing labour may lose a few pounds (Fig. 15.2). This weight loss may result from changes in estrogen and progesterone levels, causing electrolyte shifts and decreased body fluid.

 Recall Tyrese, who is at 38 weeks' gestation. Based on the information provided in the opening scenario, which signs would the nurse identify as indicating that Tyrese's labour is approaching? What additional information does the nurse need to assess?

True Versus "False" Labour

The term "false labour" has been used inaccurately to describe a situation in which women are, in fact, in prodromal or very early labour, which can last from a few hours to a few days. The contractions usually do not progress in frequency, duration, or intensity, and there is usually no progressive cervical dilation. In addition, the contractions of prodromal labour decrease with changes in position or activity.

A client experiencing prodromal labour needs anticipatory guidance and reassurance. The nurse

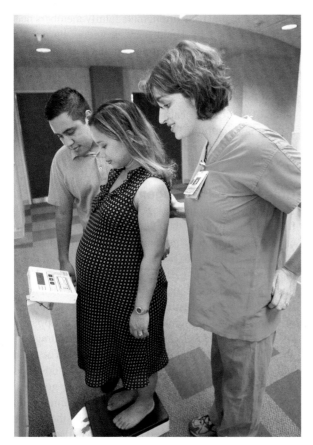

FIGURE 15.2 When labour is near, the woman may lose weight after months of steady weight gain.

● **BOX 15.1** **Characteristics of True Labour Contractions**

- Regular
- Gradually become closer together, eventually occurring every 4 to 6 minutes and lasting 30 to 60 minutes
- Strengthen with time
- Cause vaginal pressure and discomfort starting in the back and radiating to the front
- Continue regardless of position or activity

Emotional Experience of Impending Labour

Because of the many physical changes women experience late in pregnancy and before labour, restless or sleepless nights are common and may contribute to gradually mounting tension and fatigue. Increased anxiety heightens awareness; therefore, women may become more sensitive to various stimuli. If the fetus is less or more active than usual, the client may worry. The client may question whether the weight loss of 0.9 to 1.3 kg that sometimes precedes the onset of labour is normal. She may be concerned about her ability to cope with labour. During this time, the client may be preoccupied with planning last minute details for the baby. Throughout labour, nurses play a vital role in assisting the client and partner to use effective coping mechanisms to achieve a positive outcome (Simpson, 2005).

Sociocultural Aspects Related to Impending Labour and Birth

Although childbirth is a universal occurrence, cultural values and norms exert an influence on the experience. Culture forms the backdrop for all human behaviour and learning. Families bring their own beliefs, world-views, rituals, attitudes, and values about pregnancy and childbirth (Etowa, 2012; Watts & McDonald, 2007). Clients and families frequently base their coping with childbirth on cultural beliefs, rituals, and traditions (Andrews & Boyle, 2007).

Ethnic and cultural groups vary in their beliefs, values, and behaviours surrounding childbirth. A goal of perinatal nursing is to provide a culturally competent environment in which women and their families feel supported, cared for, and that their specific needs, rituals, and expectations are respected (Fuller, 2012; Greene, 2007). When working with clients from a culture that differs from his or her own, the nurse needs to remain aware of the many possibilities that may exist in that culture and avoid assuming that a particular client will automatically conform to a specific pattern or

should advise her and her partner to observe and record the characteristics of contractions, especially noting any changes with alterations in position or activity. Also, the nurse should urge the woman to obtain adequate nutrition and fluids (in case contractions become progressive). Fatigue and discouragement are common, especially if prodromal labour is lengthy or recurrent. Care providers should avoid labelling the woman's experience as "false labour" because such terminology tends to invalidate the woman's real experience. In addition, these early contractions are, in fact, helping to prepare for childbirth.

When the client moves from prodromal to true labour, contractions become rhythmic and regular. The contractions increase in frequency, duration, and intensity. The intervals between contractions are constant, and positional or activity changes do not affect them (walking may, in fact, enhance their progression.) Progressive contractions often start in the back and then radiate to the lower groin. They are usually associated with pelvic pressure, increased vaginal discharge, loss of the mucous plug (or "bloody show"), and possibly rupture of the membranes. They result in progressive cervical effacement and dilation. See Box 15.1.

tradition (Brathwaite & Williams, 2004). He or she needs to look for cues, develop skills, acquire knowledge, and maintain objectivity.

Areas that require particular cultural sensitivity from nurses include the meaning of childbirth to the client and the ways she experiences and chooses to deal with pain (Cioffi, 2004; Etowa, 2012). Understanding childbirth from the context of the birthing woman can help to improve maternity care (Varcoe et al., 2013). Western medicine tends to convey a message that childbirth is a medical problem fraught with danger and that it demands interventions, monitoring, and assistance from qualified medical professionals (Smeenk & ten Have, 2003).

For some women, however, this belief tarnishes the birth experience. Some clients view childbirth as normal, natural, and healthy, and face labour confidently, relying on their inner wisdom (Kennedy & Shannon, 2004; Lothian, 2001). Many cultures praise women for their achievement in birthing a baby. Other cultures attribute or give at least partial credit for this accomplishment to the skill of the obstetrician. For example, in Canada, people often use terminology indicating that a woman is "delivered" of her child as opposed to giving birth. In addition, certain cultures require strict adherence to rituals during labour and birth. These beliefs may influence the position the woman chooses for labour, as well as who is allowed to remain with her during birth (Andrews & Boyle, 2007).

Just as attitudes toward the meaning of birth differ among cultures, so do expressions of pain and feelings about pain management (Higginbottom et al., 2013; Jones et al., 2012; McLachlan & Waldenstrom, 2005). For some clients, crying and moaning are culturally appropriate responses to discomfort. For others, remaining stoic and nonverbal about pain is culturally expected. Cultures that view childbirth as a natural experience may prefer nonpharmacologic options for pain relief or complementary and alternative therapies (see Chapter 17). The upbringing, culture, and personal values of the nurse and other health care providers, as well as their own ability to cope with pain, may influence their attitudes toward the clients' responses and choices about the expression and relief of pain.

The intrapartum nurse should also consider his or her values and beliefs regarding family members' involvement in providing labour support (Simmonds et al., 2013). Gender-determined roles and responsibilities vary across cultures, as does family decision making. Such influences may contribute to decisions about where labour and birth will take place and who will be the support person(s) (Bashour & Abdulsalam, 2005). For cultural or religious reasons, some fathers cannot touch the woman during labour or birth. Regardless of their degree of participation, male family members need to feel accepted by health care providers during this time (Steen et al., 2012). Some women feel that exposing any part of their body is unacceptable. This may influence their choice of health care provider and who can perform procedures during labour and birth. Expectation of the role of health care providers also may vary according to culture. The nurse needs to ascertain what the woman's preferences are about care providers and procedures.

Collaborative Management

During the prelabour phase, collaborative management focuses on providing the client and her significant others with anticipatory guidance and support. The best advice for a client is to be patient and to have confidence that her body is doing exactly what it is supposed to at this time. The nurse should encourage the woman not to worry whether it is really labour. For the vast majority of women, labour eventually becomes quite apparent. As labour approaches, the nurse should encourage the client to eat, drink plenty of fluids, and rest. The client and her partner or other support people can do things that they enjoy, such as watching television, going for a walk, or visiting with friends. By surrounding herself with people with whom she is comfortable, the woman can stay positively focused and receive reassurance. Nursing Care Plan 15.1 highlights the care of a woman in prelabour.

LABOUR AND BIRTH

Labour refers to the series of events by which the products of conception are expelled from the mother's body (Cunningham et al., 2005). This technical definition does not in any way convey the wonder of the process responsible for this beautifully synchronized achievement. Nature has designed labour and birth simply and elegantly (Lothian, 2001). Although every birth is unique and unfolds in a special way, the process is remarkably consistent. Once labour begins, it normally runs its course until its purpose—the birth of the baby—is fulfilled.

The traditional definition of labour is the period when regular uterine contractions are associated with cervical effacement and dilation. This explanation, however, presents many clinical problems. Some facilities arbitrarily define the onset of labour as the time of admission to the birth unit. Other maternity care settings define labour as when a woman's cervix has achieved a dilation of 3 or 4 cm. Yet other facilities use the woman's self-reporting of the onset of symptoms as the time of onset of labour. Unfortunately, none of these interpretations are entirely adequate.

NURSING CARE PLAN 15.1

●

The Client in Prelabour

Physical examination of Tyrese reveals cervical dilation of 1 cm and effacement of 30%. Her membranes are intact. The fetus is in a cephalic presentation, vertex position at –2 station. FHR is 144 bpm. Tyrese says, "Does this mean I'm in labour? I'm not having contractions."

NURSING DIAGNOSES

- Deficient Knowledge related to prelabour signs and symptoms and upcoming labour and events
- Anxiety related to first experience with labour and uncertainty of the unknown.

EXPECTED OUTCOMES

1. The client will state the signs and symptoms of true labour.
2. The client will verbalize events related to upcoming labour and birth.
3. The client will identify areas causing her concern.

INTERVENTIONS	RATIONALES
Assess the client's level of understanding about signs and symptoms of approaching labour and the process of childbirth	Assessment provides a baseline to identify specific client needs and develop an individualized plan
Discuss her concerns, feelings, and perceptions related to labour and birth	Talking provides opportunities to emphasize positive aspects of the current situation; verbalization of concerns aids in establishing sources of stress and problem areas to address
Communicate accurate data and answer questions honestly. Reinforce facts, emphasizing that each pregnancy, labour, and birth is highly individualized	Open honest communication promotes trust and helps correct any misconceptions. Facts help to dispel unfounded fears, myths, or guilt feelings
Evaluate the client's past coping strategies to determine which have been most effective	Use of appropriate coping strategies aids in reducing anxiety
Correlate the client's current signs and symptoms with those associated with approaching labour; review the signs and symptoms of true labour and actions to take	Correlation of current status provides insight into changes occurring in preparation for labour. Having knowledge of true labour signs and symptoms and actions to take alleviates stress
Urge the client to report any spontaneous gush of fluid	Spontaneous rupture of membranes can lead to cord prolapse. If rupture is prolonged, the risk for infection increases
Teach the client what to expect relative to contraction strength and frequency and progression of labour	An understanding of what to expect reduces fear of the unknown

(continued)

NURSING CARE PLAN 15.1 ● The Client in Prelabour *(Continued)*

INTERVENTIONS	RATIONALES
Review comfort measures, such as music, distraction, hot/cold compresses, massage, and position changes that can be used	Knowledge of available measures to control pain helps reduce anxiety associated with contractions
Give the client the phone number of a person to notify when signs of true labour occur	Availability of a contact person helps reduce anxiety, providing a source for anticipatory guidance once labour begins

EVALUATION

1. The client states the signs and symptoms of true labour accurately.
2. The client identifies the progression of events associated with labour and birth.
3. The client verbalizes appropriate measures to cope with concerns related to labour and birth.

Etiology of Labour

Just what initiates labour is not definitely known (Gross et al., 2005; Ragusa et al., 2005). For many years, researchers have assumed that several factors (either alone or combined) bring about labour. For example, some have attributed labour to the withdrawal of progesterone near the end of pregnancy. Others have supported the idea that marked distention of the uterus and pituitary action lead to the release of oxytocin and thus uterine activity (Simpson, 2008).

During the past few decades, new information has challenged several proposed causes of the initiation of labour. Currently, interrelationships between mother and fetus are considered to play important roles, although these relationships are not yet well understood. The following discussion summarizes some of the most common theories of the onset of labour.

Progesterone Withdrawal

The progesterone withdrawal theory suggests that initiation of labour is related to both maternal hormones and fetal status. Progesterone is thought to suppress uterine irritability throughout pregnancy by counterbalancing the increased uterine contractility resulting from increased estrogen levels (Kamel, 2010). Changes within the fetal membranes and decidua as the placenta ages and as term approaches may be associated with increased estrogen synthesis and decreased progesterone production. Increased estrogen levels can increase oxytocin in the myometrium (uterine muscles). In addition, a compound called transforming growth factor beta may

react in a gene-specific manner that not only decreases progesterone but also increases oxytocin receptors. Research is currently being conducted in this area.

Oxytocin Production

Oxytocin is a hormone released from the posterior pituitary gland in increased amounts during labour. Release of oxytocin alone, however, does not adequately explain what initiates labour. Progesterone during labour tends to inhibit the uterine response to oxytocin. It is only after estrogen has already influenced the uterine muscles that sensitivity to oxytocin increases, as does the number of oxytocin receptors. In fact, oxytocin may be given in large amounts early in pregnancy with little or no effect, and such administration often has little influence on an unripened cervix (Blackburn & Loper, 2003). This finding has major clinical implications for the use of oxytocin as an agent for elective induction of labour. Because oxytocin performs best after oxytocin receptors in the uterus have increased, one of the best ways to determine whether a woman will respond well to labour induction is to perform a pelvic assessment for cervical ripening. A ripe cervix is likely to have many oxytocin receptors and, subsequently, favourable outcomes.

A **Bishop score** is a system for rating cervical ripeness for labour based on assessment of its position, consistency, effacement, and dilation, as well as the fetal station (Table 15.1). A favourable Bishop score indicates that even without exogenous oxytocin stimulation, labour will most likely begin soon on its own.

● TABLE 15.1 **Bishop Score System**

Score	Dilation (cm)	Effacement (%)	Station	Cervical Consistency	Cervical Position
			Factor		
0	Closed	0–30	−3	Firm	Posterior
1	1–2	40–50	−2	Medium	Midposition
2	3–4	60–70	1, 0	Soft	Anterior
3	5 or more	80 or more	+1 or more		

Each factor is given a score, and the subtotals are combined. Scores above 8 indicate cervical ripeness and a high likelihood for labour and successful induction. Canadian guidelines use >6 as an indication of cervical ripeness.

From Bishop, E. H. (1964). Pelvic scoring for elective induction. *Obstetrics and Gynecology, 24*, 266–268.

Remember Tyrese, the woman being seen at the prenatal clinic at 38 weeks' gestation. If a vaginal examination revealed cervical dilation of 1 cm, 30% effacement, −2 station, and a soft cervix at the midposition, what would be Tyrese's Bishop score?

Prostaglandin Production

Prostaglandins are agents formed from fatty acids that act as chemical mediators or local hormones. They stimulate smooth muscle contraction and probably have been the most studied compounds in the past 25 years in relation to labour's onset (Blackburn & Loper, 2003). Unlike oxytocin, administration of prostaglandins appears to initiate labour any time during gestation. The importance of prostaglandins is further enhanced by findings that women who take high doses of anti-prostaglandin drugs (e.g., aspirin, ibuprofen) may have delayed labour (Blackburn & Loper, 2003; Cunningham et al., 2005).

Estrogen Stimulation

The estrogen stimulation theory is based on an increase in estrogen levels that occur at 34 to 35 weeks' gestation. Estrogen appears to promote oxytocin production and the formation of estrogen receptors in the uterine muscles. It is also thought to stimulate prostaglandin production. Researchers have postulated that because estrogen production comes from fetal adrenal precursors, this may be an example of fetal factors contributing to labour initiation (Blackburn & Loper, 2003).

Fetal Influence

The fetus may have roles in both initiation of labour and the process of labour itself, although exact mechanisms are not well understood. For example, the fetal lungs or kidneys may transmit a signal for labour through a mediator secreted into the amniotic fluid (Cunningham et al., 2005). Theorists have suggested that fetal cortisol levels rise to a point that initiates labour. The fact that fetuses with anencephaly tend to be postterm supports this finding. Anencephalic fetuses also have adrenal dysfunction, which in turn decreases available fetal cortisol (Cunningham et al., 2005).

Other Theories

Some other explanations for initiation of labour include overdistention of the uterus and infections. According to the overdistention theory (also termed the "stretch theory"), the uterus reaches a set threshold that leads to synthesis and release of prostaglandins (Rouse & St. John, 2003). Infections may be associated with the initiation of labour, especially preterm labour. In such cases, however, it is likely that labour results not simply from the infectious process but also from the increased level of prostaglandins, which is a natural mediating response to infection.

Processes of Labour and Birth

To understand what labour and birth involve, subdividing the topic into different categories can be helpful. The traditional way of doing so has been to identify the "Ps" of labour (Rouse & St. John, 2003):

- *Powers:* uterine contractions and maternal pushing
- *Passageway:* the maternal pelvis and soft parts
- *Passenger:* fetus

Other influences on labour and birth include maternal psychological status, support from partners and others, and maternal position during labour.

Powers

Uterine Contractions. As mentioned earlier, uterine contractions are intermittent tightenings of the myometrium. Throughout labour, the muscles in the upper uterine segment are more active, contracting more intensely and for longer than those of the lower uterine

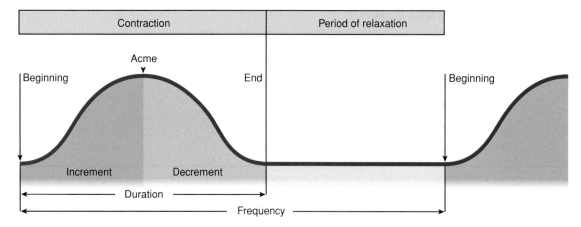

FIGURE 15.3 A uterine contraction has three phases: increment, acme, and decrement.

segment. After the muscles have contracted, they relax, pulling up the cervix and lower uterine segment. The upper segment thickens with time, while the more passive lower segment thins (Rouse & St. John, 2003).

Normal uterine contractions are like waves, composed of an *increment* (the building up or ascending portion), an **acme** (the peak), and a *decrement* (the coming down or descending portion). When describing contractions, caregivers refer to their frequency, duration, and intensity (Fig. 15.3). **Contraction frequency** means the time from the beginning of one contraction to the beginning of the next. **Contraction duration** is timed from the beginning to the end of the same contraction. **Contraction intensity** refers to strength.

Contractions, the primary power needed to accomplish labour and birth, are intermittent throughout labour, forming a regular pattern interspersed with rest periods. The intervals of rest between contractions are essential, not only for maternal comfort but also for fetal welfare, as they allow for reoxygenation of the placenta. Labour contractions are mild at first and then become increasingly more intense as labour progresses.

Pushing. In addition to contractions, the other power is the intra-abdominal force provided by the mother through pushing (Rouse & St. John, 2003). This power is reserved for the second stage of labour, after effacement and dilation are complete. It is commonly referred to as "bearing down." As labour continues, many women begin to experience an involuntary urge to push. With pushing, the woman contracts her abdominal muscles to provide an auxiliary force to the contractions, increasing the intra-abdominal pressure to force the fetus through the vagina.

For many years, it was suggested that women should push with a closed glottis (also called Valsalva manoeuvre) and under directed efforts by health care personnel. Research findings, however, questioned both the efficacy and potential harm of these measures.

Closed glottis pushing increases intrathoracic pressure and impairs blood return from the lower extremities, leading to an initial increase and then decrease in blood pressure. These changes affect uteroplacental blood flow and perfusion (Simpson, 2008). Fetal hypoxia and resultant acidosis and maternal pelvic or perineal damage have been associated with prolonged and forceful closed glottis pushing (Roberts & Hanson, 2007). In addition, some studies have shown that coached pushing resulted in only a minimal decrease in the length of the second stage of labour (Bloom et al., 2006; Sampselle et al., 2005). Efforts to implement a guideline for second stage management provide confirmation that a consistent approach to care during this stage of labour is warranted (Allen et al., 2009; Sprague et al., 2008). Nurses have observed that women push effectively by either controlled exhalations or brief breath holding when they are not instructed to do otherwise. Physiologic and spontaneous approaches to pushing avoid risks and allow women to follow their own instincts (Chalk, 2004; Karnng-Edgren, 2001; Roberts, 2002; Simpson et al., 2008).

Passageway

The passageway consists of both a hard passage (bony pelvis) and a soft passage (maternal soft tissue structures).

Maternal Bony Pelvis. The pelvis is the bony ring known as the hip girdle, which separates the lower extremity from the trunk. It transmits the body weight to the lower extremities. In women, the pelvis also serves as the passage for the fetus to be born.

Pelvic Structures. The major pelvic bones include the innominate bones (formed by the fusion of the ilium, ischium, and pubis around the acetabulum), sacrum, and coccyx. For obstetric purposes, the pelvis is arbitrarily divided into halves: the false pelvis and the true

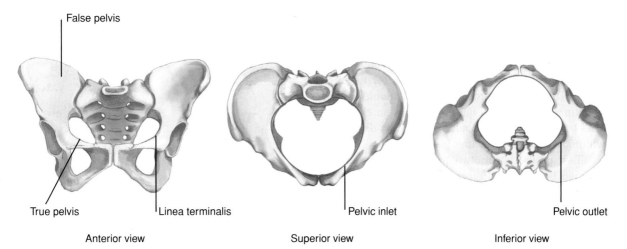

False pelvis

True pelvis   Linea terminalis

Anterior view

Pelvic inlet

Superior view

Pelvic outlet

Inferior view

FIGURE 15.4 The maternal bony pelvis: anterior, superior, and inferior view.

pelvis (Fig. 15.4). An imaginary line called the *linea terminalis*, which extends from the symphysis pubis to the sacral prominence, separates them.

The false pelvis is the wide, broad area between the iliac crests. It supports the uterus and directs the fetus into the true pelvis to engage. The true pelvis is below the linea terminalis and actually serves as the bony birth passage. The entrance to the true pelvis is called the **pelvic inlet**. The shape of the true pelvis is curved, not straight, which means that the fetus must first move down and then up over the sacrum as it descends through the **pelvic outlet**, or the lower border of the true pelvis. This has implications for the positioning of women during the expulsion stage.

Pelvic Types. Various methods have been used to predict the adequacy of a pelvis in terms of the ease of passage. Four basic types have been classified according to shape: *gynecoid, android, anthropoid,* and *platypelloid.* The features of these types are discussed in Chapters 12 and 16. In some women, the pelvis is a mixture of two types. Generally, vaginal birth is most easily accomplished with a gynecoid pelvis and is difficult or impossible with an android or platypelloid type (Rouse & St. John, 2003).

Pelvic Diameters. In addition to pelvic shape, fetal ability to pass through depends on the size of the true pelvis. To determine the size, examiners take measurements of diameters of the pelvic inlet, midpelvis, and pelvic outlet early in the antepartal period, often on the first prenatal visit (see Chapter 12).

Maternal Soft Parts. For normal labour and birth, the soft tissues of the cervix, vagina, and perineum must stretch to allow passage of the fetus. Progesterone and relaxin facilitate such softening and increase the elasticity of the muscles and ligaments. During the last few weeks of pregnancy, the cervix softens, effaces,

and becomes more elastic. Ripening also results from Braxton Hicks contractions and engagement of the fetal head, which serves as a wedge against the cervix. Already distensible, the vagina becomes even more stretchable throughout pregnancy. Estrogen promotes growth of the vaginal mucosa and underlying tissues and increases cellular glycogen. Increased vascularity helps to thicken and lengthen the vaginal walls. These changes allow the vagina to accommodate passage of the fetus. The muscles of the perineum also soften and become more stretchable.

Passenger

Fetal Head. Because the fetal head is usually the largest part that must pass through the vaginal opening, its size and relative rigidity are important factors that influence the mechanism of labour. The fetal head is divided into the face and base of the skull and the cranial vault (Fig. 15.5). The bones of the skull are well ossified and firmly united. The bones of the cranial

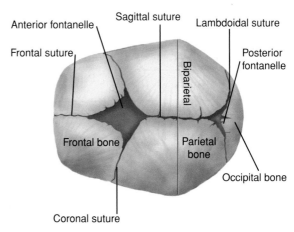

Anterior fontanelle
Frontal suture
Sagittal suture
Lambdoidal suture
Posterior fontanelle
Biparietal
Frontal bone
Parietal bone
Occipital bone
Coronal suture

FIGURE 15.5 Landmarks of the fetal skull.

vault, however, are relatively thin, poorly ossified, and loosely connected to one another by membranous attachments. At birth, flexibility of the bones of the cranial vault allows some movement and overriding, so that the fetal head can adapt to the maternal pelvis. This adaptive process is called **moulding** and sometimes manifests in the newborn as an elongated head (see Chapter 16). Moulding generally disappears within the first few days after birth.

Two frontal bones, two parietal bones, and one occipital bone make up the cranial vault. The associated diameters are important (Fig. 15.6). The biparietal diameter, or the distance between the two parietal bones, is considered the widest transverse diameter of the fetal head. It measures approximately 9.25 cm (Cunningham et al., 2005). Other important fetal diameters include the following:

- Suboccipitobregmatic—approximately 9.5 cm
- Submentobregmatic—approximately 9.5 cm
- Occipitofrontal—approximately 11.75 to 12 cm
- Occipitomental—approximately 13.5 cm (Rouse & St. John, 2003)

The membranous attachments are called *sutures*. The *sagittal suture* joins the two parietal bones. The *lambdoidal suture* joins the parietal and occipital bones. The *coronal suture* joins the parietal and frontal bones. The sutures are considerably enlarged at their point of intersection. These intersections are known as **fontanelles**. The two major fontanelles are the diamond-shaped anterior fontanelle (also known as the **bregma**) and the triangular-shaped posterior fontanelle. The anterior fontanelle does not close until a baby is approximately 18 months old. The posterior fontanelle usually closes by 6 to 8 weeks after birth.

The cranial vault is divided into three distinct sections. The **vertex** is the portion that lies between the anterior and posterior fontanelles. The **occiput** constitutes the area of the occipital bone. The *brow* is the portion lying between the large anterior fontanelle and the eye sockets.

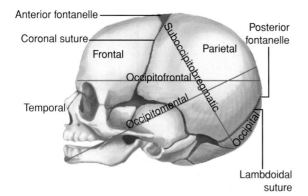

FIGURE 15.6 Diameters of the fetal skull.

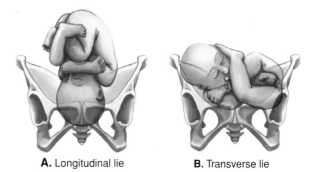

A. Longitudinal lie   **B.** Transverse lie

FIGURE 15.7 Fetal lie. **A**: Longitudinal lie. **B**: Transverse lie.

Fetopelvic Relationships. To understand the relationship between the fetus and the maternal uterus and pelvis, the nurse needs to be familiar with descriptive terminology (Rouse & St. John, 2003).

- **Lie** is the relationship of the fetal long axis (spine) to the maternal long axis (spine). Lie is *longitudinal* when the fetal spine is parallel with the maternal spine. Lie is *transverse* when the fetal spine is perpendicular to the maternal spine (Fig. 15.7).
- **Presentation** refers to the fetal part that lies over the pelvic inlet. The main presentations are *cephalic* (head first), *breech* (pelvis or buttocks first), and *shoulder*. Cephalic presentations are subdivided as vertex, military, brow, and face (Fig. 15.8).
- **Presenting part** refers to the most dependent fetal part lying nearest to the cervix. During a vaginal examination, it is the area with which the examiner's finger first makes contact.
- **Attitude** is the relation of the fetal parts to one another. The basic attitudes are *flexion* and *extension* (Fig. 15.9). The fetal head is in flexion when the chin approaches the chest. It is in extension when the occiput nears the back. The typical fetal attitude is flexion.
- **Denominator**, an arbitrarily chosen landmark on the fetal presenting part, is used when describing the position. Each presentation has its own denominator. With a cephalic presentation, the denominator is the occiput.
- **Position** means the relationship of the denominator to the front, back, or sides of the maternal pelvis and is described using the first three letters of these landmarks. To use an example, a fetus in the cephalic presentation has the denominator as the occiput, which in this case is in the right quadrant of the maternal pelvis. The abbreviation assigned is OA (occiput anterior) (Box 15.2). OA positions facilitate labour because the head acts as a dilating wedge as the contractions help propel the fetus through the smallest pelvic diameters. Occiput posterior positions tend to prolong labour and are associated with other risks (Senecal et al., 2005). The woman usually

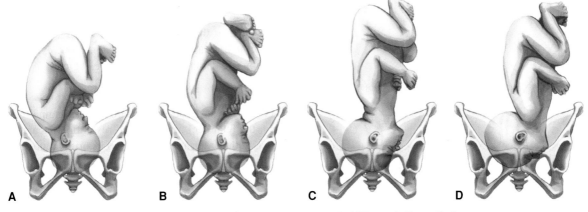

FIGURE 15.8 Cephalic fetal presentations. **A**: Vertex. **B**: Military. **C**: Brow. **D**: Face.

experiences increased back pain, especially because the fetal head is not well flexed (see Chapter 16).

Station. Station refers to the relationship of the fetal presenting part to an imaginary line drawn at the ischial spines within the maternal pelvis. When the largest diameter of the fetal presenting part has passed the pelvic inlet, **engagement** has occurred. Fetal engagement normally accompanies lightening, approximately 2 weeks before labour in a primipara. When the head is the engaged part, not only has the widest diameter passed the pelvic inlet, but also its most forward portion, the vertex, lies approximately at the imaginary line joining the ischial spines. A presenting part at the level of the spines is at 0 station. A part 1 cm below the spines is at +1 station. If it is at 2 cm below, it is at +2 station. A part 1 cm above the spines is at −1 station. See Figure 15.10.

 Yolanda arrived at the health care facility saying that she has contractions. A vaginal examination reveals that the fetus is in a cephalic presentation in right occipitoposterior (ROP) position. What assessments would be priorities?

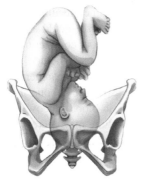

FIGURE 15.9 Full fetal flexion, with the smallest fetal diameter presenting to the maternal pelvis.

Mechanisms of Labour

While labour is causing uterine and cervical changes, the fetal presenting part goes through a series of passive movements designed to mould its smallest possible diameter to the irregular shape of the pelvic canal. In this way, the presenting part will encounter as little resistance as possible. These *cardinal movements*,

● **BOX 15.2   Terminology of Fetal Positions**

Vertex Presentation (Occiput)
● Left occipitoanterior (LOA)
● Left occipitotransverse (LOT)
● Left occipitoposterior (LOP)
● Right occipitoanterior (ROA)
● Right occipitotransverse (ROT)
● Right occipitoposterior (ROP)

Face Presentation (Mentum)
● Left mentoanterior (LMA)
● Left mentotransverse (LMT)
● Left mentoposterior (LMP)
● Right mentoanterior (RMA)
● Right mentotransverse (RMT)
● Right mentoposterior (RMP)

Breech Presentation (Sacrum)
● Complete
● Left sacroanterior (LSA)
● Left sacrotransverse (LST)
● Left sacroposterior (LSP)
● Right sacroanterior (RSA)
● Right sacroposterior (RSP)

Shoulder Presentation (Acromion)
● Left acromion dorsal anterior (LADA)
● Left acromion dorsal posterior (LADP)
● Right acromion dorsal anterior (RADA)
● Right acromion dorsal posterior (RADP)

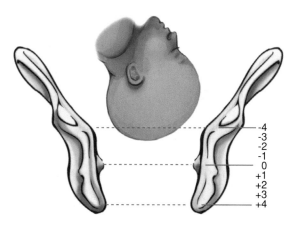

FIGURE 15.10 Fetal stations.

which usually occur in a smooth sequence, constitute the **mechanisms of labour** (Khan & Razi, 2005). Because a vertex presentation is the most common, the next discussion describes the mechanisms of labour for this type (Fig. 15.11).

Descent
When the fetal head presents, it usually enters the pelvis in a transverse position facing the mother's side. This is because the pelvic inlet is widest from side to side, and the oval-shaped fetal head fits best that way.

Descent, the downward movement of the fetus, is attributed to one or more of four forces:

* Pressure of amniotic fluid
* Direct pressure of the uterine fundus on the fetus
* Contraction of the maternal abdominal muscles during pushing
* Extension and straightening of the fetal body

Although descent is said to be continuous, it actually occurs only with contractions. In the intervals of relaxation, the presenting part recedes somewhat, thus relieving pressure on it and the maternal soft tissues, as well as restoring circulation diminished temporarily by the contraction.

Flexion
Early in the process of descent, the fetal head encounters resistance, causing it to flex so that its chin rests on its chest. The head thus presents its narrowest diameter, the suboccipitobregmatic, to the pelvic outlet.

Internal Rotation
When the occiput reaches the pelvic floor, it is rotated 45 degrees anteriorly and comes to lie beneath the symphysis pubis. In this fashion, the shoulders remain in their original position. Internal rotation of the head thus involves a twisting of the fetal neck.

Extension
During extension, the occiput passes out of the pelvis. The nape of the fetal neck moves under the maternal pubic arch, enabling the fetal scalp, brow, eyes, nose, mouth, and chin to push through the vagina.

Restitution
As soon as the head passes through the vaginal opening, the fetal neck untwists and restitution occurs. The occiput thus returns 45 degrees to its original position.

External Rotation
When the fetal anterior shoulder meets the resistance of the pelvic floor, it is shunted downward, forward, and inward to the maternal symphysis pubis. This positioning brings the shoulder into the anteroposterior diameter of the outlet and causes the head to rotate externally 45 degrees more.

Birth of the Shoulders and Expulsion
When the anterior shoulder comes into view beneath the pubic arch, it pauses while the posterior shoulder is being born by lateral flexion. Once both shoulders are out of the vagina, the rest of the baby is readily born.

Maternal Responses to Labour
Maintenance of the normal physiologic process of labour is an important goal in the care of a pregnant woman and her fetus. Identifying factors that influence normal labour and how they might be enhanced or altered is important in promoting health and achieving expected outcomes.

Cardiovascular System
Labour has major effects on maternal cardiovascular status. Generally, cardiac output, cardiac workload, heart rate, and blood pressure all increase. Cardiac output elevates as a result of the transfer of maternal blood (300 to 500 mL) from the uterus and placental vascular bed into the maternal systemic vascular system with each contraction. Blood pressure and heart rate may rise with contractions. Fear and anxiety can cause the release of catecholamines, leading to transient tachycardia. Therefore, the nurse should assess blood pressure and pulse between labour contractions.

Hematologic changes include an elevated white blood cell count, which researchers hypothesize may be related to the stress of labour. The physical work of labour may cause blood glucose levels to decrease. Blood coagulation time may decrease, whereas plasma fibrinogen levels increase. Peripheral vascular changes may result in maternal flushed cheeks (malar flush) or hot or cold feet.

Position in labour or at birth may further influence cardiovascular changes. Supine positions can lead

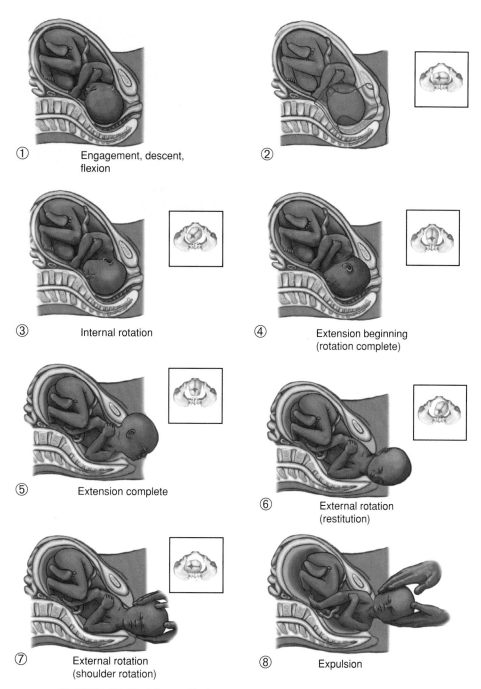

① Engagement, descent, flexion

②

③ Internal rotation

④ Extension beginning (rotation complete)

⑤ Extension complete

⑥ External rotation (restitution)

⑦ External rotation (shoulder rotation)

⑧ Expulsion

FIGURE 15.11 The cardinal movements of labour, vertex presentation.

to decreased cardiac output and stroke volume with increased heart rate from compression of the inferior vena cava and descending aorta. Extended breath holding (Valsalva manoeuvre) can increase intrathoracic pressure, decrease venous return, and increase venous pressure. This results in increased cardiac output, increased blood pressure, decreased pulse, and potential fetal hypoxia (Blackburn & Loper, 2003). Anxiety and pain also increase cardiac work and may be a major component of the changes demonstrated with a contraction.

Respiratory System

Uterine muscle activity increases oxygen consumption. Maternal respiratory rates usually rise with anxiety, pain, exertion, or the use of controlled breathing techniques for pain management. The client should try to avoid persistent hyperventilation resulting from fear or pain.

Major changes occur in acid–base relationships during labour, although these appear to quickly reverse themselves after birth. These normal alterations include mild respiratory alkalosis in early first-stage labour and mild metabolic acidosis compensated by respiratory alkalosis at the end of first-stage labour, mild respiratory acidosis during bearing down efforts, and finally metabolic acidosis uncompensated by respiratory alkalosis at birth (Blackburn & Loper, 2003).

Gastrointestinal System

During active labour, gastric motility decreases, whereas the emptying time of the stomach increases. If opioids are administered, the emptying time is likely to be even more prolonged (Cunningham et al., 2005). Traditional practice was to limit food and fluids during labour because of the risk of vomiting and possible aspiration. When the stomach remains relatively empty, however, nausea and vomiting are common intrapartal occurrences, particularly during the transition phase. In fact, an empty stomach increases gastric acidity, which may lead to nausea and vomiting. Some women also experience belching during transition. To compensate for restriction of oral fluids, administration of intravenous (IV) fluids has become routine care in many facilities. According to the findings from randomized clinical trials, however, withholding food and fluid from women at low risk in labour and giving routine IV infusions are unlikely to be beneficial (Enkin et al., 2000; Goer et al., 2007; Singata et al., 2013). Clear liquids are absorbed rapidly (Canadian Anesthesiologists' Society, 2008), so providers can encourage the woman to drink these if no apparent complications exist (Romano & Lothian, 2008). Caregivers may offer a woman in labour a light or liquid diet according to her preferences (Enkin et al., 2000; Goer et al., 2007; O'Sullivan et al., 2007). IV infusions are needed only for high-risk or special cases (e.g., use of epidural anaesthesia, administration of oxytocin).

Genitourinary and Renal System

Glomerular filtration rate increases during labour with increased cardiac output; therefore, polyuria is common. The nurse should observe the labouring woman closely for bladder distention or inability to void. These findings can result from relaxed bladder tone, analgesia or anaesthesia, fetal compression, or trauma. Along with polyuria, diaphoresis, decreased hydration, and increased respirations also can affect electrolyte balance. Proteinuria (trace to 1+) may result from the breakdown of muscle tissue.

Psychosocial Responses

Maternal emotional status before and during labour strongly influences the progression of childbirth. The psyche of a frightened, anxious, or upset client can affect the normal physiology of labour and birth (Fig. 15.12). High levels of catecholamines may interfere with the normal process (Simpson, 2008). Norepinephrine and

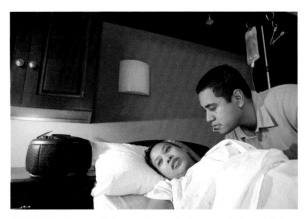

FIGURE 15.12 Fear, anxiety, or distress during childbirth can alter maternal physiology negatively and prolong labour. Support from partners and others during this time can be crucial to assisting women through this emotional time.

epinephrine may stimulate both α and β receptors of the myometrium and interfere with labour's rhythmic nature, culminating in a pattern of ineffective contractions and, consequently, prolonging childbirth (see Chapter 16). Anxiety also can increase pain perception, leading to an increased need for analgesia or anaesthesia (see Chapter 17).

Many factors contribute to the client's emotional response to birth. Lack of knowledge, fear of pain, personal or family stress, lack of labour support from a significant other, degree of self-confidence, feelings of loss of control, negative attitudes about birth, cultural background, and concerns for personal safety can all serve to block labour's progress (Goodman et al., 2004; Turley, 2004). The birth environment can influence labour as well (Hodnett et al., 2005).

Maternal psychosocial responses vary based on previous coping strategies and associated events. Early in labour, the client may be apprehensive, yet excited. As labour progresses and contractions increase in frequency and intensity, the woman tends to focus on the work at hand. As pain increases, so may discouragement and fatigue, decreasing the client's ability to effectively tolerate contractions (Simpson, 2008). For example, during the active phase, the client experiences growing discomfort, including pressure on the bladder and rectum. Strategies she used earlier in labour may be less effective when dealing with the more intense sensations. The client may respond to pain with screaming or crying. Fatigue and exhaustion may further compound these feelings. As a result, the client may fear that she will completely lose control.

Nurses play a key role in ensuring that the client in labour receives adequate support throughout the experience. Research has shown that women with strong self-esteem, as well as support from trained providers and significant others, feel more in control over the sensations and events not previously anticipated (Goodman et al., 2004; MacKinnon et al., 2005; Moore, 2001; Society of Obstetricians and Gynaecologists of Canada [SOGC], 2007). Encouraging prenatal participation in childbirth education classes helps to prepare women for labour (see Chapter 14). Once in labour, the nurse can urge the client to use techniques and strategies learned in these classes. Providing assistance in the form of emotional support, comfort measures, information, and advocacy is the key (Hodnett et al., 2002; Matthews & Callister, 2004; Simpson, 2008).

Recall Yolanda, the woman in early labour described at the beginning of the chapter. She voiced concern about whether her husband would arrive in time to attend the birth. What effects might this situation have on her labour?

Fetal Responses to Labour

In addition to caring for the mother during labour, nurses are responsible for evaluating fetal well-being throughout this time. Although most fetuses respond well to the changing intrauterine environment, the contractions, restricted mobility and positioning, and various obstetrical interventions can be potentially stressful. Thus, close monitoring of fetal health is important.

Fetal heart rate (FHR) patterns provide important insights into response to labour; alterations can signal developing problems. The goal of monitoring FHR in labour is to assist care providers to identify potential fetal decompensation that will lead to timely and effective intervention to risk the status of both the labouring woman and the fetus. The FHR can be monitored through either intermittent labour auscultation or continuous electronic fetal monitoring (EFM) (SOGC, 2007).

Auscultation of Fetal Heart Rate

For mothers and fetuses with no risk factors, intermittent auscultation provides a safe, noninvasive way to evaluate fetal well-being (Alfirevic et al., 2013). Intermittent auscultation of FHR can be done with a fetoscope or, more commonly, with an ultrasound Doppler device. Current recommendations for auscultation are as follows (SOGC, 2007):

- In low-risk pregnancies, auscultate every 15 to 30 minutes during the active phase of the first stage of labour.
- In low-risk pregnancies, auscultate every 5 minutes during the second stage of labour.
- In addition, the FHR should always be checked and recorded after any invasive procedure or potential

changes in the intrauterine environment, such as rupture of membranes, vaginal examinations, or administration of medications.

Before auscultating FHR with a fetoscope or Doppler, the examiner should first determine the location of the back of the fetus, where the heart sounds can best be heard. The examiner can determine the location of the fetal back using Leopold manoeuvres to palpate (see Chapter 12). He or she should place the fetoscope or Doppler on the maternal abdomen and listen and count for 60 seconds following a contraction (SOGC, 2007) (Fig. 15.13). Knowledge of differentiation between normal and abnormal findings is necessary (Table 15.2). In cases of suspected fetal distress, continuous EFM (discussed next) may be indicated so that providers can carefully assess the fetal response to contractions (SOGC, 2007).

Electronic Fetal Monitoring

Electronic fetal monitoring (EFM) involves ongoing evaluation of the FHR and uterine contractions through the application of either external (indirect) or internal (direct) leads. EFM provides a digital reading of the FHR and uterine contractions in a window display on the unit as well as on printed paper that records tracings over time. The FHR appears as a wavy line at the top of the paper as it prints from the monitor. Contractions appear along the bottom as a series of little hills that gradually become steeper as labour progresses. The fetal monitor printout becomes part of the woman's permanent medical record.

Use of EFM allows care providers to assess fetal well-being by examining the relationship between FHR and maternal uterine activity. The nurse is responsible for ensuring that fetal monitor tracings reflect interpretable FHR and maternal uterine activity. Knowledge of maternal and fetal physiology, understanding of the labour process, and appreciation of maternal and fetal response to labour in normal as well as abnormal circumstances enhance interpretation of fetal monitor tracings and subsequent clinical judgments.

Studies have consistently shown limited benefits in perinatal or neonatal outcomes using EFM instead of intermittent auscultation (Alfirevic et al., 2013; Thacker et al., 2001). Since its introduction into obstetrical care, fetal monitoring has not proved valuable to predicting or preventing fetal neurologic morbidity (Feinstein et al., 2000; Goodwin, 2000; Bailey, 2009). Although continuous EFM has failed to reduce fetal neurologic morbidity, it has coincided with an increase in cesarean births and instrumental vaginal births and has decreased overall maternal satisfaction with the childbirth experience (Alfirevic et al., 2013; SOCG, 2007; Thacker et al., 2001). Despite evidence questioning the benefits

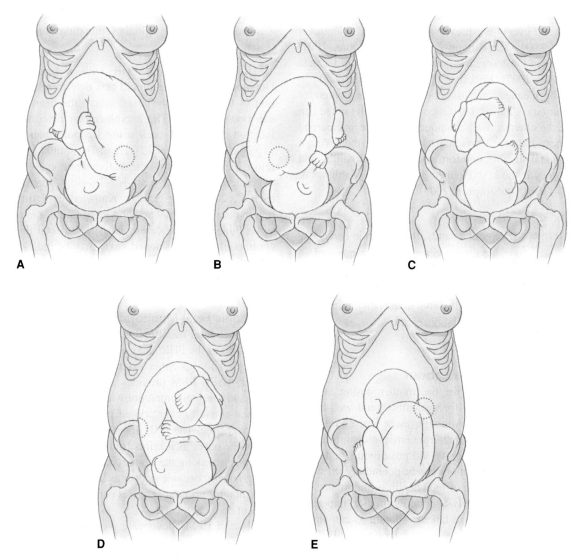

FIGURE 15.13 Sites for auscultation of the fetal heart rate based on fetal position. **A:** Left occiput anterior (LOA). **B:** Right occiput anterior (ROA). **C:** Left occiput posterior (LOP). **D:** Right occiput posterior (ROP). **E:** Left sacral anterior (LSA).

of routine continuous EFM, many Canadian and US labour and delivery units use it (Priddy, 2004). Protocols for monitoring FHR vary according to health care facility. SOGC (2007) supports the use of fetal auscultation and palpation of uterine activity as well as the judicious, appropriate application of intrapartum EFM to assess and promote maternal and fetal well-being. It does not support EFM as a substitute for appropriate and professional nursing intrapartum care.

External EFM. External EFM uses the principles of ultrasound by means of two types of leads applied to the maternal abdomen. A disk-shaped ultrasound transducer is placed over the abdomen and sends and receives FHR signals from the fetus to the device, which records these signals as waveforms. A pressure-sensitive transducer

called a tocodynamometer ("toco") is placed over the maternal uterine fundus to record uterine activity and to assess contractions. Both external transducers are held in place with elastic Velcro-like belts.

Technologic advances have led to the development of telemetry-like external EFM systems. Wireless transducers send the signals to the monitoring device, allowing the woman to be out of bed and to change positions readily throughout labour. Some systems are also waterproof, designed to enable external EFM for women using tubs for pain relief or birthing.

Some clients find the external EFM to be painless and are actually unaware of its presence during use; others find the constant sound of the FHR reassuring. Some women, however, find the belts used to hold the transducers in place uncomfortable. If appropriate, the

● TABLE 15.2   **Management of Abnormal Fetal Heart Rate by Intermittent Auscultation**

Tachycardia	Reposition woman to increase uteroplacental perfusion or alleviate cord compression Rule out fever, dehydration, drug effect, prematurity Correct maternal hypovolemia, if present, by increasing IV fluids Check maternal pulse and blood pressure
Bradycardia	Reposition woman to increase uteroplacental perfusion or alleviate cord compression Perform vaginal examination to assess for prolapsed cord or relieve cord compression Administer oxygen at 8–10 L/min Correct maternal hypovolemia, if present, by increasing IV fluids Check maternal pulse and blood pressure
Decelerations	Reposition woman Assess for passage of meconium Correct hypotension, if present Administer oxygen at 8–10 L/min
Additional measures	Continue to auscultate FHR to clarify and document components of FHR Consider initiation of electronic fetal monitoring (EFM) If abnormal findings persist despite corrective measures and ancillary tests are not available or desirable, expedited delivery should be considered

Adapted from: Feinstein, N. F., Sprague, A., & Trepanier, M. J. (2000). Fetal heart rate auscultation. Washington, DC: AWHONN (Association of Women's Health, Obstetrical and Neonatal Nurses). Source: Society of Obstetricians and Gynaecologists of Canada (SOGC). (2007). Fetal health surveillance: Antepartum and Intrapartum Consensus Guideline (SOGC Clinical Practice Guidelines Supp4). *Journal of Obstetrics and Gynaecology Canada, 29*(9), S3–S56.

transducers can be removed for a short time to allow the woman to change her position. Once she is comfortable, the transducers can be reapplied. In such an instance, the fetal position most likely will have changed; therefore, the transducers will need to be repositioned appropriately.

Although advantageous, external EFM is not as accurate a method as direct (internal) EFM (see next discussion). Changes in maternal or fetal position can interfere with recordings. In addition, obesity may affect the consistency and quality of tracings. External EFM is helpful in identifying pressure changes as the uterus tightens with a contraction; however, it cannot measure the intensity or resting tone of a contraction.

Internal EFM. When external assessment of the fetal heart is difficult, direct or internal EFM is viewed by some as the most accurate method for assessing FHR (Association of Women's Health, Obstetric and Neonatal Nurses [AWHONN], 2006). To perform internal EFM, the woman's amniotic membranes must be ruptured, and her cervix must be dilated at least 2 to 3 cm.

Internal EFM involves the insertion of an intrauterine pressure-sensitive catheter through the vagina and into the uterine cavity to record the pressure of the cavity with each contraction. The monitor records the frequency, duration, and strength (both at the beginning of the contraction and at its peak). A small spiral-shaped electrode is attached just under the skin of the fetal presenting part (most commonly, the fetal scalp) (Fig. 15.14). This electrode records the FHR and the pattern on the monitor.

Internal EFM, although highly accurate, poses some risks. Because the method is invasive, the mother and fetus are at risk for infection with use. It also requires the woman to remain in bed throughout labour and childbirth. Internal EFM is contraindicated for use in women who are HIV-positive or who have active or chronic hepatitis, herpes simplex virus, or any other known untreated sexually transmitted infection (STI) as well as in cases of placenta previa or face presentations (SOGC, 2007).

Fetal Heart Rate Patterns
Patterns of FHR generally are common and consistent. Table 15.3 compares various FHR interpretations.

Baseline Fetal Heart Rate. Baseline FHR is the typical FHR during a 10-minute period or between uterine contractions in labour. It is the average speed at which the heart is beating and normally ranges from 110 to 160 beats per minute (bpm). Counting FHR for a full 60 seconds provides most the accurate results (SOGC, 2007).

Bradycardia is an FHR less than 110 bpm and lasting greater than 10 minutes. Common causes of mild bradycardia include postterm pregnancy and persistent posterior position. Fetal hypoxia and prolonged umbilical cord compression may lead to bradycardia. **Tachycardia**, which is an FHR above 160 bpm and lasting greater than 10 minutes, may be associated with acute hypoxia, maternal or fetal fever, and use of certain β-sympathomimetic drugs.

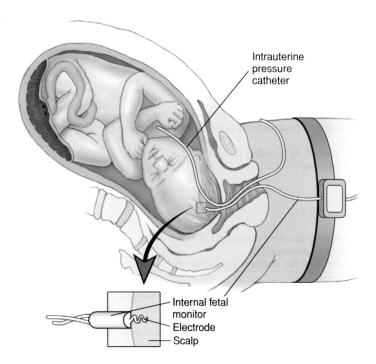

Intrauterine
pressure
catheter

Internal fetal
monitor
Electrode
Scalp

FIGURE 15.14 With internal electronic fetal monitoring, an intrauterine pressure catheter is inserted through the vagina and into the uterine cavity. An electrode is attached just under the skin of the fetal presenting part.

Baseline variability or rhythm is described as the fluctuations in baseline FHR greater than two cycles per minute within a 10-minute section. Irregular amplitude and frequency are evident. Absent variability indicates an undetectable range, minimal variability indicates the amplitude range is detectable but less than or equal to 5 bpm, moderate variability indicates the amplitude range is 6 to 26 bpm, and for marked variability, the amplitude range is greater than 25 bpm. Decreased variability is associated with fetal central nervous system depression. Fetal sleep cycles may cause the variability to decrease temporarily (30 to 60 minutes).

Periodic and Episodic Changes. Periodic changes are brief deviations above or below the baseline FHR. Such changes usually occur in relation to uterine contractions or fetal activity. Episodic changes refer to the changes above or below the baseline FHR unrelated to uterine contractions. See Figure 15.15.

An **acceleration** of the FHR is an increase of at least 15 bpm over baseline that lasts at least 15 seconds. An acceleration of FHR is often associated with fetal movement and is considered a sign of fetal well-being.

A **deceleration** of the FHR is a deviation below baseline that persists for at least 10 to 15 seconds but for less than 2 minutes. A *prolonged deceleration* lasts longer than 2 minutes. If the deceleration persists longer than 10 minutes, it becomes a new baseline.

An **early deceleration** is a decrease in the FHR that begins and ends at the same time as the uterine contraction, causing a consistent uniform U-shaped wave-form that mirrors the contraction on the EFM tracing. Early decelerations are thought to result from vagal nerve stimulation caused by compression of the fetal head during labour. They are considered a normal physiologic response to labour and need no intervention.

A **late deceleration** is a decrease in the FHR that begins after the peak of the contraction and ends after the contraction has ended. Late decelerations are thought to result from uteroplacental insufficiency or compromised uteroplacental perfusion. They are often associated with supine hypotensive syndrome or hyperstimulation of the uterus with oxytocin. Late decelerations are an indication for measures to increase uteroplacental circulation and fetal oxygenation. Maternal position changes can improve maternal venous return. Upright positions are also associated with more efficient uterine activity. Administration of oxygen by a nasal cannula or facemask may raise the mother's PO_2 and oxygen saturation, thereby making more oxygen available for transfer to the fetus. Discontinuing administration of oxytocin should reduce uterine activity and in turn increase uteroplacental perfusion.

A **variable deceleration** is a rapid decrease in the FHR and a rapid return to baseline. It may occur during or between contractions and has a characteristic V shape; prolonged variable decelerations that do not recover quickly may take on a U- or W-shaped appearance, or may not resemble other patterns (Feinstein et al., 2003). Variable decelerations are usually associated with compression of the umbilical cord. Changes in maternal position may correct variable decelerations by relieving cord compression. See Figure 15.16.

● TABLE 15.3   **Classification of Intrapartum EFM Tracings**

	Normal Tracing Previously "Reassuring"	Atypical Tracing Previously "Nonreassuring"	Abnormal Tracing Previously "Nonreassuring"
Baseline	110–160 bpm	Bradycardia 100–110 bpm Tachycardia >160 for >30 min to <80 min Rising baseline	Bradycardia <100 bpm Tachycardia >160 for >80 min Erratic baseline
Variability	6–25 bpm ≤5 bpm for <40 min	≤5 bpm for 40–80 min	≤5 bpm for >80 min ≥25 bpm for >10 min Sinusoidal
Decelerations	None or occasional uncomplicated variables or early decelerations	Repetitive (≥3) uncomplicated variable decelerations Single prolonged deceleration >2 min, but <3 min	Repetitive (≥3) complicated variables Deceleration to <70 bpm for >60 s Loss of variability in trough or in baseline Biphasic decelerations Overshoots Slow return to baseline Baseline lower after deceleration Baseline tachycardia or bradycardia Late decelerations >50% of contractions Single prolonged deceleration >3 min. but <10 min
Accelerations	Spontaneous accelerations present (FHR increases >15 bpm lasting >15 s) (<32 wks' gestation increase in the FHR >10 bpm lasting >10 s) Accelerations present with fetal scalp stimulation (<32 wks' gestation increase in the FHR >10 bpm lasting >10 s) Accelerations present with fetal scalp stimulation	Absence of acceleration with fetal scalp stimulation	Usually absent[a]
Action	EFM may be interrupted for periods up to 30 min if maternal–fetal condition stable and/or oxytocin infusion rate stable	Further vigilant assessment required especially when combined features present	ACTION REQUIRED Review overall clinical situation, obtain scalp pH if appropriate/prepare for delivery

[a]Usually absent, but if accelerations are present, this does not change the classification of tracing.

From Society of Obstetricians and Gynaecologists of Canada (SOGC). (2007). Fetal health surveillance: Antepartum and Intrapartum Consensus Guideline (SOGC Clinical Practice Guidelines Supp4). *Journal of Obstetrics and Gynaecology Canada, 29*(9), S3–S56.

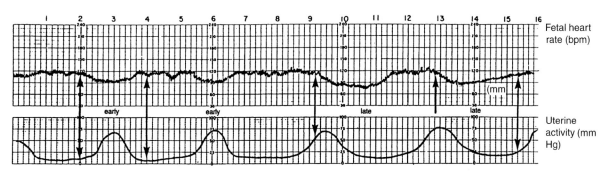

FIGURE 15.15   Electronic fetal monitoring tracing, showing early and late decelerations.

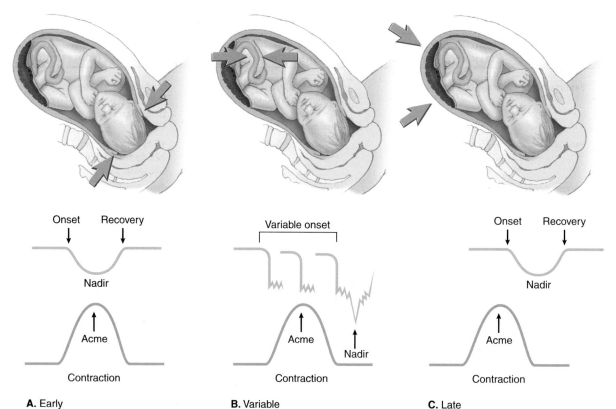

A. Early   **B.** Variable   **C.** Late

FIGURE 15.16 A: Early deceleration. **B:** Variable deceleration. **C:** Late deceleration.

Think back to Yolanda. Suppose that external EFM is being used, and the nurse notes a rapid decrease in the FHR with a rapid return to baseline. This change occurs between contractions; the waveform appears V-shaped. What should the nurse do next?

Stages and Phases of Labour

Labour is divided into distinct "stages" to portray the typical changes as it progresses. The first stage is subdivided into three "phases." In reality, most women usually move from one "phase" or "stage" to another in a fairly seamless continuum (Table 15.4). A "fourth" stage of labour generally includes the first 4 hours after delivery of the placenta, at which time the mother's body is undergoing dramatic changes (see Chapter 18).

● TABLE 15.4 **Stages and Phases of Labour**

Stage	Cervical Dilation (cm) and Effacement (%)	Duration	Contractions
First Stage			
Latent phase	0 to 3; 0–40	Nulliparas: up to 9 hr Multiparas: 5–6 hr	Occur every 5–10 min, lasting 30–45 s and mild
Active phase	4–7; 40–80	Nulliparas: 6 hr Multiparas: 4 hr	Occur every 2–5 min, lasting 45–60 s and moderate
Transition phase	8–10; 80–100	Nulliparas: 1 hr Multiparas: 30 min	Occur every 1–2 min, lasting 60–90 s and strong
Second Stage	10; 100	Nulliparas: 1 h Multiparas: 30 min	Occur every 2–3 min or less, lasting 60–90 s and strong
Third Stage	10; 100	Approximately 30 min	Mild to moderate
Fourth Stage	Gradual return to nonpregnant state	1–4 h	Dissipate

Consider Yolanda, the woman in labour described at the beginning of the chapter. Based on her report of contractions, which stage of labour should the nurse suspect at this time?

First Stage: Effacement and Dilation

The **first stage of labour** is characterized by noticeable cervical changes as a result of uterine contractions. The cervix softens, thins, shortens, and opens to a diameter of 10 cm. These cervical changes are referred to as effacement and dilation.

Effacement is the softening, thinning, and shortening of the cervical canal from a structure 1 or 2 cm long to one in which no canal exists at all. What remains is merely a circular orifice with almost paper-thin edges. During effacement, the edges of the internal os are drawn upward, so that the former cervical mucosa becomes part of the lower uterine segment.

Dilation of the cervix means that the cervical canal or "os" enlarges from an orifice a few millimetres in diameter to an opening large enough (approximately 10 cm) to permit the passage of the fetus. When the cervix can no longer be felt, dilation is said to be complete. Although the forces concerned with dilation are not well understood, several factors appear to be involved. The muscle fibres of the cervix are arranged in such a way that they pull on and tend to draw open the edges. The uterine contractions put pressure on the amniotic sac; through hydrostatic pressure, the sac burrows into the cervix in pouch-like fashion, exerting a dilating action. Without the membranes, the pressure of the presenting part against the cervix and the lower uterine segment has a similar, although less efficient, effect.

In women giving birth for the first time, effacement usually occurs before dilation. In women who have given birth before, effacement and dilation are simultaneous. In other words, the cervix of a woman who has given birth before opens or dilates with rather thick cervical edges (Cunningham et al., 2005).

The first stage of labour is divided into three phases: early (or latent), active (or accelerated), and transition. The first stage often starts slowly with short, infrequent uterine contractions. Over a period of hours or sometimes days, the contractions become stronger and closer together. As contraction intensity increases, the cervix continues to efface and dilate and the fetus descends into the pelvis. The contractions are most intense as the cervix dilates the last few centimetres. At the end of the first stage of labour, the cervix is opened or dilated fully, and the fetus is ready to be born (Fig. 15.17).

Early Labour (Latent Phase). During **early labour**, also called the latent phase of the first stage of labour,

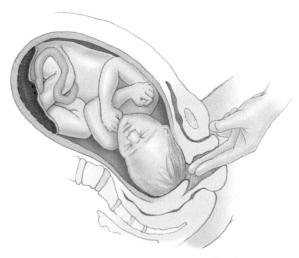

FIGURE 15.17 When performing vaginal examinations, the clinician can check to see the progress of cervical effacement and dilation to ensure that the woman is ready to give birth.

the cervix continues to thin and open, dilating to 3 to 4 cm. Contractions in early labour may feel much like the Braxton Hicks contractions that the woman experienced in late pregnancy, like an intermittent backache, or like menstrual cramps. They begin relatively mildly and do not usually interfere with the woman's activity. This phase is often a time of excitement and anticipation of the events that lie ahead. The woman may be talkative and enthusiastic. Health care providers should encourage the client and her support people to remain at home as long as possible in early labour because relaxation and mobility are easier to accomplish there. Labour is meant to be gradual, so this phase may take some time. Early labour usually accounts for approximately two thirds of the total time spent in labour.

Over several hours, contractions become longer, stronger, more regular, and closer together (approximately 5 minutes apart, each lasting 25 to 45 seconds). Several factors such as the degree of maternal fatigue, hydration, and nutrition, influence progress during this phase. Maternal emotions and attitudes about labour, as well as the availability and effectiveness of support systems, can affect this phase. In addition, sedation and regional anaesthesia may slow or even halt labour if given at this time.

Active Labour (Accelerated Phase). During **active labour**, contractions become longer and stronger, eventually occurring approximately 2 minutes apart and lasting for up to 1 minute or more. During this phase, which generally takes 2 to 6 hours, the cervix continues to efface and dilate from approximately 4 to 8 cm. These stronger contractions help the fetus rotate into a proper position for birth. The woman may experience additional physical symptoms that add to discomfort. Clients in active labour usually become serious and more focused. Labour is very hard work for women during this phase (Cunningham et al., 2005).

Transition Phase. The **transition phase**, the last phase of the first stage of labour, often starts when the cervix is 8 cm and ends when cervical dilation is complete. The maternal body makes the transition from cervical opening to pushing the fetus through the opened cervix. Contractions are now powerful and efficient, so this phase is usually quite short (Cunningham et al., 2005). Some women feel nauseous or shaky, restless, or irritable. The descent of the fetal presenting part accounts for the signs and symptoms of rectal pressure and a beginning urge to bear down. Bloody show may increase and darken.

 Think back to Yolanda, GTPAL 2-1-0-0-1, who has come to the labour and birth suite complaining of contractions. How would the nurse expect her contractions to change as she progresses through labour?

COLLABORATIVE CARE: FIRST STAGE OF LABOUR

Health care providers, including nurses, have major responsibilities and accountability during labour, birth, and the period immediately following. Clinical management depends on understanding normal physiologic and emotional responses, appreciating and watching for variations and deviations from normal, and individualizing care so that the experience is both safe and satisfying for the childbearing family (Matthews & Callister, 2004). Using the nursing process can help with the formulation of a plan of care that promotes positive labour and birth. See Nursing Care Plan 15.2.

Assessment

Assessment of a labouring woman arriving at the health care facility varies depending on her current phase. Determining how soon birth may occur is a crucial first priority. If birth is imminent, staff members should complete a focused assessment of maternal and fetal well-being and prepare the woman for childbirth. Areas of focus in such cases include the following:

- Pregnancy status (GTPAL status) and expected date of delivery, including date of last menstrual period
- Contraction frequency, intensity, and duration, including when contractions first started
- Other signs and symptoms such as bloody show, rupture of membranes, pressure, or urge to push
- Maternal vital signs and FHR
- Allergies

- Blood type and Rh status
- Oral intake, including the time and what was ingested
- Current pregnancy health care provider
- Past and present obstetric history, including outcomes and any problems encountered
- Birth plans, including personal preferences such as measures for pain relief, people for support, or photographing

Chapter 16 discusses care measures in the event of a precipitous or emergency vaginal birth.

If birth is not imminent, a more detailed assessment is performed that usually includes a maternal history, physical examination, and specimen collection. Assessment Tool 15.1 illustrates a sample assessment form on admission to the labour and birth area. Once initial evaluations are completed, assessment of maternal and fetal well-being continues throughout this stage of labour.

Maternal History

A detailed maternal history includes review of the current gestation, information about estimated date of delivery, date of last menstrual period, and progression throughout pregnancy. The nurse should ask the client about her contractions, including onset, duration, frequency, and intensity. In addition, he or she should inquire about fetal movement and any other signs and symptoms the client has experienced such as bloody show and rupture of membranes (including the time). Questions about weight gain, any problems (e.g., elevated blood pressure or blood glucose levels, excessive nausea and vomiting, bleeding, infection), and results of previous testing, such as ultrasounds or biophysical profiles, can provide clues to potential problems during labour and birth. The nurse should note the client's blood type, Rh, and group B streptococcus status.

The nurse should gather information about the maternal psychosocial condition including the woman's adjustment to this pregnancy, available support people, and possible cultural influences. He or she should review the mother's expectations, plans, and preferences for this labour and birth, such as choice of pain relief measures and presence of support people (including any of her other children), to ensure individualized care.

Past obstetric history is also essential to obtain. This information includes the numbers of previous pregnancies and their progression, problems, and outcomes (e.g., preterm birth); abortions; and living children and their birth weights. Questions about previous labour and birth experiences may help to provide clues about any preconceptions or possible factors that may influence how the woman approaches and copes this time.

Other areas to address include the woman's past health history, including any previous illnesses such as

NURSING CARE PLAN 15.2

●

The Client in Labour

Yolanda's labour has progressed slowly over the past 6 hours. She is experiencing contractions of moderate to strong intensity every 3 to 4 minutes, lasting approximately 50 to 60 seconds each. Cervical effacement is 80%, with dilation at 6 cm. The fetal presenting part is at +1 station; FHR is averaging 128 to 136 bpm.

Yolanda's husband has just arrived. She states, "I'm so glad you made it. I'm so tired and these contractions are really starting to hurt. My music doesn't seem to be helping the pain anymore."

NURSING DIAGNOSES

- Pain related to increased intensity and frequency of contractions and progression of labour
- Fatigue related to slow progression of otherwise normal labour events and anxiety about husband's arrival

EXPECTED OUTCOMES

1. The client will report a decrease in pain to a tolerable level.
2. The client will identify appropriate positions to aid in pain relief.
3. The client will demonstrate ability to participate in labour activity with support from her husband.

INTERVENTIONS	RATIONALES
Ask the client to rate her pain on a scale of 1 to 10.	Assessment provides a baseline from which to develop an individualized plan of care and to provide a basis for future comparison.
Question the client about measures she is using currently for pain relief.	Identification of current measures helps determine alternative strategies.
Encourage the client to change positions frequently, such as sitting upright or forward leaning, getting on her hands and knees, or squatting; suggest ambulation.	Sitting promotes perineal relaxation; forward leaning aids in fetal rotation and relief of back pain and pressure; hands-and-knees position enhances placental blood flow and promotes fetal rotation; squatting widens the pelvic outlet and facilitates fetal movement. Ambulation encourages fetal rotation and descent and improves contraction efficiency.
Discourage the supine position; encourage the side-lying position.	Side-lying position prevents supine hypotension syndrome and promotes uteroplacental blood flow.
Suggest use of a birthing ball with a gentle rocking or side-to-side motion.	A birthing ball helps widen the pelvis and enhances fetal descent and rotation.
Encourage the husband to assist with position changes, using stroking and light massage.	Participation promotes sharing of the experience and provides support to the client.

(continued)

NURSING CARE PLAN 15.2 ● The Client in Labour *(Continued)*

INTERVENTIONS	RATIONALES
Suggest the use of heat and cold therapy or a warm bath, if appropriate.	Heat aids in muscle relaxation; cold slows pain impulse transmission. Submersion in warm bath water relaxes muscles and promotes buoyancy, allowing the body to float.
Offer analgesics as indicated.	Analgesics alter the sensation of pain.
Give the client time to rest between position changes and contractions; balance activity and rest periods.	A balance of activity and rest reduces the risk for fatigue.
Assess maternal and fetal status before and after each strategy; continue to monitor the client's pain level for changes.	Frequent monitoring is necessary to ensure well-being and to determine the effectiveness of interventions.

EVALUATION

1. The client states contraction pain is tolerable.
2. The client uses varying positions to assist with pain relief.
3. The client and her husband participate in labour events.

---

tuberculosis, heart disease, kidney disorders, or STIs, as well as a brief family medical history. The nurse should ask the client about the use of cigarettes, alcohol, complementary and alternative therapies, and any prescribed, over-the-counter, or illicit drugs or herbal remedies. Screening for possible intimate partner violence is also important.

Physical Examination

Physical examination of the woman in labour begins with measurement of the client's height and weight. The nurse should obtain the client's vital signs (Fig. 15.18). He or she should complete a review of body systems or head-to-toe examination, as well as checking fetal status.

Maternal Status

Physical examination of maternal status involves assessing contractions and status of the amniotic membranes. The nurse should inspect the abdomen for contour changes and measure fundal height. He or she should palpate the abdomen for tightening and relaxation with contractions, and ask the client to rate current pain level to establish a baseline for future comparison. Leopold manoeuvres can assist team members to determine fetal presentation and position (see Chapter 12). These manoeuvres also help to determine the best location for auscultating fetal heart sounds.

The woman's membrane status is evaluated (Nursing Procedure 15.1). If SROM is suspected, the vaginal fluid should be tested for confirmation. Detection for rupture of membranes involves the Fern test. A small amount of amniotic fluid is placed on a clean glass slide, allowed to air dry, and then visualized under a microscope for characteristics of a "fern-like" pattern. Vaginal examinations are not performed in the presence of unexplained vaginal bleeding or rupture of the membranes (Simpson, 2008) until the women is in active labour. Vaginal examinations should not be done during a contraction.

Fetal Status

Physical examination of the fetus focuses on assessing the rate and pattern of the fetal heartbeat, either intermittently by auscultation in pregnancies that are of low risk or continuously by electronic monitoring in pregnancies with risk factors present. Nursing Procedure 15.2 describes the steps in applying an external EFM.

Specimen Collection

Collection of urine and blood specimens is part of initial intrapartal assessment. Protocols for specific testing vary among health care facilities. Generally, a clean-catch urine specimen for urinalysis is collected. Other laboratory tests may include blood specimens for hemoglobin and hematocrit, complete blood count, blood

● **ASSESSMENT TOOL 15.1** **Sample Documentation Form Used for Admission to the Perinatal Unit**

ADMISSION ASSESSMENT OBSTETRICS

▲ PATIENT IDENTIFICATION ▲

ADMISSION DATA

Date	Time	Via			
		☐ Ambulatory ☐ Wheelchair ☐ Stretcher			

Grav.	Term	Pre-term	Ab.	Living	EDC	LMP	GA

Prev. adm. date _____ Reason _____
Obstetrician _____ Pediatrician _____

Ht. _____ Wt. _____ Wt. gain _____

Allergies (meds/food) ☐ None _____ ☐ Hx latex sensitivity

BP _____ T _____ P _____ R _____

FHR _____ Vag exam _____

Reason for Admission

☐ Labour / SROM ☐ Induction _____

☐ Primary C/S _____ ☐ Repeat C/S

☐ Observation _____

☐ OB / Medical complication _____

Onset of labour: ☐ Not in labour
Date _____ Time _____
Membranes: ☐ Intact
☐ Ruptured / Date _____ Time _____
☐ Clear ☐ Meconium ☐ Bloody ☐ Foul
Vaginal bleeding: ☐ None
☐ Normal show ☐ _____

Current Pregnancy Labs   ☐ NPC

☐ POL ☐ PPROM ☐ Cerclage
☐ PIH ☐ Chr. HTN ☐ Other _____
☐ Diabetes _____ Diet _____
☐ Insulin _____
☐ Amniocentesis _____ Results _____
Bld type / RH____ Anti-D IgG ____
Antibody screen ☐Neg ☐Pos

	Pos	Neg	Tested
Hepatitis B	☐	☐	☐ No
HIV	☐	☐	☐ No
Group B strep	☐	☐	☐ No
GC	☐	☐	☐ No
Chlamydia	☐	☐	☐ No
RPR	☐	☐	☐ No

Rubella ☐Non-immune ☐ Immune
Diabetic screen ☐ Normal ☐Abnormal
Recent exposure to chick pox ☐
Current meds:_____

Previous OB History

☐ POL ☐ Multiple gestation
☐ Prev C/S type _____ Reason _____
☐ Pre-eclampsia ☐ Chronic HTN ☐ Diabetes _____
☐ Stillbirth/demise ☐ Neodeath ☐ Anomalies
☐ Precipitous labour (<3 H) ☐ Macrosomia
☐ PP Hemorrhage
☐ Hx Transfusion reaction ☐Yes ☐ No
☐ Other _____

Latest risk assessment ☐ None
1. _____ 3. _____
2. _____ 4. _____

Date _____
Signature _____ Time _____

NEUROLOGICAL

☐ WNL
Variance: ☐HA
☐ Scotoma / visual changes
Reflexes ☐ < 2 + ☐ > 2 +
☐ Clonus ___ bts
☐ Numbness ☐ Tingling
☐ Hx Seizures
☐

RESPIRATORY

☐ WNL
Variance: ☐ Hx Asthma ☐URI
Respirations: ☐< 12 ☐> 24
Effort: ☐ SOB
☐ Shallow ☐ Laboured
Auscultation:
☐ Diminished ☐ Crackles
☐ Wheezes ☐ Rhonchi   No Yes
Cough for greater than 2 weeks? ☐ ☐
Is the cough productive? ☐ ☐
Blood in the sputum? ☐ ☐
Experiencing any fever or night sweats? ☐ ☐
Ever had TB in the past? ☐ ☐
Recent exposure to TB? ☐ ☐
Weight loss in last 3 weeks? ☐ ☐
If the patient answers yes to any three of the above questions implement policy and procedure # 5725-0704.

GASTROINTESTINAL

☐ WNL
Variance: ☐ Heartburn
☐ Epigastric pain   Nausea
☐ Vomiting ☐ Diarrhea
☐ Constipation ☐ Pain
☐ Wt. Gain < 2lbs / month**
☐ Recent change in appetite of
< 50% of usual intake for > 5 days

INTEGUMENTARY

☐ WNL
Variance: ☐ Rash ☐ Lacerations
☐ Abrasion ☐ Swelling
☐ Urticaria ☐ Bruising
☐ Diaphoretic/hot
☐ Clammy/cold
☐ Scars
☐

FETAL ASSESSMENT

☐ WNL
Variance:
☐NRFS
FHR ☐ < 110 ☐ > 160
LTV ☐ Absent ☐ Minimal
☐ Increased
STV Absent
Decelerations: _____
☐ Decreased fetal movement
☐ IUGR
☐

Tobacco use	☐Denies	☐Yes	Amt _____
Alcohol use	☐Denies	☐Yes	Amt _____
Drug use	☐Denies	☐Yes	Amt type_____
Primary language	☐English	☐Spanish	

CARDIOVASCULAR

☐ WNL
Variance:
☐MVP
Heart rate: ☐< 60 ☐ > 100
B/P: Systolic: ☐< 90 ☐ > 140
Diastolic: ☐< 50 ☐ > 90
☐ Edema _____
☐ Chest pain / palpitations
☐

MUSCULOSKELETAL

☐ WNL
Variance:
☐ Numbness ☐ Tingling
☐ Paralysis ☐ Deformity
☐ Scoliosis
☐

GENITOURINARY

☐ WNL
Variance: ☐ Albumin _____
Output: ☐ < 30 cc/Hr.
☐ UTI ☐ Rx ☐ Frequency
☐ Dysuria ☐ Hematuria
☐ CVA Tenderness
☐ Hx STD _____
☐ Vag. discharge _____
☐ Rash ☐ Blisters
☐ Warts ☐ Lesions
☐

EARS, NOSE, THROAT, AND EYES

☐ WNL
Variance:
☐ Sore throat ☐ Eyeglasses
☐ Runny nose ☐ Contact lenses
☐ Nasal congestion

PSYCHOSOCIAL

☐ WNL
Variance: ☐ Hx depression
☐ Yes ☐ No
☐ Emotional behavioral care
Affect: ☐ Flat ☐ Anxious
☐ Uncooperative ☐ Combative
Living will ☐ Yes ☐ No
☐ On chart
Healthcare surrogate ☐ Yes ☐No
☐ On chart
Are you being hurt, hit, frightened by anyone
at home or in your life? ☐Yes ☐ No
Religious preference _____
_____

PAIN ASSESSMENT

1. Do you have any ongoing pain problems? ☐ No ☐ Yes
2. Do you have any pain now? ☐ No ☐ Yes
3. If any of the above questions are answered yes, the patient has a positive pain screening.
4. Patient to be given pain management education material.
   Complete pain / symptom assessment on flowsheet.
5. *Please proceed to complete pain assessment.*

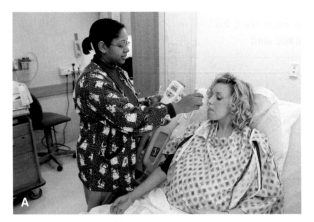
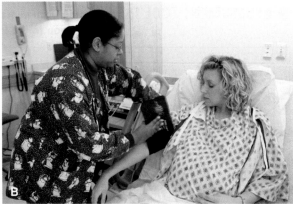

FIGURE 15.18 The nurse assesses maternal vital signs upon admission to the health care facility for childbirth.

NURSING PROCEDURE 15.1
Testing for Rupture of Membranes

PURPOSE

To determine the status of the amniotic membranes during labour and to differentiate amniotic fluid from urine and bloody show

ASSESSMENT AND PLANNING

- Assess the client's knowledge of and previous exposure to the procedure.
- Question the client about any report of a sudden gush of fluid or slow trickle of fluid.
- Inspect the fluid for colour if possible.
- Gather the necessary equipment:
  - Nitrazine test paper
  - Sterile speculum
  - Glass slide
  - Sterile cotton-tipped applicator
  - Microscope
  - Sterile gloves

IMPLEMENTATION

1. Explain the procedure to the client and answer any questions *to help allay her anxiety.*
2. Position the client for a vaginal examination.
3. Wash hands.
4. Expose the perineal area, making sure to keep the client covered as much as possible *to ensure privacy and promote adequate access to the perineum.*
5. Put on sterile gloves; obtain a small strip of Nitrazine paper, approximately 2 inches in length, making sure that bare hands do not come in contact with the paper *to prevent contaminating the test strip.*
6. Spread the labia with the nondominant hand and apply a small section of the Nitrazine paper to the vaginal opening near the cervical os until it is wet to obtain a sample of fluid. *An adequate sample is needed to ensure the accuracy of the results.*
7. Compare the colour of the test strip with the colour guide on the paper container *to determine the pH of the secretions.*

(continued)

NURSING PROCEDURE 15.1 (CONTINUED)
Testing for Rupture of Membranes

8. Interpret the findings; if the test strip turns blue (blue-green, blue-grey, or deep blue), then the pH is alkaline and suggests rupture of membranes; if the test strip is yellow, olive-yellow, or olive-green, then the pH is acidic and membranes are probably intact.
9. *Alternatively*, perform or assist with a sterile vaginal examination to obtain a specimen of fluid with a sterile cotton-tipped applicator to ensure collection of an accurate specimen *without contamination*; apply the fluid to a glass slide and allow to dry.
10. Observe the slide under the microscope for a ferning appearance, *which indicates a high estrogen content suggestive of amniotic fluid and ruptured membranes.*
11. Provide perineal care *to promote client comfort.*
12. Remove gloves and wash hands.
13. Report and document the findings.

EVALUATION

- The client tolerated the procedure without difficulty.
- Rupture of membranes confirmed.

AREAS FOR CONSIDERATION AND ADAPTATION

Perinatal Considerations

- If necessary, use a sterile cotton-tipped applicator to obtain a specimen of fluid from the posterior vagina during a sterile vaginal examination. Then apply the applicator to the test strip.
- Be aware that false test results may occur if inadequate fluid is obtained.

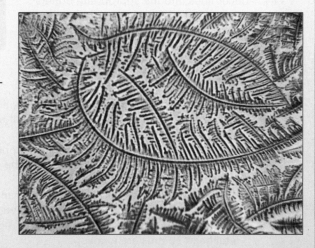

---

type and Rh factor, and serologic testing (Rouse & St. John, 2003).

Select Potential Nursing Diagnoses

Nursing diagnoses commonly included in the care of a woman experiencing the first stage of labour are as follows:

- **Pain** related to increasing intensity of uterine contractions and progression of labour
- **Risk for Injury** (maternal or fetal) related to potential complications associated with labour
- **Anxiety** related to uncertainty of the progression of labour and anticipated birth
- **Anxiety** related to first experience with labour and birth
- **Powerlessness** related to inability to cope with demands and work of labour
- **Deficient Knowledge** related to labour process and events
- **Risk for Deficient Fluid Volume** related to limited fluid intake, increased insensible fluid loss, or fluid replacement
- **Ineffective Breathing Pattern** related to inappropriate use of breathing techniques
- **Fatigue** related to duration of the labour process and energy expenditure

NURSING PROCEDURE 15.2
Applying an External Electronic Fetal Monitor

PURPOSE

To assess FHR and uterine contractions continuously during labour.

ASSESSMENT AND PLANNING

* Assess the client's knowledge of and previous exposure to the procedure.
* Auscultate FHR and maternal vital signs; assess contractions by palpation.
* Perform Leopold manoeuvers *to determine the location of the fetal back and best area to assess FHR.*
* Gather the necessary equipment:
  * Electronic fetal monitor with paper installed
  * Tocodynamometer
  * Ultrasound transducer
  * Belts or Velcro to secure transducers
  * Conductive gel

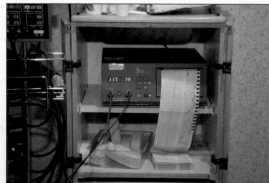

* Plug in the monitor and insert the transducer lines into the appropriate outlets on the front of the monitor.
* Turn on the monitor and run a test strip.

IMPLEMENTATION

1. Wash hands.
2. Place the client in a comfortable position, elevating the head of the bed approximately 30 degrees; if appropriate, place the client in a side lying position *to maximize uteroplacental blood flow.*
3. Place one belt under the woman at the upper part of her abdomen and the other at her lower abdomen and bring the edges of the belt out to the side *to facilitate securing the transducers once they are in place.*
4. Apply conductive gel to the ultrasound transducer *to ensure sound transmission* and place it on the client's abdomen in the area of the fetal back *to hear the FHR.*
5. Increase the volume on the monitor and reposition the transducer to the area where the fetal heart sounds are loudest.
6. Secure the transducer with the lower belt.
7. Palpate the uterine fundus to determine where it is the firmest and apply the tocodynamometer at that location.
8. Secure the tocodynamometer with the upper belt.
9. Observe the recording from the monitor *to ensure that the monitor is recording the events.* Record the date and time of initiating EFM along with the client's vital signs and identifying information.
10. If necessary, reposition the woman comfortably, making sure that the EFM is working correctly.

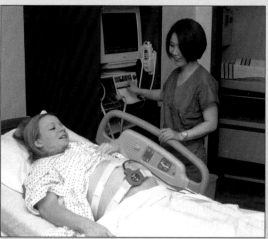

(continued)

NURSING PROCEDURE 15.2 (CONTINUED)
Applying an External Electronic Fetal Monitor

11. Place the client's call light within easy reach.
12. Wash your hands.
13. Document the procedure.

EVALUATION

- Client tolerated procedure without difficulty
- External EFM applied
- Tracing is adequate for interpretation

AREAS FOR CONSIDERATION AND ADAPTATION

Perinatal Considerations

- Be aware that telemetry-like units are available for external EFM so that the woman can ambulate and get out of bed without disrupting the monitoring.
- Warn the woman that the conductive gel may feel cold to her skin.
- Assess FHR patterns frequently for periodic and episodic changes that might indicate fetal distress.

Planning/Intervention

As with all care, goal setting and implementation need to be individualized to the client's specific circumstances. Assessment Tool 15.2 provides a sample of a chart used to document labour's progress over time.

Early Labour

During early labour, the woman may have difficulty believing that she is really in labour. The best thing for her to do is to take good care of herself. Alternating between rest and activity may be helpful (e.g., a long walk followed by a warm shower). The nurse should encourage her to eat easily digested foods (e.g., tea and toast) and to drink plenty of fluids. The SOGC (2007) recommends a light or liquid diet be offered to a woman in active labour. Examples of clear liquids include water, juice, fruit juices without pulp, carbonated beverages, clear tea, and black coffee. Offering women clear fluids during labour enhances maternal comfort and satisfaction (American Society of Anesthesiologists, 2006). A recent study found no difference in rates of medical interventions, adverse birth outcomes, or vomiting between eating and noneating groups of labouring women; however, the same study showed that eating during early labour may increase labour's total duration (Parsons et al., 2006).

Many women find that home is the best place to be during this phase because they can move about easily and do things for themselves. Findings from a Swed-ish study indicated that first-time mothers who stayed at home during the latent stage of labour felt strengthened and developed a sense of decision-making power over their bodies (Carlsson et al., 2012). When contractions become so strong that she cannot talk through them, the client should begin using relaxation and breathing techniques. She may find it comforting to have support people nearby, helping her to stay calm and confident.

Active Labour

During contractions in active labour, many women find it helpful to develop a rhythmic response, using breathing, movement, and sound, followed by rest between contractions. Birthing balls can be valuable tools (Fig. 15.19). While leaning or sitting on the ball, the woman can rock, move, or circle her hips to decrease discomfort. Movement also stimulates the release of endorphins, the body's natural painkiller (Simkin & Ancheta, 2000). When women are encouraged to respond to their own body's cues, assuming different positions, labour may progress more efficiently (Romano & Lothian, 2008).

Ambulation during labour has many benefits. It facilitates progress by stimulating more effective contractions, increases pressure of the presenting part against the cervix to facilitate effacement and dilation, and promotes fetal rotation and descent. It may promote comfort and offer diversion and stimulation. Many women find walking beneficial during early and active labour (Fig. 15.20).

(text continues on page 609)

● ASSESSMENT TOOL 15.2   Sample Labour Flow Sheet*

Labour Progress Chart
Maternal/Newborn Record System

Admit date	Admit time	Blood type and Rh	Age	G	T	Pt	A	L	EDD___/___/___	Membranes	☐ Intact	☐ Ruptured SROM AROM
___/___/___									LMP___/___/___		☐ Bulging	Date___/___/___ Time___

	Current date ___/___/___	Time →																			

Vital signs
- Temperature
- Pulse
- Respiration /O$_2$ saturation
- Blood pressure

Maternal
- Deep tendon reflexes (L/R)   / / / / / / / / / / / / /
- Urine (protein/sugar)   / / / / / / / / / / / / /
- Vaginal bleeding
- Pain
- Edema (site, extent)

Uterine activity
- Monitor mode
- Frequency
- Duration
- Peak IUP
- Resting tone
- Intensity
- MVUs

Fetal assessment
- Monitor mode (Strip #____)
- Baseline (FHR)
- STV
- LTV
- Accelerations
- Decelerations
- Membranes/fluid
- Scalp pH

Intake/output (mLs/Hr)
- IV
- PO
- Urine
- Emesis

Cont meds
- Pitocin mU/min
- Magnesium sulfate gms/hr

Intervention
- Treatments
- Teaching/support
- Touch
- Position/activity
- Physical care

Initials

Abbreviations/key

Deep tendon reflexes	Vaginal bleeding	Pain	Uterine activity monitor mode	MVUs Montevideo units	Fetal monitor mode	STV short-term variability
0 = No response +1 = Sluggish +2 = Normal +3 = Hyperactive +4 = Brisk + hyperactive C = Clonus	NS = Normal show ABN = Frank vaginal bleeding	0 = No pain ⋮ 5 = Distressing pain ⋮ 10 = Highest intensity	P = Palpation E = External I = Internal	The sum of the peak of each uterine contraction minus its resting tone, in a 10-minute period.	A = Auscultation (fetoscope) D = Doppler E = External I = Internal	+ = Present (roughness of tracing line present) ∅ = Absent (tracing line is smooth) **LTV long-term variability** ∅ = 0– 2 BPM = Absent ↓ = 3– 5 BPM = Minimal + = 6–25 BPM = Absent ↑ = greater than 25 BPM = Marked

(continued)

● **ASSESSMENT TOOL 15.2**   **Sample Labour Flow Sheet** *(Continued)*

Labour Progress Chart
Maternal/Newborn Record System

Current date	Allergy/sensitivity	☐ None	☐ Latex		
/ /	☐ Other			Chart_____ of _____	

Accelerations
++ = 15 BPM ↑X 15 sec
+ = less than 15 BPM
↑+/or less than 15 sec
0 = None
Decelerations
N = None   L = Late
E = Early   P = Prolonged
V = Variable

Membranes
I = Intact
B = Bulging
R = Ruptured
Fluid
C = Clear
M = Meconium stained
B = Bloody
F = Foul odor
NF = No foul odor

Treatments
O₂ = O₂ L/min
IVB = IV bolus
SC = Straight catheterization
FC = Foley catheterization
ABD = Abdominal hair removal

Teaching/support
O = Orient to unit
SR = Safety review
LR = Labour review
F = Focusing
BRT = Breathing/relaxation techniques
PrO = PreOp.

Touch
E = Effleurage
B = Backrub
CP = Counterpressure
M = Massage

Position/activity
W = Walking
C = Chair
SQ = Squatting
JR = Jet hydrotherapy
SH = Shower
K = Kneeling
LS = Left side
RS = Right side
KC = Knee chest
T = Trendelenburg

Physical care
MC = Mouth care
SC = Superficial cold
SH = Superficial heat
PC = Peri care
BP = Bedpan

(continued)

● **ASSESSMENT TOOL 15.2** **Sample Labour Flow Sheet** *(Continued)*

Labour Progress Chart
Maternal/Newborn Record System

COMPOSITE NORMAL DILATATION CURVES

COMPOSITE CURVES OF ABNORMAL LABOUR PROGRESS—MULTIPAROUS

Labour progress curves derived from the work of Emanuel A. Friedman, M.D.

IV Record

Start date	Time	Site	Solution	Amount (mL's)	Medication/dose added	Initials	Infused date	Time	Amount infused

Interval medications

Date, time	Medication/dose	Route	Site	Initials

Signature key

Initials	Signature

*Courtesy of Briggs Corporation.

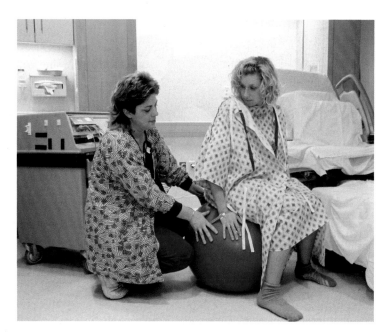

FIGURE 15.19 While leaning or sitting on the birthing ball, the labouring woman can move in various ways to ease discomfort.

Although ambulation during labour has many benefits, many women may not walk during labour. The Listening to Mothers survey consisted of phone or electronic mail interviews about women's labour and birth experiences. Of the 1,583 women who responded, 71% reported that they did not walk around even once after regular contractions began. The primary reason given for not walking was that they were "connected to things." Other reasons reported for staying in bed were pain drugs "that made them unable to support themselves," being told by care providers not to walk around, and grogginess from pain medication. Twenty percent chose to stay in one place (Declercq et al., 2002). As long as there are no maternal or fetal contraindications, the nurse is responsible for suggesting walking and providing assistance as needed, because the client in labour may not consider this option. If the woman has an IV line inserted, she can take the IV pole with her as she ambulates. If EFM is being used, the nurse can disconnect the leads for short intervals if FHR and variability are normal. An alternative is the use of wireless transducers for external EFM. Ambulation should not be advised for clients receiving medication or when there is concern about maternal or fetal status.

Labouring women may find a warm bath relaxing. The buoyancy of water helps relieve discomfort; warmth may relieve tension (Cluett et al., 2004). Relaxation and warmth may also help labour progress (Primeau et al., 2003). Using a handheld showerhead to direct water onto the abdomen also may be soothing. The tingling water stimulates the skin, resulting in less awareness of pain. Sometimes, alternating applications of warm and cold compresses is more effective than using just one or the other. Cold packs are particularly useful for musculoskeletal and joint pain; back pain usually responds particularly well to cold therapy.

As contraction strength increases, so does the woman's need for continuous support. Thus, companionship from a birth partner or family members becomes more important as labour progresses (Gilliland, 2002) (Fig. 15.21). One successful measure for reducing labour pain is the continuous presence of a professionally trained, supportive companion who focuses on the

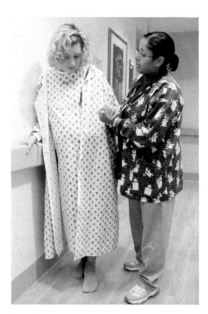

FIGURE 15.20 Walking and moving during labour can help relieve pain and may assist with moving labour forward.

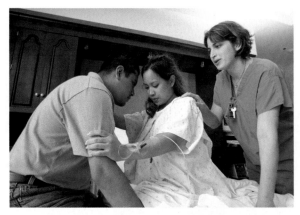

FIGURE 15.21 Ongoing assistance with breathing and pain management techniques from partners, support people, nurses, and doulas can be of great benefit to women in labour.

woman throughout each contraction. This person can softly speak words of reassurance and encouragement, stroke the client, hold her hand, walk with her, suggest position changes, instruct her, and reassure her partner. Controlled trials have shown that such a person, often called a **doula** from the Greek word meaning "woman's servant," improves obstetric outcomes and client satisfaction compared with usual hospital care (Berg & Terstad, 2006; Declercq et al., 2002; Pascali-Bonaro & Kroeger, 2004). Clear evidence demonstrates the effectiveness of physical, emotional, and psychological support for women during childbirth (Gilliland, 2002). Research has also demonstrated consistently that birth

satisfaction is linked to the amount of support a woman receives from caregivers, the quality of her relationship with them, her involvement with decision making, and her personal expectations (Goodman et al., 2004; Hodnett, 2002) (Research Highlight 15.1). The SOGC (2007) maintains that continuous available labour support by professional registered nurses is a critical component in achieving positive birth outcomes.

Changing positions frequently not only helps the woman stay more comfortable but also encourages labour to progress. Under normal circumstances, the nurse should encourage the client to adopt whatever position is most comfortable (Gupta & Hofmeyr, 2004). If progress slows, changes in position and movement may help without causing excessive pain (Table 15.5). Experienced caregivers try not to restrict clients but suggest alternatives and encourage them to seek comfortable positions (Gupta & Hofmeyr, 2004).

A peaceful and personalized environment can influence labour positively (Hodnett et al., 2005). Although a small but increasing number of Canadian labours occur in nonhospital settings, the most common birth site remains the hospital. The hospital environment may be very different from the woman's home or a free-standing birth centre. To some clients whose cultural belief is that birth is natural and best supported without medical intervention (unless complications arise), the hospital may represent illness or death. Many hospitals today provide home-like birth settings, and some have single-room labour, delivery, recovery, postpartum (LDRP) units (Fig. 15.22). Some women find that bringing favourite

---

● **RESEARCH HIGHLIGHT 15.1**   **Why Do Some Women Change Their Opinion About Childbirth Over Time?**

PURPOSE

To study women's memories of childbirth, compare their immediate feelings with recollections at various stages, and determine influential variables in changed perceptions.

DESIGN

The investigator analyzed questionnaires completed by women 2 months postpartum and 1 year postpartum and grouped findings into two subsamples: those who said childbirth was positive and those who said it was negative at 2 months postpartum. Within each sample, the researcher then compared psychosocial background, labour outcomes, infant health outcomes, and experiences of intrapartum care for those whose 1-year assessment was consistent with their 2-month report, as well as those whose views had changed.

RESULTS

Evaluations of childbirth that became more negative with time were associated with labour complications, dissatisfaction with intrapartum care, psychosocial problems, and depression. Improved assessments with time were associated with positive interactions with and support from birth attendants.

NURSING IMPLICATIONS

Supportive care from those who work with women giving birth can have long-term effects whose influence grows with time. Such assistance may also protect against negative memories and general dissatisfaction.

From Waldenstrom, U. (2004). Why do some women change their opinion about childbirth over time? *Birth, 31*(2), 102–107.

● TABLE 15.5   **Positions for Labour**

Position	Description
 Lithotomy	The woman is flat with her legs in stirrups. This position provides the birth attendant with good access to the perineum and allows him or her to control the birth. Risks for supine hypotensive syndrome and injury are increased.
 Modified dorsal recumbent	The woman is sitting up in bed with her feet placed on pedals. This position provides the birth attendant with good access to the perineum and allows him or her to control the birth. It is not comfortable for the woman and does not assist with fetal expulsion.
 Side-lying	The woman lies on her side. This position may increase maternal comfort; however, it may be awkward for the birth attendant and require assistance from a third party to hold the woman's upper leg during birth.
 Squatting	The woman squats. This position can enhance maternal comfort and relies on gravity to facilitate fetal expulsion. The woman is at risk for losing her balance and thus needs support from another person behind her or the use of a birthing bar or stool.

(table continues on page 612)

● TABLE 15.5   **Positions for Labour** (continued)

Position	Description
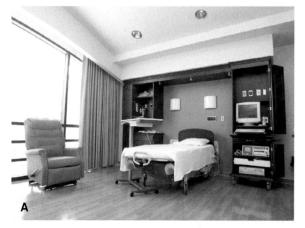 Hands and knees	The woman gets on her hands and knees with assistance from others. This position encourages rotation of the fetal head and perineal stretching and provides the best access to the perineum for the birth attendant. The woman may become tired. This position usually prohibits the use of instruments for assistance.

pictures and pillows and wearing their own nightgowns can personalize the environment. Music and dim lights also may help them cope well with labour.

Transition

During transition, the client may find it helpful to focus on one contraction at a time. She should continue breathing during contractions. Even though rest between contractions becomes shorter, the nurse should encourage the client to relax and to use the time to restore her energy. Those providing labour support should offer close, undivided attention; gentle, unwavering encouragement; and praise. As with earlier phases of this first stage, ongoing assessment of maternal and fetal well-being is crucial.

Evaluation

Interventions during the first stage of labour are effective if the client progresses without developing any complications. The fetus should demonstrate normal FHR patterns between 110 and 160 bpm. In addition, the client uses various techniques to achieve a tolerable level of pain and participates in decision making. If problems develop, appropriate interventions are instituted to ensure maternal and fetal well-being.

Second Stage: Pushing or Expulsion

Once the cervix is dilated fully, the woman is said to move into the **second stage of labour** and begins pushing (when an urge is felt). At this time, the fetus manoeuvres through the maternal pelvis, rotating and slowly descending through the birth canal. This stage can last from 15 minutes to several hours (Cunningham et al., 2005). For some women, initial contractions during this stage are strong and powerful, causing an

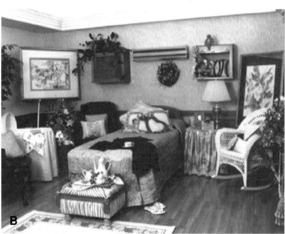

FIGURE 15.22   A: An LDRP (labour, delivery, recovery, postpartum) unit in a hospital. **B**: A home-like unit in a birthing centre. (Photos courtesy of Joe Mitchell.)

overwhelmingly strong urge to push. As they experience this feeling, many clients become very focused on the task at hand. For some women, however, second-stage contractions increase gradually, similarly to those of first-stage labour. Pressure grows as the fetus descends. Women may grunt or groan with the contractions. It is not unusual for clients to hold their breath instinctively as they bear down (Roberts, 2002).

When the fetus reaches the maternal perineum, contractions are intense and often accompanied by burning or stretching. The perineum begins to bulge outward, the labia separate, and the presenting fetal part (usually the head) gradually becomes visible. After each contraction, the fetal head recedes somewhat until the next contraction, when it bulges a little more. Eventually the fetal head reaches a point at which it no longer recedes. This is called **crowning**. As the head descends, the pelvic floor becomes thin and shiny, and the anus protrudes. When the head emerges, the woman usually experiences tremendous relief and some pressure with delivery of the shoulders. Then the rest of the fetus moves out easily (Fig. 15.23).

The time for all this to happen varies widely, depending partly on fetal size and position, as well as on the woman's freedom to move into different positions. Breathing that the woman uses for pushing (i.e., prolonged breath holding versus controlled exhalation) also can influence the effectiveness of her efforts. Fear may influence expulsion. A woman who is scared of birth or anticipated pain may be reluctant to push.

See Figure 15.24 for an illustrated sequence of a normal vaginal birth.

COLLABORATIVE CARE: SECOND STAGE OF LABOUR
Assessment
Assessment during the second stage involves monitoring of maternal vital signs. The nurse assesses, as required,

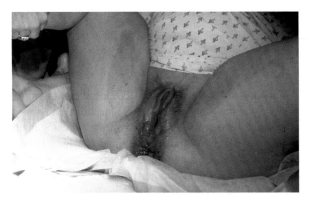

FIGURE 15.23 As the fetal head pushes down, the perineum bulges. This sign indicates that birth is imminent. (Copyright © Barbara Proud.)

cervical dilation and effacement and fetal station. The nurse should check uterine contractions frequently. At this time, the woman may voice a strong urge to push because of pressure from the fetal head.

For pregnancies considered to be low risk, FHR patterns are monitored every 15 minutes when not pushing, and every 5 minutes when pushing (SOGC, 2007). The nurse should monitor the FHR for signs of abnormal pattern and intervene as necessary to maintain the supportive physiologic goals of the maternal–fetal unit. The nurse should consider the woman's psychosocial status and ability to handle the increased physical and emotional stress of this time. Because of the increased intensity and frequency of contractions, she may find coping difficult. On the other hand, she may have less apprehension or feel relieved now that she can sense the urge to push and sees an end in sight.

Select Potential Nursing Diagnoses
Nursing diagnoses commonly associated with the care of a woman in the second stage of labour may include the following:

- **Pain** related to the increased intensity and frequency of contractions
- **Ineffective Coping** related to unfamiliar sensations and increased intensity of contractions
- **Fatigue** related to prolonged efforts of pushing
- **Risk for Injury** (maternal or fetal) related to inappropriate pushing techniques, umbilical cord compression

Planning/Intervention
The health care team must individualize second-stage management. Nevertheless, certain universal interventions are recommended (AWHONN, 2006).

- Teach women prenatally about the benefits of upright positions.
- During labour, encourage women to change positions frequently. Suggested positions include squatting, semirecumbent, standing, and upright kneeling.
- Allow women to rest until they feel an urge to push.
- Encourage spontaneous bearing down.
- Support, rather than direct, the client's involuntary pushing efforts.
- Discourage prolonged maternal breath holding (more than 6 to 8 seconds).
- Validate the normalcy of sensations and sounds the woman is voicing.

During the second stage, the urge to push usually feels strongest at the peak of the contraction and then fades toward the end. Women should follow along and do what feels right. Evidence from a recent systemic review supports spontaneous pushing and suggests that

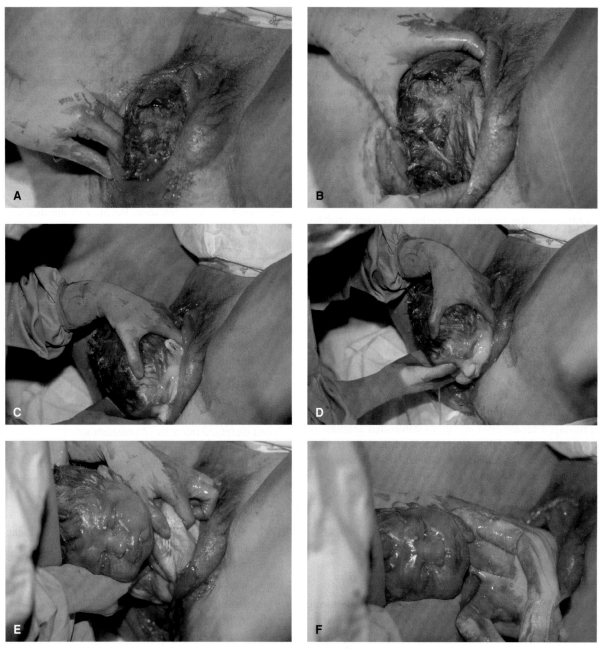

FIGURE 15.24   Normal vaginal birth sequence. **A**: Early crowning. **B**: Late crowning. The fetal head is face down in normal occiput anterior position. **C, D**: Extension of the fetal head (right occiput anterior position). **E**: Birth of the shoulders. **F**: Emergence of the rest of the fetal body, including the umbilical cord.

women follow the feelings of their bodies, and using bearing-down efforts and urges to push that work for them under the guidance and assistance of the nurse (Prins et al., 2011). For most clients, this means taking normal breaths as the contraction builds and then pushing when the urge becomes irresistible (Hansen et al., 2002). Some women find it helps to make sounds in response to what they are feeling. Low-pitched groaning, sighing, and moaning may help release tension, which may assist

in coping with pain (Roberts, 2002). Labour supporters should validate the normalcy of sensations and sounds she makes and provide quiet, reassuring encouragement. Some women may find cheering and coaching helpful, but this behaviour may annoy others. Individualized support for the client and her partner is most important (Bloom et al., 2006). If progress is slow, the nurse can encourage the client to change positions. For example, benefits of upright or lateral positions compared to supine

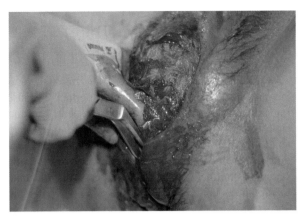

FIGURE 15.25 Episiotomy.

or lithotomy positions include reduced duration of second-stage labour, reduced assisted deliveries, reduced episiotomies, and smaller increases in second-degree perineal tears (Carroli & Mignini, 2009; Eason et al., 2000). The nurse should urge the client to release tension in the perineum. Warm compresses may help with relaxing this area. It is most important for the woman to rest between contractions. Pushing is hard work.

Episiotomy is a surgical incision into the perineum to enlarge the outlet (Fig. 15.25). It was introduced as an obstetric intervention in the late 1800s based on a belief that it would protect the perineum from severe lacerations. Historically, obstetricians also proposed that the use of episiotomy improved future sexual function and reduced urine and fecal incontinence. Research findings, however, suggest otherwise. Episiotomy is associated with increased third- and fourth-degree lacerations and greater postpartum pain compared with spontaneous lacerations (Eason & Feldman, 2000; Hartmann et al., 2005). Research shows no reliable evidence that routine use of episiotomy has any beneficial maternal effect (Carroli & Mignini, 2009). On the contrary, clear evidence shows that it may cause harm, such as greater need for surgical repair and poorer future sexual capacity (Nager & Helliwell, 2001). Although hospitals vary widely in their use of episiotomies, in recent years it appears that the number of routine episiotomies has decreased (Goldberg et al., 2002; Webb & Culhane, 2002).

Although there is no maternal indication for routine episiotomy, sometimes there are fetal indications for the procedure. Because episiotomy does shorten the second stage of labour, it may be indicated in cases of fetal distress.

Evaluation

Interventions during the second stage of labour are effective when the woman pushes successfully without experiencing fatigue and maternal and fetal well-being are maintained in preparation for birth.

QUOTE 15-2
"It was hard work. Really, really tough. But look at my little one! Yes, it was worth it."

From a woman who just gave birth after 13 hours of labour

Third Stage: Afterbirth

The **third stage of labour** refers to the separation and expulsion of the **afterbirth**, or placenta and membranes. This stage usually occurs spontaneously within 5 to 30 minutes of the fetus emerging from the birth canal (Smith & Brennan, 2004). After this time, the uterus relaxes for a few minutes. Then contractions begin again. This causes the placenta to fold and separate from the uterus. Bleeding on the maternal side of the placenta occurs, further helping the placenta to separate. Separation leads to movement of the placenta to the lower uterus or upper vagina.

Indications that placental expulsion is imminent include the following:

- Lengthening of the umbilical cord
- A sudden gush of blood
- Change in uterine shape to globular and ascent into the abdomen

These signs usually occur within 5 to 10 minutes of birth. Maternal bearing-down efforts may lead to actual expulsion of the placenta. When examined, the placenta may present with the shiny, glistening fetal side (indicating separation first at the centre and then at the edges; called Schultze mechanism), or the red, raw, rough-shaped maternal side (indicating that the placenta separated at the edges first; called Duncan mechanism). See Figure 15.26.

Contractions during third-stage labour are mild to moderate. They usually feel like strong menstrual cramps. Many women overlook them because they are focused on seeing their babies. Some women experience generalized shivering during this stage, which may result from a low environmental temperature, the sudden release of pressure on the pelvic nerves, or excess epinephrine production during labour (Smith & Brennan, 2004). The woman also may experience a range of other physical symptoms such as hunger, thirst, exhaustion, or bladder distention.

After expulsion of the placenta, the birth attendant examines the woman's cervix, vaginal tract, and perineum for lacerations. Lacerations are common in women who experience a difficult or precipitate birth, a birth of a baby weighing more than 4.1 kg, or a birth that involves the use of the lithotomy position and instrumentation, such as forceps (see Chapter 16). Lacerations may occur anywhere along the birth canal, commonly affecting the perineum. Perineal lacerations are classified as first, second, third, or fourth degree,

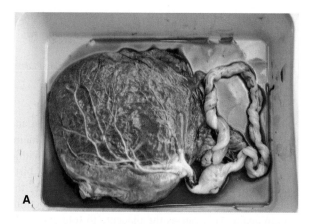

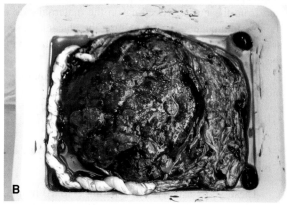

FIGURE 15.26 Placenta. **A**: Schultze mechanism—fetal side. **B**: Duncan mechanism—maternal side.

depending on the extent and depth of tissue involvement. See Table 15.6.

One of the most important issues during this time is protecting the woman against the dangers of postpartum hemorrhage. Active management of the third stage of labour, consisting of administration of IV or IM oxytocin after delivery of the anterior shoulder, contributes to a significant decrease in the incidence of postpartum hemorrhage (SOGC, 2009). Postpartum hemorrhage is discussed in detail in Chapters 18 and 19.

● TABLE 15.6 **Lacerations**

Degree	Characteristics
First degree	Involve the fourchette, perineal skin, and vaginal mucous membrane, but no muscle
Second degree	Involve all of the above and the muscles of the perineum, but not the rectal sphincter
Third degree	Involve all of the above and the rectal sphincter
Fourth degree	Involve all of the above and extend through the rectum

COLLABORATIVE CARE: THIRD STAGE OF LABOUR
Assessment

Assessment continues throughout the third stage of labour and becomes especially important because, immediately after birth, nurses are frequently responsible for both the woman and her newborn (see Chapter 20). When the placenta has been delivered in the third stage of labour, the birth attendant assesses the status of uterine contractility, inspects the placenta, membranes, and cord, and inspects and repairs any episiotomy or lacerations of the cervix, vagina, or perineum. The umbilical cord should contain two arteries and one vein. Blood samples from the umbilical cord arteries or vein may be drawn promptly after delivery of the placenta and sent for cord blood analysis. Analysis of cord blood may be done for blood typing should the newborn require emergency blood replacement therapy. In newborns who demonstrated abnormal FHR patterns during labour, exhibited respiratory depression or low Apgar scores at birth, or had meconium-stained amniotic fluid, cord blood may be used to evaluate for acidemia secondary to possible cord compression or placental hypoperfusion. An umbilical cord blood sample also may be obtained for a direct Coombs test to detect the presence of maternal Rh-positive antibodies (see Chapter 22).

Select Potential Nursing Diagnoses

Nursing diagnoses that may be applicable during the third stage of labour are similar to those for the second stage of labour, with the following additions:

1. **Risk for Injury** (maternal and newborn) related to birth process, possible hemorrhage
2. **Risk for Deficient Fluid Volume** related to blood loss during birth
3. **Deficient Knowledge** related to birth and body system changes after birth
4. **Risk for Infection** related to perineal lacerations, creation of episiotomy
5. **Readiness for Parenting** related to birth of newborn and immediate bonding

Planning/Intervention

After birth of the baby, the woman needs continued support for delivery of the placenta, examination of the genital tract, and repair of the episiotomy or lacerations. Ongoing assessment of the uterine fundus is essential. Relaxation techniques and breathing strategies she used throughout first-stage labour will be helpful at this time as well to deal with any discomforts.

Evaluation

The desired outcomes associated with the third stage of labour include birth of a healthy newborn, expulsion of an intact placenta, and evidence of beginning uterine involution. In addition, the woman experiences blood loss less than 500 mL and reports a significant decrease in pain (Cunningham et al., 2005). Moreover, the mother and her partner demonstrate beginning bonding behaviours with their newborn.

Fourth Stage: Immediate Postpartum

The **fourth stage of labour** refers to the period immediately after delivery of the placenta. It typically lasts 1 to 4 hours and may be referred to as the recovery phase (Cunningham et al., 2005). During this period, the woman's body begins to undergo several major physiologic changes as it starts returning to a nonpregnant state. Intra-abdominal pressure decreases markedly from birth of the baby and delivery of the placenta. The uterus should be well contracted, in the midline of the abdomen, and between the symphysis and umbilicus. Uterine contraction is a major means of achieving hemostasis. If inadequate, postpartum hemorrhage can occur. Therefore, frequent continued assessment of the uterine fundus is essential.

Major hemodynamic changes result from normal blood loss at delivery and decreased intra-abdominal pressure. With placental expulsion, blood flow to the placenta is no longer needed. As a result, blood is shunted to the maternal systemic venous circulation. In addition, blood volume decreases because of the blood loss and diuresis. Cardiac output initially increases, most likely from increased stroke volume related to the increased venous return. It then gradually returns to prelabour levels within 1 hour after birth.

In addition to mild uterine cramping, some women experience generalized shivering. They may experience urinary retention, especially if they received regional anaesthesia. Women may also feel fatigue, muscle aches, and hunger and thirst. Emotional reactions vary from overwhelming joy and relief to temporary disbelief and withdrawal.

Chapter 18 discusses in detail care of the family during the fourth stage of labour. See Chapter 19 for discussion of maternal complications during the postpartum period.

SUMMARY

- Prelabour refers to the period before the actual onset of labour, associated with signs such as lightening, Braxton Hicks contractions, backache, bloody show, SROM, a spurt of energy, and weight loss.
- Labour is typically defined as the series of processes that result in the expulsion of the products of conception from the mother's body. The exact cause of labour is not known, but several theories have attempted to explain the cause. Some of the more common theories include progesterone withdrawal, oxytocin production, prostaglandin production, estrogen stimulation, and fetal influence.
- The process of labour and birth involves powers (uterine contractions and maternal pushing), passageway (maternal pelvis and soft parts), and passenger (fetus). In addition, psychosocial factors play a role.
- Normal uterine contractions are composed of an increment, acme, and decrement. Frequency refers to the time from the beginning of one contraction to the beginning of the next. Duration is measured from the beginning to the end of the contraction. Intensity refers to the strength of the contraction.
- The four basic shapes of the female pelvis are gynecoid, android, anthropoid, and platypelloid. Vaginal birth is most easily accomplished with a gynecoid pelvis.
- Fetal lie, presentation, attitude, and position are key factors involved in the relationship between the fetus and the maternal pelvis.
- A fetus is engaged when the presenting part is at station 0, at the level of the ischial spines. Measurements of the presenting part above the ischial spines are identified as a negative station (e.g., −1, −2); measurements below are identified as a positive station (e.g., +1, +2).
- For birth, the fetus goes through a series of passive movements so that the smallest diameter of the presenting part presents to the irregular shape of the pelvis. These movements are called the cardinal movements or mechanisms of labour: descent, flexion, internal rotation, extension, restitution, external rotation, and birth of the shoulders and expulsion.
- During labour, the woman's body undergoes physiologic and psychological changes to meet the demands of labour. The fetus also must respond to the changing intrauterine environment.
- FHR can be monitored by auscultation or electronic monitoring, depending upon the risk status of the woman and fetus. Electronic monitoring may be external (indirect) or internal (direct).
- Baseline FHR is the typical FHR during a 10-minute period or between uterine contractions in labour. It normally ranges from 110 to 160 bpm. Variability refers to the fluctuations in baseline FHR greater than two cycles per minute within a 10-minute section. Irregular amplitude and frequency are evident. Decreased variability is associated with fetal central nervous system depression.

- Periodic changes involve brief deviations in FHR above or below the baseline, usually in response to uterine contractions or fetal activity. Episodic changes are deviations above or below baseline, unrelated to uterine contractions.
- Accelerations of FHR are associated with fetal activity and are usually considered signs of fetal well-being. Early decelerations are thought to result from vagal nerve stimulation from fetal head compression during labour and are considered a normal physiologic response. Late decelerations are thought to result from uteroplacental insufficiency or compromised uteroplacental perfusion and require intervention to increase uteroplacental circulation and fetal oxygenation. Variable decelerations are usually associated with compression of the umbilical cord and typically require a change in maternal positioning.
- Labour is divided into four stages based on the degree of cervical dilation, cervical effacement, and contraction pattern.
- The first stage of labour is further divided into three phases: early (latent) phase, active phase, and transition phase. During the first stage of labour, the cervix softens, thins, shortens, and dilates to a diameter of 10 cm. Contractions become regular, frequent, and intense.
- Care of the woman during the first stage of labour focuses on assessing maternal and fetal well-being, assisting the woman to cope with the increased contraction frequency and intensity, providing support to the woman and her partner, and ensuring adequate pain relief.
- The second stage of labour involves the woman's pushing efforts and movement of the fetus through the birth canal, resulting in the birth of a newborn.
- During the second stage of labour, care focuses on more frequent assessment of maternal and fetal well-being, position changes, and support of pushing efforts.
- The third stage of labour involves separation and expulsion of the placenta. Care focuses on continued support of the woman as the placenta is delivered.
- The fourth stage of labour refers to the period immediately after delivery of the placenta, typically lasting from 1 to 4 hours. At this time, care focuses on monitoring the woman and her newborn, promoting maternal comfort, providing adequate education and support, and facilitating attachment behaviours.

Questions to Ponder

1. A client, pregnant for the first time, comes to the labour and birth suite stating, "I think I'm in labour." After several hours, her contractions continue to be mild and irregular with no increase in frequency, duration, or intensity. Her cervical dilation remains at 1 cm and membranes are intact. She is discharged home to wait. What information would the nurse include in the discharge teaching?

2. A couple in the fourth stage of labour is inspecting their newborn. The father says, "His head looks so funny. It's so oblong." How would the nurse explain this condition?

3. A nurse is teaching a childbirth education class to a group of expectant parents. As part of this class, the nurse is planning to describe how the fetus moves through the pelvic canal for birth. Develop a teaching plan that explains these movements.

REVIEW QUESTIONS

1. During a sterile vaginal examination of a woman in labour, the nurse identifies the buttocks as lying over the pelvic inlet. The nurse should document this presentation as
   A. cephalic.
   B. breech.
   C. shoulder.
   D. transverse.

2. Examination reveals that the presenting part of the fetus in the cephalic presentation has passed the pelvic inlet and is at the level of the ischial spines. The nurse interprets this to mean that the presenting part is
   A. engaged.
   B. floating.
   C. at −1 station.
   D. crowning.

3. Which method would be most effective for the nurse to use when assessing the intensity of a client's uterine contractions?
   A. Auscultating with a Doppler ultrasound
   B. Observing the woman's facial expression
   C. Asking the woman to rate the intensity
   D. Palpating the uterine fundus

4. When assessing contractions by the recording from an EFM, the nurse measures from the beginning of the contraction to the end of that contraction to determine
   A. frequency.
   B. duration.
   C. acme.
   D. intensity.

5. A woman in labour states, "I think my water just broke." On inspection, the nurse notes a large amount of clear straw-coloured fluid on the bed. Which action should the nurse do first?
   A. Test the fluid with Nitrazine paper
   B. Call the primary care provider

C. Provide perineal care

D. Assess FHR

6. The nurse is preparing to auscultate the FHR with a Doppler device. Assessment reveals that the fetal back is toward the mother's left side, fetal arms are toward the mother's right side, and the fetus is in a vertex presentation. Where should the nurse position the device initially?

A. Left upper quadrant

B. Left lower quadrant

C. Right upper quadrant

D. Right lower quadrant

7. EFM reveals a baseline FHR of 144 bpm, which slows to 128 bpm as the client's contraction peaks. The FHR then returns to baseline by the end of the contraction. The nurse interprets this finding as indicating

A. compression of the fetal head.

B. uteroplacental insufficiency.

C. umbilical cord compression.

D. uterine hyperstimulation.

8. A woman admitted to the labour and birth suite is accompanied by her partner and a doula. The nurse includes the doula in the client's plan of care based on the understanding that the doula's primary role is to

A. assist the primary care provider in the birth.

B. provide for client comfort and continuous support.

C. act as major decision maker during labour.

D. care for the client's partner during labour.

9. A woman arrives at the labour and birth area. Assessment reveals moderate contractions every 5 minutes and lasting approximately 45 seconds. Cervical dilation is 3 cm, cervical effacement is approximately 50%. The nurse determines that the client is in which stage of labour?

A. First stage, latent phase

B. First stage, transition phase

C. Second stage

D. Third stage

10. The labour and birth record of a client who gave birth to a healthy newborn approximately 45 minutes ago indicates that she had an episiotomy. The nurse explains this to the client, describing it as which of the following?

A. Artificial rupture of the membranes

B. Use of medication to enhance contractions

C. A perineal incision to enlarge the outlet

D. Thinning of the cervical tissue

REFERENCES

Alfirevic, Z., Devane, D., & Gyte, G. M. L. (2013). Continuous cardiotocography (CTG) as a form of electronic fetal monitoring (EFM) for fetal assessment during labour. *Cochrane Database of Systematic Reviews*, doi:10.1002/14651858.CD006066.pub2

Allen, V., Baskett, T., O'Connell, C. McKeen, D., & Allen, A. (2009). Maternal and perinatal outcomes with increasing duration of the second stage of labor. *Obstetrics and Gynecology, 113*, 1248–1258.

American Society of Anesthesiologists (ASA). (2006). *Practice guidelines for obstetrical anesthesia*. Available at the American Society of Anesthesiologists website: http://www. asahq.org

Andrews, M., & Boyle, J. (2007). *Transcultural concepts in nursing care* (5th ed.). Philadelphia, PA: Lippincott Williams & Wilkins.

Association of Women's Health, Obstetric and Neonatal Nurses (AWHONN). (2006). *AWHONN position statement, issue: Professional nursing support of laboring women*. Washington, DC: Author.

Bailey, E. (2009). Intrapartum fetal monitoring. *American Family Physician, 80*(12), 1388–1396.

Bashour, H., & Abdulsalam, A. (2005). Syrian women's preferences for birth attendant and birth place. *Birth, 32*(1), 20–26.

Berg, M., & Terstad, A. (2006). Swedish women's experiences of doula support during childbirth. *Midwifery, 22*(4), 330–338.

Blackburn, S., & Loper, D. (2003). *Maternal, fetal, and neonatal physiology: A clinical perspective* (2nd ed.). Philadelphia, PA: W.B. Saunders.

Bloom, S. L., Casey, B. M., Schaffer, J. I., McIntire, D. D., & Leveno, K. J.. (2006). A randomized trial of coached versus uncoached maternal pushing during the second stage of labor. *American Journal of Obstetrics and Gynecology, 194*(1), 10–13.

Brathwaite, S., & Williams, C. (2004). Childbirth experiences of professional Chinese Canadian women. *Journal of Obstetric, Gynecologic, and Neonatal Nursing, 33*(6), 748–755.

Bryanton, J., Gagnon, A., Johnston, C., & Hatem, M. (2008). Predictor of women's perceptions of the childbirth experience. *Journal of Obstetrics, Gynecologic, and Neonatal Nursing, 37*(1), 24–34.

Canadian Anesthesiologists' Society. (2008). *Guidelines for obstetrical regional analgesia*. Retrieved August 24, 2008, from http://www.cas.ca/members/sign_in/guidelines/ default.asp?load = ora

Carlsson, I., Ziegert, K., Sahlberg-Blom, E., & Nissen, E. (2012). Maintaining power: Women's experiences from labour onset before admittance to maternity ward. *Midwifery, 28*(1), 86–92.

Carroli, G., & Mignini, J. (2009). Episiotomy for vaginal birth. In: *The Cochrane Library*. doi:10.1002/14651858.CD00008.1.pub2.

Chalk, A. (2004). Spontaneous versus directed pushing. *British Journal of Midwifery, 12*, 626–630.

Cioffi, J. (2004). Caring for women from culturally diverse backgrounds: Midwives' experiences. *Journal of Midwifery and Women's Health, 49*(5), 437–442.

Cluett, E., & Burns, E. (2009). Immersion in water in labour and birth. *Cochrane Database Systematic Review*, (2), CD000111.

Cunningham, F. G., Gant, N. F., Leveno, K. J., Bloom, S. L., Hauth, J. C., Gillstrap, L. C., III, et al. (2005). *Williams obstetrics* (22nd ed.). New York, NY: McGraw-Hill.

Declercq, E., Sakala, C., Corry, M., Applebaum, S., & Risher, P. (2002). *Listening to mothers: Report of the first national U.S. survey of women's childbirth experiences*. New York, NY: Maternity Center Association.

Dilbaz, B., Ozturkoglu, E., Dilbaz, S., Ozturk, N., Sivaslioglu, A. A., & Haberal, A. (2006). Risk factors and perinatal outcomes associated with umbilical cord prolapse. *Archives of Gynecology and Obstetrics, 274*(2), 104–107.

Eason, E., & Feldman, P. (2000). Clinical commentary. Much ado about a little cut: Is episiotomy worthwhile? *Obstetrics and Gynecology, 95*(4), 616–618.

Eason, E., Labrecque, M., Wells, G., & Feldman, P. (2000). Preventing perineal trauma during childbirth: A systematic review. *Obstetrics & Gynecology, 95*(93), 464–471.

Enkin, M., Keirse, M., Renfrew, M., & Neilson, J. (2000). *A guide to effective care in pregnancy and childbirth* (3rd ed.). New York, NY: Oxford University Press.

Etowa, J. (2012). Becoming a mother: The meaning of childbirth for African-Canadian women. *Contemporary Nurse, 41*(1), 28–40.

Feinstein, N., Sprague, A., & Trepanier, M. (2000). Fetal heart rate auscultation. *AWHONN Life-lines, 4*(3), 35–44.

Feinstein, N., Torgersen, K. L., & Atterbury, J. (2003). *AWHONN's fetal heart monitoring principles and practices* (3rd ed.). Dubuque, IA: Kendall-Hunt Publishing Company.

Fuller, O. (2012). Assessing cultural and spiritual practices for the childbearing family. *International Journal of Childbirth Education, 27*(1), 43–45.

Gilliland, A. (2002). Beyond holding hands: The modern role of the professional doula. *Journal of Obstetric, Gynecologic, and Neonatal Nursing, 31*(6), 762–769.

Goer, H., Leslie, M., & Romano, A. (2007). The Coalition for Improving Maternity Services: Evidence basis for the ten steps of mother-friendly care: Step 6: Does not routinely employ practices, procedures unsupported by scientific evidence. *Journal of Perinatal Education, 16*(1), 32S–64S.

Goldberg, J., Holtz, D., Hyslop, T., & Tolosa, J. (2002). Has the use of routine episiotomy decreased: Examination of episiotomy rates from 1983 to 2000. *Obstetrics and Gynecology, 99*(3), 395–400.

Goodman, P., Mackey, M. C., & Tavakoli, A.S. (2004). Factors related to childbirth satisfaction. *Journal of Advanced Nursing, 46*(2), 212–219.

Goodwin, L. (2000). Intermittent auscultation of the fetal heart rate: A review of general principles. *Journal of Perinatal and Neonatal Nursing, 14*(3), 53–61.

Greene, M. (2007). Strategies for Incorporating Cultural Competence Into Childbirth Education Curriculum. *Journal of Perinatal Education, 16*(2), 33–37.

Gross, M. M., Drobnic, S., & Keirse, M. J. (2005). Influence of fixed and time-dependent factors on duration of normal first stage labor. *Birth, 32*(1), 27–33.

Gross, M. M., Hecker, H., Matterne, A., Guenter, H. H., & Keirse, M. J. (2006). Does the way that women experience the onset of labour influence the duration of labour? *British Journal of Obstetrics and Gynaecology, 113*(3), 289–294.

Gupta, J. K., & Hofmeyr, G. J. (2004). Positions for women during second stage of labour. *Cochrane Database of Systematic Reviews,* (1), CD002006.

Hannah, M.E., Hodnett, E.D., Willan, A., Foster, G.A., Di Cecco, R., & Helewa, M. (2000). Prelabor rupture of the membranes at term: Expectant management at home or in hospital? The TermPROM Study Group. *Obstetrics and Gynecology, 96*(4), 533–538.

Hansen, S., Clark, S., & Foster, J. (2002). Active pushing versus passive fetal descent in the second-stage of labor: A randomized controlled trial. *Obstetrics & Gynecology, 99*(1), 29–34.

Hartmann, K., Viswanathan, M., Palmieri, R., Gatlehner, G., Thorp, J., Jr., & Lohr, K. N. (2005). Outcomes of routine episiotomy: A systematic review. *The Journal of the American Medical Association, 293*(17), 2141–2148.

Higginbottom, G., Salipour, J., Murntaz, Z., Chiu, Y. Paton, P., & Pillay, J. (2013). "I have to do what I believe": Sudanese women's beliefs and resistance to hegemonic practices at home and during experiences of maternity care in Canada. *BMC Pregnancy and Childbirth, 13*, 51.

Hodnett, E. (2002). Caregiver support for women during childbirth. In: *The Cochrane Library, Issue 4.* Oxford, UK: Update Software.

Hodnett, E. D., Downe, S., Edwards, N., & Walsh, D. (2005). Home-like versus conventional institutional settings for birth. *Cochrane Database of Systematic Reviews,* (1), CD000012.

Hodnett, E., Lowe, N. K., Hannah, M. E., Willan, A. R., Stevens, B., Weston, J. A., et al. (2002). Effectiveness of nurses as providers of birth labor support in North American hospitals. *The Journal of the American Medical Association, 288*(11), 1373–1381.

Jones, L., Othman, M., Dowswell, T., Alfirevic, Z., Newburn, M., Jordan, S., et al. (2012). Pain management for women in labour: An overview of systematic reviews. *Cochrane Database Systematic Reviews, 14*(3), CD009234. Retrieved from http://www.ncbi.nlm.nih.gov/pubmed/22419342

Kamel, R. (2010). The onset of human parturition. *Archives of Gynecology and Obstetrics, 281*, 975–982.

Karnng-Edgren, S. (2001). Using evidence-based practice to improve intrapartum care. *Journal of Obstetric, Gynecologic, and Neonatal Nursing, 30*(4), 371–375.

Kennedy, H. P., & Shannon, M. T. (2004). Keeping birth normal: Research findings on midwifery care during childbirth. *Journal of Obstetrical, Gynecological, and Neonatal Nursing, 33*(5), 554–560.

Khan, F. O., & Razi, M. S. (2005). Normal labor and delivery. *E-medicine.* Retrieved from http://www.emedicine.com/med/topic3239.htm

Lee, C. J., & Lamp, J. K. (2005). The birth story interview: Enhancing student appreciation of the personal meaning of pregnancy and birth. *Nurse Educator, 30*(4), 155–158.

Lothian, J. (2001). Back to the future: Trusting normal birth. *Journal of Perinatal Education, 15*(3), 13–22.

Lund, K., & McManaman, J. (2008). Normal labor, delivery, newborn care, and puerperium. In: R. S. Gibbs, et al., Eds., *Danforth's obstetrics and gynecology* (10th ed., pp. 23–42). Philadelphia, PA: Lippincott Williams and Wilkins.

Lundgren, I. (2004). Releasing and relieving encounters: Experiences of pregnancy and childbirth. *Scandinavian Journal of Caring Sciences, 18*(4), 368–375.

Lundgren, L. (2005). Swedish women's experience of childbirth 2 years after birth. *Midwifery, 21*(4), 346–354.

MacDonald, T., & Saurette, K. (2010). Management of prelabour rupture of membranes at term. *Clinical Practice Guideline No.13, Association of Ontario Midwives.* Retrieved from http://www.ontariomidwives.ca/images/uploads/guidelines/No13CPG_PROM_final.pdf

MacKinnon, K., McIntyre, M., & Quance, M. (2005). The meaning of the nurse's presence during childbirth. *Journal of Obstetric, Gynecologic, and Neonatal Nursing, 34*(1), 28–36.

Matthews, R., & Callister, L. C. (2004). Childbearing women's perceptions of nursing care that promotes dignity. *Journal of Obstetric, Gynecologic, and Neonatal Nursing, 33*(4), 498–507.

McLachlan, H., & Waldenstrom, U. (2005). Childbirth experiences in Australia of women born in Turkey, Vietnam, and Australia. *Birth, 32*(4), 272–282.

Mercer, R. (2006). Nursing support of the process of becoming a mother. *Journal of Obstetric, Gynecologic, and Neonatal Nursing, 35*(5), 649–51.

Moore, M. (2001). Adopting birth philosophies to guide successful birth practices and outcomes. *Journal of Perinatal Education, 10*(2), 43–45.

Nager, C., & Helliwell, J. (2001). Episiotomy increases perineal laceration length in primiparous women. *American Journal of Obstetricians and Gynecologists, 185*(2), 444–450.

O'Sullivan, G., Liu, B., & Shennan, A. (2007). Oral intake during labor. *International Anesthesiology Clinics, 45*(1), 133–147.

Parsons, M., Bidewell, J., & Nagy, S. (2006). Natural eating behavior in latent labor and its effect on outcomes in active labor. *Journal of Midwifery and Women's Health, 51*(1), e1–e6.

Pascali-Bonaro, D., & Kroeger, M. (2004). Continuous female companionship during childbirth: A crucial resource in times of stress or calm. *Journal of Midwifery and Women's Health, 49*(4 Suppl. 1), 19–27.

Pennick, V., & Liddle, S. (2013). Interventions for preventing and treating pelvic and back pain in pregnancy. *The Cochrane Library.* doi:10.1002/14651858.CD001139.pub3

Pillitteri, A. (2014). *Maternal and child health nursing* (7th ed.). Philadelphia, PA: Lippincott Williams & Wilkins.

Priddy, K. D. (2004). Is there logic behind fetal monitoring? *Journal of Obstetric, Gynecologic, and Neonatal Nursing, 33*(5), 550–553.

Primeau, M. R., Lucey, K. A., & Crotty, P. M. (2003). Managing the pain of labor. *Advance for Nurses, 4*(12), 15–19.

Prins, M., Boxem, J., Lucas, C., & Hutton, E. (2011). Effect of spontaneous pushing versus Valsalva pushing in the second stage of labour on mother and fetus: A systematic review of randomized trials. *BJOG: An International Journal of obstetrics and Gynecology, 118*(6), 662–670.

Ragusa, A., Mansur, M., Zanini, A., Musicco, M., Maccario, L., & Borsellino, G. (2005). Diagnosis of labor: A prospective study. *Medscape General Medicine, 7*(3), 61.

Roberts, J. (2002). The push for evidence: Management of the second-stage. *Journal of Midwifery and Women's Health, 47*(1), 2–15.

Roberts, J., & Hanson, L. (2007). Best practices in second stage labor care: Maternal bearing down and position. *Journal of Midwifery and Women's Health, 52*(3), 238–245.

Romano, A., & Lothian, J. (2008). Promoting, protecting, and supporting normal birth: A look at the evidence. *Journal of Obstetric, Gynecologic, and Neonatal Nursing, 37*(1), 94–105.

Rouse, D. J., & St. John, E. (2003). Normal labor, delivery, newborn care, and puerperium. In J. R. Scott, R. S. Gibbs, B. Y. Karlan,

& A. F. Haney (Eds.), *Danforth's obstetrics and gynecology* (9th ed., pp. 35–56). Philadelphia, PA: Lippincott Williams & Wilkins.

Sampselle, C. M., Miller, J. M., Luecha, Y., Fischer, K., & Rosten, L. (2005). Provider support of spontaneous pushing during the second stage of labor. *Journal of Obstetric, Gynecologic, and Neonatal Nursing, 34*(6), 695–702.

Senecal, J., Xiong, X., & Fraser, W. D. (2005). Effect of fetal position on second-stage duration and labor outcome. *Obstetrics and Gynecology, 105*(4), 763–772.

Simkin, P., & Ancheta, R. (2000). *The labor progress handbook: Early interventions to prevent and treat dystocia.* Malden, MA: Blackwell Science.

Simmonds, A., Peter, E., Hodnett, E., & McGillis-Hall, L. (2013). Understanding the moral nature of intrapartum nursing. *Journal of Obstetrics, Gynecology and Neonatal Nursing, 42*, 148–156.

Simpson, K., Morin, K., Morin, T., & Snelgrove-Clarke, E. (2008). *Evidence-based guidelines for second stage management.* Philadelphia, PA: Lippincott.

Simpson, K. R. (2005). The context and clinical evidence for common nursing practices during labor. *MCN—American Journal of Maternal/Child Nursing, 30*(6), 356–363.

Simpson, K. R. (2008). Labor and birth. In: K. R. Simpson & P. A. Creehan (Eds.), *AWHONN's perinatal nursing.* (3rd ed., pp. 300–398). Philadelphia, PA: Lippincott Williams & Wilkins.

Singata, M., Tranmer, J., & Gyte, G. (2013). Restricting oral fluids and food intake during labour. *The Cochrane Library,* doi:10.1002/14651858.CD003930.pub3

Smeenk, A., & ten Have, H. (2003). Medicalization and obstetric care: An analysis of developments in Dutch midwifery. *Medicine, Health Care and Philosophy, 6*(2), 153–165.

Smith, J. R., & Brennan, B. G. (2004). Management of the third stage of labor. *E-Medicine.* Retrieved August 25, 2008, from http://www.emedicine.com/med/topic3569.htm

Society of Obstetricians and Gynaecologists of Canada. (SOGC). (2007). Fetal health surveillance; Antepartum and intrapartum consensus guideline. (SOGC Clinical Practice Guidelines).

Journal of Obstetrics and Gynaecology Canada, 29(9 Suppl. 4), S3–S56.

Society of Obstetricians and Gynaecologists of Canada. (SOGC). (2009). Active management of labour: prevention and treatment of postpartum haemorrhage. *Journal of Obstetrics and Gynaecology Canada, 31*(10),980–993.

Sprague, A., Oppenheimer, L., McCabe, L., Graham, I., & Davies, B. (2008). Knowledge to action. Implementing a guideline for second stage labor. *MCN: American Journal of Maternal Child Nursing, 33*, 179–186. doi:10.1097/01.NMC.0000318354.00859.41

Steen, M., Downe, S., Bamford, N., & Edozien, L. (2012). Non-patient and not-visitor: A metasynthesis fathers' encounters with pregnancy, birth and maternity care. *Midwifery, 28*, 422–431.

Thacker, S. B., Stroup, D., & Chang, M. (2001). Continuous electronic heart rate monitoring for fetal assessment during labour. *Cochrane Database of Systematic Reviews*, (2), CD000063.

Turley, G. M. (2004). Essential forces and factors in labour. In: S. Mattson, & Smith, J.E. (Eds.), *AWHONN: Maternal–newborn nursing* (3rd ed., pp. 227–270). Philadelphia, PA: Elsevier.

Varcoe, C., Brown, H., Calam, B., Harvey, T., Tallio, M. (2013). Help bring back the celebration of life: A rural community-based participatory study of rural Aboriginal women's maternity experiences and outcomes. *BMC Pregnancy and Childbirth, 13*, 26.

Vedham, S., Schummers, L., Stoll, K., Rogers, J., Klein, M., Fairbrother, N., et al. (2012). The Canadian birth place study: Describing maternity practice and providers' exposure to home birth. *Midwifery, 28*, 600–608.

Vincent, P. (2002). *Baby catcher: Chronicles of a modern midwife.* New York, NY: Scribner.

Waldenstrom, U. (2004). Why do some women change their opinion about childbirth over time? *Birth, 31*(2), 102–107.

Watts, N., & McDonald, C. (2007). The beginning of life (the perinatal period). In Srivastava, R. H. (Ed.), *Guide to clinical cultural competence* (pp. 203–226). Toronto, ON: Mosby.

Webb, D., & Culhane, J. (2002). Hospital variation in episiotomy use and the risk of perineal trauma during childbirth. *Birth, 29*(2), 132–136.

CHAPTER 16

High-Risk Labour and Childbirth

Nancy Watts

Beverly, a 35-year-old client (GTPAL 3-2-0-0-2) at 39 weeks' gestation, arrives at the labour and birth suite with her partner, Chris. She is experiencing contractions approximately every 5 minutes. On examination, she is found to be 3 cm dilated and 50% effaced. Beverly states, "I have a lot of pain in my back. It feels like the baby is pressing on my spine. This happened with my last pregnancy, too."

Carlotta (GTPAL 1-0-0-0) is at the end of her 41st week gestation. She and her boyfriend have come to the labour and birth area for a scheduled induction of labour. Carlotta appears tired, saying, "I really haven't slept much because I've been a bit worried about what's next." She adds that she is really hoping to use the whirlpool during labour and that she won't need an epidural.

You will learn more about these stories later in this chapter. Nurses working with these and similar clients need to understand the material in this chapter to manage care and address issues appropriately. Before beginning, consider the following points:

- Does anything about either case qualify as an emergency? Explain your answer.
- Would you consider each client to be at high risk during labour and birth? Why or why not?
- How might each client's specific situation influence the nurse's approach to care?

● What details will the nurse need to investigate with Beverly about her complaints? What about Carlotta?

● What areas of teaching would the nurse need to address with both women and their families?

LEARNING OBJECTIVES

On completion of this chapter, the reader should be able to:
● Explain what is meant by dystocia or abnormal progress in labour.
● Identify the general causes of problems with the powers of labour and ways that health care providers collaborate with women/families to resolve them.
● Discuss common fetal positions, presentations, and circumstances that may halt the progress of labour and appropriate related nursing measures to address them.
● Identify problems with the maternal pelvis or vaginal outlet that may pose risks during childbirth.
● Describe the risks associated with preterm labour, contributing factors, and associated management parameters.
● Explain complications that can accompany postterm pregnancy and alternatives for resolving these circumstances.
● Identify conditions that can result in hemorrhage during labour and childbirth.
● Discuss why quick interventions for cord prolapse and amniotic fluid embolism are important.
● Describe necessary adaptations during labour in cases of multiple gestation, maternal obesity, and women who have undergone circumcision.
● Outline the process of labour induction and related nursing care.
● Identify indications for amnioinfusion.
● Explain when forceps or a vacuum extractor might be used, related processes, and appropriate nursing care.
● Discuss general reasons for increasing rates of cesarean birth.
● Outline the process of cesarean birth and appropriate nursing interventions during the preoperative, intraoperative, and postoperative stages.

KEY TERMS

amnioinfusion	hypotonic uterine contractions
amniotic fluid embolism	macrosomia
arrest disorder	moulding
breech presentation	occipitoposterior (OP) positioning
cephalopelvic disproportion (CPD)	pathologic retraction ring
constriction rings	Piper forceps
cord prolapse	postterm pregnancy
dystocia	precipitous labour
external cephalic version	preterm labour
failure to progress	protraction disorder
forceps	shoulder dystocia
hydrocephalus	uterine rupture
hyperstimulation	vacuum extractor
hypertonic uterine contractions	vaginal birth after cesarean (VBAC)

his chapter focuses on those conditions that pose risks during the process of labour and birth. It explores difficulties related to abnormal progress in labour and problems with the timing of labour—either too early or too late in gestation. The chapter covers hemorrhagic problems in labour, as well as difficulties with the umbilical cord and amniotic fluid. It focuses on some special conditions that require adaptations in labour, such as maternal obesity, female circumcision, and multiple gestation. The last section focuses on common interventions employed when labour and birth are at risk, including cervical ripening and labour induction, amnioinfusion, assisted birth, and cesarean birth.

RISK ASSESSMENT AND IDENTIFICATION

A fundamental component of quality perinatal care is the identification of pregnancies at increased risk for complications, whether maternal, fetal, or both (Herzig et al., 2006). Various systems have been used to determine such risks. As discussed in Chapter 13, previous obstetric history, medical health, current pregnancy, anxiety, social support, age, and socioeconomic background are critical components of assessment for each pregnant woman.

Risk factors related specifically to labour and birth may be identified early in pregnancy when the mother has an established health problem, such as pre-existing cardiac disease or diabetes (see Chapter 13). Other circumstances of concern can be known before the onset of labour, but do not pose significant problems until then. Examples include breech presentation and placenta previa. Still other problems manifest only during labour and birth, such as shoulder dystocia and hypotonic uterine contractions. Regardless of when the situation is determined to be at high risk, the nurse's role involves multidisciplinary collaboration to facilitate health and healing for the client and her family. The goal is to minimize fetal, maternal, and neonatal complications (Gilbert, 2011).

Although pregnancy is always a situational stressor, high-risk gestation, labour, and childbirth pose greater concerns for all family members. Expectant parents normally complete several developmental tasks and psychological adjustments to facilitate their future attachment with the newborn. When parents are anxious about maternal and fetal safety, health, well-being, and outcomes, bonding processes may be delayed or impeded (Sittner et al., 2005). Common emotions include ambivalence, anxiety, frustration, low self-esteem, decreased preparation for the newborn, increased unmet expectations, and increased risk for postpartum depression (Gilbert, 2011). The client and her partner or support person may feel guilty about an inability to protect the fetus, which also may compromise bonding. See Research Highlight 16.1.

Alternatively, women who have had a previous loss, defined by early or late miscarriage, stillbirth, or death of an infant within the first 28 days of life, may

---

● **RESEARCH HIGHLIGHT 16.1**   **Effects of High-Risk Pregnancies on Families**

PURPOSE

To describe the psychosocial effects that high-risk gestation can have on the entire family and to examine what strengths can assist families to cope with the special challenges inherent in such situations

SAMPLE AND DESIGN

Researchers employed a descriptive study with naturalistic inquiry to interview pregnant women who had various high-risk concerns. They collected data using semistructured, one-on-one audiotaped interviews, observations, and autobiographical profiles directly from the participants. The researchers then transcribed, examined, and clustered data to arrive at specific themes.

RESULTS

The participants consistently identified having mixed emotions throughout their pregnancies. Family strengths

that assisted them through the experience included an ability to manage stress and crisis, commitment, appreciation, affection, spiritual well-being, and enjoyable time together. The least common strength identified was positive communication.

CONCLUSIONS

Nurses can help families coping with high-risk pregnancies to identify strengths and to use them during difficult stages, including the labour and birth itself.

From Sittner, B. J., DeFrain, J., & Hudson, D. B. (2005). Effects of high-risk pregnancies on families. *MCN. The American Journal of Maternal Child Nursing, 30*(2), 121–126.

perceive this label of "high risk" differently (Simmons & Goldberg, 2011). Having a previous loss increases anxiety for women in a subsequent pregnancy. A greater number of antenatal visits, with increased assessment (eg, ultrasound), and access to health care providers who previously had not been available to them can all contribute to an increased sense of control for women with a previous loss and a greater ability to cope with this subsequent pregnancy (Simmons & Goldberg, 2011).

The nurse needs to consider the client's and family's response to a high-risk diagnosis and develop a plan of care to support them. Assessment of stress level and support systems is important (Denis et al., 2012; Sittner et al., 2005). Formulating diagnoses based on individual needs facilitates patient and family-centred care and a mutual decision making process (Behruzi et al., 2010). Encouraging family members to express concerns regarding the high-risk status, providing explanations regarding the normal process of labour, teaching how the high-risk problem might alter the course of labour and birth, and clarifying misconceptions can be supportive interventions. Keeping the client informed of her progress and the results of any testing or assessments that she and the fetus are receiving are encouraging and helpful. Advocating on the family's behalf for appropriate goals may alleviate any feelings of ambivalence members may have. Referrals, as appropriate, to social workers, public health nurses, advanced practice nurses, obstetricians, or physicians with other services may be critical for appropriate follow-up.

 Think back to Carlotta, the client with a postterm pregnancy scheduled for induction of labour. What types of stress might she and her family be experiencing?

DYSTOCIA

Dystocia (inadequately progressing labour) can happen for many reasons. It occurs in approximately 10% of all labours and is the leading cause of cesarean births (Ressel, 2004). Dystocia can develop during any of the phases of labour (see Chapter 15). Normal progress in labour was originally studied in the 1950s by Friedman who developed a graph that plots cervical dilatation and station across time. Using this graph, the latent phase is seen to last an average of 5 to 9 hours; a latent phase beyond 14 to 20 hours is considered prolonged (Dudley, 2008). The active phase of labour begins once the cervix is dilated 3 to 4 cm and normally lasts 2 to 5 hours. Currently, the definition of progress in labour is broader than

Friedman's, with the time for active labour (4 to 10 cm dilatation) averaging 5.5 hours or 1.1 cm/hour (Shields et al., 2007). Up to 4 hours of labour can have as little as 0.5 cm/hour of progress and still be considered normal, to accommodate individual patterns of progress particularly early in the active phase. The definition of dystocia, therefore, is considered to be greater than 4 hours in active labour of less than 0.5 cm of dilatation per hour, or greater than 1 hour in the second stage with no fetal descent (Neal et al., 2010; Society of Obstetricians and Gynaecologists of Canada [SOGC], 2005).

One classification of dysfunctional labour is a **protraction disorder**, which is characterized by delayed cervical dilatation and slowed descent of the fetal head. Protraction disorders may develop in the latent phase, active phase, or second stage of labour. In some women who experience a protracted latent phase, cervical dilatation can progress normally once they receive supportive fluids, reassurance, and minimum sedation, although some providers opt to manage labour in such cases more aggressively with augmentation or induction (Dudley, 2008).

Arrest disorders generally happen during active labour and are characterized by the following:

* *Prolonged deceleration phase* (at least 3 hours in a nullipara and 1 hour in a multipara)
* *Secondary arrest of cervical dilatation* (no progress for more than 2 hours)
* *Arrest of the descent of the fetal head* (more than 60 minutes in a nullipara and 30 minutes in a multipara)
* *Failure of the descent of the fetal head* (none during the first stage, deceleration phase, or second stage of labour) (Dudley, 2008)

Arrest disorders frequently are associated with **cephalopelvic disproportion (CPD)**, or inability of the fetal head to pass through the maternal pelvis because of shape, size, or position (Cunningham et al., 2010).

When the cervix does not dilate despite adequate uterine contractions and without CPD, the condition is called **failure to progress**. When early labour fails to progress despite adequate uterine contractions, the health care team should evaluate carefully whether the client is experiencing true or prodromal labour.

As discussed in Chapter 15, several elements must interact successfully for labour and birth to progress normally. The *powers* (contractions and pushing) must be sufficient for the cervix to thin and open and to propel the fetus through the birth canal. The *passage* (pelvis) and *passenger* (fetus) must be sized, shaped, and positioned in such a way as to allow the fetus to pass through. Causes of dystocia can involve any of three "Ps":

* *Powers.* During the first stage of labour, uterine contractions are too weak or uncoordinated to facilitate

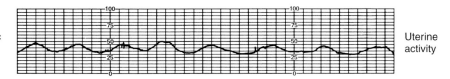

FIGURE 16.1 With hypertonic uterine contractions, tracings will show a high resting pressure (35 to 40 mm Hg).

Uterine activity

adequate cervical effacement and dilatation. During the second stage, contractions and pushing are insufficient to promote fetal descent. Another problem involves uterine contractions that are so rapid and strong that labour progresses more quickly than normal.

- *Passenger.* These problems include such issues as fetal malpresentation, malposition, or macrosomia.
- *Passageway.* Difficulties related to the passageway involve abnormalities of maternal pelvic shape or size.

PROBLEMS WITH THE POWERS

When problems with uterine contractions or maternal bearing-down efforts lead to prolonged labour, maternal and fetal complications can ensue. For example, risks for intrauterine infection are increased if labour continues for an extended time after the membranes have ruptured (Cunningham et al., 2010). Other potential difficulties include exhaustion and dehydration. Examples of problems with the powers include hypertonic and hypotonic contractions, inadequate expulsion forces, pathologic retraction and constriction rings, and precipitous birth.

Hypertonic Uterine Contractions

Normally, contractions start at the superior aspect of the uterus and proceed downward to the cervix. In contrast, **hypertonic uterine contractions** are distorted. The uterine midsegment may contract with more force than the fundus, or the impulses in each upper corner of the uterus may not be synchronized (Fig. 16.1). This problem is associated most commonly with a prolonged latent phase (Dudley, 2008).

Hypertonic uterine contractions fail to promote normal cervical dilatation and can interfere with placental function and reoxygenation. They can be extremely painful, leading to uterine tenderness even between contractions. A common contributing factor is placental abruption, which must be considered and ruled out or managed aggressively, depending on the findings.

Treatment usually involves fluid administration to maintain hydration and electrolyte balance, as well as rest. Intramuscular morphine may be administered to inhibit the uncoordinated contraction pattern. A short-acting barbiturate may be given to promote rest. Oxytocin is usually contraindicated because it could compound uterine resting tension, which might interfere with fetal oxygenation. When this pattern of contractions persists despite the above interventions, cesarean birth is usually indicated, especially if an atypical or abnormal fetal heart rate tracing is observed (Cunningham et al., 2010).

Hypotonic Uterine Contractions

Hypotonic uterine contractions have no basal tone, have insufficient intensity, are infrequent, and fail to dilate the cervix satisfactorily (Fig. 16.2). They usually appear during the active phase of labour; however, this pattern may also develop during the second stage. Common causes include uterine overdistension (eg, multiple gestation, macrosomic fetus), fetal malposition, incorrect timing of analgesic administration, and use of regional anaesthesia (see Chapter 17).

Treatment generally involves pinpointing and managing the underlying cause. For example, if the problem is uterine overdistension related to macrosomia, a cesarean birth might be elected. If no cause can be found, the next step, following diagnosis of dystocia, is clinical rupture of the membranes to facilitate labour progression. Oxytocin may be administered as well following rupture of the membranes. Labour that fails to progress despite adequate contractions achieved with these measures generally indicates consideration of the need for cesarean birth.

Pathologic Retraction and Constriction Rings

When the membranes have ruptured and labour is prolonged, a **pathologic retraction ring** (Bandl ring) may develop in the uterus. This finding manifests as an exaggeration of the normal physiologic retraction ring found

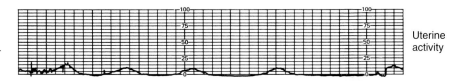

FIGURE 16.2 With hypotonic uterine contractions, tracings reflect a low resting pressure (less than 10 mm Hg).

Uterine activity

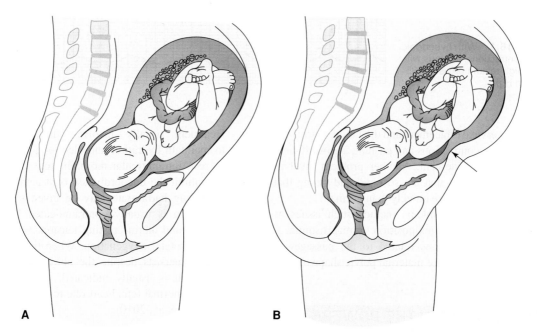

FIGURE 16.3 **A:** In normal labour, the upper uterine segment thickens, whereas the lower segment thins. **B:** With a pathologic retraction (Bandl) ring, the abdomen shows an indentation where the wall below the ring is thin. Unrectified, this problem can lead to uterine rupture.

at the junction of the upper and lower uterine segments (Fig. 16.3). The area above the ring thickens, whereas the lower segment thins. A pathologic retraction ring is a medical emergency because the lower segment will rupture unless the obstruction is relieved. An immediate cesarean birth is usually indicated.

Constriction rings are rare and usually conform to a narrowing of the diameter of the fetus, such as in the neck or abdomen. They do not extend all the way around the uterus. The area of spasm is thick, but the lower uterine segment does not become stretched or thinned. Cesarean birth is usually the treatment of choice with constriction rings.

Inadequate Voluntary Expulsive Forces

During uterine contractions, most women with a fully dilated cervix and fetal presenting part at spines or lower cannot resist the urge to push. Under normal circumstances, the force of the maternal abdominal muscles helps propel the fetus through the birth canal. Certain factors, however, can interfere with sensing or responding to the urge to push. Examples include fatigue, pain, fear, and anxiety. Pharmacologic agents used to manage labour pain also may pose problems due to decreased maternal sensation, particularly if administered at the wrong time or in an incorrect dose (see Chapter 17). In some situations, spinal cord injury or other physical problems render maternal expulsive efforts inadequate.

A lengthy second stage, that is, greater than 3 hours, is associated with maternal morbidity, such as

postpartum hemorrhage due to uterine atony, fever, as well as significant perineal trauma (Rouse et al., 2009). Treatment measures aimed at achieving vaginal birth without increasing morbidity vary and depend on the underlying cause. For example, the client whose pushing efforts are inhibited because of pain may require analgesia. Conversely, if a client has received too strong a dose of epidural anaesthesia, time may be needed to decrease the effects of the anaesthetic while still providing pain relief, to enable pushing. Notification of the health care provider after 2 hours in the second stage and then hourly thereafter regarding progress is beneficial for implementation of treatment measures if needed (Sprague et al., 2008).

Waiting for the fetal presenting part to descend in second stage without pushing for a period of time, if fetal and maternal health are assessed to be normal, can also facilitate working with the sensations of pushing. Women who are coached to push when the fetal presenting part is at a high fetal station (above a +1 or +2) become fatigued more easily and are less satisfied with their birth experience. Waiting for the fetal presenting part to descend and then initiating nondirected pushing, open glottis pushing, or physiologic management of the second stage will decrease the duration of this stage by as much as half (Kelly et al., 2010). This approach can also decrease the incidence of third and fourth degree tears and provide greater oxygenation to the baby, decreasing neonatal morbidity (Mahlmeister, 2008).

Precipitous Labour

With **precipitous labour**, uterine contractions are so frequent, intense, or both that labour progresses very quickly. The total duration of a precipitous labour is generally less than 3 hours. Clients prone to precipitous labour tend to have soft, stretchable perineal tissue, facilitating rapid fetal descent. Complications may include perineal lacerations and postpartum hemorrhage. The biggest problems tend to arise when precipitous labour occurs outside of or on the way to a health care facility. In addition, even within a health care institution, the labour and birth can be so rapid that staff members may be unprepared or may lack the equipment to handle the event. Figure 16.4 presents an algorithm for nurses to follow in cases of emergency birth.

PROBLEMS WITH THE PASSENGER

Fetal presentation and position are two important conditions that influence the course of labour and birth. As discussed in Chapter 15, the fetus moves most easily through the birth canal when the head is well flexed, with the chin resting on the thorax, and the occipital area of the skull presenting anterior to the maternal pelvis. These conditions allow the smallest diameter of the fetal head to enter the maternal pelvis, while enabling the most flexible part of the fetal body, the back of the neck, to adapt to the curve of the birth canal (Gilbert, 2011). When fetal presentation or position deviates from normal, labour becomes more difficult or even impossible. Other problems in labour may result when the fetus is large or has abnormalities that significantly alter body size or shape.

Breech Presentation

In a **breech presentation**, the fetal buttocks or feet are the presenting part, a circumstance that develops in approximately 3% to 4% of all births (Fischer, 2006; RCOG, 2010). The following different attitudes are variations of a breech presentation:

- *Frank breech:* the hips are flexed and the legs lie alongside the fetal body.
- *Complete breech:* the legs are flexed at the thighs and the feet present with the buttocks.
- *Footling (incomplete) breech:* one foot (single) or both feet (double) present before the buttocks (Fig. 16.5).

Factors that increase the risk for incidence of breech presentation include prematurity, intrauterine growth restriction (IUGR), congenital anomalies (eg, hydrocephaly), multiple pregnancy, previous breech position, and oligohydramnios (Fischer, 2006; Klatt & Cruikshank, 2008; RCOG, 2010).

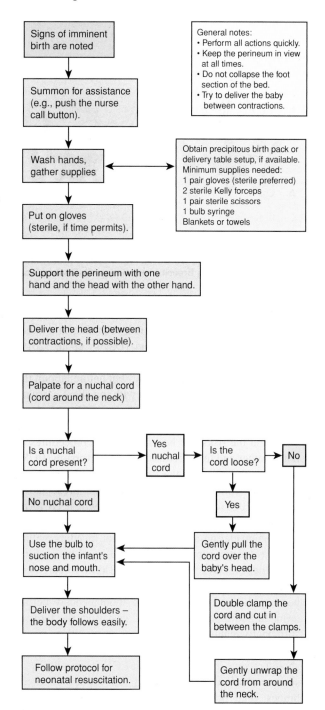

FIGURE 16.4 An algorithm for emergency birth in the case of precipitous labour.

The Term Breech Trial has changed the guidelines for labour and birth in cases of breech presentation. Results have indicated that vaginal birth of a fetus presenting as breech increases risks for overall morbidity and mortality; thus, cesarean birth is recommended as part of the care in such circumstances (Ghosh, 2005). This opinion remains controversial, however, and some obstetricians attempt vaginal breech births depending

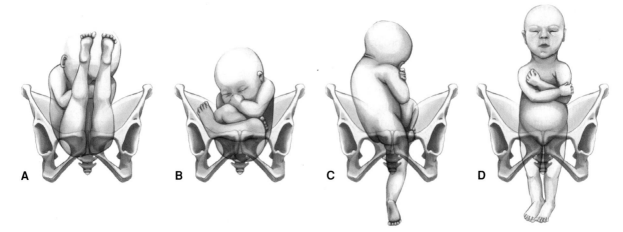

FIGURE 16.5 A: Frank breech presentation. **B:** Complete breech presentation. **C:** Single footling breech presentation. **D:** Double footling breech presentation.

on the specific attitude involved, collaboration with the woman/family regarding risks/benefits, and other maternal and fetal risk factors (Daviss et al., 2010; Doyle et al., 2005).

Close to the end of pregnancy but before labour, the health care team should discuss with the client carrying a fetus with breech presentation the possibility of **external cephalic version**, the need to schedule a cesarean birth, and the risks and benefits of these procedures to both mother and fetus. External cephalic version (ECV) is the manipulation of the fetus, through the maternal abdomen, from a breech to a cephalic presentation (RCOG, 2010). The woman's history will need to be reviewed for the presence of any contraindications such as a major uterine anomaly, antenatal bleeding within the last 7 days, ruptured membranes, and major fetal anomalies (RCOG, 2010). The ideal time to carry out the procedure is after 36 completed weeks' gestation because the fetus may still turn spontaneously before term. In addition, by 37 weeks' gestation, the fetus is sufficiently mature if complications develop that require emergency cesarean birth. The client and her family should receive information about ECV, its possibility of success (30% to 80%), its risks (eg, rupture of membranes, fetal bradycardia), and discomfort associated with the procedure (Hutton & Hofmeyr, 2006). ECV should be performed in a hospital setting with staff and resources to accommodate emergency cesarean birth as necessary. The fetus is assessed prior to the procedure with a 20-minute fetal monitor strip and a nonstress test following the version. Maternal vital signs are assessed every 15 minutes for 30 to 45 minutes post procedure. During the procedure, the fetus is turned so that he or she "follows its nose" (Fig. 16.6). Ultrasound is used appropriately throughout the procedure to assess the effectiveness of efforts and to evaluate the position of the cord and the volume of amniotic fluid (Skupski

et al., 2003). Following the procedure, it is important to provide information to the woman/family on when to return to the hospital (eg, presence of contractions, bright red bleeding, fluid leakage, or decreased fetal movement).

Occasionally, a woman presents in labour and during abdominal palpation the fetus is found in breech presentation. In such an event, the woman's primary care provider should be contacted as soon as possible so that appropriate interventions and adjustments can be enacted. For a woman with a multiple pregnancy, one or both fetuses may be breech. Ultrasound imaging may assist in this determination before birth; again, development of an individualized plan of care is essential.

COLLABORATIVE CARE: BREECH PRESENTATION
Assessment

If a breech presentation has not been identified previously by ultrasound or other methods, indications in a labouring client include a palpable head in the uterine fundus during Leopold maneuvers, fetal heart tones audible slightly above the umbilicus, palpable buttocks during a vaginal examination, and passage of meconium after rupture of the membranes. Once ultrasound confirms breech presentation, the nurse continues to monitor maternal and fetal status while the team makes decisions about the method of birth. The nurse usually plays an important role in communicating information among team members and with the client and family during this time. Continuous fetal assessment is especially important because breech presentation increases the possibility of cord prolapse (see later discussion). Electronic fetal monitoring is usually used in cases of breech presentation.

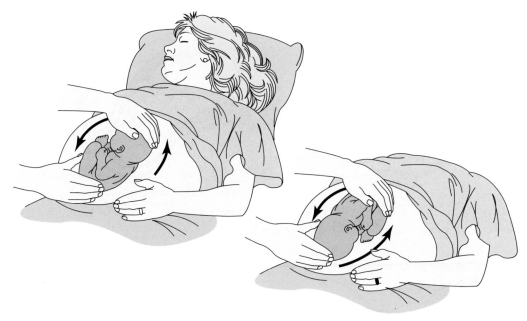

FIGURE 16.6 To perform external cephalic version, the provider uses external pressure to rotate the fetus to a cephalic lie.

Select Potential Nursing Diagnoses

The following nursing diagnoses are likely:

- **Risk for Injury (Maternal)** related to invasive monitoring
- **Risk for Injury (Maternal)** related to cesarean birth
- **Risk for Injury (Fetal)** related to potential prolapsed cord
- **Anxiety** related to concern about birth method

Planning/Intervention

The nurse should work with the client and other team members to outline appropriate goals and to implement identified interventions. Common nursing activities at this time include beginning monitoring techniques, reporting the status of maternal and fetal well-being and any changes, preparing the client for the chosen birth method (vaginal or cesarean), and discussing with the client and her support people what is happening. Explanations and reassurance may be particularly helpful because anxiety and fear related to concern over a breech presentation may compromise the woman's ability to participate effectively during labour.

Pudendal or epidural anaesthesia may be used during vaginal breech births because they do not interfere with labour and facilitate the client's active participation. With a vaginal breech birth, the mechanism of labour is similar to that for vertex presentations (see Chapter 15 and Fig. 16.7). Although some vaginal breech births are spontaneous, they usually require assisted methods, generally to extract the fetal head. An example is the application of Piper forceps, which is discussed later in this chapter.

The procedure for cesarean birth is described and illustrated in detail toward the end of this chapter.

Evaluation

Desired outcomes with a breech presentation include the following:

- The client and fetus show no indications of distress.
- The client verbalizes minimal anxiety and fear.
- The client demonstrates positive coping strategies.
- The client verbalizes understanding of the chosen method of birth.
- The client gives birth to a healthy newborn.

Other Malpresentations

Other abnormal fetal presentations that affect the progress of labour include shoulder, face, brow, and compound presentations.

- *Shoulder presentation* (transverse lie) occurs when the fetus lies crosswise rather than longitudinally in the uterus. The shoulder usually is in the brim of the inlet. Depending on positioning, the back, abdomen, ribs, or flank can also be the presenting part. Common risk factors include multiparity, prematurity, placenta previa, and contracted pelvis (Cunningham et al., 2010). This serious complication increases risks for uterine rupture and perinatal mortality for both mother and child. ECV in late pregnancy or

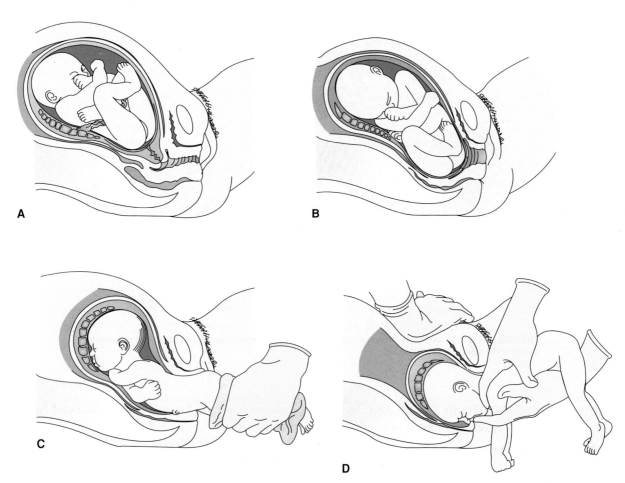

FIGURE 16.7 Steps in a vaginal breech birth. **A:** The fetus is in the left sacroposterior position. **B:** The fetus begins to descend and rotate internally. **C:** The birth attendant uses a cloth to hold the fetal legs below the horizontal, helping to turn the shoulders. **D:** Using gentle pressure, the attendant flexes the fetal head fully and applies traction to move the shoulders upward and outward. The nurse may apply suprapubic pressure to help facilitate flexion of the fetal head.

early labour occasionally is successful in alleviating this problem (Klatt & Cruikshank, 2008). Generally, however, this presentation in a client in active labour is an indication for cesarean birth.

- With *face presentation*, the chin usually enters the pelvic inlet first. A contracted pelvis is the most common cause. If labour is effective and the maternal pelvis is adequate, spontaneous vaginal birth is possible. A cesarean birth is indicated when the fetus shows signs of distress or the maternal pelvis is contracted.
- In *brow presentation*, the largest diameter of the fetal head presents at the pelvic inlet. Again, the underlying factor usually is a contracted pelvis. Unless the fetus is small and the pelvis is large, vaginal birth is impossible. Frequently, however, this unstable presentation spontaneously converts to an occiput or face presentation. Principles of management are the same as for face presentations. Labour progressing normally without fetal distress requires no intervention.

Erratic or hyperactive labour and failure of the presentation to change are indications for cesarean birth.
- *Compound presentations* occur when an extremity prolapses and enters the pelvis with the presenting part. The most common development is for a fetal arm to prolapse with the head. The major complication is increased incidence of prolapsed umbilical cord. Many compound presentations correct themselves spontaneously. If the progress of labour is arrested, the birth attendant may attempt to reposition the prolapsed part. If such attempts are unsuccessful or contraindications to a vaginal birth exist, a cesarean birth is performed (Klatt & Cruikshank, 2008).

Occipitoposterior Position

Occipitoposterior (OP) positioning has the fetus lying with the occiput toward the mother's spine and face toward the mother's pubic symphysis (Shields et al., 2007) (Fig. 16.8). During labour, OP position

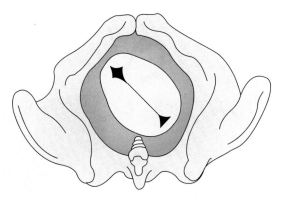

FIGURE 16.8 View from the vaginal outlet of a fetus in the left occipitoposterior position with a cephalic presentation.

may resolve to the anterior position; however, the fetus remains in OP position for 10% of labouring women, and 5% of babies are in OP position at birth (Cheng et al., 2006). This position is associated with a prolonged second stage, and less than 30% of nulliparous women with a fetus in this position will have a spontaneous vaginal birth (Shields et al., 2007). Clients with a previous history of pregnancies with OP position are at increased risk for carrying another fetus in this position. The fetal head may be poorly applied to the cervix, and labour may be slow. Labour induction or augmentation with oxytocin may have limited success (see later discussion). Risk factors associated with persistent OP position include a 5-minute Apgar score less than 7, meconium-stained amniotic fluid, birth trauma, and longer neonatal stay in the hospital (Cheng et al., 2006).

COLLABORATIVE CARE: OP POSITION

When labour occurs with a fetus in OP position, the major finding generally is maternal back pain with contractions. The underlying cause is internal pressure from the fetal skull against the maternal spine. Monitoring of this woman's progress in labour and the ongoing position of the fetus is critical to care.

Assessment

When a client arrives at the obstetrical unit describing her labour primarily as "back pain," health care providers should suspect that the fetal position is OP. They can use abdominal palpation for verification. A space or dip at the maternal umbilicus might indicate the space between the fetal arms and legs. Palpating the fetal back may be difficult; the fetal heart rate may be auscultated at the level of the umbilicus or laterally. The fetal head may not be felt deep in the pelvis because engagement may or may not occur before labour (Robbins, 2011).

Select Potential Nursing Diagnoses

Appropriate nursing diagnoses may include the following:

- **Pain** related to fetal position centred in the maternal back as well as abdomen
- **Anxiety** related to the possibility of an extended labour and its effects on fetal health
- **Risk for Injury (Trauma)** related to increased risk for an operative birth, cesarean birth, or both

Planning/Intervention

For the woman, it is essential to encourage ambulation and different positions that may allow the pelvis to open further and promote a fetal rotation (Fig. 16.9). Specifically, asking the woman to lie on the side in which the fetal spine is located is helpful. For example, if the fetus is in right occiput posterior position, the woman would lie on her right side. Gravity will then assist the fetal occiput and trunk toward the right occiput transverse and then right occiput anterior positions. On her side, the woman has a pillow wedged between her back and the bed, with another under the abdomen for support (Bianchi & Adams, 2009). Using the hands-and-knees, side-lying, or sitting position, walking, or trying the birthing ball may help to spontaneously turn the fetus. Pain management may include use of a Jacuzzi, analgesics, or epidural (Fig. 16.10). Discussion of the client's preferences for labour would be important to assist her in choosing such elements of her plan of care. Providing information regarding the fetal position and explanations for different strategies may facilitate willingness of the client and her family to try alternative positions. See Nursing Care Plan 16.1.

Evaluation

Desired outcomes include normal progress in labour, fulfillment of the client's wishes according to her birth plan, and achievement of a spontaneous vaginal birth.

 Remember Beverly, the client from the beginning of the chapter who is complaining of back pain. Assessment reveals that the fetus is in the OP position. What measures might the care team use to help turn the fetus?

Shoulder Dystocia

Shoulder dystocia is defined as a birthing process that requires additional obstetric maneuvers after gentle downward traction on the fetal head fails to enable delivery of the shoulders (Beck, 2013). It occurs

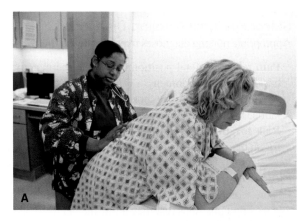

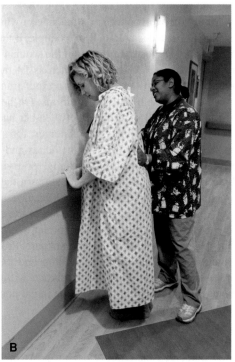

FIGURE 16.9 To help ease the pain of back labour and facilitate a fetal shift in position, the nurse may encourage the woman to (**A**) try different positions and (**B**) ambulate.

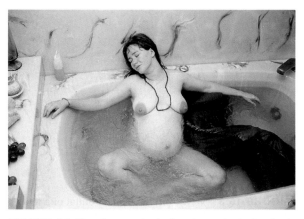

FIGURE 16.10 One method of easing pain during back labour may include the use of a Jacuzzi or bath. (Photo courtesy of Kaye Bullock, CPM.)

COLLABORATIVE CARE: SHOULDER DYSTOCIA

Once shoulder dystocia is diagnosed, the health care team usually tries several steps to assist with birth. It is crucial for members to remain calm, attempt different strategies in a timely fashion, and move on at the right point. Potential maternal complications include vaginal, cervical, or perineal lacerations requiring extensive repair; bladder injury; hematoma; uterine rupture; and postpartum hemorrhage (see Chapter 19). Potential fetal complications include brachial plexus injury, fractures, and asphyxia (Politi et al., 2010).

Assessment

Nursing assessment of the second stage of labour includes awareness of the descent of the fetal head and time. If the client has received epidural anaesthesia (see Chapter 17), she may not push until after her cervix has become fully dilated and her fetus has "laboured down" to a lower station prior to initiating pushing. This facilitates the woman having an "urge to push" to ensure that her efforts work with her body sensations. The nurse assesses fetal health as well as maternal vital signs to ensure stability. Once pushing efforts begin, it is important to monitor duration and to communicate with the client's care provider if progress, fetal descent, or both are not occurring.

Select Potential Nursing Diagnoses

Common nursing diagnoses in the care of shoulder dystocia include the following:

- **Anxiety** related to unexpected emergency measures required to facilitate birth
- **Deficient Knowledge** related to measures being done to assist with this birth
- **Risk for Injury (Trauma)** related to fetal and maternal measures required to facilitate birth

in 0.2% to 3% of all births (Beck, 2013). Risk factors include maternal diabetes, maternal obesity, postterm pregnancy, fetal macrosomia, previous history of shoulder dystocia, and multiparity (Sheiner et al., 2006). Often, shoulder dystocia is unexpected and presents only as slow extension of the fetal head with the chin remaining tight against the maternal perineum. The fetal head may appear to retract against the perineum ("*turtle sign*").

Care of all labouring women during the second stage includes identification of shoulder dystocia. Clear, ongoing communication among team members enhances assessment of the client's progress and of the appropriate interventions.

NURSING CARE PLAN 16.1

●

The Client in Labour With Significant Back Pain

 Beverly, the client in labour, is complaining about significant back pain. Assessment reveals that her fetus is in the OP position. "My second baby was also this way, but he turned pretty quickly. I had back pain for a bit, but not like now. This is not what I expected. I'm worried. What if he doesn't turn?" The client rates her pain as 9 out of 10.

NURSING DIAGNOSES

- **Pain** related to fetal OP position
- **Anxiety** related to continued pain, unexpected events of labour, and failure of the fetus to turn to the anterior position for birth

EXPECTED OUTCOMES

1. The client will verbalize that pain is reduced to a tolerable level.
2. The client will state that her anxiety level has decreased.
3. The client will participate in decision making about preferences for labour.

INTERVENTIONS	RATIONALES
Frequently assess the client's level of pain, asking her to rate it on a scale of 1 to 10	Ongoing assessment provides valuable indicators for effectiveness of relief strategies
Discuss with the client her concerns, feelings, and perceptions related to changes in expectations about labour and birth and current pain level	Discussion allows the nurse to emphasize positive aspects of the current situation; verbalization of concerns helps to identify sources of stress and problem areas
Communicate accurate data and answer questions honestly. Reinforce facts, emphasizing that each pregnancy, labour, and birth is highly individualized	Open communication promotes trust and helps correct any misconceptions. Facts can dispel unfounded fears, myths, misconceptions, and feelings of guilt
Evaluate the client's past coping strategies to determine which have been effective	Use of appropriate coping strategies aids in reducing anxiety
Explain to the client and her partner measures that facilitate spontaneous turning of the fetus. Encourage frequent position changes and ambulation. Suggest the use of a birthing ball, hands-and-knees position, or sitting	Different maternal positions and ambulation can help open the pelvis and facilitate fetal turning
Teach the client's partner how to provide pressure or massage to the lower back. Suggest applying ice or heat to the area	Fetal head rotation may compress the sacral nerve. Pressure, massage, or heat or cold may help alleviate this painful sensation
Offer pharmacologic measures for pain relief	Medications can reduce or decrease pain
Frequently assess the abdomen for fetal position; perform Leopold maneuvers; monitor fetal and maternal status as indicated	Leopold maneuvers aid in determining fetal presentation and position. Frequent monitoring provides information about maternal and fetal well-being

(continued)

NURSING CARE PLAN 16.1 • The Client in Labour With Significant Back Pain *(Continued)*

INTERVENTIONS	RATIONALES
Update the couple regularly about the progress of labour and the fetus. Offer them continuing support and guidance	Frequent communication promotes the couple's participation and reinforces the effectiveness of their activities, thus enhancing a sense of accomplishment

EVALUATION

1. The client verbally rates pain as tolerable.
2. The client states that she is more comfortable.
3. The client identifies preferences and choices for labour and birth.
4. The client progresses through labour without additional problems.

Planning/Intervention

The sense of urgency present in any obstetrical emergency accompanies shoulder dystocia. The nurse should begin by calling for additional help and then working with the obstetrician and other team members to facilitate birth.

1. The first step is usually to use McRoberts maneuver (Fig. 16.11). This procedure involves hyperflexing the woman's legs into a knee-chest position, allowing elevation of the anterior fetal shoulder while flexing the fetal spine. The woman's legs may need to be supported if she has had an epidural. This maneuver alone often results in resolution of the shoulder dystocia.

2a. If McRoberts maneuver alone is unsuccessful, the next step is application of suprapubic pressure (Fig. 16.12). This steady pressure with the palm or heel of the hand against the fetal back directs the

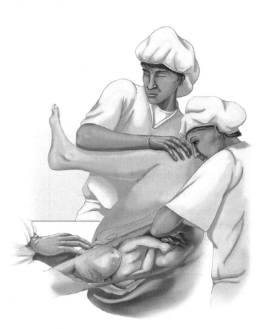

FIGURE 16.11 McRoberts maneuver.

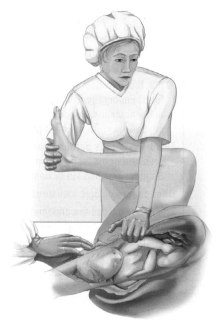

FIGURE 16.12 Application of suprapubic pressure.

pressure toward the fetal midline. The nurse and all care providers must know the difference between fundal and suprapubic pressure to apply suprapubic pressure appropriately. Generally, McRoberts maneuver and suprapubic pressure resolve 50% to 91% of cases of shoulder dystocia when the episiotomy has been adequate (Kwek & Yeo, 2006).

2b. Another alternative is to assist the woman into a hands-and-knees position with the objective of dislodging the shoulder. This may be an early consideration or may be attempted after the Wood's maneuver. (This measure is not possible with an epidural in place.)

3. The next attempt is the Wood's screw rotational maneuver, which is to move the posterior fetal shoulder through a 180-degree turn, allowing the anterior fetal shoulder to present for birth.

After birth is complete, examinations for maternal injury and hemorrhage and appropriate neonatal resuscitation efforts are crucial, as well as assessment of the infant for injury. Documentation of all appropriate medical and nursing interventions is vital, as is communication with the family to describe what was done and why.

Evaluation

Birth without extensive injury to either mother or infant is the desired outcome of care. Team members who work together in a calm and organized fashion can assist in decreasing stress perceived by the client and her family under these circumstances. Shoulder dystocia can be mild, with only repositioning required to free the fetal shoulders, or it can become traumatic, with many health care providers involved and increasing concern over the health of the woman and fetus. If the woman and the nurses are feeling shaken, stunned, or anxious, it is important to provide care to everyone. The obstetrician or health care provider can be encouraged to talk with the woman and family, explaining what occurred and describing the next steps. The nurse can report his or her emotional state to the charge nurse and request an opportunity to debrief, particularly if this is a new experience (Beck, 2013).

Excessive Fetal Size or Fetal Abnormalities

Other passenger-related problems include excessive fetal size and fetal abnormalities. Usually, these problems are determined *in utero* based on ultrasound findings and Leopold maneuvers. In many cases, however, these complications are not suspected unless the client has a condition increasing her risk (eg, diabetes). When such problems are diagnosed early enough, the health care team can plan with the client for a cesarean birth. If diagnosis is uncertain or not made, the client may progress

through labour with attempts for vaginal birth. Risks for cervical lacerations, prolapsed uterus, and other problems are increased, however, and many obstetricians elect to proceed with surgical birth when problems with fetal size or other circumstances are detected early enough.

Macrosomia

A newborn is considered to have **macrosomia** (excessive size) when he or she weighs more than 4,500 g at birth, a complication in approximately 10% of pregnancies (Jazayeri & Contreras, 2007). Macrosomia usually results from uncontrolled diabetes, genetics, multiparity, or a combination of these factors. Postterm pregnancy also may be responsible. Fetuses weighing more than 4,900 g are rare.

Macrosomia can cause cephalopelvic disproportion. It can also cause uterine overdistention, reducing the strength of contractions, prolonging labour, and increasing the risk for overall maternal and fetal complications. When the fetal biparietal diameter (usually 9.5 to 9.8 cm at term) of a macrosomic fetus attempts to fit through the maternal pelvis, **moulding** (overlapping of the skull bones at major suture lines) occurs, decreasing the biparietal diameter up to 0.5 cm without fetal injury (Fig. 16.13). Severe moulding may lead to tearing, intracranial hemorrhage, or scalp edema. Moulding generally disappears within the newborn's first few days, but severe pressure between fetus and pelvis may cause skull fracture.

Birth trauma frequently associated with macrosomia increases risks for fetal or newborn mortality. Macrosomic newborns may have a difficult extrauterine transition because of problems during labour and birth, such as bruising, cephalohematoma, and brachial plexus injury.

Fetal Abnormalities

Fetal abnormalities that can contribute to dystocia include such problems as hydrocephalus, neck masses,

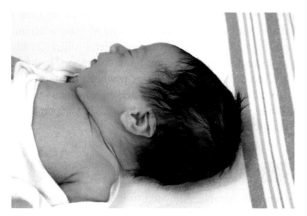

FIGURE 16.13 A macrosomic newborn may have cranial moulding if the presenting part is too big for the maternal outlet.

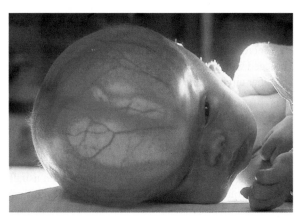

FIGURE 16.14 One problem with the passenger that may cause dystocia is hydrocephalus.

a large and swollen fetal abdomen from excessive bladder distention, enlarged liver or kidneys, and, rarely, conjoined twins. Any of these problems can interfere with fetal descent or passage through the birth canal.

The most common fetal anomaly causing dystocia is **hydrocephalus**, or excess accumulation of cerebrospinal fluid in the brain ventricles and subsequent cranial enlargement (Fig. 16.14). Hydrocephalus accounts for approximately 12% of all birth-related malformations (Cunningham et al., 2010) and is frequently associated with other congenital defects (eg, spina bifida) (see Chapter 22). Breech presentations are common with cases of hydrocephalus because the distended cranium cannot fit into the pelvic inlet.

Obstructed labour associated with hydrocephalus may lead to uterine rupture, particularly if the problem is not detected before labour begins. The nurse should suspect hydrocephalus when palpation for the fetal head reveals an enlarged symmetric mass in the uterine fundus. Such detection can be challenging, however, because excessive amniotic fluid commonly makes such palpation more difficult.

When ultrasound reveals hydrocephalus in advance of labour and birth, a cranial shunt may be inserted *in utero* to minimize brain damage and to delay birth until gestation advances closer to term. Fetal surgery to treat hydrocephalus is becoming more common. The labour will be difficult, and risks for newborn morbidity and mortality are high. Nursing interventions focus on providing significant maternal support. See Chapter 22 for additional information.

PROBLEMS WITH THE PASSAGE

Generally, problems related to the passage involve the maternal pelvis. Many of these concerns can be predicted and prepared for when a woman has received adequate prenatal care; however, if a woman arrives at the health care facility for the first time in labour, problems with the passage may need to be addressed as an obstetric emergency.

Pelvic Shape Problems

As discussed in Chapter 12, the maternal pelvis is one of four types: gynecoid, anthropoid, android, and platypelloid. Vaginal birth is usually successful when the maternal pelvis is gynecoid or anthropoid. The chances for vaginal birth are usually poor for women with the other two pelvic types, generally indicating a need for cesarean birth.

Contracted Pelvis

With a contracted pelvis, one or more of the pelvic diameters are reduced to the point of interference with the progress of labour. Pelvic contraction can occur at the inlet, midpelvis, or outlet.

- *Inlet contraction.* The pelvic anteroposterior diameter is less than 10 cm, the pelvic transverse diameter is less than 12 cm, or both. This problem may result from small maternal body size, rickets, or delayed maternal development. It is difficult for the fetal presenting part to fit well at the cervix, leading to the complications inherent with prolonged labour.
- *Midpelvic contraction.* The distance between the ischial spines is less than 9 cm or the sum of the interspinous and posterior sagittal distance is less than 13.5 cm. The presenting part can engage in the pelvis, making this problem harder to recognize and manage than inlet contraction.
- *Outlet contraction.* The distance between the ischial tuberosities is less than 8 cm. Although this problem increases the risks for perineal tears and forceps-assisted birth, vaginal birth can usually be accomplished.

Measurement of the pelvis in comparison to the fetal head size has been studied recently with the aim of predicting labour dystocia and the need for cesarean birth. Use of magnetic resonance imaging has potential for assessment of the bony pelvis as well as the soft tissue in the pelvis. Unfortunately, the results identify the women at risk for dysfunctional labour but cannot accurately predict those who will require a cesarean birth, because the variability of uterine activity and molding of the fetal head cannot be foreseen (Zaretsky et al., 2005).

PRETERM LABOUR

Preterm labour is considered true labour that begins before 37 completed weeks of gestation. The rate of preterm birth in Canada is approximately 7.9% (PHAC, 2011).

This rate is much higher in multiple pregnancies, with a rate of 6.4% in twins, 55% in triplets, and 98% in quadruplets (PHAC, 2011). Avoidance, early detection, and management of this problem are major foci of prenatal and antepartal care.

In Canada, the approximate lifetime cost for each surviving preterm infant with a birth weight less than 2,500 g is $600,000. A conservative estimate is that $250,000,000 is spent annually in Canada on problems associated with low-birth-weight infants (Canadian Institute for Health Information [CIHI], 2006). IUGR is increased in women who present with preterm labour and progress to premature childbirth (Gilbert & Danielsen, 2003). Other complications include neurodevelopmental delay, respiratory complications (eg, bronchopulmonary dysplasia), and blindness (Rosenberg, 2008).

Etiology and Risk Factors

The causes of preterm labour are not well identified or clear. Common contributing factors include history of a previous preterm birth, polyhydramnios, placental abruption or previa, short cervix, preterm prelabour rupture of membranes (PPROM) (see Chapter 13), multiple pregnancy, uterine malformation, and maternal infection. Frequently, the cause remains unknown. Research has shown several conditions to increase risks for preterm labour. See Box 16.1.

In all pregnancies, health care providers exert significant effort to detect and treat any risk factors

● **BOX 16.1   Risk Factors for Preterm Labour**

- Adolescent pregnancy
- Alcohol or drug use, especially cocaine
- Anemia
- Bacterial vaginosis
- Cervical insufficiency
- Chorioamnionitis
- Cigarette smoking
- Closely spaced pregnancies
- Diabetes mellitus
- Intimate-partner violence
- History of previous preterm birth
- Hydramnios
- Hypertension
- Low socioeconomic status
- Malnutrition
- Multiple gestation
- Periodontal disease
- Placental problems
- Sexually transmitted infections
- Stress
- Urinary tract infections
- Uterine abnormalities

aggressively. Although actual cervical changes are necessary for preterm labour to be diagnosed, any premature uterine activity requires immediate evaluation to ensure that nothing more serious is developing. The anticipated success rate of delaying labour in such instances depends on the stage of labour at which interventions are implemented. Ideally, however, labour is postponed for as long as possible to advance the gestation closer to 37 weeks. See the section Preterm Premature Rupture of the Membranes in Chapter 13 for more discussion of measures commonly used to halt labour. Also see Teaching Tips 16.1.

The cervix has been described as a "purse string" that closes the lower segment of the uterus, formed by cartilaginous connective tissue that begins softening during pregnancy, with further effacement in the 4 to 8 weeks prior to labour (Taylor, 2011). This process begins in the inner os of the cervix, with "funneling," and moves to the external os over time. Cervical length and funneling can be accurately measured using transvaginal ultrasound, and this is helpful when a woman is assessed for symptoms of preterm labour, or has a history of previous preterm labour. Average length of the cervix shortens as pregnancy continues, with an average length of 40 mm before 22 weeks, 35 mm at 22 to 32 weeks, and 30 mm after 33 weeks. The shorter the cervix, the higher the risk of preterm birth (Taylor, 2011). The majority of women with symptoms will not go on to preterm labour, so use of ultrasound to measure length can assist with a diagnosis.

Fetal fibronectin testing is also an assessment for the risk of preterm birth. Fibronectin is a glycoprotein found between the fetal membranes and the uterine decidua, and is released as the cervix prepares for labor. A negative test indicates a high probability that labour will not occur within the next 1 to 2 weeks. A positive test is less predictive but indicates a possibility of preterm labour within the week. A pelvic examination, vaginal ultrasound, or vaginal intercourse within 24 hours of testing can make the test inaccurate.

Cervical length assessment and collection of cervical fluid for fetal fibronectin testing can be used together to more accurately predict the likelihood of preterm labour and birth.

Bacterial infection of the lower genital tract may contribute to preterm labour (Denney & Culhan, 2009). Thus, experts have recommended prenatal screening of urine and cervical cultures for group B Streptococcus, with appropriate antibiotics and follow-up cultures for those women who test positive (see Chapter 13). Abstinence from sexual intercourse is another preventive measure in clients susceptible to preterm labour. Tocolytic agents are used for management of early preterm labour because the effectiveness of these drugs decreases as labour advances.

● TEACHING TIPS 16.1 Preventing Premature Birth

Babies born before 37 weeks' completed gestation can suffer lifelong health consequences such as chronic lung disease, cerebral palsy, and blindness. Being born too soon is the leading cause of death in newborns. Because ways to prevent preterm labour are not clearly established, the best approach is for pregnant women to try to preserve and maintain their overall health and to know the signs of pre-term labour. Early treatment may reduce problems.

Measures to preserve and to optimize maternal health include the following:

- Schedule and attend regular prenatal appointments.
- Take a prenatal vitamin daily throughout pregnancy.
- Give the health care provider a comprehensive medical history including any other instances of preterm labour and birth.
- Quit smoking or cut back as much as possible.
- Stop drinking alcohol.
- Avoid illegal drugs; inform the health care provider of any over-the-counter medications or herbal remedies used.

- Avoid stress as much as possible; talk to family and friends about ways that they can help.
- Call the health care provider if any burning or pain accompanies urination or if vaginal discharge is increased and whitish.
- Be aware of the signs of preterm labour; call the health care provider if they develop.

Signs for women to be aware of and to report to providers are as follows:

- Contractions every 10 minutes or more often
- Clear, pink, or brownish fluid (water) leaking from the vagina
- The feeling that the baby is pushing down
- A low, dull backache
- Menstrual-like cramps
- Cramps with or without diarrhea

Assessment Findings

Early diagnosis is often difficult. Possible signs and symptoms include menstrual-like cramps or abdominal pain, diarrhea, pressure in the pelvis or lower back, and increased vaginal discharge. Because these symptoms are nonspecific, however, they may not concern the woman until a real problem has developed. Diagnosis of preterm labour occurs with regular uterine contractions and rupture of the membranes.

COLLABORATIVE CARE: PRETERM LABOUR

Health care providers must work together to assess a client who presents to the labour and birth area before term to identify her risk factors for preterm labour, establish her gestation, and evaluate her contractions. If she is found to be in true labour, limited activity, intra-venous (IV) fluid administration, and tocolytic medications (eg, indomethacin) may be used; however, there is little evidence to show that these measures effectively arrest labour. Nevertheless, even moderate prolongation of pregnancy can be beneficial and provide sufficient time to administer antenatal steroids that can assist with fetal lung maturity. SOGC recommends two 12-mg doses of IM betamethasone given 24 hours apart or four 6-mg doses of IM dexamethasone given 12 hours apart (SOGC, 2003). Tocolytics whose use has been or continues to be investigated through research include indomethacin, progesterone, and transdermal nitroglycerin (Smith et al., 2007; SOGC, 2010a, 2010b; Tan et al., 2006) (Table 16.1).

Health care providers need to determine the best location for this client, depending on gestation and other risk factors. If true labour is diagnosed, admission of the client to a centre with advanced neonatal facilities may be necessary. If a fetal fibronectin test produces a negative result, the need to transfer the client would be significantly decreased, as a negative result indicates a less than 1% risk of delivery within the following 14 days.

Assessment

The nurse who first sees this client and her family in the obstetrical assessment area should approach them calmly to decrease anxiety. Depending on institutional policy, labour assessment may include vaginal examination; evaluation of contraction frequency, intensity, and duration; and monitoring of fetal well-being. The nurse records the presence of amniotic fluid, vaginal bleeding, or bloody show, along with information about the onset of contractions, maternal well-being, and past medical history.

Select Potential Nursing Diagnoses

Nursing diagnoses commonly included in the care of the woman experiencing preterm labour are as follows:

- **Deficient Knowledge** related to treatment plan for preterm labour

● TABLE 16.1   **Common Medications Used in Preterm Labour**

Drug	Action	Nursing Considerations
Betamethasone (Celestone)	Stimulates production of surfactant, which promotes fetal lung maturity and protects against respiratory distress (in fetuses younger than 34 weeks' gestation)	Teach the client and family about the medication's potential benefits to the fetus. Monitor the client for any signs of edema or infection. Regularly assess maternal lung sounds.
Indomethacin (Indocin)	Inhibits uterine activity	Continuously assess vital signs, fetal heart rate, and uterine activity. Administer the oral form with food to reduce gastric irritation. Be alert for adverse maternal effects, including rash, nausea and vomiting, heartburn, oligohydramnios, and hypertension; and adverse fetal effects, including heart problems, pulmonary hypertension, and necrotizing enterocolitis. Administration should be limited to those pregnancies of less than 32 weeks' gestation and should not be given for more than 72 hours to prevent premature closure of the ductus arteriosus and secondary pulmonary hypertension.
Transdermal nitroglycerin	Appears to inhibit uterine activity	Administration of normal saline bolus prior to administration of transdermal nitroglycerin may decrease incidence of hypotension. Assess for maternal headache.
Progesterone	May have a limited role in hormonal control of contractions	Recommended for use exclusively in women with history of previous preterm labour or who have a short cervix of <15 mm detected by transvaginal ultrasound at 22–26 weeks Women should be encouraged to participate in research studies investigating the use of progesterone.

- **Anxiety** related to maternal and fetal health
- **Risk for Injury (Trauma)** related to preterm labour and birth (particularly fetal)

Planning/Interventions

Once the nurse has collected assessment information, he or she notifies the client's primary obstetric provider as soon as possible. Depending on the stage and progress of labour, staff members may need to arrange transport to another location to facilitate the safest care for the newborn.

Indications for labour tocolysis involve considerations related to gestational age. Because fetal lungs are usually mature by 36 completed weeks, the baby born between 36 and 38 weeks and weighing more than 2,500 g usually does not need pulmonary support. Tocolytic therapy for a fetus older than 35 weeks is unlikely to be instituted. Tocolytic therapy generally is employed in the following situations:

- Preterm labour has been diagnosed definitively.
- Gestational age is more than 20 but less than 36 weeks.
- Fetal weight is estimated as less than 2,500 g.
- Fetal lung profile shows signs of immaturity (inadequate alveolar surfactant) (SOGC, 2000).

If tocolytic management stops labour, drug administration may need to continue until contractions have decreased or ceased according to medication recommendations, the health care provider's preferences, and the client's ability to tolerate the medications. Antenatal steroids should be administered during this time per normal dosages. If labour stops spontaneously, the client needs ongoing monitoring in the assessment area (based on facility protocol), with plans made about when to return.

- If contractions begin again
- If she experiences low backache
- With any presence of show, rupture of the membranes, vaginal bleeding, or a combination of these problems

In early labour (cervical dilatation of 2 to 3 cm), limited activity, hydration, and sedation may stop uterine activity by increasing intravascular volume and uterine blood flow, as well as by reducing pressure of the fetal head on the cervix. Tocolytic therapy (eg, indomethacin) further enhances success.

If the client gives birth spontaneously, staff must be available to care for the newborn. Ideally, personnel from the neonatal intensive care unit (NICU) attend the birth. Explaining to the family the procedures employed and the care provided helps alleviate anxiety. If transport of the newborn is required following birth, taking pictures with the baby, holding the baby, or even briefly touching the baby can assist parents with bonding. Establishing communication with the transport team and the institution where the baby will be transferred for care is essential; if possible, the mother should be transported to the same site as the baby.

Evaluation

Ideal outcomes include early diagnosis of labour and identification and treatment of the cause. If preterm labour cannot be controlled or delayed, desired outcomes are having appropriate resources and personnel present during the birth and a healthy newborn and mother.

POSTTERM PREGNANCY AND LABOUR

Establishment of an accurate due date is a critical element in effective prenatal care. A woman's last menstrual period, together with her obstetric history, including the length of her menstrual cycle, and an initial ultrasound (the ultrasound associated with genetic screening may be done at 11 to 13 weeks with the morphologic ultrasound scheduled for sometime between 16 and 20 weeks of pregnancy) helps primary care providers determine an accurate due date (see Chapter 12). The earliest ultrasound is the most accurate predictor of an accurate due date. The fetal biparietal diameter obtained at the initial ultrasound normally is accurate to within 5 days (Schmidt, 1999).

Approximately 90% of women give birth within 14 days after their due date (Butler & Wilkes, 2006). Significant concern arises with **postterm pregnancy** (a pregnancy that extends beyond 41 completed weeks' gestational age) (Moore & Martin, 2003):

- After 40 weeks, the overall fetal mortality rate of 1% to 2% begins to increase.
- By 42 weeks, the mortality rate doubles.
- Morbidity increases exponentially as gestation exceeds 40 weeks, particularly when other risk factors (eg, gestational diabetes) exist.
- Placental function peaks at 36 weeks and begins to deteriorate by 38 weeks. This deterioration may lead to inadequate fetal nutrition and IUGR, oligohydramnios, and inadequate fetal oxygenation. Efficient placental function beyond 38 weeks may contribute to macrosomia and subsequent birth trauma.
- Meconium in the amniotic fluid occurs in 25% to 30% of all prolonged pregnancies (twice the rate of term pregnancies). Causes include hypoxic events or maturity of the fetus with vagal reflex. Fresh meconium

occurs most often with umbilical cord compression and impaired maternal–fetal blood flow. With oligohydramnios, meconium thickens and increases the risk for aspiration.

Consider Carlotta, who is at 42 weeks' gestation and scheduled for induction of labour. What would be the rationale for inducing her labour?

Women with postterm pregnancy generally experience various emotions. Impatience, frustration, fatigue, depression, and pressure from family and friends may cause them to become anxious about labour and birth and concerned for fetal safety and health. These emotions may accumulate with ongoing prenatal visits and questions from interested others. Setting a date for induction of labour and then having to change that date (eg, because of an unexpected increase in activity at the birthing centre) may lead to anger and sadness. Allowing the client to express her feelings, come to the health care facility for a fetal health evaluation (nonstress test), and reschedule at the soonest available time may help mitigate negative feelings in such circumstances. Scheduling of induction for physician or patient convenience has led to an increase in near-term infant births (35 to 37 weeks' gestation) and cesarean births (Zwelling, 2008).

Factors to consider in deciding whether to induce labour include the following:

- Cervical ripeness
- Fetal pulmonary maturity
- Fetal ability to tolerate labour
- Uterine sensitivity to the proposed induced method
- Maternal condition
- Gestational age
- Fetal size

Contraindications to labour induction include the following:

- Complete placenta previa or vasa previa (see Chapter 13)
- Classical uterine incision from a previous cesarean birth
- Pelvic structural deformities
- Active genital herpes infection
- Abnormal fetal presentation (eg, transverse lie)

Labour is most likely to occur when the cervix displays readiness to progressively efface and dilate. The Bishop score is used to assess cervical readiness (see Chapter 15). Low numbers indicate an unfavourable cervix and an increased likelihood of prolonged labour and cesarean birth. A score greater than 6 indicates an increased likelihood of a successful induction of labour. Studies have shown a significantly increased risk of cesarean birth after induction of labour, particularly in nulliparous women or women with an unfavourable Bishop score at the initiation of the induction (Zwelling, 2008).

Detailed discussion of the methods of labour induction is found later in this chapter.

 The health care provider obtained the following scores when evaluating Carlotta's cervical readiness: dilatation = 2, effacement = 2, station = 2, cervical consistency = 1, position = 2. What would these findings indicate?

HEMORRHAGIC PROBLEMS

Vaginal bleeding at any time during pregnancy is physically and emotionally stressful for clients and their health care providers. Pregnant women are repeatedly told during childbirth education classes, prenatal appointments, and preadmission visits to be vigilant for this problem. The nurse in the labour and birth area must be aware of the different causes of vaginal bleeding so that he or she can assess and communicate other appropriate signs and symptoms to the obstetrician or midwife if this is noted at the time of presentation. Initial assessment focuses on the severity of bleeding and stability of the woman and fetus. Optimal management of bleeding in the third trimester relies on accurate identification of the cause and timely intervention related to the severity of the bleeding (Sakornbut et al., 2007).

PLACENTAL PROBLEMS

Bleeding associated with labour may involve the placenta and its membranes. Problems of placental attachment are presented in detail in Chapter 13; they are described briefly here in terms of their role in labour and birth.

Placenta Previa

Painless, bright red vaginal bleeding is the defining characteristic of *placenta previa* which occurs in 1 out of every 200 pregnancies (see Chapter 13). If such bleeding has not been identified or does not develop until after labour starts, bloody show and uterine contractions may further confuse the situation (Oyelese & Smulian, 2006). Accurate identification depends on

thorough assessment of the extent of vaginal bleeding. In cases of hemorrhage, blood loss is not difficult to diagnose. When the amount of bleeding is ambiguous, review of the prenatal history for placental location, vaginal bleeding, or maternal–fetal tachycardia can assist with a diagnosis. The nurse immediately reports any excessive vaginal bleeding during labour. Vaginal examination in clients with vaginal bleeding should be avoided until placenta previa is ruled out.

Evaluations during labour would include the following:

- Bleeding: amount, presence of clots, colour, and ability to stop spontaneously
- Pain and contractions
- Vital signs: pulse, temperature, respiratory rate, and blood pressure
- Fetal heart rate
- Leopold maneuvers to determine fetal position and presentation

The nurse reports any findings outside of the normal range to the client's health care provider. Other communication issues include progress in labour and need for pain management. If the woman has a history of cesarean birth and presents with placenta previa or a placenta located at the site of the previous incision, an evaluation for potential placenta accreta with colour-flow Doppler studies should be done, if at all possible. The risk of placenta accreta, increta, or percreta increases with the number of previous cesarean births (Sakornbut et al., 2007).

A cesarean birth should be anticipated with placenta previa at or beyond 36 weeks' gestational age (Rao et al., 2012). General anaesthesia is likely if the client is hypovolemic, bleeding, or both; spinal anaesthesia would be considered if bleeding stops and volume status is within normal limits. The mother will need close monitoring during the postpartum period for signs of hemorrhage.

Placental Abruption

As discussed in Chapter 13, *placental abruption* (premature separation of a normally implanted placenta) can be a minor or life-threatening problem. Smoking, uterine malformation, previous cesarean section, and history of placental abruption are significant risk factors for placental abruption in a subsequent pregnancy (Tikkanen et al., 2006). Because of the pregnant state, maternal vital signs may not be valid indicators of the degree of blood loss or shock.

Care of the client and family depends on the gestational age and maternal and fetal status. The goal is to stabilize both mother and fetus; if the fetus is alive, the team focuses on a cesarean birth as quickly as possible. Blood loss may be substantial during birth; medications

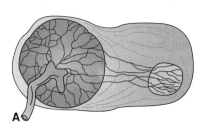 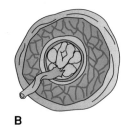 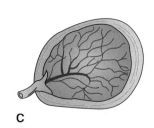 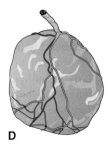

FIGURE 16.15 A: Succenturiate placenta. **B:** Circumvallate placenta. **C:** Battledore placenta. **D:** Velamentous placenta.

such as oxytocin, ergometrine, and Hemabate should be readily available at this time (Palmer, 2002). Collection of cervical fluid for fetal fibronectin testing and ongoing assessment of vital signs, pain, bleeding, and fetal monitoring for reassuring signs are essential components of the plan of care. In some cases of severe abruption, the fetus dies *in utero*. In such cases, the decision for vaginal or cesarean delivery is based on the risks for hemorrhage or other complications related to optimizing maternal health.

Other Placental Anomalies

Some placental problems are not identified until labour begins or until after birth (Fig. 16.15):

- With *succenturiate placenta*, one or more small accessory lobes develop in the membranes at a distance from the main placenta. Connecting vessels may tear during birth or when the membranes rupture. After placental expulsion, one or more lobes may be retained in the uterus, resulting in maternal postpartum hemorrhage (see Chapter 19).
- In *circumvallate placenta*, the membranes are folded back on the fetal surface of the placenta, exposing part of the umbilical cord. Such exposure increases risks for small prenatal hemorrhages leading to preterm birth, as well as of retained placenta leading to postpartum hemorrhage.
- In a *battledore placenta*, the umbilical cord inserts at the placental margin rather than in the centre. This variation is not considered clinically significant.
- With a *velamentous cord insertion* into the placenta, umbilical blood vessels course unprotected for long distances through the membranes to insert into the placental margin. The vessels may be at risk for compression by the fetus and decreased oxygen. If they pass over the internal cervical os, they are at risk for rupture and this is described as a vasa previa. This is a situation in which there can be a fetal hemorrhage at the time of membrane rupture that can cause exsanguination within 10 minutes. An emergent cesarean birth is required immediately if an Apt test confirms the presence of fetal blood with any hemorrhage (Rao et al., 2012).

UTERINE RUPTURE

Uterine rupture is a full thickness disruption of the uterine wall with or without fetal expulsion (Harper et al., 2012). Spontaneous uterine rupture is rare and is typically associated with scar dehiscence or incomplete rupture, usually secondary to a previous cesarean birth at a risk of <1% in clients with a prior low-transverse cesarean (Harper et al., 2012). This risk is increased if the time between the previous surgery and the current labour is less than 18 months (Cunningham et al., 2010). A woman who has had a classical uterine incision (vertical scar), which involves the contractile portion of the uterus, has an increased risk. Other contributing factors include the following:

- Induction or augmentation of labour with potential for hypertonic contractions
- Instrument-assisted birth
- Manipulation during pregnancy (eg, ECV)
- Shoulder dystocia
- Use of fundal pressure in the second stage of labour
- Multiparity
- Placental implantation over a previous uterine scar

Common signs and symptoms include severe abdominal pain that continues between contractions, fresh vaginal bleeding, abnormal fetal heart rate pattern (eg, complicated variables or late decelerations, tachycardia, or bradycardia), cessation of labour contractions, maternal hemodynamic instability, and hematuria. Team members must be aware of the need to palpate the contractions of a woman in labour receiving epidural anaesthesia whose resting tone is not present between contractions. Assessment for resting tone ensures that the uterus is contracting, with relaxation between uterine activity. A recent study has also pointed to a dystocia in active labour, particularly after 7 cm of dilatation, as a warning sign of a possible future rupture of the uterus (Harper et al., 2012).

As soon as a diagnosis of uterine rupture is established, preparations for emergency abdominal surgery must begin. A cesarean birth usually occurs, and

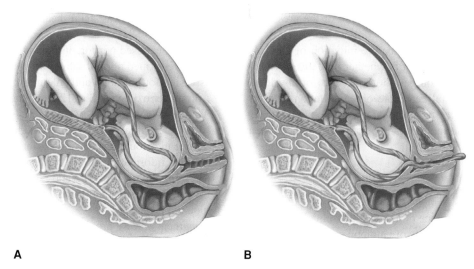

A   **B**

FIGURE 16.16   Cord prolapse may be (**A**) contained within the uterus or (**B**) visible at the vulva.

neonatal well-being largely depends on the age of gestation when the rupture happened and how quickly the surgery occurs. In most cases, the client must undergo a hysterectomy. Depending on the woman's condition, age, and desire for additional children, debridement of the rupture site and primary closure may be attempted. Blood transfusions and IV fluids to replace lost blood and to alleviate shock will be ordered and given. The client receives antibiotics to prevent or to combat infection.

PROLAPSED UMBILICAL CORD

When a portion of the umbilical cord falls in front of, lies beside, or hangs below the fetal presenting part following rupture of membranes, it is defined as **cord prolapse** (Fig. 16.16). This development occurs in 0.1% to 0.6% of births (Lin, 2006). Cord prolapse is an obstetric emergency occurring as one of two types:

- *Occult or hidden:* The cord is alongside the presenting part and is confirmed by palpation on pelvic examination, visualization on speculum examination, or by abnormal or atypical fetal surveillance.
- *Overt:* The umbilical cord precedes the fetal head or feet and can be seen protruding from the maternal vagina or at the introitus.

Cord prolapse may be related to an abnormally long umbilical cord, and is often related to those conditions that result in the fetus not filling the maternal pelvis (eg, malpresentation such as transverse lie and breech presentation). Other risk factors include preterm labour, fetal abnormalities, polyhydramnios, amniotomy (particularly if the presenting part is high), premature rupture of the membranes, multiparity, low birth weight, and obstetric procedures such as ECV (Dilbaz et al., 2006).

COLLABORATIVE CARE: CORD PROLAPSE

Perinatal mortality associated with cord prolapse is at least 10% to 20% and is related to the interval between detection and birth (Baskett, 2004). Rapid action is most likely to have a favourable outcome. Compression of the umbilical cord between the presenting part and maternal pelvis decreases or cuts off fetal circulation. Fetal hypoxia can occur quickly; if uncorrected, umbilical cord compression leads to damage to the fetal central nervous system, fetal death, or both.

Prevention of cord prolapse is the best form of management and includes bed rest for a woman with ruptured membranes if the presenting part is high (unengaged). Amniotomy should not be done until the presenting part is engaged. If prolapse occurs while providing care, preparations for prompt cesarean birth should begin immediately (unless the maternal cervix is fully dilated, in which case vaginal birth may be attempted). Oxygen is administered, and continuous fetal monitoring is begun. Saline-soaked gauze at room temperature can be applied to any portion of the umbilical cord outside the vagina (a vagal response can be stimulated with chilling of the cord). The priority should be to keep pressure off the cord until birth. To do so, the Trendelenburg or knee chest position is employed to elevate the presenting part from the pelvis, or the maternal bladder may be filled to tolerance (approximately 500 mL), which raises the presenting part off the compressed cord. The health care provider may need to insert his or her fingers in the vagina to assist with elevation of the presenting part until delivery.

If the cord prolapses before initiation of care, the first question to consider is whether the fetus is viable. Viability depends on gestation, presence of any lethal anomaly, and fetal heart rate on auscultation or ultrasound. This assessment should occur as quickly as possible, and information should be provided to the woman and family members.

Assessment
Assessment findings may include the following:

- Sudden appearance of a loop of umbilical cord at the introitus after rupture of amniotic membranes
- Complicated variable or prolonged fetal heart decelerations following rupture of amniotic membranes that does not resolve with position change (spontaneous or with an amniotomy)
- Fetal bradycardia in conjunction with rupture of amniotic membranes
- Presence of the umbilical cord in the vagina on vaginal examination
- Any combination of these factors

A perinatal nurse working in a triage or admission area of a birthing unit should be alert to any risk factors for cord prolapse when assessing each labouring woman. Determining fetal station and status of the amniotic membranes is important and should be documented for each client. Regular observations of the perineum should be part of every woman's assessment, particularly after rupture of the membranes.

Select Potential Nursing Diagnoses
Common nursing diagnoses in cases of cord prolapse include the following:

- **Deficient Knowledge** related to the unexpected, emergent nature of care required to ensure maternal and fetal well-being
- **Anxiety** related to maternal and fetal well-being
- **Ineffective Tissue Perfusion** related to cord compression causing decreased placental circulation to the fetus

Planning/Implementation
Interventions focus on relieving pressure of the fetal presenting part from the cord and increasing fetal oxygenation. They include the following measures:

- Assist the woman into a knee-chest, Trendelenburg, or Sims lateral position, using pillows to elevate the buttocks.
- Place a hand into the vagina to elevate the presenting part and separate the cord from the presenting part and pelvis.

- Continuously assess fetal heart rate for ominous changes.
- Keep the exposed portion of the umbilical cord moist with prewarmed normal saline (do not reinsert) while assessing for pulsation and colour.
- Administer oxygen at 8 to 12 L/minute.
- Administer IV fluids.
- Notify the primary health care provider.
- Initiate ultrasound or real-time scanning as needed.
- Provide information to the woman and her family regarding the plan for care and rationales.
- Provide constant emotional and physical support (nursing presence).
- Document all care provided.
- An emergency cesarean birth may be required.

Evaluation
Ongoing evaluation of care is based on fetal vital signs and maternal pain and anxiety and continues until birth, usually cesarean, is completed. Desired outcomes are as follows:

- Fetal gas exchange is normal, as evidenced by normal fetal heart rate patterns (average variability, no decelerations, and baseline within normal limits).
- The client and family verbalize understanding of the condition and the plan of care.
- The client expresses a decrease in pain and anxiety.
- A healthy infant is born.

AMNIOTIC FLUID EMBOLISM

With **amniotic fluid embolism**, a tear in the amnion and chorion provides a mechanism by which amniotic fluid can enter the maternal circulation and reach the pulmonary capillaries, causing an embolism (Schoening, 2006). This rare complication, which occurs between 1 in 8,000 and 1 in 80,000 births, has a high maternal mortality rate of approximately 10% of all maternal deaths in developed countries (Benson, 2011; Gist et al., 2009). Morbidity is also significant, with survivors having neurologic sequelae or septicemia and 94% needing admission to an intensive care unit (Benson, 2011). It is most likely to occur during a difficult labour, induced or augmented labour, or during or just after birth of the newborn. Predisposing factors include multiparity, advanced maternal age, macrosomia, intrauterine fetal death, and meconium in the amniotic fluid.

Signs and symptoms include cyanosis, hypotension, dyspnea, tachypnea, and chest pain. Seizures develop in some clients. Pulmonary edema is common in those women who survive the initial cardiovascular insult, and many of these clients subsequently develop coagulopathy, which may manifest as postpartum hemorrhage. Diagnostic tests include arterial blood gases, complete blood count, and disseminated intravascular coagulation profile.

The general goals of management are to maintain oxygenation, blood pressure, and cardiac output and to manage any coagulopathy (Moore & Baldisseri, 2005). Treatment may include intubation and mechanical ventilation with 100% oxygen if the client is unconscious. Monitoring of central venous pressure and blood transfusions may be implemented as necessary. IV fluids in normotensive clients should be restricted to avoid pulmonary edema (Perozzi & Englert, 2004).

The nurse monitors the client's responses, anticipates possible therapies, and provides supportive care for her and her family. The nurse places the client in Fowler position and administers oxygen, medication, and blood products, as ordered. The nurse regularly monitors intake and output and does not leave the client alone. If the client has not yet given birth, the nurse is responsible for monitoring the fetal heart rate and preparing for emergency birth. Because risk for maternal mortality is high with this condition, the nurse may also need to prepare to help the family through the grieving process (Perozzi & Englert, 2004).

MULTIPLE PREGNANCY

As discussed in Chapter 13, the number of multiple pregnancies is increasing for various reasons, including increased maternal age, increased use of reproductive-assisted technologies, and hereditary factors (Healy & Gaddipati, 2005; Sultana et al., 2011). During labour and birth, the care of clients carrying more than one fetus can be particularly challenging. Potential perinatal complications include PPROM, preeclampsia, anemia, placental dysfunction, cesarean delivery, cord abnormalities, congenital anomalies, IUGR, and low birth weight (Boyle et al., 2013; Dodd & Crowther, 2005; Wen et al., 2004).

During pregnancy, ultrasounds are used to determine fetal chorionicity as early as possible in the pregnancy which will assist in determining care and pregnancy outcome (Taylor, 2006). Ultrasound is also used to determine gestation, fetal growth, and amniotic fluid volume. Planning for the birth of multiple fetuses usually occurs during pregnancy and includes education regarding the many possibilities and options that may become part of the care of the client and her family. A birth plan should be flexible enough not only to include interventions such as cesarean birth as necessary, but also to allow as much choice and decision making as possible over such things as feeding method, support people, and early labour comfort measures. The team providing care should give realistic information that dispels any myths regarding labour and birth, such as

amount of pain and time between births of the newborns. The nurse openly discusses with the client fears and concerns and documents findings for team members to review upon admission (Ramsey & Repke, 2003).

Labour requires ongoing assessment and may progress differently than with a single gestation (Dodd & Crowther, 2005). The myometrium in a multiple pregnancy is exposed to a greater degree of stretch and distension created by the addition of an extra fetus (Turton et al., 2009), which may impact on the oxytocin receptors affecting labour progress. The early first stage may be shorter and the active stage longer because of uterine overdistention, malpresentation, or both. The second stage of labour also may be longer than with a singleton pregnancy because of a slower descent of the first presenting fetus (Silver et al., 2000).

Method of childbirth depends on the position of the first fetus. If the presenting fetus is in the cephalic position, vaginal birth would most likely be the plan. If the first fetus is in a breech position, a cesarean birth would be most likely. The presenting fetus may be in a transverse position or malposition; in this case, cesarean birth usually is the plan of care. If the second fetus is in a breech position, the health care team may discuss with the client the best plan for the birth. Concerns may include size of the fetuses and the ability to complete ECV at some point in labour.

Assessing the client's preference for pain medication or nonpharmacologic relief options is important at the beginning of labour. An epidural may be beneficial if conditions exist that require an operative or cesarean birth (SOGC, 2000).

Throughout labour, the nurse monitors the presence of show; evaluates contraction frequency, intensity, and duration; and assists with vaginal examinations. Ensuring that the client is comfortable is important, as is encouraging her to voice her fears and concerns. Enabling her support person to stay with her and assist with comfort measures and encouragement is beneficial.

Care between births of the fetuses is also important because of increased risk for cord entanglement, fetal compromise, and placental abruption. Continuing to monitor subsequent fetuses after the birth of the first, as well as maternal bleeding and vital signs, is important to ensure maternal and fetal health.

Each infant must be identified clearly, as must each cord blood sample. Times of birth of each infant must be recorded and documented. Average time between vaginal births of multiple gestations is 30 minutes, whereas it is approximately 1 minute if the birth is cesarean (Ellings et al., 1998).

The SOGC (2000) recommends that health care providers' workshops and educational sessions focus on the special needs of families with twins and higher order multiples (Research Highlight 16.2). Achievement

● **RESEARCH HIGHLIGHT 16.2** **Mothering Multiples: A Metasynthesis of Qualitative Research**

PURPOSE

To assist nurses to develop "a richer understanding" and to successfully apply clinical knowledge when working with women who give birth to multiple newborns.

SAMPLE AND DESIGN

The researchers synthesized findings from six separate qualitative studies focused on mothering multiples in the first year of life. They performed a seven-stage process to extract and compare themes from these studies in a documented format.

RESULTS

Many of the participants reported that providing child care 24 hours a day, 7 days a week was simply overwhelming. Emotions fluctuated from wonder and gratitude to depression and despair. Many of these mothers identified a need for a support network. They also expressed concern that they would not always be able to treat their children equally and reported challenges in learning how to adapt to the differences in their children.

CONCLUSIONS

While clients are pregnant and during postpartum teaching in cases of multiple gestation, nurses should be aware of the unique needs of this experience and assist families to develop supportive networks. Community resources may be helpful. Further research is needed with women of different cultural and demographic groups.

From Beck, C. (2002). *Journal of Maternal Child Nursing, 27,* 214–221.

of healthy infants and ongoing maternal health are the desired care outcomes.

MATERNAL OBESITY

The woman in labour who is obese (BMI >30) (Smith et al., 2008) faces some special challenges. Her care includes all normal admission blood work, assessments, and information. Depending on her weight, the team may need to review the safety and weight restrictions of certain pieces of equipment such as labour beds, chairs in the birthing room, and stretchers. Correct assessments regarding whether such equipment can support the woman are vital for safety; however, it is critical that team members make such assessments factually and with sensitivity to avoid communicating judgement or negative reactions about the woman's weight to her and her family.

Accurate weight assessment is also important for ensuring that doses of analgesics and anaesthesia are sufficient. An increased dose is particularly encouraged with cesarean section to prevent the risk of infection and ensure pain management to promote ambulation and therefore recovery. Determining the size of monitoring equipment to use is also critical; for example, an appropriately sized blood pressure cuff is essential to obtain correct readings.

Because obese women are at increased risk for prolonged labour, macrosomia, a very low–birth-weight infant, neural tube defects, preterm birth, blood loss, cesarean birth, or other problems, regular assessments of the progress of labour and early communication about any abnormalities are essential (Gunatilake & Perlow, 2011; Smith et al., 2008). Obese women also have an increased risk for an unsuccessful VBAC. Any significant blood loss during labour should be reviewed for colour, amount, and cause.

Accurate assessments of uterine activity, auscultation, and position changes may be challenging. Obesity has been associated with a tendency to have longer first stages of labour and inadequate uterine contractility, which may be related to an altered lipid profile (Nodine & Hastings-Tolsma, 2012). The client may require internal monitoring. Ideally, the client is placed in an upright or semi-Fowler position to increase her lung capacity and decrease her cardiac workload (Cesario, 2003). Macrosomia or very low birth weight should be anticipated by assisting the client into a hyperflexed position for birth and ensuring that newborn resuscitative equipment and neonatal/pediatric staff are available and ready if needed (Ehrenberg et al., 2004).

If the client requires a cesarean birth, the anaesthetic of choice is epidural or spinal. Insertion of the needle may be difficult, however, because of adipose tissue. Helping the client curl her back as tightly as possible for insertion is important. Attempting to intubate her for general anaesthesia is difficult because of her weight; however, it may be necessary if emergency complications develop. Placing a folded blanket under her head may facilitate access to her airway and more rapid intubation (Soens et al., 2008). Goals for care include sensitive treatment, accurate weights, regular assessment of vital signs and progress of labour, and a healthy mother and newborn.

FEMALE GENITAL MUTILATION (FEMALE CIRCUMCISION)

As discussed in Chapter 6, female circumcision has a history estimated to date back more than 5,000 years (Box 16.2). It continues to be practiced in many countries. Long-term and short-term health problems associated with female circumcision include hemorrhage, infection, increased risk for HIV, urinary retention, and frequent urinary tract infections. Circumcised women may experience dysmenorrhea, pelvic inflammatory disease, incontinence, depression, and sexual dysfunction.

With the increasing cultural diversity in Canada, encounters with clients who have undergone female circumcision are becoming more frequent (Whitehorn et al., 2002). In caring for circumcised women, the nurse should try to view these clients within the context of their culture, values, and beliefs to provide empathetic and nonjudgemental care. The first time that a nurse sees the external genitalia of such a client, she may be shocked, upset, or angry. Nurses must remember, however, that the client may not have been part of the decision making about the procedure. Or, the client may value the procedure and see it as positive.

Many cultures that practice female circumcision tend to encourage women to receive information about pregnancy, labour, and birth from other women in their community. Such clients who receive antepartal care in a health facility may arrive in labour with normal anxiety inherent to the unknown, as well as additional fear because of a lack of familiarity with the hospital environment or Western health care practices.

Clients who have not been defibulated before labour require immediate assessment. The scar may be opened early in labour or during the second stage to facilitate progress toward birth. Evaluation of the client's anxiety and knowledge regarding labour and birth is important. Discussing her wishes regarding labour support people, pain medications, comfort measures, and health care providers can decrease anxiety and increase culturally competent care provision.

If preferred or necessary, interpretative services should be arranged to enhance communication, which is key to culturally sensitive care. Normal vaginal examinations are extremely difficult to perform in infibulated women, so an experienced practitioner should modify the procedure to use a single finger with extensive lubrication. The nurse should pay close attention to the progression of labour because female circumcision may increase the risk for dysfunctional labour. The nurse should rely on behavioural cues instead of vaginal examinations to assess progress such as expressions of an "urge to push," increased number or length of contractions, increased maternal focus, and presence of "show." The nurse explains all procedures and how they will be completed while the woman is in labour. Labour support according to the woman's wishes should be provided.

Perineal tears can occur or an episiotomy may be necessary, depending on the degree of circumcision. The nurse should explain about this process (Elnashar & Abdelhady, 2007). Postpartum explanations regarding anatomy and repair may help the client understand and be comfortable with her recovery. The client needs preparation for postpartum pain that results from reversal of the infibulation. Pain management interventions may include analgesics and sitz baths.

BIRTH-RELATED PROCEDURES COMMON IN HIGH-RISK LABOUR AND BIRTH

Cervical Ripening and Labour Induction

During pregnancy and labour, the uterine cervix goes through changes in physical appearance and biochemical composition (Hadi, 2000). Cervical ripening is a series of events similar to those seen with tissue inflammation (Arias, 2000). A ripe cervix is shortened, softened, partly dilated, and centred. This type of cervix is necessary for the full dilatation needed to accommodate passage of the fetus. See Chapter 15 for a review of Bishop scoring.

● **BOX 16.2** **Types of Female Genital Mutilation (Female Circumcision)**

Female genital mutilation is classified into four major types:

- Clitoridectomy: partial or total removal of the clitoris
- Excision: partial or total removal of the clitoris and the labia minora, with or without excision of the labia majora
- Infibulation: narrowing of the vaginal opening through the creation of a covering seal. The seal is formed by cutting and repositioning the inner, and sometimes outer, labia, with or without removal of the clitoris.
- Other: all other harmful procedures to the female genitalia for nonmedical purposes, eg, pricking, piercing, incising, scraping, and cauterizing the genital area (WHO, 2008).

Methods of Cervical Ripening

Various methods can be used to ripen the cervix (Tenore, 2003). For example, the client may be advised to try sexual intercourse, breast stimulation, or both to promote the release of endogenous oxytocin. Current research, however, has not validated the safety or effectiveness of these methods (Kavanagh & Kelly, 2005; Kavanagh et al., 2005). Some clients use herbal treatments such as black and blue cohosh or evening primrose oil. Such agents have not been studied, and nurses need to document the client's use of these or any other complementary/alternative modalities.

Mechanical Methods. One mechanical method of cervical ripening involves the insertion of an indwelling (Foley) catheter (with the bulb inflated with 30 to 60 mL of water) into the endocervical canal, with direct pressure from the balloon applied to the lower uterine segment (Rai & Schreiber, 2008). Another method is the use of hydroscopic dilators such as laminaria and synthetic products containing magnesium sulfate. These dilators can be inserted on an outpatient basis because they provide slow progressive cervical ripening over 12 to 24 hours. Although use of the Foley catheter for induction appears to be effective for cervical ripening, neither of these methods are recommended for induction of labour because of lack of evidence about their effectiveness in comparison to other methods (SOGC, 2001). The use of hydroscopic dilators has also been associated with increased risk of infection.

Cervical ripening also can be done by "stripping" the membranes. With stripping of the membranes, the care provider inserts a finger through the cervical os and moves it in a circular direction to detach the membranes. Although results of some studies indicate promotion of the onset of labour, there have not been clinically important benefits to maternal or neonatal outcomes demonstrated for this procedure that may produce maternal discomfort, bleeding, and increased uterine irritability (SOGC, 2001).

Pharmacologic Methods. Prostaglandins are frequently used to help ripen the cervix and have been shown to ripen the cervix, increase the likelihood of being delivered before 24 hours, and decrease the use of oxytocin for augmentation (Baxley, 2003; SOGC, 2001). Currently, two types of prostaglandin E_2 preparations (PGE_2) are administered:

- Intracervical
- dinoprostone (Prepidil) 0.5 mg into the cervical canal
- Intravaginal
- dinoprostone (Prostin) 1 or 2 mg into the posterior fornix
- dinoprostone (Cervidil) 10 mg into the posterior fornix

Because there is insufficient evidence about the ideal dose, route, and frequency of the prostaglandin E_1 (misoprostol), its use should be restricted to clinical trials (SOGC, 2001) (Pharmacology Box 1).

Oxytocin Pharmacology

Oxytocin is a synthetic octapeptide used as a potent uterotonic agent to increase uterine contractility by increasing the circulation of free intracellular calcium. There are two types of oxytocin: endogenous (naturally secreted by the fetus and woman in labour) and exogenous (synthetic hormone used to induce or augment labour) (Clayworth, 2000). Oxytocin receptors in the smooth muscle of the uterus, the myometrium and decidua, increase during pregnancy, particularly in the third trimester and during the latent phase of labour as a result of the hormonal influences of estrogen, progesterone, and prostaglandin. With the increased number of receptors, the amount of oxytocin required to produce uterine contractions decreases. Uterine activity is rhythmic and coordinated but not constant.

● PHARMACOLOGY 16.1   Misoprostol (Cytotec)

INDICATION

Misoprostol is a synthetic prostaglandin.

ACTION

It produces dilatation of the cervix.

PREGNANCY RISK CATEGORY

X

DOSAGE

25 to 50 μg orally or placed intravaginally in the posterior fornix

POSSIBLE ADVERSE EFFECTS

Abnormal fetal heart rate patterns, uterine hyperstimulation, nausea, headache, diarrhea

NURSING IMPLICATIONS

- Ensure that the client does not have any problems or risk factors that would contraindicate use of this drug.
- Continuously monitor uterine activity and fetal heart rate.
- Check that a tocolytic agent and an IV fluid line are readily available in the event of uterine hyperstimulation.

From Karch, A. (2013). *2013 Lippincott's nursing drug guide.* Philadelphia: Lippincott Williams & Wilkins.

● PHARMACOLOGY 16.2 Oxytocin

INDICATION

Oxytocin is a synthetic form of the naturally occurring hormone.

ACTION

It is used to facilitate uterine contractions.

PREGNANCY RISK CATEGORY

C

DOSAGE

Initially 1 to 2 mU/minute by IV infusion, increased at a rate of no more than 1 mU/minute every 30 minutes until a regular contraction pattern is established

POSSIBLE ADVERSE EFFECTS

Cardiac dysrhythmia, uterine hypertonicity, nausea and vomiting, fetal bradycardia, water intoxication.

NURSING IMPLICATIONS

- Use an infusion pump to ensure accuracy of administration.
- Monitor the frequency, duration, and strength of each contraction.
- Assess maternal vital signs, especially blood pressure for signs of hypotension. If hypotension develops, the oxytocin needs to be discontinued, and the primary health care provider needs to be alerted.
- Check the fetal heart rate regularly for any abnormal characteristics.

From Karch, A. (2013). *2013 Lippincott's nursing drug guide*. Philadelphia: Lippincott Williams & Wilkins.

In normal spontaneous labour, the highest concentrations of oxytocin are found in the umbilical cord blood. Maternal blood levels reach what would be achieved with an exogenous oxytocin infusion of 2 to 4 mU/minute, whereas the fetus secretes another 2 mU/minute. These levels increase in the second stage of labour to accomplish birth. Therefore, the total oxytocin concentration is in the range of 4 to 6 mU/minute.

Exogenous oxytocin is the drug of choice when the cervix is ripe and labour is being induced or augmented. A continuous IV infusion of oxytocin is administered at an ordered starting dose (Pharmacology Box 2). Then, the dose is increased until an adequate contraction pattern is achieved (Clayworth, 2000). Reassessment should occur if the rate reaches 20 mU/minute. A continuous oxytocin infusion raises the circulating blood level slowly: 20 to 40 minutes are required to reach a steady state (Smith & Merrill, 2006). The client may feel a uterine response within 3 to 5 minutes (increase in uterine contractions) (Fig. 16.17). The half-life of oxytocin is approximately 5 minutes, so its effect is diminished quickly if it is discontinued or decreased.

Oxytocin was added to the Institute for Safe Medication Practices' (ISMP) high alert list of medications that have a heightened risk of harm, indicating that safeguards that reduce risk of error are beneficial (Pearson, 2011). Use of this medication has been a large part of litigation throughout Canada and the United States.

Goal of Oxytocin Administration. The goal of oxytocin administration is to produce uterine contractions with a frequency of every 2 to 3 minutes, lasting 40 to 60 seconds. The desired intrauterine pressure (IUP) is 50 to 60 mm Hg above baseline, with a palpated resting tone between contractions (less than 20 mm Hg).

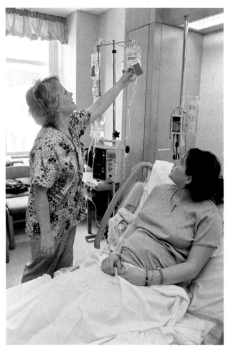

FIGURE 16.17 During IV infusion of oxytocin, the nurse uses an infusion pump to regulate flow, which has been piggybacked into the main IV line.

Formula for Calculation of an Oxytocin Dosage. The following formulas can be used to calculate dosages of oxytocin:

1. Determine mU oxytocin/mL by
$$\frac{\text{Units of oxytocin}}{\text{mL of IV fluid}} \times 1{,}000 = \text{milliunits per (mU/mL)}$$

2. Determine mU of oxytocin/minute by
$$(\text{mU/mL})/1 \times (\text{mL/hour})/60 \text{ minute} = \text{milliunits per minute (mU/minute)}$$

3. Confirm administration rate in mL/hour by
$$(\text{mU/minute} \times 60 \text{ minute/hour})/\text{mU/mL}$$
$$= \underline{\quad} \text{ mL/hour}$$

 Suppose the health care provider initially orders an IV infusion of oxytocin at 2 mU/minute. The pharmacy supplies an infusion that contains 10 mU/mL. How much solution would Carlotta receive in 1 hour?

Associated Complications. Several complications are associated with the use of oxytocin to induce or augment labour.

- Uterine **hyperstimulation** or tachysystole is defined as more than five uterine contractions occurring within a 10-minute time period. In addition, other abnormal uterine contraction patterns of concern include a series of single contractions lasting 2 minutes or more or contractions of normal duration occurring within 1 minute of each other (Doyle et al., 2011; Kunz et al., 2012). Tachysystole results in an absence of uterine relaxation between contractions, causing a decreased oxygen level to the fetus. Excessive uterine contractions also can lead to uterine rupture or abruptio placentae. Problems may stem from an overdosage of oxytocin, increased sensitivity to oxytocin by increased number of oxytocin receptors, or increased exogenous oxytocin production by maternal or fetal components. During labour, the exchange of oxygen and carbon dioxide for the fetus occurs primarily between contractions. Placental function decreases when IUPs are greater than 35 mm Hg and severely reduced when IUPs are at 50 to 60 mm Hg. This means that there is some reduction of maternal fetal blood flow in almost all contractions. Fetal compromise from hypoxia, uterine rupture, or both may occur with uterine hyperstimulation or tachysystole, particularly with a uterine resting tone above 20 mm Hg (Clayworth, 2000).
- Continuing oxytocin through a dysfunctional pattern is a myth and does not increase the likelihood of effective labour or decrease the length of the induction. Contraction patterns with low amplitude or high frequency or doubling tripling are caused by saturated

oxytocin receptors and decreasing the oxytocin is more likely to improve the pattern (Doyle et al., 2011).
- Oxytocin administered over long periods, at high dosages, or both, can result in hyponatremia (water intoxication), confusion, convulsion, and congestive heart failure. Detailed records of intake and output are essential to prevent these problems or manage them if they develop.
- Oxytocin administered for a prolonged period has a hypotensive effect; blood pressure monitoring is required in the nursing care management.
- Initiation of induction of labour can lead to a variety of other interventions described by some as a "cascade" that includes need for IV fluids, epidural pain management, continuous fetal monitoring, amniotomy, and immobility due to bed rest for these interventions (Romano & Lothian, 2008).

Collaborative Management. Nursing care of the client before oxytocin infusion begins includes the following:

- Assess baseline vital signs and fetal heart rate.
- Explain the physiology of uterine contractions and pharmacology of oxytocin.
- Describe the process of induction to the woman and family.
- Assess for uterine contractions and rupture of membranes.
- Ensure the presence of written orders for the oxytocin.
- Complete an obstetrical nursing history of the woman before starting the induction.

During oxytocin infusion, the nurse performs the following interventions:

- Continuously monitor fetal heart rate and uterine activity.
- Palpate the abdomen for uterine activity (the goal is contractions every 2 to 3 minutes lasting 45 to 60 seconds with adequate resting tone). If an IUP catheter is in place, resting tone should not be above 20 mm Hg; contraction intensity should not exceed 60 mm Hg.
- Assess blood pressure and pulse hourly or more often if these values are increasing.
- Maintain records of intake and output.
- Communicate with the woman and her support people and other care providers about labour progress.
- Provide encouragement and support as the woman progresses through labour.
- Provide comfort measures and pain management according to the woman's wishes.
- Encourage ambulation, if at all possible, and with appropriate monitoring devices (Romano & Lothian, 2008)
- Continue oxytocin infusion with increases per the contraction pattern and the health care provider orders if no tachysystole and fetal heart rate pattern remains normal.

- Document oxytocin dosages, uterine activity, fetal heart rate, vital signs, and the woman's response.
- Notify the health care provider of identified concerns related to uterine activity, fetal heart rate, labour progress, or presence of meconium. If uterine hyperstimulation or tachysystole is noted, decrease or discontinue the oxytocin (as per hospital policy), notify the health care provider, and provide measures such as changing position, monitoring of maternal and

fetal vital signs, and increased IV fluids. Document all assessments and interventions.

See Nursing Care Plan 16.2 for more information.

Amnioinfusion

With **amnioinfusion**, a volume of warmed, sterile, Ringer lactate solution or normal saline is infused

(text continues on page 656)

NURSING CARE PLAN 16.2

●

The Client Undergoing Labour Induction

 Recall Carlotta, who is at the end of her 41st week of pregnancy and undergoing labour induction. Four hours after induction begins, oxytocin is being administered at 12 mU/minute. Carlotta reports that the contractions are becoming more painful and rates them as 7 on a scale of 1 to 10. They are approximately 3 minutes apart and lasting 90 seconds each. Her cervix is 4 cm dilated. An amniotomy was performed with the last vaginal examination; clear fluid was obtained. Fetal heart rate ranges from 134 to 146 beats/minute with a normal pattern.

NURSING DIAGNOSES

- **Deficient Knowledge** related to process of induction, labour and birth experience, and pain relief measures
- **Anxiety** related to fear of the unknown and lack of familiarity with labour progression

EXPECTED OUTCOMES

1. The client will demonstrate understanding of the events associated with induction, labour, and birth.
2. The client will identify appropriate options for comfort during labour and birth.
3. The client will verbalize specific areas of concern.
4. The client will identify positive strategies to cope with her concerns.

INTERVENTIONS	RATIONALES
Assess the client's level of understanding about induction, labour, and birth	Such data provide a baseline for identifying specific client needs and developing an individualized plan
Discuss concerns, feelings, and perceptions with the client/family related to labour and birth and expectations about pain	Discussion allows the nurse to emphasize positive aspects of the current situation; verbalization of concerns can establish sources of stress and problem areas
Communicate accurate facts; answer questions honestly. Reinforce information, emphasizing that each pregnancy, labour, and birth is highly individualized	Open, honest communication promotes trust and helps correct misinformation. Facts help dispel unfounded fears, myths, misconceptions, or guilt feelings

(continued)

NURSING CARE PLAN 16.2 ● The Client Undergoing Labour Induction *(Continued)*

INTERVENTIONS	RATIONALES
Evaluate the client's past coping strategies to determine which have been effective	Use of appropriate coping strategies aids in reducing anxiety
Review measures used during labour and birth to monitor maternal and fetal well-being	Knowledge of ongoing fetal surveillance aids in alleviating stress related to the unknown
Encourage the client to include her partner in this experience	The partner's participation promotes sharing and provides support
Teach the client and partner about oxytocin, preparing them for what to expect relative to contraction strength and frequency	Understanding the need for monitoring related to use of oxytocin will facilitate appropriate choices of pain management
Explain the need for continuous monitoring of maternal and fetal well-being	Continuous monitoring allows for early detection and prompt intervention, should problems arise
Review comfort measures, such as music, distraction, hot/cold compresses, massage, and position changes that the client can employ	Pharmacologic and nonpharmacologic measures can help control pain
Provide opportunities for the client and partner to practice various comfort measures; allow the client to select the methods best for her	Practice reinforces learning. Allowing the client to choose the best methods for her promotes decision making and feelings of control
Assist the client and partner to adapt measures or try alternatives for pain relief should previous choices prove ineffective	Events and pain level vary throughout labour. Adapting methods or selecting alternatives helps to ensure effectiveness
Continually update the client and partner about the client's progress. Provide positive reinforcement related to methods used and labour progression	Ongoing information helps prevent unnecessary fear and anxiety about the unknown and promotes progress toward the goal of a healthy newborn. Positive reinforcement promotes the couple's involvement and feelings of control, thereby enhancing self-esteem

EVALUATION

1. The client verbalizes accurate information related to events of induction and labour.
2. The client identifies nonpharmacologic and pharmacologic options for pain relief.
3. The client states that her concerns and fears have decreased.
4. The client demonstrates use of appropriate coping strategies to deal with anxiety and fear.

NURSING DIAGNOSES

- **Risk for Injury** related to the use of oxytocin and effects on mother and fetus
- **Pain** related to increased uterine contractions

(continued)

NURSING CARE PLAN 16.2 ● The Client Undergoing Labour Induction *(Continued)*

EXPECTED OUTCOMES

1. The client will remain free of adverse effects of oxytocin administration.
2. The client will progress through labour without complications.
3. The client will report a decrease in pain to a tolerable level.
4. The client will demonstrate use of appropriate pain-relief measures.

INTERVENTIONS	RATIONALES
Assess vital signs, especially blood pressure, fetal heart rate and pattern, and contractions	Assessment provides a baseline for comparisons and allows for early detection of problems
Reinforce explanations about oxytocin infusion, equipment, and monitoring	Anxiety can contribute to pain perception. Continued explanations help to reduce anxiety
Assess the oxytocin infusion rate by infusion pump; gradually increase rate as ordered. Ensure that oxytocin is administered as a secondary infusion piggybacked into the main IV line	The goal of oxytocin administration is to produce uterine contractions lasting 45 to 60 seconds approximately every 2 to 3 minutes. Administering oxytocin as a secondary infusion allows for prompt discontinuation if complications develop
Palpate the abdomen between contractions; note resting tone	Increased resting tone can cause decreased placental perfusion. Oxytocin use can lead to hypertonic uterine contractions
Encourage the client to lie on her side	A side-lying position promotes placental perfusion
Assess pain level; ask the client to rate it	Such rating objectively quantifies the level of pain
Review options for pain relief; assist the client with measures per her request; administer pharmacologic agents as indicated and ordered	Increased pain may compound anxiety and tension, leading to enhanced pain perception. Immediate assistance to control pain is important at this time
Continue to assess pain level and vital signs, as well as fetal heart rate and patterns	Ongoing assessment provides indicators about the effectiveness of chosen pain relief methods and oxytocin administration
Monitor intake and output closely; obtain laboratory tests as ordered; assess for changes in mental status (such as confusion); be alert for signs and symptoms of heart failure	Oxytocin can lead to hyponatremia, confusion, convulsion, and congestive heart failure. Close monitoring is essential to prevent these problems

EVALUATION

- The client exhibits vital signs and other assessment findings (including fetal heart rate and pattern and uterine contractions) within acceptable parameters.
- The client progresses through the stages of labour without incident.
- The client states that pain is tolerable, with appropriate pain relief measures.

through an IUP catheter to increase fluid volume. The infusion improves fetal and placental oxygenation, helps cushion the umbilical cord, and dilutes any meconium that may be found. Indications for amnioinfusion include complicated variable decelerations resulting from cord compression, oligohydramnios (decreased amniotic fluid), postmaturity, preterm labour with rupture of the membranes, and thick meconium fluid (Gramellini et al., 2003). Contraindications to this procedure include cord prolapse, vaginal bleeding of unknown cause, hypertonic uterine contractions, amnionitis, and severe fetal distress.

The client must be given an explanation of the procedure that includes risks and benefits. Informed consent must be obtained. The client will need to remain on bed rest during the procedure. The health care provider performs a vaginal examination to establish dilatation, confirm presentation, and ensure that the umbilical cord has not prolapsed. An infusion pump is used to instill 250 to 500 mL of the chosen solution over 20 to 30 minutes. Close monitoring of fluid volume and uterine contractions is required to prevent uterine overdistention or increased uterine tone. Team members regularly assess maternal vital signs, pain, and intake and output, as well as the fetal heart rate pattern. The team and the client should be prepared to begin the procedure for cesarean birth if fetal heart rate does not improve after the amnioinfusion.

Forceps-Assisted Birth

Instrumental or assisted birth occurred as part of 13.5% of births in Canada in 2010/2011 (PHAC, 2011) and is used for many reasons. Forceps may be used for maternal exhaustion following prolonged labour, failure to progress in the second stage of labour, and medical conditions such as preeclampsia, abruption, or congenital heart disease. Fetal distress in the second stage is also a common reason for an assisted birth (O'Mahony et al., 2010). **Forceps** are stainless steel instruments that look like tongs; they can fit around the head of the fetus to help pull the baby through the vaginal outlet (Fig. 16.18). Forceps consist of two parts that cross each other like a pair of scissors. Each part has a handle,

lock, shank, and blade (Belfort, 2003). The lock may be of a sliding type or a screw type. The blade usually consists of two curves. The cephalic curve conforms to the shape of the fetal head, whereas the pelvic curve conforms to the shape of the birth canal. The two blades are designated as left and right. The left blade is placed into the vagina on the mother's left side; the right blade is inserted on the right side.

Criteria for Use

Certain criteria are necessary to ensure the safe use of forceps (Ross et al., 2007).

- The woman is having uterine contractions. Her membranes have ruptured, and the cervix is dilated fully.
- The maternal bladder is empty. (Urinary catheterization may be used to drain the bladder as necessary before forceps are implemented.)
- The woman is receiving adequate anaesthesia. Type of anaesthesia depends on the forceps used, which is related to fetal position and presentation.
- The team providing care has determined that birth is mechanically feasible based on an adequate maternal pelvis and engaged fetal head.
- The presenting part is vertex, or after-coming head in breech.
- The fetal head position is known.
- Under no circumstances should forceps be applied to an unengaged presenting part or when the cervix is not fully dilated.

Types of Applications

The following types of applications are appropriate according to the station and position of the fetal presenting part at the time of application (Hook & Damos, 2008; SOGC, 2004):

- *Outlet forceps:* The fetal skull has reached the pelvic floor, with the fetal head at the perineum and the fetal scalp visible at the introitus without spreading the labia. Rotation of 45 degrees or less is required. The sagittal suture is in the anteroposterior diameter or the right or left anterior or posterior position.
- *Low forceps:* The leading point of the fetal skull is at or lower than station +2 and not on the pelvic floor. This category is subdivided into rotation requiring less or more than 45 degrees.
- *Mid forceps:* These are applied when the fetal head is engaged but the leading point of the skull is above station +2.

Collaborative Management

When use of forceps is indicated and the type has been selected, the client is assisted into a lithotomy position. The health care provider explains the procedure and its risks and benefits to the client and family and obtains informed consent. He or she tells the woman that she

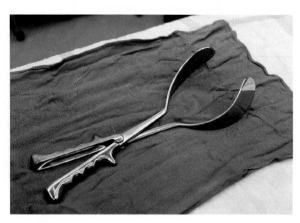

FIGURE 16.18 Forceps.

will feel pressure and pulling, but should not feel any pain with adequate regional or spinal anaesthesia. The nurse encourages the client to use any breathing techniques and other labour-coping mechanisms she has learned to prevent muscle tensing during application of the forceps. Usually, an episiotomy is performed to provide adequate room for maneuvering the forceps without tearing the maternal tissues (see Chapter 15).

The birth attendant performs a vaginal examination to check the exact position of the fetal head. He or she then introduces two or more fingers of one hand into the left side of the vagina to guide the left blade of the forceps into place while protecting the maternal vagina and cervix from injury. The attendant uses the other hand to gently place the left blade of the forceps into the left side of the vagina between his or her fingers and the fetal head. The attendant then carries out the same procedure on the right side. He or she attaches the blades together at the shank, applying traction intermittently with contractions, not continuously (Fig. 16.19). Between traction, the attendant partly disarticulates the blades of the forceps to ease pressure on the fetal head. During application, the nurse monitors uterine contractions and reports findings, so that the birth attendant can coordinate the timing of the contractions with forceps traction. Team members encourage the mother to continue with pushing efforts as traction is applied.

Fetal bradycardia is common with forceps-assisted birth, generally related to the increased pressure of the fetal head, umbilical cord compression, or both. Continuous fetal monitoring is thus required, and appropriate newborn resuscitation equipment should be available.

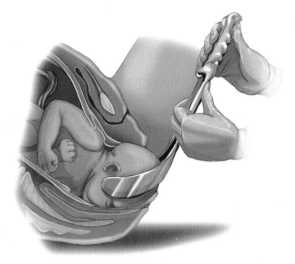

FIGURE 16.19 Application of the forceps to the fetal head.

An individual trained in neonatal resuscitation or team should be present at the birth to provide appropriate steps immediately after birth as needed.

Piper forceps (a special type of forceps used in breech presentations with an after-coming head) are applied after the shoulders have been delivered and after gentle traction combined with suprapubic pressure has brought the fetal head into the maternal pelvis (Locksmith et al., 2001). The body and arms are suspended with a towel to facilitate application of the blades (Fig. 16.20). The birth attendant introduces the left blade upward along the fetal head on the left side and then applies the right blade in the same fashion. After locking the forceps in place, the attendant uses palpation to confirm their position on the head.

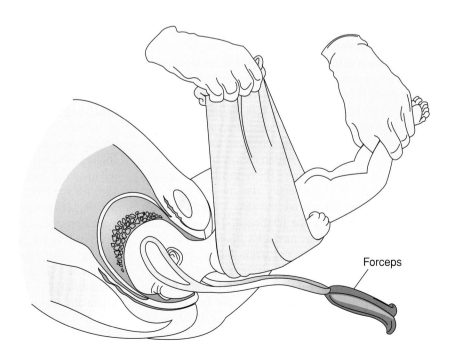

Forceps

FIGURE 16.20 The Piper forceps are occasionally used to assist with vaginal breech births.

Following an episiotomy, traction is applied, and the chin, mouth, and nose emerge over the perineum.

Complications

Forceps-assisted birth can pose risks for both mother and newborn. Forcible rotation can injure the maternal uterus, vagina, or cervix, potentially causing lacerations and bleeding, increased episiotomy rates, and need for additional maternal analgesia. Injury to the anal sphincter is also common (Christianson et al., 2003; O'Mahony et al., 2010). If forceps are applied incorrectly and one blade overlies the fetal face, the newborn may exhibit bruising and/or facial or scalp lacerations which usually disappear after a few days. Excessive force may cause more serious injury to the newborn's head, including skull fracture, or subdural hematoma (Patel & Murphy, 2004).

Women who have had forceps-assisted birth have a greater risk of developing anxiety, depression or post-traumatic stress disorder postpartum related to their experience of labour and birth. Their labours may have been longer; there may have been concern about their labour or their infant, lack of control, and worry that contributes to these ongoing psychological symptoms. Many of these women speak with their health care providers about their birth and report that it helps while others identify that they wish that they had. Perinatal nurses who work in labour and birth can assist these women postpartum in talking about their concerns about their birth, answering their questions and clarifying any misunderstandings (Rowlands & Redshaw, 2012).

QUOTE 16-1

"Although I understood the rationale for the use of forceps in giving birth to my baby, I was so terrified while it was happening. I kept worrying they would scrape the baby's face or hurt us in some way."

A client who required a forceps-assisted birth

Vacuum-Assisted Birth

The **vacuum extractor** is a cup-shaped device attached to a suction pump and applied to the fetal head to assist with birth (Fig. 16.21). Cups come in various sizes; usually, the birth attendant selects the largest cup that can be applied with ease of use. The vacuum is built up slowly to create negative pressure, and the suction creates an artificial caput within the cup, providing firm attachment to the fetal scalp. The birth attendant applies traction until the head emerges from the vagina.

Indications for use are the same as with forceps, except for rotation of the fetal head. The rate of vacuum-assisted births has increased from 6.8% to 9.6% (PHAC, 2011). Vacuum extraction has progressively replaced forceps as the delivery instrument of choice for many practitioners (O'Grady, 2008). Some believe that vacuum extractors are safer because they pose less risk for maternal injury, although findings also show the

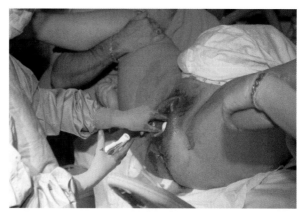

FIGURE 16.21 Application of the vacuum extractor.

use of forceps to pose fewer risks to the fetus (Caughey et al., 2005).

Criteria for Use

Criteria for using the vacuum extractor are the same as those for using forceps, with the following exceptions:

- The vacuum extractor can be used in multiparous women who have only a very small rim of cervix that is stretched easily over the remaining fetal head.
- The vacuum extractor should never be used in cases of preterm birth because the suction cup can injure the fetal head and scalp.
- It should never be used in cases of breech presentation.

Collaborative Management

When a vacuum extractor is being used, the health care provider briefly explains the procedure and its necessity to the client and family and obtains informed consent. He or she advises the woman that she will feel pressure and pulling; however, with adequate regional or spinal anaesthesia, the client should not feel pain. The client should employ breathing techniques and other labour management techniques she has learned to cope with labour.

After the birth attendant assembles the appropriate-size cup and sterile tubing, the nurse attaches the distal end to suction. Once the cup has been applied to the fetal head, the suction is activated. Other suction devices are disposable and hand-held and operated solely by the health care provider. To prevent damage to the maternal tissues, suction must be released if the cup slips off the fetal head. The team encourages maternal pushing efforts during contractions, whereas the birth attendant applies the device (Fig. 16.22).

Fetal heart rate during the procedure requires ongoing monitoring. Newborn resuscitation equipment should be available, and a health care provider trained in neonatal resuscitation should be present and prepared to initiate initial steps at the time of birth. Team members advise the parents that the newborn's head will have

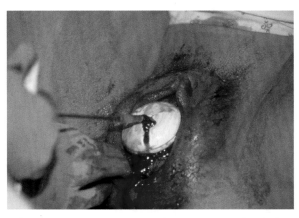

FIGURE 16.22 When a birth is being assisted with the use of a vacuum extractor, the woman is encouraged to continue pushing to facilitate movement of the fetal head out of the vaginal outlet.

edema or bruising where the cup was applied, but that this will disappear within a few days (McQuivey, 2004).

Complications

As with forceps, use of the vacuum extractor can result in maternal and fetal injuries (Johnson et al., 2004). One measure to prevent vaginal lacerations is to perform a digital examination of the entire circumference of the suction cup after application but before initiation of the vacuum. Use of the device should be kept as brief as possible to prevent fetal scalp injuries. Generally, if traction on the suction cup during three contractions does not produce descent of the fetal head, the suction cup has popped off three times without obvious cause, or 20 minutes have passed and delivery is not imminent, the team should abandon the use of vacuum extraction and move to plans for a cesarean birth. Subgaleal hemorrhage is a fetal complication specific to the use of the vacuum extractor and is evidenced by a gradual swelling of the head circumference in the first 24 hours after birth.

Cesarean Birth

Indications for cesarean birth include previous cesarean birth, dystocia, malpresentation, and compromised fetal status (SOGC, 2005). The public view of cesarean birth has moved away from being considered surgery with significant risks for maternal morbidity and mortality to surgery that some women are actively requesting. The number of cesarean births is rising (Campbell, 2011), with the Canadian cesarean rate ranging from 21.9% to 27.8% in different areas across Canada (PHAC, 2011). The primary cesarean rate has increased from 16.1% to 19.7% with women 35 years of age and older at 23.1%. The repeat cesarean rate is approximately 82% (PHAC, 2011). The increase is based on many factors, including greater use of assisted reproductive technologies, multiple gestation, and maternal age greater than 35 years. Reasons a woman may want to undergo cesarean birth without trying vaginal birth include fear of labour pain, fetal morbidity, or concern about the future health of her pelvic floor, as well as finding it more convenient to have a planned date of birth and greater control over the whole process (Mayberry, 2006). Although the American College of Obstetricians and Gynecologists supports maternal request as an indication for cesarean birth, the SOGC in Canada does not support this (Pakenham et al., 2006). Other factors that may be contributing to the rising incidence of cesarean birth include the use of electronic fetal monitoring, which decreases maternal mobility and provides earlier indications than in the past of fetal heart rate tracings that cause concern, and more frequent use of labour induction and augmentation (Campbell, 2011).

Cesarean birth involves complications such as hemorrhage requiring transfusion, infection, pneumonia, increased length of stay, decreased breastfeeding, and an increase in NICU admissions. Subsequent pregnancies also carry risks such as placental problems (eg, previa, percreta, as well as abruption). Increased risk of cesarean birth complications are seen particularly with a pregnancy weight gain of greater than 40 lb (15 to 18 kg), diabetes during pregnancy, gestational hypertension, and chronic hypertension (Campbell, 2011).

When working with clients undergoing cesarean birth, perinatal nurses must be skilled in providing care during surgery, either in the scrubbing or circulating role. The client being cared for may be having an anticipated or an emergency or urgent cesarean birth. Reasons for an emergency cesarean birth may include failure to progress in labour, abnormal fetal heart rate tracings, breech presentation, placenta previa, and fetal malposition (Kolas et al., 2003).

Classification

Classification refers to the type of uterine incision (Fig. 16.23). A *transverse incision* in the lower uterine segment is usually chosen for several reasons. The lower segment is the thinnest portion of the uterus with the least activity. Thus, an incision at this site minimizes blood loss. The area is easier to repair than the upper portion, and chances of rupture of the scar in subsequent pregnancies are minimized. Use of this type of incision also has a decreased risk for paralytic ileus, peritonitis, and bowel adhesions. After opening the abdominal cavity, the surgeon makes the initial incision transversely across the uterine peritoneum, where it is attached loosely just above the bladder. He or she then dissects the lower peritoneal flap and bladder from the uterus and incises the uterine muscle. The membranes are ruptured, the fetus is removed, the placenta is extracted, and IV oxytocin is administered to facilitate

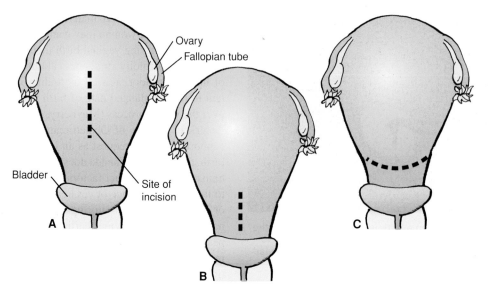

FIGURE 16.23 **A:** The classical cesarean incision is vertical and used in emergencies when quick removal of the fetus is critical or when the fetus is so large that this method is the only way to enable delivery. **B:** The low cervical vertical approach is used rarely. **C:** The most common method is the low transverse approach because the scar has a decreased risk for rupture during subsequent pregnancies.

uterine contractions. Suturing of the uterine wall occurs in two layers, which seals off the incision and helps prevent lochia from entering the peritoneal cavity. A layer of absorbable suture is used to reapproximate the visceral peritoneum. Packs are removed from the abdominal cavity, with the abdomen closed in layers.

With a classic cesarean, the surgeon makes a vertical incision directly into the wall of the uterine body. After extraction of the uterine contents, three layers of absorbable sutures are used to close the incision. This approach requires cutting into the full thickness of the uterine corpus. Indications for this type of incision are extensive adhesions involving the bladder and lower uterine segment from previous cesarean births, transverse lie, or anterior placenta previa. Because it provides rapid access to the fetus, it may be chosen in cases of acute hemorrhage or other emergencies that threaten maternal or fetal safety. Other conditions that may warrant a classic incision include a fetus of less than 34 weeks who presents by breech, maternal fibroids that restrict the lower uterine segment, need for maternal hysterectomy immediately following the birth, invasive maternal cervical cancer, and cesarean birth being performed to rescue a living fetus from a dead woman.

A rare type of incision is the low (cervical) vertical approach. It is generally used only if the surgeon is having difficulty extracting the fetus through other methods.

Collaborative Management

Standards of care for clients undergoing cesarean birth should be included within each institution's perioperative and obstetric program. A family-centred approach is vital and should accommodate involvement of the client's support person. Preadmission should include discussion of postoperative pain management, realistic understanding of pain and surgical recovery, and warning signs of infection.

Preoperative Management. Even if the cesarean birth is an elective procedure, the experience of surgery can be anxiety-producing for the client and her family. Such anxiety can be heightened when the cesarean birth is unanticipated or an emergency. Team members need to concentrate on alleviating fears, correcting misperceptions, teaching normal procedures and likely outcomes, and communicating findings. If the surgery is elective, providers should verify the pregnancy's gestation and review the maternal and pregnancy history.

Preparation for the surgery is extensive. Common diagnostic studies performed to ensure maternal and fetal well-being include complete blood count, urinalysis, blood type and cross match (in case blood for transfusion is needed), and ultrasound to evaluate fetal position and placental location. If the gestation is preterm, an amniocentesis may be needed to check fetal lung maturity. The health care provider usually discusses the need for the surgery, the risks, and the type of anaesthesia that will be used (spinal, epidural, or general) (see Chapter 17). Spinal anaesthesia is used most frequently for elective cesarean births so that the mother can remain awake and aware of the birth experience.

The nurse documents the mother's last oral intake and what was eaten. He or she assists with preparing the necessary equipment, including newborn resuscitation

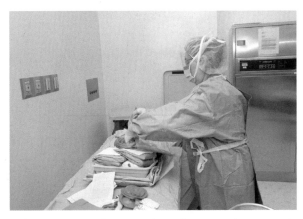

FIGURE 16.24 The nurse is setting up equipment and material in preparation for an impending cesarean birth.

equipment and a warm crib (Fig. 16.24). The nurse can begin teaching interventions that reduce postoperative complications, including use of deep-breathing exercises and ambulation within 8 to 12 hours postoperatively. Team members will prepare the surgical site and begin an IV infusion for fluid replacement therapy, as ordered. Antibiotics will also be provided with the surgery, with a single dose of a first-generation cephalosporin as the recommended medication. It is recommended that, for women with a BMI greater than 35, a double dose be given. Clindamycin or erythromycin can be used if the woman has a penicillin allergy. This can be given 15 to 60 minutes prior to initiation of the surgery or skin incision (SOGC, 2010a, 2010b).

The client will need an indwelling (Foley) catheter, which will remain in place for approximately 24 hours. The nurse administers any ordered preoperative medications and record when they were given, as well as any unexpected side effects. He or she also may assist the woman's partner or other support person to be gowned and prepared appropriately if this person will be attending the birth.

Intraoperative Management. Typically, the team involved in a cesarean birth includes the obstetrician, surgical assistant, anaesthesiologist, registered nurses, and pediatrician/neonatologist, depending on the reason for the cesarean birth and degree of acuity. Nurses are particularly helpful during this time at providing comfort, information, and reassurance to the client and her support people.

The presence of a pediatrician/neonatalogist or team to care for the infant helps to ensure adequate care of the newborn so that the obstetrician and his or her supports can focus on giving attention to the woman following the surgery. Neonatal nurses also may be in attendance, depending on the newborn's condition and need for treatment or transport. After removal from the uterus, the newborn who is experiencing no complications may be shown to the mother or given to the support person to hold before general newborn care procedures are initiated (see Chap. 20). Figure 16.25 depicts a cesarean birth sequence.

Postoperative Management. Maternal postpartum care is similar to that for women who have undergone vaginal birth. The experience of major surgery, however, necessitates some added measures. The nurse checks the client's vital signs and lochia flow every 15 minutes for the first hour, every 30 minutes for the next hour, and every 4 hours thereafter, if stable. If the client received sedation, her level of consciousness needs to be monitored; if she received regional anaesthesia, the nurse needs to document motor and sensory assessments. The client should cough, and perform deep-breathing exercises, as required.

The client will likely be in the health care facility for 2 to 3 days longer than the client who has a vaginal

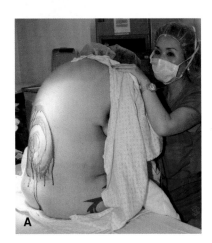
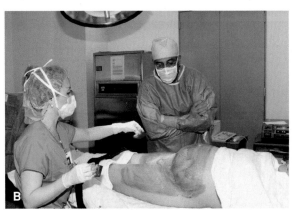

FIGURE 16.25 A cesarean birth sequence. **A:** The client is receiving anaesthesia. **B:** The surgical area is being cleaned and prepared.

(continued)

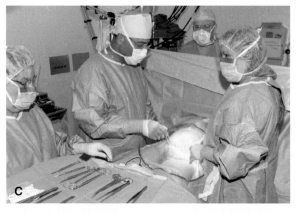

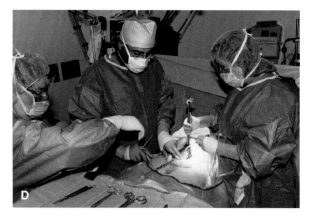

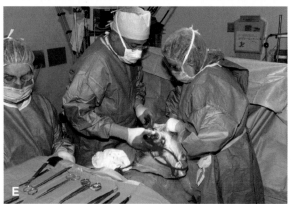

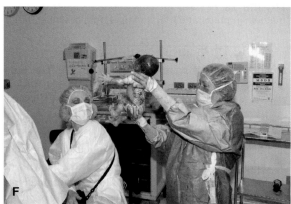

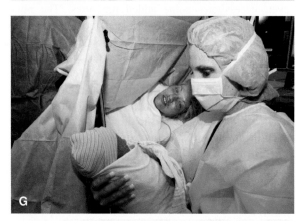

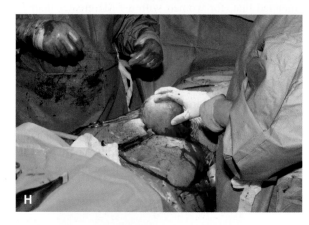

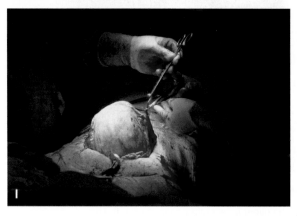

FIGURE 16.25 *(Continued)* **C:** The obstetrician begins cutting. **D:** The uterus has been opened. **E:** Team members begin extracting the fetus from the uterus. **F:** The newborn emerges successfully. **G:** The nurse holds the newborn and shows her to the mother. **H:** The uterus is being pushed back into the woman's body. **I:** The surgeon is repairing the uterus.

(continued)

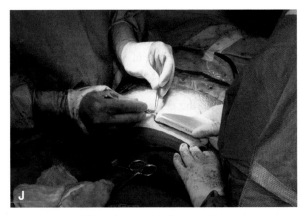

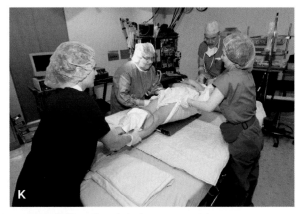

FIGURE 16.25 *(Continued)* **J:** The incision site is sutured. **K:** The client is being prepared for transfer from the operating area to a recovery area.

birth. During this time, regular assessments will be done of her abdominal dressing and drainage, uterine fundus for firmness, urinary output, and lochia. The client will likely receive a regimen of pain medication that will be adjusted as the incision heals. The client may need assistance with moving in bed and turning from side to side. The nurse will need to check any IV infusions and monitor intake and output. Although standards of introducing solid foods vary, some clients are able to eat regular food within 12 to 18 hours post partum.

One major difference between vaginal and cesarean births is that the surgery may impose a forced separation between mother and newborn in the first few hours. Depending on the condition of mother and baby, team members should make every effort possible to reunite the family quickly and to facilitate early touching and holding of the newborn to promote bonding. Clients who intend to breastfeed may require extra support, because post-operative pain and recovery from surgery may make the initial experience more challenging. Special involvement from a lactation consultant and extra attention to this area may be helpful. Early ambulation is important to prevent cardiovascular and respiratory problems. If the surgery was unanticipated, follow-up regarding the disparity between the family's expectations (ie, vaginal birth) and actuality and how they are adjusting to it is an important emotional consideration.

Discharge teaching focuses on ensuring adequate rest, and adhering to restrictions about lifting and performing household tasks, like vacuuming. Emphasis would appropriately be placed on knowing the signs of infection, such as fever, chills, burning with urination, or redness or draining from the surgical site. The risk of infection, whether urinary tract or wound, is 5 to 20 times greater with a cesarean than with a vaginal delivery, affecting up to 25% of women who have this surgery (SOGC, 2010a, 2010b). The teaching would most appropriately include who to call and when or where to

go to seek help (eg, health care provider's office, public health nurse visit, etc.). The client should avoid sexual intercourse until lochia has ceased and she no longer has any abdominal or perineal discomfort. As with all postpartum clients, contraception education should be provided. Protocols for follow-up appointments vary, but many clients who undergo cesarean birth are seen 6 weeks after discharge from the hospital, which is similar to women who undergo vaginal birth.

Vaginal Birth After Cesarean

Vaginal birth after cesarean (VBAC) is the term used for a vaginal birth after the client has undergone at least one previous cesarean birth. Factors associated with a positive VBAC experience include spontaneous labour, an initial favourable pelvic examination, and no use of oxytocin (Durnwald & Mercer, 2004). Several factors, including prior vaginal birth, gestational age, and maternal obesity, are also included in the individual care planning (Smith & Merrill, 2006). VBAC is recommended as safe and the best practice for the majority of women and is associated with a lower maternal mortality than repeat surgery and less morbidity for mothers and infants (Lundgren et al., 2012). Although many health care providers emphasize the possibility of VBAC to clients who have had transverse incisions (Fig. 16.26), a variety of factors contribute to a woman's decision about whether to try a VBAC or schedule a repeat cesarean birth. Women have expressed the opinion that a balanced approach by their health care provider in explaining the benefits—such as improved recovery, better rates of breastfeeding and its initiation closer to when they gave birth, as well as increased empowerment— would have been beneficial to the discussion about having a VBAC. Arguments against VBAC focus on the increased risks of uterine rupture (approximately 1%) (Smith & Merrill, 2006) and hemorrhage. In most

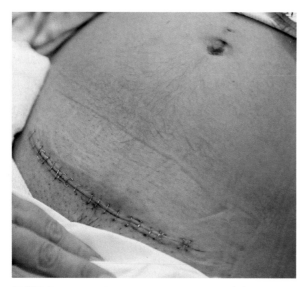

FIGURE 16.26 A low-transverse incision for a cesarean birth provides options for future attempts at a vaginal birth in subsequent pregnancies.

cases of attempted VBAC, women go through a trial of labour to see how they progress; such a trial must occur in an environment capable of managing an acute emergency in the event of uterine rupture.

Contraindications to VBAC include a prior classic cesarean birth, prior myomectomy, uterine scar other than low transverse cesarean scar, contracted pelvis, and inadequate staff or facility available should emergency cesarean birth be required (SOGC, 2005). Pharmacologic methods of cervical ripening increase the risk for uterine rupture; thus, this procedure is contraindicated in clients attempting VBAC (SOGC, 2005). Other means of labour induction, such as use of a Foley catheter or amniotomy, may be considered appropriate and safe. Labour induction in a woman who has experienced previous cesarean birth also poses risk for uterine rupture and needs to be discussed with the client before the induction takes place (Dauphinee, 2004; Kayani & Alfirevic, 2005).

The client attempting VBAC must give fully informed consent before labour begins and express a clear understanding of the risks and benefits. The nurse must keep detailed and accurate records of the client's plan of care, the timing of interventions, the client's response, and fetal status. Such records provide the details necessary to ensure that prompt attention is given to any emergency development. An abnormal fetal heart rate is an indication of potential uterine rupture and should lead the team to begin the process of emergency cesarean birth. Upon recommendations for a safe trial of labour for VBAC, the obstetrician, anaesthesia provider, and operating room team must be immediately available (Dauphinee, 2004; SOGC, 2005).

SUMMARY

- Dystocia is abnormal or dysfunctional labour. It can develop at any point in labour and may involve a problem with the powers of labour, passenger (fetus), or passage (maternal birth canal).

- Problems with the powers of labour usually involve uterine contractions or maternal bearing-down efforts. Examples include hypertonic and hypotonic contractions, inadequate expulsion forces, pathologic retraction and constriction rings, and precipitous birth. Many of these conditions necessitate surgical birth.

- Breech presentation means that the fetal buttocks or feet are the presenting part. In most cases, a breech presentation is an indication for cesarean birth. If the fetus is between 35 and 37 weeks, providers may initiate ECV to rotate the fetus and facilitate vaginal birth. Vaginal breech birth is less common, but happens in discussion with the woman/family under appropriate circumstances and may require the use of forceps.

- In addition to the buttocks in breech presentation, other abnormal fetal presentations include shoulder, face, brow, and compound presentations.

- With OP positioning, the fetal occiput lies in the posterior part of the maternal pelvis. As a result, the fetal head is not well applied to the cervix, which may delay the progress of labour. This problem also can result in significant back pain for the mother. To resolve the problem, the client might try changes in position or ambulation to encourage the fetus to move.

- When shoulder dystocia develops, the fetal shoulders cannot move through the maternal pelvis after the fetal head has emerged. A calm cooperative team approach to intervention is necessary and requires a stepwise approach. Techniques to alleviate shoulder dystocia include McRoberts maneuver, suprapubic pressure, assisting the woman into a hands-and-knees position to dislodge the shoulder, and the Woods screw rotational maneuver.

- Other problems with the fetus that may pose risks for labour and childbirth include macrosomia and fetal abnormalities.

- Many problems with the maternal pelvis can be anticipated if a woman has received adequate prenatal care.

- True labour that starts before 37 completed weeks of gestation is considered preterm. This occurrence is responsible for most neonatal deaths unrelated to congenital anomalies. Health care providers focus heavily on teaching clients the signs of preterm labour and, when it occurs, working to possibly halt or at least delay progress for as long as possible to provide corticosteroids to the baby to develop the lungs and/or get the gestation closer to 37 weeks.

- Postterm pregnancy is pregnancy that extends beyond 42 completed weeks' gestation. This situation poses significant risks for fetal morbidity and mortality and usually necessitates labour induction.

- Hemorrhage during labour can result from problems with the placenta or because of a ruptured uterus. Excessive bleeding is always a medical emergency requiring prompt and focused interventions.

- Cord prolapse occurs when part of the umbilical cord falls in front of, lies beside, or hangs below the fetal presenting part. It can cause fetal death and thus mandates emergent management.

- Amniotic fluid embolism can occur during labour or postpartally and poses significant risks for maternal mortality. General treatment goals include maintaining oxygenation, blood pressure, and cardiac output and managing any coagulopathy. Continuous accurate monitoring of the fetus and woman is essential.

- The birth process in cases of multiple gestation may require some adjustments based on the number of fetuses and their individual presentations, weights, and other factors.

- The obese woman in labour requires special considerations such as monitoring her vital signs, ensuring equipment can accommodate her safely, and regularly checking the progress of her labour.

- Growing diversity in North America is exposing more health care providers to women in labour who have previously undergone various forms of female circumcision. Nurses and other caregivers need to treat circumcised women with sensitivity and respect and assist them through their labour process with enhanced attention to managing their pain and risks for hemorrhage and infection.

- Various factors may require assisted labour through cervical ripening and induction. Methods to ripen the cervix include mechanical and pharmacologic interventions.

- Exogenous administration of oxytocin is used to increase uterine contractility. Administration of a continuous IV infusion of oxytocin begins with a starting dose that is increased until an adequate contraction pattern is achieved. Nursing care during oxytocin administration focuses on monitoring maternal vital signs and fetal heart rate, explaining to the client and family how oxytocin facilitates uterine contractions, monitoring the progress of uterine contractions, checking for any complications, providing comfort and assistance with pain management, and documenting findings.

- Amnioinfusion may be used in cases of cord compression, oligohydramnios, postmaturity, preterm labour with rupture of the membranes, and thick meconium fluid to improve fetal and placental oxygenation, help cushion the umbilical cord, and dilute any meconium that may be found.

- Rates of cesarean births are increasing for several reasons. Regardless of whether the surgery is planned or unexpected, this type of birth requires expert nursing care during all phases of the birth to protect maternal and fetal health and to optimize long-term outcomes for the family.

- Women who receive low-transverse incisions during cesarean birth may be candidates for vaginal birth in future pregnancies.

Questions to Ponder

1. A client is attending a regular prenatal visit. She is at 24 weeks' gestation. During a discussion with the nurse, the client reports that a few weeks ago, she had some light pink vaginal spotting that lasted for 1 day only. She says, "It went away, and I can still feel the baby moving, so I didn't think it was anything to worry about."
   - What is your reaction to this scenario? How would you respond to the client?
   - What teaching needs do you identify? What would be your next steps?

2. One of your close family members is in the 14th week of a second pregnancy that is progressing as expected. Her first pregnancy ended with a low-transverse cesarean birth of a healthy baby. The surgery was unplanned and occurred because of failure to progress after several hours of labour. Your relative says to you, "My obstetrician has been telling me that I can attempt a vaginal birth with this pregnancy, but I'm really not sure if that would be for the best. It seems in some ways that it would be easier and more convenient for me to just schedule another surgery—at least I'll know what to expect! What do you think?"
   - How do you feel about the growing rates of cesarean births? When do you think they should be indicated for clients?
   - What risks and benefits of both vaginal and cesarean birth in these circumstances can you outline for your relative? What things would you consider in responding to her statements?

REVIEW QUESTIONS

1. A woman in labour is experiencing hypertonic uterine contractions. The nurse would be least likely to prepare the client for which intervention?
   A. Intravenous fluid therapy
   B. Intramuscular morphine
   C. Administration of short-acting barbiturate
   D. Intravenous oxytocin

2. A client has undergone external cephalic version successfully. Which of the following would the nurse do next?
   A. Prepare the client for an ultrasound
   B. Plan for an immediate cesarean birth
   C. Have the client undergo a nonstress test
   D. Perform McRoberts maneuver

3. Which finding would lead the nurse to suspect that the fetus of a client in labour is in OP position?
   A. Client reports significant back pain with contractions
   B. Auscultation of fetal heart sounds in the lower abdomen
   C. Fetal back easily palpated with Leopold maneuvers
   D. Fetal buttocks identified as the presenting part

4. Which of the following assessment findings would indicate the need for tocolytic therapy in a client with preterm labour?
   A. Fetus at 37 weeks' gestation
   B. Immature fetal lung profile
   C. Fetal weight of 2,700 g
   D. Intact membranes

5. A woman who is at 41 weeks' gestation is being evaluated for possible labour induction. The nurse assesses the client's cervical readiness using the Bishop scoring method. Which score would indicate that the cervix is favourable for labour induction?
   A. 3
   B. 5
   C. 6
   D. 9

6. After teaching a group of students about placental anomalies, the instructor determines that the teaching was successful when the students identify which anomaly as least problematic?
   A. Battledore placenta
   B. Velamentous placenta
   C. Circumvallate placenta
   D. Succenturiate placenta

7. Which position would be least effective for a pregnant woman in labour who is experiencing umbilical cord prolapse?
   A. Knee-chest
   B. Trendelenburg
   C. Semi-Fowler
   D. Sims lateral

8. A client is to receive a continuous intravenous infusion of oxytocin. The nurse determines that the client is receiving the intended effect as evidenced by:
   A. Uterine resting tone of 35 mm Hg.
   B. Contractions occurring every 2 to 3 minutes.
   C. Contractions lasting approximately 2 minutes.
   D. Contraction intensity of 70 mm Hg.

9. The nurse is describing the types of uterine incisions that may be used with a client who is to have an elective cesarean birth. Which of the following should the nurse include as characteristics of a transverse incision?
   A. Reduces the amount of blood lost during the procedure
   B. Promotes rapid access to the fetus if problems develop
   C. Allows for birth of a fetus younger than 34 weeks in breech presentation
   D. Uses three layers of absorbable sutures to close the incision

REFERENCES

Arias, R. (2000). Pharmacology of oxytocin and prostaglandins. *Clinical Obstetrics and Gynecology, 43*, 455–468.

Baskett, T. (2004). *Essential management of obstetric emergencies* (4th ed.). Bristol: Clinical Press Ltd.

Baxley, E. G. (2003). Labour induction: A decade of change. *American Family Physician, 67*(10), 2076–2080.

Beck, C. (2013). The obstetric nightmare of shoulder dystocia: A tale of two perspectives. *MCN. The American Journal of Maternal Child Nursing, 38*(1), 34–40.

Behruzi, R., Hatem, M., Goulet, L., Fraser, W., Leduc, N., & Misago, C. (2010). Humanized birth in high risk pregnancy: Barriers and facilitating factors. *Medicine, Health Care and Philosophy, 13*, 49–58.

Belfort, M. A. (2003). Operative vaginal delivery. In J. R. Scott, R. S. Gibbs, B. Y. Karlan, & A. F. Haney (Eds.), *Danforth's obstetrics and gynecology* (9th ed., pp. 419–447). Philadelphia: Lippincott Williams & Wilkins.

Benson, M. (2011). Current concepts of immunology and diagnosis in amniotic fluid embolism. *Clinical and Developmental Immunology, 2012*, 1–7.

Bianchi, A., & Adams, E. (2009). Labor support during second stage labor for women with epidurals: Birth in this era is technology driven. Many women giving birth in hospital settings have epidurals for pain management. Yet laboring women need more than technology–they have basic needs that can't be addressed by technology alone. *Nursing for Women's Health, 13*(1), 38–47.

Boyle, B., McConkey, R., Garne, E., Loane, M., Addor, M., Bakker, M., et al. (2013). Trends in the prevalence, risk and pregnancy outcome of multiple births with congenital anomaly: A registry-based study in 14 European countries 1984–2007. *An International Journal of Obstetrics & Gynaecology, 120*(6), 707–716.

Butler, J., & Wilkes, P. (2006). Postterm pregnancy. Retrieved September 7, 2008, from http://www.emedicine.com/med/topic3248.htm

Campbell, C. (2011). Elective cesarean delivery: Trends, evidence and implications for women, newborns and nurses. *Nursing for Women's Health, 15*(4), 308–318.

Canadian Institute for Health Information (CIHI). (2006). *Giving birth in Canada: The costs*. Retrieved September 7, 2008, from http://dsp-psd.pwgsc.gc.ca/Collection/H118-38-2006E.pdf

Caughey, A. B., Sandberg, P. L., Zlatnik, M. G., Thiet, M. P., Parer, J. T., & Laros, R. K., Jr. (2005). Forceps compared with vacuum: Rates of neonatal and maternal morbidity. *Obstetrics and Gynecology, 106*(5 Pt 1), 908–912.

Cesario, S. (2003). Obesity in pregnancy: What every nurse needs to know. *AWHONN Lifelines, 7*(2), 118–125.

Cheng, Y. W., Shaffer, B. L., & Caughey, A. B. (2006). The association between persistent occiput posterior position and neonatal outcomes. *Obstetrics and Gynecology, 107*(4), 837–844.

Christianson, L. M., Bovbjerg, V. E., McDavitt, E. C., & Hullfish, K. L. (2003). Risk factors for perineal injury during delivery. *American Journal of Obstetrics and Gynecology, 189*(1), 255–260.

Clayworth, S. (2000). The nurse's role during oxytocin administration. *MCN. The American Journal of Maternal Child Nursing, 25*, 80–85.

Cunningham, F. G., Gant, N. F., Leveno, K. J., Bloom, S. L., Hauth, J. C., Gilstrap, L. C., III, et al. (2010). *Williams obstetrics* (23rd ed.). New York: McGraw-Hill.

Dauphinee, J. D. (2004). VBAC: Safety for the patient and the nurse. *Journal of Obstetric, Gynecologic, and Neonatal Nursing, 33*(1), 105–115.

Daviss, A., Johson, K., & LaLonde, A. (2010). Evolving evidence since the trem breech trial: Canadian response, European dissent, and potential solutions. *Journal of Obstetrics and Gynaecology Canada, 32*(2), 217–224.

Denney, J., & Culhan, J. (2009). Bacterial vaginosis: A problematic infection from both a perinatal and neonatal perspective. *Seminars in Fetal and Neonatal Medicine, 14*(4), 200–203.

Denis, A., Michaux, P., & Callahan, S. (2012). Factors implicated in moderating the risk for depression and anxiety in high risk pregnancy. *Journal of Reproductive and Infant Psychology, 30*(2), 124–134.

Dilbaz, B., Ozturkoglu, E., Dilbaz, S., Ozturk, N., Sivaslioglu, A. A., & Haberal, A. (2006). Risk factors and perinatal outcomes associated with umbilical cord prolapse. *Archives of Gynecology and Obstetrics, 274*(2), 104–107.

Dodd, J. M., & Crowther, C. A. (2005). Evidence-based care of women with a multiple pregnancy. *Best Practice & Research. Clinical Obstetrics & Gynaecology, 19*(1), 131–153.

Doyle, J., Kenny, T., Burkett, A., & von Gruenigen, V. (2011). A performance improvement process to tackle tachysystole. *Journal of Obstetric, Gynecologic and Neonatal Nursing, 40*(5), 512–519.

Doyle, N. M., Riggs, J. W., Ramin, S. M., Sosa, M. A., & Gilstrap, L. C., 3rd. (2005). Outcomes of term vaginal breech delivery. *American Journal of Perinatology, 22*(6), 325–328.

Dudley, D. J. (2008). Complications of labour. In J. R. Scott, R. S. Gibbs, B. Y. Karlan, & A. F. Haney (Eds.), *Danforth's obstetrics and gynecology* (10th ed., pp. 431–551). Philadelphia: Lippincott Williams & Wilkins.

Durnwald, C., & Mercer, B. (2004). Vaginal birth after cesarean delivery: Predicting success, risk of failure. *Journal of Maternal-Fetal, and Neonatal Medicine, 15*(6), 388–393.

Ehrenberg, H. M., Mercer, B. M., & Catalano, P. M. (2004). The influence of obesity and diabetes on the prevalence of macrosomia. *American Journal of Obstetrics and Gynecology, 191*(3), 964–968.

Ellings, J., Newman, R., & Bowers, N. (1998). Intrapartum care for women with multiple pregnancy. *Journal of Obstetric, Gynecologic, and Neonatal Nursing, 27*(4), 466–472.

Elnashar, A., & Abdelhady, R. (2007). The impact of female genital cutting on health of newly married women. *International Journal of Gynaecology and Obstetrics, 97*(3), 238–244.

Fischer, R. (2006). Breech presentation. *E-Medicine.* Retrieved September 7, 2008 from http://www.emedicine.com/med/topic3272.htm

Ghosh, M. K. (2005). Breech presentation: Evolution of management. *Journal of Reproductive Medicine, 50*(2), 108–116.

Gilbert, E.,(2011). *Manual of high risk pregnancy and delivery* (4th ed.). St. Louis: Mosby.

Gilbert, W., & Danielsen, B. (2003). Pregnancy outcomes associated with intrauterine growth restriction. *American Journal of Obstetrics and Gynecology, 188*(6), 1596–1601.

Gist, R., Stafford, I., Leibowitz, A., & Beilin, Y. (2009). Amniotic fluid embolism. *Anesthesia & Analgesia, 108*(5), 1599–1602.

Gramellini, D., Fieni, S., Kaihura, C., Faiola, S., & Vadora, E. (2003). Transabdominal antepartum amnioinfusion. *International Journal of Gynaecology and Obstetrics, 83*(2), 171–178.

Gunatilake, R., & Perlow, J. (2011). Obesity and pregnancy: Clinical management of the obese gravid. *American Journal of Obstetrics and Gynecology, 204*(2), 106–119.

Hadi, H. (2000). Cervical ripening and labour induction: Clinical guidelines. *Clinical Obstetrics and Gynecology, 43*, 524–536.

Harper, L., Cahill, A., Roehl, K., Odibo, A., Stamilio, D., & Macones, G. (2012). The pattern of labor preceding uterine rupture. *American Journal of Obstetrics and Gynecology, 207*, 210e1–210e6.

Healy, A. J., & Gaddipati, S. (2005). Intrapartum management of twins: Truths and controversies. *Clinics in Perinatology, 32*(2), 455–473.

Herzig, K., Danley, D., Jackson, R., Petersen, R., Chamberlain, L., & Gerbert, B. (2006). Seizing the 9-month moment: Addressing behavioral risks in prenatal patients. *Patient Education and Counseling, 61*(2), 228–235.

Hook, C., & Damos, R. (2008). Vacuum-assisted vaginal delivery. *American Family Physician, 78*(8), 953–960.

Hutton, E. K., & Hofmeyr, G. J. (2006). External cephalic version for breech presentation before term. *Cochrane Database of Systematic Reviews, 10*, CD000084.

Jazayeri, A., & Contreras, D. (2007). Macrosomia. *E-Medicine.* Retrieved September 7, 2008, from http://emedicine.com/med/topic3279.htm

Johnson, J. H., Figueroa, R., Garry, D., Elimian, A., & Maulik, D. (2004). Immediate maternal and neonatal effects of forceps and vacuum-assisted deliveries. *Obstetrics and Gynecology, 103*(3), 513–518.

Kavanagh, J., & Kelly, A. J. (2005). Sexual intercourse for cervical ripening and induction of labour. *Cochrane Database of Systematic Reviews,* (2), CD003093.

Kavanagh, J., Kelly, A. J., & Thomas, J. (2005). Breast stimulation for cervical ripening and induction of labour. *Cochrane Database of Systematic Reviews,* (2), CD003092.

Kayani, S. I., & Alfirevic, Z., (2005). Uterine rupture after induction of labour in women with previous caesarean section. *British Journal of Obstetrics and Gynaecology, 112*(4), 451–455.

Kelly, M., Johnson, E., Lee, V., Massey, L., Purser, D., Ring, K., et al. (2010). Delayed vs. immediate pushing in second stage of labor. *MCN. The American Journal of Maternal Child Nursing, 35*(2), 81–88.

Klatt, T. E., & Cruikshank, D. P. (2008). Breech, other malpresentations, and umbilical cord complications. In R. S. Gibbs, B. Y. Karlan, A. F. Haney, & I. Nygaard (Eds.), *Danforth's obstetrics and gynecology* (10th ed., pp. 400–416). Philadelphia: Lippincott Williams & Wilkins.

Kolas, T., Hofoss, D., Daltveit, A. K., Nilsen, S. T., Henriksen, T., Hager, R., et al. (2003). Indications for cesarean deliveries in Norway. *American Journal of Obstetrics and Gynecology, 188*(4), 864–870.

Kunz, M., Loftus, R., & Nichols, A. (2012). Incidence of uterine tachysystole in women induced with oxytocin. *Journal of Obstetric, Gynecologic, and Neonatal Nurses, 41*(1), 12–18.

Kwek, K., & Yeo, G. S. (2006). Shoulder dystocia and injuries: Prevention and management. *Current Opinion in Obstetrics and Gynecology, 18*(2), 123–128.

Lin, M. G. (2006). Umbilical cord prolapse. *Obstetrical and Gynecological Survey, 61*(4), 269–277.

Locksmith, G. J., Gei, A. F., Rowe, T. F., Yeomans, E. R., & Hankins, G. D. (2001). Teaching the Laufe-Piper forceps technique at cesarean delivery. *Journal of Reproductive Medicine, 46*(5), 457–461.

Lundgren, I., Begley, C., Gross, M., & Bondas, T. (2012). Groping through the fog: A metasynthesis of women's experiences on VBAC (Vaginal Birth after cesarean Section). *BMC Pregnancy and Childbirth, 12*, 85.

Mahlmeister, L. (2008). Best practices in perinatal nursing: Implementing safe and effective practices for second-stage labor. *Journal of Perinatal and Neonatal Nursing, 22*, 183–185.

Mayberry, L. (2006). Cesarean delivery on maternal request. *MCN. The American Journal of Maternal Child Nursing, 31*(5), 286–289.

McQuivey, R. W. (2004). Vacuum-assisted delivery: A review. *Journal of Maternal-Fetal, and Neonatal Medicine, 16*(3), 171–180.

Moore, J., & Baldisseri, M. R. (2005). Amniotic fluid embolism. *Critical Care Medicine, 33*(10 Suppl), S279–S285.

Moore, L., & Martin, J. N., Jr. (2003). Prolonged pregnancy. In J. R. Scott, R. S. Gibbs, B. Y. Karlan, & A. F. Haney (Eds.), *Danforth's obstetrics and gynecology* (9th ed., pp. 219–223). Philadelphia: Lippincott Williams & Wilkins.

Neal, J., Lowe, N., Patrick, T., Cabbage, L., & Corwin, E. (2010). What is the slowest-yet-normal cervical dilation rate among nulliparous women with spontaneous labor onset? *Journal of Obstetric, Gynecologic and Neonatal Nurses, 39*, 361–369.

Nodine, P., & Hastings-Tolsma, M. (2012). Maternal obesity: Improving pregnancy outcomes. *MCN. The American Journal of Maternal Child Nursing, 37*(2), 110–115.

O'Grady, J. (2008). Vaccuum extraction. Retrieved September 7, 2008, from http://www.emedicine.com/med/topic3389.htm

O'Mahony, F., Hofmeyr, G., & Menon, V. (2010). Choice of instruments for assisted vaginal delivery. *Cochrane Database of Systematic Reviews,* (11), CD005455.

Oyelese, Y., & Smulian, J. C. (2006). Placenta previa, placenta accreta, and vasa previa. *Obstetrics and Gynecology, 107*(4), 927–941.

Pakenham, S., Chamberlain, S. M., & Smith, G. N. (2006). Women's views on elective primary caesarean section. *Journal of Obstetrics and Gynecology Canada, 28*(12), 1089–1093.

Palmer, C. (2002). Obstetric emergencies and anesthetic management. *Current Reviews for Perianesthesia Nurses, 24*(11), 121–132.

Patel, R. R., & Murphy, D. J. (2004). Forceps delivery in modern obstetric practice. *British Medical Journal, 328*(7451), 1302–1305.

Pearson, N. (2011). Oxytocin safety: Legal implications for perinatal nurses. *Nursing for Women's Health, 15*(2), 110–117.

Perozzi, K. J., & Englert, N. C. (2004). Amniotic fluid embolism: An obstetric emergency. *Critical Care Nurse, 24*(4), 54–61.

Politi, S., D'Emidio, L., Cignini, P., Gioriandino, M., & Gioriandino, C. (2010). Shoulder bdystocia: An evidence-based approach. *Journal of Perinatal Medicine, 4*(3), 35–42.

Public Health Agency of Canada. (2011). *Perinatal Birth Indicators for Canada: 2011*. Ottawa, ON: Author.

Rai, J., & Schreiber, J. R. (2008). Cervical ripening. *E-Medicine*. Retrieved September 7, 2008 from http://www.emedicine.com/med/topic3282.htm

Ramsey, P. S., & Repke, J. T. (2003). Intrapartum management of multifetal pregnancies. *Seminars in Perinatology, 27*(1), 54–72.

Rao, K., Belogolovkin, V., Yankowitz, J., & Spinnato, J. (2012). Abnormal placentation: Evidence-based diagnosis and management of placenta previa, placenta accreta, and vasa previa. *Obstetrical and Gynecological Survey, 67*(8), 503–519.

Ressel, G. W. (2004). ACOG releases report on dystocia and augmentation of labour. *American Family Physician, 69*(5), 1290–1291.

Robbins, J. (2011). Malpresentations and malpositions. In M. Boyle (Ed.), *Emergencies around childbirth: A handbook for midwives* (2nd ed., pp. 63–82). Oxon, UK: Radcliffe Medical Press.

Romano, A., & Lothian, J. (2008). Promoting, proteching, and supporting normal birth: A look at the evidence. *Journal of Obstetric, Gynecologic & Neonatal Nursing, 37*(1), 94–105.

Rosenberg, A. (2008). The IUGR newborn. *Seminars in Perinatology, 32*(3), 219–224.

Ross, M. G., Beall, M. H., & Bonni, A. (2007). Forceps delivery. *E-Medicine*. Retrieved September 7, 2008, from http://www.emedicine.com/med/topic3284.htm

Rouse, D., Weiner, S., Bloom, S., Varner, M., Spong, C., Ramin, S., et al. (2009). Second stage labor duration in nulliparous women: Relationship to maternal and perinatal outcomes. *American Journal of Obstetrics and Gynecology, 201*(4), 357.e1–357.e7.

Rowlands, I., & Redshaw, M. (2012). Mode of birth and women's psychological and physcial wellbeing in the postnatal period. *BMC Pregnancy and Childbirth, 12*, 138.

Royal College of Obstetricians and Gynecologists. (2010). *External cephalic version and reducing the incidence of breech presentation: Guideline #20*. Retrieved from www.nice.org

Sakornbut, E., Leeman, L., & Fontaine, P. (2007). Late pregnancy bleeding. *American Family Physician, 75*(8), 1199–1206.

Schmidt, J. (1999). Prolonged pregnancy. In L. Mandeville & N. Troiano (Eds.), *High-risk and critical care intrapartum nursing* (2nd ed., pp. 123–138). Philadelphia: Lippincott Williams & Wilkins.

Schoening, A. M. (2006). Amniotic fluid embolism: Historical perspectives and new possibilities. *MCN. The American Journal of Maternal Child Nursing, 31*(2), 78–83.

Sheiner, E., Levy, A., Hershkovitz, R., Hallak, M., Hammel, R. D., Katz, M., et al. (2006). Determining factors associated with shoulder dystocia: A population-based study. *European Journal of Obstetrics, Gynecology, and Reproductive Biology, 126*(1), 11–15.

Shields, S., Ratcliffe, S., Fontaine, P., & Leeman, L. (2007). Dystocia in nulliparous women. *American Family Physician, 75*(11), 1671–1676.

Silver, R. K., Haney, E. I., Grobman, W. A., MacGregor, S. N., Casele, H. L., & Neerhof, M. G. (2000). Comparison of active phase labour between triplet, twin, and singleton gestations. *Journal of the Society for Gynecologic Investigation, 7*(5), 297–300.

Simmons, H., & Goldberg, L. (2011). "High-Risk" pregnancy after perinatal loss: Understanding the label. *Midwifery, 27*, 452–457.

Sittner, B. J., DeFrain, J., & Hudson, D. B. (2005). Effects of high-risk pregnancies on families. *MCN. The American Journal of Maternal Child Nursing, 30*(2), 121–126.

Skupski, D., Harrison-Restelli, C., & Dupont, R. (2003). External cephalic version. *Gynecologic and Obstetric Investigation, 56*, 83–88.

Smith, G. N., Walker, M. C., Ohlsson, A., O'Brien, K., & Windrum, R. (2007). Randomized double-blind placebo-controlled trial of transdermal nitroglycerin for preterm labor. *American Journal of Obstetrics and Gynecology, 196*(37), 37.e1–37.e8.

Smith, J., & Merrill, D. (2006). Oxytocin for induction of labour. *Clinical Obstetrics & Gynecology, 49*(3), 594–606.

Smith, S., Hulsey, T., & Goodnight, W. (2008). Effects of obesity on pregnancy. *Journal of Obstetric, Gynecologic & Neonatal Nursing, 37*(2), 176–184.

Society of Obstetricians and Gynaecologists of Canada. (2000). *Advances in labour and risk management* (7th ed.). Ottawa, ON: Author.

Society of Obstetricians and Gynaecologists of Canada. (SOGC). (2001). Induction of labour at term. *Journal of Obstetricians and Gynaecologists Canada, 23*(8), 717–728.

Society of Obstetricians and Gynaecologists of Canada. (SOGC). (2003). Antenatal corticosteroid therapy for fetal maturation. *Journal of Obstetricians and Gynaecologists Canada, 25*(1), 45–48.

Society of Obstetricians and Gynaecologists of Canada. (2004). *SOGC clinical practice guidelines: Guidelines for operative vaginal birth*. Retrieved September 7, 2008, from http://www.sogc.org/guidelines/public/148E-CPG-August2004.pdf

Society of Obstetricians and Gynaecologists of Canada. (2005). SOGC clinical practice guidelines. Guidelines for vaginal birth after previous caesarean birth. Number 155 (replaces guideline Number 147), February 2005. *International Journal of Gynaecology and Obstetrics, 89*(3), 319–331.

Society of Obstetricians and Gynecologists of Canada. (2010a). The use of progesterone for prevention of preterm birth. *Journal of Obstetrics & Gynecology in Canada, 30*(1), 67–71.

Society of Obstetricians and Gynecologists of Canada. (2010b). Clinical practice guidelines: Antibiotic prophylaxis in obstetric procedures. *Journal of Obstetrics and Gynecology in Canada, 247*, 878–884.

Soens, M., Birnbach, D., Ranasinghe, J., & Van Zundert, A. (2008). Obstetric anesthesia for the obese and morbidly obese patient: An ounce of prevention is worth more than a pound of treatment. *Acta Anaesthesiologica Scandinavica, 52*, 6–19.

Sprague, A., Oppenheimer, L., McCabe, L., Graham, I., & Davies, B. (2008). Knowledge to action: Implementing a guideline for second stage labour. *MCN. The American Journal of Maternal Child Nursing, 33*(3), 179–186.

Sultana, R., Chen, X., Lee, C., & Hader, J. (2011). Outcomes in multiple gestation pregnancies among Canadian women age 35 years and older. *Healthcare Quarterly, 14*(4), 22–24.

Tan, T. C., Devendra, K., Tan, L. K., & Tan, H. K. (2006). Tocolytic treatment for the management of preterm labour: A systematic review. *Singapore Medical Journal, 47*(5), 361–366.

Taylor, B. (2011). Sonographic assessment of cervical length and the risk of preterm birth. *Journal of Obstetric, Gynecologic and Neonatal Nursing, 40*, 617–631.

Taylor, M. J. (2006). The management of multiple pregnancy. *Early Human Development, 82*(6), 365–370.

Tenore, J. L. (2003). Methods for cervical ripening and induction of labour. *American Family Physician, 67*(10), 2123–2128.

Tikkanen, M., Nuutila, M., Hiilesmaa, V., Paavonen, J., & Ylikorkala, O. (2006). Prepregnancy risk factors for placental abruption. *Acta Obstetricia et Gynecologica Scandinavica, 85*(1), 40–44.

Turton, P. Neilson, J., Quenby, S., Burdyga, T., & Wray, S. (2009). A short review of twin pregnancy and how oxytocin receptor expression may differ in multiple pregnancy. *European Journal of Obstetrics & Gynecology and Reproductive Biology, 144* (Suppl 1), S40–S44.

Wen, S. W., Demissie, K., Yang, Q., & Walker, M. C. (2004). Maternal morbidity and obstetric complications in triplet pregnancies and quadruplet and higher-order multiple pregnancies. *American Journal of Obstetrics and Gynecology, 191*(1), 254–258.

Whitehorn, J., Ayonrinde, O., & Maingay, S. (2002). Female genital mutilation: Cultural and psychological implications. *Sexual and Relationship Therapy, 17*(2), 161–170.

World Health Organization. (2008). Female genital mutilation. Retrieved September 7, 2008, from http://www.who.int/mediacentre/factsheets/fs241/en/

Zaretsky, M., Alexander, J., McIntire, D., Hatab, M., Twickler, D., & Leveno, K. (2005). Magnetic resonance imaging pelvimetry and the prediction of labor dystocia. *Obstetrics & Gynecology, 106*(5 Pt 1), 919–926.

Zwelling, E. (2008). The emergence of high-tech birthing. *Journal of Obstetric, Gynecologic & Neonatal Nursing, 37*(1), 85–93.

CHAPTER 17

Pharmacologic Pain Management of Labour

Kimberley T. Jackson, Lorraine Jarvie, and Judy Kaye Smith*

Marnie is a 20-year-old GTPAL 1-0-0-0-0 client admitted to the labour and delivery unit. She is experiencing contractions that last approximately 30 seconds every 5 to 6 minutes. She denies taking any drugs or medications during the pregnancy except for prenatal vitamins. Marnie is using relaxation breathing that she learned during her prenatal education classes, but states, "When my contractions get stronger, I definitely want something for the pain."

Felicia, 36 years old, is admitted to the health care facility in active labour. Her husband, Chuck, is with her. This is Felicia's third pregnancy. Her cervix is 80% effaced and 5 cm dilated. She is experiencing moderately strong contractions that last for 60 seconds every 4 minutes. Past medical history reveals the use of pudendal blocks during her two previous vaginal births.

You will learn more about these stories later in this chapter. Nurses working with these clients and others like them need to understand this chapter to manage care and address issues appropriately. Before beginning, consider the following points related to the above scenarios.

- What care is appropriate for clients experiencing pain related to uterine contractions during labour?
- What aspects of the two clients' histories and pregnancies are similar? What components are different?
- What factors might be contributing to each client's pain?
- What behavioural manifestations might each client exhibit in response to pain?
- What medications would be most appropriate for Marnie? For Felicia?

LEARNING OBJECTIVES

On completion of this chapter, the reader should be able to:
- Define the relevant terms that describe pain management strategies within a multicultural perspective.
- Describe the two major theories related to pain.
- Identify methods of pharmacologic pain management.
- Compare and contrast the different methods used to achieve analgesia and anaesthesia.
- Discuss complications of regional anaesthesia.
- Describe the processes involved in the administration of general anaesthesia.
- Describe collaborative care related to specific forms of pain management.

KEY TERMS

ambulatory epidural pump
analgesia
anaesthesia
epidural anaesthesia block
epidural blood patch
general anaesthesia
local anaesthesia
narcotic agonist–antagonists
narcotic antagonist

pain threshold
pain tolerance
patient-controlled analgesia
referred pain
sedative hypnotics
somatic pain
spinal anaesthesia
transition
visceral pain

Over the years there have been dramatic changes in the pharmacologic options available for pain management during labour and birth. In order to promote the comfort and pain management of clients during labour and birth, nurses need to be knowledgeable about current, evidence-based information regarding pain management interventions. With this knowledge, nurses can provide appropriate information that will enable their clients to make informed decisions about which pain-relieving modalities will be most effective and acceptable. This chapter describes the most commonly utilized pharmacologic interventions for pain relief during labour and birth, and the associated nursing care management of the woman in labour and her fetus.

Pain is a multidimensional experience that varies from person to person. What one woman may describe as mildly cramping, another might describe as the most excruciating feeling she has ever known. Because pain is a highly subjective experience shaped by individual and cultural factors, nurses and clients need to discuss expectations and plans regarding pain management. Ideally, discussions regarding pain management will occur at or before the client's admission to the health care facility. Through assessment of the client's under-standing of the different methods of relief, nurses can identify areas for which additional education and collaborative care may be necessary. As client advocates, nurses provide accurate and understandable information regarding the various methods of pain relief. If clients express interest in having epidural anaesthesia during labour, informed consent is essential, with thorough explanations. Agencies may require the client's signature on the facility's consent form to confirm understanding.

PHYSIOLOGY OF LABOUR PAIN

The International Association for the Study of Pain (IASP) defines pain as "an unpleasant sensory and emotional experience associated with actual or potential tissue damage, or described in terms of such damage" (International Association for the Study of Pain [IASP], 2012). This universally recognized phenomenon is typically caused by some type of noxious stimuli and is a frequent and compelling reason for seeking health care. From a behavioural perspective, pain is a pattern of responses that functions to protect a person from harm.

Pain Terminology

Pain threshold is the point at which a person physically perceives a sensation as painful. **Pain tolerance** is the maximum amount of pain that a person is willing to endure (IASP, 2012).

Pain associated with labour and birth can be classified as visceral, somatic, or referred. **Visceral pain** is associated with the affected organ. It is usually diffuse or poorly localized, and is often described as aching. An example is the pain most clients experience with contractions during the first stage of labour (see Chapter 15), starting over the lower portion of the abdomen and radiating to the lumbar region and down the thighs. **Somatic pain** is associated with actual or potential musculoskeletal or cutaneous tissue damage and is usually described as intense, aching, and/or gnawing. Somatic pain usually occurs during the late phases of the first stage of labour and the second stage of labour and results from the stretching of the perineal tissues to allow passage of the fetus. **Referred pain** is felt at a site different from the damaged or diseased organ or tissues. An example is pain during labour that a woman may feel in the back, flank, or thighs.

Variations in Labour Pain

Although labour pain is considered a ubiquitous phenomenon regardless of age, culture, or parity, the description and severity of pain varies widely among women. Labour pain is an example of acute pain, which generally results from normal physiologic processes and obstetrical factors, including progressive cervical dilation, perineal distention, intensity of contractions, and fetal position and size.

First Stage of Labour

During the first stage, the cervix dilates and the lower uterine segment stretches (Fig. 17.1). Hypoxia develops as a result of the contractions and lactic acid accumulates in the uterine muscle. Cervical dilation and lower uterine stretching create traction on the ovaries, fallopian tubes, and uterine ligaments. Pressure on the maternal pelvis causes afferent pain impulses to travel along the sympathetic nerves that terminate in the dorsal horn of the spinal cord between the 10th thoracic and first lumbar spinal segment (Simpson, 2008). Stimulation of these nerves causes chemical mediators to release substances into the extracellular fluid surrounding the pain fibres. In the dorsal horn of the spinal column, somatostatin, cholecystokinin, and substance P serve as neurotransmitters for the pain impulse across the synapse between the peripheral and spinal nerves. The sensation then ascends the spinal column to the brain cortex, which interprets the sensation as pain (Fig. 17.2).

The degree of pain in labour changes as dilation progresses; in addition, the client's ability to tolerate the changes varies with the duration of labour. Exhaustion from lack of sleep or prolonged labour can contribute to increased pain perception. If the fetal presenting part is descending in the occipital posterior position, the force

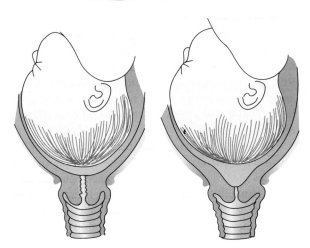

FIGURE 17.1 During the first stage of labour, progressive cervical dilatation and lower uterine stretching create traction on the maternal reproductive structures, which can lead to pain.

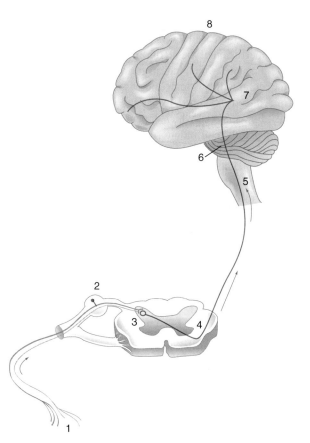

FIGURE 17.2 *(1)* Pain receptors transmit the sensation of pain through sensory nerves into the dorsal root ganglia. *(2)* The pain impulse enters the spinal cord. *(3, 4)* Signals cross the cord and ascend to *(5)* the reticular formation, *(6)* midbrain, *(7)* thalamus, and *(8)* cerebral cortex.

of the contractions may push the presenting part into the client's sacrum and coccyx, producing lower back pain.

Think back to Marnie, the client in labour from the beginning of the chapter, who is using breathing techniques to help manage her discomfort. How might Marnie's pain level change as she progresses through the first stage of labour?

Second Stage of Labour

During the second stage of labour, descent of the fetal presenting part exerts pressure on the pelvic floor muscles, vagina, perineum, and vulva. This pressure also places stress on the urethra, bladder, and rectum. As a result, pain may be perceived in any of these areas (Fig. 17.3).

In response to the physical discomfort produced by labour contractions, physiologic responses to the pain occur over which the woman has little control. Labour pain often causes anxiety (Hodnett et al., 2011; Kukulu & Demirok, 2008). When anxiety is unrelieved, cortisol, glucagons, and catecholamines naturally multiply, leading to increased metabolism and oxygen consumption. The increased levels of catecholamines also cause hypoperfusion of the uterus and decreased blood flow to the placenta, which can in turn lead to increased uterine contractility. Such increased contractility results in reduced oxygen delivery and can place the fetus at risk for asphyxia, which appears as abnormal heart rate changes on fetal monitoring (The Society of Obstetricians and Gynaecologists of Canada [SOGC], 2007). As labour continues, the period between uterine contractions gradually becomes shorter. As the client prepares to push, intervals between contractions may be only a few seconds. The point at which the cervix is at 7 to 10 cm and uterine contractions are occurring most frequently and for the longest duration is known

as **transition** and is likely to be the peak intensity of labour pain.

Third and Fourth Stages of Labour

At birth, afferent pain impulses travel along the sympathetic nerve fibres that enter the neuroaxis between the second and fourth sacral spinal segments and follow much the same pathway as outlined in the first stage of labour. Although pushing can be exhausting and taxing, many clients find the experience of pushing a relief from pain. Obviously, the amount of pain will be related to how quickly the client moves from crowning to expulsion, whether the birth needs to be assisted through use of forceps or other devices, whether lacerations occur or an episiotomy is necessary, and other variables. In addition, these and other aspects are likely to influence the client's experience of pain during the fourth stage of labour (the first hour after childbirth). At this time, however, the client's recovery may also be facilitated by distraction and stronger emotions as she interacts with her newborn for the first moments of life (Fig. 17.4).

QUOTE 17-1

"My mother always told me that you forget the pain of childbirth once your baby is born. I wouldn't say I've forgotten it, but holding my little one in my arms and interacting with her every day definitely make up for the pain!"

A client recounting her experiences with labour, childbirth, and post partum

PSYCHOLOGY OF PAIN

All pain involves both physical and psychological components. A person's attention, thoughts, feelings, prior experiences, memories, and beliefs are interconnected with her perceptions of pain (Fig. 17.5). People may experience more pain when they focus on it, if they have been told to expect one thing but experience something different, or if they expect a high level of pain and are tense as well as being under stress (Choi et al., 2012). Researchers believe the limbic-hypothalamic system and the frontal cortex in the brain influences rational interpretation and emotional response to pain (Hansen & Streltzer, 2005).

Acute pain, such as labour pain, is primarily physical in nature. It usually has a finite duration and can be alleviated by various nonpharmacologic methods (see Chapter 14) and pharmacologic agents. Chronic pain has a distinctly significant psychological component that needs both physical and psychological interventions. Clients usually develop emotional symptoms when medical treatment does not eliminate pain. Chronic pain following labour and childbirth is unlikely, unless a client's circumstances leads to a

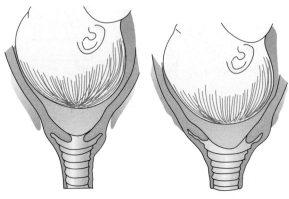

FIGURE 17.3 In the second stage of labour, much pain comes from pressure of the fetal presenting part on the maternal pelvis, genitalia, and perineum.

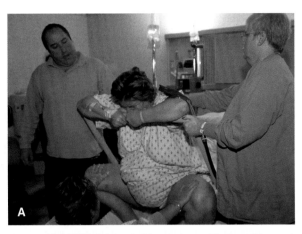
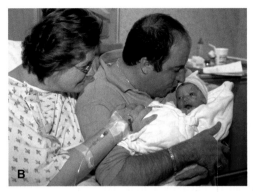

FIGURE 17.4 **A**: Many women find pushing to be a relief of pain, although it is challenging and exhausting. **B**: During the postpartum recovery period, initial bonding with the newborn and the positive emotions it engenders can help mitigate residual pain and discomfort from childbirth.

problem or abnormality requiring special intervention. This does not mean, however, that all pain or discomfort associated with pregnancy and childbirth will disappear as soon as the baby is born. The maternal body makes many adjustments over the postpartum weeks and months, and exhaustion and other emotions during that time actually may decrease her tolerance of pain during this time.

Emotional stress can increase pain intensity. Secondary factors such as the degree of disability, financial stress, or loss of work are also part of a client's pain experience, and treatment must be designed to address all relevant issues. Psychological treatment goals can help clients to learn how to predict and manage the pain cycle, use coping skills to minimize pain, and maximize active involvement in positive life experiences, despite pain.

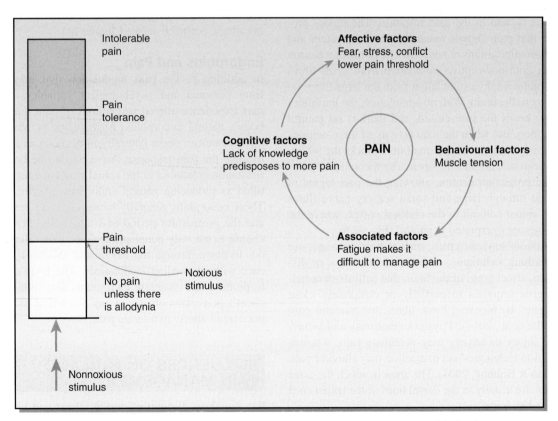

FIGURE 17.5 Many factors at various levels can interact to produce an individual pain response.

PAIN THEORY

Each client's experience with pain is different; furthermore, each pain experience for that particular client also may be unique. For example, a woman may experience significant pain during labour in her first pregnancy, but less pain in a subsequent pregnancy. A host of variables influence pain experiences, including physiologic, psychosocial, cultural, and environmental factors. Understanding what causes pain perception is important for nurses because it can help them to ensure that pain management strategies are employed during times and in ways that can be most effective for clients. Much of what is understood about pain has been built upon the principles of the gate control theory introduced by Melzack and Wall in 1965. Gate control theory led to further research that contributed to our current understanding of pain mechanisms such as sensitization and central nervous system plasticity (DeLeo, 2006).

Gate Control Theory

The gate control theory was the first pain theory proposing the integration of the physical and psychological aspects of the pain response, whereby the experience of pain does not just result from tissue damage. Rather, pain is a highly subjective experience shaped by various individual factors (Melzack, 1999). In addition, the gate control theory focused on the role of the central nervous system in the pain response. The theory proposed that pain signals reach the nervous system and excite smaller groups of neurons. The projection neuron carries both nociceptive stimulation from small fibres and nonnociceptive stimulation from the large fibres on the way to the brain. With no stimulation, the inhibitory neuron keeps the gate closed, and there is no painful perception. But when the total activity of these neurons reaches a certain level, the small fibre blocks the inhibitory neuron. This in turn opens the theoretical "gate" for the projection neuron, allowing the pain signal to proceed through large and small sensory nerve fibres in the spinal column to the cerebral cortex, where the impulses are interpreted as painful (Fig. 17.6).

Actions to reduce pain, such as light massage, use of breathing techniques, ambulation, positions, or distraction, affect areas of the brain that activate descending nerve impulses to partially or completely close the "gate" by blocking those fibres that transmit pain (Chaillet et al., 2014). Physical, emotional, and behavioural injury or anxiety may potentiate pain, whereas relaxation techniques and distraction may alleviate pain (Simkin & Bolding, 2004). The areas in which the gates operate are usually in the dorsal horn of the spinal cord and the brainstem.

Since the gate control theory was introduced, our understanding of pain has evolved significantly. Another

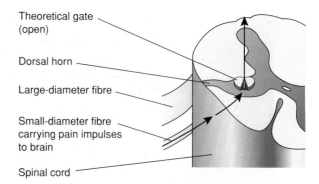

Theoretical gate (open)

Dorsal horn

Large-diameter fibre

Small-diameter fibre carrying pain impulses to brain

Spinal cord

FIGURE 17.6 In the gate control theory, the small fibre blocks the inhibitory neuron that normally preserves a pain-free state. In turn, the theoretical "gate" for the projection neuron opens, allowing the pain signal to proceed through large and small sensory nerve fibres in the spinal column to the cerebral cortex, where the impulses are interpreted as painful.

process in the gate control theory deals with the memory and cognitive processes of pain. Previous experiences, cultural influences, the amount of perceived anxiety, understanding of the birth process, and the meaning that the situation may have for the woman influence the way in which the cerebral cortex interprets painful stimuli. Just as anxiety may enhance pain, feelings of confidence and control may decrease pain (Green & Baston, 2003). Prenatal education and one-to-one labour support are effective methods of pain management from a nonpharmacologic perspective (see Chapter 14).

Endorphins and Pain

In addition to the pain modulation that may result from personal and psychological variables, women may experience altered perceptions of pain due to the body's natural endorphins. *Endorphins,* or morphine-like substances, occur naturally in the body and help to mediate the pain response. Areas within the brain and substantia gelatinosa of the spinal cord have been identified as producing natural endorphins (Yerby, 2000). These endorphins generally increase during pregnancy and the postpartum period and may help clients who choose to use only nonpharmacologic pain relief methods to move through the labour and childbirth experience without needing medications. The body's ability to produce and maintain endorphins also influences a client's perception of pain at any given time as well as her overall ability to tolerate pain.

INFLUENCES ON PAIN AND PAIN MANAGEMENT

For centuries, discomfort during labour and birth was considered inevitable and something that women simply had to endure. Nevertheless, people searched for many remedies to provide labour pain relief. Early Chinese writings mention the use of opiates and herbs such as hemp and mandrake; Persian writings discuss the drinking of wine by women in labour; and wine, beer, and brandy were commonly self-administered in Europe during the Middle Ages (Yerby, 2000). The greatest strides in labour pain management, however, occurred during the past 200 years.

In the mid-19th century, the use of anaesthesia was introduced in Great Britain and the United States. The early use of ether and chloroform in obstetrical practice has been credited to Dr. James Young Simpson, professor of midwifery at Edinburgh University (Cohen, 1996). During this period, the American Medical Association Committee on Obstetrics justified the use of anaesthesia during labour and birth (Morrison et al., 1996); however, great debate existed over its validity. The earliest record of pain management in obstetrical practice in Canada was on March 22, 1848, when James Frazer of Pictou County in Nova Scotia used chloroform during a cesarean section (Ramsay, 2006). Some physicians felt that anaesthesia masked the mother's response to labour, which was considered to be a valuable guide in determining labour progress. Religious objections also were prominent, based on the interpretations of God's decree to Eve in the Garden of Eden (Genesis Chapter 3, Verse 16) that pain for women shall be greatly multiplied during childbirth (Cohen, 1996). The controversy was minimized, however, when Dr. John Snow administered chloroform to Queen Victoria during the birth of the last two of her nine children, Prince Leopold in 1853 and Princess Beatrice in 1857 (Ramsay, 2006). By 1862, chloroform and ether had become widely used anaesthetics in obstetric practice.

During this same period, other methods of pain relief, including parenteral opioids (e.g., morphine and meperidine [Demerol]), as well as parenteral and inhalation anaesthesia, were being developed. In the early 1900s, twilight sleep produced by the addition of scopolamine to morphine became an accepted method for pain relief during childbirth. A high incidence of neonatal respiratory distress following its administration, however, led to its discontinuation (Morrison et al., 1996).

In the 1930s, a focus on natural childbirth techniques began with the work of Dr. Grantley Dick-Read, who believed that women could use *psychoprophylaxis* (mind over physical matter) to control the pain of childbirth (Yerby, 2000). Dick-Read felt that relief of fear and tension could diminish pain to a level at which women would be able to cope, or that the pain would possibly even cease. In the 1960s, the Lamaze method of patterned breathing techniques to promote relaxation during labour became popular. These and other nonpharmacologic methods of pain control are discussed in more detail in Chapter 14.

More recently, agonist–antagonist drugs such as nalbuphine (Nubain) and butorphanol (Stadol) have been used to produce sedation and relaxation during the latent phase of the first stage of labour. More refined techniques of epidural anaesthesia administration, however, have led to the widespread contemporary use of drugs for pain during active labour.

Cultural Considerations

When clients are asked if any cultural or religious beliefs affect their health care, their response is frequently "No." Nurses should recognize that every client has cultural beliefs and values that influence her perceptions, whether or not she recognizes these factors. Cultural factors associated with a person's pain experience include pain expression, pain language, meaning of pain and suffering, social roles, traditional remedies for pain, perceptions, and expectations (Shipton, 2013). For example, culture often dictates what a person considers appropriate verbal behaviour or body language in response to pain (Munoz & Luckmann, 2005). Understanding these various cultural responses to pain can assist nurses to recognize and support individual client responses.

Client responses to pain can be classified into two broad categories: stoic and emotive. Stoic responses are characterized by fewer verbal and nonverbal expressions, with clients seldom making verbal comments or showing emotion. Conversely, emotive responses are frequent, often verbal, and expressive.

First- and second-generation immigrants to Canada and the United States tend to respond to pain in ways that are conventional within their culture or family origin. Later generations who may have assimilated the values of the culture into which they have moved, however, are less likely to retain traditional views about pain (Munoz & Luckmann, 2005). Some clients consider pain a natural part of labour, whereas others view it as excruciating and inhumane. Additional information on cultural health assessment is provided in the reference list at the end of this chapter.

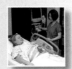 Remember Felicia, the woman in labour with her third child described at the start of the chapter. How might the pain she experienced in previous labours currently influence her perception of her pain?

Legal and Ethical Perspectives

Because methods of pain relief available during labour are constantly evolving, clients need to be sufficiently informed about their options so that they are equipped to make informed decisions about their care. The real challenge for health care providers is to provide optimal care, enabling clients to feel satisfaction with the birth experience, while ensuring that they attain the maximum relief possible. Satisfaction with pain management is difficult to measure, however, because each woman is unique.

Nurses should understand that a client's personal, ethical, or moral views, shaped through past events, life experiences, thoughts, and actions, need to be considered as influences on her decision making relative to pain management modalities. Clients have the right to make informed decisions based on their ability to take personal responsibility for their decisions, to understand the consequences of their actions, and to make choices apart from coercive or obstructive controlling influences (Lowe, 2004). Informed choice and consent are key factors in the partnership between clients and health care providers.

Choice of pain management methods is personal. Obtaining informed consent, however, is a legal requirement, especially in relation to invasive procedures such as epidural or spinal anaesthesia. Three main elements must be present for consent to be considered truly informed.

- The client must receive unbiased information before giving consent.
- Consent must be a voluntary decision (made free of coercion).
- The client must be mentally competent and capable of accepting responsibility for the selected decision.

The timing for providing information about pain relief can be challenging. Obviously, giving information during active labour would be least effective. When at all possible, health care providers must ensure that they give adequate information to the client before she reaches the active phase of labour. Ideally, such discussion occurs well in advance of labour, and at least as soon as labour is suspected. For example, ideal times to discuss and plan for pain management options would be during prenatal appointments. Effective collaborative communication and a trusting relationship provide support for women to effectively cope with pain during labour (Leap et al., 2010).

QUOTE 17-2

"During appointments with clients, I really try to discuss with them the different options and techniques available for managing pain in labour. It's much easier with women who have already been through the experience, but many first-time parents can be overwhelmed by the options, risks, and benefits. Still, I find those clients who have been educated about labour pain management tend to have better experiences during the actual event, regardless of what specific methods they choose to employ."

A nurse practitioner/midwife

Pharmacologic Pain Management

There are classically three pharmacologic choices for analgesia in labour in Canadian facilities, with availability being dependent on the resources of the facilities providing care. These include epidural analgesia, systemic opioids, and inhaled nitrous oxide. In 2010 to 2011, epidural analgesia was used in 55.2% of all vaginal births in Canada (Canadian Institute of Health Information [CIHI], 2012). The range of epidural use varies greatly across Canada, with rates as low as 21% in the Territories and as high as 70% in Québec (CIHI, 2012). The use and type of parenteral opioids vary from province to province. Nitrous oxide has been used widely since the 1840s as a labour analgesia, and although its efficacy varies, it is recommended as a pharmacologic pain management option when used with an appropriate waste anaesthetic gas scavenging system.

Drug Pharmacokinetics

Pharmacokinetics refers to drug absorption, metabolism, distribution, and excretion in the body. Physiologic changes during pregnancy and childbirth, such as increased cardiac output, alter a woman's normal pharmacokinetics. Depending on the stage of pregnancy and the medication being utilized, the function of drug-metabolizing enzymes and transport of drugs may be altered (Isoherranen & Thummel, 2012). In addition, weight gained during pregnancy as a result of changes in fluid balance within the body compartments alters the distribution and plasma concentrations of drugs.

The optimum goal of pharmacologic pain management during labour is to provide maximum pain relief to the mother while ensuring minimum risks to both mother and fetus. Three factors must be considered when determining whether analgesic medications are appropriate for use during labour.

- *Possible effects on the woman.* The effect of pharmacologic agents in labour on the woman poses the greatest concern because fetal well-being depends on adequate functioning of the maternal homeostatic mechanism that maintains adequate oxygenation and circulation to the fetus.
- *Possible effects on the fetus.* All drugs given for pain relief during labour cross the placental barrier by simple diffusion. Some drugs cross more readily than others. The action of drugs depends on the rate at which the medication is metabolized by liver enzymes and excreted by the kidneys. Because the fetal liver and kidneys are too immature to metabolize analgesics, high doses of medications may remain active in the fetal circulation for prolonged periods.
- *Possible effects on the strength and frequency of labour contractions.* Incorrect dosages or medications given at the wrong time can negatively affect the course of labour and childbirth.

TYPES OF PHARMACOLOGIC PAIN MANAGEMENT

Knowledge of the changes that occur during pregnancy, labour, and birth enables health care providers to determine which pharmacologic methods to use as well as the proper dosage to relieve pain without causing severe maternal or fetal side effects. Pain control methods work best when administered as soon as possible after the pain is recognized as uncomfortable.

Inhaled Nitrous Oxide

The 50/50 mix of oxygen and nitrous oxide is a central nervous system depressant thought to alter pain stimuli, resulting in a decreased perception of pain (Rooks, 2012). Nitrous oxide is self-administered by women with a mask or a mouthpiece. Women should be instructed on proper use of the mask or mouthpiece to prevent contamination of the labour room. Inhalation of nitrous oxide should commence as soon as the woman experiences a contraction starting and should stop when the contraction has neared completion. The maximum therapeutic effect occurs approximately 50 seconds after continuous inhalation is commenced.

Nitrous oxide use is inexpensive, easy to deliver, and has rapid onset and termination. Nitrous oxide is relatively safe in both term and preterm labour with little or no neonatal effects, and does not affect uterine activity. Despite the advantages of nitrous oxide use, studies are conflicting as to its efficacy as a pain-relieving modality (Likis et al., 2014). The most common side effects include nausea, vomiting, and light-headedness.

Sedative Hypnotics

Sedative hypnotics relieve anxiety and aid sleep. They are not a specific drug classification but a description of the effects produced by this group of drugs. In low doses, they cause sedation and rest; higher doses produce a hypnotic effect. There are three classifications of sedative hypnotics that have been used in obstetric practice. These are barbiturates, histamine-1 (H₁) receptor antagonist (antihistamine) ataractics, and benzodiazepines.

Barbiturates

Barbiturates include secobarbital sodium (Seconal) and pentobarbital (Nembutal). Such medications do not relieve pain, but may be given during early labour (when birth is unlikely for another 12 to 24 hours) to induce sleep and decrease anxiety. Barbiturates cross the placenta and cause central nervous system depression in the neonate (Rice Simpson & Creehan, 2008). Due to the high risk of neonatal and maternal respiratory and vasomotor depression, these drugs are very rarely, if ever, used in Canada.

Histamine-1 Receptor Antagonist Ataractics

Promethazine hydrochloride (Phenergan) and dimenhydrinate (Gravol) are H₁ receptor antagonist ataractics frequently administered with narcotics during labour to relieve anxiety, increase sedation, to potentiate the effects of systemic opioid use, and to decrease the narcotic side effects of nausea and vomiting. Promethazine is absorbed readily from the gastrointestinal tract and has an onset of action within 20 minutes when administered by the intramuscular (IM) route and within 5 minutes when administered by the intravenous (IV) route. The effect lasts up to 12 hours after administration, and most clients describe feeling sedated or groggy after administration (Karch, 2008). Promethazine is metabolized in the liver and excreted in urine and feces. It crosses the placental barrier and can cause cardiorespiratory depression in the newborn if birth occurs soon after administration.

Benzodiazepines

Benzodiazepines, such as lorazepam (Ativan) and clonazepam (Rivotril), are a class of psychoactive drugs considered minor tranquilizers, with varying hypnotic, sedative, anxiolytic, anticonvulsant, muscle relaxant, and amnesic properties, which are mediated by slowing down the central nervous system. Benzodiazepines are useful in treating anxiety and restlessness throughout labour, which may allow the woman to participate more actively in labouring processes. The dosage of benzodiazepines should be individualized and carefully titrated to avoid excessive sedation and mental or motor impairment. Benzodiazepines depress the central nervous system in both the mother and neonate. As such, the lowest effective dose should be used and the need for continued therapy reassessed frequently through the woman's labour.

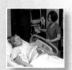 Think back to Felicia, the woman in labour with her third child, at the beginning of the chapter. What if Felicia received promethazine 3 hours ago and now requests to go to the bathroom to urinate: should the nurse support this request?

Analgesic Compounds

Analgesia means the use of agents to reduce or decrease awareness of pain. Opioid analgesics possess properties derived from or similar to morphine. The other commonly used form of analgesia is narcotic agonist–antagonist compounds. Table 17.1 summarizes the most common analgesics used during labour and childbirth.

Opioid Analgesics

Morphine provides excellent analgesia, but its long duration of action (up to 7 hours) after administration and its

TABLE 17.1 Pain Control Medications During Labour

Analgesia Medication and Drug Classification	Usual Dosage/Routes	Optimal Time for Administration and When to Stop Medication	Indication for Use/ Desired Effects/ Nursing Implications	Maternal–Fetal Side Effects
Secobarbitol sodium (Seconal) or pentobarbital (Nembutal) Barbiturate Sedative hypnotic	100–200 mg PO	Early prodromal labour	Sedation to induce sleep, decrease anxiety, CNS depression	Maternal paradoxical apprehension, hyperactivity, and disorientation Neonatal CNS depression Decreases neonatal ability to suck
Promethazine hydrochloride (Phenergan) or hydroxyzine (Vistaril, Atarax) Histamine-1 receptor antagonist (antihistamines) ataractics	12.5–25 mg IM/IV 25–50 mg IM	Early phases of labour	Adjunct therapy to decrease nausea and vomiting associated with opioid narcotic analgesics	Maternal sedation Neonatal cardiopulmonary sedation if birth occurs too soon after administration
Benzodiazepines Benzodiazepines include lorazepam (Atavan), and clonazepam (Rivotril) class of psychoactive drugs considered minor tranquilizers with varying hypnotic, sedative, anxiolytic, anticonvulsant, muscle relaxant, and amnestic properties, which are mediated by slowing down the central nervous system.	The dosage of benzodiazepines should be individualized and carefully titrated to avoid excessive sedation and mental or motor impairment. The lowest effective dose should be used and the need for continued therapy reassessed frequently throughout the woman's labour Lorazepam: 0.5–1 mg PO or SL PRN not to exceed 3 mg per day. Clonazepam: In selective cases as longer acting 0.5–1 mg PO not to exceed 3 mg per day	Throughout labour	To treat anxiety and restlessness	
Meperidine (Demerol) Opioid agonist analgesic/narcotic analgesic	25–50 mg IV, 50–100 mg IM Usually given with promethazine IV or hydroxyzine IM, which potentiate the narcotic effects and decrease nausea and vomiting	Early labour during the first phase of the first stage Pain relief after cesarean birth	Decreases pain impulse transmission by opioid receptors Effective analgesic that produces a sense of well-being Promotes relaxation, which possibly aids cervical relaxation Have Narcan readily available to reverse adverse effects	Can slow labour contractions if given too soon in labour Nausea, vomiting, sedation, neonatal respiratory depression Decreased beat-to-beat variability of the fetal heart rate
Morphine sulfate (Morphine) Opioid narcotic analgesic	Intrathecally 0.2–1 mg; 5 mg epidurally	After client is in active labour or in preparation for a cesarean birth	Effective analgesia, relaxation, and pain relief Have Narcan available	Itching, respiratory depression, nausea and vomiting, hypotension Can possibly slow labour progress
Nalbuphine (Nubain) or butorphanol tartrate (Stadol) Mixed agonist–antagonist analgesics	10–20 mg IM; 5–10 mg slow IV push 1–2 mg IV/IM	Usually given during the early stages of labour when birth is not imminent	Effective for relief of mild to moderate pain Have Narcan readily available	Mild maternal sedation and some neonatal respiratory depression Dizziness, weakness, nausea and vomiting

Source: From Karch, A. M. (2008). 2008 Lippincott's nursing drug guide. Philadelphia, PA: Lippincott Williams & Wilkins.

• PHARMACOLOGY 17.1   Meperidine (Demerol)

ACTION

Meperidine acts as an agonist at specific opioid receptors in the central nervous system to produce analgesia, sedation, and euphoria.

PREGNANCY CATEGORY

C

DOSAGE

When contractions are regular, 50 to 100 mg IM or SC every 1 to 3 hours.

POSSIBLE ADVERSE EFFECTS

Light-headedness, dizziness, facial flushing, irregular heart beat, palpitations, pruritus, nausea, vomiting, sweating

NURSING IMPLICATIONS

- Have opioid antagonist and facilities for assisted or controlled respirations available with parenteral administration.
- Use with extreme caution in patients with renal problems.

From: Karch, A. (2008). *2008 Lippincott's nursing drug guide.* Philadelphia: Lippincott Williams & Wilkins.

depressive effects on the newborn limit its use to the latent phase of labour, when birth is not anticipated for several hours. Side effects frequently include nausea, vomiting, possible histamine release that causes orthostatic hypotension, and occasional bradycardia (Karch, 2008).

A synthetic morphine-like compound, *meperidine* (Demerol), was once the most commonly used opioid analgesic in labour (Pharmacology Box 17.1). Meperidine has been found to be effective in relieving severe, persistent, or recurrent pain. In labour, it helps to relax the cervix and stimulates a feeling of maternal euphoria and well-being. Meperidine is metabolized by the liver into an active form, normeperidine, and excreted through the urine. Peak effect usually occurs 40 to 50 minutes after IM administration. With IV administration, onset of action is rapid (within 30 seconds), reaching peak effects in 5 to 10 minutes. Effects can last up to 3 hours (Karch, 2008).

Meperidine may also be administered in low doses by **patient-controlled analgesia**, which is a system of drug dispensing in which a preset IV dose of narcotic agent is delivered when the client presses a button. Use of patient-controlled analgesia facilitates more frequent dosing (Fig. 17.7).

The most frequent side effects of meperidine are nausea and vomiting. To minimize them, promethazine (Phenergan) or dimenhydrinate (Gravol) are often given prophylactically with meperidine. Studies have demonstrated deleterious effects on fetal heart rate when women receive meperidine during labour (Sekhavat & Behdad, 2009). If birth occurs soon after administration or during peak effect periods, the newborn may experience respiratory depression and lower APGAR scores (Rooks, 2012). Therefore, 0.1 mg/kg of a **narcotic antagonist** (a drug primarily used to treat narcotic-induced respiratory depression) must be readily available for administration to the newborn after birth (Karch, 2008). A commonly used narcotic antagonist is naloxone (Narcan) (Pharmacology Box 17.2). Naloxone can be given intramuscularly, intravenously, or subcutaneously. Its duration of effect is considerably shorter than the analgesic medication for which it is being given. Therefore, nurses should remain alert for the return of respiratory depression and the need for repeated doses of naloxone.

When meperidine is used during labour, implications for breastfeeding mothers during the postpartum period are significant because it may take 2 to 3 days for the body to excrete 95% of the medication. The meperidine that remains within the mother's system is transferred to the baby through the breast milk (Karch, 2008). Because the newborn liver is immature and cannot readily metabolize the residual medication, the baby tends to exhibit neurobehavioural depression for at least 3 days (see Chapters 20 and 22). Manifestations include general sleepiness and increased problems with latching on for breastfeeding (Anderson, 2011). Infants who have been exposed to high doses of meperidine are more likely to cry when handled. In addition, the ability to self-console is reduced for as long as 3 to 6 weeks after administration (Anderson, 2011). Thus, before administration, the nurse should find out whether the

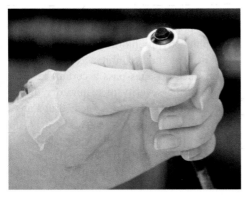

FIGURE 17.7   Client-controlled analgesia.

● **PHARMACOLOGY 17.2** Naloxone Hydrochloride (Narcan)

ACTION

Naloxone hydrochloride is a narcotic antagonist that counteracts the effect of narcotic analgesics.

PREGNANCY CATEGORY

B

DOSAGE

0.01 mg/kg, administered either IV by umbilical vein, SC, or IM; repeated at 2- to 3-minute intervals until response is obtained.

POSSIBLE ADVERSE EFFECTS

Hypotension, hypertension, tachycardia, diaphoresis, tremors

NURSING IMPLICATIONS

● Anticipate the need for resuscitative measures; have resuscitative equipment and emergency drugs readily available.
● If no IV access is available, prepare for possible administration by endotracheal tube.
● If no response is seen after two or three doses, question whether respiratory depression is caused by narcotics.
● Continuously monitor all vital signs for changes.
● Remember that the pain-relieving effect of narcotics will be reversed; assess for pain in the neonate.

Source: Karch, A. M. (2008). *2008 Lippincott's nursing drug guide*. Philadelphia, PA: Lippincott Williams & Wilkins.

---

client intends to breastfeed and advocate for the use of drugs with fewer residual effects.

Fentanyl. Fentanyl is a highly potent opioid which should be administered intravenously slowly over a period of 1 to 2 minutes; onset occurs in around 3 to 5 minutes with peak action between 5 and 15 minutes. Fentanyl has a maternal half-life of less than 1 hour and therefore produces less maternal sedation, nausea, and vomiting than morphine; it also has a low placental transfer rate and a neonatal half-life of between 1 and 6 hours.

As with other opioids, fentanyl is a potent respiratory depressant and no initial dose or subsequent dose should be administered to women with less than eight breaths per minute or an oxygen saturation rate of less than 94%. Naloxone (Narcan) should be readily available for administration to the mother or neonate as an antidote against respiratory depression (Kattwinkel et al., 2010). Fentanyl can be administered either intravenously or by IV patient-controlled analgesia (PCA) or via epidural or spinal infusion.

Remifentanil. Remifentanil is a relatively new opioid with a very short life of less than 3 minutes, which has benefits for both mother and fetus. The main advantage of remifentanil is that due to the short life of the drug the labouring woman can continue using it until delivery and, even if the newborn is depressed at birth, it will rapidly recover with minimal resuscitation. Naloxone is rarely required (Volikas et al., 2005).

Remifentanil has a rapid onset, peaks between 60 and 90 seconds, and rapidly crosses the placenta where it is quickly metabolized and redistributed. Remifentanil is given mainly via IV PCA. As with fentanyl, remifentanil

is a very potent opioid, and women can rapidly develop respiratory depression; therefore, respiratory rate and oxygen saturation must be closely monitored.

Suppose Marnie, described at the beginning of the chapter, received meperidine for pain during labour. She is breastfeeding her newborn and asks why the newborn is sleepy. How should the nurse respond?

Narcotic Agonist–Antagonist Compounds

Narcotic agonist–antagonists are analgesic agents that stimulate opiate receptors, resulting in pain relief, and block-specific opiate receptors, alleviating the severity of maternal and neonatal respiratory depression. The latter antagonist property, however, could lead to withdrawal symptoms in opioid-dependent clients and their newborns. Two narcotic agonist–antagonists becoming increasingly popular are butorphanol tartrate (Stadol) and nalbuphine hydrochloride (Nubain). Their major advantage is that they exhibit a *ceiling effect,* which means that once dosages pass a certain level, there is no increase in the severity of respiratory distress as a newborn side effect. Therefore, these drugs are considered safer alternatives for clients. There is, however, a negative ceiling effect on the analgesic level, which means that once dosages are given beyond a certain level, there is no further increase in the amount of pain relief obtained from them. However, some of the side effects may increase with increased dosages despite the ceiling effect it has on pain. Major side effects include drowsiness, dizziness, weakness, nausea, and vomiting. In some clients, these drugs can cause a psychomimetic reaction of dysphoria and unease.

Butorphanol (Stadol). Butorphanol (Stadol) has an analgesic potency 30 to 40 times that of meperidine and seven times that of morphine (Wilson et al., 2010). It can be given through IM or IV administration, usually in dosages of 1 to 2 mg. Butorphanol takes effect in approximately 5 minutes, peaks in 30 to 60 minutes, and has duration of action of approximately 3 to 4 hours. This drug may cause both maternal and neonatal respiratory depression, but effects may be reversed by administration of naloxone. Butorphanol also has been shown to produce a sinusoidal fetal heart rate pattern before birth (Wilson et al., 2010). Less risk for nausea and vomiting is associated with administration of butorphanol than with meperidine. Butorphanol is considered safer for women who intend to breastfeed because it is metabolized more readily than meperidine.

Butorphanol should not be used with clients who have a known dependence on opiates; it should be used with caution in cases of suspected drug dependence, because it may precipitate withdrawal symptoms. Urinary retention, although not common, may occur. Therefore, the nurse should be vigilant in assessing for bladder distention. Butorphanol should be stored at room temperature and away from light (Wilson et al., 2010).

Nalbuphine (Nubain). Nalbuphine (Nubain) can be given by IM, subcutaneous, or IV push routes in doses of 10 to 20 mg. With IV administration, the drug produces effects in approximately 2 to 3 minutes, peaks within 15 to 20 minutes, and lasts approximately 3 to 6 hours. IV administration should occur over 3 to 5 minutes; therefore, it should be given over two contractions (Wilson et al., 2010). Adverse effects include drowsiness, dizziness, crying, blurred vision, diaphoresis, and urinary urgency. Respiratory depression, nausea, and vomiting also may occur but to a lesser degree than noted with meperidine and other narcotic agents. Nurses need to review the client's history to identify the possibility of contraindications. Examples include a history of past or current drug dependence, sensitivity to sulfites, and asthma (Karch, 2008). If there are no contraindications, the IV route is used most commonly.

As with other narcotics and synthetic narcotic derivatives, health care providers should evaluate the client's respiratory status and the fetal heart rate characteristics carefully after administration. Common side effects include dizziness, sedation, confusion, and respiratory depression. Naloxone may be used to reverse the effects of both maternal and neonatal respiratory depression. Nalbuphine is metabolized more readily than meperidine, and therefore is safe for clients who intend to breastfeed.

Anaesthesia

When analgesics are no longer effective in the management of labour pain or when labour progresses to the second stage, alternative methods of relief may need to be considered. These methods involve anaesthesia. **Anaesthesia** means the use of agents that cause partial or complete loss of sensation with or without loss of consciousness.

Table 17.2 summarizes the most common anaesthetic agents used during labour and childbirth. The various categories of anaesthesia have different applications, actions, effects, and requirements. The obstetrician or certified midwife initiates local and pudendal anaesthesia, whereas an anaesthesiologist is responsible for administration of regional (epidural) and general anaesthesia. Regardless of the type of anaesthesia used, the single most important aspect of care is to ensure client safety. The most optimum way to avert complications involves adequately and thoroughly assessing the client in advance of administering any anaesthetic medications.

Local Anaesthesia

Local anaesthesia is used during vaginal birth to induce loss of sensation in the perineum and vagina during cutting, repair, or both of the episiotomy. Local anaesthetic agents injected into the perineum and posterior vagina block the conduction of nerve impulses between the perineum and the central nervous system. The types of nerve fibres react differently to various anaesthetic agents. The smaller nerve fibres (small C- and A-delta fibres) are more sensitive to local anaesthetics, whereas the larger A-alpha, A-beta, and A-gamma fibres continue to retain pressure sensation, muscle tone, sense of position, and motor function.

Absorption of anaesthetic agents depends primarily on the vascularity of the area being injected. Such anaesthetic agents also increase blood flow to the injected area by causing vasodilation. If the client is healthy or has a high metabolic rate, absorption is expedited. If the client is malnourished, dehydrated, has an electrolyte imbalance, or has a history of cardiovascular or pulmonary problems, toxic side effects are possible. If the anaesthetic agent contains a vasoconstrictor such as epinephrine, absorption is delayed and the anaesthetic effect is prolonged. Agents containing vasoconstrictors decrease uteroplacental blood flow, however, which makes them undesirable additives in most situations. The liver and plasma esterase break down local anaesthetics and the byproduct is excreted by the kidneys. The drug is administered in the weakest possible concentration and the smallest amount necessary to

● TABLE 17.2   Obstetric Anaesthesia

Analgesia Medication and Drug Classification	Usual Dosage/Routes	Optimal Time for Administration and When to Stop Medication	Indication for Use/Desired Effects/Nursing Implications	Maternal–Fetal Side Effects
Fentanyl (Sublimaze) Opioid Analgesic/narcotic analgesic	50–100 mcg or 25–50 mcg IV; can also be continuously administered epidurally with bupivacaine	Generally given epidurally after the client has reached 4–5 cm dilation and is in active labour	For epidural of intrathecal analgesia, usually given in combination with a local anaesthetic or given IV to induce relaxation for general anaesthesia. Monitor client vital signs closely. Preload client with IV fluids.	Maternal hypotension; maternal, fetal respiratory depression; slowing of labour if given too early
Remifentanil Opioid	IV-PCA Currently not enough information available to make recommendations as to optimal dosage—SHOULD ALWAYS BE PRESCRIBED BY AN ANAESTHESIOLOGIST WHO IS IMMEDIATELY AVAILABLE TO DEAL WITH MATERNAL SIDE EFFECTS	Generally given after the patient is in active labour 3–4 cm and can continue until delivery	Normally used when an epidural is contraindicated One-to-one nursing care is indicated due to the possibility of rapid development of respiratory depression. Pulse oximetry monitoring will be required and the availability of O_2	Rapid onset maternal respiratory depression
Bupivacaine (Marcaine) Local anaesthetic	Administered with fentanyl or morphine as a continuous epidural agent in titrated doses based on client's weight	Generally given epidurally after the client has reached 4–5 cm dilation and is in active labour	Rapid onset; loss of pain perception	Maternal hypotension; slowing of labour if given too early; may obliterate pushing sensation; possibly prolongs the second stage of labour
Xylocaine (Lidocaine)	Local anaesthetic	Administered just before birth	Produces perineal anaesthesia of the perineum, vagina, and vulva in pudendal anaesthesia or for local infiltration of perineum just before episiotomy incision	None apparent
Pentothal (thiopental) Short-acting barbiturate	Administered IV by an anaesthesiologist	Just before a cesarean birth to obtain to achieve a rapid anaesthetic effect to enable placement of an endotracheal tube and inhalation anaesthetic administration	Emergency cesarean birth when it is imperative to deliver the neonate quickly. Position client in left lateral tilt to prevent vena caval compression. Oxygenate client at 100%.	Maternal pulmonary aspiration, pneumonitis, pulmonary edema, uterine atony postpartum
Anectine (succinylcholine) Depolarizing muscle relaxant	Administered IV by an anaesthesiologist	Same as above	Same as above	Same as above; triggering mechanism in clients with hereditary tendency for developing malignant hyperthermia

Source: Karch, A. M. (2008). 2008 Lippincott's nursing drug guide. Philadelphia, PA: Lippincott Williams & Wilkins.

produce the desired numbness. Most agents used for local anaesthesia are rapidly metabolized and have little or no effect on the mother or breastfeeding newborn after birth.

Three local anaesthetics are currently available for use.

- **Esters**. These include chloroprocaine hydrochloride (Nesacaine). These are rapidly metabolized, thereby reducing the potential for maternal toxicity and preventing placental transfer to the fetus. They are very rarely used within Canada.
- **Amides**. Examples include lidocaine hydrochloride (Xylocaine), mepivacaine hydrochloride (Carbocaine), bupivacaine hydrochloride (Marcaine), and the newer agent, ropivacaine (Naropin). These agents are more powerful and longer acting than the esters. They readily cross the placenta and enter fetal circulation.
- **Opiates**. Generally, opiates are reserved for epidural anaesthesia, but may be used as adjuncts to local anaesthetics in spinal and epidural anaesthesia. They include morphine (Duramorph) and fentanyl (Sublimaze). When opiates are used in isolation, the amount of pain relief is less effective than when they are combined with a low-dose local anaesthetic.

The mechanism of action is specific to opiate receptors in the spinal column (Datta, 2006).

Reactions to local anaesthetics range from mild, transient symptoms to total cardiovascular collapse. Mild side effects generally include heart palpitations, ringing in the ears, itching, apprehension, and confusion. The client may also complain of a metallic taste in the mouth. High concentrations can cause a local reaction, with tissue edema forming on the perineum. Moderate reactions are characterized by more intense degrees of the mild symptoms. In addition, nausea, vomiting, hypotension, and muscle twitching that can possibly progress to convulsions with a loss of consciousness can occur. The severest reaction involves laryngeal edema, joint pain, swelling of the tongue, bronchospasm, sudden loss of consciousness, coma, severe hypotension, and potentially, cardiac arrest.

Systemic lethal reactions are most common when an excessive dose (either too great a concentration or too large a volume) has been administered. Accidental injection into the venous system may cause vasomotor and respiratory depression as well as depression of the medullary centres in the brain. With a massive intravascular dose, sudden circulatory collapse can occur within 1 minute of administration. Therefore, close monitoring of the client following administration of any local anaesthetic is essential. To ensure that resuscitative medications can be administered readily in the event of a systemic reaction, anaesthetic agents should never be given without having an IV access in place.

With mild symptoms of toxicity, oxygen is administered by face mask. If the client develops convulsions, maintenance of a patent airway and administration of 100% oxygen are essential. Thiopental (Pentothal) or diazepam (Valium) may be used to stop convulsions.

Pudendal Anaesthesia

Pudendal anaesthesia is typically administered during the second stage of labour to anaesthetize the lower vagina, vulva, and perineum. The obstetrician or certified midwife injects the anaesthetic agent, such as lidocaine, bupivacaine, or ropivacaine, through the lateral vaginal walls into the area near both the right and left pudendal nerve behind the sacrospinous ligament at the level of the ischial spines (Fig. 17.8). The injection is made through the vagina with the woman in lithotomy or dorsal recumbent position. Pudendal anaesthesia can provide pain relief within 2 to 10 minutes after administration that lasts for approximately 1 hour. The procedure provides adequate anaesthesia for vaginal births, application of outlet forceps or vacuum extraction, and perineal repair. Frequently, local infiltration of the perineum is combined with pudendal anaesthesia because it is possible for pudendal anaesthesia to be ineffective if that is the only area of injection. Although the injection is localized to the involved area and does not usually impact maternal vital signs or fetal heart rate, the fetal heart rate and the mother's blood pressure are checked immediately after the injection to identify possible hypotension.

Neuraxial Analgesia

Neuraxial analgesia techniques are considered the most effective methods of pain relief for women during labour and childbirth. They are the only pharmacologic intervention that can offer the potential of complete analgesia without the side effect of maternal

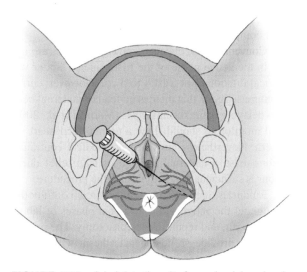

FIGURE 17.8 Administration site for pudendal analgesia.

or fetal sedation. While many women would be eligible for neuraxial analgesia, there are a few contraindications, which include refusal by the patient, signs of infection at the catheter insertion site, and some pre-existing coagulopathies. Women having hemorrhage or hypovolemia, any systemic infection, or lumbar spine pathology would need to be assessed for suitability by an anesthesiologist before receiving an epidural (Wong, 2010). Among the neuraxial techniques available, the most commonly utilized in Canada include epidural anaesthesia block and combined spinal–epidural. Continuous spinal, single-shot spinal, and caudal analgesia are used less commonly (Wong, 2010).

Epidural Anaesthesia Block. Epidural anaesthesia block is a common method of intrapartum pain management currently used in Canada, and the rate of epidural use is increasing, with 57% of women receiving an epidural prior to vaginal delivery. However, it is important to note that epidural rates vary dramatically among provinces. In 2010 to 2011, vaginal births were preceded by an epidural for approximately two thirds of women in Ontario and Quebec compared with less than one third of women in Newfoundland and Labrador and British Columbia (CIHI, 2012). Although many clients now go into labour and childbirth expecting to receive an epidural block, many may not be offered this treatment, especially those residing in rural or remote areas. Epidural administration requires continuous availability of an anesthesiologist in addition to having nurses who are sufficiently educated on the care of women receiving such services (Canadian Anesthesiologists' Society, 2010).

Although it is possible for an epidural to be unsuccessful or only partly successful in providing relief, generally it is considered the most effective and flexible method of pain management during labour (Simpson, 2008). Epidurals usually cause less depression of the central nervous system for the mother and fetus than do sedative hypnotics, opioids, and narcotic agonist–antagonist compounds.

Conventionally, clients receiving epidurals are usually in the active phase of the first stage of labour with cervical dilation of at least 4 to 5 cm. However, current literature suggests that there is no fetal or maternal benefit to delaying neuraxial analgesia (Marucci et al., 2007). Fetal monitoring should show a normal fetal heart rate pattern. Nevertheless, provided no medical contraindications exist, a maternal request for pain relief during labour is sufficient reason to initiate the procedure.

Epidurals are usually administered continuously throughout the active and transitional phases of labour, vaginal birth, and repair of the episiotomy. The primary goal is to provide sufficient anaesthesia with as little blockage to the sensory and motor nerves as possible. Ideally, pain relief is balanced with maternal need to ambulate during the first stage of labour, and retaining the ability to sense pressure in the vagina and to push during the second stage of labour.

The epidural block alters the client's physiologic responses to pain, but enables her to be fully awake during labour and birth. It promotes good relaxation. In addition, airway reflexes remain intact, gastric emptying is not delayed, and blood loss during birth is not excessive. The continuous method allows for variation in the blocking for the later stages of labour, which allows for the internal rotation of the fetus. In many cases, the dose of anaesthetic agents can be adjusted to preserve the client's reflex urge to push during the second stage of labour.

The anaesthesiologist injects epidural anaesthesia through a small catheter into the client's back. The tip of the catheter lies in the epidural space located between the dura mater and the ligamentum flavum, generally between the third and fourth or the fourth and fifth lumbar vertebrae (Fig. 17.9). The client may be placed on either her right or left side with her knees flexed upward near her abdomen and her head tucked down toward her chest, or in a sitting position on the side of the bed with her head tucked down toward the chest. A small pillow may be placed in front of her chest and abdomen for support to help the client maintain positioning. Such positioning facilitates the opening of the epidural space between the vertebrae and minimizes the risk for inadvertent puncture of the spinal column.

Initially, an epidural needle makes the puncture for insertion. Then, a small catheter is threaded through the needle into the space, and the needle is removed, leaving the catheter in place for administration of medications. Once the needle has been inserted into the client's back, she must be encouraged and supported to remain in as stable a position as possible until the Silastic catheter has been threaded and the needle has been removed.

Epidurals are used most frequently to provide continuous analgesia and anaesthesia from the T10 to the S5 levels, which is necessary for relieving pain during the remainder of labour and vaginal birth. For a cesarean birth, the block must extend from at least T8 to S1 to be effective. The diffusion of epidural anaesthesia depends on the location of the catheter tip, the dose and volume of the anaesthetic agent used, and the woman's position.

Epidurals may be administered in various ways. Blocks can be administered as a one-time single dose through an epidural needle that is inserted and then removed; as a single dose through an epidural catheter, with additional doses given periodically if the client begins to experience discomfort; or as a continuous infusion. One form of continuous infusion is an **ambulatory epidural pump**, in which the pump is connected to the catheter and titrated doses of pain medication are delivered to the client based on her height and weight until she has given birth. Some types of administration

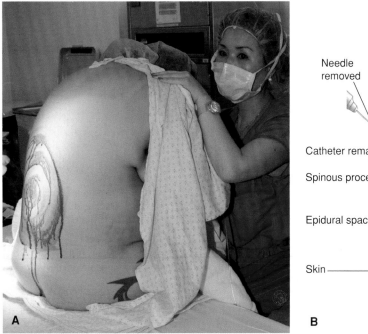
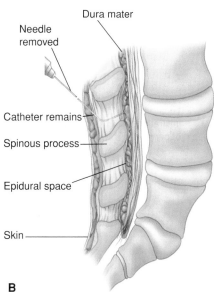

Dura mater

Needle
removed

Catheter remains

Spinous process

Epidural space

Skin

A

B

FIGURE 17.9 A, B: Administration of epidural anaesthesia.

require that the client remain in bed, whereas ambu-latory epidurals allow the client with sufficient motor control to be out of bed.

QUOTE 17-3

"When my labour wasn't progressing and the obstetrician decided to do a C-section, I felt so sad, because I thought I would not be able to experience the actual birth. I was so pleased to know that my birth could be done with epidural anaesthesia and that I would be able to see him when they pulled him out. I crashed for a few hours as soon as he was born, and I don't remember much about the initial recovery, but I remember the important part!"

A woman who had epidural anaesthesia during cesarean birth

Combined Spinal Epidural Anaesthesia. Combined spinal epidural anaesthesia may be accomplished through much the same procedure as for epidural anaes-thesia, except that a needle is inserted through the epi-dural needle, past the dura to first deliver an injection of fentanyl (Sublimaze) and bupivacaine (Marcaine) into the subarachnoid space. The spinal needle is removed and the Silastic epidural catheter is threaded through the epidural needle.

Combined spinal epidural anaesthesia has several benefits over epidural analgesia. Combined spinal epi-dural anesthesia has a faster onset of pain relief than epidural anaesthesia. This is especially beneficial for women at advanced stages of labour or where labour seems to be progressing rapidly. The synergistic effect of opioids and local anaesthesia, in addition to a lower total dose of required medication, reduces the motor blockade response and the risk of hypotension, thus

allowing the woman to ambulate. This method also enables the woman to feel pressure and have the sensa-tion needed to push during the second stage of labour. Finally, combined spinal epidural anesthesia may offer lower rates of failed analgesia when compared with epi-dural anaesthesia (Pan, Bogard, & Owen, 2004). Occa-sionally, especially when combined spinal epidural anaesthesia is used during cesarean births, a one-time injection of an opioid, such as morphine (Duramorph), into the epidural space immediately after birth provides analgesia for approximately 24 hours. Morphine takes effect within 30 to 60 minutes after the injection and peaks at approximately 14 to 16 hours. Side effects are possible, however, including respiratory depression, itching, rash, nausea, vomiting, and urinary retention.

If the client has received epidural morphine imme-diately after birth, vital signs are monitored hourly for 24 hours. No narcotic medications can be given to the client because they will potentiate the narcotic effect of the morphine. If the client develops itching and a rash, comfort measures, such as back rubs, the use of lotion, cool or warm compresses, and diversional activities are implemented. If the itching cannot be tolerated, diphen-hydramine hydrochloride (Benadryl) can be given.

Spinal Anaesthesia. In **spinal anaesthesia**, a local anaes-thetic agent is injected directly into the subarachnoid space between the dura and the spinal cord (Fig. 17.10). Here the agent mixes with the cerebrospinal fluid to provide anaes-thesia from the region of T10 (hip) to the feet for a vaginal birth, and from the region of T6 (nipples) to the feet for a cesarean birth. Whether the spinal is continuous or single

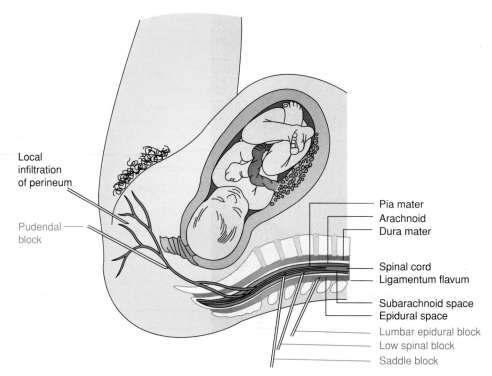

FIGURE 17.10 Injection of spinal anaesthesia directly into the subarachnoid space between the dura and the spinal cord.

shot will depend upon whether the woman is delivering vaginally or by cesarean section.

The advantages of spinal anaesthesia include the immediate onset of effect, relative ease of administration, need for a smaller dose volume to produce anaesthesia, excellent muscle relaxation, and retention of the drug in the mother's body (i.e., no passage through the placenta). The onset of action is usually within 1 to 2 minutes after administration, lasting approximately 1 to 3 hours, depending on the type of agent used.

Despite the advantages, spinal anaesthesia has some disadvantages and is not considered useful for most parturients due to its short duration and considerable risk of side effects (Wong, 2010). First, spinal analgesia carries a high risk of postdural puncture headache (PDPH) (Basurto et al., 2013). PDPHs, although not life threatening, can be severely painful and may be accompanied by neck stiffness, hearing loss, photophobia, nausea, and severely limits activity. Second, the client cannot sense the urge to push, which results in the need for an episiotomy, low forceps, or vacuum extraction. Finally, the incidence of bladder and uterine atony is also higher than that associated with epidural anaesthesia (see later discussion).

General Anaesthesia

Occasionally, life-threatening complications such as severe preeclampsia, abruptio placentae, abnormal fetal heart rate patterns, or hemorrhagic conditions in obstet-

rics arise that necessitate an expeditious emergency cesarean birth to facilitate the best possible outcome. The procedure for spinal and epidural anaesthesia generally takes several minutes to perform properly. Then it takes several more minutes to achieve maximum pain control. As a result, precious minutes can be lost during which the fetus could suffer irreparable damage or even die in utero. Therefore, general anaesthesia is often the method of choice for emergency births. **General anaesthesia** involves rendering the client totally unconscious.

General anaesthesia does not come without serious risks. As a result of physiologic and anatomical changes during pregnancy, expectant women have a higher risk of hypoxemia, have reduced diameter of the pharyngolaryngeal tract, and a higher risk of inhaling gastric contents (Boutonnet et al., 2011). The changes in the pharyngolaryngeal tract make intubation especially difficult and may result in increased risk of vomiting and aspiration (Munnur & Suresh, 2009). In addition to the maternal risks, all anaesthetic agents cross the placenta and can result in fetal depression.

Induction is accomplished through IV injection. The drugs of choice for induction are as follows:

- Thiopental sodium (Pentothal), an ultrashort-acting barbiturate
- Succinylcholine chloride (Anectine), a neuromuscular blocking agent that usually exerts its effect rapidly but has a brief duration of action

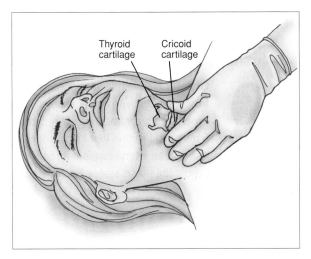

FIGURE 17.11 Technique of cricothyroid pressure.

After induction, the anaesthesiologist inserts a cuffed endotracheal tube into the trachea. During the insertion of the endotracheal tube, the nurse should occlude the esophagus by applying and maintaining cricoid pressure just below the "Adam's apple." The nurse should use the thumb and forefinger to firmly compress the cricoid ring (the first and only tracheal cartilage ring that is a complete circle) 2 to 3 cm posteriorly. This pressure prevents passive regurgitation and possible aspiration during the procedure (Fig. 17.11). The pressure is maintained until the anaesthesiologist has inserted the endotracheal tube, inflated the cuff, and confirmed proper placement or has indicated that the pressure can be released.

After securing the airway, the obstetrician proceeds with the cesarean birth. The use of inhalation anaesthetics such as isoflurane, desflurane, or sevoflurane, and oxygen maintains maternal unconsciousness throughout the procedure. After childbirth, nitrous oxide is often added to enhance the anaesthetic effect. Additional doses of muscle relaxants may be given as needed to maintain appropriate surgical conditions.

COLLABORATIVE CARE: PHARMACOLOGIC PAIN MANAGEMENT

Clients in labour have many choices available for pain management. Some clients prefer to use nonpharmacologic methods (see Chapter 14). Others choose to use only pharmacologic methods, and the discussions that follow focus on collaborative care oriented toward the various types available. Some women use a combination of nonpharmacologic and pharmacologic techniques. Nurses must be continuously aware of and sensitive to individual variations that influence the client's choices for dealing with pain.

If a client asks for a pharmacologic pain intervention, the nurse should inform her of what to expect about the onset, duration, and side effects that she may experience after administration. Determining the optimum time for administration depends on a thorough assessment of numerous factors. If given too early in labour, contractions may become less frequent, thus prolonging labour, or result in depression of the fetal central nervous system. If given too late, the woman has no or minimal pain relief, and the newborn may experience respiratory depression.

Assessment

Because of pain's highly subjective nature, the two most reliable sources for determining the existence and severity of pain are the client's vital signs and the client's self-report. In addition, the nurse should assess the client's typical pain relief measures, including the use of drugs and complementary/alternative therapies.

Adequately assessing the level of pain and the extent to which it is affecting the client are key to the proper administration of medications. Factors to include when determining whether analgesics are necessary for pain relief are whether the client is willing to take medications and whether the client's vital signs are stable and within normal limits. The nurse should listen very closely to what the client is saying about her level of pain and remain alert for more subtle signs of discomfort. Assessment of the fetal heart rate must reveal a normal pattern with a baseline between 110 and 160 beats per minute (bpm), with no decelerations present. The client should be in active labour with a well-established contraction pattern and demonstrated progression in cervical dilation and fetal descent. In addition, before any medication is given, the nurse should ascertain whether the woman has any history of drug reactions or allergies. The nurse should also ensure that activities such as changing position or assisting the client to the bathroom to urinate are completed before the administration of any analgesic.

Vital Signs

Usually, when pain is present, the client demonstrates changes in her vital signs. Pulse rate, respiratory rate, and blood pressure may significantly increase above the client's baseline. Once pain is relieved, the vital signs generally return to baseline (Fig. 17.12).

Client Self-Report

Various scales that rely on a client's self-reports have been developed to assist nurses and other health care providers to uniformly measure levels of pain. These pain-rating scales provide a measure for quantifying the severity of pain. Commonly used rating scales include

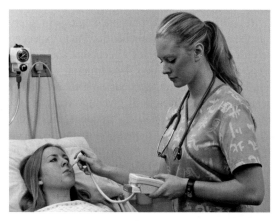

FIGURE 17.12 The nurse should regularly assess the client's vital signs to evaluate the effectiveness of pain-relieving measures.

shows the scale to the client and asks her to choose which face best represents her level of pain.

 Consider Marnie, the young woman from the beginning of the chapter experiencing contractions every 5 to 6 minutes. Imagine that Marnie does not speak English and an interpreter is not readily available. How could the nurse assess Marnie's pain?

Medication Use

Assessment to determine appropriate selection of pharmacologic agents also includes obtaining a thorough history of medication use at home, including legal prescription drugs, illicit drugs, and complementary/alternative therapies. When clients have used certain drugs, interactions with analgesics and anaesthetics that may be administered during labour can have serious implications. Although not recommended for pregnant women because of mutagenic effects to developing cells in early pregnancy, clients at times elect to take illicit and herbal drugs without discussing the ramifications of such use with their physician or nurse midwife. For example, St. John's Wort (*Hypericum perforatum*), to treat mild to moderate depression, can decrease the sedative effects of barbiturates, increase the sedative effects of narcotics, and prolong the bleeding time of clients receiving general anaesthesia, increasing the risk for hemorrhage during a surgical procedure such as cesarean birth (Springhouse Corporation, 2006). Most anaesthesiologists generally prefer that the woman discontinue medications and herbs that pose problems in labour and birth for at least 30 days before having an invasive procedure performed.

the 0 to 10 numeric rating scale (NRS) and the visual analog descriptive pain intensity scale (VAS). Both scales ask the client to rate her level of pain between 0 (no pain) and 10 (excruciating, the worst pain that can be imagined). The NRS and VRS are commonly used to assess acute pain. They are simple to use, easy for patients to understand, and are considered among the most effective pain measurement tools available (Australian and New Zealand College of Anaesthetists, 2010). Assessment Tool 17.1 illustrates the numerical pain-rating scale.

The Wong-Baker FACES pain-rating scale is a pictorial representation used to assess pain (Assessment Tool 17.2). This tool contains a series of six faces that depict six levels of pain. The first face is a happy face. Subsequent faces increase in intensity to the last face, depicting tears. Each face is numbered from 0 to 5 with a corresponding description ranging from "no hurt" to "hurts worst." The tool is easy to use, especially with non–English-speaking clients. The health care provider

● ASSESSMENT TOOL 17.1 Pain Distress Scales

SIMPLE DESCRIPTIVE PAIN DISTRESS SCALE[a]

None	Annoying	Uncomfortable	Dreadful	Horrible	Agonizing

0–10 NUMERIC PAIN DISTRESS SCALE[a]

No pain   Distressing pain   Unbearable pain

0	1	2	3	4	5	6	7	8	9	10

VISUAL ANALOG SCALE (VAS)[b]

No distress _____ Unbearable distress

[a]If used as a graphic rating scale, a 10-cm baseline is recommended.
[b]A 10-cm baseline is recommended for VAS scales.
(From AHCPR, Acute Pain Management Guide Panel, 1992.)

● **ASSESSMENT TOOL 17.2** *Wong-Baker Faces Rating Scale*

1. Explain to the client that each face is for a person who feels happy because she has no pain (hurt, or whatever word the client uses) or feels sad because she has some or a lot of pain.
2. Point to the appropriate face and state, "This face...":
   0—"is very happy because she doesn't hurt at all."
   1—"hurts just a little bit."
   2—"hurts a little more."
   3—"hurts even more."

4—"hurts a whole lot."
5—"hurts as much as you can imagine although you don't have to be crying to feel this bad."
3. Ask the client to choose the face that best describes how she feels. Be specific about which pain (e.g., "shot" or incision) and what time (e.g., Now? Earlier before lunch?)

From Hockenberry, M. J. (2005). *Wong's essentials of pediatric nursing* (7th ed.). St. Louis, MO: Mosby.

Drugs such as butorphanol (Stadol) and nalbuphine (Nubain) should be used with extreme caution in clients with a recent history of substance use because they can precipitate a withdrawal type of reaction. To collaborate with the client's primary care provider regarding the methods of pain management and to provide a safe, therapeutic environment, nurses should refer to appropriate resources such as drug handbooks and the *Nursing Herbal Medicine Handbook* (Springhouse Corporation, 2006) when the client's history reveals drugs or herbs not commonly used in pregnancy.

Select Potential Nursing Diagnoses

The most obvious nursing diagnosis for the woman in labour is **pain** related to increasing intensity and frequency of uterine contractions and perineal tissue pressure and stretching. Other appropriate nursing diagnoses may include the following:

- **Deficient Knowledge** related to lack of familiarity with pain relief methods
- **Anxiety** related to stress of labour progression and concern about fetal well-being
- **Ineffective Coping** related to stress of labour and pain
- **Situational Low Self-Esteem** related to feelings of inadequacy and lack of control over pain

Planning/Intervention

Outcomes are highly individualized based on the woman's situation. Ideally, the outcome for the woman in pain is relief of that pain. Nursing Care Plan 17.1 provides information about a general approach to managing pain in labour. The following sections focus on specific collaborative interventions and considerations for each type of pharmacologic pain relief available.

Administering Sedative Hypnotics and Analgesic Compounds

When medications are administered, the nurse should document the name of drug, dose, route, site, time administered, and effect according to the agency's policy. In addition, he or she should document the client's vital signs and fetal heart rate (Fig. 17.13). When medications begin to take effect, the client may sleep between contractions. This short period of rest can facilitate relaxation and restore the client's energy level. In some cases, the client's pain may be so intense that she may not want to do anything except get the medication. Subsequently, drug administration should be facilitated as expeditiously as possible to be helpful. The nurse also should caution any family members or other support people that the client might become disoriented and confused after administration of analgesic medications.

Managing Care During Epidural Anaesthesia

Before the administration of epidural analgesia, the anaesthesiologist must obtain the client's informed consent, with all potential side effects fully explained. IV access is established to provide a route for administration of resuscitative drugs should the epidural create an adverse reaction. Most anaesthesiologists prefer that the client receive a preparatory loading dose of solution, usually a minimum of 500 to 1,000 mL of IV-lactated Ringer or normal saline solution over 15 to 30 minutes before epidural administration. If at all possible, this

(text continues on page 692)

NURSING CARE PLAN 17.1

●

The Client Experiencing Pain During Labour

 Recall Marnie, the client described at the beginning of the chapter. Marnie has progressed in labour and is now experiencing moderately strong contractions every 3 minutes, lasting 60 seconds. She is now 6 cm dilated and 90% effaced. She is holding on tightly to the side rail of the bed, crying softly, and grimacing. She states, "I'm really uncomfortable." Her vital signs are stable; the fetal heart rate is 140 bpm.

NURSING DIAGNOSIS

Acute Pain related to increased contraction intensity and frequency and increased perineal pressure and stretching

EXPECTED OUTCOMES

1. The client will state that she is experiencing decreased pain.
2. The client will demonstrate no nonverbal indicators of pain.
3. The client will remain free from any adverse effects of analgesia administration.

INTERVENTIONS	RATIONALES
Thoroughly review the client's history for use of prescription, illegal, herbal, or homeopathic medications.	Certain medications interact with analgesics and anaesthetics, with serious implications for client care.
Ask the client to rate her pain using a rating scale of 0–10 (with 0 being no pain and 10 being the worst pain imaginable). Assess for evidence of behavioural responses to pain such as grimacing, crying, or wringing of hands. Assess pain location and characteristics.	These data provide information about the etiology and characteristics of pain. Rating allows for objective reassessment of the client's pain.
Accept the client's interpretation of pain; assess for possible factors influencing the pain level.	Pain is a unique experience for each person. Physical, social, psychological, cultural, and spiritual norms influence the expression of pain.
Promote a comfortable environment with one-to-one support for the client.	A comfortable environment reduces stressors that influence pain. One-to-one support assists the client to use techniques learned in any childbirth education classes to cope with discomfort during labour.
Reinforce and encourage her use of breathing and nonpharmacologic methods of pain relief during early labour.	
Explain the physiology of the client's discomfort (e.g., back labour). Explain pharmacologic methods of pain management, including advantages and disadvantages of each option.	Explanations decrease fear and anxiety as well as assist the client to cope with discomfort. Information empowers the client to make some decisions when she may feel that she has little control over anything.
Administer analgesia as ordered.	Administration of analgesia promotes pain relief.

(continued)

NURSING CARE PLAN 17.1 ● The Client Experiencing Pain During Labour (Continued)

INTERVENTIONS	RATIONALES
Monitor maternal and fetal responses to medications. Observe for adverse reactions.	All drugs given to the mother potentially carry risks for the client and also cross the placental barrier and can adversely affect the fetus. Prompt recognition and treatment to minimize maternal–fetal responses to medications is critical to producing an optimum outcome.
Re-evaluate the client's perception of pain after drugs have been administered.	Re-evaluation helps determines the effectiveness of the method of pain relief employed.
Monitor the mother's vital signs and the fetal heart rate as ordered.	Medications can pass through the placenta and affect the fetus.
Change the client's position frequently as tolerated. Assist with ambulation if allowed.	Position changes promote comfort. Ambulation helps to reduce pain. Because of possible central nervous system depression with pharmacologic agents such as sedatives and narcotics, the client needs assistance with balance and ambulation to promote safety.
If the client wants an epidural or spinal anaesthesia, ensure that she is fully informed of all potential complications and that she signs a consent form. Notify appropriate personnel if the client desires such pain relief.	Informed consent is necessary for any invasive procedure. All consents should be signed in advance of receiving sedatives, hypnotics, opioids, and agonist–antagonist medications, which can cause sedation and drowsiness. Early notification facilitates organization of the anaesthesia provider's time to promote the quickest administration of the epidural possible when the client is ready for one.
Continually reassess the client's level of pain, vital signs, and fetal status. Administer additional doses of analgesia as ordered.	Continued reassessment is necessary to determine the effectiveness of interventions and to identify possible adverse effects on mother and fetus. Additional medication may be necessary to achieve desired results.

EVALUATION

1. The client states that pain is tolerable and that she is comfortable.
2. The client rates her pain as 2 to 3 or less on a pain rating scale of 0 to 10.
3. The client demonstrates no crying, grimacing, or other nonverbal indicators of pain.
4. The client's vital signs and fetal heart rate are within acceptable parameters.

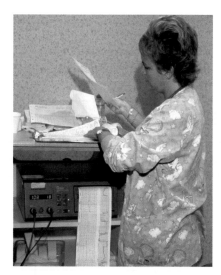

FIGURE 17.13 Following the administration of analgesic medications for labour pain, the nurse should document maternal vital signs and fetal heart rate.

loading dose should be given early, when beginning to provide care for the client, rather than waiting until just before the epidural is going to be administered. See Nursing Care Plan 17.2 for care of the client receiving epidural anaesthesia.

Some clients have difficulty maintaining the stable position required during epidural anaesthesia because of the severity and duration of their contractions. The nurse, along with the client's support person (if possible), should be diligent in providing stable support for the client during the procedure as well as in encouraging the client to remain calm. Catheter insertion is performed between contractions as often as possible to prevent movement during this time, which can increase the risk for inadvertent perforation of the subarachnoid space containing the cerebrospinal fluid.

Ongoing Monitoring. Regardless of how the epidural is administered, close observation of both the maternal vital signs and fetal heart patterns and rates are essential components of care. The nurse should assess vital signs every 2 minutes initially for the first 20 to 30 minutes, and then every 5 to 15 minutes depending on the client's status and agency policy. Oxygen saturation levels are monitored by pulse oximetry. In addition to frequent blood pressure readings, the pulse oximeter reading may reveal one of the first signs of a complication related to the epidural anaesthesia. The client may be placed in a semireclining position tilted laterally to keep the gravid uterus from compressing the ascending vena cava and descending aorta, which can impair venous return and decrease placental perfusion. The nurse should change the woman's position every 15 to 30 minutes to facilitate even dispersion of the anaesthetic

agent and to prevent a one-sided dose effect. The nurse should keep in mind that onset of anaesthesia can take 20 to 30 minutes to be effective. Therefore, ongoing provision of comfort measures and encouragement in relaxation techniques are essential.

Often, a period of continuous electronic fetal monitoring of between 30 and 60 minutes depending on facility policy, is recommended following commencement of epidural anaesthesia to assess for reflexive decelerations in the fetal heart rate in relation to maternal hypotension. However, the SOGC indicates that intermittent auscultation may be used, provided that a protocol is in place that ensures frequent intermittent auscultation assessment throughout labour, that is, every 5 minutes for the first 30 minutes after epidural administration and following each bolus top-up, as long as maternal vital signs are within normal range (SOGC, 2007).

Addressing Adverse Reactions and Complications. Although their incidence is relatively low, the client receiving epidural anaesthesia is at risk for possible adverse reactions and complications. Therefore, nurses should be thoroughly prepared to handle any and all potential complications.

Maternal hypotension is one of the most frequent effects of epidural anaesthesia. If the client's blood pressure drops significantly, fetal distress can occur. Rapid administration of the loading dose of the IV solution, however, generally can minimize this effect. Continuous IV access is maintained throughout labour to allow for repeated bolus doses of fluids as needed to maintain maternal homeostasis. The IV access also provides a means for drug administration should an emergency arise. If hypotension occurs, the anesthesiologist is notified, oxygen is administered by face mask, and a bolus of IV fluid is given. If these measures fail to stabilize the client's blood pressure, ephedrine, a vasopressor, should be readily available for administration and the epidural infusion may need to be discontinued.

Epidurals are at risk for failure because the catheter has to be placed properly within the epidural space to produce adequate anaesthesia. Potentially distressing complications include an inadequate block, an one-sided block, and a hot spot. In an *inadequate block*, the epidural fails to minimize the client's pain sufficiently. If the block is inadequate, the anaesthesiologist can inject a bolus dose of medication through the catheter, possibly increase the continuous ordered dose, or both. With a *one-sided block*, pain is managed only on one side. In such cases, the nurse can turn the woman to the unaffected side. In rare cases, the anaesthesiologist may have to readminister the drug through the catheter with the client lying on her unaffected side. With a *hot spot* (window of pain), the epidural provides effective

(text continues on page 695)

NURSING CARE PLAN 17.2

●

The Client Who Receives Epidural Anaesthesia

 Recall Felicia, the client from the beginning of the chapter admitted to the health care facility in active labour. During the interview, she states, "I tried natural childbirth with my other two children, but eventually I needed something for pain. The contractions were just too strong. Chuck and I talked this over with our physician, and we all agreed that I would get an epidural for the pain."

NURSING DIAGNOSIS

Risk for Injury related to the effects of epidural anaesthesia, including hypotension, prolongation of labour, neurologic injuries, and systemic toxicity

EXPECTED OUTCOMES

1. The client will experience relief of discomfort with minimal to no adverse effects.
2. The client will demonstrate progression through the stages of labour within expected timelines following the initiation of epidural anaesthesia.
3. The client will exhibit a return of sensation and ability to void in the postpartum period after epidural anaesthesia is discontinued.

INTERVENTIONS	RATIONALES
Obtain baseline maternal vital signs and fetal heart rate before the procedure.	Baseline assessment ensures that the client's values are within normal limits and allows for comparison with future assessments to detect changes.
Check to make sure that the client has signed an informed consent.	Informed consent is necessary because the procedure is invasive and the client is at risk for potential adverse effects. A signed informed consent indicates that the client understands the procedure and associated risks.
Provide adequate hydration, including a 500–1000-mL bolus of fluid before the procedure.	Adequate hydration ensures adequate intravascular fluid volume, which minimizes the risk for hypotension after administration.
Assist the client to assume either a sitting or side-lying position with the back arched to open the spaces between the spinal vertebrae.	Such positioning facilitates opening of the epidural space and minimizes the risk for inadvertent puncture of the spinal column.
Provide ongoing encouragement and support, assisting the client to remain stable during the procedure.	Proper positioning minimizes the potential for spinal cord injury from inadvertent client movement during the critical point when the spinal needle has been inserted into the client's back.

(continued)

NURSING CARE PLAN 17.2 ● The Client Who Receives Epidural Anaesthesia *(Continued)*

INTERVENTIONS	RATIONALES
Monitor blood pressure, pulse, and respirations every 2 min after initial injection of an anaesthetic agent for a minimum of 20 min and then every 5–15 min until stable. Repeat monitoring of vital signs every 2 min after additional doses for 20 min. Evaluate results against the baseline readings.	Changes in vital signs, especially blood pressure, indicate a possible adverse reaction. Blocking of the sympathetic nerve fibres in the epidural space causes decreased peripheral resistance, resulting in hypotension. Systolic blood pressure less than 100 mm Hg can lead to fetal hypoxia.
Monitor maternal temperature every 2 hr until birth.	Epidural anaesthesia can temporarily elevate the mother's temperature.
Observe for signs of local anaesthetic/analgesic toxicity: tinnitus, tingling, or unexplained confusion. If toxicity occurs, medications should be discontinued, and emergency interventions should be implemented.	Such observation aids in early detection and prompt intervention should any problems occur, minimizing risks to mother and fetus.
Monitor maternal oxygen saturation levels by pulse oximetry.	Adequate maternal oxygenation promotes adequate fetal oxygenation. Changes in oxygen saturation levels aids in detecting hypoxia related to suppression of respirations secondary to high anaesthesia.
Assist the client to a semi-reclining position in a lateral tilt.	Proper positioning promotes a more even distribution of the medication bilaterally and prevents the anaesthetic effect from rising too high; lateral tilt aids in keeping the gravid uterus from compressing the ascending vena cava and the descending aorta, which can impair venous return and decrease placental perfusion.
Assess the level of anaesthesia.	The higher the level of anaesthesia, the greater the risk for respiratory depression from paralysis of the diaphragm.
Monitor uterine contractions closely. Carefully check the fetal heart rate and progress of labour; notify the health care provider if the second stage becomes prolonged (more than 3 hr in a primipara or more than 2 hr in a multipara).	No contractions may indicate that the anaesthesia is rising too high. The client may not be able to feel the pressure of the fetal head descending in the pelvis. Fetal distress is rare after an epidural but can occur if the medication is absorbed rapidly or with severe maternal hypotension. Epidural anaesthesia is associated with an increased risk for prolonged second stage of labour.
Check to ensure that the pump is functioning properly and that tubing is not kinked or compressed by maternal weight or positioning. Assess for hot spots and breakthrough pain. Notify anaesthesiology personnel of any of these problems.	A patent infusion is necessary to provide adequate pain relief. Hot spots may require removal of the catheter and reinsertion. Breakthrough pain typically indicates the infusion is below the therapeutic dose or interrupted integrity of the epidural line.

(continued)

NURSING CARE PLAN 17.2 ● The Client Who Receives Epidural Anaesthesia *(Continued)*

INTERVENTIONS	RATIONALES
Anticipate use of an intermittent catheter as required.	Use of a catheter prevents bladder distention, which may interfere with fetal descent.
Provide comfort measures for nausea, vomiting, and shivering.	Comfort measures are important to provide relief from troublesome effects.
If hypotension is noted, administer oxygen by face mask at the prescribed rate and increase IV fluids. Reposition the client as necessary to maintain adequate oxygenation to the fetus.	Oxygen administration ensures that maternal blood is well oxygenated, leading to adequate fetal oxygenation. Increasing IV fluids helps to restore intravascular fluid volume, thereby increasing blood pressure.
Elevate the client's legs on a pillow for 2 to 3 min but avoid a Trendelenburg position.	Placing the client in the left lateral tilt position improves placental blood flow. Elevating the legs can increase venous blood return from the extremities to the heart and circulation to the brain. The Trendelenburg position should be avoided following an epidural because it can cause the anaesthesia level to rise too high, leading to possible respiratory paralysis.
Notify the health care provider and anaesthesia personnel if measures are ineffective.	If the above measures are ineffective, the anaesthesiologist may need to administer ephedrine to increase the client's blood pressure.
After birth, remove the epidural catheter, verifying that the tip of the catheter is intact.	Confirmation of the catheter tip ensures that all the catheter has been removed and hasn't broken off.
Maintain the client on bed rest with use of a Foley catheter in place (if necessary) until effects of epidural anaesthesia have worn off. Assess for return of sensation, range of motion, and ability to control lower extremities.	Bed rest helps to ensure client safety with ambulation after birth; the catheter aids in reducing the risk for bladder distention that can interfere with uterine involution, which can lead to postpartum hemorrhage.

EVALUATION

1. The client remains free of any adverse effects of epidural anaesthesia.
2. The client gives birth to a healthy newborn.
3. The client demonstrates a return of bodily functions upon discontinuation of epidural anaesthesia after birth.

relief, except for one small area of the abdomen in which pain is intense; this is referred to as a "missed segment." If this occurs, the anaesthesiologist should be notified. The catheter may need to be removed and reinserted.

Breakthrough pain can occur any time the epidural infusion is below the therapeutic dose required or the integrity of the epidural line is interrupted. The nurse should first ascertain whether the infusion pump is functioning properly and check that maternal body weight or positioning is not kinking or compressing the tubing. If nursing care measures fail to rectify the problem, the anaesthesiologist may need to provide a bolus injection of the anaesthetic agent.

Itching and rash can occur during the epidural infusion. Typically, these begin on the client's face, neck, or torso and usually result from the anaesthetic agent used. If an allergic reaction occurs, comfort measures such as back rubs, application of lotion, cool or warm compresses, and diversion are implemented. If the itching becomes too uncomfortable for the client, an order for diphenhydramine hydrochloride (Benadryl) may be obtained from the anaesthesiologist. The usual dose is 25 to 50 mg every 4 to 6 hours, as needed to control the symptoms.

Epidural anaesthesia may slow the progress of labour and extend the duration of the second stage. The health care team working with the client needs to monitor the client's motor and sensory function carefully as she prepares to start pushing. If the client lacks motor and sensory function, pushing should be delayed until some of the sensation returns, thus facilitating her ability to push effectively.

Short-term localized tenderness at the puncture site and backache are common during the first postpartum week. The discomfort is thought to result from muscle tension during stressful times in labour as well as the required positioning during the administration of the epidural.

Other possible complications include urinary retention, shivering, nausea, and vomiting. After relief of the client's discomfort has been achieved through the administration of the epidural, a catheter may need to be inserted to prevent bladder distention from inadvertently impeding fetal descent. The nurse should monitor urinary output hourly. Shivering is commonly experienced by labouring women and it is theorized that there may be a relationship between shivering and the receipt of the epidural agent (Oliver et al., 1999). Covering the client with a warm blanket may help reduce the shivering. The nurse should reassure the client that the shivering should resolve spontaneously shortly after delivery. If the client becomes nauseous and experiences vomiting, application of a cool cloth to the forehead or throat may help. If nausea and vomiting persist, the nurse should give an antiemetic if one is ordered.

Neurologic injuries also may result from epidural anaesthesia. Because of the resulting relaxation and decreased pain sensation, the client's legs may be excessively flexed when positioned during pushing. Overstretching of the pelvic nerves may result. Clients may report numbness, tingling, and paresthesia in one foot or leg that can be severe or last long enough to require the use of a cane or a walker for weeks to months. Any report of such symptoms that last longer than the expected duration for an epidural should be referred to the anaesthesiologist for further evaluation.

A rare but serious complication of epidural anaesthesia is a systemic toxic reaction. This may result from inadvertent injection of anaesthetic agents into the spinal column, excessive doses of medications injected into the epidural space, or accidental intravascular injection of medications. The client who experiences a toxic reaction generally complains of numbness and tingling that rises progressively higher to the arms and chest. If the reaction is severe, the nerves supplying the respiratory muscles may be blocked, thus causing severe respiratory depression or arrest, oxygen desaturation, and loss of consciousness. Such clients may require endotracheal intubation and emergency resuscitation measures until their condition stabilizes. If respiratory stability is achieved, a vaginal birth may still be possible.

The effect of epidural anaesthesia on postpartum breastfeeding is controversial. Some observers suggest that epidurals are safer than other forms of analgesia and anaesthesia with minimal long-term side effects (Wilson et al., 2010). Breastfeeding also may be hampered, however, by drugs used during epidural anaesthesia (Bell et al., 2010). The "amide" anaesthetic agents enter the maternal circulation by diffusion and cross the placenta to the fetus. The newborn's liver is too immature to break down the medication, so the effects can linger for prolonged periods, often causing the newborn to be sleepy, have difficulty latching on, and have an inefficient, disorganized sucking and swallowing ability. When such problems occur, mothers may become discouraged, which may lead to early unintentional weaning. The nurse should work to provide additional assistance and support to the mother and the baby to promote and acquire successful, efficient breastfeeding skills. See Research Highlight 17.1.

Discontinuing Use. After childbirth, the epidural infusion and pump are discontinued, and the catheter is removed from the client's back. The intactness of the black tip of the catheter must be confirmed with a physician or another nurse. The epidural amount administered through the pump is calculated and charted on the appropriate agency flow sheet such as a narcotic control record. Client ambulation is usually delayed until the effects of the anaesthesia have worn off and the client has full sensation and the ability to control leg movements. The obstetrician may elect to leave the urinary catheter in place until full sensation has returned. Doing so helps to prevent urinary retention because the client may be unable to determine when her bladder is full as a result of residual anaesthetic effects. Adequate bladder emptying also promotes effective uterine contraction.

Managing Care During Spinal Anaesthesia

When spinal anaesthesia is used, the client is positioned in much the same way as for epidural anaesthesia to ensure that the intravertebral space is widened. After

● RESEARCH HIGHLIGHT 17.1   Epidural Analgesia During Labour and Delivery: Effects on the Initiation and Continuation of Effective Breastfeeding

OBJECTIVES

Epidural anaesthesia used frequently during labour is commonly regarded as a safe procedure. The purpose of this study was to determine whether epidural anaesthesia is associated with problems initiating or continuing breast-feeding in newborns.

DESIGN

The research design was a prospective cohort study examining a sample of women who gave vaginal birth to healthy infants. One group received epidural analgesia. The other group did not. Each mother in both groups was assessed 8 to 12 hours postpartum and in a telephone follow-up interview 4 weeks after childbirth.

RESULTS

No significant differences were found in either group relative to immediate success at the beginning of breastfeeding or in the number of women who continued breastfeeding at 4 weeks postpartum.

NURSING IMPLICATIONS

The findings of this study indicate that epidural anaes-thesia should not negatively influence the outcomes of breastfeeding. In evaluating the causes of problems with breastfeeding after administration of epidural anaesthe-sia, health care providers should carefully assess all the specific dynamics of the client's situation to help address problems and facilitate an effective experience.

From Chang, Z. M., & Heaman, M. I. (2005). Epidural analgesia during labor and delivery: Effects on the initiation and continu-ation of effective breastfeeding. *Journal of Human Lactation*, 21(3), 305–314.

---

insertion, the client may be positioned upright to pro-vide anaesthesia to the desired level for a vaginal birth, or more supine if the level desired is for a cesarean birth. Because spinal anaesthesia is generally used during cesarean births, positioning the client flat in bed with a small, flat pillow under her head for at least 8 hours after administration is highly recommended.

Addressing Adverse Reactions and Complications. Marked hypotension, decreased cardiac output, decreased placental perfusion, and respiratory distress may occur during spinal anaesthesia. Systemic allergic drug reactions and respiratory paralysis resulting in the need for cardiopulmonary resuscitation are more severe potential complications. If signs of serious maternal distress, fetal compromise, or both occur, emergency care must be implemented. The client is turned to the left side or placed in a left lateral tilt position. Oxygen is administered through face mask according to the agency's protocol. The nurse should monitor maternal vital signs and fetal heart rate every 2 to 5 minutes until stable. In addition, the nurse should notify the anaesthesiologist and the primary care provider.

Hematoma in the spinal column is a rare compli-cation that can result in spinal cord compression or ischemia. Neurologic damage may range from sensory or motor weakness to quadriplegia and death. Present-ing symptoms generally include lower-body motor weakness, back pain, and sensory deficits. Delays in symptom identification, diagnosis, and treatment can result in more severe damage. Concern about hematoma in the spinal column is one of the primary reasons that epidural and spinal anaesthesia methods are contraindi-cated in cases of severe coagulopathy.

Addressing Postdural Spinal Headache. Headaches after childbirth are not unusual and can be from several causes, including dehydration, prolonged labour, pushing, or regional anaesthesia. The distinguishing characteristic of a postdural spinal headache is the association between the client's position and headache severity. A true postdural spinal headache causes severe pain when the client is upright (i.e., sitting or standing), but the pain is minimal or disappears completely when the client is recumbent. A postdural spinal headache usually begins within 5 days after the procedure. The headache can last for several days and is usually unresponsive to minor analgesics.

Leakage of cerebrospinal fluid from the inadvert-ent puncture or actual puncture into the spinal column is thought to be the major cause of a postdural spinal head-ache. With postural changes during the postpartum period, the diminished volume of cerebrospinal fluid allows the brain to shift more than usual. This shifting exerts traction on the pain-sensitive structures of the brain, resulting in a severe headache with visual and auditory disturbances when the client is upright. Left untreated, the problem may persist for days to several weeks.

The likelihood of a postdural spinal headache can be minimized if the anaesthesiologist uses a small-gauge spinal needle and avoids puncturing the meninges. If a postdural headache does occur, treatment generally includes hydration measures. The nurse should encourage the client to increase her intake of water and caffeinated beverages. In addition, an IV infusion of lactated Ringer solution may be administered at 150 mL/hour to assist the body in replacing the cerebrospinal fluid loss. Caffeine is encouraged because it causes cerebral vasoconstriction. The client is placed on bed rest. Analgesics for the headache may be beneficial in some instances. Such therapy, however, is not always effective in relieving a postdural spinal headache. Sometimes, the leakage of the cerebrospinal fluid is excessive to the point that an **epidural blood patch** may be required. However, this invasive procedure carries additional risks. The spinal column may be punctured again, which will result in worsening of the headache and arachnoiditis if the blood is inadvertently injected into the subarachnoid space.

The technique for an epidural blood patch involves insertion of an epidural needle, preferably in the same vertebral interspace as the original puncture. A venipuncture is performed, and 20 mL of the client's blood is obtained using a sterile technique. The autologous blood, without an anticoagulant present, is then injected through the epidural needle into the epidural space by an anaesthesiologist.

The epidural blood patch seems to work in two ways. First, the blood clots and plugs the hole in the spinal column to stop the leakage of cerebrospinal fluid. Second, the volume of the blood in the epidural space exerts pressure within the spinal column, which increases the cerebrospinal fluid level surrounding the brain.

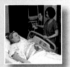 Think back to Felicia from the beginning of the chapter and Nursing Care Plan 17.2. Suppose Felicia develops a postdural headache following epidural anaesthesia during labour. What measures would the nurse implement?

Managing Care During General Anaesthesia

Before induction of general anaesthesia, the nurse should place a wedge under the client's right hip to displace the uterus to the left, which prevents compression of the vena cava. The client is then preoxygenated for 3 to 5 minutes with 100% oxygen. This is followed by induction.

Addressing Adverse Reactions and Complications. Although general anaesthesia is an expeditious method of providing pain control, it is never the preferred method during childbirth because it carries added risks for both mother and fetus. Increased pressure on the stomach from the weight of the gravid uterus, in conjunction with more production of gastric acid and pepsin, places pregnant clients at risk for gastric reflux. In addition, physiologic changes in the gastrointestinal system during labour increase the likelihood of regurgitation and aspiration. These changes also include decreased bowel motility, delayed stomach emptying, and decreased barrier pressure at the gastroesophageal junction. As a result, the client receiving general anaesthesia has an increased risk for possible aspiration of vomitus and hypoxia during administration. Pulmonary aspiration of gastric contents can cause lower airway obstruction, pneumonitis, pulmonary edema, and death. Therefore, before receiving general anaesthesia, the client should receive a nonparticulate antacid such as sodium citrate (Bicitra). Additional medications such as histamine-2 blockers, for example, cimetidine (Tagamet), or ranitidine (Zantac), also may be given to help decrease the gastric pH level and volume of stomach acid.

Thiopental (Pentothal) and inhalation anaesthetics rapidly cross the placenta. Therefore, the obstetrician has only an extremely short window from induction of anaesthesia to birth to get the fetus out without causing severe respiratory depression. Infants born to women under general anaesthesia may be slow to respond at birth and may require resuscitative measures. Therefore, adequate equipment and personnel, including a pediatrician, must be present during birth.

Two other complications of general anaesthesia include awareness during the procedure and uterine atony. It is possible for some clients to have some degree of awareness during the procedure, which may be attributed to an attempt to minimize drug-induced respiratory depression of the newborn. The addition of nitrous oxide after birth of the infant can decrease maternal awareness. If the client describes instances of awareness, the nurse should explore the implications and notify the anaesthesiologist so that the client can receive further assessment and explanation of the incident. In some cases, women experience flashbacks or nightmares as a result of awareness of events during surgery. These types of posttraumatic symptoms necessitate a referral for counselling.

Uterine atony is a potential complication in all births regardless of whether analgesia or anaesthesia is used. With general anaesthesia, the use of inhalation anaesthetic agents can produce decreased uterine contractility and tone after birth. Therefore, IV oxytocin (Pitocin) is administered to facilitate uterine contraction. Checking fundal firmness and lochia each time vital signs are taken is imperative during the postoperative period.

Controlling Malignant Hyperthermia. Malignant hyperthermia is an uncommon but dangerous complication of general anaesthesia. This autosomal-dominant inherited disorder of the skeletal muscles is characterized by a hypermetabolic response triggered by commonly used inhalation anaesthetics, such as halothane, and depolarizing muscle relaxants, such as succinylcholine chloride (Wappler, 2001). The exact mechanism by which different substances initiate malignant hyperthermia is essentially unknown; however, research has shown that a genetic mutation results in abnormal proteins in muscle cells. When triggered, calcium is released from the cellular endoplasmic reticulum, resulting in sustained muscle contraction and increased metabolism and heat production (Malignant Hyperthermia Association of the United States [MHAUS], 2014). Family history generally reveals unexplained or sudden deaths during surgery as well as history of cardiac disease. When anaesthesiologists interview clients before administering anaesthesia, this is a key point that they assess before determining which method of pain control will be the most beneficial during the surgical procedure.

The clinical syndrome of malignant hyperthermia includes muscle rigidity, jaw rigidity, hypercapnia, tachycardia, hyperpyrexia, and myoglobinuria. Hypoxia results from increased carbon dioxide production, oxygen consumption, and muscle membrane breakdown. The disruption of the cell membranes leads to electrolyte imbalances (hyperkalemia). Malignant hyperthermia is suspected when the client displays the following:

- Temperature greater than 38.7°C
- Difficulty with intubation from muscle rigidity, jaw rigidity, and laryngospasm
- Oxygen desaturation
- Blood loss that changes in colour from bright red to dark maroon
- Cyanosis
- Tachycardia
- Dysrhythmias
- Cardiac arrest
- Respiratory and metabolic acidosis

Once malignant hyperthermia is recognized, volatile inhaled anaesthetics and depolarizing muscle relaxants must be discontinued. In addition, all the breathing circuits and IV lines need to be changed immediately. Primary care measures include reversing the muscle rigidity with dantrolene sodium (Dantrium). Dosages are generally 2 to 3 mg/kg initially to a total of 10 mg/kg until rigidity is absent. Other measures include the symptomatic relief of the elevated temperature by placing the client on a cooling blanket, placing ice packs at the axillary and groin areas, continuously monitoring core

body temperature, correcting acidosis with administration of sodium bicarbonate, 1 to 2 mEq/kg, and restoring electrolyte balance. In addition, intake and output are closely assessed. Cooled isotonic IV solutions are used instead of lactated Ringer solution, which may worsen the acidosis rather than correcting it. Cooling measures are stopped when core body temperature reaches 38°C to prevent hypothermia. IV furosemide (Lasix) and continuous infusion of glucose and insulin are used to force diuresis, which is geared to 1 to 2 mL/kg of body weight. Arterial and central venous catheters are inserted to monitor hemodynamic status. Specimens obtained periodically for laboratory testing include arterial blood gases, electrolyte levels, complete blood count, coagulation studies, and renal function tests. Low-dose heparin therapy should also be initiated as soon as possible (MHAUS, 2014). After stabilization is accomplished, the client is transferred to the intensive care unit for follow-up.

Discontinuing Use. After general anaesthesia is completed, the client is awakened. Once she is responsive and spontaneously breathing with sufficient rate and tidal volume, and has the protective airway reflexes of swallowing, the mouth is suctioned, the endotracheal cuff is deflated, and the client is extubated. Once the tube has been removed, the client is transferred to the recovery room.

Clients who have received general anaesthesia require close observation and monitoring after giving birth. Nurses should thoroughly assess all major body systems and prepare to provide immediate responses to any problems encountered.

Respirations should be observed closely for rate and depth. Oxygen can be administered by nasal cannula or face mask (when higher concentrations are needed). Pulse oximetry is used to determine oxygen saturation. Frequent monitoring of all vital signs is performed until the woman is stable. Suction equipment must be readily available for use should the client vomit. The client must not be left alone during the critical point of recovery, which is the first hour after birth. The client should be stimulated and oriented to time and place frequently to prevent her from being too sleepy and hypoventilating. Vigilance by the nursing staff is the most important aspect in promoting a safe recovery period after administration of general anaesthesia.

Evaluation

The nurse should monitor to ensure that the client's pain is managed effectively during labour and birth and that complications or problems postpartally are minimized. Each client's outcomes are further individualized based on the particulars of her situation.

SUMMARY

- Pain, a truly unique experience, varies for each woman.
- Because pain is subjective, nurses need to understand not only the physiology and psychology of pain, but also the pharmacology of pain relief methods and how cultural beliefs affect client perceptions of pain.
- Factors that produce pain during labour include the progression of cervical dilation, perineal distention, intensity and duration of contractions, and fetal position and size.
- During the first stage of labour, the uterine muscle experiences hypoxia and lactic acid accumulation from cervical dilation and stretching of the lower uterine segment. These in turn create traction on the ovaries, fallopian tubes, and uterine ligaments. Pressure on the maternal pelvis causes afferent pain impulses to travel along the sympathetic nerves that enter the spinal column.
- During the second stage of labour, descent of the fetal presenting part exerts pressure on the pelvic floor muscles, vagina, perineum, and vulva, which in turn exerts pressure on the urethra, bladder, and rectum. The pain impulses ascend the spinal column in the same manner as during the first stage of labour.
- The gate control theory suggests that pain signals reach the nervous system and excite small groups of neurons. When the total activities of these neurons reach a certain level, a theoretical gate opens up and allows the pain signal to proceed through large and small sensory nerve fibres in the spinal column to the cerebral cortex, where the impulses are interpreted. Depending on the influence of physical, emotional, and behavioural factors, the gate also can close, which blocks the pain impulse from reaching the brain.
- Endorphins are naturally occurring pain-moderating substances in the spinal column, which generally increase during pregnancy and the postpartum period. This may explain why various forms of massage, water therapy, or transcutaneous electrical nerve stimulation (TENS) may reduce the discomfort of pain.
- The real challenge for health care providers is to give optimum care, which enables clients to feel satisfaction with the birth experience while attaining the maximum pain relief possible.
- Choice of pain management methods is based on personal beliefs. Implementation of a client's desired methods is an ethical responsibility for health care providers, whereas informed consent is the prevailing legal consideration, especially related to invasive procedures such as epidural or spinal anaesthesia.
- Three main elements must be present to be considered a truly informed consent: unbiased information should be given before giving consent, consent must be a voluntary decision, and the client must be competent and capable of accepting responsibility for the selected decision.
- Pharmacokinetics is the study of drug absorption, metabolism, distribution, and excretion in the body. The increased cardiac output of pregnancy and childbirth and its concomitant physiologic changes alter these processes.
- For centuries, discomfort during labour and birth has been considered inevitable and something to be endured. The desire for pain relief during childbirth has led to the trial of many remedies; however, the greatest strides in pain management have occurred during the past 200 years.
- Inhaled nitrous oxide is an inexpensive, easy-to-deliver, self-administered intervention that may provide analgesia for women having either preterm or term labour. Maximum therapeutic effect takes up to 50 seconds after continuous inhalation has occurred. Timing of inhalation is important for optimal effect.
- Determining the optimum time for giving analgesics depends on a complete assessment of various factors. If given too early in labour, contractions may become less frequent, thus prolonging labour, or it may cause fetal central nervous system depression. If given too late, the woman will experience minimal or no pain relief, and the newborn may experience respiratory depression.
- Analgesia reduces or decreases awareness of pain, whereas anaesthesia can cause partial or complete loss of sensation with or without loss of consciousness.
- Sedative hypnotics relieve anxiety and induce sleep. Common sedative hypnotics include promethazine (Phenergan), dimenhydrinate (Gravol), lorazepam (Atavan), midazolam (Versed), and clonazepam (Rivotril).
- Common opioid drugs include morphine and meperidine (Demerol). Common narcotic agonist–antagonists include butorphanol (Stadol) and nalbuphine (Nubain). Naloxone (Narcan) is a narcotic antagonist used to reverse the effects of opioid and narcotic agonist–antagonist agents. Fentanyl and remifentanil are newer emerging potent opioids with shorter maternal and neonatal half-lives.
- Local anaesthesia is used in obstetrics to induce a loss of sensation in the perineum and vagina during a vaginal delivery to facilitate the cutting, repair, or both of the episiotomy.
- An epidural block is the injection of local anaesthetic agents into the epidural space between the dura mater and the ligamentum flavum between the third and fourth or fourth and fifth lumbar vertebrae through a small catheter inserted into the client's back by an anaesthesiologist. The catheter may be connected to a pump, which delivers titrated doses of pain medication until birth is accomplished.

Common drugs used with epidurals are bupivacaine (Marcaine) and fentanyl (Sublimaze).

- With spinal anaesthesia, a local anaesthetic agent is injected directly into the subarachnoid space between the dura and the spinal cord, where it mixes with the cerebrospinal fluid to provide anaesthesia from the T10 region (hip) to the feet for a vaginal delivery and from the T6 region (nipples) to the feet for a cesarean birth.

- General anaesthesia renders the client unconscious with short-acting IV sedation followed by endotracheal intubation and the use of inhalation anaesthetics such as nitrous oxide, isoflurane, desflurane, sevoflurane, and oxygen.

- The two most reliable sources for determining the existence of pain and its severity are the client's vital signs and the client's self-report.

- Client self-report of pain can be determined through the use of various measurement scales, including the Wong-Baker FACES scale, the numerical rating scale (0 to 10), and the visual analogue scale.

- Assessment to determine appropriate selection of analgesic and anaesthetic agents also entails obtaining a thorough history of medication use at home, including legal prescription drugs, illegal drugs, homeopathic remedies, and herbal derivatives. When homeopathic, herbal, or illicit drugs have been used, interactions with analgesics and anaesthetics can occur that may have serious implications for client care.

- The most common complication of epidural anaesthesia is maternal hypotension. Failure to correct hypotension in the mother can result in fetal hypoxia.

- Postdural spinal headache is a frequent complication of spinal anaesthesia. It also can be a result of an inadvertent spinal administration occurring during epidural insertion. The postdural spinal headache causes severe pain when the client is in an upright position such as sitting or standing, but is minimal or disappears completely when the client assumes a recumbent position.

- Common complications of general anaesthesia include nausea, vomiting, and aspiration. A less common complication is malignant hyperthermia.

Questions to Ponder

1. A woman is admitted to labour and birth area in active labour. She is quiet and reserved, but looks apprehensive. You note that she is Asian and does not speak or understand English.
   - What strategies would you use to assess this woman's level of pain?
   - What would be the most therapeutic way to assist the client in managing her pain during labour?

2. A client received epidural anaesthesia 15 minutes ago, and her systolic blood pressure drops from a baseline of 120 to 88 mm Hg.
   - What complication is the client most likely experiencing?
   - How would you expect to intervene?
   - What follow-up nursing care measures would be appropriate?

REVIEW QUESTIONS

1. The nurse should be alert for the development of malignant hyperthermia in a client who has received
   A. epidural anaesthesia.
   B. general anaesthesia.
   C. pudendal anaesthesia.
   D. local anaesthesia.

2. Three hours after giving vaginal birth to a healthy newborn with the aid of epidural anaesthesia, a client complains of a headache unrelieved by medication. The nurse suspects that the client is possibly suffering from
   A. exhaustion and needs more rest in a quiet environment.
   B. dehydration and needs to drink more decaffeinated fluids.
   C. migraine with a low tolerance for pain and needs stronger medication.
   D. effects of an inadvertent spinal anaesthetic requiring additional intervention.

3. A client in the first phase of labour whose cervix is dilated to 3 cm states she is having pain. The nurse would anticipate an order for pain management at this point in time that involves
   A. continuing nonpharmacologic pain relief techniques.
   B. giving secobarbital by mouth.
   C. giving nalbuphine and promethazine by IV push.
   D. assisting with epidural anaesthetic administration.

4. The nurse identifies the pain occurring during the late phase of the first stage and second stage of labour that results from stretching of the perineal tissues to allow passage of the fetus as which of the following?
   A. Somatic pain
   B. Visceral pain
   C. Referred pain
   D. Psychosomatic pain

5. Effective pain management of labour involves the nurse
   A. recommending the use of nonpharmacologic techniques.
   B. informing the woman that all pharmacologic techniques are similar.

C. being sensitive to the individual woman's choice for managing her pain.

D. recommending the use of pharmacologic pain interventions.

6. One reliable source for determining the existence of pain and severity are the client's vital signs and

A. observing the client's behaviours.

B. subjective client observation using the Wong-Baker FACES pain scale.

C. self-report of the client using a 0- to-10-point NRS for the level of pain.

D. evaluating the client's verbal statements about pain.

7. The health care provider administers an injection of local anaesthetic into a space between the dura mater and the ligamentum flavum. The nurse documents this

A. pudendal block.

B. spinal block.

C. local block.

D. epidural block.

8. If used for analgesia in labour, which drug has a significant impact on breastfeeding during the postpartum period?

A. Fentanyl

B. Meperidine (Demerol)

C. Remifentanil

D. Nalbuphine (Nubain)

9. Following an epidural, the client's systolic blood pressure drops from a baseline of 118 to 75 mm Hg. The nurse's most immediate response should be to

A. administer ephedrine IV.

B. inform the anaesthesiologist.

C. increase the IV fluid rate.

D. administer oxygen by nasal cannula.

REFERENCES

Anderson, D. (2011). A review of systemic opioids commonly used for labor pain relief. *Journal of Midwifery and Womens Health, 56*(3), 222–239. doi:10.1111/j.1542-2011.2011.00061.x

Basurto, O. X., Uriona, T. S. M., Martinez, G. L., Sola, I., & Bonfill, C. X. (2013). Drug therapy for preventing post-dural puncture headache. *The Cochrane Library,* (2), CD001792.

Baumgarder, D. J., Muehl, P., Fischer, M., & Pribbenow, B. (2003). Effect of labor epidural anesthesia on breast-feeding of healthy full-term newborns delivered vaginally. *Journal of the American Board of Family Practice, 16*(1), 7–13.

Beech, B. (1999). Drugs in labour: What effect do they have twenty years hence? *Midwifery Today, 50,* 31–33, 65.

Bell, A. F., White-Traut, R., & Medoff-Cooper, B. (2010). Neonatal neurobehavioral organization after exposure to maternal epidural analgesia in labor. *Journal of Obstetric, Gynecologic and Neonatal Nursing, 39,* 178–190.

Boutonnet, M., Faitot, V., & Keita, H. (2011). Airway management in obstetrics. *Annales Francaises d'Anesthesie et de Reanimation, 30*(9), 651–664.

Canadian Institute of Health Information. (2012). Highlights of 2010–2011 selected indicators describing the birthing process in Canada. Retrieved from https://secure.cihi.ca/free/Childbirth_Highlights_2010-11_EN.pdf

Chang, Z. M., & Heamon, M. I. (2005). Epidural analgesia during labor and delivery: Effects on the initiation and continuation of effective breastfeeding. *Journal of Human Lactation, 21*(3), 305–314.

Chaillet, N., Belaid, L., Crochetiere, C., Roy, L., Gagne, G., Moutquin, J., Rossignol, M., et al. (2014). Non-pharmacologic approaches for pain management during labor compared with usual care. *Birth, 41*(2), 122–137.

Choi, J. C., Chung, M. I., & Lee, Y. D. (2012). Modulation of pain sensation by stress-related testosterone and cortisol. *Anaesthesia, 67*(10), 1146–1151. doi:10.1111/j.1365–2044.2012.07267.x

Cohen, J. (1996). Doctor James Young Simpson, Rabbi Abraham De Sola, and Genesis Chapter 3, verse 16. *Obstetrics and Gynecology, 88,* 895–898.

Datta, S. (2006). *Spinal opiates in obstetrics* (4th ed.). New York: Springer.

Gaiser, R. R. (2005). Labor epidurals and outcome. *Best Practice and Research: Clinical Anaesthesiology, 19*(1), 1–16.

Green, J. M., & Baston, H. A. (2003). Feeling in control during labor: Concepts, correlates, and consequences. *Birth, 30*(4), 235–247.

Hansen, G., & Streltzer, J. (2005). The psychology of pain. *Emerg Med Clin North America, 23,* 339–348.

Hodnett, E. D., Gates, S., Hofmeyr, G. J., Sakala, C., & Weston, J. (2011). Continuous support for women during childbirth (Review). *The Cochrane Database of Systematic Reviews,* (2), CD003766.

International Association for the Study of Pain (IASP). (2012). IASP taxonomy. Retrieved from http://www.iasppain.org/Education/Content.aspx?ItemNumber = 1698&navItemNumber = 576

Karch, A. M. (2008). *2008 Lippincott's nursing drug guide.* Philadelphia, PA: Lippincott Williams & Wilkins.

Kattwinkel, J., Perlman, J. M., Aziz, K., Colby, C., Fairchild, K., Gallagher, J., et al. (2010). Part 15: Neonatal resuscitation: 2010 American Heart Association Guidelines for Cardiopulmonary Resuscitation and Emergency Cardiovascular Care. *Circulation, 122*(18 suppl 3), S909–S919.

Kukulu, K., & Demirok, H. (2008). Effects of epidural anesthesia on labor progress. *Pain Management Nursing, 9*(1), 10–16.

Leap, N., Sandall, J., Buckland, S., & Huber, U. (2010). Journey to confidence: Women's experiences in pain in labour and relational continuity of care. *Journal of Midwifery and Women's Health, 55*(3), 234–242.

Likis, F. E., Andrews, J. C., Collins, M. R., Lewis, R. M., Seroogy, J. J., Starr, S. A., et al. (2014). Nitrous oxide for the management of labor pain: A systematic review. *Anesthesia and Analgesia, 118*(1), 153–167.

Lowe, N. K. (2004). Context and process of informed consent for pharmacologic strategies in labor pain care. *Journal of Midwifery and Women's Health, 49*(3), 250–259.

Macintyre, P. E., Schug, S. A., Scott, D. A., Visser, E. J., Walker, S. M.; APM:SE Working Group of the Australian and New Zealand College of Anaesthetists and Faculty of Pain Medicine (2010). *Acute pain management: Scientific evidence* (3rd ed.). ANZCA & FPM, Melbourne.

Malignant Hyperthermia Association of the United States of America (MHAUS). (2014). What causes a malignant hyperthermia episode? Retrieved from http://www.mhaus.org/faqs/about-mh

Marucci, M., Cinella, G., Perchiazzi, G., Brienza, N., & Fiore, T. (2007). Patient-requested neuraxial analgesia for labor. *Anesthesiology, 106,* 1035–1045.

Melzack, R., & Wall, P. D. (1965). Pain mechanisms: A new theory. *Science, 150,* 971–979.

Merchant, R., Bossenberg, C., Brown, K., Chartrand, D., Dain, S., Dobson, J., et al. (2010). Guidelines to the practice of anesthesia, revised edition 2010. *Canadian Journal of Anesthesia, 57,* 58–87. doi:10.1007/s12630-009-9209-4

Morrison, L. M., Wildsmith, J. A., & Ostheimer, G. W. (1996). History of pain in childbirth. In A. Van Zundert & G. W. Ostheimer (Eds.), *Pain relief and anesthesia in obstetrics.* New York: Churchill Livingstone.

Munnur, U., & Suresh, M. S. (2009). Difficult airway management in the pregnant patient. In B. A. Bucklin, D. R. Gambling, & D. Wlody (Eds.). *A practical approach to obstetric anesthesia.* Philadelphia, PA: Lippincott, Williams & Wilkins.

Munoz, C., & Luckmann, J. (2005). *Transcultural communication in nursing* (2nd ed.). Albany, NY: Thompson Delmar Learning.

Nystedt, A., Edvardsson, D., & Willman, A. (2004). Epidural analgesia for pain relief in labour and childbirth: A review with a systematic approach. *Journal of Clinical Nursing, 13*(4), 455–466.

Panzer, O., Ghazanfari, N., Sessler, D. I., Yucel, Y., Greher, M., Akca, O., et al. (1999). Shivering and shivering-like tremor during labor with and without epidural analgesia. *Anesthesiology, 90*(6), 1609–1616.

Ramsay, M. A. (2006, January). John Snow MD: Anaesthetist to the Queen of England & Pioneer epidemiologist. *Proceedings (Baylor University Medical Center), 19*(1), 24–28.

Reproductive Care Programme of Nova Scotia. (2004). *Labour analgesia guidelines for obstetrical practice.* Halifax, Nova Scotia: Author.

Rice Simpson, K., & Creehan, P. A. (2008). *Perinatal Nursing.* Philadelphia, PA: AWHONN & Lippincott Williams & Wilkins.

Rooks, J. P. (2011). Safety and risks of nitrous oxide labor analgesia: A review. *Journal of Midwifery and Womens Health, 56,* 557–565.

Rooks, J. P. (2012). Labor pain management other than neuraxial: What do we know and where do we go next? *Birth, 39*(4), 318–322.

Rosen, M. (2002). Nitrous oxide for relief of labor pain: A systematic review. *American Journal of Obstetrics and Gynecology, 186*(5), S110–S126.

Sekhavat, L., & Behdad, S. (2009). The effects of meperidine analgesia during labor on fetal heart rate. *International Journal of Biomedical Science, 5*(1), 59–62.

Shipton, E. (2013). The pain experience and sociocultural factors. *The New Zealand Medical Journal, 126*(1370), 7–9.

Simkin, P., & Bolding, A. (2004). Update on nonpharmacologic approaches to relieve labor pain and prevent suffering. *Journal of Midwifery and Women's Health, 49*(6), 489–504.

Simpson, P. A. (2008). Pain relief and comfort measures in labor. In K. R. Simpson & P. A. Creehan (Eds.), *AWHONN's perinatal nursing* (3rd ed. pp. 443–472). Philadelphia, PA: Lippincott Williams & Wilkins.

Springhouse Corporation. (2006). *Nursing herbal medicine handbook* (3rd ed.). Philadelphia, PA: Lippincott Williams & Wilkins.

The Society of Obstetricians and Gynaecologists of Canada (SOGC). (2007). Fetal health surveillance: Antepartum and intrapartum consensus guideline. *Journal of Obstetrics and Gynaecology Canada, 29*(9 suppl 5), S1–S53.

Volikas, I., Butwick, A., Wilkinson, C., Pleming, A., & Nicholson, G. (2005). Maternal and neonatal side-effects of Remifentanil patient-controlled analgesia in labour. *British Journal of Anaesthesia, 95,* 504–509.

Volmanen, P., Valanne, J., & Alahuhta, S. (2004). Breast-feeding problems after epidural analgesia for labour: A retrospective cohort study of pain, obstetrical procedures and breast-feeding practices. *International Journal of Obstetric Anesthesia, 13*(1), 25–29.

Wappler, F. (2001). Malignant hyperthermia. *European Journal of Anaesthesiology, 18,* 632–652.

Wilson, B. A., Shannon, M. T., & Shields, K. L. (Eds.) (2010). *Nurse's drug guide: 2010.* Upper Saddle River, NJ: Prentice Hall.

Wilson, M. J., MacArthur, C., Cooper, G. M., Bick, D., Moore, P. A., & Shennan, A. (2010). Epidural analgesia and breastfeeding: A randomised controlled trial of epidural techniques with and without fentanyl and a non-epidural comparison group. *Anaesthesia, 65*(2), 145–153. doi:10.1111/j.1365-2044.2009.06136.x

Wong, C. A. (2010). Obstetric pain. In S. M. Fishman, J. C. Ballantyne, & J. P. Rathmell (Eds.), *Bonica's management of pain* (4th ed.). Baltimore, MD: Lippincott, Williams & Wilkins.

POSTPARTUM PERIOD AND NEWBORN CARE

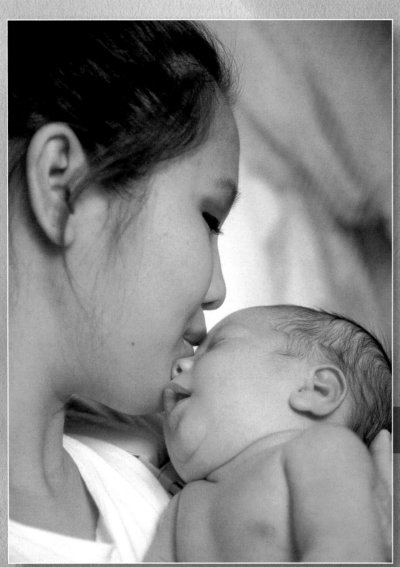

UNIT 5

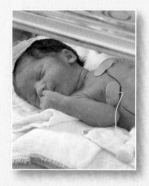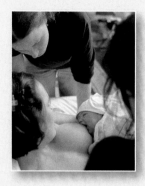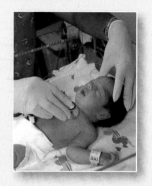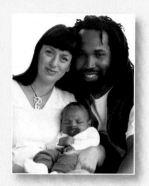

Rapid changes mark the first days and weeks after a baby enters the world, both for mother and newborn, as well as for their family and support people. The maternal body begins its gradual return to the nonpregnant state, the duration of which is influenced by the choice of newborn feeding method, the woman's own unique physiology, the conditions under which she is making the transition to motherhood, and other factors. Under normal circumstances, the newborn is embarking on a series of rapid and remarkable changes that allow him or her to not only survive but also to thrive in the extrauterine environment.

This unit describes normal and unexpected maternal physiologic and psychological changes throughout the first 6 weeks after childbirth, as well as collaborative care provisions for the new family. It explores the healthy baby's immediate postbirth transitions, as well as topics of importance to new parents for their child's initial weeks of life. The unit reviews important details about newborn feeding for both nursing and nonnursing families. It also covers common problems that newborns can face as a result of size, gestational age, congenital or acquired conditions, or other factors, and collaborative strategies for managing them.

CHAPTER 18

Fourth Stage of Labour and Postpartum Period

Robin J. Evans

Nadia, 27 years old, has just given vaginal birth to a viable, healthy boy after 18 hours of labour. Nadia required a midline episiotomy. The placenta was delivered intact. Nadia's life partner, Chelsea, is in the labour suite attending the birth. Chelsea asks, "What happens now?"

Jody, 32 years old, is single and gave birth to her first child 3 days ago in the local hospital. Jody and her daughter were discharged home on the second postpartum day. The nurse from the health care facility's early discharge program arrives at Jody's house for a routine follow-up visit 4 days later. A tearful Jody states, "The baby's been really fussy and has hardly slept since we got home. I don't know how to make her stop crying." Jody also reports that her "bottom" is sore and that her breasts "hurt a fair amount."

Nurses working with these and similar clients need to understand this chapter to care for clients immediately after they have given birth and in the weeks that follow. Before beginning, consider the following points related to the above scenarios.

- What care is appropriate for the maternal client immediately after giving birth? How can health care providers appropriately involve spouses, partners, and other support people?
- What physical, psychological, emotional, and other effects might early discharge from health care facilities have on new mothers and their families? How can nurses help prepare clients for the challenges ahead?
- What behaviours and responses by clients and their families during the postpartum period would you consider "normal" reactions? What behaviours and responses would require nursing intervention?

On completion of this chapter, the reader should be able to:
- Discuss expected physiologic and psychological variations during the fourth stage of labour and postpartum.
- Identify the etiologies of physical and psychological changes during the fourth stage of labour and postpartum.
- Summarize the areas of focus in assessment during the fourth stage of labour.
- Explain comprehensive collaborative care of the woman during the postpartum period.
- Discuss teaching strategies to enhance the health, comfort, and psychological well-being of the postpartum woman.

afterpains
boggy uterus
colostrum
engorgement
episiotomy
erythroblastosis fetalis
family-centred maternity and newborn care
fourth stage of labour
hemolytic disease of the newborn
hemorrhoids
involution

Kegel exercises
Lesbian, gay, bisexual, transgender (LGBT)
lochia
lochia alba
lochia rubra
lochia serosa
postpartum blues
postpartum weight retention
puerperium
subinvolution
uterine atony

The birth of an infant signals the beginning of a new chapter in the life of the mother and her significant others. It also initiates several changes within the client's body, with both physiologic and psychological effects.

In this chapter we focus on maternal physiologic and psychological changes during the fourth stage of labour and puerperium (postpartal period). The fourth stage of labour begins after delivery of the placenta and lasts until 1 hour postpartum (see Chapter 15). The **puerperium** consists of the first 6 weeks following childbirth. The content in this chapter provides information important in assisting nurses to conduct appropriate assessments and interventions for prevention of maternal complications and promotion of a healthy mother and baby. Chapter 19 describes care in high-risk postpartum situations in detail.

PHYSIOLOGIC CHANGES

During pregnancy, all maternal body systems experience many progressive changes over 9 months. Starting with the fourth stage of labour and for several weeks to months after, these changes revert as the client's body returns to a nonpregnant state.

Weight

Immediately following birth, clients lose approximately 5 to 6 kg, which is largely a combination of uterine contents and blood (Cunningham et al., 2010). Weight loss then tends to fluctuate in the first 2 to 3 weeks postpartum, plateauing over the remainder of the 6 weeks postpartum (Walker et al., 2006).

By 6 to 18 months postpartum, women weigh an average of 3.6 kg more than they did before pregnancy (Gore et al., 2003; Olson et al., 2003). This phenomenon has now been coined "**postpartum weight retention**," and defined as "the difference between weight at 'some time after delivery' and weight prior to pregnancy" (Slotkin & Herbold, 2010, p. 256). Recent studies (Lipsky et al., 2012) have suggested that this weight gain is more likely to have occurred between 1 and 2 years postpartum. Factors associated with increased postpartum weight include excess weight prior to pregnancy, smoking cessation during pregnancy, reduced postpartum physical activity, lifestyle changes that may contribute to obesity, stress, weight gain during pregnancy, and health problems such as depression (Biesmans et al., 2013; Olson et al., 2003; Slotkin & Herbold, 2010). It is often a challenge to balance the demands of postpartum life, such as lack of sleep, time, and differing levels of support, with weight management (Montgomery et al., 2011; Montgomery et al., 2013) (see Research Highlight 18.1). Studies have not shown lactation to have statistically significant effects on postpartum weight loss, contrary to a popular notion (Dewey, 2004; Goldberg, 2005; Montgomery et al., 2013).

Cardiovascular System

Once the fetus and placenta are delivered, the maternal body begins to return to its prepregnant state. The blood flow to the uteroplacental unit that increased during pregnancy is diverted to the systemic maternal circulation immediately after delivery of the placenta (James, 2014). The woman loses approximately 500 mL of blood with a vaginal birth, and 1000 mL or more with a cesarean birth (Gabel & Weeber, 2012; James, 2014; Leduc et al., 2009). Plasma volume decreases initially by as much as 1,000 mL from this blood loss, but increases again by the third postpartum day as fluid shifts from the extracellular space into the vascular space (James, 2014). Overall blood volume in the postpartum client is decreased, resulting from blood loss during birth and diuresis in the first postpartum week (James, 2014). Blood volume returns to prepregnant values by approximately 1 week postpartum (Cunningham et al., 2010).

Cardiac output, which increases by as much as 40% during pregnancy, remains elevated for approximately 48 hours postpartum. The cause is thought to be primarily increased stroke volume from venous return (Cunningham et al., 2010). Cardiac output returns to prepregnancy values by 1 to 3 weeks postpartum (Cunningham et al., 2010).

Pulse rate remains stable or decreases following birth (James, 2014). A pulse rate higher than 100 beats/minute may indicate postpartum hemorrhage or infection (see Chapter 19). A rise in blood pressure is common in the first 4 to 5 days postpartum (Magee & von Dadelszen, 2013). Blood pressure may remain elevated, however, in women who had gestational hypertension or preeclampsia, hypertension before pregnancy, or late onset preeclampsia (see Chapter 13).

● RESEARCH HIGHLIGHT 18.1   Postpartum Weight Loss: Weight Struggles, Eating, Exercise, and Breastfeeding

OBJECTIVE

To gain a better understanding of women's experiences and struggles in losing weight gained from pregnancy.

DESIGN

This qualitative study used the phenomenology method to understand the experience from the women's perspectives.

PARTICIPANTS AND SETTING

Twenty-four women who were between 25 and 35 years with one to four children between the ages of 2 months and 5 years were interviewed in a private location following informed consent. A second brief interview, lasting about 15 minutes, provided an opportunity to ensure the information obtained from the first interview was correct and complete. The researcher also used the second interview to reinforce the emerging themes. All interviews were analyzed simultaneously with data collection.

RESULTS

Overall, the experience of trying to lose weight was described by the women as achieving balance between their various life roles and other life and family demands. Common themes were weight struggles, exercise, breastfeeding, healthier food consumption choices, and pregnancy contributions to weight gain.

The themes identified were consistent with the triad of nutrition, weight, and physical activity; each influences the others. Women identified that they struggled to lose weight during the postpartum period. Identified practice implications included the need for anticipatory guidance about the realities of postpartum weight loss; individualized strategies that consider the woman's feelings, assist her to remove barriers, and encourage her to make healthy choices in diet and exercise; and programs based on her interest in, and readiness to, make a change.

CONCLUSION

Women struggle to balance successes and setback in losing weight during the postpartum period. Nurses are in a key position to assist these women in their transition to parenthood, including weight maintenance, healthy eating behaviors, and sufficient physical activity.

From Montgomery, K. S., Best, B., Aniello, T. B., Phillips, J. D., & Hatmaker-Flanigan, E. (2013). Postpartum weight loss: Weight struggles, eating, exercise, and breast-feeding. *Journal of Holistic Nursing, 31*(2), 129–138. doi:10.1177/0898010112464120.

Within the puerperium, clients have increased blood coagulability; plasma fibrinogen and sedimentation rate remain elevated, especially in the first week (Cunningham et al., 2010; James, 2014). This increased coagulability corresponds with an increased risk for thromboembolism in the puerperium.

Hematologic System

Following birth, the client's hemoglobin and hematocrit values fluctuate. By 6 weeks postpartum, hemoglobin rises to nonpregnant values (120 to 160 g/L) (Cunningham et al., 2010). Any significant blood loss during labour and birth results in a decreased hemoglobin value that will take longer to return to normal (Cunningham et al., 2010).

Most women regain normal serum iron levels (7 to 32 mmol/L) by the second week of the puerperium (James, 2014). The most common causes of postpartum anemia are iron deficiency and hemorrhage (Cunningham et al., 2010). These causes may be linked in that significant hemorrhage in one pregnancy with subsequent depletion of iron stores may contribute to iron-deficiency anemia in a later pregnancy (Cunningham et al., 2010). Clients who had iron-deficiency anemia and took a prenatal iron supplement may need to continue the supplement for some time postpartum.

Abruptio placentae, placenta previa, and **uterine atony** (failure of the uterus to contract) are all significant causes of postpartum hemorrhage (see Chapter 19). Because of the risk for decreased perfusion to vital organs, hemorrhage requires aggressive collaborative management. Once hypovolemia is under control, the primary health care provider usually orders the administration of iron supplements for the resulting anemia.

Leukocytosis is common in the postpartum period, with white blood cell (WBC) counts elevated to 25,000 to 30,000 × 10^9/L (Cunningham et al., 2010; James, 2014). This leukocytosis is nonpathologic, with granulocytes predominant. The relative lymphopenia (decreased lymphocytes) and absolute eosinopenia (decreased eosinophils) that may be seen, along with an elevated erythrocyte sedimentation rate (ESR), may complicate assessment of infections. A 30% increase in WBC count over a 6-hour period requires further investigation for possible infection.

Respiratory System

Following childbirth, maternal progesterone levels, intra-abdominal pressure, and diaphragmatic pressure all decrease. These changes result in the respiratory system returning quickly to a prepregnant state. Breathing becomes easier as the client expels the uterine contents. With more cesarean births being done with spinal or epidural anaesthesia, effects on the respiratory system that previously resulted from the use of general anaesthesia are decreasing.

Gastrointestinal System

After birth, maternal abdominal muscles that were stretched during pregnancy remain relaxed. This relaxation, combined with decreased gastrointestinal motility that may result from labour and birth, may lead to gaseous distention (James, 2014). This finding may be especially prevalent in women who have had a cesarean birth, as a result of manipulation of the abdominal contents. Decreased motility may predispose the woman to paralytic ileus. Thus, clients who undergo cesarean birth usually receive only clear fluids until bowel sounds are present, followed by solids. Heartburn during pregnancy usually resolves by approximately 6 weeks postpartum as pressure on the esophageal sphincter and stomach decrease following birth.

Women may continue to experience constipation in the postpartum period, although the underlying reasons for it differ from those during the antepartum period. Postpartally, fear of pain or tearing of sutures may lead to reluctance to defecate, increasing the incidence of constipation. Other contributing factors may include dehydration, immobility, and use of medications such as iron preparations and codeine. **Hemorrhoids** (rectal varicose veins that protrude from the anus or are hidden internally) during pregnancy may be more prominent following labour and birth. They may cause discomfort and also contribute to constipation. Women usually have a bowel movement within the first several days after childbirth. Normal bowel function returns in approximately 2 weeks.

Integumentary System

Following childbirth, skin hyperpigmentation that resulted in chloasma (mask of pregnancy) disappears. Chloasma may reappear, however, if the woman experiences excessive sun exposure or takes oral contraceptives (Tunzi & Gray, 2007). Striae gravidarum, or "stretch marks," begin to fade to a silvery white.

Abdominal muscle distention during pregnancy that results in separation of the rectus muscles may persist after birth. With proper exercise and limited stress placed on these muscles, they usually reapproximate and heal by the late postpartum period.

Endocrine System

During pregnancy, the placenta produces large amounts of estrogen and progesterone, causing significant elevations of these hormone levels from the nonpregnant state. With delivery of the placenta, estrogen and progesterone levels sharply decrease (Cunningham et al., 2010; James, 2014). Prolactin, a hormone secreted by the anterior pituitary gland, promotes milk secretion

(Hall, 2011). The concentration of prolactin begins to rise in the fifth week of pregnancy and continues until birth, when it reaches a level 10 to 20 times that of the nonpregnant level (Hall, 2011). The high levels of estrogen and progesterone during pregnancy inhibit secretion of milk; their decrease at birth initiates the client's ability to lactate (Hall, 2011). Plasma prolactin levels fall to the prepregnant state over the first few weeks following birth; however, the levels surge and rise with each act of suckling by the infant (Cunningham et al., 2010; Hall, 2011).

Remember Nadia, who has just given birth to a son. What hormonal changes would the nurse expect Nadia to be experiencing at present?

During pregnancy, the thyroid gland increases up to 50% from its prepregnancy state, with a corresponding rise in production of thyroxine, primarily from placental secretion of human chorionic gonadotropin (hCG) (Hall, 2011). Thyroid hormone levels normally return to prepregnancy values approximately 4 to 6 weeks postpartum (James, 2014). Immunosuppression, a normal physiologic consequence of pregnancy, may result in the development of transient thyroiditis and hypothyroidism, which can become permanent (Sarvghadi et al., 2005). Accompanying symptoms include memory loss, lack of concentration, and depression (Lazarus, 2005). The basal metabolic rate (BMR), which was elevated during pregnancy partly because of increased adrenocortical hormones and increased thyroxin levels, returns to normal within 7 to 14 days postpartum.

Postpartum glucose levels often fall as a result of delivery of the placenta and the resulting loss of its hormones, such as human placental lactogen (hPL). As the client loses the insulin resistance produced by hPL, her blood glucose levels also decrease. The client with type 1 diabetes mellitus experiences reduced insulin requirements postpartum and will need adjustments to her insulin dosages. Breastfeeding may contribute to hypoglycemia.

Reproductive System

The reproductive system probably experiences the greatest postpartum changes of all. As during pregnancy, the most noticeable changes occur in the uterus (see Chapter 12).

Uterus

The uterine body consists primarily of myometrium covered by serosa and lined by basal decidua (Cunningham et al., 2010). Once its contents are expelled with birth

of the newborn and delivery of the placenta, the uterine cavity collapses. The uterus contracts and the myometrial cells begin to shrink (Cunningham et al., 2010; James, 2014). This process of contraction and shrinkage is referred to as **involution**.

The uterus weighs approximately 1,000 g after birth. With involution, it decreases to 500 g by 1 week postpartum, 300 g at 2 weeks postpartum, and finally to 100 g or less by 6 weeks postpartum (Cunningham et al., 2010; James, 2014). Immediately after birth, the uterine fundus is palpable slightly below the level of the umbilicus. After the first 2 days, the fundus descends into the pelvis at a rate of approximately 1 cm/day until it returns to its previous prepregnant size by approximately 4 to 6 weeks postpartum (Cunningham et al., 2010; James, 2014). This rate is highly individualized, however, and thus may not follow a specific schedule (Marchant, 2009) (Fig. 18.1).

During the first few days postpartum, the uterus continues to contract. In primiparas, contractions are usually tonic, that is, continuous. In multiparas, the uterus periodically contracts vigorously, causing cramps referred to as **afterpains**. Although seen primarily in multiparas, some primiparas also experience afterpains (Cunningham et al., 2010; Marchant, 2009). Women tend to feel afterpains more severely during breastfeeding, probably because the process of nursing stimulates the release of oxytocin from the posterior pituitary gland (Cunningham et al., 2010).

The decidua basalis separates into two layers: basal and superficial (Cunningham et al., 2010; James, 2014). As the superficial layer is sloughed off, vaginal discharge, termed **lochia**, results (Cunningham et al., 2010). Erythrocytes, shreds of decidua, epithelial

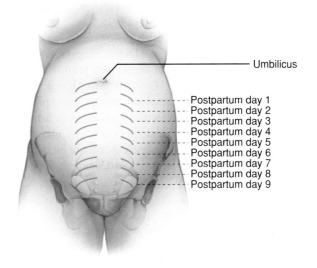

Umbilicus
Postpartum day 1
Postpartum day 2
Postpartum day 3
Postpartum day 4
Postpartum day 5
Postpartum day 6
Postpartum day 7
Postpartum day 8
Postpartum day 9

FIGURE 18.1 Progression of uterine involution during the postpartal period.

cells, and bacteria are visible microscopically in lochia (Cunningham et al., 2010). For the first 3 to 4 days, enough blood is in the lochia to make it appear dark red (**lochia rubra**). By 4 to 5 days, less blood is present and the lochia becomes progressively paler (**lochia serosa**). By approximately the 10th day, increased leukocytes and decreased fluid content combine to give the lochia a white or yellowish white appearance (**lochia alba**). Lochia may continue for up to 4 weeks postpartum (Cunningham et al., 2010). The total volume of lochia is approximately 150 to 400 mL (James, 2014). Its flow may increase concurrently with breastfeeding and after-pains, probably from the secretion of oxytocin, which stimulates uterine contractions.

 Think back to Jody, the single mother who was discharged home on her second postpartum day and is receiving routine follow up 4 days later. Where would the nurse expect to assess Jody's uterine fundus? What type of lochia would be expected?

The endometrium regenerates by the third week postpartum, and the placental site takes approximately 6 weeks to heal (Cunningham et al., 2010). Immediately after birth, the site measures approximately 8 to 10 cm, decreasing rapidly until the end of the second week, when it is approximately 3 to 4 cm in diameter (James, 2014). The placental site heals from the margins, preventing the formation of scar tissue. During this process, necrotic tissue is exfoliated and sloughed off, sometimes resulting in a slightly increased vaginal flow that lasts only 1 to 2 hours (Cunningham et al., 2010). If the site does not heal properly, postpartal hemorrhage may occur (see Chapter 19).

Subinvolution, an arrest or slowing of involution, is characterized by prolonged lochia, irregular or excessive uterine bleeding, and sometimes profuse hemorrhage (Cunningham et al., 2010; MacMullen et al., 2005). The primary cause of subinvolution is failure of the uterus to contract effectively, resulting in a **boggy uterus**. The main contributors to a boggy uterus are retention of placental tissue and exposure of large blood vessels after placental separation (Cunningham et al., 2010; MacMullen et al., 2005).

Cervix

The cervix and lower uterine segment remain thin after birth. Cervical lacerations may be present, especially along the lateral outer margin, which corresponds with the external os (Cunningham et al., 2010). Women who have had a precipitous labour, an instrument-assisted

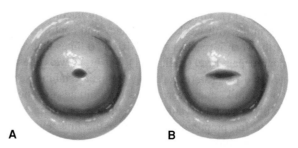

FIGURE 18.2 The cervical os in a client who has never been pregnant **(A)** and after giving birth **(B)**.

birth (e.g., forceps or vacuum extractor) are at greatest risk for cervical lacerations (Melamed et al., 2009). It is unclear whether or not cervical cerclage during pregnancy is also a risk factor, as research has resulted in contradictory results (Melamed et al., 2009; Seravalli et al., 2013).

The cervical os contracts slowly, continuing to admit two fingers until the end of the first postpartum week, when it narrows to 1 cm. By this time, the cervix has begun to thicken and elongate. Cervical edema may be present for several months after childbirth (James, 2014).

The cervix never returns to its pregravid state (Fig. 18.2). The os continues to be slightly wider than previously, with depressions where lacerations occurred (Cunningham et al., 2010). The lower uterine segment contracts much less forcefully than does the remainder of the uterus. It does, however, eventually return to a smaller isthmus between the uterine body and the internal cervical os (Cunningham et al., 2010).

Ovaries

For the first several weeks following birth, there is minimal gonadotropin activity (James, 2014). Menstruation usually returns approximately 6 to 10 weeks postpartum for the nonlactating client and 8 weeks to 18 months postpartum for the breastfeeding client. Ovulation can occur as early as 25 days postpartum, although it may not occur in lactating women until several weeks after cessation of nursing (Cunningham et al., 2010; Hall, 2011; James, 2014). Researchers hypothesize that elevated prolactin levels suppress secretion of gonadotropic hormones in lactating women, which partly accounts for the delayed return of menstruation (Hall, 2011; James, 2014). Approximately 25% of women ovulate before the first menses (James, 2014); the remainder do not ovulate until after menses returns. Ovulation will occur in 20% of lactating women within the first 6 months postpartum (Bouchard et al., 2012).

Vagina

The vagina and vaginal wall may appear smooth and bruised in the early postpartum period. The bruising tends to disappear quickly, partly from decreased pelvic congestion. Rugae reappear in the vagina approximately 3 weeks postpartum (James, 2014). The voluntary muscles of the pelvic floor, often lax in the early puerperium, regain their tone after approximately 6 weeks. Because the lactating woman often has a high circulating estrogen level as a result of ovarian suppression, the return of rugae may be delayed.

Breasts

Postpartum changes in the breasts are primarily related to the client's newborn feeding decision. Delivery of the placenta and the subsequent sudden decrease in circulating progesterone and estrogen stimulate the anterior pituitary to secrete prolactin (see Chapter 21). Repeated sucking by the infant stimulates the release of prolactin and affects the intensity and duration of lactation (Cunningham et al., 2010; Hall, 2011). Prolactin levels are high for approximately the first 10 days postpartum before declining slowly over the next 6 months (Janke, 2014).

The neurohypophysis secretes oxytocin, which stimulates contractions of the uterus, myoepithelial cells in the alveoli, and small milk ducts (Cunningham et al., 2010; Hall, 2011) (Fig. 18.3). Women sometimes feel the "let-down reflex," the sensation that accompanies the release of oxytocin and contractions of the alveoli and small milk ducts in the breast, as a tingling or heaviness in the breast (Janke, 2014). It is stimulated primarily by the infant sucking on the breast, but it also may be stimulated by the sound of the infant's cry. See Chapter 21 for further discussion of breastfeeding.

Production of milk is closely related to the infant's demands. Efficient nursing, in which the breasts are emptied with each feeding, results in a quicker synthesis of milk with a higher fat content. Milk production is slower in the client whose infant does not empty the breast completely at each feeding.

Clients may experience breast discomfort, leakage, and **engorgement** (swelling of breast tissue caused by congestion and increased vascularity). This tends to peak at approximately 3 to 5 days postpartum. In clients who choose not to breastfeed, the engorgement will recede because of lack of breast stimulation (Janke, 2014).

Urinary System

Diuresis occurs between postpartum days 2 and 5 as the body reverses the increased extracellular fluid

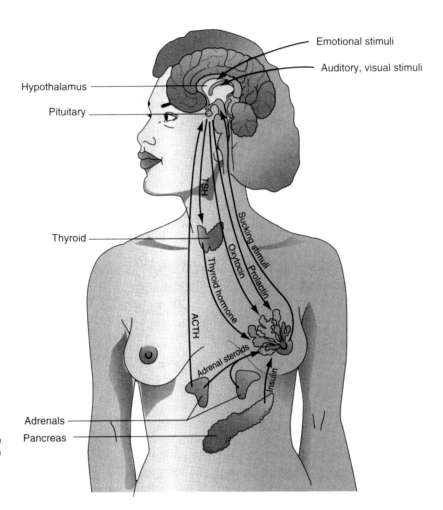

FIGURE 18.3 Stimulation of the hormones responsible for lactation by the newborn's suckling. ACTH, adrenocorticotropic hormone; TSH, thyroid-stimulating hormone.

that accumulated during the pregnancy (Datta et al., 2010). The bladder often has an increased capacity and decreased sensation to intravesical fluid pressure, leading to problems of urinary retention and overdistention. Other contributing factors include any anaesthesia used during labour and birth, perineal lacerations, hematomas, generalized swelling and bruising of the perineum, as well as alterations in bladder neural function. Urinary retention can lead to uterine atony and the possibility of postpartum hemorrhage (see Chapter 19). Bladder distention is evident when the fundus is found higher in the abdomen and off to the right as the full bladder displaces the uterus. Spontaneous voiding should resume within 8 hours after birth. Bladder tone should return by postpartum day 5 to 7. Carpal tunnel syndrome that the woman may have experienced during pregnancy resolves as diuresis reverses the edema that caused pressure on the median nerve (Pazzaglia et al., 2005).

The dilated ureters and renal pelves that accompany pregnancy return to the prepregnant state by approximately 2 to 8 weeks postpartum (Cunningham et al., 2010). Glomerular filtration rate (GFR) and renal blood flow return to normal prepregnant values within 6 weeks (James, 2014).

Postpartum clients may develop or continue to have stress incontinence. This finding occurs primarily in clients who experienced stress incontinence during pregnancy, had a vaginal delivery, a prolonged second stage of labour, a perineal injury, or a delivery by vacuum or forceps, or who required an **episiotomy** (see Chapter 15) that resulted in impaired muscle function around the urethra (Glazener et al., 2006; Svare et al., 2013; Wesnes et al., 2012).

Glycosuria disappears; creatinine clearance is usually normal by 1 week postpartum. Mild proteinuria, however, may persist for the first day or two. Blood urea nitrogen (BUN) may be increased because of the sloughing of necrotic tissue during involution (James, 2014).

PSYCHOLOGICAL CHANGES AND MATERNAL ADJUSTMENT

Many primiparous clients anticipate that life following birth will be a modified version of their usual circumstances. Adequately preparing for the physical, psychological, social, and emotional changes they will undergo, particularly during the early postpartal period, is challenging. Even a client with previous children who is somewhat prepared for what to expect after a new baby arrives, may sense expectations from others to quickly "pick up the pieces" and carry on with her life, experiencing only joy and delight in her baby (O'Reilly, 2004). While many clients relish their new roles and responsibilities, several challenges, both physiologic and psychological, influence reactions. Various factors can cause the postpartum period to unfold differently than initially expected. Regardless of how much the client and her family may have prepared for the baby, the reality of parenthood is still a significant change. This is true for first-time parents as well as for those who have been parents before.

The time that a postpartum client spends in hospital following childbirth has decreased over recent years, from 2.6 days (5 days for cesarean delivery) in 1995 to 1996 to 2.2 days (3.9 days for cesarean delivery) in 2004 to 2005, the last year this data was collected (Public Health Agency of Canada, 2008). Shorter hospital stays have significant implications for both the care provided in the hospital and the care provided in the community. During her time in the hospital, the mother is expected to demonstrate that she can care for both herself and her baby competently at the same time as she is recovering physically (Bowman, 2005). Because this shortened hospital stay provides little time for new teaching, prenatal classes and appointments have assumed a larger role as opportunities for discussion of care for both mother and infant; evidence shows that often, information provided during prenatal classes about postpartum care is not retained (Razurel et al., 2011). Established discussions during the prenatal period allow teaching directed toward the postpartum client in the hospital to serve as reinforcement of prior learning. Nevertheless, not all pregnant clients participate in prenatal classes or receive adequate prenatal care, so the potential for substantial learning needs is high.

Immediate Reactions

Immediately following birth, the mother often views her newborn in wonderment, closely inspecting and counting fingers and toes (Fig. 18.4). If she intends to breastfeed, initiation at this point is beneficial to both her and

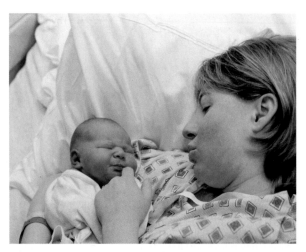

FIGURE 18.4 The new mother bonds with her baby immediately after giving birth.

the baby. The newborn is in a quiet wakeful state, usually ready to feed. Success in initiating breastfeeding at this time provides positive feedback to the client and instils feelings of confidence.

Theories of Change

Development of the maternal role begins during pregnancy and continues in the early postpartum period. Over time, the profile of childbearing women has evolved from one in which most women remained at home, assuming primary responsibility for child care, to that of the contemporary woman who more typically delays childbearing, is employed outside of the home, and is older at the time of a first birth (Emmanuel et al., 2008; Public Health Agency of Canada, 2008). Dominant theories of postpartum change suggest that the process is composed of distinct phases through which the client progresses in a linear fashion, completing each before moving into the next. More contemporary studies indicate that the processes clients experience are much more fluid, complex, and may not be complete until a significant time has elapsed following the birth (Darvill et al., 2010; Emmanuel et al., 2008; Fahey & Shenassa, 2013). Some researchers (Darvill et al., 2010) have found that women report a "roller coaster" type of experience; nearly every aspect of their life is disrupted (Fahey & Shenassa, 2013). Experiences with the transition have an impact on women's self-concept, which changes over the same time. Confounding factors that may interfere with maternal role development include older maternal age, marital status, insufficient social support, and short partner relationships (Emmanuel et al., 2008). Other concerns such as fatigue, pain, self-care deficits (often related to lack of time for self), and care of the infant, house, and family may be significant enough to interfere with activities of daily living, but may be issues for which the women do not seek assistance (Fahey & Shenassa, 2013; Fenwick et al., 2005; Waldenstrom, 2004).

Rubin's theory, developed in 1961, identified that in the first three postpartum days, the new mother often wants to share her experiences of labour and birth with others in an effort to understand and resolve inconsistencies between expectations and reality. However, this generalization does not apply to all women. Some clients may need to discuss and resolve developments during the labour and birth that did not happen as they had anticipated (e.g., the client who anticipated a vaginal birth but instead had a cesarean birth).

Psychosocial tasks that require adaptation include changes in the parental role, alterations in self-perception and body image, and changes in family relationships (Fahey & Shenassa, 2013). Women spend the first few postpartum days focusing on regaining control of their lives and adjusting to the responsibilities of caring for

their infants. Because clients may spend only a small part of this time in a hospital where support is directly available to assist with caring for self and baby, the availability of support in the home and community after discharge assumes new importance (Jack et al., 2005). There may be a correlation between maternal distress and maternal role development (Emmanuel et al., 2011). Other areas of stress are often common "hassles," which may include breastfeeding that is more difficult than the mother expects (Razurel et al., 2011). Contact with other new mothers and pregnant women is an important source of support, although it may be difficult for the woman to achieve (Darvill et al., 2010; Razurel et al., 2011).

Think back to Nadia and her partner Chelsea who have just become parents of a new baby boy. Chelsea asks, "What happens now?" How would you respond?

Sleep Deprivation and Exhaustion

While the mother is working to accept her new reality, she also is concerned with her newborn. Depending on the length and timing of labour and birth, the new mother may be coping with sleep deprivation, which may be aggravated as she contends with multiple interruptions and expectations while tending to her baby's and her needs. Sleep deprivation (including sleep fragmentation) may lead to such problems as seeming disinterest in the baby, mood swings, and difficulty coping (Dennis & Ross, 2005; George, 2005; Park et al., 2013; Ross et al., 2005). Health care providers need to critically assess for signs of sleep deprivation to differentiate behaviours resulting from exhaustion from those caused by true attachment problems. The health care provider may seek information about the amount of sleep that the client is getting, both during the night and with any naps taken during the day. If behaviours such as disinterest or excessive crying are evident despite sufficient sleep, the health care provider may consider alternative reasons for challenges to attachment with the baby.

Emotional State

Society, in general, often has unrealistic expectations of motherhood that are difficult, if not impossible, to attain. The client may expect to be a perfect mother, happy with her child, and able to cope with the baby and all the changes with little or no help; in short, the fairy-tale mother. She or others close to her may assume that the client will have no difficulty in adapting to her multiple roles, bonding with her baby, or coping with the amount of time and the unpredictability of caring for the tiny, helpless newborn. Such expectations tend to be inconsistent with reality (George, 2005). Clients who

● **RESEARCH HIGHLIGHT 18.2**   **Culture and Postpartum Mood Problems: Similarities and Differences in the Experiences of First- and Second-Generation Canadian Women**

OBJECTIVE

To explore the role of culture in experiences of postpartum mood problems (PPMP) between first- and second-generation Canadian women.

DESIGN

The researchers used an exploratory qualitative design.

PARTICIPANTS AND SETTING

Using semistructured interviews, the researchers interviewed nine first-generation and eight second-generation English-speaking women who were clients of a Women's Health Centre in Toronto, Canada. Purposive sampling was used to ensure that participants were from a variety of countries of origin.

RESULTS

Four themes emerged that reflected cultural issues: stigma of PPMP, relationships with parents and/or in-laws, society's expectations of motherhood, and identity issues.

CONCLUSION

The study results contribute to the limited amount of literature on factors that might contribute to PPMP and can inform development of resources for delivering culturally appropriate mental health care for women who experience PPMP. Limitations of the study include a small sample, with recruitment from a single setting.

From Mamisachvili, L., Ardiles, P., Mancewicz, G., Thompson, S., Rabin, K., & Ross, L. E. (2013). Culture and postpartum mood problems: Similarities and differences in the experiences of first- and second-generation Canadian women. *Journal of Transcultural Nursing 24*(2), 162–170.

believe that they should meet these expectations are at risk for compromising their mental health (Mazzeo et al., 2006). Culturally appropriate mental health care should be incorporated into plans for postpartum care (see Research Highlight 18.2).

Estimates are that 26% to 84% of women experience **postpartum blues** (feelings that cause them to cry frequently, often for what they consider no reason), usually within 2 to 3 weeks after giving birth (O'Hara et al., 2014). Symptoms are mild and may include increased emotional lability, crying, emotional sensitivity, loss of appetite, and irritability (O'Hara et al., 2014). Lack of sleep can compound the woman's inability to cope with these symptoms; conversely, the associated emotional lability and crying may affect the woman's ability to achieve a satisfactory amount and quality of sleep to meet her needs. Thus, health care providers should urge women to nap and rest as much as possible whenever the baby is quiet.

Postpartum depression is a more serious condition that is independent of postpartum blues, although the blues are a risk factor for development of depression (O'Hara et al., 2014). Women with postpartum depression experience many emotions including anger, guilt, anxiety, irritability, loneliness, sleep disorders, feelings of being overwhelmed, a sense of failure, and feelings of wanting to harm themselves or their babies (Gaillard et al., 2013; O'Hara et al., 2014). There seems to be no absolute set of symptoms that any woman experiences; each woman's combination of feelings and emotions is unique. Other psychological problems during the postpartum period include postpartum psychosis and postpartum anxiety disorders. See Chapters 5 and 19 for more detailed discussion.

COLLABORATIVE CARE: THE FOURTH STAGE OF LABOUR AND POSTPARTUM PERIOD

Care provided during the fourth stage of labour and the early postpartum period is family centred, where mothers and infants are cared for as a unit and separated only if absolutely necessary (Health Canada, 2000). This is in contrast to previous models of care that separated mothers and newborns for extended periods. The **family-centred maternity and newborn care** model provides the mother and significant others with time to interact with the infant, becoming attuned to his or her schedules and habits (Fig. 18.5).

Most facilities employ one of two models of care for the overall process of labour through postpartum. The first model is referred to as *labour, delivery, recovery, and postpartum (LDRP)*. In LDRP, the client remains in the same room throughout all four phases. In the second model, the client is in one room to experience labour, childbirth, and recovery. She then moves to another room, often on another unit, for her postpartum stay.

Immediate Assessment

Health care providers conduct a focused maternal assessment during the **fourth stage of labour**, the

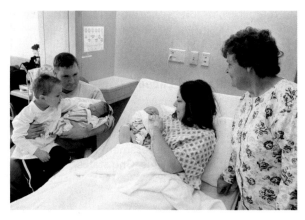

FIGURE 18.5 Family-centred maternity and newborn care allows the family to bond with the newborn during recovery period in the health care facility.

period from delivery of the placenta until 1 hour after birth (Table 18.1). Vital signs, including pulse and blood pressure, are assessed every 15 minutes for the first hour following delivery of the placenta (James, 2014; Weathersby et al., 2008). More frequent monitoring may be required if the woman's condition is unstable. Nursing Care Plan 18.1 highlights the assessment and care of a client in the fourth stage of labour.

The nurse assesses the client's temperature at least once in this first hour. Many clients develop generalized shaking and teeth chattering, as though they were cold, even though temperature remains stable during this time. This response is normal following the stress of labour and birth; a warmed blanket can provide comfort. If the client underwent a cesarean birth with general anaesthesia, assessment of her vital signs also includes evaluation of her respiratory rate.

The nurse assesses the client's uterus every 15 minutes during the fourth stage of labour for fundal height and tone (Nursing Procedure 18.1). The examiner places one gloved hand just above the symphysis pubis, either with the medial side of the hand or the area between the thumb and other fingers in a "V" shape against the client's skin. This positioning guards the uterus and prevents any downward displacement that may result in prolapse or inversion. With the other gloved hand, using the flat side of the fingers and hand and beginning above the umbilicus, the nurse firmly palpates the abdomen and feels for the uterine fundus. The fundus will feel like a hard round object within the abdominal cavity. In the period immediately following birth, the fundus is easily palpable. The examiner assesses the position of the fundus in relation to the umbilicus and measures it in fingerbreadths (e.g., one fingerbreadth above the umbilicus). Immediately following birth, the uterus should be one to two fingerbreadths under the umbilicus, although it is normal to find it up to the height of the umbilicus. The fundus should be in the midline of the abdomen.

During palpation for tone, the fundus should feel hard as a result of uterine contraction. If the uterus is not well contracted, the fundus will feel boggy, soft, or will be difficult to find. The nurse gently massages a boggy fundus with his or her hand, maintaining the position of the second hand that is guarding the uterus until the uterus returns to firm. Once the fundus regains firmness, the nurse discontinues massage. The postpartum woman is at greatest risk for hemorrhage within the first hour following birth because of the exposure of large venous sinuses after placental separation (James, 2014; Weathersby et al., 2008).

(text continues on page 720)

● **TABLE 18.1** **Expected Findings and Alterations During the Fourth Stage of Labour**

Assessment	Expected Findings	Alterations	Possible Causes
Pulse	May be slightly decreased from labour	Rate > 100 beats/min	Postpartum hemorrhage
Blood pressure	Mild rise of approximately 6 mm Hg systolic, 4 mm Hg diastolic	Increases above levels mentioned	Gestational hypertension, preeclampsia, hypertension before pregnancy, late-onset preeclampsia
Temperature	May be slightly increased	>38 °C	Early postpartum infection
Uterus	Fundus usually approximately one to two fingerbreadths below umbilicus, firm and midline	Fundus above umbilicus, deviated from midline	Distended bladder, clots retained in uterus
		Fundus boggy	Uterine atony, retained placental fragments
Lochia	Moderate rubra	More than two pads saturated in 1 hr	Bleeding from lacerations, uterine atony, postpartum hemorrhage
Bladder	Should not be palpable	Distention	Urinary retention
Perineum	Pink, no signs of bruising or edema	Bruising, edema, hematoma	Tissue trauma during delivery

NURSING CARE PLAN 18.1

●

The Postpartum Mother During the Fourth Stage of Labour

Recall Nadia and her partner, Chelsea, the new parents of a healthy baby boy. Nadia is in the fourth stage of labour and Chelsea is at her bedside. They have decided that Nadia will breastfeed the newborn. Maternal assessment reveals that Nadia's fundus is firm and midline at the level of her umbilicus. She states, "I feel cold and tired. I'm a bit sore." Chelsea asks, "Is this normal?"

NURSING DIAGNOSIS

Risk for Injury related to possible complications associated with the fourth stage of labour

EXPECTED OUTCOMES

1. The client will remain free of injury during the fourth stage of labour.

INTERVENTIONS	RATIONALES
Assess vital signs every 15 minutes, including temperature at least once during the first hour.	Fluctuating vital signs provide clues to changes in the client's physiologic status.
Palpate fundus for height, location, and firmness every 15 minutes.	After childbirth, the uterus should be firm and located at the midline.
Massage the uterus if it feels boggy, soft, or difficult to locate; administer medications such as oxytocin as ordered.	A uterus that is not well contracted can predispose the client to hemorrhage. Oxytocin aids in contracting the uterus.
Inspect the lochia for amount, colour, and clots every 15 minutes.	Saturation of more than two perineal pads during this time suggests hemorrhage; clots may suggest uterine atony or retention of placental fragments, predisposing the client to hemorrhage.
Inspect the perineum every 15 minutes for edema, appearance of episiotomy, and possible evidence of lacerations; inspect the episiotomy for intactness and approximation.	Perineal inspection provides clues to possible areas of infection or hematoma formation or unsuspected areas of bleeding. The episiotomy should be intact with well-approximated edges to prevent possible complications.
Apply ice to the perineum.	Ice provides comfort and promotes vasoconstriction.
Palpate the client's bladder for distention; encourage her to void if possible.	A distended bladder interferes with uterine involution, increasing risk for hemorrhage.
Offer the client a warm blanket; change bed clothes and linens frequently.	A warm blanket promotes comfort; chilling and shaking are common after childbirth. Frequent linen changes prevent further chilling from diaphoresis, also common postpartally.

(continued)

NURSING CARE PLAN 18.1 ● The Postpartum Mother During the Fourth Stage of Labour *(Continued)*

INTERVENTIONS	RATIONALES
Provide the client with fluids (intravenously or orally as indicated); provide diet as tolerated and ordered.	The postpartum client is often hungry after childbirth because of energy expended during labour and limited oral intake. Fluids aid in maintaining fluid balance.
Assess the lower extremities for redness, swelling, and warmth.	Postpartum clients are at risk for thrombophlebitis and thrombus formation from an increased hypercoagulable state.
Encourage the client to put the newborn to her breast to feed.	Breastfeeding in this early period helps stimulate milk production and promote attachment.

EVALUATION

1. The client exhibits vital signs and assessment findings within acceptable parameters.
2. The client remains free of any signs and symptoms of complications.

NURSING DIAGNOSIS

Lack of Knowledge related to client's and partner's inexperience with labour, birth, and parenthood

EXPECTED OUTCOMES

1. The client and partner will verbalize understanding of events associated with labour and birth.
2. The client and partner will demonstrate beginning attachment behaviours with the newborn.

INTERVENTIONS	RATIONALES
Assess understanding of postpartum events and care; recognize the client, partner, and newborn as a family unit.	Assessment provides a baseline from which to develop appropriate interventions.
Explore the family's exposure to postpartum and newborn care; ascertain their participation in perinatal education classes; correct any misconceptions or myths related to these methods; allow time for questions.	Information about exposure provides additional foundation for teaching and provides opportunities to clarify or correct misinformation and teach new information.
Explain the various assessments and monitoring that will be done and the information that each can reveal.	This information will help alleviate anxiety about unknown aspects of the process.
Review the measures to facilitate physiologic adjustment during the postpartum period, including self-care measures and the need for adequate rest and nutrition.	Numerous physiologic changes occur during the postpartum period as the client's body returns to her prepregnancy state.

(continued)

NURSING CARE PLAN 18.1 ● The Postpartum Mother During the Fourth Stage of Labour *(Continued)*

INTERVENTIONS	RATIONALES
Assist the family with initial efforts at putting the newborn to the breast; encourage en face positioning, touching, stroking, and talking.	Breastfeeding immediately after birth and interaction with the newborn promote bonding and attachment.
Encourage the partner to assist the client with measures and provide necessary support; discuss ways the partner can participate in breastfeeding, such as the client pumping her breasts and the partner feeding the newborn.	Partner participation promotes sharing of the experience and feelings of control over the situation.
Begin teaching the family newborn care measures as appropriate; when possible, have them demonstrate care.	Initial teaching helps foster independence and self-esteem; return demonstration aids in determining the effectiveness of the teaching.
If necessary, initiate referral for community services to assist with transition.	Additional support from community services may be necessary to promote a positive experience for the family.

EVALUATION

1. The client and partner verbalize understanding of events associated with labour and birth.
2. The client and partner use appropriate behaviours to interact with the newborn.
3. The client and partner verbalize positive statements about their newborn and about themselves as parents.
4. The client and partner demonstrate beginning ability to care for their newborn.

The nurse assesses the woman's lochia every 15 minutes during the fourth stage of labour for colour, amount, and any clots. During this first hour, the expected finding is moderate lochia rubra with no clots. Saturation of more than two pads within this first hour is abnormal (Weathersby et al., 2008). Excessive lochia may indicate uterine atony, retention of placental fragments, or lacerations of the perineum, vagina, or cervix. Assessment of the uterine fundus reveals whether uterine atony is the cause of the excessive bleeding; if atony is present, the nurse begins to massage the fundus. If clots are present and the fundus is found higher than expected, the nurse massages it carefully to expel any clots. If massage does not result in firming of the fundus, health care personnel administer medications often ordered routinely during the fourth stage of labour, such as oxytocin, carboprost, carbetocin, misoprostol, or methylergonovine (Leduc et al., 2009).

Methylergonovine elevates blood pressure and should not be used in any woman with pre-existing high blood pressure. If bleeding continues, the nurse notifies the physician. Bleeding that continues with a contracted uterus may indicate cervical lacerations that have not been repaired adequately or a previously undiagnosed bleeding disorder such as von Willebrand disease (James, 2014).

The nurse assesses the perineum every 15 minutes during the fourth stage of labour. He or she identifies any edema or signs of hematoma (a swollen, discoloured area). If they are present, the nurse applies ice to the affected area. In addition, the nurse evaluates the site of episiotomy or laceration for edema and approximation.

Ongoing Assessment

Ongoing assessments involve those measures performed during the first hour postpartum as well as several

NURSING PROCEDURE 18.1

Assessing the Uterus, Lochia, and Perineum after Vaginal Childbirth

PURPOSE

To evaluate uterine involution after vaginal birth and reduce the risk for postpartum hemorrhage

ASSESSMENT AND PLANNING

- Review the client's intrapartal record for time of childbirth and any possible complications during labour and birth, including the presence of episiotomy.
- Assess the amount of blood loss during birth.
- Determine the time of the last uterine assessment.
- Ask the client about any pain.
- Gather equipment
    - Clean gloves
    - Perineal pads (if not at the client's bedside)
    - Light source (overhead light, penlight, or flashlight)
    - Waterproof linen saver pad

IMPLEMENTATION

1. Explain the procedure and rationale to the client, informing her that she may feel some discomfort, *to aid in alleviating anxiety*.
2. Ask the client when she last voided; have her empty her bladder *to prevent bladder from interfering with uterine involution*; help the client ambulate to the bathroom or offer a bedpan as indicated.
3. Provide for client privacy by drawing the curtain, closing the door, and covering the client with a bath blanket or sheet.
4. Have the client lie supine with her head flat or on a pillow *to assist in accurate assessment of fundal height*. Allow the client to flex her knees if appropriate *to help relax the abdominal muscles*.
5. Put on gloves and expose the abdominal and perineal areas.
6. Place the nondominant hand in a slightly cupped position at the lower fundus just above the symphysis pubis *to help stabilize and support the uterus*.
7. Working from the umbilicus down, gently move the dominant hand down the abdomen until the top of the fundus is located. It should be at the midline and feel hard and round.
8. If the fundus does not feel firm, gently massage the uterus using the dominant hand while maintaining the position of the nondominant hand on the lower uterus *to stimulate uterine contraction and prevent uterine inversion*. Continue to massage the uterus until it becomes firm; avoid massaging that is too vigorous or overmassaging *to prevent uterine muscle exhaustion*.

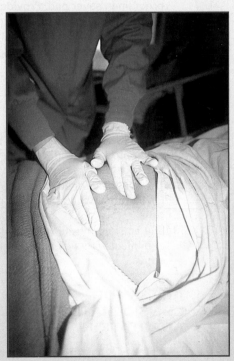

(continued)

NURSING PROCEDURE 18.1 (CONTINUED)
Assessing the Uterus, Lochia, and Perineum after Vaginal Childbirth

9. Using the fingers as a guide, measure the distance from the umbilicus to the top of the fundus in fingerbreadths *to determine the progression of involution.*

10. Remove and inspect the client's perineal pad; note the amount, colour, and character of the drainage.

11. Check under the client's buttocks *to evaluate for any blood that may be pooling there.*

12. Assist the woman to turn on her left side; lift the upper buttock to reveal the perineal area. Inspect the area for changes.

13. Inspect the perineal area *to assess for possible complications.* Include the episiotomy line as appropriate. Note the approximation of the episiotomy edges and the appearance of any drainage. Report any redness, edema greater than minimal, ecchymosis, or hematomas.

14. Assist the client back to the supine position and provide or assist with perineal care. Replace the waterproof linen saver pad. Provide the woman with a clean perineal pad.

15. Remove gloves and discard all used equipment and supplies appropriately.

16. Document findings.

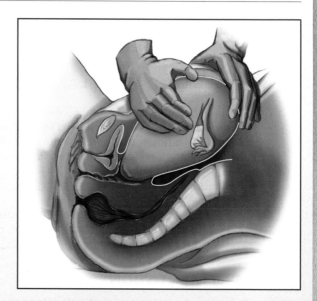

EVALUATION

1. Fundus was firm and midline at the appropriate height for the client's postpartum day.

2. The client exhibited moderate lochia rubra, with minimal to no clots.

3. The episiotomy site was clean, dry, and intact with well-approximated edges.

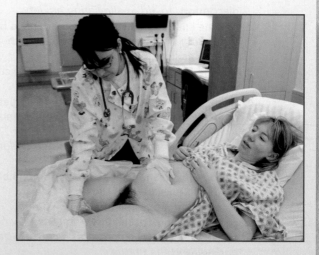

AREAS FOR CONSIDERATION AND ADAPTATION

Perinatal Considerations

- Encourage the client to void before palpation of the fundus. A full

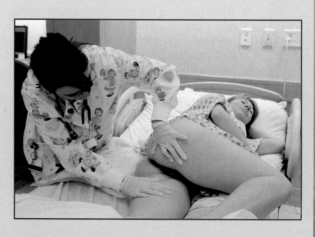

(continued)

NURSING PROCEDURE 18.1 (CONTINUED)

Assessing the Uterus, Lochia, and Perineum after Vaginal Childbirth

bladder can interfere with uterine involution. A uterus that feels boggy and is displaced from midline suggests a full bladder. If the client cannot void after a designated time (e.g., 6 to 8 hours), anticipate the need for catheterization.

- Closely assess the fundus of a client who has given birth to more than one newborn or to a large baby. Uterine overdistention may result, placing the client at risk for uterine atony and subsequent hemorrhage.
- Be alert for other risk factors that may lead to uterine atony and postpartum hemorrhage, including prolonged or difficult labour, placenta previa or abruption, labour induction or augmentation with oxytocin, and use of tocolytics.

Lifespan Considerations

- Closely assess the fundus and lochia of a multiparous client because multiparity is a predisposing risk factor for postpartum hemorrhage.

Community-Based Considerations

- Expect to continue to assess a client's fundus, lochia, and perineum at home visits. The fundus should no longer be palpable by the 10th day postpartum.
- Teach the client how to massage her uterus, inspect her episiotomy site, and monitor her lochia.
- Review signs and symptoms associated with uterine subinvolution, which may lead to late postpartum hemorrhage.
- Instruct the client to notify her primary care provider about any changes in lochia amount, characteristics, and odour or if she experiences any fever.

---

additional components (Table 18.2). Following a systematic regimen that the nurse can repeat multiple times for many clients is most efficient. One of the most common methods is to use the acronym BUBBLES to organize a head-to-toe assessment (Assessment Tool 18.1). When working with postpartum clients, it is important for the nurse to recognize not only any alterations and their significance, but also the interrelationship between changes in body systems and their different manifestations in different assessments.

Vital Signs

Protocols for assessment of pulse and blood pressure vary among institutions; however, most include a schedule of more frequent assessments for the first 24 hours postpartum, which is when the client is at greatest risk for hemorrhage (James, 2014) (Fig. 18.6). An example may include assessment of vital signs every 30 minutes for 1 hour after the first hour of assessments, then every 4 to 6 hours for the remainder of the first 24 hours postpartum. Indications for more frequent monitoring will dictate any necessary variations.

Nurses usually take the client's temperature every 4 to 6 hours postpartum. Temperature may increase minimally in the initial 24 hours postpartum as a result of the dehydration that accompanies prolonged labour. The nurse instructs the client to report any elevation in temperature above 38 °C once she is at home. This finding may indicate a postpartum infection, especially if it occurs in the first 10 days.

Breasts

Assessment of the breasts is related primarily to the client's decision about newborn feeding. For example, slight engorgement in a client who has chosen to breastfeed has different significance than in a client who has chosen to formulafeed. The subsequent plan for nursing actions also differs for each.

The nurse assesses any postpartum client's breasts for symmetry, consistency, and lumps. If the client is breastfeeding, the breasts initially are soft, usually for approximately the first 48 to 72 hours. After this time, milk begins to form, and the breasts fill. As milk production increases, the breasts become fuller and firmer. Veins become more prominent. Some clients experience engorgement, in which the breasts and/or nipples become hard and distended. Engorged breasts are usually extremely uncomfortable and may create breastfeeding difficulties because the infant may have trouble latching onto the nipple.

● TABLE 18.2 **Expected Findings and Alterations in the Postpartum Period**

Assessment	Expected Findings	Alterations	Possible Causes
Pulse, blood pressure, and temperature	Within normal limits	Increased pulse Increased or decreased blood pressure Increased temperature	Postpartum hemorrhage Puerperal infection Late-onset preeclampsia
Breasts	Soft for first 48 to 72 hr If breastfeeding, fuller, firmer breasts, intact nipples If not breastfeeding, breasts may be engorged and leaking by the third day	Engorgement if breastfeeding Painful, reddened, bruised nipples	Incorrect latch Tongue tie
Uterus	Fundus firm, midline, height decreasing approximately one fingerbreadth below umbilicus each day	Fundus higher in abdomen than expected Fundus boggy	Full bladder Retention of placental fragments Subinvolution Uterine atony
Bladder	Voiding, not palpable, diuresis	Decreased sensation to void	Prolonged effects of anaesthesia Altered bladder neural function
Bowels	Bowel sounds Bowel movements	Absent or decreased bowel sounds Constipation	Decreased motility Paralytic ileus Fear of pain, tearing of any sutures Hemorrhoids Dehydration Immobility Medications
Lochia	Gradually decreasing amount, which may increase after breastfeeding or rising from recumbent position Rubra for 3 to 4 d, serosa until day 10, then alba	Increased amount from expected or previously assessed	Uterine atony Retention of placental fragments Postpartum hemorrhage
Episiotomy/perineum	No ecchymosis or edema, sutures (if present) intact and well approximated	Ecchymosis, edema, sutures missing, episiotomy reddened, with discharge, dehiscence, or both	Trauma to tissues during delivery Infection of episiotomy/laceration
Psychosocial	Shares experiences of labour and birth Looks directly at infant (en face position) Touches and talks to baby Interprets baby's behaviour appropriately May have increased emotional lability and sensitivity and cry more between day 3 and week 2	Interacts very little with infant Rarely talks or touches infant Feels angry, guilty, anxious, irritable, lonely, overwhelmed Has difficulty sleeping Feels sense of failure Has thoughts of harming self or baby Palpitations	Fatigue Thyroid dysfunction Postpartum depression Anxiety disorder Postpartum psychosis

● **ASSESSMENT TOOL 18.1**
Postpartum Assessment Guide

B—breasts
U—uterus
B—bladder
B—bowel
L—lochia
E—episiotomy/perineum
S—psychosocial

If the client is breastfeeding, the nurse assesses the nipples for intactness. He or she notes any signs of redness, bruising, or cracking. Bruising appears as black or blue patches, often toward the periphery of the nipple. Cracking usually develops following redness as the nipple is subjected to continued suction from an incorrectly positioned infant's mouth. Assessment of the latch during feeding may reveal reasons for these conditions and provide cues to the nurse for additional teaching that may assist the woman to correct latching issues. See Chapter 21 for further discussion.

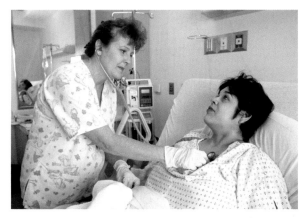

FIGURE 18.6 The nurse checks the client's vital signs as part of postpartum assessment.

If the client is formulafeeding, the nurse checks the nipples for any discharge and the breasts for any lumps or hardness. The client may experience some fullness of her breasts and leaking 1 to 4 days following the birth of her baby (Janke, 2014). The swelling is usually less pronounced than in the mother who is breastfeeding; however, it can be equally painful and disturbing.

Uterus

As discussed earlier, the nurse assesses the client's uterus for fundal height and tone. He or she checks the position of the fundus in relation to the umbilicus and measures it in fingerbreadths (e.g., one fingerbreadth above the umbilicus). By approximately 12 hours after childbirth, the fundus is found at about 1 cm above the level of the umbilicus (Weathersby et al., 2008). It usually decreases by approximately one fingerbreadth per day beginning on day 2 until it can no longer be palpated by approximately day 8 to 10. By that time, it is too low in the abdomen to be felt. The nurse should feel the fundus in the midline of the abdomen. A fundus palpable above the level of the umbilicus and to the right is most frequently the result of a full bladder. For this reason, it is advantageous for the nurse to encourage the client to void before assessment.

Other factors the nurse considers when assessing and interpreting uterine findings include vital signs, particularly the pulse and blood pressure, lochia, and the bladder.

Bladder

The nurse assesses the client's bladder function for amount of urine, frequency of voiding, and any difficulties initiating voiding or emptying the bladder. Some women experience problems with retention, either an inability to void at all or retaining residual urine. Such difficulties may relate to pressure on the bladder during labour and birth, perineal trauma and resulting edema; these may result from a vacuum-assisted delivery, prolonged second state of labour, mediolateral episiotomy, or uterine fundal pressure during the second stage of labour (Pifarotti et al., 2014). If the course of childbirth suggests a risk for these problems, the nurse measures the client's initial voidings until output is adequate.

Urinary frequency typically accompanies diuresis. It also may be present, however, as overflow if the woman does not empty the bladder completely. The nurse palpates the bladder to assess for adequate emptying. A full bladder usually pushes the uterus up in the abdomen, resulting in a fundus higher than expected and shifted to the client's right side. A full bladder is implicated in uterine atony and increased vaginal discharge. Critical thinking in performing any postpartum assessment includes ensuring that the woman has voided prior to the assessment.

Bowel Function

Bowel function is the next area for assessment. The nurse auscultates the client's abdomen for bowel sounds, especially after cesarean birth, during which manipulation of abdominal contents may cause an increase in the potential for an ileus. Sounds should be audible in all four abdominal quadrants. The nurse asks the client whether she has had a bowel movement and if any problems or complications accompanied it. Clients may have some apprehension about having a bowel movement. Concerns are often related to fear of associated discomfort or pain and, for women with episiotomy or lacerations, of "ripping my stitches." Teaching about potential effects of postponing elimination—that is, that retaining feces in the large intestine promotes further absorption of water leading to more difficult passage—may provide the information necessary to make an informed decision. Information also may have the added benefit of providing reassurance.

Lochia

Assessment of lochia is closely tied to assessment of the fundus, bladder, and vital signs, particularly pulse and blood pressure. The nurse assesses the lochia for colour, amount, odour, and presence of clots (see Nursing Procedure 18.1 and Fig. 18.7). The significance of these findings is assessed contextually according to the stage of the postpartum period. Although the greatest risk for postpartum hemorrhage is within the first hour after birth, clients may develop late postpartum hemorrhage between 24 hours and 6 weeks postpartum. Typically, flow decreases over time. The colour of lochia changes from rubra (red) to serosa (pink) by approximately postpartum day 4 or 5. The serosa lochia changes to alba (yellowish white) by approximately day 10.

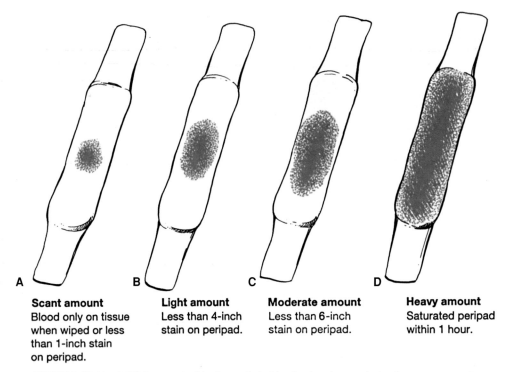

A	**B**	**C**	**D**
Scant amount Blood only on tissue when wiped or less than 1-inch stain on peripad.	**Light amount** Less than 4-inch stain on peripad.	**Moderate amount** Less than 6-inch stain on peripad.	**Heavy amount** Saturated peripad within 1 hour.

FIGURE 18.7 **A:** With scant lochia, just a little bit of colouring or darkening appears to be on the top. **B:** With light lochia, approximately one third of the pad is covered centrally. **C:** With moderate lochia, approximately two thirds of the pad is covered centrally. **D:** With heavy lochia, the whole pad is covered.

If the woman has changed her perineal pad just prior to the assessment, the nurse will not be able to make an accurate assessment. The nurse can either ask the client to refrain from discarding the pad in the garbage and to leave it in the bathroom for assessment, or ask the client to describe her flow. The nurse's decision should be individualized—more likely to visually assess the lochia of the client who has very recently given birth and more likely to consult with the client who is several days postpartum and familiar with the characteristics of her flow.

During the fourth stage of labour, lochia is usually rubra, moderate in amount, and without clots. The client should not saturate more than two pads in the first hour. If the client's flow is heavier or contains clots, the fundus may be atonic, and further interventions would be necessary. The nurse looks for clots, including size and consistency, and differentiates between true clots and tissue. If the material can be easily separated using gloved hands or tongue depressors, it is likely a clot. If separation is difficult or impossible, the nurse suspects the presence of tissue. In this case, the specimen is sent to the laboratory for histologic examination.

Perineum

Before assessing the perineum, the nurse collects information about whether the client had an episiotomy, a laceration, or an intact perineum. If the client received an episiotomy, the nurse also checks whether it was midline or mediolateral. If midline, the nurse may ask the client to lie on either side for the assessment. If the episiotomy is either right mediolateral (RML) or left mediolateral (LML), the client should lie on the side that puts the episiotomy next to the bed. For example, if a client had an LML episiotomy, she should lie on her left side for the assessment; if the client had an RML, she should lie on her right side. Such positioning prevents tension on the episiotomy and sutures, as the nurse lifts the upper cheek of the buttocks to facilitate inspection.

Collection of information about any perineal laceration, including the degree assigned, prepares the nurse for what will be seen. Cervical, first-degree, and second-degree lacerations are rarely visible because the sutures are usually hidden within the vagina, making direct assessment impossible. Visible lacerations, most frequently third and fourth degree, involve structures that the nurse can assess more easily.

To check the episiotomy or lacerations, the nurse dons clean gloves and asks the client to assume a side-lying position on the bed. The nurse lifts the client's upper buttock cheek to allow for adequate light and visualization. Assessment of episiotomy and lacerations follows the same guidelines as for any incision. These include evaluations for redness, edema, ecchymosis, discharge, and approximation (REEDA). The nurse also checks to ensure that any sutures are intact. See Nursing Procedure 18.1.

If the client has no episiotomy or laceration, the nurse assesses the perineum for edema and bruising. Even though the perineum is intact, the client may still experience edema, resulting from prolonged pushing during the second stage or from a large baby. Cool compresses or ice packs are most effective in reducing edema and promoting comfort if applied during the first 24 hours postpartum (Weathersby et al., 2008). The nurse ensures that the cold is not applied directly to the skin, but that a barrier is used for application. After 24 hours, warmth is more appropriate. The nurse encourages the client to use a tub bath to provide warm, moist heat. Alternatively, for the same outcome, the client may use a sitz bath.

Lower Legs

Because the postpartum woman is at increased risk for thrombophlebitis and subsequent development of a thrombus (Jackson et al., 2011), the nurse directs assessment toward early detection of these problems. He or she checks the client's lower legs for any redness, swelling, or warmth that may indicate early thrombophlebitis. Although some agencies have included the use of Homans sign in assessing for thrombophlebitis, it is unreliable and nonspecific and is therefore not recommended (Urbano, 2001).

Psychological and Emotional State

The nurse may perform psychological assessment during the formal assessment as well as during any later interactions (James, 2014). He or she monitors the mother and infant for evidence of attachment behaviours: holding the baby to enable looking directly at him or her ("en face" position), touching and talking to the baby, and interpreting infant behaviour appropriately. The nurse assesses the mother's emotional lability as well as her level of fatigue (Beck & Indman, 2005). Her state of fatigue can have direct implications for behaviours that may be incorrectly assessed as emotional lability. The nurse evaluates the client's teaching needs on an ongoing basis, taking opportunities to educate whenever needs are apparent.

Rectus Muscle

The nurse assesses the client's rectus muscle at least once in the early postpartum period for diastasis or separation. This diastasis may result from the growing uterus and fetus during pregnancy that forces the muscles apart. The client lies supine on the bed without a pillow under her head. The nurse places the index and middle fingers across the muscle and asks the woman to raise her head. This movement results in the rectus abdominis muscles becoming more prominent (Bickley, 2012), making any separation in the muscles easily palpable. The effect of exercise in the presence of diastasis is unclear if nonspecific exercise helps to prevent or reduce the diastasis (Benjamin et al., 2014). Therefore, if the nurse feels a separation of more than two fingers' width, or if "peaking" of the abdominals is visible, it may be prudent to caution the client to avoid exercises that put stress on the abdominal muscles and to avoid any heavy lifting or vacuuming for at least 6 weeks until the muscle can heal. A hernia may result from a diastasis that does not heal.

Rh Status

The Rh antigen is inherited as a dominant factor. The potential for Rh incompatibility exists when the mother is Rh negative (lacks Rh antigen) and the biologic father is Rh positive. If the couple's first fetus is Rh positive, the mother may be sensitized by exposure to the Rh antigen through mixing of fetal and maternal blood. The woman's body recognizes the antigens as foreign and thus begins to make antibodies against them (isoimmunization). Because this process takes time, the first fetus is usually not at any risk for complications. Problems may develop, however, with subsequent pregnancies. If the fetus is Rh positive, the antibodies can cross the placenta, attach to fetal RBCs, and begin to hemolyze them (Liumbruno et al., 2010). This can lead to a fetal anemia called **erythroblastosis fetalis** or **hemolytic disease of the newborn**. Hemolytic disease of the newborn may be possible in a first fetus if the mother was exposed to the antigen because of a fetal maternal hemorrhage during a miscarriage or abortion (Cunningham et al, 2010; Liumbruno et al., 2010).

To prevent hemolytic disease of the newborn, 300 µg of anti-D IgG is given routinely to all Rh-negative women when the fetal blood type is either unknown or known to be Rh positive at 28 weeks' gestation (Fung & Eason, 2003). After any invasive procedures that could result in mixing of maternal and fetal blood (e.g., amniocentesis; chorionic villus sampling; percutaneous blood sampling; induced, spontaneous, or threatened abortion; ectopic pregnancy; or molar pregnancy) women who are Rh negative and nonsensitized should be given 300 µg of anti-D IgG (Cunningham et al., 2010; Fung & Eason, 2003). If the abortion, ectopic pregnancy, or chorionic villous sampling occurs prior to 12 weeks' gestation, 120 µg is given.

Since the introduction of routine prophylaxis with anti-D IgG in Canada in 1976, the incidence of erythroblastosis fetalis has decreased to 0.4 per 1,000 births (Fung & Eason, 2003). Nevertheless, isoimmunization can still happen in clients who either receive an inadequate dose or do not receive the prophylaxis at all. For this reason, the nurse reviews the client's Rh status and administer anti-D IgG as appropriate (see Nursing Procedure 18.2).

NURSING PROCEDURE 18.2
Administering Anti-D IgG

PURPOSE

To prevent Rh isoimmunization in future pregnancies for a woman who is Rh negative with an Rh-positive newborn

ASSESSMENT AND PLANNING

- Assess the maternal blood type to determine whether the client is a candidate for therapy. A candidate for therapy is RhD-negative and has never been sensitized to RhD-positive blood (evidenced by a negative result on the indirect Coombs test), and has given birth within the past 72 hours to an Rh-positive newborn who is not sensitized (as evidenced by negative direct Coombs test).
- Verify the time of newborn birth.
- Check for any possible allergies to immunoglobulins, blood, or blood products.
- Ascertain that the client has signed an informed consent, if required by the health care facility.
- Gather the necessary equipment:
    - Anti-D IgG (standard dose [300 μg])
    - Appropriate-sized syringe and needle for intramuscular injection
    - Alcohol wipes
    - Assess the deltoid site for appropriateness of injection; if the client is extremely thin or a dose larger than standard is ordered, the ventrogluteal or gluteal site may be used.

IMPLEMENTATION

1. Explain the purpose of the anti-D IgG. Inform the client that it is a blood product; answer any questions.
2. Inform the client that the drug is given by intramuscular injection.
3. Prepare the standard dose as ordered in syringe.
4. Confirm the client's identity *to ensure that the right drug is being administered to the right client*.
5. Identify the proper site for injection *to promote optimal absorption*.
6. Prepare the site for injection by wiping with an alcohol wipe using a circular direction *to ensure cleanliness*.
7. Administer the dose intramuscularly into the appropriate site.
8. Discard syringe and needle into sharps container.
9. Document administration of injection, including vial identification number, route, dose, and the client's response.
10. Attach the top copy of the triplicate form to the client's chart; send the remaining two copies back to the laboratory or blood bank with the empty vial.
11. Give the client an identification card identifying her Rh status and use of anti-D IgG; encourage her to keep it with her or in a convenient location.

EVALUATION

1. The client demonstrated understanding of the need for anti-D IgG administration.
2. The client tolerated the injection without incident.

(continued)

NURSING PROCEDURE 18.2 (CONTINUED)
Administering Anti-D IgG

AREAS FOR CONSIDERATION AND ADAPTATION

Perinatal Considerations

- Administer a standard dose of anti-D IgG routinely at 28 weeks' gestation to all women who are Rh negative as prophylaxis to prevent isoimmunization.
- Expect to administer larger than standard doses as ordered in situations involving large amounts of bleeding, such as severe abruptio placentae.
- Administer microdoses of anti-D IgG after spontaneous abortion, elective abortion, ectopic pregnancy, and gestational trophoblastic disease occurring during the first trimester.
- Give anti-D IgG after any maternal trauma, chorionic villi sampling, amniocentesis, and percutaneous umbilical blood sampling.

Community-Based Considerations

- If the client has been discharged early from the health care facility, check to ensure that she has received anti-D IgG before discharge. If not, expect to administer anti-D IgG on the first home visit, which must occur within 72 hours of childbirth.

Select Potential Nursing Diagnoses

The following are examples of commonly applicable diagnoses during the fourth stage of labour and postpartal period:

- **Pain** related to engorgement and nipple discomfort
- **Ineffective Breastfeeding** related to maternal anxiety, lack of knowledge, or difficulty with latch
- **Risk for Decreased Fluid Volume** related to postpartum hemorrhage secondary to uterine atony, retention of placental fragments, or subinvolution
- **Pain** related to continued uterine contractions secondary to involution after delivery
- **Risk for Urinary Retention** related to decreased sensation secondary to pressure on the bladder during labour and childbirth or lingering anaesthesia
- **Risk for Infection** related to urinary retention
- **Risk for Stress Incontinence** related to weak pelvic muscles
- **Risk for Injury** related to possible hemorrhage secondary to uterine atony and resulting increased lochia
- **Risk for Infection** related to organism invasion of placental site, episiotomy, or laceration
- **Pain** related to edema, bruising, hematoma, episiotomy, or laceration
- **Fatigue** related to sleep deprivation during labour and postpartum

- **Risk for Impaired Parent–Infant Attachment** related to fatigue, unrealistic expectations, and depression

Planning/Intervention

Expected outcomes for the postpartum woman are highly individualized and are based on her particular circumstances. Certain outcomes are appropriate for any postpartum woman, however, during the fourth stage of labour and then throughout the postpartum period:

- The client will remain free of any signs and symptoms of infection or injury after delivery.
- The client will exhibit vital signs, uterine involution, and lochia within acceptable parameters.
- The client will rate her pain as tolerable.
- The client will void within 8 hours of childbirth without any signs or symptoms of urinary retention or fluid imbalance.
- The client will demonstrate ability to provide care for herself and her newborn.
- The client will exhibit ability to provide adequate nutrition to the newborn.
- The client will demonstrate appropriate bonding and attachment behaviours with the newborn.

Initially, the client most likely needs close, frequent assessments, and additional instruction and support to achieve these outcomes during the fourth stage of labour. As the postpartum period progresses, the nurse expects that the client will develop increasing independence in caring for herself and her newborn and will demonstrate continued behaviours to foster attachment and bonding with the newborn, thereby promoting the development of trust. In addition, expectations will include the client who demonstrates a return to her prepregnancy level of function, incorporating healthy lifestyle practices to address any prepregnancy areas of concern and measures to balance the need for activity and rest. See Nursing Care Plan 18.2, which addresses the care of a new mother in the postpartum period.

Caring for the Breasts in the Breastfeeding Client

For the breastfeeding client, engorgement often results from vascular congestion and milk stasis, primarily

---

NURSING CARE PLAN 18.2

●

The Postpartum Mother and Newborn at Home

 Recall Jody and her newborn, who were presented at the beginning of this chapter. On inspection, the nurse notices that Jody's episiotomy area is reddened and edematous. Her uterus is firm and approximately 6 cm below the umbilicus. Lochia is moderate and reddish pink. The client's breasts are firm and tender on palpation. Other findings of the physical examination are normal.

Jody is bottlefeeding her newborn. Jody's mother, Olivia, has just arrived to stay at the home for the next 2 weeks. Olivia tells the nurse that she is concerned about Jody and wants to know what she can do to best help her.

NURSING DIAGNOSES

- **Pain** related to breast engorgement and episiotomy
- **Lack of Knowledge** related to measures to promote comfort

EXPECTED OUTCOMES

1. The client will state that breast and episiotomy discomfort has decreased.
2. The client will identify two strategies to decrease discomfort.

INTERVENTIONS	RATIONALES
Ask the client to rate her breast pain on a scale of 1 to 10, with 1 being no pain and 10 being the worst pain; have the client rate her perineal pain in the same manner.	Use of a pain rating scale helps quantify subjective information about the client's pain and provides a baseline from which to plan interventions.
Explain the current physiologic changes and how the body is attempting to heal.	Information about the underlying events associated with pain helps the client understand the normal processes and helps alleviate fears that something is wrong.
Inform the client that breast engorgement typically subsides within 2 to 3 days from the lack of breast stimulation; instruct the client in measures to decrease discomfort, such as applying cool compresses and using a supportive, well-fitting bra.	Knowledge that breast engorgement is a short-term problem along with strategies to promote comfort can assist the client to cope with the situation.

(continued)

NURSING CARE PLAN 18.2 ● The Postpartum Mother and Newborn at Home (Continued)

INTERVENTIONS	RATIONALES
Suggest strategies to alleviate episiotomy discomfort, such as perineal care with warm-water sitz baths or tub baths; encourage the client to perform perineal care after each voiding or bowel movement; assist her to plan time for the use of sitz or tub baths during the day.	The warmth and moisture provided by the baths increase circulation to the area, which facilitates healing and decreases edema. These measures also will help keep the area clean and prevent infection, which could prolong healing and increase discomfort.
Assist the client to identify ways to decrease discomfort, such as tightening the buttocks before sitting. Urge the client to avoid using inflated rings or similar devices.	Tightening the buttocks before sitting will prevent placing direct pressure on the episiotomy. Avoiding the use of an inflated ring will prevent circulatory compromise to the perineum.
Instruct the client in signs and symptoms to report to her health care provider: elevated temperature, foul-smelling vaginal drainage, or change in colour or amount of lochia.	Knowledge of potential signs and symptoms of complications promotes early detection and prompt intervention.
Contact the client within 2 days (either by phone or in person) to assess if pain is decreased.	Follow-up client contact aids in determining the success of strategies and if further planning and intervention are necessary. If pain is unchanged or worsened, further assessment is warranted to rule out infection or other complications.

EVALUATION

1. The client verbalizes understanding of the body's healing process.
2. The client demonstrates strategies to decrease discomfort.
3. The client reports that pain is controlled at a tolerable level.

NURSING DIAGNOSES

- **Fatigue** related to demands of caring for newborn, early discharge, and postpartal status
- **Health-Seeking Behaviours** related to fatigue, discomfort, and anxiety
- **Risk for Ineffective Parent–Infant Attachment** related to fatigue and unrealistic expectations

EXPECTED OUTCOMES

1. The client will identify measures to relieve fatigue and obtain adequate rest.
2. The client will verbalize activities to promote positive interactions with her newborn.
3. The client will identify areas for additional support.

(continued)

NURSING CARE PLAN 18.2 ● The Postpartum Mother and Newborn at Home (Continued)

INTERVENTIONS	RATIONALES
Question the client about her usual day, including the newborn's typical routine; assess the client's emotional state and interaction with the newborn.	Assessment provides a baseline from which to develop appropriate individualized interventions. Evaluation of the client's emotional state is important to identify evidence of postpartum blues and to differentiate this from postpartum depression or psychosis.
Teach the client about behaviours to watch for in the newborn that can assist in anticipating routines.	Knowledge of the newborn's developing routines aids in improved anticipation of, and planning for, time for herself and the baby's needs.
Use both oral and written materials to assist the client to identify common behaviours in newborns.	Helping the client understand newborn behaviours and their causes fosters realistic expectations of both baby and herself.
Assist the client to identify newborn patterns of sleeping and waking; help her identify times when she can plan for rest or naps; involve the client's mother in the discussion.	Understanding the newborn's patterns helps the client plan times to obtain additional rest; short naps throughout the day will assist the client to supplement sleep she may be missing at night. Including the client's mother in the discussion allows her to provide support.
Question the client about any measures she uses to promote sleep; encourage her to use these measures.	Drinking warm milk, listening to soothing music, and maintaining a dark room can help promote sleep.
Assist the client to identify things that her mother can do that will help her.	Doing so will allow the client to maintain control but receive support that will promote coping and adequate rest.
Monitor the client and newborn for evidence of attachment behaviours; reinforce using the en face position, touching, and talking to the newborn during interactions.	Fatigue can directly affect the client's ability to interact with her newborn. Positive interactions with the newborn foster attachment and promote a sense of well-being in the mother.
Provide the client and her mother with available community resources and encourage their use.	Additional support can be effective in helping the client adapt to her new role.
Plan a follow-up telephone call to the client in the next few days and a return home visit within 3 days to evaluate status.	Follow-up is essential to determine the effectiveness of interventions and to determine the need for additional instruction and possible referrals.

EVALUATION

1. The client verbalizes understanding of infant sleep–wake cycles.
2. The client identifies times during the day when she can nap while her mother assumes care of the newborn.
3. The client participates in a community support group for new single parents.
4. The client demonstrates positive attachment behaviours with her newborn.

caused by the infant not fully emptying the mother's breasts at each feeding. Encouraging the infant to feed every 2 or 3 hours may help prevent or decrease engorgement. Application of warm compresses to the breasts may also be helpful. The client can avoid lumps that result from milk stasis in the ducts by ensuring that the infant empties the breast at feedings. Expressing a small amount of breast milk may help to soften the breasts enough to allow the infant to latch on successfully (Bergman et al., 2014).

The client who is nursing may experience some nipple tenderness that may progress to redness, bruising, or cracking. Some nipple pain in the first week postpartum is common, but pain beyond this time usually indicates a problem requiring significant intervention (Bergman et al., 2014; McClellan et al., 2012; Morland-Schultz & Hill, 2005). The most common cause of nipple pain is improper positioning and latch (Bergmann et al., 2014; McClellan et al., 2012; Morland-Schultz & Hill, 2005). The client who is breastfeeding for the first time often needs support and teaching when starting. Although most babies latch on and nurse well from the beginning, many take time to be able to nurse efficiently. Breastfeeding is a learned activity for mother and infant, a fact that clients don't always recognize or internalize. Clients whose newborns are not feeding well need additional support because their difficulties are inconsistent with their image of what the breastfeeding experience should be like. See Chapter 21 for a discussion of positioning for breastfeeding.

Pain or bruising on the upper portion of the nipple may result from the infant pinching the nipple with his or her gums. The mother can correct this problem by lifting the infant's head up so that he or she faces the nipple directly. It is commonly suspected that if the infant has received a pacifier or bottle nipple, he or she may repeat the different action required to suck on these when returning to feed at the breast. The different sucking action may lead to nipple pain when the infant uses the same actions to breastfeed. Failure to revert back to the necessary sucking motions may require suck training. However, recent research has not demonstrated a causal relationship between pacifiers and breastfeeding difficulties (Jaafar et al., 2012; Kair et al., 2013). A short frenulum, or "tongue tie," prevents the infant from using the proper sucking motions, again leading to sore nipples. Health care professionals may have limited knowledge about the difficulties in breastfeeding the infant with a tongue tie, leading to a lack of support and resulting in early discontinuation of breastfeeding (Edmunds et al., 2013). Early identification may facilitate early management, which may include "clipping" the baby's tongue tie to allow the movement necessary to feed (Edmunds et al., 2013; Wallace & Clarke, 2006).

Infectious organisms also may cause nipple pain, the most common being *Candida albicans*. Nipples infected with Candida appear bright red and shiny and are extremely sore during breastfeeding. Women often describe the pain as shooting or burning. The nurse notifies the physician of this development; treatment consists of application of an antifungal cream to the nipples following feedings and administration of oral nystatin to the infant (Wiener, 2006).

McClellan et al. (2012) found that women may experience nipple pain with or without visible trauma. The pain experienced by both groups is often severe and prolonged, leading to interference with breastfeeding, mood, general activity, and sleep. While the pain may be associated with infectious organisms, it may also be associated with infants who have a very strong suck, creating significant vacuum pressure (McClellan et al., 2012).

Several remedies for nipple pain have been suggested, including the application of a small amount of expressed **colostrum** or breast milk to traumatized nipples; this has subsequently been found to be less effective than highly purified lanolin cream (Bergman et al., 2014). Other suggested remedies include tea bags, warm-water compresses, and air drying the nipples after feedings (Morland-Schultz & Hill, 2005).

Caring for the Breasts in the Formulafeeding Client

The client who is not breastfeeding may experience some engorgement at approximately 1 to 4 days postpartum, with the problem peaking at 3 to 5 days postpartum (Janke, 2014). Application of cool compresses will assist with vasoconstriction, which can help eliminate discomfort. Another helpful measure is to wear a well-fitting bra. This engorgement usually disappears approximately 48 to 72 hours later as the lack of stimulation prevents the production of milk (Janke, 2014). Avoiding nipple or breast stimulation may assist in comfort.

Recall Jody, the single mother discharged home with her newborn on the second postpartum day. She is experiencing breast discomfort. Jody states, "I thought since I wasn't breastfeeding, I wouldn't have this problem." How should the nurse respond?

Monitoring the Fundus

If the examiner finds the uterine fundus boggy or cannot feel it, he or she initially should gently massage the fundus, which should become firm within a short time. If this does not happen, the nurse should notify the primary care provider. Intravenous administration of 10 to 20 units of oxytocin added to 1,000 mL crystalloid often is ordered routinely in the immediate postpartum period, when the client is at highest risk for hemorrhage. Carboprost, misoprostal, or methylergonovine may also be ordered.

If the fundus continues to remain uncontracted, other factors may be contributing to atony. Retained placental fragments could be the cause. In addition to uterine atony, the client may pass pieces of tissue vaginally. The examiner can differentiate tissue from blood clots by attempting to tear them apart with gloved hands or tongue depressors. Blood clots are easily pulled apart; tissue does not readily tear. If the woman passes tissue, the examiner puts it into a container with a preservative and sends the material to the laboratory for analysis. If the client continues to present with uterine atony, the nurse notifies the primary care provider. In some instances, clients require surgical removal of placental fragments.

There may be several causes for a fundus found above the expected height in relation to the length of time postpartum. The underlying cause would dictate the appropriate intervention. The most common cause is a distended bladder or blood clots within the uterus (Weathersby et al., 2008). The nurse encourages the woman to empty her bladder. Some women have difficulty voiding postpartum as a result of anaesthesia used intrapartally or alterations in neural function of the bladder. Catheterization may be indicated in these instances. Fundal massage may be used to dispel uterine clots.

Remember Nadia, the new mother from the beginning of the chapter. Initially the nurse assessed her fundus midline immediately below the umbilicus. Her lochia was moderate and dark red, without any clots. Now, 30 minutes later, assessment reveals a fundus that is 2 cm above the umbilicus, boggy, and displaced to the right. What would the nurse suspect? How should the nurse intervene?

Assisting With Elimination

The nurse assists the client to the bathroom (unless contraindicated by her condition), which often helps initiate voiding. The nurse assesses the client's first voiding postpartum, which should occur within 8 hours of childbirth, to ensure that it is sufficient (Cunningham et al., 2010; James, 2014). A client who cannot void and who has a distended bladder requires catheterization. A distended bladder can lead to loss of muscle tone and

continued difficulty voiding. At the same time, catheterization should not be used indiscriminately because it increases the risk for urinary tract infection.

The client may continue to experience stress incontinence postpartum, primarily because of loss of pelvic muscle tone. Routinely doing **Kegel exercises**, in which the woman alternately contracts and relaxes the perineal muscles as though stopping urination, may assist with preventing incontinence (see Chapter 24).

Monitoring Lochia

If the nurse assesses that a woman's lochia is excessive, he or she also evaluates the uterus and bladder. The nurse checks the uterus for tone and position to rule out atony as the cause of the increased lochia. If the nurse finds that the client's uterus is atonic, he or she institutes actions to reverse this problem, which will ideally result in decreased lochia to expected amounts. The nurse also checks the bladder for distention.

The nurse informs the client about expected changes in the colour and amount of lochia throughout the postpartum period. Education includes the importance of contacting the health care provider immediately if flow significantly increases or returns to rubra after changing to serosa.

The nurse assesses the odour of the lochia. Normal lochia is not foul smelling. Foul-smelling lochia usually indicates endometritis and is frequently accompanied by an elevation in the woman's temperature, most commonly after the third postpartum day (James, 2014).

Caring for the Perineum and Episiotomy

The nurse plans interventions for the perineal area based on the client's point in the postpartum period and the presence of edema, hematoma, or episiotomy. Shortly after childbirth, perineal care with warm water provides a feeling of comfort and facilitates visualization of the area. If the postpartum client develops perineal edema during the first 24 hours, she can apply ice to the perineum to decrease swelling. Ice is also soothing when applied after repair of episiotomy or laceration.

For edema that appears or continues after the first 24 hours, warmth, especially moist heat, is appropriate. Methods of heat application include the use of a tub or sitz bath. Both cause vasodilation, increasing circulation to the area that aids in comfort, healing, and cleanliness. A client whose perineum is quite tender, or who has either a laceration or episiotomy repair, should use such baths two or three times a day.

Educating the Client and Family

Women and their significant others often have many learning needs as they seek information to care for themselves and the new baby. The short time that many new families spend in the hospital, however, often prevents many questions and issues from being addressed adequately. Prenatal education has begun to incorporate many aspects of postpartum and newborn care in an effort to ensure that families are informed before childbirth. Information is also readily available in books, on the internet, and in classes (see Chapter 14). Nevertheless, it remains important for nurses to assess learning needs of mothers. Research has shown that new mothers may identify different learning needs than do nurses during the early postpartum period (Wagner et al., 2011). A positive relationship between the nurse and mother, especially when client autonomy and mutual decision making are present, increases client satisfaction with care (Peterson et al., 2007; Wagner et al., 2011) Prenatal and postpartum support groups are available to provide instruction and discussion. Nurses keep in mind that hormonal changes, fatigue, and discomfort, which may affect a woman's attention span and thinking, compounded by the large volume of new information that she is exposed to and expected to learn and remember, may compromise her learning abilities.

The new mother needs support to get enough rest to meet her needs. Learning needs may differ among postpartum women, although satisfaction with the method of teaching may be less significant (Wagner et al., 2011). Education, therefore, focuses on needs identified by the client and her significant others; the nurse implements teaching at the time of identification (Fig. 18.8). Rather than attempting to cover everything

that the new mother might need to know, the nurse may find it more appropriate to concentrate on a few essential topics, keeping explanations simple, and reinforcing learning through repetition. The nurse tries to individualize teaching to the client's preferred learning style and usual problem-solving strategies. He or she informs the client of available community resources and provide supplementary data in a written format. These may include support such as a visiting program offered from the public health offices for mothers who are discharged early from the hospital, La Leche League support for breastfeeding, parenting groups and hotlines, and other similar resources that may be available in the community. It may also be helpful for the nurse to assist the woman to recognize the need to sort through all the available information and advice that she may obtain and assist her to develop strategies to match selections to her lifestyle and problem-solving approaches.

As mothers are in the hospital for short periods following birth, the time available to complete teaching is decreased. The shorter time frame has implications for both the amount of information that the nurse can provide and the amount that the client can take in and remember. The role of the nurse as educator within the acute-care setting is evolving to focus on facilitating information that centres on essential material. The role of the community nurse in educating is continuing to evolve. Provision of information about support services—as well as support in developing skills in evaluating information and advice that is provided in and by a multitude of sources—assists the new mother to cope.

Assisting LGBT Parents

Expectations attached to the concepts of family and motherhood in Canadian society may be linked to traditional Euro-American values in which families include children with two parents of the opposite sex. Many health care providers share this expectation. However, there are increasing numbers of parents, that is, those who are LGBT, who do not fit within the traditional concept of parenthood (Statistics Canada, 2012). Health care providers can easily avoid acknowledging the existence of these clients and hence any recognition of their needs, creating feelings of discomfort, invisibility, limited contact, and lack of emotional support (Dahl et al., 2012; McManus et al., 2006). This may be manifested by a demonstrated lack of sensitivity and respect on the nurse's part, as well as disparaging remarks (Dahl et al., 2012).

Dahl et al. (2012) found that one of the first decisions a lesbian woman needs to make, once she is pregnant, is whether to "come out" to her health care provider; it is important for the woman to be in control of this as it can be "risky." This dilemma continues not only throughout pregnancy, but also following birth. Many women have

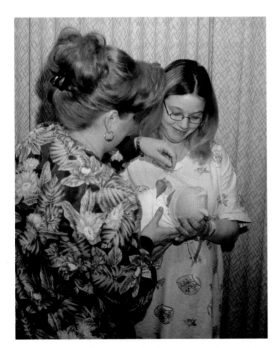

FIGURE 18.8 The nurse provides teaching according to the new mother's learning readiness and needs.

found that forms and questions within the health care environment enforce invisibility, placing the burden to explain (often repeatedly) on the woman, creating stress (Dahl et al., 2012).

Lesbian women want understanding of their needs from their health care providers as well as inclusion of their partners, just as do heterosexual women (Dahl et al., 2012). Lesbian women, unlike heterosexual women, have to decide whether disclosure would facilitate or impede this. Additional concerns are whether this knowledge will affect the quality of care provided and whether the information will produce a prejudiced reaction. Regardless of their decision, most women want to be able to share this information.

Another stressor that lesbian women have identified during the postpartum period is the lack of support provided to their partners. In some cases, clinicians have not recognized partners as part of the family unit and have mistreated them accordingly (Dahl et al., 2012; Goldberg et al., 2011). This leads to anxiety for the postpartum woman (and her partner) as well as depriving her of her source of support. Some lesbian mothers want to be treated the same as all mothers, regardless of sexual orientation (Lauderdale, 2003); others feel particular attention should be paid to the needs of the lesbian mother and her partner (Goldberg et al., 2011). For example, some may feel that the difference between the two groups of mothers needs to be acknowledged and respected rather than ignored (Goldberg et al., 2011).

Acknowledging the partner as a support for the mother and recognizing the family unit are essential nursing activities, whether in the hospital or community setting. Nurses must be careful with the language that they use. The mother and nurse may assign different meanings to "partner" and "parent." Health care providers are sensitive to all women's right to have their choice of partner and family unit respected. They facilitate inclusion of partners and encourage their participation.

Evaluation

Evaluation of changes in assessment and the effectiveness of interventions are important to ensuring appropriate maternal progress in the postpartum period. Nursing mothers should attend to any nipple pain quickly; such pain can progress rapidly to tissue breakdown and cracking of the nipples. This causes increased discomfort, potential for infection, and prolonged healing. All these potential outcomes can have a discouraging effect on the mother and may result in discontinuing breastfeeding. The nurse provides assistance to all clients experiencing difficulties with breastfeeding or problems with the breasts postpartum. If lactation consultants are available in the hospital and community, nurses and clients consult them when problems persist or are exacerbated.

The uterus should remain well contracted and be found further down in the abdomen over time. The client should understand how her flow will change over time and be advised to notify her health care practitioner immediately if the flow changes inappropriately.

An empty bladder should not be palpable above the symphysis pubis. The client should be able to sense a full bladder and have no difficulty emptying her bladder. Burning or increased frequency, which may indicate a urinary tract infection, should not accompany urination. The client may, however, experience some increase in frequency as diuresis takes place in the early postpartum.

In some instances, a transient increase in lochia is normal, such as following breastfeeding, as a reaction to uterine contraction caused by the release of oxytocin stimulated by the infant sucking. Women's lochia may also increase when they initially rise after having been recumbent for some time. Such positioning can result in lochia pooling in the uterus; when the client sits or stands, the lochia then flows. In other instances, increased lochia or a return to lochia rubra from lochia serosa requires investigation to rule out late postpartum hemorrhage.

Sutures, if present, should remain intact. The nurse tells the client that the sutures are dissolvable and will not need removal. Signs that an episiotomy or laceration is not healing properly include redness, edema, ecchymosis, and discharge. With normal healing, the edges are well approximated.

SUMMARY

- Women lose approximately 5 to 6 kg of weight following childbirth. By 6 to 18 months postpartum, clients tend to weigh 3.6 kg more than they did before pregnancy.
- Approximately 500 mL of blood is lost with a vaginal birth, and approximately 1,000 mL with a cesarean birth. Plasma volume decreases by as much as 1,000 mL. Blood volume returns to prepregnant values by approximately 1 week postpartum.
- Cardiac output remains elevated for 48 hours. The pulse rate remains stable or decreases slightly. A mild rise in blood pressure is a common phenomenon in the first 4 days postpartum.
- Hemoglobin and hematocrit values fluctuate and then rise to nonpregnancy values by 6 weeks postpartum. Normal serum iron levels are regained by the second week postpartum. Nonpathologic leukocytosis is seen in the postpartum period.
- After childbirth, intra-abdominal pressure decreases, as does diaphragmatic pressure. Abdominal muscles remain in a relaxed state. Gaseous distention and

decreased motility may result. Constipation may be a problem related to fear, dehydration, immobility, or medications. Hemorrhoids may be present.

- Chloasma disappears after delivery. Striae gravidarum fade to a silvery white.
- Estrogen and progesterone levels decrease. Plasma prolactin level falls lower than during pregnancy, but increases with each act of sucking by the infant. Thyroid hormone levels return to prepregnant levels by 6 weeks postpartum. BMR returns to normal approximately 7 to 14 days postpartum. Glucose levels fall as a result of delivery of placenta.
- The uterus weighs approximately 1,000 g after birth and decreases to 100 g or less by 6 weeks postpartum. The fundus is felt one fingerbreadth below the umbilicus immediately after childbirth, decreasing approximately one fingerbreadth each day following. The uterus remains contracted.
- Lochia is sloughed off up to 4 weeks postpartum. Lochia rubra is dark red and lasts for the first 3 to 4 days. Lochia serosa is paler and lasts from day 4 or 5 until day 9. Lochia alba is yellowish white and lasts from the 10th day until the flow stops.
- The endometrium regenerates by the third week postpartum. The placental site takes approximately 6 weeks to heal.
- Subinvolution may occur because of failure of the uterus to contract, most commonly caused by retention of placental tissue or exposed blood vessels after placental separation.
- The cervical os contracts slowly. Cervical edema may be present for several months. The cervix never returns to the pregravid state.
- Menstruation returns for the woman who is not breastfeeding by approximately 6 to 10 weeks postpartum, and from the eighth week to 18 months postpartum for the woman who is breastfeeding. Approximately 25% of women ovulate before the first menses.
- Rugae reappear in the vagina approximately 3 weeks postpartum. The voluntary muscles of the pelvic floor regain their tone approximately 6 weeks postpartum.
- Changes in the breasts are related primarily to the decision of whether or not to breastfeed.
- Diuresis occurs between the second and fifth day postpartum. Spontaneous voiding should resume within 8 hours after birth. Bladder tone should return by 5 to 7 days.
- Many clients experience postpartum blues, usually between 3 and 14 days postpartum. Symptoms may include increased emotional lability, crying, and sensitivity. Postpartum depression and psychosis are more serious, but have significantly lower incidences.

- A focused assessment is done during the fourth stage of labour, including vital signs, uterus, lochia, and perineum.
- A more complete assessment is done less frequently for the remainder of the postpartum. This assessment includes breasts, uterus, bladder, bowels, lochia, episiotomy and perineum, and psychological state.

Questions to Ponder

1. A client who gave birth to her first baby 14 hours ago asks to be discharged home. She indicates that her mother and mother-in-law are both at home to help.
   - What are your personal feelings about a first-time mother going home early in the puerperium?
   - What additional information might be helpful for the nurse to have before responding?
   - What specific supports might the nurse want to ensure are in place before discharge?

REVIEW QUESTIONS

1. A client who is 2 days postpartum tells the nurse that she is voiding frequently. Further assessment reveals that the client's temperature is 37.8 °C, her fundus is at the umbilicus and firm, and she is voiding 500 mL at a time. Which of the following would the nurse recognize as a potential cause for urinary frequency?
   A. Urinary overflow
   B. Postpartum diuresis
   C. Urinary tract infection
   D. Trauma to pelvic muscles

2. A client just gave birth to her second child 30 minutes ago. The newborn boy weighs 3,800 g. The client is currently breastfeeding. Which of the following findings would the nurse recognize as most significant in her next assessment?
   A. Lochia is moderate rubra.
   B. Pulse rate has decreased by 10 beats/minute.
   C. The client reports abdominal pains.
   D. The fundus is two fingerbreadths above the umbilicus.

3. The nurse is examining the results of laboratory blood testing for a client who is 2 days postpartum. Which of the following findings would the nurse recognize as most significant?
   A. WBC count = $27,000 \times 10^9$/L
   B. Hematocrit = 0.4
   C. Hemoglobin = 100 g/L
   D. Serum iron = 9 mmol/L

4. The nurse is assessing a client who is 2 days postpartum. During attempted examination of the fundus, the nurse cannot find it. Which of the

following nursing actions would be most appropriate next?

A. Assess the lochia.

B. Massage the fundus.

C. Administer ordered oxytocin.

D. Nothing, it is probably already too low to be felt.

5. A postpartum client who is breastfeeding asks when she can expect menses to return. Which response from the nurse would be most appropriate?

A. "Your menses will return at 8 weeks postpartum whether you breastfeed or formulafeed."

B. "Women who breastfeed can expect menstruation to return at 6 weeks postpartum."

C. "Women who breastfeed can expect menstruation to return at 8 weeks postpartum."

D. "Women who breastfeed may not experience menstruation until 18 months postpartum."

6. A client who is 3 days postpartum is breastfeeding her baby girl. The client reports that her breasts are very swollen and sore. Which of the following interventions would be the most appropriate for the nurse to recommend?

A. Lanolin ointment

B. Warm compresses

C. Cool compresses

D. Expression of the excess milk

7. During a home visit to a postpartum client, the nurse suspects early signs of postpartum depression based on initial conversation. Which intervention would be most important to consider when completing a full assessment?

A. Assess for signs of bipolar disorder.

B. Assess for shortness of breath and sensations of smothering.

C. Consider that the client may show unique signs.

D. Refrain from questions to which the client might be sensitive.

8. A nurse is admitting a client from the labour and delivery unit who gave birth to a baby girl 3 hours ago. During initial assessment, the client reports that she is LGBT with a supportive female partner. Which of the following would be most important for the nurse to include as part of her care?

A. Ask the client how she got pregnant.

B. Include the client's partner in all care.

C. Act as though there is nothing different about her.

D. Tell the other nurses to promote sensitivity.

9. The nurse is teaching a new mother who is 1 day postpartum. The client indicates that she is planning to go home the next day. Which of the following principles would be most important?

A. Implement teaching whenever the nurse is with the client.

B. Sit with the client to review everything she will need to go home.

C. Identify what the client thinks she needs to know.

D. Reinforce information every time the nurse has an opportunity.

10. During a routine assessment, the nurse finds that the fundus of a client who is 14 hours postpartum is two fingerbreadths above the umbilicus and slightly boggy. The flow is large rubra. Which of the following actions would the nurse consider taking next?

A. Notify the physician.

B. Palpate the bladder for distention.

C. Massage the uterus to expel clots.

D. Administer oxytocin to stimulate uterine contractions.

REFERENCES

Beck, C. T., & Indman P. (2005). The many faces of postpartum depression. *Journal of Obstetrical, Gynecological, and Neonatal Nursing, 34*(5), 569–576.

Benjamin, D. R., van de Water, A. T., & Peiris, C. L. (2014). Effects of exercise on diastasis of the rectus abdominis muscle in the antenatal and postnatal periods: A systematic review. *Physiotherapy, 100*, 1–8. doi:10.1016/j.physio.2013.08.005

Bergman, R. L., Bergmann, K. E., von Weizsacker, K., Berns, M., Henrich, W., & Dudnhausen, J. W. (2014). Breastfeeding is natural but not always easy: Intervention for common medical problems of breastfeeding mothers-a review of the scientific evidence. *Journal of Perinatal Medicine, 42*(1), 9–18. doi:10.1515/jpm-2013-0095

Bickley, L. S. (2012). *Bates' guide to physical examination and history taking* (11th ed.). Philadelphia, PA: Lippincott Williams & Wilkins.

Biesmans, K., Franck, E., Ceulemans, C., Jacquemyn, Y., & Van Bogaert, P. (2013). Weight during the postpartum period: What can health care workers do? *Maternal Child Health Journal, 17*, 996–1004.

Bouchard, T., Fehring, R. J., & Schneider, M. (2012). Efficacy of a new postpartum transition protocol for avoiding pregnancy. *Journal of the American Board of Family Medicine, 26*, 35–44. doi:10.3122/jabfm.2013.01.120126

Bowman, K. G. (2005). Postpartum learning needs. *Journal of Obstetrical, Gynecological, and Neonatal Nursing, 34*(4), 438–443.

Cunningham, F. G., Leveno, K. J., Bloom, S. L., Hauth, J. C., Rouse, D. J., & Sprong, C. Y. (2010). *Williams obstetrics* (23rd ed.) New York, NY: McGraw-Hill.

Dahl, B., Fylkesnes, A. M., Sorlie, V., & Malterud, K. (2012). Lesbian women's experiences with healthcare providers in the birthing context: A meta-ethnography. *Midwifery, 29*, 674–681. doi:org/10.1016/j.midw.2012.06.008

Darvill, R., Skirton, H., & Farrand, P. (2010). Psychological factors that impact on women's experiences of first-time motherhood: A qualitative study of the transition. *Midwifery, 26*, 357–366. doi:10.1016/j.midw.2008.07.006

Datta, S., Kodali, B. S., & Segal, S. (2010). *Obstetric anesthesia handbook* (5th ed.) New York, NY: Springer. doi:10.1007/978-0-387-88602-2

Dennis, C. L., & Ross, L. (2005). Relationships among infant sleep patterns, maternal fatigue, and development of depressive symptomatology. *Birth, 32*(3), 187–193.

Dewey, K. G. (2004). Impact of breastfeeding on maternal nutritional status. *Advances in Experimental Medical Biology, 554*, 91–100.

Edmunds, J. E., Fullbrook, P., & Miles, S. (2013). Understanding the experiences of mothers who are breastfeeding an infant with tongue-tie: A phenomenological study. *Journal of Human Lactation, 29*(2), 190–195. doi:10.1177/0890334413479174

Emmanuel, E., Creedy, D. K., St John, W., & Brown, C. (2011). Maternal role development: The impact of maternal distress and social support following childbirth. *Midwifery, 27,* 265–272. doi:10.1016/j.midw.2009.07.003

Emmanuel, E., Creedy, D. K., St John, W., Gamble, J., & Brown C. (2008). Maternal role development following childbirth among Australian women. *Journal of Advanced Nursing, 64*(1), 18–26. doi:10.1111/j.1365-2648.2008.04757.x

Enakpene, C. A., Morhason-Bello, I. O., Enakpene, E. O., Arowojolu, A. O., & Omiqbodun, A. O. (2007). Oral misoprostol for the prevention of primary post-partum hemorrhage during third stage of labor. *Journal of Obstetrics and Gynaecology Research, 33*(6), 810–817.

Fahey, J. O., & Shenassa, E. (2013). Understanding and meeting the needs of women in the postpartum period: The perinatal maternal health promotion model. *Journal of Midwifery and Womens Health, 58,* 613–621. doi:10.1111/jmwh.12139

Fenwick, J., Hauck, Y., Downie, J., & Butt, J. (2005). The childbirth expectations of a self-selected cohort of Western Australian women. *Midwifery, 21*(1), 23–35.

Fung Kee Fung, K., & Eason, E. (2003). SOGC clinical practice guidelines: Prevention of Rh alloimmunization. *Journal of Obstetrics and Gynecology of Canada, 25*(9), 765–773.

Gabel, K. T., & Weeber, T. A. (2012). Measuring and communicating blood loss during obstetric hemorrhage. *Journal of Obstetric, Gynecologic and Neonatal Nursing, 41*(4), 551–558.

Gaillard, A., Le Strat, Y., Mandelbrot, L., Keïta, H., & Dubertret, C. (2013). Predictors of postpartum depression: Prospective study of 264 women followed during pregnancy and postpartum. *Psychiatry Research, 215,* 341–346. doi:10.1016/j.psychres.2013.10.003

George, L. (2005). Lack of preparedness: Experiences of first-time mothers. *MCN. The American Journal of Maternal and Child Nursing, 30*(4), 251–255.

Glazener, C. M., Herbison, G. P., MacArthur, C., Lancashire, R., McGee, M. A., Grant, A. M., et al. (2006). New postnatal urinary incontinence and other risk factors in primiparae. *British Journal of Obstetrics & Gynecology, 113*(2), 208–217.

Goldberg, G. (2005). Maternal nutrition in pregnancy and the first postnatal year—2. After the birth. *Journal of Family Health Care, 15*(5), 137–138, 140.

Goldberg, L., Harbin, A., & Campbell, S. (2011). Queering the birthing space: Phenomenological interpretations of the relationships between lesbian couples and perinatal nurses in the context of birthing care. *Sexualities, 14*(2), 173–192. doi:10.1177/1363460711399028

Gore, S. A, Brown, D. M., & West, D. S. (2003). The role of postpartum weight retention in obesity among women: A review of the evidence. *Annals of Behavioral Medicine, 26*(2), 149–159.

Hall, J. E. (2011). *Guyton and Hall textbook of medical physiology* (12th ed.). Philadelphia, PA: W. B. Saunders.

Health Canada. (2000). *Family-centred maternity and newborn care: National guidelines.* Ottawa: Minister of Public Works and Government Services.

Jaafar, S. H., Jahanfar, S., Angolkar, M., & Ho, J. J. (2012). Effect of restricted pacifier use in breastfeeding term infants for increasing duration of breastfeeding. *Cochrane Database of Systematic Reviews, 7,* CD007202. doi:10.1002/14651858.CD007202.pub3

Jack, S. M., DiCenso, A., & Lohfeld, L. (2005). A theory of maternal engagement with public health nurses and family visitors. *Journal of Advanced Nursing, 49*(2), 182–190.

Jackson, E., Curtis, K. M,. & Gaffield, M. E. (2011). Risk of venous thromboembolism during the postpartum period: A systematic review. *Obstetrics & Gynecology, 117*(3), 691–703. doi:10.1097/AOG.0b013e31820ce2 db

James, D. C. (2014). Postpartum care. In Simpson, K. R., & Creehan, P. A. (Eds.), *AWHONN's perinatal nursing* (4th ed., pp. 530–580). Philadelphia, PA: Lippincott Williams & Wilkins.

Janke, J. (2014). Newborn nutrition. In Simpson, K. R., & Creehan, P. A. (Eds.), *AWHONN's perinatal nursing* (4th ed., pp. 626–661). Philadelphia, PA: Lippincott Williams & Wilkins.

Kair, L. R., Kenron, D., Etheredge, K., Jaffe, A. C., & Phillipi, C. A. (2013). Pacifier restriction and exclusive breastfeeding. *Pediatrics, 131*(4), e1101–e1107. doi:10.1542/peds.2012-2203

Lauderdale, J. (2003). Transcultural perspectives in childbearing. In Andrews, M. M., & Boyle, J. S. (Eds.), *Transcultural concepts in nursing care* (4th ed., pp. 95–131). Philadelphia, PA: Lippincott Williams & Wilkins.

Lazarus, J. H. (2005). Thyroid disorders associated with pregnancy: Etiology, diagnosis, and management. *Obstetrics and Gynecology Survey, 4*(1), 31–41.

Leduc, D., Senikas, V., & Lalonde, A. B. (2009). SOGC clinical practice guideline: Active management of the third stage of labour: Prevention and treatment of postpartum hemorrhage. *Journal of Obstetrics and Gynecology of Canada, 235,* 980–993.

Lipsky, L. M., Strawderman, M. S., & Olson, C. M. (2012). Maternal weight change between 1 and 2 years postpartum: The importance of 1 year weight retention. *Obesity, 20,* 1496–1502. doi:10.1038/oby.2012.41

Liumbruno, G. M., D'Allessandro, A., Rea, F., Piccinini, V., Catalano, L., Calizzani, G., et al. (2010). The role of antenatal immunioprophylaxis in the prevention of maternal-foetal anti-Rh(D) alloimmunisation. *Blood Transfusion, 8*(1), 8–16. doi:10.2450/2009.0108-09

MacMullen, N. J., Dulski, L. A., & Meagher, B. (2005). Red alert: Perinatal hemorrhage. *MCN. The American Journal of Maternal and Child Nursing, 30*(1), 46–51.

Magee, L., & von Dadelszen, P. (2013). Prevention and treatment of postpartum hypertension. *Cochrane Database of Systematic Reviews, 4,* 4CD004351. doi:10.1002/14651858.CD004351.pub3

Marchant, S. (2009). Physiology and care in the puerperium. In Fraser. D. M., & Cooper. M. A. (Eds.), *Myles textbook for midwives* (15th ed., pp. 651–664). Philadelphia, PA: Churchill Livingstone.

Mazzeo, S. E., Slof-Op't Landt, M. C., Jones, I., Mitchell, K., Kendler, K. S., Neale, M. C., et al. (2006). Associations among postpartum depression, eating disorders, and perfectionism in a population-based sample of adult women. *International Journal of Eating Disorders, 39*(3), 202–211.

McClellan, H. L., Hepworth, A. R., Garbin, C. P., Rowan, M. K., Deacon, J., Hartmann, P. E. et al. (2012). Nipple pain during breastfeeding with or without visible trauma, *Journal of Human Lactation, 28*(4), 511–521. doi:10.1177/0890334412444464

McManus, A. J., Hunter, L. P., & Renn, H. (2006). Lesbian experiences and needs during childbirth: Guidance for health care providers. *Journal of Obstetric, Gynecologic, and Neonatal Nursing, 35*(1), 13–23.

Melamed, N., Ben-Haroush, A., Chen, R., Kaplan, B., & Yogev, Y. (2009). Intrapartum cervical lacerations: Characteristics, risk factors, and effects on subsequent pregnancies. *American Journal of Obstetrics and Gynecology, 200*(4), 388.e1–e4.

Montgomery, K. S., Aniello, T. D., Phillips, J. D., Kirkpatrick, T., Catledge, C., Braveboy, K. et al. (2013). Experiences accompanying postpartum weight loss: Benefits, successes and well-being. *Health Care for women International, 34,* 577–591. doi:10.1080/07399332.2012.736568

Montgomery, K. S., Best, M., Aniello, T. B., Phillips, J. D., & Hatmaker-Flanigan, E. (2013). Postpartum weight loss; Weight struggles, eating, exercise, & breastfeeding. *Journal of Holistic Nursing, 31,* 129–138. doi:10.1177/0898010112464120

Montgomery, K. S., Bushee, T. D., Phillips, J. D., Kirkpatrick, T., Catledge, C., Braveboy, K. et al. (2011). Women's challenges with postpartum weight loss. *Maternal Child Health Journal, 15,* 1176–1184. doi:10.1007/s10995-010-0681–9

Morland-Schultz, K., & Hill, P. D. (2005). Prevention of and therapies for nipple pain: A systematic review. *Journal of Obstetrical, Gynecological, and Neonatal Nursing, 34*(4), 428–437.

O'Hara, M. W., Wisner, K. L., & Asher, H. (2014). Perinatal mental illness: Definition, description and aetiology. *Best practice & Research Clinical Obstetrics and Gynaecology, 28.* 3–12. doi:10.1016/j.bpobgyn.2013.09.002

O'Reilly, M. M. (2004). Achieving a new balance: Women's transition to second-time parenthood. *Journal of Obstetrical, Gynecological, and Neonatal Nursing, 33*(4), 455–462.

Olson, C. M., Strawderman, M. S., Hinton, P. S., & Pearson, T. A. (2003). Gestational weight gain and postpartum behaviors associated with weight change from early pregnancy to 1 y postpartum. *Journal of Obesity and Related Metabolic Disorders, 27*(1), 117–127.

Park, E. M., Meltzer-Brody, S., & Stickgold, R. (2013). Poor sleep maintenance and subjective sleep quality are associated with postpartum maternal depression symptom severity. *Archives of Womens Mental Health, 16*, 539–547. doi:10.1007/s00737-013-0356-9

Pazzaglia, C., Caliandro, P., Aprile, I., Modelli, M., Foschini, M., Tonali, PA., et al. (2005). Multicenter study on carpal tunnel syndrome and pregnancy incidence and natural course. *Archives of Womens Mental Health, 92*, 35–39.

Peterson, W. E., Sword, W., Charles, C., & DiCenso, A. (2007). Adolescents' perceptions of inpatient postpartum nursing care. *Qualitative Health Research, 17*(2), 201–212.

Pifarotti, P., Gargasole, C., Folcini, C., Gattei, U., Nieddu, E., Sofi, G., et al. (2014). Acute post-partum urinary retention: Analysis of risk factors, a case-control study. *Archives of Gynecology and Obstetrics.* Advance online publication. doi:10.1007/s00404-014-3144-5

Public Health Agency of Canada. (2008). *Canadian perinatal health report 2008 edition.* Ottawa: Author.

Razurel, C., Bruchon-Schweitzer, M., Dupanloup, A., Irion, O., & Epiney, M. (2011). Stressful events, social support and coping strategies of primiparous women during the postpartum period; A qualitative study. *Midwifery, 27*, 237–242. doi:10.1016/j.midw.2009.06.005

Ross, L. E., Murray, B. J., & Steiner, M. (2005). Sleep and perinatal mood disorders: A critical review. *Journal of Psychiatry and Neuroscience, 30*(4), 247–256.

Sarvghadi, F., Hedayati, M., Mehrabi, Y., & Azizi, F. (2005). Follow up of patients with postpartum thyroiditis: A population-based study. *Endocrine, 27*(3), 279–282.

Seravalli, V., Potti, S., & Berghella, V. (2013). Risk of intrapartum cervical lacerations in women with cerclage. *The Journal of Maternal-Fetal & Neonatal Medicine, 26*(3), 294–298.

Slotkin, E., & Herbold, N. (2010). Influences on weight status of female adults at 6 months postpartum. *Topics in Clinical Nutrition, 25*(3), 256–263.

Statistics Canada. (2012). *Portrait of families and living arrangements in Canada.* (Catalogue no. 98–312-X2011001). Retrieved from http://www12.statcan.gc.ca/census-recensement/2011/as-sa/98–312-x/98–312-x2011001-eng.cfm.

Svare, J. A., Hansen, B. B., & Lose, G. (2013). Risk factors for urinary incontinence 1 year after the first vaginal delivery in a cohort of primiparous Danish women. *International Urogynecology Journal, 25*, 47–51. doi:10.1007/s00192-013-2233-5

Tunzi, M., & Gray, G. R. (2007). Common skin conditions during pregnancy. *American Family Physician, 75*(2), 211–218.

Urbano, F. L. (2001). Homans sign in the diagnosis of deep vein thrombosis. *Hospital Physician, 23*, 22–24.

Wagner, D. L., Bear, M., & Davidson, N. S. (2011). Measuring patient satisfaction with postpartum teaching methods used by nurses within the interaction model of client health behavior. *Research and Theory for Nursing Practice: an International Journal, 25*(3), 176–190. doi:10.1891/1541-6577.25.3.176

Waldenstrom, U. (2004). Why do some women change their opinion about childbirth over time? *Birth, 31*(2), 102–107.

Walker, L. O., Sterling, B. S., Kim, M., Arheart, K. L., & Timmerman, G. M. (2006). Trajectory of weight changes in the first 6 weeks postpartum. *J Obstet Gynecol Neon Nurs, 35*(4), 472–481.

Wallace, H., & Clarke, S. (2006). Tongue tie division in infants with breast feeding difficulties. *International Journal of Pediatric Otorhinolaryngology, 70*(7), 1257–1261.

Weathersby, A. M., Waugh, P., & Rodgers, E. (2008). Assessment of the newborn and newly delivered mother. In Kennedy, B.B., Ruth, D.J., & Martin, E. J. (Eds.), *Intrapartum management modules: A perinatal education program* (4th ed., pp. 407–431). Philadelphia, PA: Lippincott Williams & Wilkins.

Wesnes, S. L., Hunskaar, S., & Rortveit, G. (2012). Epidemiology of urinary incontinence in pregnancy and postpartum. In Alhasso. A. (Ed.) *Urinary Incontinence.* Croatia: InTech.

Wiener, S. (2006). Diagnosis and management of Candida of the nipple and breast. *Journal of Midwifery and Women's Health, 51*(2), 125–128.

CHAPTER 19

The High-Risk Postpartum Woman

Wendy Hall, Debbie Raines*, and Della Campbell*

Rosanna, 36 years old, gave birth vaginally to her fourth child, a healthy boy, 6 hours ago. She received oxytocin to augment her labour, which was prolonged. She appears quite anxious and her extremities are cool. She states, "I think something might be wrong. I haven't urinated yet, but I feel like I have to. And I've been changing my pad frequently. I don't remember this happening after giving birth to my other children."

Ten days ago, Leslie, 26 years old, underwent a planned cesarean birth. Her recovery in the health care facility was unremarkable, and she was discharged home with her healthy daughter on postpartum day 5. Today, she calls the health care provider to report that she has had a fever ranging from 38.2° to 38.6°C for the past 2 days. She also states that her incision is reddened and very sore. "I have little energy and feel shaky," she reports.

You will learn more about Rosanna's and Leslie's stories throughout this chapter. Nurses working with clients experiencing postpartum complications need to understand the content in this chapter to adequately assess them and provide care. Before beginning, consider the following points related to the above scenarios:

- What issues are similar for each client? What issues are different?
- What additional information would the nurse need to obtain from each client?
- What factors might be contributing to each client's risk for developing a postpartum complication?
- How can you help to prevent maternal postpartum complications?
- How would you respond to each woman? What steps would you take?

*Contributor to first U.S. edition.

On completion of this chapter, the reader should be able to:

- Distinguish potential maternal complications following childbirth.
- Identify congenital and acquired factors that place clients at risk in the postpartum period.
- Apply components of the nursing process (assessment, diagnosis, planning, intervention, and evaluation) to specific maternal postpartum conditions.
- Explain perinatal nurses' roles in assisting clients and their families in acute and long-term resolution of maternal postpartum complications.
- Acknowledge effects of maternal postpartum complications on women's and family members' psychological well-being.

cystocele	postpartum depression
deep venous thrombosis	postpartum hemorrhage
early postpartum hemorrhage	puerperal infection
endometritis	pulmonary embolism
hematoma	rectocele
late postpartum hemorrhage	superficial venous thrombosis
mastitis	thromboembolic disorder
parametritis	uterine displacement
pelvic relaxation	uterine inversion
peripartum cardiomyopathy	uterine prolapse
peritonitis	

Maternal postpartum complications can occur for any new mother and may be related to problems that started before or during pregnancy, during labour and birth, or after birth. For example, they may be related to pre-existing or coexisting medical problems such as diabetes, cardiac disease, HIV infection, or hypertension (see Chapters 4 and 13). Complications may have resulted from the birth itself, such as in cases of hemorrhage or infection. Psychological complications, which may not manifest until weeks or months after the birth, may be influenced by factors including teenage or mature motherhood, homelessness, intimate partner violence, or drug use (Apgar et al., 2005; Escribà-Agüir et al., 2013). Maternal postpartum physiologic and psychological complications affect not only the health status of the mother but also the newborn's condition by potentially interfering with the maternal–newborn attachment process. Complications can also disrupt the family dynamics through health-related, fiscal, and emotional effects and costs (Box 19.1).

Short stays in health facilities preclude detection of many infections and other postpartum complications until after the mother and newborn have been discharged. Rehospitalization of the new mother may be required, which can separate her from her newborn. Nurses' teaching about the signs and symptoms of potential postpartum problems and the importance of contacting the health care provider in case they develop

● **BOX 19.1 Postbirth Mortality and Severe Morbidity**

- In Canada, there were 7.8 maternal deaths per 100,000 live births between 2008 and 2010.
- Postpartum hemorrhage with transfusion accounts for 398.4/100,000 cases of severe maternal morbidity with a case fatality rate of 3.2/1,000.
- Cardiac arrest, cardiac failure, or myocardial infarction account for 104.5/100,000 cases of severe maternal morbidity with a case fatality rate of 22.2/1,000.
- Puerperal sepsis accounts for 112.5/100,000 cases of severe maternal morbidity with a case fatality rate of 2.7/1,000.

From Maternal Health Study Group of the Canadian Surveillance System (2010), and Public Health Agency of Canada (2011) Maternal mortality fact sheet. Retrieved from http://www.phac-aspc.gc.ca/rhs-ssg/maternal-maternelle/mortality-mortalite/index-eng.php

is vital to discharge planning and family health and well-being.

Nurses differentiate normal variations from true postpartum complications and educate clients and families about potential alterations following hospital discharge. Many conditions described in this chapter occur in clients who had no complications during pregnancy or childbirth. Therefore, ongoing assessment of all postpartum clients is essential to the quality of your nursing care.

FOCUSED ASSESSMENTS FOR CLIENTS WITH POSTPARTUM COMPLICATIONS

General nursing assessment of postpartum clients who develop a complication involves comprehensive health history taking and physical examination (see Chapter 18). The nurse should carefully review the woman's pregnancy, intrapartum, and birth histories and events to identify potential risk factors and to implement strategies that promote the safety and well-being of the client and her newborn and family (Box 19.1).

Areas of particular focus include the following:

- Pregnancy factors (e.g., high parity)
- Infections, especially urinary tract infections (UTIs)
- Preterm labour or preterm rupture of membranes
- Abnormal placental implantation (i.e., placenta previa, placenta accreta, placenta increta)
- Intrapartal and birth factors
- Length of labour (e.g., rapid or prolonged labour)
- Mode of birth (e.g., cesarean section)
- Use of invasive technologies: internal uterine and fetal monitoring, fetal pulse oximetry, urinary catheterization, frequent vaginal examinations
- Type of analgesia and anaesthesia
- General health status factors (e.g., maternal obesity)
- Chronic pre-existing disease states such as hypertension or diabetes (see Chapter 4)
- Nutritional status
- Use of drugs, alcohol, and other substances
- Access to health care systems

BLEEDING COMPLICATIONS

Bleeding complications are a leading cause of postpartum morbidity and mortality; more than 50% of all maternal deaths occur within 24 hours of childbirth, most frequently from excessive bleeding (Rath, 2011). Awareness of risk factors for postbirth bleeding complications, early identification of assessment parameters indicating such alterations, and prompt intervention are important to promote client safety and well-being.

Clients can generally tolerate a certain amount of blood loss following birth because the body uses compensatory mechanisms related to the normal expansion of blood volume during pregnancy (see Chapters 12 and 18). *Postpartum hemorrhage* is defined as blood loss greater than 500 mL with vaginal delivery, or 1000 mL with cesarean section (Rath, 2011), although reliance on volume estimation without incorporating clinical signs has been criticized; any blood loss with the potential to result in hemodynamic instability should be viewed as a postpartum hemorrhage (Leduc et al., 2009; Rath, 2011). Identifying the etiology of the hemorrhage enables the nurse and health care team to initiate prompt and effective interventions to eliminate it and halt the blood loss. A delay in initiation of appropriate management of postpartum hemorrhage increases the incidence of adverse outcomes (Rath, 2011).

The anatomic origin of postpartum hemorrhage can be the contractile tissue of the upper uterine segment at the site of placental implantation, or the non-contractile or poorly contractile tissue of the lower uterine segment, cervix, vagina, or broad ligament. Cases of postpartum hemorrhage can be avoided or limited in severity with the active management of the third stage of labour (Leduc et al., 2009). Active management of the third stage includes the administration of oxytocin (IM, IV push, or IV infusion) with the delivery of the anterior shoulder, delayed cord clamping, controlled cord traction with uterine palpation, uterine massage, and inspection of both the placenta and the lower genital tract for intactness (Leduc et al., 2009).

Postpartum hemorrhage can occur with little warning; risk factors predict only about 40% of cases (Rath, 2011). For women who present with risk factors, it is prudent for the nurse and health care team to initiate IV access, coagulation studies, and crossmatching of blood. Risk factors can be categorized using the "4Ts" mnemonic (Leduc et al., 2009) including tone, tissue, trauma, and thrombin (Table 19.1.)

Postpartum hemorrhage can be further classified as early (within the first 24 hours of birth) or late (24 hours or more after birth). Figure 19.1 depicts the various problems leading to early and late postpartum hemorrhage.

Consider Rosanna, the 36-year-old woman who has given birth to her fourth child. What factors might be contributing to her increased risk for postpartum hemorrhage? What are some clinical signs of early postpartum hemorrhage?

● TABLE 19.1   **Risk Factors in Postpartum Hemorrhage**

	Etiology Process	Clinical Risk Factors
Abnormalities of uterine contraction *(Tone)*	Overdistended uterus Uterine muscle exhaustion Intra-amniotic infection Functional/anatomic distortion of the uterus Uterine-relaxing medications	Polyhydramnios Multiple gestation Macrosomia Rapid labour Prolonged labour High parity Oxytocin use Fever Prolonged ROM Fibroids Placenta previa Uterine anomalies Halogenated anesthetics Nitroglycerin
Retained products of conception *(Tissue)*	Retained products Abnormal placenta Retained cotyledon or succenturiate lobe Retained blood clots	Incomplete placenta at delivery Previous uterine surgery High parity Abnormal placenta on ultrasound Atonic uterus
Genital tract trauma *(Trauma)*	Lacerations of the cervix, vagina, or perineum Extensions, lacerations at cesarean section Uterine rupture Uterine inversion	Precipitous delivery Malposition Deep engagement Previous uterine surgery High parity Fundal placenta Excessive cord traction

Abnormalities of coagulation *(Thrombin)*	Pre-existing states
	  Hemophilia A
	  von Willebrand disease
	acquired in pregnancy
	  Idiopathic thrombocytopenia purpura
	  Thrombocytopenia with preeclampsia
	  DIC
	    Gestational hypertensive disorder of pregnancy with adverse conditions
	    Dead fetus in utero
	    Severe infection
	    Abruption
	    Amniotic fluid embolus
	    Therapeutic anticoagulation
		History of hereditary coagulopathies
		History of liver disease
		Bruising
		Elevated BP
		Elevated blood pressure
		Fetal demise
		Fever, neutrophilia/neutropenia ante-partum hemorrhage
		Sudden collapse
		History of thrombotic disease

Reprinted with permission of the Society of Obstetricians & Gynaecologists of Canada from Leduc, D., Senikas, V., Lalonde, A. B., Ballerman, C., Biringer, A., Delaney, M., et al. (2009). SOGC clinical practice guidelines: Active management of the third stage of labour: Prevention and treatment of postpartum hemorrhage. *Journal of Obstetrics and Gynaecology Canada, 31*(10), 980–993.

Early Postpartum Hemorrhage

Early postpartum hemorrhage occurs within 24 hours of birth, usually resulting from uterine atony and continued bleeding from the placental implantation site. Early postpartum hemorrhage presents with heavier bleeding and greater morbidity than late postpartum hemorrhage. After noting excessive vaginal bleeding, further assessment is necessary to identify the cause, estimate the blood loss, and control the bleeding. Identification and interventions need to be focused, organized, and implemented quickly to manage this obstetrical emergency and decrease the risk of morbidity and mortality (Leduc et al., 2009).

COLLABORATIVE CARE: EARLY POSTPARTUM HEMORRHAGE
Assessment

Although estimating the blood loss is critical to ongoing assessment of the client's hemodynamic status, blood loss is typically underestimated (Rath, 2011). To better

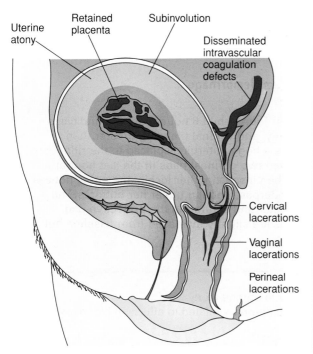

Uterine atony

Retained placenta

Subinvolution

Disseminated intravascular coagulation defects

Cervical lacerations

Vaginal lacerations

Perineal lacerations

FIGURE 19.1 Postpartum hemorrhage can develop from various causes.

estimate blood loss, the nurse may weigh the perineal pads and convert weight to milliliters of blood (1 g = 1 mL of blood). Bleeding may be concealed if it occurs as a hematoma: clinical signs of hypovolemia may be slow to develop if secondary to retained tissue or trauma (Ramanathan & Arulkumaran, 2006). The nurse should assess a woman's level of consciousness, vital signs, and skin colour, warmth, and promptness of capillary refill. Changes in vital signs, particularly blood pressure, develop slowly and are a late sign of blood loss related to postpartum hemorrhage (Leduc et al., 2009)

(Table 19.2). The increased blood volume in pregnancy, which remains during the first 24 to 48 hours postpartum, decreases the rate of change in maternal heart rate and blood pressure until a significant volume of blood has been lost. Frequent monitoring of maternal vital signs and uterine firmness and contraction, as well as other signs of hemodynamic instability, is important during the first 2 hours after birth because only careful surveillance reveals hemodynamic instability.

Select Potential Nursing Diagnoses

The following nursing diagnoses may be appropriate in cases of early postpartum hemorrhage:

- **Ineffective Tissue Perfusion** related to decreased oxygen-carrying capacity and oxygen transport to vital organs and tissues
- **Deficient Fluid Volume** related to excessive blood loss
- **Risk for Injury** related to decreased circulating volume
- **Impaired Tissue Integrity** related to laceration
- **Fear** related to excessive blood loss
- **Fear** related to lack of understanding of what is happening

Planning/Intervention

The goal of interventions is to control the bleeding and decrease the risk of morbidity and mortality (Rath, 2011). See Nursing Care Plan 19.1.

In addition to vital signs, attention to behaviour, and estimation of blood loss, the nurse must assess the uterus to determine if it is firm and contracted. If it feels boggy or is difficult to palpate, the nurse should implement fundal massage (see Chapter 18) (Leduc et al., 2009).

(text continues on page 748)

● TABLE 19.2   **Clinical Findings in Postpartum Hemorrhage**

DEGREE OF SHOCK				
	Compensation	**Mild**	**Moderate**	**Severe**
Blood loss	500–1,000 mL 10–15%	1,000–1,500 mL <20%	1,500–2,000 mL 40%	2,000–3,000 mL >40%
Blood pressure change (systolic pressure)	None	Slight fall		
Symptoms and signs		Diaphoresis Increased capillary refilling Cool extremities Anxiety	Left plus Tachycardia Tachypnea Postural hypotension Oliguria	Left plus Hypotension Agitation/confusion Hemodynamic instability

Reprinted with permission of the Society of Obstetricians & Gynaecologists of Canada from Leduc, D., Senikas, V., Lalonde, A. B., Ballerman, C., Biringer, A., Delaney, M., et al. (2009). Active management of the third stage of labour: Prevention and treatment of postpartum hemorrhage. *Journal of Obstetrics and Gynaecology, 31*(10), 980–993.

NURSING CARE PLAN 19.1

●

The Client With Postpartum Hemorrhage

 Recall Rosanna, who gave birth to her fourth child 6 hours ago. She indicates an inability to void, a feeling of anxiety, and vaginal bleeding greater than expected. Further assessment reveals a boggy uterus displaced to the right with a distended bladder. She has saturated two perineal pads in the last hour and her hands and feet are quite cool. When inspecting her lochia, the nurse notices moderate blood on the protective underpad, pooling under her buttocks. The area is approximately 25 cm in diameter and saturating the protective pad. Rosanna's pulse and respiratory rates are slightly increased from baseline but within acceptable parameters.

NURSING DIAGNOSES

- **Postpartum Hemorrhage** secondary to uterine atony
- **Ineffective Tissue Perfusion: Cardiopulmonary** related to effects of blood loss from postpartum hemorrhage

EXPECTED OUTCOMES

1. The client will remain free of injury from postpartum hemorrhage.
2. The client will exhibit a firm uterus with moderate lochia rubra.
3. The client will demonstrate vital signs and cardiopulmonary status within acceptable parameters.

INTERVENTIONS	RATIONALE
Continue to assess uterine fundus and lochia for changes. Inspect the perineal area. Check for evidence of clots.	Ongoing assessment is necessary to determine effectiveness of interventions and identify signs and symptoms of possible hypovolemic shock. Lochia may contain some clots that will interfere with uterine involution. Bleeding that occurs in the presence of a contracted uterus may be a result of other factors such as previously undetected lacerations.
Reposition the client to inspect for pooling of blood.	Blood may pool in the lower uterine segment and become evident only with positional changes.
Encourage voiding; monitor amounts voided. If necessary, insert a urinary catheter.	Urinary retention leads to bladder distention, which interferes with uterine involution. Urinary catheterization can help keep the bladder empty.
Massage the uterus gently but vigorously until firm.	Uterine massage aids in uterine contraction. Too vigorous massage can overstimulate the uterine muscle, leading to uterine relaxation and further bleeding.
Anticipate bimanual compression by the midwife or obstetrician.	Bimanual compression promotes uterine contraction.

(continued)

NURSING CARE PLAN 19.1 ● The Client With Postpartum Hemorrhage *(Continued)*

INTERVENTIONS	RATIONALE
Insert a large-bore IV line if one is not already in place; administer fluid replacement as ordered.	Fluid replacement helps to maintain vascular volume.
Administer 5–10 international units oxytocin IV bolus or 100 µg carboprost/hemabate IM as ordered.	Oxytocin and carboprost/hemabate stimulate uterine contraction.
Monitor vital signs frequently for changes	Continued blood loss can lead to hypovolemic shock. Recognize that changes in vital signs are often a later sign and may not be representative of the actual blood loss
Administer oxygen as ordered.	Oxygen administration ensures adequate tissue perfusion.
Provide emotional support and teaching to the client and family about what is happening, including measures to prevent further problems.	Emotional support and information help to reduce anxiety and fear.

EVALUATION

1. The client demonstrates reduced bleeding to within acceptable parameters.
2. The client exhibits moderate lochia rubra with a uterus that remains firm and contracted.
3. The client demonstrates vital signs and cardiopulmonary status within acceptable limits.
4. The client and family verbalize understanding of events.

NURSING DIAGNOSIS

Difficulty voiding related to effects of vaginal birth

EXPECTED OUTCOMES

1. The client will use measures to promote voiding.
2. The client will provide a measured voiding.

INTERVENTIONS	RATIONALE
Assess the abdomen for bladder distention	Bladder distention indicates urinary retention and interferes with uterine involution
Assist the client to the bathroom to sit on the toilet to void; provide privacy	Sitting on the toilet helps the client maintain the normal anatomic position for urination

(continued)

NURSING CARE PLAN 19.1 ● The Client With Postpartum Hemorrhage *(Continued)*

INTERVENTIONS	RATIONALE
Run water in the sink, run warm water over the perineum, or place client's hand in a basin or sink filled with warm water; if necessary, fill a sitz bath or tub with warm water and have the client immerse her perineum in the water	The sound of running water or the sensation of warm water stimulates urination and also helps promote client relaxation
Allow the client sufficient time to void	Rushing increases anxiety and contributes to urinary retention
If the client cannot void, prepare to catheterize her	Bladder distention must be relieved to prevent further interference with uterine involution
Measure the amount of urine voided	Voiding less than 100 mL suggests incomplete bladder emptying

EVALUATION

1. The client used water to stimulate voiding.
2. The client voided at least 100 mL clear yellow urine.

Fundal massage may also be helpful in expressing any clots or placental fragments that may be retained in the uterus, interfering with the ability of the uterus to contract. Manual removal of placental fragments may be necessary (Leduc et al., 2009). Urinary retention resulting from edema and soft tissue damage to the urethra may result in excessive blood loss. The nurse can assist the mother to empty her bladder because a full bladder interferes with uterine contractility. If the uterus does not respond to fundal massage, more aggressive interventions are used.

 Think back to Rosanna, the client who gave birth to her fourth child 6 hours ago. Fundal assessment reveals a boggy uterus displaced to the right. She indicated a need to void. How should the nurse intervene?

If the fundus remains atonic, uterotonics can be administered concurrently with fundal massage (Table 19.3). These include oxytocin as an IV bolus and IV maintenance infusion, and/or carboprost/hemabate, ergonovine, and/or misoprostal (Leduc et al., 2009). An IV bolus of oxytocin is recommended for postpartum hemorrhage prevention for vaginal birth but not elective cesarean section. Carbetocin as an IV bolus should be used instead of continuous oxytocin infusion following elective cesarean section (Leduc et al., 2009). It may be necessary for the primary care provider to utilize bimanual uterine massage in a further attempt to stimulate uterine contraction. Exploration of the genital tract may be indicated, especially if bleeding continues in the presence of a contracted uterus (Leduc et al., 2009). Lacerations need to be carefully visualized and repaired. After surgical repair of a genital tract laceration, nursing care is similar to episiotomy care: application of an ice pack for 12 to 24 hours to minimize swelling, followed by sitz baths to enhance circulation and healing. Maintaining perineal hygiene decreases the risk for a secondary infection at the site of the tissue damage. See Box 19.2.

Uterine inversion needs to be corrected by promptly replacing the uterus in the abdominal cavity prior to further administration of oxytocic drugs. Uterine rupture should prompt arrangements to be made for timely laparotomy. If bleeding continues in spite of a well-contracted uterus and retained tissue or trauma has been ruled out, a coagulation disorder should be suspected and appropriate treatment initiated (Leduc et al., 2009).

● TABLE 19.3   **Drugs Used to Control Postpartum Hemorrhage**

Drug	Action/Indication	Nursing Implications
Oxytocin	Stimulates the uterus to contract to control bleeding from the placental site	Assess fundus for evidence of contraction and compare amount of bleeding every 15 minutes or according to orders. Monitor vital signs every 15 minutes. Monitor uterine tone to prevent hyperstimulation. Reassure client about the need for uterine contraction and administer analgesics for comfort. Offer explanation to client and family about what is happening and the purpose of the medication. Provide nonpharmacologic comfort measures to assist with pain management. Set up the IV infusion to be piggybacked into a primary IV line. This ensures that the medication can be discontinued readily if hyperstimulation or adverse effects occur while maintaining the IV site and primary infusion.
Prostaglandin (PGF-2 a, carboprost/hemabate)	Stimulates uterine contractions to treat postpartum hemorrhage due to uterine atony when not controlled by other methods	Assess vital signs, uterine contractions, client's comfort level, and bleeding status as per protocol. Offer explanation to client and family about what is happening and the purpose of the medication. Monitor for possible adverse effects, such as fever, chills, headache, nausea, vomiting, diarrhea, hypertension, flushing, restlessness, oxygen desaturation, and bronchospasm.
Misoprostal	Stimulates the uterus to contract	Assess baseline bleeding, uterine tone, and vital signs every 15 minutes or according to protocol. Offer explanation to client and family about what is happening and the purpose of the medication. Monitor for possible adverse effects, such as shaking, palpitations.

Most women experiencing early postpartum hemorrhage respond to these interventions. If there is no response, blood loss needs to be minimized by compression (manually and/or with tamponade (i.e., balloon catheters). If angiographic embolization is available, it may be implemented. Surgery may be indicated and may include laparotomy with ligation of the uterine vessels, uterine compression sutures, or hysterectomy (Leduc et al., 2009).

Evaluation

Successful outcomes include immediate decreased bleeding. Ongoing assessment is necessary to detect developing signs of hypovolemic shock and infection.

● BOX 19.2   **Good Perineal Hygiene**

Frequent perineal care
Sitz or tub baths
Frequent pad changes
Warm compress to area
Good handwashing technique
Wipe or pat perineal area front to back

Even after resolution of the acute bleeding episode, clients who experience postpartum hemorrhage are at risk for anemia. In cases of mild hemorrhage, dietary counselling and iron supplements are used to rebuild the client's blood volume and hemoglobin stores. Fatigue associated with anemia, combined with exhaustion resulting from the newborn's round-the-clock demands interfere with women's coping and adjustment. Therefore, support in the home environment and assistance with infant care activities are essential components of the follow-up plan. If anemia is severe or results in symptoms of hypovolemia, a blood transfusion may be ordered.

Hematoma

A **hematoma** is a localized collection of blood that results from bleeding into the connective tissue beneath the vaginal mucosa or vulvar skin as a consequence of tissue injury or trauma. It can develop rapidly with no visual evidence of external bleeding.

Types. The most common type is a *vulvar hematoma*, which results when blood from ruptured arteries and veins in the superficial fascia seeps into the nearby tissue. Because the bleeding is into an enclosed area, localized pressure, discolouration, and pain result. Trauma to the

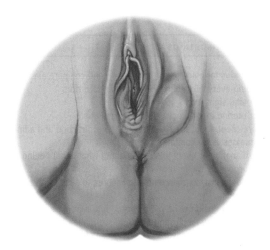

FIGURE 19.2 With a hematoma, the area is ecchymotic, and an outline of the swollen area is visible.

soft tissue during birth may result in a *vaginal hematoma,* which can obstruct the urethra, making urination difficult. *Retroperitoneal hematomas* are rare, but extremely dangerous. Because of their location, they may not be evident until a large amount of blood loss results in hypotension and hypovolemic shock.

The characteristic sign of a hematoma is severe, localized pain, which does not diminish despite administration of analgesics and other supportive measures. Other indicators include difficulty voiding or inability to void and complaints of rectal pressure similar to the sensation during second stage labour. On inspection, the vulvar area may appear ecchymotic, and an outline of the hematoma is visible, if it is located there (Fig. 19.2).

Hematomas present as tense, fluctuant masses. Vaginal hematomas may require vaginal examination for visualization. Changes in vital signs and blood work are unlikely to identify acute bleeding because of pregnancy-related physiologic adaptations and expansion of total blood volume.

Collaborative Management. The priority goal is prevention of hematoma. The best method of prevention of a vulvar hematoma is application of ice to the perineum following a difficult or traumatic birth. When a hematoma has already developed, the goals become cessation of the bleeding, reabsorption or drainage of the blood mass, and attention to the client's need for pain management and elimination care.

Small vulvar hematomas often absorb spontaneously. Comfort measures including localized ice and heat application may help reduce swelling and discomfort and facilitate reabsorption of the hematoma. Large hematomas that may be increasing in size need incision, evacuation, and drainage of the blood and clots. Any vessels that continue to bleed are sutured to

prevent reformation of the hematoma. After incision, the area may be packed for 12 to 18 hours to promote hemostasis and drainage. The packing is then removed before it becomes a reservoir for bacterial proliferation. A Foley catheter is often inserted to promote urinary elimination.

The amount of blood may be significant but difficult to estimate because of the enclosed nature of a hematoma. Fluid and blood replacement may be necessary to prevent hypovolemic shock. In addition, broad-spectrum antibiotics are often prescribed to prevent secondary infection.

Comprehensive and ongoing inspection of the perineal tissue facilitates early identification and intervention. Indicators of effective interventions are resolution of the bleeding as evidenced by decreasing size of the mass, decreasing pain, returning perfusion to area, and no secondary infection.

Late Postpartum Hemorrhage

Late postpartum hemorrhage is excessive vaginal bleeding that occurs 24 hours or more after birth. It most frequently develops 7 to 14 days following birth but can occur as late as 1 month. Late hemorrhage is associated with subinvolution of the uterus, which may be caused by retained placental fragments (see Chapter 18) (Cunningham et al., 2010; James, 2014). Placental fragments, which remain attached to the uterine wall, begin to undergo necrosis as the uterine blood supply decreases. As retained placental fragments necrose, a fibrin deposit and placental polyp form. Eventually, the polyp detaches from the uterine wall, resulting in hemorrhage (Cunningham et al., 2010). A typical scenario is a new mother at home beginning to regain energy and resume daily activities who suddenly experiences a gush of foul-smelling lochia rubra and uterine cramping, which may or may not be accompanied by uterine tenderness and low-grade fever.

COLLABORATIVE CARE: LATE POSTPARTUM HEMORRHAGE

Because late postpartum hemorrhage usually occurs post discharge the woman is responsible for recognition of the symptoms. Therefore, it is important to teach postpartum women about normal patterns and changes in uterine involution and lochial flow and the symptoms that require immediate follow-up.

Assessment

A woman who experiences sudden bright red bleeding; excessive passage of clots; persistent lochia rubra; foul-smelling lochia; pain or tenderness in the lower abdomen, back, or perineum; or a low-grade, persistent fever should see her health care provider immediately.

The uterine fundus may be palpable beyond the first 7 to 10 days after birth as a result of subinvolution. When palpable, the fundus is usually tender. Bimanual examination confirms a uterus larger than expected for the specific stage of the postpartum recovery period. A uterine ultrasound can identify remnants of tissue in the uterine cavity.

A complete blood count (CBC) is important, because the white blood cell (WBC) count and differential are used to assess for infection, and the hemoglobin and hematocrit are examined for the quantity of blood lost.

Select Potential Nursing Diagnoses

Appropriate nursing diagnoses in cases of late postpartum hemorrhage may include the following:

* **Deficient Fluid Volume** related to excessive blood loss
* **Ineffective Maternal Role Performance** related to rehospitalization and sick role
* **Infection** related to retention of necrotic tissue and bacterial proliferation
* **Risk for Injury** related to blood loss, infection, and altered hemodynamics
* **Impaired Parenting** related to rehospitalization of mother and potential separation from infant

Planning/Intervention

The client experiencing late postpartum hemorrhage needs treatment at a health care facility. Physiologic needs related to blood loss resulting in potential hemodynamic changes are the highest priority; however, these clients also have significant psychological needs related to the unexpected emergency. Nursing care focuses on measures to provide a sense of maternal safety and well-being, as well as methods to help the woman deal with any separation from her newborn.

On admission, the client should have a large-bore IV started to infuse crystalloid solutions (e.g., normal saline, Ringer's lactate) to expand circulating volume. Pharmacologic agents such as oxytocin, ergonovine, or a prostaglandin analog such as misoprostal or carboprost may be administered to stimulate uterine contraction, which is necessary to decrease bleeding as well as to stimulate expulsion of any remaining necrotic tissue. If bleeding continues despite pharmacologic interventions and uterine massage, bimanual compression may be necessary.

Curettage of the uterine lining is used only when nonsurgical interventions are ineffective (Cunningham et al., 2010). Surgical curettage further traumatizes the uterine lining, which may result in increased bleeding. When surgical intervention is used, the client and her family need to be aware that a hysterectomy may be necessary if the bleeding cannot be controlled with less invasive measures.

Evaluation

Elimination of the causative factors and resolution of the bleeding are indicators of effective treatment. Decreases in uterine size and lochia indicate involution. Nursing follow-up includes evaluation of hematocrit and hemoglobin for signs of anemia and treatment with dietary counselling and iron supplementation, as needed.

POSTPARTUM INFECTIONS

The classic definition of **puerperal infection** is a temperature of 38°C or higher on any two of the first 10 days following birth, exclusive of the first 24 hours (James, 2014; Maharaj, 2007a). In addition, a temperature of 38°C or higher during the first 24 hours is considered a parameter for identification of early infection.

The timing of pyrexia provides cues about the source and cause of the infectious process. Pyrexia during the first 24 hours indicates infections that are pre-existing or began before the birth. For example, a client who had premature rupture of membranes (PROMs) 7 days before birth has increased susceptibility to ascending infection and may manifest signs of endometrial infection in the first 24 hours after birth. Infections directly related to the birth generally appear 24 to 72 hours later. The most common sites for infection are the uterus and vagina. Finally, infections related to an incision (episiotomy or cesarean section), blood clots, or the breasts usually do not develop until 4 days or more after birth. Infections can be classified according to site as shown in Box 19.3.

Although pyrexia is the primary finding suggestive of postpartum infection, increased temperature can indicate other problems such as dehydration during the first 24 hours or breast engorgement at postpartum days 3 to 5. Therefore, comprehensive assessment and critical analysis of collected data are essential to making such determinations.

Infection of the Uterus and Surrounding Tissues

Endometritis is the primary cause of postpartum infections (Cunningham et al., 2010). During pregnancy, the uterine cavity and endometrial lining are sterile when the intact amniotic membrane protects them from bacterial organisms. After membranes rupture, anaerobic and aerobic bacteria normally residing in the cervix, vagina, perineum, and bowel can ascend into the uterus and contaminate its lining. The introduction of these bacteria, combined with an open wound in the decidua at the site of placental attachment, results in a favourable environment for bacterial growth and infection. When endometritis presents 1 to 2 days after birth the causative organism is usually group A streptococcus (Cunningham et al., 2010). Caesarian delivery is the most significant risk factor for the development of a uterine infection (Cunningham et al., 2010; James, 2014). Without the use of prophylactic antibiotics, 2% to 8% of patients may develop pelvic infection after vaginal delivery, and 18% to 25% after operative delivery (Maharaj, 2007a).

Known risk factors for endometritis include cesarean birth, PROM, long labour, multiple vaginal examinations, placement of intrauterine catheters, fetal scalp electrodes, or fetal pulse oximetry, intrapartum chorioamnionitis, and manual removal of the placenta (Cunningham et al., 2010; James, 2014). These risk factors enhance the opportunity for introduction of bacterial organisms into the uterine cavity. Other risk factors include lower socioeconomic status, young maternal age, nulliparity, smoking, diabetes, and obesity (Cunningham et al., 2010; James, 2014).

COLLABORATIVE CARE: UTERINE INFECTIONS
Assessment

Classic signs of endometritis are a temperature of 38°C or greater, tachycardia, and fundal tenderness. In cases of severe infection, the pattern of temperature elevation is characterized by jagged, irregular spikes, with peaks usually in the evening (Fig. 19.3). Clients present with initial characteristics that include generalized symptoms of fever, chills, anorexia, malaise, tachycardia, and "just not feeling well." Subsequent assessment findings, consistent with postpartum endometritis, include lower abdominal pain, subinvolution of the uterus, tenderness on fundal palpation, malodorous lochia, and prolonged or painful afterpains.

Necessary laboratory data include a CBC with differential; lochial, cervical, and endometrial cultures; and a blood culture. To provide accurate data, all cultures need to be collected before antimicrobial therapy begins. Blood work that shows an elevated leukocyte count with a shift to the left is consistent with endometritis.

 Think back to Leslie, the client described at the beginning of the chapter who had a cesarean birth 1 week ago. What assessment information is needed to determine the likelihood of endometritis?

Select Potential Nursing Diagnoses

The following nursing diagnoses may be appropriate for the client with infection of the uterus and surrounding tissues:

- **Impaired Tissue Integrity** related to bacterial invasion of endometrial tissue
- **Imbalanced Body Temperature** related to intrauterine infection
- **Impaired Parenting** related to lack of energy to engage in child care activities
- **Impaired Parenting** related to maternal–newborn separation
- **Risk for Impaired Urinary Elimination** related to decreased bladder sensation secondary to pain and inflammation
- **Risk for Impaired Bowel Elimination** related to decreased activity and dietary intake

Planning/Intervention

Because the highest risk for infection is associated with cesarean birth, antibiotic prophylaxis is typically administered for these clients, whether this route of delivery is

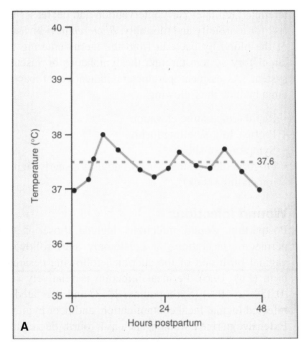

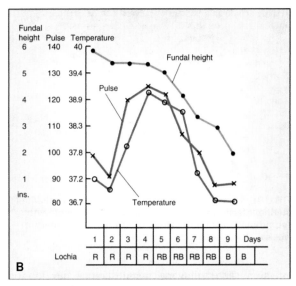

FIGURE 19.3 **A:** In normal postpartum recoveries, the client's temperature shows characteristic resolution within 48 hours of childbirth. **B:** With endometritis, temperature remains elevated for several days. Other signs of endometritis include increased pulse, uterine subinvolution, and malodorous lochia, which remains red. (R, red; B, brown.)

planned or not. Research supports the administration of a single dose of ampicillin or a first-generation cephalosporin, given prior to skin incision; for women colonized with methicillin-resistant *Staphylococcus aureus* (MRSA), vancomycin is given in addition to the cephalosporin (Cunningham et al., 2010).

For the client who has a puerperal infection, after the collection of blood, tissue, and lochia for cultures, the nurse initiates IV antibiotic treatment as prescribed. Initially, the client receives a combination of antibiotics effective against a broad range of aerobic and anaerobic organisms known to cause endometritis, including piperacillin and tazobactam, ampicillin and gentamicin, clindamycin or metronidazole (Cunningham, 2010; Faro, 2005). Most endometrial infections respond to these types of IV antibiotics within 48 hours of initiation of treatment (Faro, 2005; James, 2014). If a client's fever and other symptoms persist despite 48 hours of antimicrobial treatment, other causes of the symptoms need investigation or the antibiotic needs to be changed. IV antimicrobial therapy usually continues until the client has been afebrile for 24 to 48 hours, the WBC returns to normal, and the client is ambulating without difficulty (Faro, 2005; James, 2014).

Nursing care for a client with postpartum endometritis includes use of semi-Fowler position to encourage uterine drainage, good perinatal hygiene to prevent reintroduction of bacterial organisms, and gen-

eral care and support of the client with a fever and generalized infection, such as hydration, rest, nutrition, and comfort management. Inflammation and pain from the infected uterus may lead to incomplete bladder emptying, urinary retention or infection, and sluggish peristalsis. Thus, fluid status and urine and bowel elimination should be monitored and interventions used to prevent secondary complications.

Evaluation

Expected outcomes reflecting effective collaborative treatment include afebrile status, normal uterine involution and lochial changes, and enhanced client feelings of well-being. Most clients respond to antimicrobial treatment within 24 to 48 hours as evidenced by resolution of symptoms.

Sequelae of unresolved endometritis include peritonitis, gastrointestinal tract compromise or paralytic ileus, and septic shock. Ongoing assessment and client education are critical to identifying any recurrence of endometritis, which requires aggressive management to prevent long-term morbidity and mortality.

Other Genital Tract Infections

Parametritis or parametrial cellulitis is the extension of a uterine infection into the broad ligament (Fig. 19.4). Lymphatic transmission of bacteria or direct exposure of the tissue to the invading organism disseminates the

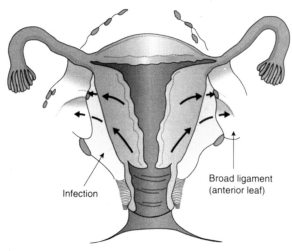

FIGURE 19.4 With parametritis (parametrial cellulitis), uterine infection spreads into the broad ligament, with symptoms developing usually after the first postpartum week.

infection. The following manifestations develop on approximately the 10th postpartum day:

- Prolonged fever with fluctuations
- Lateral extension of abdominal pain
- Uterine subinvolution, hypotension, chills, decreased bowel sounds, nausea, and vomiting
- Positive rebound tenderness on abdominal palpation
- Pain and tenderness in both iliac fossae
- Firm, tender mass felt in one adnexum, or both adnexa pushing the uterus to the opposite side or restricting its mobility

Peritonitis, infection of the peritoneum or abdominal cavity, is a life-threatening postpartum complication (Fig. 19.5). The client with peritonitis exhibits assessment findings such as the following:

- Temperature as high as 40°C
- Severe abdominal pain
- Paralytic ileus
- Abdominal rigidity
- Vomiting leading to dehydration
- Excessive thirst and anxiety

Treatment of both parametritis and peritonitis involves administration of antibiotics. With persistent fever, antimicrobials effective against organisms such as *Peptostreptococcus, Peptococcus, Bacteroides,* and *Clostridium* species, as well as aerobic coliforms, are added. If a paralytic ileus is present, gastric decompression is required. Clients with these conditions require vigilant nursing care focused on the regulation of body temperature, balancing fluids and electrolytes, management of nutrition, and administration of antibiotics.

Ongoing nursing assessment, which focuses on the possible development of septic shock caused by bac-

teremia, facilitates early intervention and decreases the risk for morbidity and mortality. *Bacteremia* is invasion of the blood by bacteria from the uterus entering the circulatory system through the lymphatics or vascular system. Assessment parameters indicative of bacteremia include the following:

- Rapid temperature elevation
- Profuse foul-smelling lochia
- Symptoms of shock
- Oliguria (decreasing urinary output is an early sign of impending shock)

Wound Infections

Postpartum wound infections include those of the perineum (lacerations or episiotomy site) following vaginal birth and of the abdomen following cesarean birth (Fig. 19.6). Perineal infection is relatively rare (0.35% to 10%) (Spiliopoulos, 2013) and is related to infected lochia, fecal contamination, and poor hygiene. Extensive perineal trauma, such as a fourth-degree laceration, and instrument-assisted births, such as forceps and vacuum extractions, place the woman at increased risk for perineal infection. Abdominal incision infection (3% to 15%) usually results from contamination of the wound with organisms from the vaginal flora; however, *S. aureus* from the skin or other sources is identified in 25% of cases (Spiliopoulos, 2013). The

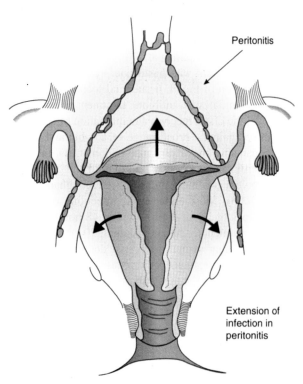

FIGURE 19.5 Life-threatening peritonitis can develop from spread of a postpartum uterine infection into the abdominal cavity.

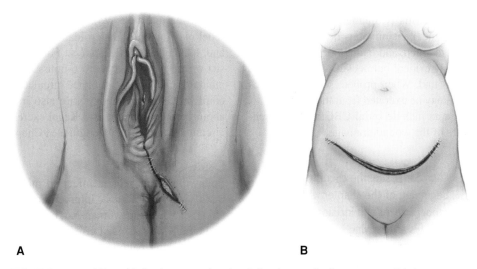

A   **B**

FIGURE 19.6 Wound infections can develop following vaginal or cesarean births. **A:** Postpartum vaginal wound infection may stem from the episiotomy site. **B:** Postpartum cesarean wound infection may arise at the site of the surgical incision.

most common complication of a wound infection is prolonged hospitalization.

A meta-analysis demonstrated that disruption of the skin incision post cesarean section occurs in 2.5% to 16% of procedures; the rate is significantly lowered with antimicrobial prophylaxis (Chelmow et al., 2004; Cunningham et al., 2010). Risk factors for abdominal wound dehiscence include infected abdominal incisions and/or tissue necrosis that then lead to additional surgical intervention, hemorrhage or anemia, obesity, immunosuppression, complex wound care therapies, or prolonged healing time that may be associated with underlying medical conditions such as diabetes (Chelmow et al., 2004; Cunningham et al., 2010; James, 2014). Primary prevention of wound infections includes prophylactic antimicrobial administration, and keeping incisions clean and dry to eliminate the opportunity for bacterial growth and proliferation. See Teaching Tips 19.1.

COLLABORATIVE CARE: WOUND INFECTIONS
Assessment

Erythema, induration, warmth, tenderness, and purulent drainage at the site, with or without fever, are indicative of a wound infection (James, 2014; Maharaj, 2007b). A draining wound often presents without fever. Early clues of a developing wound infection include edema, skin discolouration, or poor approximation of the skin edges.

Clients with a perineal infection frequently complain of excruciating pain, malodorous discharge, and vulvar edema. On inspection, the perineal area is edematous and red. Thorough inspection is necessary to determine the coexistence of a hematoma or perineal abscess as the reservoir of the infection.

Abdominal wound infections do not typically present until 4 to 5 days postoperatively, and are often

● TEACHING TIPS 19.1   Postpartum Infections

The nurse teaches the client recovering from postpartum infections the following:

- Follow the antibiotic regimen exactly as described. Self-administer the medication precisely as described. Even if you begin to feel better, be sure to finish the entire set of drugs.
- Monitor your temperature at least once daily; report to your health care provider any reading above 38°C.
- Report to your health care provider any abdominal pain, chills, changes in the odour or colour of lochia,

or abnormalities at a specific site, such as warmth, redness, or swelling.
- Wash your hands thoroughly before and after eating, newborn care, using the bathroom, or wiping/touching the genitals and anal area.
- Use a front-to-back motion when changing your perineal pad.
- Drink adequate fluids; follow a diet that is high in protein and vitamins.
- Get as much rest as possible (e.g., sleep when the baby sleeps).

preceded by endometritis (Cunningham et al., 2010). On examination, the incision may be erythematous, warm and tender to touch, and indurated. Drainage may not be immediately evident but pockets of fluid may be found near the wound. When probed, serosanguineous or purulent fluid may be excreted from the pockets.

Laboratory data include serial CBC with differentials and cultures of the wound drainage.

 Consider Leslie, the client from the beginning of the chapter who called to report a fever and incisional complaints 10 days after giving birth. The nurse instructs Leslie to come to the health care facility for an evaluation because she might have an incisional infection. What assessment elements would the nurse undertake for Leslie?

Select Potential Nursing Diagnoses

The following nursing diagnoses may be appropriate for the client with a wound infection:

- **Impaired Skin Integrity** related to fluid accumulation or open incision
- **Disturbed Body Image** related to draining wound or wound healing by secondary intention
- **Pain** related to wound care procedures

Planning/Intervention

Treatment is based on facilitating drainage of the infected area. An infected incision may dehisce spontaneously and begin to drain; in other cases, the skin incision must be opened to allow drainage. After the infected area is drained and cleaned, antibiotic treatment is initiated to eradicate the causative bacterial organism. Ongoing nursing care of an infected abdominal incision also involves efforts to keep the area clean. Most infected wounds are left open and heal by secondary intention, packed with saline-moistened gauze pads. Client and family teaching about ongoing wound care at home and potential referral for home care and support are also necessary components of the nursing plan of care. Nursing Care Plan 19.2 highlights the care of a woman with an infection of an incision.

Pharmacologic treatment of perineal and abdominal wound infections includes antibiotics to eradicate the bacterial organism. Antimicrobials are selected based on the culture of the organism and its sensitivity to the specific class of antibiotic. The health care provider will initiate a broad-spectrum antibiotic until this laboratory report has been received (24 to 48 hours). Probiotics may also be used; there is limited but promising evidence

supporting their use (Wong et al., 2013). Symptomatic relief may include nonsteroidal anti-inflammatory drugs and local anaesthetic sprays. For perineal infections sitz or tub baths every 4 to 6 hours facilitate drainage, maintain cleanliness, enhance circulation, and provide comfort. Ongoing nursing care also includes teaching about perineal hygiene and Kegel exercises to enhance circulation and tissue strength (see Chapter 23).

Evaluation

Following drainage of the infection, most clients respond rapidly to antibiotics. Interventions are considered effective when the woman has been afebrile for 24 to 48 hours. Other signs of effective nursing interventions are decreasing pain and inflammation. If the wound is left open, the base and surrounding tissue should appear pink and healthy throughout healing. Ongoing evaluation after discharge is important for monitoring wound healing and identifying early indicators of a secondary infection.

Urinary Tract Infection (UTI)

UTIs are a common medical complication during pregnancy; incidence in the postpartum period is increased for women who have had an antepartum UTI (See Chapter 12) (James, 2014). Postpartum clients are at increased risk for UTI for several reasons:

- Trauma to the bladder from passage of the fetus from uterus to perineum
- The dilation of the ureters and pelves during pregnancy takes 2 to 8 weeks to return to prepregnancy size.
- Hypotonicity of the lower urinary tract leading to overdistention, incomplete emptying, and resultant urinary stasis
- Frequency of urinary catheterization (primary cause) and vaginal examinations during labour (associated with a higher incidence of UTIs)
- Instrument-assisted births, including cesarean, forceps, and vacuum births, and induction of labour

A UTI is diagnosed when a pathogen is detected in the presence of clinical symptoms; asymptomatic bacteriuria is diagnosed if the upper limit of 100,000 cfu/mL is exceeded in two consecutive midstream urine samples collected appropriately (Schmiemann et al., 2010). The majority of UTIs are caused by gastrointestinal organisms; *Escherichia coli* account for 80% to 90% of infections (Maharaj, 2007b).

Obtaining a clean-catch urine culture during the postpartum period is difficult because of lochial discharge, which contaminates the urine specimen. A catheterized specimen increases the risk for introducing bacteria into the urinary tract and promoting an ascending infection. The benefits and limitations of each specimen collection

NURSING CARE PLAN 19.2

●

The Postpartum Client Who Develops a Wound Infection

 Remember Leslie, who had a cesarean birth approximately 1 week ago. She reported to the emergency department at the nurse's instructions. Assessment reveals that the client's temperature is 38.4°C. Other vital signs are within acceptable parameters. Her low transverse incision is reddened, edematous, and warm to the touch. A 3.8-cm area at the right end of her incision is bulging and tense. On palpation, the area opens and drains approximately 45 mL of serosanguineous and purulent drainage.

NURSING DIAGNOSES

- **Potential Injury** related to postpartum wound infection
- **Decreased Knowledge** related to wound care

EXPECTED OUTCOMES

1. The client will exhibit decreased redness, warmth, and inflammation at the incision site.
2. The client will care for her wound to promote healing.

NURSING ACTIVITY	RATIONALE
Assess the incisional wound closely; note drainage amount, colour, and character	This information provides a baseline from which to determine appropriate interventions
Assess the client's temperature at least every 4 hours for changes	Temperature assessment provides information about the client's current infection
Obtain a culture of the wound and send it to the laboratory	Wound culture identifies the causative organism for initiating appropriate antibiotic therapy
Clean the wound using aseptic technique; pack the open area with saline-moistened gauze pads	Wound cleansing and packing promote healing and prevent abscess formation
Administer prescribed antibiotics	Antibiotic therapy is necessary to treat the underlying cause of the wound infection
Institute wound care, such as irrigation, as ordered	Specific wound care measures help to promote healing
Teach the client about consuming a diet high in protein	She needs additional protein for wound healing
Instruct the client in the wound care procedure with her participation	Client participation enhances learning and feelings of control over the situation
Request the client return demonstrate the procedure for wound care	Return demonstration of the procedure indicates client learning
Arrange referral for home care services after discharge	Home care provides opportunities for additional teaching, follow-up, and care
Administer antipyretics as ordered	Antipyretics aid in reducing fever
Encourage fluid intake	Fluid intake helps to replace fluids lost from fever
Institute measures to promote rest and relaxation	Fever and infection can stress the body's reserves

EVALUATION

1. The client exhibits a clean dry wound with pink base and surrounding tissue.
2. The client demonstrates the procedure for wound care appropriately.

procedure need to be evaluated based on the individual client situation and client-specific data.

Inflammation of the lower urinary tract (bladder and urethra) is known as *cystitis,* whereas inflammation of the upper urinary tract (kidneys and ureters) is known as *pyelonephritis.*

COLLABORATIVE CARE: POSTPARTUM URINARY TRACT INFECTIONS

Assessment

The primary early sign of postpartum cystitis is elevated temperature. Consequently, when the client has a temperature of 38°C or higher, a UTI should be considered. UTIs are often characterized by a lingering low-grade fever. Clients may also report symptoms of urinary frequency, urgency, dysuria, hematuria, and suprapubic or lower abdominal pain. Bacteriuria is often asymptomatic with only 21% women with positive cultures reporting symptoms (Maharaj, 2007b). Moreover, many typical symptoms are difficult to distinguish from some expected renal system adaptations during the early postpartum period.

On inspection, the urine is frequently dark with particulate matter and a foul odor. Relevant laboratory assessments include urinalysis, CBC, and urine culture. Voided urine specimens are likely to be contaminated with lochial discharge and other vaginal secretions.

Cystitis can appear anytime during the puerperium. Pyelonephritis does not usually appear until the end of the first postpartum week. The client with pyelonephritis exhibits an extremely high temperature (40°C) accompanied by chills, anorexia, and flank pain, and feels extremely ill. In addition to signs of urinary frequency and dysuria, there is costovertebral angle tenderness over the kidney area. Pyelonephritis is more common in the right kidney and results from bacteria ascending from the lower urinary tract.

Select Potential Nursing Diagnoses

The following nursing diagnoses may apply to the client with postpartum UTI:

- **Difficulty voiding** related to infection and pain
- **Ineffective Thermoregulation** related to bacterial infection
- **Pain** related to dysuria
- **Risk for Fluid Volume Deficit** related to elevated body temperature and decreased oral intake to avoid painful urination

Planning/Implementation

The best treatment is prevention, beginning with teaching self-care practices and encouraging healthy behaviours, such as good perineal hygiene, wiping from urinary meatus to rectum to prevent bacterial contamination, and frequent bladder emptying.

Once a UTI is diagnosed, medical treatment consists of antimicrobial therapy and analgesia. A broad-spectrum antibiotic is usually started before urine culture and sensitivity results are available, but when the culture results identify the causative organism the appropriate antibiotic must be prescribed. Initially, most antibiotics are administered intravenously and switched to an oral form for the remainder of a 10-day course. Urinary tract analgesics are prescribed to relieve symptoms of dysuria. In addition, the woman needs to maintain high fluid intake to help to flush the bacteria from the bladder.

Clients with pyelonephritis are acutely ill and require bed rest, IV fluids for hydration, parenteral antimicrobial therapy, and a cooling blanket for a high fever until a woman is afebrile (Maharaj, 2007b). Follow-up diagnostic procedures such as a renal ultrasound or IV pyelogram may be indicated for those with continuing urinary tract problems.

Evaluation

At the completion of treatment, the client should have a follow-up urine culture to evaluate effectiveness. Bacteria counts will be decreased if the treatment is effective. Continuing high counts may indicate a persistent infection. Following the treatment of UTI, the nurse should teach self-care practices to prevent future infections:

- Good perineal and bladder hygiene
- Adequate fluid intake, including cranberry juice
- Kegel exercises

Mastitis

Mastitis is inflammation of the mammary glands caused by milk stasis and bacterial invasion of breast tissue. It is most commonly caused by *S. aureus;* other common pathogens include *Group A and B Hemolytic Streptococci, E. coli, Hemophilus organisms,* or community-acquired methicillin-resistant *S. aureus* (CA-MRSA) (Cunningham et al., 2010; Maharaj, 2007b). Cracked nipples provide a portal of entry for the organism; once the bacteria enter the breast tissue milk, stasis provides a medium for proliferation.

Proper self-care and breastfeeding technique prevent mastitis (see Chapter 21). Primary prevention strategies include the following:

- Wash hands before breastfeeding
- Breastfeed frequently to prevent engorgement and milk stasis
- Avoid constant pressure on the breast tissue, such as tight clothing, poorly fitting bras, or pressure on the nipple or areola that stops milk flow

- Latch the infant to areola and nipple and change positions to prevent sore and cracked nipples
- If the woman experiences distended breasts before feeding, apply warm, moist heat to the breast, gently massage the area, and change the infant's nursing position to ensure emptying of the breast after each feeding

COLLABORATIVE CARE: MASTITIS
Assessment

Identification of mastitis is based entirely on clinical presentation. The onset is usually sudden and may mimic influenza. Common symptoms include a short history of fever, chills, and localized warmth, swelling, and tenderness of the breast (Maharaj, 2007b).

Mastitis does not usually develop until the third to fourth week after birth (Cunningham et al., 2010). On inspection, a painful, hardened, red area is seen on the breast (Fig. 19.7). The axillary glands may be enlarged on the affected side and the breast may be engorged. Mastitis is usually unilateral; however, if left untreated, it can progress to abscess formation and systemic infection, including toxic shock syndrome (Cunningham et al., 2010). Blood work reveals leukocytosis, consistent with an infection, but does not provide specific indicators of the source of infection. Cultures of breast milk may be obtained to identify the causative organism.

Select Potential Nursing Diagnoses

The following nursing diagnoses may be appropriate for the client with mastitis:

- **Ineffective Breastfeeding** related to pain or discomfort, malaise, and fear of transmitting infection to the infant
- **Imbalanced Infant Nutrition** related to interrupted breastfeeding because of maternal illness and discomfort
- **Decreased Self-Image** related to self-perceived inability to meet basic infant feeding needs

Planning/Intervention

The nurse's primary goals are treating the infection, preventing milk stasis (incomplete emptying of the breast), and maintaining nipple integrity. The primary care provider generally prescribes a penicillinase-resistant penicillin (i.e., dicloxacillin); erythromycin may be prescribed in the presence of penicillin sensitivity, and vancomycin if the causative organism is CA-MRSA (Cunningham et al., 2010; Maharaj, 2007b). Most antimicrobials used to treat mastitis are safe during breastfeeding. The infection usually resolves following 48 hours of treatment with an appropriate antibiotic.

To prevent milk stasis, it is important to encourage continued breastfeeding. The infant suckling at the breast is a more effective means of emptying the breast than is a breast pump or manual expression. Analgesics, application of intermittent ice packs to the affected breast followed by a warm pack immediately before feeding, and a supportive bra are useful adjuncts in decreasing maternal discomfort (Maharaj, 2007b).

The nurse also assesses and evaluates the infant for signs and symptoms of bacterial colonization. If the infant is colonized, additional treatment is indicated.

It is important to educate the woman about avoiding practices that place pressure on the breast tissue and impede milk flow, such as wearing tight clothing or underwire bras, gripping the breast tightly when nursing, using pressure on the breast tissue to move it away from the infant's nose while nursing, sleeping on her stomach, and stopping milk flow by applying pressure to the areola. Finally, the nurse or health care provider teaches clients about the importance of good hygiene, complete emptying of the breast, and care of nipples to prevent cracking as measures that can prevent mastitis.

Evaluation

Resolution of the maternal febrile state and elimination of breast pain and inflammation are indicators of effective treatment. In addition, the nurse evaluates breastfeeding technique, specifically infant positioning, latch-on technique, and sucking behaviour (see Chapter 21).

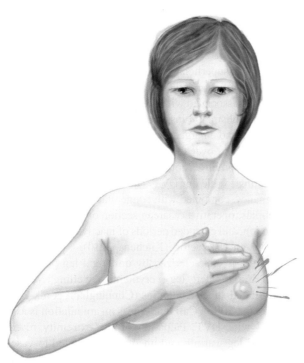

FIGURE 19.7 Mastitis is characterized by a hard, reddened, and painful area on an engorged breast.

THROMBOEMBOLIC COMPLICATIONS

The hypercoagulability associated with pregnancy places the postpartum client at increased risk for thromboembolic disorders. A **thromboembolic disorder** is the formation of a clot or clots inside a blood vessel and is caused by inflammation or partial obstruction of the vessel (Fig. 19.8). Thromboembolic disorders of concern during the postpartum period include the following.

- **Superficial venous thrombosis:** Inflammation, clot formation, and resulting flow obstruction are confined to the superficial saphenous venous system. This condition is also referred to as *phlebitis* because it is associated with inflammation of the vascular structures.
- **Deep venous thrombosis (DVT):** This involves the deep veins of the legs and can extend from the foot to the iliofemoral region. This condition is not associated with inflammation, but with obstruction and clot formation.

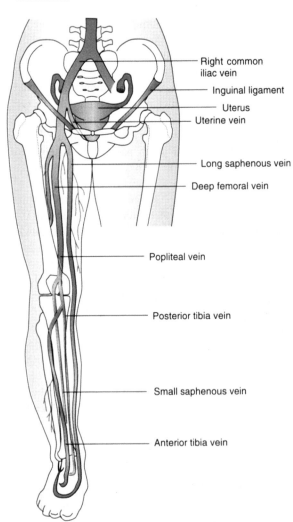

FIGURE 19.8 Common sites of postpartum thrombophlebitis.

- **Pulmonary embolism:** A rare complication of DVT, this occurs when a portion of the clot (emboli) breaks free and is carried through the circulatory system until it lodges in the pulmonary artery, where it occludes the vessel and obstructs pulmonary blood flow.

The pathophysiology of thromboembolic disease is based on the presence of Virchow triad: (1) venous stasis resulting in decreased blood flow; (2) vascular mechanical, chemical, or traumatic injury; and (3) hypercoagulability (Cunningham et al., 2010).

Specific risk factors that increase the incidence of clot formation during the postpartum period include the following (Cunningham et al., 2010; James, 2014):

- Route of birth (increased risk with cesarean births)
- Immobility, particularly prolonged bed rest or travel
- History of venous thrombosis or varicosities
- Obesity
- Dehydration
- Multiparity
- Maternal age older than 35 years
- Pre-existing cardiopulmonary disease or diabetes
- Hemorrhage and anemia

COLLABORATIVE CARE: THROMBOEMBOLIC COMPLICATIONS

The incidence of thromboembolic complications decreases with early ambulation (Cunningham et al., 2010; Morrison, 2006). However, the incidence of venous thromboembolism and pulmonary embolism has been found to be significantly higher during both pregnancy and the postpartum period (Chan et al., 2014; Helt et al., 2005).

Assessment

Phlebitis or superficial venous thrombosis is characterized by unilateral pain and tenderness in the lower extremity. It may be associated with deep vein thrombosis or pulmonary embolism. On inspection, the affected area appears reddened and enlarged. Palpation reveals warmth and an enlarged vein over the site of the thrombus. Superficial venous thromboses above the knee need further diagnostic testing to rule out DVT. The hypercoagulable state of pregnancy, combined with congenital or acquired thrombophilias, operative cesarean section or vaginal delivery, infection, and extended periods of inactivity, bed rest, and obesity, are risk factors (Kitchens, 2010).

DVT is characterized by unilateral leg pain (often involving the left leg), erythema, swelling, warmth, and dilated superficial veins (Cunningham et al., 2010; Morrison, 2006). Calf tenderness on ambulation is associated with DVT. Palpation of the extremity reveals unequal leg warmth and unequal size related to vascular congestion in the affected leg. Clinically observable signs may be absent in some clients with DVT.

Assessment for potential thrombophlebitis should include assessment of the calves of the legs for redness, swelling, and heat (see Chapter 18). Because of the highly variable presentation of thromboembolic disorders and the inaccuracy of clinical symptoms alone, additional diagnostic testing is needed. Although venogram remains the gold standard, it is cumbersome and associated with complications (Cunningham et al., 2010). Vascular ultrasound has replaced the venogram (Chan et al., 2014; Morrison, 2006). There are mixed views about whether serum D-dimer assay can predict DVT development in the early postpartum period, some positive (Yoshiiwa et al., 2011) and some negative (McClintock, et al., 2012).

Doppler studies and impedance plethysmography are noninvasive diagnostic tests that may be used to confirm DVT. Doppler studies use a combination of ultrasound and Doppler technology to visualize the veins and to detect their compressibility. If the vein is not compressible, thrombosis is likely. Impedance plethysmography measures the rate of emptying of the deep veins in the calf after occlusion of the deep veins in the thigh (Cunningham et al., 2010).

Signs of pulmonary embolism include dyspnea, tachypnea, sudden chest pain, tachycardia, cardiac dysrhythmia, apprehension, and hemoptysis (Cunningham et al., 2010; James, 2014). Without prompt intervention, death may result from cardiac failure and hypoxia. Laboratory tests include indirect measures such as serial blood gases, blood coagulation studies, electrocardiogram, and chest x-ray, but the definitive diagnostic procedure is a ventilation–perfusion scan of the lung using radioisotopes.

Select Potential Nursing Diagnoses
The following nursing diagnoses may be appropriate for the client with thromboembolic disorders:

- **Pain** related to venous obstruction and altered tissue oxygenation
- **Impaired Tissue Integrity** related to obstructed blood flow and tissue oxygenation
- **Impaired Mobility** related to bed rest
- **Impaired Gas Exchange** related to clot in pulmonary artery
- **Risk for Injury** related to the clot dislodging and becoming a pulmonary embolus and bleeding secondary to anticoagulation administration
- **Impaired Parenting** related to pain, and treatment plan

Planning/Intervention
Low molecular weight heparin is preferred over unfractionated heparin for prophylaxis in those antepartum women at identified risk for thromboembolism (Chan et al., 2014). It is not recommended for isolated pregnancy related risk factors (Chan et al., 2014). Postpartum thromboprophylaxis, recommended for women having one or more risk factors, includes administration of low molecular weight heparin (Chan et al., 2014). Women who have had an emergency caesarian section should receive thromboprophylaxis only in the presence of one other risk factor; in the case of an elective caesarian section, there should be a minimum of two other risk factors (Chan et al., 2014). Superficial venous thrombosis is treated conservatively with nonsteroidal anti-inflammatory drugs (e.g., ibuprofen) for pain. There is some controversy with regards to activity. Although a recent meta-analysis indicated that early ambulation has been supported over bed rest to prevent development of a new deep vein thrombosis or progression to a deep vein thrombosis (Aissaoui et al., 2009), other sources continue to recommend graded ambulation after symptoms have abated (Cunningham et al., 2010). Elastic compression stockings are used to support the venous structures and prevent further stasis. Local application of heat may enhance circulation and comfort and relieve inflammation.

When a DVT is diagnosed, anticoagulation therapy is added. Initially, IV heparin therapy is started, usually with a bolus dose followed by a continuous infusion. Heparin administration is adjusted to coagulation studies; the aim is to obtain an activated partial thromboplastin time (aPTT) that is 1.5 to 2.5 times the control (Cunningham et al., 2010). The nurse also monitors the client's platelet count to assess for the development of heparin-induced thrombocytopenia.

After stabilization of her condition and evidence of adequate anticoagulation, the postpartum patient will be switched to oral warfarin sodium therapy. Warfarin therapy should overlap with intravenous heparin for 4 to 5 days, until the international normalized ratio (INR) is in the therapeutic range of 2 to 3 (Cunningham et al., 2010). Ideally, the postpartum woman will continue on oral therapy for 3 to 6 months. Warfarin sodium is contraindicated during pregnancy because it crosses the placenta and has potential teratogenic effects (McClintock et al., 2012). It is, however, safe during the postpartum period. The drug is considered safe during breastfeeding (Cunningham et al., 2010).

Clients using any type of anticoagulant therapy need monitoring. The nurse teaches clients the signs and symptoms of hemorrhage, including epistaxis, blood in urine or stool, ecchymosis, and petechiae. In the immediate postpartum period, the nurse evaluates the effect of anticoagulant therapy on uterine bleeding. He or she also cautions clients receiving anticoagulation therapy to avoid products containing aspirin, which inhibits the synthesis of clotting factors and can further prolong clotting time and precipitate bleeding. Assessment of the client receiving heparin also includes platelet counts, since heparin-induced thrombocytopenia can be a complication in the first 15 days of therapy; the risk is decreased with the use of unfractionated heparin (Cunningham et al., 2010).

Prompt intervention is required if a pulmonary embolism is suspected. Heparin and oxygen therapy are initiated. A large embolism can block pulmonary blood, resulting in right-sided cardiac failure and death. The client with a pulmonary embolism requires intensive nursing care as well as continuous support throughout the crisis.

Evaluation

Indicators of effective intervention are decreased pain and restoration of vascular flow. When the client is receiving heparin therapy, maintaining the aPTT at 1.5 to 2.5 times the control is considered effective. When a client is receiving oral warfarin sodium therapy, the INR is the measure of anticoagulation effectiveness. Dosing is individualized and titrated to achieve a target INR range of 2 to 3 (Cunningham et al., 2010).

Clients treated for thromboembolic disorders are at increased risk for recurrence, especially during subsequent pregnancies (Morrison, 2006). Therefore, client teaching about exercises and behaviours to prevent future clot formation is important. Women should perform leg exercises such as flexion and extension of the feet and pushing the back of the knees into the mattress and then flexing slightly. Other appropriate preventive measures include avoiding crossing the legs, avoiding pressure at the back of the knees, and wearing support hose or antiembolic stockings.

PERIPARTUM CARDIOMYOPATHY

Peripartum cardiomyopathy is a rare but serious complication. It may present between the last month of pregnancy and 6 months after birth; most cases appear in the early postpartum period. Clients with peripartum cardiomyopathy have a 25% to 50% risk for dying within the first 3 months (Dorbala et al., 2005). The exact etiology is unknown, but risk factors include African ethnicity, age, pregnancy-induced hypertension or preeclampsia, multiparity, multiple gestation, obesity, chronic hypertension, or prolonged use of tocolytics (Shah et al., 2013). Recent experimental work suggests that an unprotected increase in oxidative stress levels leads to increased expression and proteolytic activity of cardiac cathepsin D, which converts prolactin to a form with detrimental effects on coronary microvasculature (Elkayam et al., 2012). Other mechanisms could include an autoimmune response to pregnancy or unmasking of familial cardiomyopathy by hemodynamic stress

(increases in cardiac output, intravascular volume, and stroke volume) of pregnancy (Stewart, 2012).

COLLABORATIVE CARE: PERIPARTUM CARDIOMYOPATHY

Assessment

Assessment findings are consistent with acute heart failure and hemodynamic compromise. Common presenting symptoms are shortness of breath, orthopnea, and paroxysmal nocturnal dyspnea. Fatigue is also a common but frequently overlooked finding that may be confused with normal discomfort during the postpartum adjustment.

Chest x-rays reveal pulmonary venous congestion and occasionally pulmonary edema and pleural effusion. Electrocardiogram findings include left ventricular hypertrophy and conduction abnormalities, sinus tachycardia, and nonspecific ST-segment and T-wave changes (Elkayam et al., 2012). On laboratory testing, B-type natriuretic peptide levels increase significantly in symptomatic patients (Elkayam et al., 2012). The absence of fever and leukocytosis eliminates the diagnosis of myocarditis secondary to sepsis. An echocardiogram is used to evaluate left ventricular function (Elkayam et al., 2012).

Select Potential Nursing Diagnoses

The following nursing diagnoses may be appropriate for the client with peripartum cardiomyopathy:

- **Decreased Cardiac Output** related to heart failure
- **Ineffective Tissue Perfusion** related to hemodynamic changes

Planning/Intervention

Medical management is similar to that for other forms of heart failure. When peripartum cardiomyopathy presents in late pregnancy, health care personnel also need to consider the risk that the management protocol poses to the fetus.

Angiotensin-converting enzyme (ACE) inhibitors are the main medical therapy for postpartum clients. ACE inhibitors are contraindicated during pregnancy because of an increased association with fetal toxicity, especially in late pregnancy, secondary to fetal hypotension resulting from maternal hypotension and decreased uteroplacental perfusion. Limb malformation, growth restriction, patent ductus arteriosus, and pulmonary hypoplasia are other toxic effects (Stewart, 2012). During the postpartum period, captopril and enalapril have the most evidence for safety during breastfeeding (Stewart, 2012).

Like other forms of heart failure, peripartum cardiomyopathy can lead to thrombotic and embolic complications. Thus, clients often are started concurrently on anticoagulant therapy until the ejection fraction improves to more than 35% (Stewart, 2012); appropriate nursing care and teaching are indicated. These may include lifestyle recommendations about restriction of dietary sodium to less than 2 g and fluid to less than 2 L in 24 hours if heart failure is present (Stewart, 2012). Bed rest is not usually recommended. Identifying and providing sources of psychosocial support are important (Stewart, 2012).

The client's functional status determines her activity level. She should refrain from aerobic activities and heavy lifting during the first few months after diagnosis (Stewart, 2012). Lactation increases metabolic demands and many of the pharmacologic agents used to manage peripartum cardiomyopathy cross into breast milk. Therefore, breastfeeding must be evaluated carefully.

Evaluation

There is no "cure" for peripartum cardiomyopathy. The outcomes and need for further treatment vary. Some clients remain stable for long periods, some deteriorate gradually, and some deteriorate rapidly and may be candidates for a heart transplant.

Between 45% and 78% of women return to an ejection fraction of >50% within 6 months; however, there is a high risk of relapse. Heart failure symptoms are more common in women without normalized ejection fractions prior to a subsequent pregnancy; women with an ejection fraction of <25% should be advised against pregnancy (Stewart, 2012).

REPRODUCTIVE ANATOMIC COMPLICATIONS

Anatomic complications usually begin soon after childbirth and have long-term consequences. They include problems such as loss of urine when laughing or sneezing (stress incontinence) or prolapse of the bladder, uterus, or rectum. Working in jobs involving hard manual labour can lead to prolapse (Hagen & Stark, 2011).

Pelvic Problems

Pelvic relaxation is a broad term encompassing the stretching, pushing, and straining of the structures supporting the organs of reproduction and elimination. Pelvic relaxation is actually a complex problem due to weaknesses that can occur in various support structures, relative to the vaginal walls. Pregnancy and birth, and menopause when anatomic changes accompany the loss of ovarian hormone function, make these key times for discovery of pelvic relaxation anomalies (Fig. 19.9).

During pregnancy, elevated progesterone levels facilitate relaxation of the pelvic support structures to prepare the lower reproductive tract for expulsion of the fetus (Hock et al. 2008). Etiology of pelvic organ prolapse is complex and multifactorial. Risk factors include pregnancy, childbirth, congenital or acquired

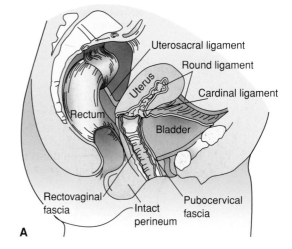

A

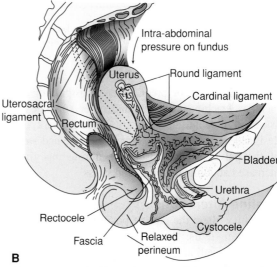

B

FIGURE 19.9 **A:** Normal support of the vagina and uterus. **B:** Problems of relaxation and support in the female reproductive system.

connective tissue abnormalities, denervation or weakness of the pelvic floor, ageing, menopause, and factors associated with chronically raised intra-abdominal pressure (e.g., heavy lifting) (Hagen & Stark, 2011).

During pregnancy, labour, and birth, the female reproductive organs undergo anatomic and physiologic adaptations, stresses, and traumas. The increased volume and weight of the uterus during pregnancy displaces and stretches the supporting structures and adjacent organs. A large infant, prolonged labour, or precipitous birth can result in excessive stretching of tissue and injury to the vaginal wall. In addition, the descending fetal head can exert downward pressure on the bladder neck and urethra, resulting in soft tissue damage. Structural changes related to pregnancy and birth may be present after birth, but they may be asymptomatic until later, often during the perimenopausal years. These conditions alter the position and function of the uterus, bladder, and rectum.

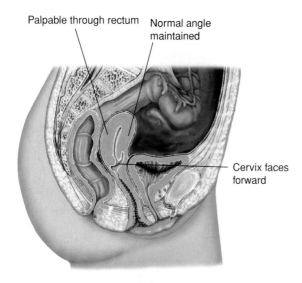

Palpable through rectum   Normal angle maintained

Cervix faces forward

FIGURE 19.10 Uterine retroversion can be a normal anatomic variant or can develop as a complication after childbirth.

Nursing care of pregnant and postpartum clients includes teaching exercises and other strategies such as pelvic floor muscle training (Hagen & Stark, 2011), designed to maintain and support the tone and strength of the pelvic support structures during this time of increased abdominal weight and stress.

Uterine Alterations

Pregnancy alters the uterine position to accommodate the growing fetus. The round ligaments attached to the uterine sidewall and the uterosacral ligaments extending from the cervix support the uterus and influence the position. In the nonpregnant state, the position of the uterus is anteverted, with the cervix positioned posterior and upward. During pregnancy, the uterus becomes retroverted to facilitate the enlarging size, and the cervix is positioned anteriorly to create a physical barrier between the flora of the posterior vaginal fornix of the female genital tract and to facilitate birth. The enlarging uterine contents stretch and create tension on the round and uterosacral ligaments. Usually by 2 months postpartum, these ligaments have regained their tone and the uterus returns to the non-pregnant position.

In a small percentage of women, the uterus remains retroverted following birth; this condition is known as **uterine displacement**. The most common types of uterine displacement are retroversion (Fig. 19.10) and anterior displacement. Uterine displacement is associated with anterior positioning of the cervix; secondary infertility is often the first sign.

Uterine prolapse is a more serious type of uterine displacement and results in the cervix and body of the uterus protruding through the vagina. The degree of prolapse is described as mild, moderate, or severe or as first degree, second degree, or third degree, depending on the amount of the uterine body protruding into the vagina (Fig. 19.11). As more of the uterus is descended, the vagina becomes inverted.

COLLABORATIVE CARE: UTERINE DISPLACEMENT OR PROLAPSE
Assessment

Uterine displacement can block the flow of blood, lymph, and nerve impulses through the pelvic structures. Altered circulation is manifested by symptoms, including dysmenorrhea (painful periods), irregular periods, low back pain, infertility, recurrent vaginal infections, urinary incontinence, constipation, and dyspareunia (painful intercourse) (Hagen & Stark, 2011).

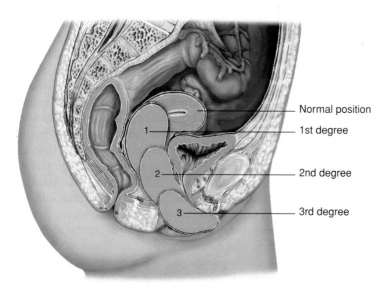

Normal position

1   1st degree

2   2nd degree

3   3rd degree

FIGURE 19.11 Uterine prolapse. In first-degree or mild prolapse, the cervix remains in the vagina. In second-degree or moderate prolapse, the cervix is at the vaginal introitus. In third-degree or severe prolapse, the cervix and uterus bulge out of the vagina entirely.

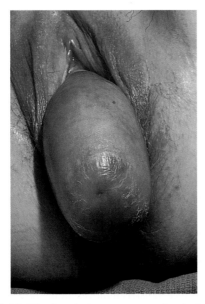

FIGURE 19.12 Physical appearance of a uterine prolapse.

Uterine prolapse is seen more often during perimenopause as the effects of ovarian hormones on the tissue decrease, resulting in decreased tone of pelvic supports and atrophic tissue changes. The most common complaints are a sensation of fullness or protrusion into the vagina, as well as low back pain and fatigue. Prolonged periods of standing and deep penetration during intercourse aggravate symptoms.

On physical examination, the protruding mass is palpable and visible in the vaginal vault (Fig. 19.12). Vaginal discharge is often present, and the upper vagina appears beefy red on visualization during speculum examination.

Select Potential Nursing Diagnoses

The following nursing diagnoses may apply to the client with postpartum uterine alterations:

- **Decreased Self-Esteem** related to change in reproductive organs and sexual function
- **Impaired urinary or bowel elimination** related to anatomic changes in the pelvic structures
- **Sexual Dysfunction** related to anatomic changes in vaginal area and sensations during coitus

Planning/Intervention

Extensive damage to the supporting structures may be identified and repaired immediately after birth. Most symptoms of uterine relaxation do not appear until perimenopause. Preventative nursing care includes teaching the client to perform pelvic-strengthening exercises, such as Kegel exercises, and pelvic floor muscle bracing against increased intra-abdominal pressure throughout the childbearing years (Hagen & Stark, 2011) (see Chapter 23).

Evaluation

Evaluation is based on the client's presenting symptoms and situation. The effectiveness of interventions is indicated by elimination of symptoms through successful repositioning of the prolapsed organ. In premenopausal clients who wish future pregnancy, fertility interventions such as artificial insemination may be useful to assist in conception (see Chapter 10).

Cystocele and Rectocele

A coexisting finding with uterine prolapse may be a cystocele or rectocele (see Chapter 4) (Fig. 19.13). A **cystocele** occurs when the wall between the bladder and vagina weakens and the bladder drops into the vagina. A **rectocele** is a weakening between the front wall of the rectum and vagina, resulting in the rectum ballooning into the vagina during defecation. The underlying cause of both cystocele and rectocele is weakening of the pelvic supports. Contributing factors include birth trauma, prolonged second stage, instrument-assisted births (forceps or vacuum extractions), and lacerations or episiotomies that extend into the rectum or anal sphincter. Related factors not specific to pregnancy include heavy lifting, obesity, repeated straining during bowel movements, low estrogen levels, and congenital vaginal wall weakness. Cystocele appears to be a phenomenon common to parous women (Law & Fiadjoe, 2012).

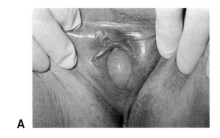

A

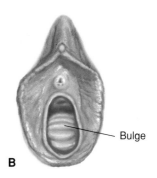

Bulge

B

FIGURE 19.13 Weakened pelvic supports can lead to cystocele and rectocele. **A:** With cystocele, the bladder drops into the vagina. **B:** In rectocele, the rectum bulges into the vagina during defecation.

COLLABORATIVE CARE: CYSTOCELE AND RECTOCELE

Assessment

The client with a cystocele frequently identifies discomfort and problems emptying the bladder. Bulging of the bladder into the vagina results in a feeling of fullness or a bearing-down sensation. Urinary symptoms include frequency and retention, resulting in numerous and recurrent UTIs. If there is damage to the bladder neck, the client may experience incontinence. The loss of support of the bladder neck (where the bladder and urethra meet) is the most common cause of female urinary incontinence. With increased abdominal pressure, such as during lifting, coughing, sneezing, or even just laughing, the natural mechanism for holding urine is lost, so the urine leaks. On pelvic examination, palpation of the anterior vaginal wall reveals a bulge when the client is asked to bear down. A cystocele is graded on a scale of 1 to 3, based on severity of the protrusion into the vagina (Box 19.4). If a cystocele is suspected, a voiding cystourethrogram may be ordered to show the shape of the bladder and any obstructions to urinary flow.

Rectoceles are often asymptomatic. If present, vaginal symptoms are similar to those of uterine or bladder prolapse: fullness and pain on intercourse. Rectal symptoms include bleeding, constipation, and difficult evacuation with straining. Usually, symptoms are associated with a large rectocele, which is uncommon in the immediate postpartum period. The exception is the client who experiences a fourth-degree laceration or extension of the episiotomy; she has a high potential for a weakened area at the suture line.

Select Potential Nursing Diagnoses

The following nursing diagnoses may apply to the woman with a cystocele or rectocele:

- **Impaired Urinary or Bowel Elimination** related to anatomic position of bladder or rectum
- **Risk for Infection** related to incomplete emptying of body's waste products providing a reservoir of bacterial proliferation.
- **Social Isolation** related to changes in anatomy and elimination functions

● BOX 19.4   Subjective Grading of Cystoceles

Grade 1: Mild—bladder creates bulging into the vagina
Grade 2: Severe—bladder has reached the opening of the vagina
Grade 3: Advanced—bladder bulges out through the opening of the vagina

- **Decreased Self-Esteem** related to loss of control of basic elimination functions
- **Anxiety** related to fear of loss of control of bodily fluids in public (i.e., stress or urge incontinence)

Planning/Intervention

Treatment for a cystocele ranges from none to surgery. In the immediate postpartum period, women may experience mild vaginal wall relaxation. The nurse instructs these clients in the use of levator muscle exercises (Kegel exercises) to restore pelvic floor muscle tone and pelvic floor muscle bracing against increased intra-abdominal pressure. He or she also instructs clients to avoid heavy lifting or straining, which could aggravate the loss of support.

Asymptomatic rectoceles are treated supportively. Activities to avoid constipation, such as a high-fibre diet and attention to hydration, are recommended. Fibre keeps the stool moist as it moves along the colon, resulting in stools that are larger, softer, and easier to pass. The nurse should instruct the client with a rectocele to avoid prolonged straining during defecation to minimize additional strain and protrusion. The client at high risk for development of a rectocele, based on contributing factors during birth or a fourth-degree episiotomy or laceration, will also benefit from teaching about diet and avoiding straining during the postpartum period when the body is healing and restoring tone.

Evaluation

Evaluation focuses on the degree of anatomic alteration and the prescribed treatment. Priority nursing concerns focus on success for control of elimination functions, comfort, and strategies to enhance the client's sense of well-being and participation in activities of daily living.

PSYCHOLOGICAL COMPLICATIONS

Because the postpartum client is at increased risk for various psychological disorders, nurses need to be familiar with their prevalence and onset, especially in the time surrounding childbirth. Onset of depressive symptoms is highest between 20 and 40 years of age for women, the usual age range for childbearing (see Chapter 5) (Muzik et al., 2009).

The birth of a child is not always a happy event for a new mother. The postpartum client with depressive feelings may be filled with loneliness. She may experience significant changes in eating, sleeping, and activity patterns, loss of interest or pleasure in activities of daily living, loss of energy, and impaired functioning (Doucet et al., 2009; Patel et al., 2012). This experience contrasts with idealized societal images of the happy mother and infant and growing family unit.

All clients need to understand that following childbirth, they are likely to experience physiologic and psychological changes that will affect daily life (see Chapter 18) (George, 2005). Normal experiences during the postpartum period that may affect daily life include the following:

- Fatigue as a result of getting up repeatedly in the middle of the night to tend to the infant
- Breast discomfort or leakage as a result of lactation and breastfeeding
- Pain and discomfort related to episiotomy, hemorrhoids, or healing of cesarean section incisions
- Uncertain time of the return of menses
- Pressure to be a good mother and wife or partner and to meet everyone's expectations

New mothers have been known to make comments such as, "Nobody told me it would be like this" and "I didn't realize it was going to be every minute of the day and night." In addition to the above physical alterations, many clients report experiencing tension, anxiety, and negative thinking (Muzik et al., 2009). Women more likely to be affected by postpartum depression are adolescents, mothers with premature infants, mothers living in urban areas, and mothers with limited support (Muzik et al., 2009).

Because of the numerous and dramatic individual and family changes during this period and failure to detect and treat postpartum depression (Muzik et al., 2009) nurses must be aware of the common postpartum psychological conditions that signify a problem beyond the normal adjustment period. Several screening tools are available for psychological alterations during the postbirth period. Nurses use these tools in the practice setting to identify clients with indicators of evolving conditions (Assessment Tool 19.1).

As these clients recover and regain energy, they often begin to recognize that their relationship with the newborn, other children, or both may have been affected as a result of the illness. In a systematic review, Kingston et al. (2012) indicated that maternal psychological distress (anxiety, depression, and stressful life events) negatively affects infants' cognitive and social–emotional development. Postpartum psychiatric conditions are family illnesses; the condition and the resulting changes in family dynamics affect everyone in the family. Therefore, the entire family needs support.

● ASSESSMENT TOOL 19.1 Postpartum Depression Screening Tools

Tool	Purpose	Format	Scoring	Interpretation	Critique
Beck Depression Inventory (BDI)	To measure behavioural manifestations of postpartum depression	21 multiple-choice items, each with four options	Item scoring: 0 = neutral score 3 = maximum score Tool score: range, 0–63	Score of 10 or higher indicates postpartum depression	Acceptable reliability and validity Widely used in the depression literature Poor sensitivity A generalized depression scale that doesn't address all the specifics of postpartum depression
Edinburgh Postnatal Depression Scale (EPDS)	To detect postpartum depression through self-report. The scale will not detect mothers with anxiety neuroses, phobias, or personality disorder	10 short statements regarding common depressive symptoms with four replies matched to the statement	Each statement is scored on a scale of 0 to 3. Total possible score ranges from 0 to 30	Scores above a threshold of 12/13 indicate the woman is suffering a depressive illness of varying severity	Simple to complete Acceptable to women who do not consider themselves unwell Does not provide mothers with an opportunity to fully describe their symptoms Obstacles to use include limited literacy and writing skills
Postpartum Depression Checklist (PDC)	A checklist of symptoms arranged in order of severity and used to make a diagnosis of postpartum depression	11 symptoms of postpartum depression arranged in a checklist format	No score is calculated. Positive responses indicate the need for further assessment and possible referral	Women contemplating harming herself or others need immediate referral to a psychiatric facility	Mothers may give "socially acceptable answers" to conform with societal expectations

The most common psychiatric conditions specific to the postbirth period are postpartum blues, postpartum depression, postpartum panic disorders, and postpartum psychosis.

Postpartum Blues

"Postpartum blues" is the term used for a self-limited, transitory mood disorder that affects about 70% of women; symptoms usually peak by 4 days post birth and abate by 10 days to 2 weeks post birth (Doucet et al., 2009; Muzik et al., 2009). Several causes of postpartum blues, including biochemical, psychological, social, and cultural factors, have been investigated, but none has been identified as the etiology. Some new mothers experience a loss of support from family and friends as the focus of attention and concern shift from the previously pregnant woman to the newborn. Others mourn the special relationship between the pregnant woman and her unborn child, whereas others experience a feeling of being let down when the excitement of labour and birth are over. A systematic review reported that welcomed social support is likely the most important aspect of any culturally prescribed postpartum rituals; such rituals may be difficult to maintain in new environments (Grigoriadis et al., 2009).

The societal norm of many cultures is that *all* new mothers should be happy and welcome and celebrate the birth of a child. When a woman does not experience overwhelming feelings of joy, she may feel depressed and/or guilty, assuming "something is wrong with her." Husbands, partners, family, and friends expect her to be happy; they may not recognize the mother's sadness and progressive changes in behaviour. The client's thoughts of not being a "good mother" may undermine her confidence, causing her to feel unable to meet the generally accepted expectations of her family. Feelings of sadness and requests for help in caring for her needs are inconsistent with the norms and expectations for the new family. Nurses can help eliminate these barriers by asking new mothers, "How was your birth experience and how are you feeling now?" and providing a safe and trusting environment for women to seek help and counselling.

COLLABORATIVE CARE: POSTPARTUM BLUES
Assessment

Emotional swings, frequent crying that often occurs for no reason, feelings of restlessness, fatigue, difficulty sleeping, headache, anxiety, loss of appetite, decreased ability to concentrate, irritability, sadness, and anger are common findings in women who experience postpartum blues. These clients are physically healthy, and the onset of the blues is believed to be unrelated to their own or their babies' health or well-being. Symptoms are typi-cally mild and transient, usually beginning a few days after delivery (Doucet et al., 2009).

Perinatal nurses can initiate conversations that encourage new mothers to openly discuss their feelings. A therapeutic communication approach from the nurse might be, "Many women have shared with me that they have a difficult time with their feelings following their births. Are you having any feelings that you would like to talk about?" With this simple question, the nurse not only attempts to assess a woman's emotional state but also to provide her with information that not all new mothers are happy. It can validate her emotions and contribute to a relationship based on freedom to share emotions without fear or shame.

Select Potential Nursing Diagnoses

The following nursing diagnoses may apply to the woman with postpartum blues:

- **Anxiety** related to new role expectations and responsibilities
- **Ineffective Coping** related to fatigue, physical discomforts, and demands of caring for infant
- **Disturbed Sleep Pattern** related to physiologic changes of the immediate postbirth period and demands of caring for a newborn

Planning/Intervention

Primary interventions related to postpartum blues are anticipatory guidance, providing opportunities for the client to share and express her emotions about her birth experience, and identifying and activating support systems. One of the most important postbirth educational strategies is to provide the client and family with information about the normality of the postpartum blues, signs and symptoms, and expected course of symptoms. The nurse emphasizes the importance of encouragement and support for the new mother. For example, a suggestion might be having family members, friends, or support people assist with the laundry, fixing meals, and performing other household tasks so the new mother can rest and care for the infant which may help decrease the client's fatigue and the severity of the blues.

Evaluation

Most cases of postpartum blues resolve spontaneously. Having support and assistance with household responsibilities will assist the client to make a successful transition. Indicators of resolution of the "blues" are increased energy and feeling more in control of the situation and her role as mother.

Postpartum Depression

Postpartum depression is more serious and persistent than postpartum blues. Unlike the limited nature of postpartum blues, postpartum depression may last for weeks or months. It usually begins between 4 and 6 weeks postpartum and evolves slowly over several weeks (Serhan et al., 2012). Symptoms of postpartum depression can develop anytime in the first year after childbirth. Although postpartum depression is considered underreported, about 7% of women have been reported to experience a major depressive episode in the first 12 weeks postpartum, increasing to 19% when minor depression is included (Gavin et al., 2005). In Canadian women, rates of about 8% are reported during the first 12 weeks postpartum (Dennis et al., 2012).

Although the exact etiology remains unclear, it appears to be a multifactorial disorder. The rapid decrease in estrogen and progesterone, and the altered cytokines profile that occurs following birth have been implicated in the development of depression (Doucet et al., 2009). A higher incidence has been observed in clients with a past personal or family history of psychiatric disorders, a history of depression or anxiety during pregnancy, poor maternal health, pronounced or lingering postpartum blues; or life-event problems (Bloch et al., 2006; Dennis et al., 2012; Doucet et al., 2009). Other factors linked to postpartum depression include the following:

- Prenatal anxiety or depression
- Child care stress
- Fatigue
- Low household income
- Stressful life events or low self esteem
- Unstable relationships with husband or partner, parents, or both
- Interpersonal violence
- Lack of social support. Women who lack sufficient social support are more than three times as likely to experience postpartum depression (Dennis et al., 2012; Doucet et al., 2009; Wylie et al., 2011).

Clients who have experienced postpartum depression have described a feeling of being in a downward spiral; an emotionally painful experience for themselves and their families (Edhborg et al., 2005). Feeling depressed at a time when family and friends anticipate happiness further intensifies anxiety and a sense of lost support. Societal norms idealizing the birth of a new family member as a joyous event may contribute to clients' reluctance to discuss their symptoms or feelings toward the infant (Morgan & Yount, 2012). The woman may experience thoughts of harming her baby or feelings of guilt about being a poor mother (Doucet et al., 2009; Patel et al., 2012). Over time, the woman may avoid the infant in an attempt to minimize these thoughts of harm. Clients rarely share these feelings because of embarrassment or fear of negative reactions from family, friends, and health care professionals (Morgan & Yount, 2012).

COLLABORATIVE CARE: POSTPARTUM DEPRESSION
Assessment

Clients who continue to show signs and symptoms of postpartum blues beyond 7 to 10 days after giving birth, those with a history of depression in pregnancy or the postpartum period, and those with a previous depressive episode are at increased risk of developing postpartum depression (Doucet et al., 2009; Muzik et al., 2009; Patel et al., 2012). Universal screening is recommended for all women (Toohey, 2012). Assessment, which may not be addressed by some practitioners, should focus on early detection and treatment (Morgan & Yount, 2012). During pregnancy, the nurse performs a comprehensive health history focused on family and personal history of psychiatric or depressive conditions. Exploring feelings about a previous birth can reveal important clues. The nurse should document risk factors or altered perceptions related to pregnancy and communicate findings to care providers during the postbirth period.

During birth and the immediate postpartum period, the nurse engages in assessment and evaluation of mother–baby attachment behaviours (how she holds, talks to, and interacts with the baby, and how she describes the infant to others), the interactions between the parents or mother and other family members, availability of support systems, and identification of community resources.

The Edinburgh Postnatal Depression Scale is an example of a tool widely available to practitioners as well as the public (Assessment Tool 19.2). This simple 10-item questionnaire can assist in identifying mothers suffering from postpartum depression. Clinical evaluation must be carried out to confirm a diagnosis and initiate intervention.

The nurse assesses clients for the following signs of postpartum depression:

- Inability to sleep or rest
- Crying that is uncontrollable and unprovoked
- Change in appetite, especially a craving for carbohydrates
- Decreased energy and fatigue
- Feelings of worthlessness and a negative outlook on the future
- Sense of isolation
- Lack of concern for personal appearance
- Feelings of uncontrollable anxiety, irritability, and loss of control; obsessive thoughts of being a failure
- Hostility or anger directed toward others
- Problems with maternal–infant interaction, perception of the infant as difficult, and feeling guilty about not being able to care for the baby
- Feeling of being an inadequate mother and of being trapped

● **ASSESSMENT TOOL 19.2** **Edinburgh Postnatal Depression Scale (EPDS)**

INSTRUCTIONS FOR USERS

1. The mother is asked to underline the response that comes closest to how she has been feeling in the previous 7 days.
2. All 10 items must be completed.
3. Care should be taken to avoid the possibility of the mother discussing her answers with others.
4. The mother should complete the scale herself, unless she has limited English or has difficulty with reading.
5. The EPDS may be used at 6 to 8 weeks to screen postnatal women. The child health clinic, postnatal checkup, or a home visit may provide suitable opportunities for its completion.
   Name: _____
   Address: _____
   Baby's Age: _____

As you have recently had a baby, we would like to know how you are feeling. Please UNDERLINE the answer that comes closest to how you have felt IN THE PAST 7 DAYS, not just how you feel today.

1. I have been able to laugh and see the funny side of things.
   As much as I always could
   Not quite so much now
   Definitely not so much now
   Not at all
2. I have looked forward with enjoyment to things.
   As much as I ever did
   Rather less than I used to
   Definitely less than I used to
   Hardly at all
3. *I have blamed myself unnecessarily when things went wrong.
   Yes, most of the time
   Yes, some of the time
   Not very often
   No, never
4. I have been anxious or worried for no good reason.
   No, not at all
   Hardly ever
   Yes, sometimes
   Yes, very often

5. *I have felt scared or panicky for no very good reason.
   Yes, quite a lot
   Yes, sometimes
   No, not much
   No, not at all
6. *Things have been getting on top of me.
   Yes, most of the time I haven't been able to cope at all
   Yes, sometimes I haven't been coping as well as usual
   No, most of the time I have coped quite well
   No, I have been coping as well as ever
7. *I have been so unhappy that I have had difficulty sleeping.
   Yes, most of the time
   Yes, sometimes
   Not very often
   No, not at all
8. *I have felt sad or miserable.
   Yes, most of the time
   Yes, quite often
   Not very often
   No, not at all
9. *I have been so unhappy that I have been crying.
   Yes, most of the time
   Yes, quite often
   Only occasionally
   No, never
10. *The thought of harming myself has occurred to me.
    Yes, quite often
    Sometimes
    Hardly ever
    Never

Response categories are scored 0, 1, 2, and 3 according to increased severity of the symptoms. Items marked with an asterisk are reverse scored (i.e., 3, 2, 1, and 0). The total score is calculated by adding together the scores for each of the ten items.

Source: Cox, J. L., Holden, J. M., & Sagovsky, R. (1987). Edinburgh Postnatal Depression Scale (EPDS). *British Journal of Psychiatry, 150.*

Initial symptoms of postpartum depression may be subtle. Health care providers, especially in health care settings, where clients bring their infants for ongoing care, should be attuned to assessing women for signs of postpartum depression and identifying subtle signs and symptoms (Fig. 19.14). Maternal nursing assessment through the first year after childbirth needs to include asking clients, "How are you feeling about interests and pleasures in your daily activities?" (Muzik et al., 2009) and providing a safe and trusting environment for them to seek help and counselling. For prevention of postpartum depression, professionally based postpartum home visits, lay or peer-based telephone support, and interpersonal psychotherapy are promising interventions (Dennis & Dowswell, 2013).

Select Potential Nursing Diagnoses

The following nursing diagnoses may apply to the woman with postpartum depression:

• **Impaired Parenting** related to negative feelings about the infant and mothering role

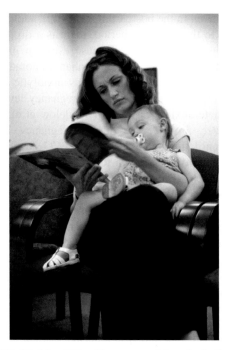

FIGURE 19.14 All health care providers, including nurses working in general practice, family health, and pediatric settings, should remember to ask about signs and symptoms of postpartum depression in mothers throughout the child's first year of life.

- **Anxiety** related to overwhelming demands of motherhood and meeting the newborn's needs
- **Self-Care Deficit** related to changes in nutrition, sleep, hygiene, and other activities of daily living secondary to depression
- **Risk for Injury:** Harm to self, infant, or both

Planning/Intervention

Early referrals for clients with a history or evidence of depression are essential. However, the client with postpartum depression may lack the energy to follow through on information that the nurse provides. Therefore, simply giving the client the name or phone number of a support group or provider is not enough. A critical component of nursing intervention is actually getting her to the support group or involved with the appropriate mental health professional. Assisting the client to make contact and conscious follow-up to be certain she keeps appointments and attends support sessions is an important responsibility.

Standard treatment includes a combination of antidepressant medications, exercise, psychotherapy, and psychosocial (support groups) modalities (Morgan & Yount, 2012; Muzik et al., 2009). Before the initiation of pharmacologic treatment, other physiologic parameters such as thyroid dysfunction (which can mimic the signs of postpartum depression) and anemia must be ruled out (Morgan & Yount, 2012).

Pharmacotherapeutics

Tricyclics and selective serotonin reuptake inhibitors are effective for treatment of postpartum depression (Muzik et al., 2009). For the breastfeeding mother, these drugs are considered safe (based on limited scientific studies) because little of the medication passes into the breast milk. An exception is fluoxetine, which has been linked to infant symptoms of distress (Sie et al., 2012). Providers need to balance the risk for drug ingestion through breast milk with the benefits of the maternal–infant attachment gained through the closeness of continued breastfeeding. Women who take SSRIs have been found to be significantly less likely to breastfeed, regardless of whether they discontinue use prior to delivery or continue to take the medication (Gorman et al., 2012). If medication is the treatment of choice, the client must continue it for at least 6 months, even if depressive symptoms improve (Muzik et al., 2009).

Complementary/Alternative Medicine Modalities

Complementary/alternative medicine refers to treatments that are considered additional to (complementary), or in place of (alternative), standard or established practice in Western medicine (Deligiannidis & Freeman, 2010; Gossler, 2010). Complementary/alternative medicine has been growing in popularity in Canada. Clients may pursue various complementary/alternative medicine treatments for postpartum depression (Complementary/Alternative Medicine 19.1) for a variety of reasons. They may want to explore every option available, want a more naturalistic approach to health care, or may be concerned about the side effects of traditional treatments; many postpartum women are concerned about the transmission of medications through breast milk (Deligiannidis & Freeman, 2010; Gossler, 2010; Zauderer & Davis, 2012).

For clients with mild postpartum depression, complementary/alternative medicine is complementary to standard treatment modalities, not a replacement (Deligiannidis & Freeman, 2010). The client needs to discuss the use of all complementary/alternative medicine modalities with the nurse or other health care provider, particularly if she is breastfeeding her newborn. Zauderer and Davis (2012) reviewed a number of alternative treatments for postpartum mood disorders: most alternative treatments have not been subjected to well-designed studies. Some herbs or herbal preparations may create potential interactions with, or inhibit the effectiveness of, other medications the woman may be taking. Some may actually be harmful. Some have been documented to create side effects in the newborn. Purity and strength of herbal preparations may be of concern, as these may not be known and are not regulated; serious side effects may result. Honest, open dialogue is important for both the woman and the health care practitioner (Gossler, 2010; Zauderer & Davis, 2012).

Psychosocial

Individual counselling, cognitive behavioural therapy, interpersonal therapy, and group therapy are interventions that have been shown to achieve success (Goodman & Santangelo, 2011; Muzik et al., 2009). Group therapy sessions are often attractive, as they can be delivered at a lower cost and encourage support from others. Women have reported feeling "safer," not as judged, and able to be more "authentic" when they share their experiences and concerns with other group members (Goodman & Santangelo, 2011; Pessagno & Hunker, 2012). The client's feelings are recognized as real and these sessions help to identify coping strategies and provide an avenue for sharing experiences. In addition, they provide many clients with an opportunity to interact with other women as a means to decrease social isolation. The client is encouraged to identify and verbalize her fears and concerns regarding her mothering role and responsibilities. She should also be asked about suicidal or homicidal thoughts during each session. If the couple is having difficulties in their relationships, counselling may also be indicated to deal with these challenges.

Evaluation

Some clients require hospitalization to protect them from harm but most are treated in the community setting. Evaluation is a long-term and ongoing process. The client with postpartum depression needs continuous support and care. Signs of effective interventions include decreased depressive symptoms and increased coping abilities concurrent with resumption of the mothering role and activities of daily living.

Postpartum Panic Disorder

Sudden terror and a sense of impending doom are characteristic of postpartum panic disorders. These disorders involve full-blown panic attacks and extreme anxiety during the postpartum period. While pregnancy is associated with improvements in panic symptoms, they worsen in the postpartum period (Bandelow et al., 2006). In the postbirth period, there is a drop in progesterone and estradiol. Because estrogen influences serotonin transporter sites and enhances noradrenergic transmission, and progesterone has anxiolytic and sedative properties, the drop from pregnancy levels may accentuate anxiety disorders (Bandelow et al., 2006). Moreover, progesterone during pregnancy leads to hyperventilation and a decrease in PCO_2 levels, which reduces the distance from thresholds and may induce panic attacks (Bandelow et al., 2006). Physical symptoms accompanying the sense of terror include shortness of breath, dizziness, nausea, palpitations, and chest pain (Zauderer, 2009). Individuals with a panic disorder are struck with fears that they know are irrational and illogical, but that cause them to drastically change their lives to avoid situations that they fear (Canadian Mental Health Association, 2014). Panic attacks often have no identifiable trigger; the onset is sudden and unanticipated.

Typical signs and symptoms that women with panic disorders exhibit include the following:

• Extreme anxiety
• Heart palpitations
• Chest pain and sensation of choking or suffocation
• Hot or cold flashes, trembling
• Restlessness, agitation, irritability
• Fear of losing control or going crazy
• Sudden awakening from sleep
• Excessive or obsessive worry or fears

Treatment of panic disorders includes a combination of cognitive and behavioural therapies. Medications are also appropriate in some cases, for example, tricyclic antidepressants (Bandelow et al., 2006). The most important aspect is supporting the client in seeking and following through with treatment. Initial treatment focuses on helping her understand what a panic disorder is and that having one does not mean she is going crazy. Cognitive therapy can assist the client to identify possible triggers for attacks and to understand that the attack is separate from the trigger event. Cognitive restructuring or changing ways of thinking may assist the client to become more comfortable with frightening

---

● **COMPLEMENTARY/ALTERNATIVE MEDICINE 19.1**

Common Complementary/Alternative Medicine Modalities for Perinatal Depression

• Folate
• Aerobic exercise
• Massage
• Aromatherapy

• Omega-3 fatty acids
• Bright light therapy
• SAMe (naturally occurring molecule in the body)
• Acupuncture (Deligiannidis & Freeman, 2012).

situations and anxiety management (Canadian Mental Health Association, 2014). Relaxation techniques can help some clients manage an attack. Useful relaxation techniques include patterned or paced breathing and positive visualization.

When clients are using antidepressants and antianxiety agents it is important for the nurse to understand and communicate the implications of the chosen medication on lactation, if the client is breastfeeding. Finally, these clients need assistance with referral to a support group as an adjunct to the previously described therapies. Commitment and follow-through are essential to success. A decrease in attacks will not occur after only one or two sessions; an extended treatment programs of 6 to 9 months may be necessary (Family Doctor.org, 2014).

Postpartum Psychosis

Postpartum psychosis is a severe condition occurring in less than 2% of postpartum clients (Doucet et al., 2009; Muzik et al., 2009). Often, a rapid presentation occurring between 48 hours and 2 weeks postpartum, the clinical picture is usually mania with rapid fluctuations into depression (Doucet et al., 2009). Most women experience psychotic symptoms, including delusions and auditory or visual hallucinations, which may include commands to hurt themselves or their babies (Doucet et al., 2009).

Psychosis arising for the first time in pregnancy is uncommon; psychosis is a condition occurring most frequently within the context of an underlying psychiatric disorder such as bipolar affective disorder, schizophrenia, or major depression (Doucet et al., 2009; Doucet et al., 2011). For some clients, postpartum psychosis is the only psychotic episode they will experience. For others, postpartum psychosis may be the first episode of a psychiatric disorder. Approximately 25% to 50% of women who give birth and have a history of bipolar disorder will experience an episode of postpartum psychosis, with rates up to 74% for women with a family history of postpartum psychosis (Doucet et al., 2011). Prophylactic approaches, such as using olanzapine or lithium within 24 hours of delivery, have prevented relapse with postpartum psychosis (Doucet et al., 2011).

During a psychotic episode, the client losses touch with reality. She may experience the following:

- Hallucinations (e.g., hearing voices when nobody is around)
- Delusions, or ideas she believes despite all proof that they are false (e.g., that someone is trying to harm her, or that her baby is the devil)
- Disordered thoughts or illogical or chaotic thought processes
- Psychosis is a very frightening condition and needs immediate treatment.

COLLABORATIVE CARE: POSTPARTUM PSYCHOSIS
Assessment

Signs and symptoms of postpartum psychosis may develop at any time from immediately after birth to 3 months later but they usually occur about 2 weeks postpartum (Muzik et al., 2009). They include the following:

- Disturbed sleep
- Emotional lability
- Confusion and disorientation
- Disorganized thoughts and behaviour
- Hallucinations (hearing voices when there is no one there)
- Delusions (thinking that people are trying to harm her or that she has special powers)
- Withdrawal

The client may be unable to stand, move, or work. As the condition progresses, she exhibits suspicious and incoherent behaviour, confusion, irrational statements, and obsessive concerns about the baby's health and welfare. Delusions, which are often specific to the infant, are common in the condition (Muzik et al, 2009).

Select Potential Nursing Diagnoses

The following nursing diagnoses may apply to the client with postpartum psychosis:

- **Disturbed Thought Processes** related to perception of hallucinations and delusional thoughts
- **Risk for Violence** related to delusional thinking

Planning/Intervention

Postpartum psychosis is a medical emergency and requires immediate hospitalization and treatment. These clients need to be hospitalized for their own safety and to prevent potential harm to the infant. Because of confusion, the client may not have the insight to recognize how ill she is and the need for treatment. Treatment options for women with postpartum psychosis include the following:

- Biologic approach: rule out medical conditions that may present as psychosis (e.g., infection, seizure disorder, electrolyte disturbance)
- Use of antipsychotic and mood-stabilizing medications. There is some evidence to support the value of electroshock therapy (Doucet et al., 2011)
- Psychological approach: interpersonal therapy, supportive psychotherapy (individual or group), couple counselling
- Social support in sharing child care responsibilities with partners, friends, and family; teaching the client how to build social networks and supports; creating a supportive living environment

Evaluation

Following treatment, most clients can return to their daily activities but may fluctuate between remissions and exacerbations. Clients may have difficulty managing during exacerbations. The presence of an ongoing support network is invaluable.

SUMMARY

- Postpartum maternal complications can develop in any pregnancy from conditions that existed before or during pregnancy, during labour, or during or after birth.
- Risk factors for postpartum complications include infections, history of preterm labour or preterm rupture of membranes, abnormal placental implantation, prolonged labour, assisted labour, cesarean section, chronic conditions or pre-existing disease states, poor nutritional status, substance use, and inadequate prenatal care.
- Postpartum hemorrhage is associated with a blood loss greater than 500 mL (vaginal birth) or 1,000 mL (cesarean birth) during or after the third stage of labour. It can develop early (within the first 24 hours of birth) or late (24 hours or more after birth).
- Causes of early hemorrhage include uterine atony, retention of placental fragments, lacerations of the genital tract, hematomas, uterine inversion and coagulopathies. The goals of care in all cases are to identify the underlying cause and to stop the bleeding.
- Late postpartum hemorrhage is usually associated with infection or retained placental fragments, both of which lead to uterine subinvolution. The client will need care for this problem in a health care facility to manage the bleeding, eliminate the cause, and treat any infection.
- Puerperal infections involve a temperature of 38°C or higher on any 2 of the first 10 days following birth exclusive of the first 24 hours. Infection can occur in the uterus and surrounding tissues (endometritis), the broad ligament of the uterus (parametritis), peritoneum or abdominal cavity (peritonitis), wounds of the perineum or abdomen, urinary tract, or breasts (mastitis).
- Pregnancy-related hypercoagulability increases the client's risk for thromboembolic disorders.
- A rare but serious postpartum complication is peripartum cardiomyopathy, which requires extensive treatment.
- Reproductive anatomic complications can have long-term consequences. Pelvic relaxation, uterine displacement, uterine prolapse, cystocele, and rectocele can interfere with a woman's urinary and bowel elimination, enjoyment of intercourse, future fertility, and other areas. In some cases, surgical repair is necessary.
- Psychological complications can range from the mild and self-limited postpartum blues to the more concerning diagnoses of postpartum depression, postpartum panic disorder, and postpartum psychosis. Ongoing assessment and evaluation of the client's mood starting in pregnancy and continuing throughout the infant's first year of life is necessary to prevent unfortunate consequences related to emotional instability.

Questions to Ponder

1. A client comes to the health care facility for her 6-week postpartum checkup. She looks sad, tired, and pale. The nurse asks the client how her mood is and how well she has been coping with the changes having a newborn brings. The client shrugs and says she's doing "as well as could be expected." When the nurse tries to gather more information, the client's responses are similarly unrevealing.
   - What other methods could the nurse employ to gather more information?
   - If the nurse determines evidence of a postpartum mood disorder, what methods might prove effective in working with this client?
   - What things might be happening, other than postpartum depression?

REVIEW QUESTIONS

1. Which of the following factors would be least likely to contribute to the development of endometritis?
   A. Use of fetal scalp electrodes
   B. Prolonged rupture of membranes
   C. Urinary catheterization
   D. Manual removal of the placenta
2. The nurse should suspect a laceration of the genital tract in a postpartum client who exhibits
   A. Dark red, steady bleeding.
   B. Spurting of bright red blood.
   C. Purulent lochia.
   D. Boggy uterus.
3. What would be the nurse's first intervention for Rosanna who is saturating her pads and indicating she thinks she needs to void?
   A. Provide Rosanna with a clean pad
   B. Give Rosanna extra fluids
   C. Assist Rosanna to void
   D. Hang 10 IU of oxytocin in an IV
4. Inspection of the perineum of a postpartum client reveals ecchymosis and a tense fluctuant mass of the vulva. The nurse interprets this finding as consistent with
   A. Uterine prolapse.
   B. Parametritis.

C. Vulvar hematoma.

D. Uterine inversion.

5. Which of the following interventions would be a priority for a client who is readmitted to the health care facility with a diagnosis of late postpartum hemorrhage?

A. Administration of broad-spectrum antibiotics to prevent infection

B. Intravenous fluid therapy to expand circulating volume

C. Preparation for surgical curettage to remove the source of bleeding

D. Application of ice to the perineum to promote vasoconstriction

6. What primary factor would the nurse recommend to support Leslie, the client who had given birth by cesarean section and been treated post discharge in emergency for a wound infection?

A. Suggest she increase her activity level at home.

B. Request that she purchase antipyretics to decrease her temperature

C. Organize home visits by nurses to change her dressing

D. Request Leslie to increase her protein intake

7. After teaching a postpartum client about measures to prevent UTIs, which statement would lead the nurse to suspect that the client needs additional teaching?

A. "I will drink plenty of fluids throughout the day to flush out my bladder."

B. "I will try to limit the number of times that I go to the bathroom to urinate."

C. "I will change my perineal pad often, keeping the area as clean as possible."

D. "I will use a front-to-back wiping motion when cleaning my perineal area."

8. A client diagnosed with mastitis asks the nurse, "Should I continue to breastfeed my baby?" Which response, if made by the nurse, would be the most appropriate?

A. "We had better ask your health care provider if you should continue to breastfeed."

B. "Well, that's really a decision for you to make. But, you can stop, if you like, for now."

C. "Continuing to breastfeed will keep your breasts empty so that organisms can't grow."

D. "You are receiving an antibiotic that could be transmitted to the baby, so you shouldn't breastfeed right now."

9. Which of the following should the nurse expect to find when assessing a postpartum woman with DVT?

A. Dyspnea

B. Sudden chest pain

C. Hemoptysis

D. Calf tenderness on ambulation

10. Which agent would the nurse expect to administer as the first drug of choice to a postpartum woman diagnosed with peripartum cardiomyopathy?

A. ACE inhibitors

B. Nonsteroidal anti-inflammatory drugs (NSAIDs)

C. Anticoagulant therapy

D. Cephalosporin antibiotics

11. Assessment of a client with postpartum depression would reveal which of the following?

A. Hallucinations

B. Delusions

C. Uncontrolled crying

D. Confusion

REFERENCES

Aissaoui, N., Martins, E., Mouly, S. Weber, S., & Meune, C. (2009). A meta-analysis of bed rest versus early ambulation in the management of pulmonary embolism, deep vein thrombosis, or both. *International Journal of Cardiology, 137*, 37–41. http://dx.doi.org/10.1016/j.ijcard.2008.06.020

Apgar, B. S., Serlin, D., & Kaufman, A. (2005). The postpartum visit: Is six weeks too late? *American Family Physician, 72*(12), 2443–2444.

Bandelow, B., Sojka, F., Broocks, A., Hajak, G. Bleich, S., & Rüther, E. (2006). Panic disorder during pregnancy and postpartum period. *European Psychiatry, 21*, 495–500. doi:10.1016/j.eurpsy.2005.11.005

Bloch, M., Rotenberg, N., Koren, D., & Klein, E. (2006). Risk factors for early postpartum depressive symptoms. *General Hospital Psychiatry, 28*(1), 3–8.

Canadian Mental Health Association. (2014). *Phobias and panic disorder.* Retrieved from http://www.cmha.ca/mental_health/phobias-and-panic-disorders/#.U2mvOCihPa4

Chan, W. S., Rey, E., & Kent, N. E. (2014). Venous thromboembolism and antithrombotic therapy in pregnancy. *Journal of Obstetrics and Gynaecology Canada, 36*(6), 527–553.

Chelmow, D., Rodriquez, E. J., & Sabatini, M. M. (2004). Suture closure of subcutaneous fat and wound disruption after cesarean delivery: A meta-analysis. *Obstetrics and Gynecology, 103*(5), 974–980.

Cunningham, F. G., Leveno, K. J., Bloom, S. L., Hauth, J. C., Rouse, D. J., & Spong, C. Y. (2010). *Williams obstetrics.* 23rd ed. New York: McGraw-Hill.

Deligiannidis, K. M., & Freeman, M. P. (2010). Complementary and alternative medicine for the treatment of depressive disorders in women. *Psychiatric Clinics of North America, 33*(2), 441–463. doi:10.1016/j.psc.2010.01.002

Dennis, C. L., & Dowswell, T. (2013). Psychosocial and psychological interventions for preventing postpartum depression. *The Cochrane Database of Systematic Reviews, 2,* doi:10.1002/14651858./cd001134.

Dennis, C. L., Heaman, M., & Vigod, S. (2012). Epidemiology of postpartum depressive symptoms among Canadian women: Regional and national results from a cross-sectional survey. *Canadian Journal of Psychiatry, 57*(9), 537–546.

Dorbala, S., Brozena, S., Zeb, S., Galatro, K., Homel, P., Ren, J. F., et al. (2005). Risk stratification of women with peripartum cardiomyopathy at initial presentation: A dobutamine stress echocardiography study. *Journal of the American Society of Echocardiography, 18*(1), 45–48.

Doucet, S., Dennis, C. L., Letourneau, N., & Blackmore, E. R. (2009). Differentiation and clinical implications of postpartum depression and postpartum psychosis. *Journal of Obstetric, Gynecologic & Neonatal Nursing, 38*(3), 269–279.

Doucet, S., Jones, I., Letourneau, N., Dennis, C. L., & Blackmore, E. R. (2011). Intervention for the prevention and treatment of postpartum psychosis. *Archives of Women's Mental Health, 14,* 89–98. doi:10.1007/s00737-010-0199-6

Edhborg, M., Friberg, M., Lundh, W., & Widstrom, A. M. (2005). "Struggling with life": Narratives from women with signs of postpartum depression. *Scandinavian Journal of Public Health, 33*(4), 261–267.

Elkayam, U., Jalnapurkar, S., & Barakat, M. (2012). Peripartum cardiomyopathy. *Cardiology Clinics, 30*, 435–440. doi:10.1016/j.ccl.2012.04.009

Escribà-Agüir, V., Royo-Marqués, M., Artazcoz, L., Romito, P., & Ruiz-Pérez, I. (2013). Longitudinal study of depression and health status in pregnant women: Incidence, course, and predictive factors. *European Archives of Psychiatry and Clinical Neuroscience, 263*, 143–151. doi:10.1007/s00406–012–0336–5

Family Doctor.Org. (2014). *Panic Disorder.* Retrieved from http://familydoctor.org/familydoctor/en/diseases-conditions/panic-disorder/symptoms.html

Faro, S. (2005). Postpartum endometritis. *Clinics in Perinatology, 32*(3), 803–814.

Gavin, N. I., Gaynes, B. N., Lohr, K. N., Meltzer-Brody, S., Gartlehner, G., & Swinson, T. (2005). Perinatal depression: A systematic review of prevalence and incidence. *Obstetrics and Gynecology, 106*(1), 1071–1083. doi:10.1097/01.AOG.0000183597.3163d6

George, L. (2005). Lack of preparedness: Experiences of first-time mothers. *MCN. The American Journal of Maternal/Child Nursing, 30*(4), 251–255.

Goodman, J. H. & Santangelo, G. (2011). Group treatment for postpartum depression: A systematic review. *Archives of Women's Mental Health, 14*(4), 277–293.

Gorman, J. R., Kao, K. & Chambers, C. D. (2012). Breastfeeding among women exposed to antidepressants during pregnancy. *Journal of Human Lactation, 28*(2), 181–188.

Gossler, S. M. (2010). Use of complementary and alternative therapies during pregnancy, postpartum, and lactation. *Journal of Psychosocial Nursing and Mental Health Services, 48*(11), 30–36.

Grigoriadis, S., Robinson, G. E., Fung, K., Ross, L. E., Dennis, C. L., & Romans, S. (2009). Traditional postpartum practices and rituals: Clinical implications. *Canadian Journal of Psychiatry, 54*(12), 834–840.

Hagen, S., & Stark, D. (2011). Conservative prevention and management of pelvic organ prolapse in women (review). *The Cochrane Database of Systematic Reviews, 11*, 1–68.

Helt, J. A., Kobbervig, C. E., James, A. H., Petterson, T. M., Bailey, K. R., & Melton, L. J. (2005). Trends in the incidence of venous thromboembolism during pregnancy or postpartum: A 30-year population-based study. *Annals of Internal Medicine, 143*, 697–706.

Hock, M., Kránicz, J., Kries, Z., Kirszbacher, I., Sebestyen, A., Boncz, I., et al. (2008). Changes in pelvic floor muscle strength during pregnancy. *Value in Health, 11*(6), A420–A421. doi:10.1016/s1098–3015(10)66422–4

James, D. C. (2014). Postpartum care. In K. R, Simpson, & P. A, Creehan. (Eds.) *Perinatal Nursing* (4th ed). Philadelphia, PA: Wolters Kluwer LWW.

Kingston, D., Tough, S., & Whitfield, H. (2012). Prenatal and postpartum maternal psychological distress and infant development: A systematic review. *Child Psychiatry and Human Development, 43*, 683–714. doi:10.1007/s10578–012–0291–4

Kitchens, C. S. (2010). How I treat superficial venous thrombosis. *Blood: Journal of The American Society of Hematology, 117*(1). Accessed from http://bloodjournal.hematologylibrary.org/content/117/1/39.full

Law, H., & Fiadjoe, P. (2012). Urogynaecological problems in pregnancy. *Journal of Obstetrics and Gynaecology, 32*, 109–112. doi:10.3109101443615–2011.635227

Leduc, D., Senikas, V., Lalonde, A. B., Ballerman, C., Biringer, A., Delaney, M.,et al. (2009). Active management of the third stage of labour: Prevention and treatment of postpartum hemorrhage. *Journal of Obstetrics and Gynaecology of Canada, 31*(10), 980–993.

Maharaj, D. (2007a). Puerperal pyrexia: A review Part I. *Obstetrical and Gynecological Survey, 62*(6), 393–399. doi:10.10971010gx.0000265998.40912.5e

Maharaj, D. (2007b). Puerperal pyrexia: A review Part II. *Obstetrical and Gynecological Survey, 62*(6), 400–406. doi:10.10971010gx.0000266063.8457.1 fb

McClintock, C., Brighton, T., Chunilal, S., Dekker, G., McDonnell, N., McRae, S., et al. (2012). Recommendations for diagnosis and treatment of deep venous thrombosis and pulmonary embolism in pregnancy and the postpartum period. *Australian and New Zealand Journal of Obstetrics and Gynaecology, 52*, 14–22. doi:10.1111/j.1479–828x.2011.01361.x

Morgan, J. P., & Yount, S. R. (2012). Postpartum depression in a primary-care setting. *The Clinical Advisor, 15*(12), 28–40.

Morrison, R. (2006). Venous thromboembolism: Scope of the problem and the nurse's role in risk assessment and prevention. *Journal of Vascular Nursing, 24*, 82–90. doi:10. 1016/j.jvn.2006.05.002

Muzik, M., Marcus, S. M., Heringhausen, J. E., & Flynn, H. (2009). When depression complicates childbearing: Guidelines for screening and treatment during antenatal and postpartum obstetric care. *Obstetric and Gynecologic Clinics of North America, 36*, 771–788. doi:10.1016/j.ogc.2009.10.006

Patel, M., Bailey, R. K., Jabeen, S., Ali, S., Barker, N. C., & Osiezagha, K. (2012). Postpartum depression: A review. *Journal of Health Care for the Poor and Underserved, 23*(2), 534–542.

Pessagno, R. A., & Hunker, D. (2012). Using short-term group psychotherapy as an evidence-based intervention for first-time mothers at risk for postpartum depression. *Perspectives in Psychiatric Care, 49*(3), 202–209.

Ramanathan, G., & Arulkumaran, S. (2006). Postpartum hemorrhage. *Current Obstetrics and Gynaecology, 16*, 6–13.

Rath, W. H. (2011). Postpartum hemorrhage: Update on problems of definition and diagnosis. *ACTA Obstetricia et Gynecologica Scandinavica, 90*(5), 421–428. doi:10.1111/j.1600–0412.2011.01107.x

Schmiemann, G., Kniehl, E., Gebhardt, K., Matejczyk, M. M., & Hummers-Pradier, E. (2010). The diagnosis of urinary tract infection. *Deutsches Arzteblatt International, 107*(21). Accessed from http://www.ncbi.nlm.nih.gov/pmc/articles/PMC2883276

Serhan, N., Ege, E., Ayranci, U., & Kosgeroglu, N. (2012). Prevalence of postpartum depression in mothers and fathers and its correlates. *Journal of Clinical Nursing, 22*(1–2), 279–284.

Shah, T., Ather, S., Bavishi, C., Bambhroliya, A., Ma, T., & Bozkurt, B. (2013). Peripartum cardiomyopathy: A contemporary review. *Methodist Debakey Cardiovascular Journal, 9*(1), 38–43.

Sie, S. D., Wennink, J. M., van Driel, J. J., te Winkel, A. G., Boer, K., Casteelen, G., et al. (2012). Maternal use of SSRIs, SNRIs and NaSSAs: Practical recommendations during pregnancy and lactation. *Archives of Diseases in Childhood: Fetal and Neonatal Edition, 97*, F472–F476. doi:10.1136/archdischild-2011–214239

Spiliopoulos, M. (2013). Normal and abnormal puerperium: Infections. *Medscape.* Retrieved from http://emedicine.medscape.com/article/260187-overview#aw2aab6b5

Stewart, G. C. (2012). Management of peripartum cardiomyopathy. *Current Treatment Options in Cardiovascular Medicine, 14*(6), 622–636. doi:10.1007/s11936–012–0210–9

Toohey, J. (2012). Depression during pregnancy and postpartum. *Clinical Obstetrics and Gynecology, 55*(3), 788–797.

Wong, V., Martindale, R., Longaker, M., & Gurtner, G. From germ theory to germ therapy: Skin microbiota, chronic wounds, and probiotics. *Plastic and Reconstructive Surgery, 132*(5), 854e–871e.

Wylie, L., Hollins Martin, C. J., Marland, G., Martin, C. R., & Rankin, J. (2011). .The enigma of post-natal depression: An update. *Journal of Psychiatric and Mental Health Nursing, 18*(1), 48–58.

Yoshiiwa, T., Miyazaki, M., Takita, C., Itonaga, I., & Tsumura, H. (2011). Analysis of measured D-dimer levels for detection of deep venous thrombosis and pulmonary embolism after spinal cord surgery. *Journal of Spinal Disorder Technology, 24*(4), E35–E39.

Zauderer, C. (2009). Postpartum depression: How childbirth educators can help break the silence. *The Journal of Perinatal Education, 18*(2), 23–30.

Zauderer, C. & Davis, W. (2012). Treating postpartum depression and anxiety naturally. *Holistic Nursing Practice, 26*(4), 203–209.

CHAPTER 20

The Healthy Newborn

Debbie Fraser and Jeannette Zaichkin*

Thomas was born 8 hours ago at 40 weeks' gestation to a 34-year-old primipara. His mother had ongoing prenatal care and experienced no complications during pregnancy, labour, or birth. Upon entering the room during a routine assessment, the nurse finds Thomas lying on the bed, clothed in a shirt and diaper. His mother sits on the bed next to him. As the nurse begins to take vital signs, Thomas has a small emesis of breast milk. He gags and coughs; mucus comes through his nose. His mother is visibly upset. "What is happening?" she asks, worriedly. "Is he choking?"

William is a 2-day-old, 37-week newborn who is having a serum bilirubin done. The nurse is providing the parents with information about bilirubin screening and follow-up. William's father seems concerned about whether or not jaundice can cause brain damage. He tells the nurse that he read something on the Internet about jaundice causing harm to the developing brain.

You will learn more about these clients as the chapter progresses. Nurses working with these and similar families need to understand the material in this chapter to manage care effectively and address issues appropriately. Before beginning, consider the following points related to the above scenarios:

- How should the nurse individualize care to ensure that each family's needs are met—not only in terms of physical care, but also in terms of emotional and psychological care?

*Contributor to first U.S. edition.

- What factors may be contributing to parental behaviour and reactions in these scenarios?
- Is there need for any additional assessment data or questions?
- What teaching might be appropriate for each family?
- What other health care personnel might assist in these scenarios?

LEARNING OBJECTIVES

On completion of this chapter, the reader should be able to:
- Identify the major differences between fetal circulation and newborn circulation.
- List three cardiopulmonary changes that must occur at birth for successful extrauterine transition.
- Discuss immediate nursing interventions at birth for active and healthy full-term newborns who are breathing and have pink mucous membranes.
- Describe appropriate calculation and use of Apgar scores.
- Identify signs of abnormal newborn transition.
- Describe collaborative strategies to promote normal newborn transition.
- Discuss the relationship between birth weight and gestational age.
- Describe normal and abnormal physical examination findings in newborns.
- Discuss four types of heat loss in newborns and preventive interventions for each.
- Identify two classifications of newborns at risk for hypoglycemia and six signs of neonatal hypoglycemia.
- Explain why most healthy full-term newborns experience jaundice in the first week of life.
- Explain why newborns are susceptible to infection.
- Identify infant behavioural states and cues.
- Identify risk factors for Sudden Infant Death Syndrome (SIDS).
- Describe an approach for assessing cultural differences in newborn care.
- List newborn care topics for parent education.

KEY TERMS

acid mantle	ductus arteriosus
acrocyanosis	foramen ovale
Apgar score	free-flow oxygen
apnea	functional residual capacity
approach cues	grunting
appropriate for gestational age (AGA)	hypoglycemia
avoidance cues	hypoxemia
Ballard Gestational Age Assessment Tool	hypoxia
bilirubin	indirect (conjugated) bilirubin
bradycardia	jaundice
brick dust spots	lanugo
brown adipose tissue	large for gestational age (LGA)
circumcision	low birth weight (LBW)
cyanotic	meconium
	meconium-stained amniotic fluid

nasal flaring	retractions
neutral thermal environment	small for gestational age (SGA)
nonshivering thermogenesis	sudden infant death syndrome (SIDS)
occipital–frontal circumference	surfactant
periodic breathing	tachycardia
petechiae	tachypnea
phototherapy	term
physiologic jaundice	total bilirubin
pink	unconjugated bilirubin
plethoric	vagal reflex
postterm	vernix caseosa
preterm, premature	very low birth weight (VLBW)
pseudomenses/pseudomenstruation	witch's milk
radiant warmer	

T he birth of a baby is a significant life event influenced by cultural norms and expectations. Nurses responsible for newborn care need to balance the expectations of the new mother and her family with astute assessment and timely interventions.

Nursing care for newborns begins with critical examination of the maternal prenatal and intrapartal history. At birth, the nurse assesses the newborn's well-being and ensures that critical extrauterine adaptations are happening. During the complete physical examination, the nurse distinguishes normal findings and variations from abnormalities. He or she evaluates the newborn continuously thereafter, taking every opportunity to monitor the infant's condition, as well as teaching the parents how to care for their baby and appreciate his or her innate abilities.

FROM FETUS TO NEWBORN

The newborn's cry signifies the beginning of life outside the uterus. New mothers, their families, and health care providers of all cultures eagerly anticipate this cry as an initial signal of wellness. The more complex mechanisms underlying a successful transition from intrauterine to extrauterine life are discussed later. Knowledge of them provides a foundation for understanding the principles of neonatal resuscitation and anticipating abnormalities.

Review of Fetal Circulation

To understand newborn's pulmonary physiology, the nurse needs to appreciate the differences between fetal circulation and extrauterine circulation. In Chapter 11, we discussed and illustrated details of fetal anatomy and physiology. The next paragraphs provide a quick review.

In utero, the placenta acts as a low-resistance circulatory pathway for gas exchange. The fetal lungs do not oxygenate tissues or excrete carbon dioxide; they are not filled with air, but with fluid consisting of secretions from the alveolar epithelium. The blood vessels that perfuse the fetal lungs are tightly constricted.

Two shunts (detours) within the fetal heart are essential to fetal circulation (see Chap. 11, Fig. 11.12). The **foramen ovale** and **ductus arteriosus** divert oxygenated blood away from the fetal lungs to the brain and other vital organs. The foramen ovale allows blood to pump directly from the right to the left ventricle. The ductus arteriosus connects the pulmonary artery and descending aorta, causing most of the blood to detour the fetal lungs (Blackburn, 2013).

The fetal lungs maintain a state of pulmonary arterial vasoconstriction. The small amount of relatively hypoxic blood that reaches the fetal lungs helps maintain this constricted state. In addition, fetal pulmonary arteries have smaller lumens and more muscle mass than adult pulmonary arteries, limiting blood flow through them. As the fetus matures, these blood vessels prepare for extrauterine life by becoming increasingly reactive to changes in oxygenation and acid–base levels (Blackburn, 2013).

Finally, resistance to blood flow is different in the fetal pulmonary blood vessels. Blood flows most easily from areas of high pressure to areas of low pressure. Fetal circulation functions so that the high pulmonary vascular resistance in the lungs encourages blood to bypass them and shunt from the right side of the heart to the left. The blood passes through the foramen ovale and ductus arteriosus to the fetal aorta and returns to the low-pressure placenta for gas exchange. In contrast, adult pulmonary vascular resistance is low to permit easy blood circulation from the pulmonary arteries into the lungs. In the adult, systemic vascular resistance is fairly high, allowing the aorta to distribute oxygenated blood throughout the body (Blackburn, 2013).

Respiratory and Circulatory Transitions at Birth

The fetal system of high pulmonary vascular resistance and low aortic systemic vascular resistance allows the placenta to be a low-resistance medium for gas exchange, which works well for the fetus. Critical transitions must occur within moments of birth, however, if transition to extrauterine life is to be successful (Fig. 20.1). If all goes correctly, the following three critical changes happen:

- Respiration begins and continues effectively.
- Fluid is cleared from the airways.
- Systemic vascular resistance increases, shunts close, and blood circulates through the lungs (Blackburn, 2013; Kattwinkel, 2011).

Respiration

Several factors induce respiration. During vaginal birth, the maternal birth canal compresses the fetal chest. As

the chest emerges, the thorax recoils and air is sucked into the lung fields. Additionally, clamping of the umbilical cord affects chemoreceptors sensitive to changes in arterial oxygen and carbon dioxide content, contributing to the onset of respirations.

Temperature also is influential. The sudden cooling of the wet newborn as he or she emerges from the warm intrauterine environment stimulates respiration (Blackburn, 2013). Finally, normal handling and drying of the newborn stimulates respirations; however, tactile stimulation does not always induce respirations in a newborn compromised at birth (Kattwinkel, 2011).

Clear Airways

First breaths must be strong enough to move the thick fluids that fill the fetal airway from the trachea to the terminal air sacs. Fetal lungs hold approximately 20 to 25 mL of fluid/kg of fetal body weight. Thus, the lungs of a newborn weighing 3,000 g hold approximately 60 to 75 mL of fluid (Steinhorn & De Ungria, 2008).

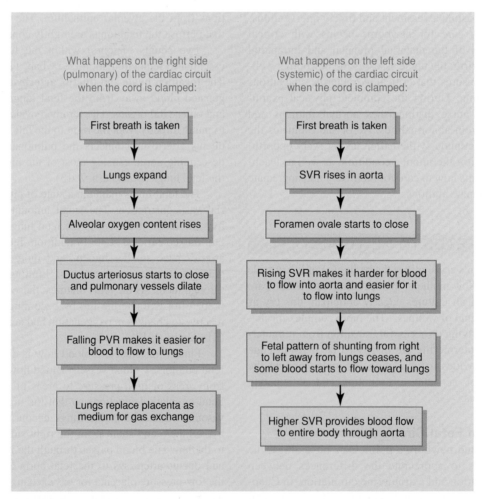

What happens on the right side (pulmonary) of the cardiac circuit when the cord is clamped:

First breath is taken

↓

Lungs expand

↓

Alveolar oxygen content rises

↓

Ductus arteriosus starts to close and pulmonary vessels dilate

↓

Falling PVR makes it easier for blood to flow to lungs

↓

Lungs replace placenta as medium for gas exchange

What happens on the left side (systemic) of the cardiac circuit when the cord is clamped:

First breath is taken

↓

SVR rises in aorta

↓

Foramen ovale starts to close

↓

Rising SVR makes it harder for blood to flow into aorta and easier for it to flow into lungs

↓

Fetal pattern of shunting from right to left away from lungs ceases, and some blood starts to flow toward lungs

↓

Higher SVR provides blood flow to entire body through aorta

FIGURE 20.1 Transition from fetal to neonatal circulation. PVR, pulmonary vascular resistance; SVR, system vascular resistance. (From Lockridge, T. [1999]. Persistent pulmonary hypertension of the newborn. *Mother Baby Journal*, 4[2], 22.)

Fortunately, production of fetal lung fluid begins to decrease before labour begins (Blackburn, 2013). Release of catecholamines is associated with labour and stimulates the lungs to begin absorbing fluid (Tutdibi et al., 2010), so that the baby must clear only a fraction of the original lung fluid volume at birth (Blackburn, 2013). In those cases in which the mother does not experience labour and exposure to catecholamines, the newborn is at risk for retaining lung fluid and developing transient tachypnea (Polin & Fox, 2011; Tutdibi et al., 2010) (see Chapter 22).

For breathing to begin, liquid in the lungs must be replaced with an equal volume of air, and **functional residual capacity** must be established (Blackburn, 2013). This means that the newborn's first breaths must be deep enough to displace the liquid in the airways and retain some air in the alveoli so that subsequent breaths are less difficult. A fatty substance functions as a **surfactant** and causes retention of air in the lungs, decreasing surface tension at the air–liquid interface (Blackburn, 2013). The surfactant consists of phospholipids and proteins produced by type II cells in the lining of the alveoli and secreted onto the alveolar surface. This surfactant is essential to normal lung function because it allows the alveoli to remain open instead of collapsing completely during exhalation. By 28 to 32 weeks' gestation, the number of type II cells increases. Surfactant production peaks at about 35 weeks' gestation. By 32 weeks, 60% of fetuses have adequate surfactant to support extrauterine respiration. Surfactant deficiency results in respiratory distress syndrome (Blackburn, 2013) (see Chapter 22).

With the first few breaths, alveolar fluid is absorbed into the lung tissue and the alveoli are filled with air. The lymphatic system reabsorbs 10% to 20% of the lung fluid (Blackburn, 2013). Aeration and increased oxygen tension increase alveolar blood flow and the capillaries' ability to remove fluid. When these systems work efficiently, they disperse lung fluid in the first few hours after birth (Blackburn, 2013). This explains why newborns have audible crackles for a short time after birth. Residual air is retained in the lungs from the early breaths; within 1 hour after birth, 80% to 90% of functional residual capacity is created (Blackburn, 2013).

Blood Circulation

Clamping of the umbilical cord shuts off the placental circuit and causes rapid changes in pulmonary vascular resistance and systemic vascular resistance. With the low-resistance pathway removed, systemic vascular resistance increases. Other contributors include increased arterial blood volume, because the blood that previously had a placenta to return to remains in the vascular system (Blackburn, 2013).

This increased systemic vascular resistance reduces right-to-left shunting and sends blood through the lungs rather than allowing it to detour through the foramen ovale and ductus arteriosus. The foramen ovale closes and seals as changes in circulatory pressures reduce pressure on the right side of the heart and increase pressure on the left side. Rise in oxygen levels causes the other fetal shunt, the ductus arteriosus, to begin to constrict almost immediately after birth of a healthy newborn. In most cases, the ductus arteriosus is functionally closed by 96 hours of life; full anatomic closure with formation of a fibrous strand known as the *ligamentum arteriosus* is complete within 2 to 3 months (Blackburn, 2013). The ductus can reopen, however, in response to **hypoxia** (abnormally low oxygen concentration in tissues) or increased pulmonary vascular resistance. This return to fetal circulation, called pulmonary hypertension, results in a dangerous cycle of hypoxia and pulmonary vasoconstriction (Fig. 20.2). Thus, attaining and maintaining adequate ventilation and oxygenation in newborns and avoiding procedures that cause hypoxia, such as deep suctioning, are important concerns (see Chapter 22).

With gaseous distention and increased oxygen in the alveoli, the pulmonary blood vessels begin to dilate and relax. Vasodilation of these arterial vessels decreases pulmonary vascular resistance in the newborn by nearly 80%, which increases blood flow through the lungs and minimizes blood flow through the fetal shunts (Blackburn, 2013). Adequate oxygen is now available from the lungs and enters the bloodstream. As the baby continues to take deep breaths, adequate oxygen moves from the lungs into the bloodstream. The baby changes from a grey-blue colour to pink. Note that this chapter uses the term **pink** to denote adequate oxygenation and perfusion for newborns of all racial and ethnic backgrounds. In newborns with dark complexions, pink mucous membranes (lips, tongues, and gums) denote adequate oxygenation and perfusion. In light-skinned newborns, providers assess the colour of the face, trunk, and mucous membranes.

IMMEDIATE NURSING MANAGEMENT OF THE NEWBORN

Most pregnancies result in the birth of a healthy, full-term newborn who requires little assistance from health care personnel. Nevertheless, nurses are prepared for any deviation from normal. Nursing actions in a compromised newborn's first moments can have lifetime consequences (Kattwinkel, 2011). Therefore, nurses who attend births and are responsible for newborn resuscitation and admission carefully assess prenatal and intrapartal history to determine risk factors for receiving a compromised newborn, ensure that all equipment for resuscitation and admission is available

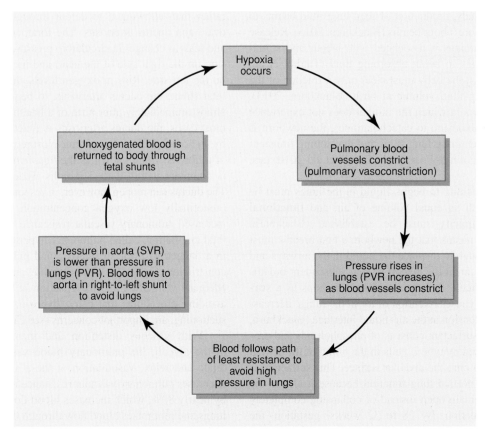

FIGURE 20.2 Cycle of inadequate ventilation/oxygenation at or shortly after birth. PVR, pulmonary vascular resistance; SVR, system vascular resistance. (From Lockridge, T. [1999]. Persistent pulmonary hypertension of the newborn. *Mother Baby Journal, 4*[2], 23.)

and working, possess skills and knowledge for competent assessment and intervention, and communicate with colleagues and the newborn's family to ensure that the plan of care incorporates any special circumstances.

Prenatal and Intrapartal History

The nurse responsible for newborn admission assesses the prenatal and intrapartal history for any risk factors. Many maternal conditions, such as diabetes, hypertension, infection, and so on, can influence the course of labour and birth, the initial transition period, and beyond. After checking the history, the nurse will have an understanding of whether to prepare for admission of a healthy newborn or to anticipate complications that will require interventions to stabilize an at-risk or sick newborn.

Preparedness for Resuscitation

At least 90% of newborns make a smooth extrauterine transition; approximately 5% to 10% need some assistance to begin breathing; rarely, 1% require complex resuscitation procedures to survive (Saugstad, 2012). Although the need for resuscitation is usually evident before birth, a newborn may require resuscitation for an unanticipated reason. Therefore, all equipment necessary for complete resuscitation must be available and operational at all births. Supplies that are visible and arranged identically in every room will help ensure that any member of the resuscitation team can always find them in the same location (Zaichkin, 2011).

Ideally, every birth is attended by at least one person whose primary responsibility is the baby and who is capable of initiating resuscitation. Either that person or someone else who is immediately available possesses the skills required to perform a complete resuscitation (Assessment Tool 20.1). This means that the person designated to attend the newborn has no other responsibilities at this time, is capable of assessing the need for resuscitation, and can competently perform initial steps of resuscitation, bag-and-mask ventilation, and chest compressions. If complex resuscitation is necessary, someone who is competent to perform procedures such as endotracheal intubation or medication administration should be immediately available (Kattwinkel, 2011).

If a high-risk birth is anticipated, the nurse follows the health care facility's protocol for assembling a team of skilled resuscitation providers to attend the birth. Team composition varies, but may include a pediatrician, neonatologist, neonatal nurse practitioner, respiratory

● **ASSESSMENT TOOL 20.1**   **Algorithm for Neonatal Resuscitation**

Birth

Term gestation?
Breathing or crying?
Good tone?

Yes—stay with mother →

Routine Care
• Provide warmth
• Clear airway if necessary
• Dry
• Ongoing evaluation

Assessment

No ↓

Warm, clear airway if necessary, dry, stimulate

Ⓐ

30 sec

HR below 100 bpm, gasping, or apnea? → No → Labored breathing or persistent cyanosis? → No → (Routine Care)

Evaluation

Yes ↓   Yes ↓

PPV, SPO₂ monitoring   Clear airway SPO₂ monitoring Consider CPAP

Ⓑ

60 sec

HR below 100 bpm? → No →

Evaluation

Yes ↓

Take ventilation corrective steps   Post-resuscitation care

HR below 60 bpm?

No (loop back)

Yes ↓

Consider intubation
Chest compressions
Coordinate with PPV

Ⓒ

HR below 60 bpm?

Evaluation

Yes ↓

IV epinephrine

Ⓓ

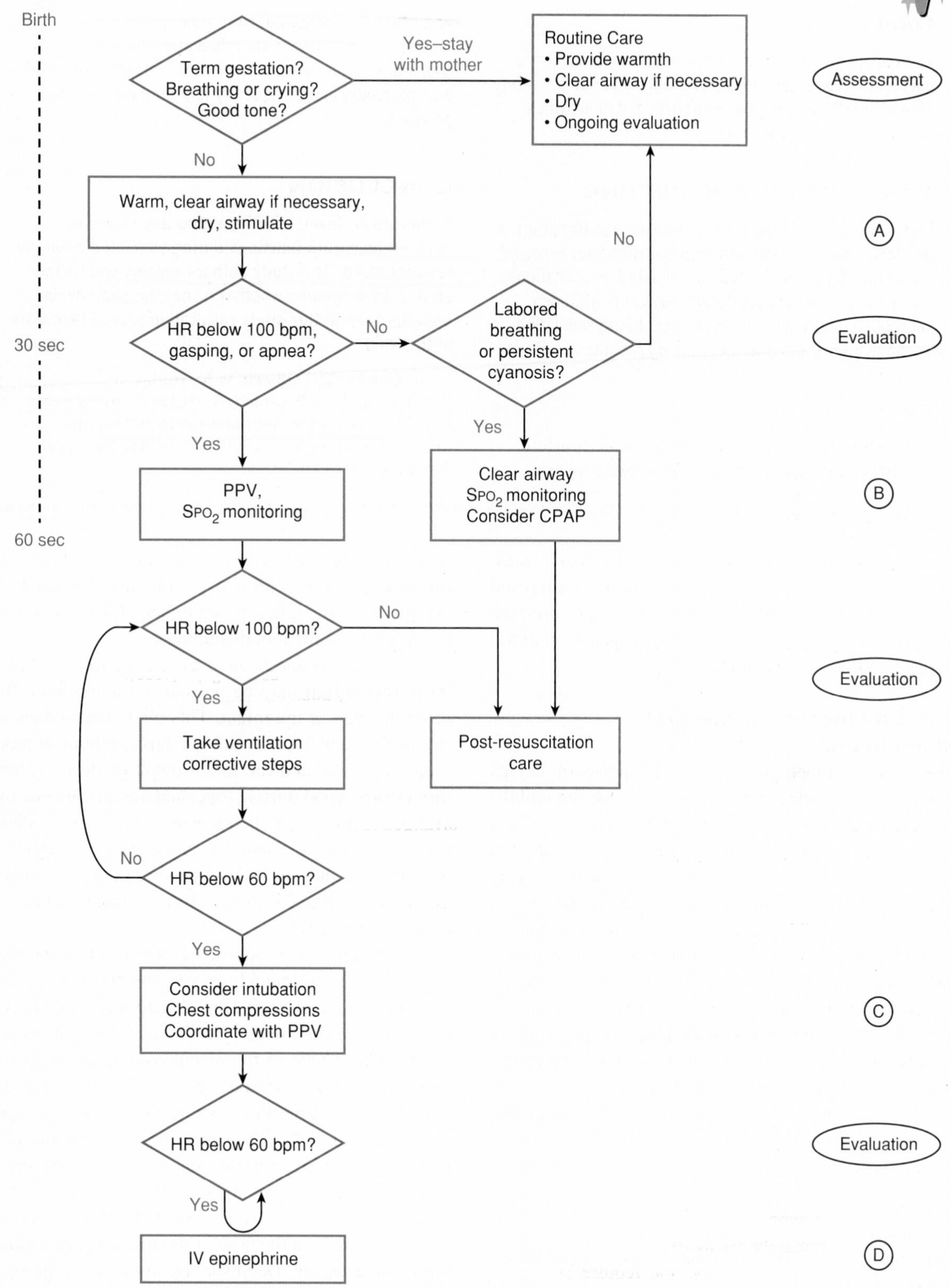

Used with permission of the American Academy of Pediatrics. (2011). *Neonatal Resuscitation Textbook* (6th ed.). American Academy of Pediatrics/American Heart Association p.12.

● **RESEARCH HIGHLIGHT 20.1** **Teamwork During Resuscitation**

OBJECTIVE

To examine the effects of interprofessional Team Strategies and Tools to Enhance Performance and Patient Safety (TeamSTEPPS) training on teamwork-related activities during neonatal resuscitation.

PARTICIPANTS AND SETTING

Forty-two nurses, respiratory therapists, and physicians in one level-three hospital with high-risk deliveries received TeamSTEPPS training, including simulated resuscitations. Using a pre- and posttest design, teamwork attitudes, knowledge, and skills were measured during simulation sessions before and after the training program.

RESULTS

There were significant improvements in team structure, leadership behaviours, communication, and support and situation monitoring. More potential medication errors were identified after the training program and incorrect chest compressions were also corrected more frequently following the training program.

CONCLUSION

In this study, TeamSTEPPS training was shown to improve teamwork functions during simulated neonatal resuscitations. The study authors recommend further studies to determine whether or not the short-term benefits seen in this study result in improved teamwork in the NICU.

From Sawyer, T., Laubach, V. A., Hudak, J., Yamamura, K., & Pocrnich, A. (2013) Improvements in teamwork during neonatal resuscitation after interprofessional TeamSTEPPS training. *Neonatal Network. 32*(1), 26–33.

therapist, and neonatal nurses. Interdisciplinary teamwork is emphasized during resuscitation training and has been found to enhance patient safety and improve the quality of the resuscitation process (Katakam et al., 2012). See Research Highlight 20.1.

Assessment During the First Moments After Birth

The nurse assigned to care for the newborn begins assessment as soon as the baby emerges and the umbilical cord is clamped and cut. This time frame may be a minimum of 1 minute or until the cord stops pulsating in the term infant, at least 30 seconds or following milking of the cord in the preterm infant (Garafalo & Abenhaim, 2012) (see Chapter 13). There is insufficient evidence to support a delay in cord clamping in a non-vigorous infant requiring resuscitation (Garafalo & Abenhaim, 2012). Although most newborns require no assistance to begin breathing, the newborn admission nurse assesses each baby in the first seconds and decides if he or she requires assistance (Kattwinkel, 2011).

When the baby is born and the umbilical cord cut, the nurse considers three questions to assess the need for intervention (Kattwinkel, 2011):

1. Is the baby full term (38 to 42 weeks' gestation)?
2. Is the baby breathing or crying?
3. Is the baby demonstrating good muscle tone (flexed position and active)?

If the answers to all three of the above questions are "yes," the newborn requires little nursing assistance. Most mothers welcome their infant onto their chest or abdomen, where a health care provider dries him or her off with a towel, continually removing the wet linen, and positions the infant prone to help drain any remaining fluids from the mouth and nose.

In some instances, such as fetal distress or breech birth, **meconium** may be present in the amniotic fluid or on the skin of the infant. This thick, dark-green first stool of the newborn is released during labour. If meconium is present and the infant displays strong respiratory efforts, good muscle tone, and has a heart rate over 100 beats/min, he or she receives routine care with the mother (Canadian Paediatric Society [CPS], 2011). If meconium is present and the newborn does not display all of these characteristics, further interventions are needed (CPS, 2011).

If the answer to any of the three initial questions is "no," the nurse quickly moves the baby to the radiant warmer for resuscitation. A **radiant warmer** is a mattress on a cart, with a heat source above it, used to warm the newborn or to prevent cooling during procedures that require exposure (Fig. 20.3). Following drying and stimulation, the nurse places the infant supine with the head in "sniffing position," the optimal position for opening the airway, and uses a bulb syringe or suction to clear the mouth first, then the nose as necessary. If the baby is not making gurgling sounds or draining fluid from the nose or mouth, repeated suctioning is unnecessary. Deep suction, by placing the tip of the bulb syringe or suction catheter deep in the throat, may elicit a gag and **vagal reflex**. This leads to apnea, **bradycardia** (heart rate less than 100 beats/min), and resulting hypoxia, which unnecessarily complicate the

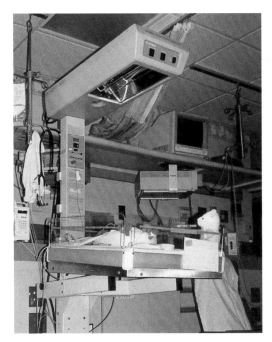

FIGURE 20.3 The newborn is placed under the radiant warmer to assist with thermoregulation.

baby's transition. All that is required to ensure that the newborn's airway is clear is wiping both mouth and nose clear with a towel or suctioning the mouth first and then the nose (Kattwinkel, 2011) (Fig. 20.4).

The nurse assesses respiratory efforts and heart rate following drying and stimulation. If the newborn is breathing and has a heart rate of more than 100 beats/min but remains dusky or **cyanotic** at 5 minutes of age, the nurse attaches an SpO_2 oximeter (a device that measures the saturation of hemoglobin with oxygen) to the infant's right hand or wrist to assess the possible need for supplemental oxygen; studies have shown that clinical assessment of skin color is not reliable (Kattwinkel, 2011). Infants transitioning normally to the extra-uterine environment often take several minutes after birth to increase their SpO_2 to over 90% from the 60% that is normal in the intrauterine environment (Kattwinkel, 2011). Supplemental oxygen has a higher concentration than room air and blows passively through oxygen tubing, an oxygen mask, or the mask of a flow-inflating oxygen bag or T-piece resuscitator. Ideally the oxygen is blended with air and the concentration delivered determined by oximetry. If the newborn has grunting respirations, intercostal retractions, or persistent central cyanosis or hypoxia confirmed by oximetry, it may be appropriate to administer supplemental oxygen through continuous positive airway pressure (Kattwinkel, 2011).

If the newborn is apneic following drying and stimulation, does not respond to oxygen with an increasing SpO_2 level, remains limp, displays signs of respiratory distress, or has a heart rate below 100 beats/min, the

nurse begins bag-and-mask ventilation and activates the emergency response system to assemble additional members of a resuscitation team. Most babies begin to breathe spontaneously within 30 seconds of effective bag-and-mask ventilation. If, after 30 seconds of effective bag-and-mask ventilation, the newborn remains apneic and/or the heart rate is below 60 beats/min, chest compressions are initiated. At this point, complex resuscitation is under way, and the newborn is not considered healthy. Any newborn needing bag-and-mask ventilation or more complex interventions requires post-resuscitation care and a closely monitored transition. The location of this care is determined by unit protocol (CPS, 2012) (see Chapter 22).

Vaginal Birth

A newborn doing well following vaginal birth requires only routine care (Kattwinkel, 2011). The nurse provides warmth, clears the airway, and dries the baby quickly and thoroughly. Unless the mother has emergent medical needs or requests otherwise, there is no reason to separate her from her healthy newborn. A policy of taking a healthy newborn immediately to a radiant warmer or other location for observation and admission is outmoded and hinders attachment. The nurse can place the

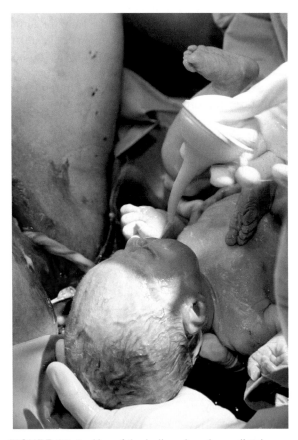

FIGURE 20.4 Use of the bulb syringe immediately after birth to suction the newborn.

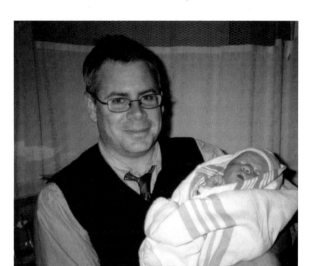

FIGURE 20.5 This father is preparing to present his newborn to the baby's mother following a cesarean birth.

baby directly on the mother's abdomen or chest, covering both with a dry, warm blanket. Skin-to-skin contact will maintain warmth (Kattwinkel, 2011).

Cesarean Birth

The nurse follows the same resuscitation and admission procedures in cases of cesarean birth. He or she immediately receives the newborn at the radiant warmer and suctions, dries, and positions the baby for further assessment. If the newborn requires no special care, the father or birth partner may use warm blankets to hold and show the newborn to the mother (Fig. 20.5).

Skin-to-skin care may be initiated by either the mother or birth partner in the OR or recovery room.

Apgar Scoring

While handling the newborn and assessing progress in the first minute of life, the nurse also assesses the 1-minute **Apgar score** (Assessment Tool 20.2). Created by anaesthesiologist Virginia Apgar in 1952, the Apgar score has become the standard of practice for assessing and documenting the infant's response to birth (Apgar, 1953). In 1962, the acronym APGAR was proposed to recall the components of the scoring system (Butterfield, 1962):

- **A:** Appearance (colour)
- **P:** Pulse (heart rate)
- **G:** Grimace (reflex irritability)
- **A:** Activity (muscle tone)
- **R:** Respiration (respiratory effort)

Each component is assigned a value of 0, 1, or 2; the five numbers are then added. Scoring is done at 1 minute and 5 minutes after birth. To help ensure accuracy, scoring should occur at the 1-minute and 5-minute marks, not retrospectively (Apgar, 1966). The Apgar score does not determine resuscitation efforts; therefore, resuscitative efforts are not delayed while waiting for the 1-minute Apgar to be determined. If the newborn does not attain a 5-minute score of at least 7, additional scores are assigned every 5 minutes up to 20 minutes (Kattwinkel, 2011).

Because Apgar scoring should be objective, Dr. Apgar suggested that an impartial observer, not the delivering practitioner, assigns the scores (Apgar, 1966). In most cases, the person responsible for newborn resuscitation and admission assigns the Apgar scores of a healthy newborn. If the newborn requires resuscitation, a collaborative effort from all resuscitation team members, in conjunction with narrative documentation of interventions and their timing, ensures an accurate record of events.

Most healthy full-term newborns receive 1-minute scores of 7 to 9 and 5-minute scores of 8 or 9. Because pink hands and feet are rare in the first few minutes of life, a perfect score of 10 is unusual.

The Apgar score alone is not sufficient evidence to predict neurologic outcomes in term newborns. The difference between 1-minute and 5-minute Apgar scores reflects the effectiveness of any resuscitation efforts. An Apgar score of 0 to 3 at 5 minutes may correlate with neonatal mortality but does not necessarily predict later neurologic dysfunction (Wheeler, 2011).

Apgar scoring is standard practice and a useful tool for documenting the newborn's responses to the extrauterine environment and resuscitation efforts. In addition

● **ASSESSMENT TOOL 20.2 Apgar Scoring System**

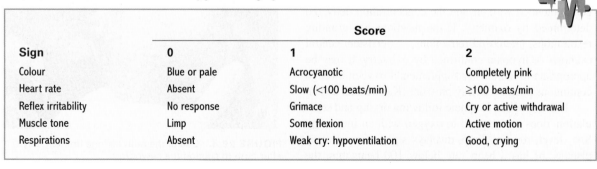

Sign	Score		
	0	**1**	**2**
Colour	Blue or pale	Acrocyanotic	Completely pink
Heart rate	Absent	Slow (<100 beats/min)	≥100 beats/min
Reflex irritability	No response	Grimace	Cry or active withdrawal
Muscle tone	Limp	Some flexion	Active motion
Respirations	Absent	Weak cry: hypoventilation	Good, crying

to Apgar scores, complete documentation, including a narrative description of the newborn's behaviour and responses to interventions, is essential to a complete medical record.

 Recall Thomas, the 8-hour-old newborn described at the beginning of the chapter. Suppose he had an Apgar score of 5 at 1 minute and 6 at 5 minutes. How would the nurse proceed?

COLLABORATIVE CARE: IMMEDIATE NEWBORN CARE

The team responsible for the newborn needs to ensure that the plan of care is clear and agreed upon before birth and well in advance of the final moments of labour. The nurse who has been involved in maternal intrapartum care and who shifts his or her responsibilities to the newborn will already have assessed family preferences for involvement in the first few minutes after birth. The nurse assigned to perform newborn admission may need to clarify the plan with the family and the labour and delivery team; he or she checks the prenatal and intrapartal history and clarifies any risk factors. The newborn admission nurse usually asks the labour nurse if there are any new risk factors with implications for the newborn, such as abnormalities in fetal heart rate, meconium in the amniotic fluid, maternal fever, prolonged rupture of membranes, or recent maternal narcotic administration.

Family preferences may include the partner's wish to cut the umbilical cord, the mother's preference to receive the newborn on her chest immediately after birth, or the family's desire to wait to hold the baby until he or she has been dried. A client giving her newborn to an adoptive family may have specific wishes about seeing and holding the baby. The nurse asks the family about cultural or spiritual beliefs that influence admission procedures and adapts routine policies to accommodate reasonable requests. The nurse's responsibility to facilitate integration of the newborn into the family begins immediately at birth; however, if the newborn requires resuscitation or intervention, nursing and medical care take precedence. Following such an emergency, the nurse ensures the inclusion of the mother and support partners in the newborn's plan of care.

Assessment

At birth, the nurse assesses many parameters simultaneously (Kattwinkel, 2011):

- Breathing
- Muscle tone

- Heart rate (by palpating the umbilical pulse)
- Any meconium on the newborn's skin
- Reflex irritability (grimacing response to bulb suction or gagging on mucus)
- Approximate gestational age
- Colour

The experienced neonatal nurse also assesses approximate weight and, by doing so, compares it to gestational age. If the newborn appears smaller or larger than appropriate, the nurse is prepared to address risk factors requiring immediate intervention, before a complete physical examination. He or she also quickly inspects the baby, scanning for unusual variances or congenital anomalies that might interfere with normal transition.

Select Potential Nursing Diagnosis

The following nursing diagnosis may be appropriate during the first few moments after birth:

- **Ineffective Breathing Pattern** related to obstructed airway, neuromuscular immaturity, perinatal compromise, or physiologic inability to make the transition to extrauterine circulation.

Planning/Intervention

The nurse ensures that the baby's airway is clear and dries fluids from the skin. The following findings and interventions may be appropriate:

- Breathing but not pink with decreased Sp_{O_2}—provide free-flow oxygen.
- Limp or having acute respiratory distress—take the infant to a radiant warmer for more thorough assessment, remembering that ventilation is the most important intervention.
- Apneic—stimulate the baby by drying or flicking the soles of the feet. If there is no response after 30 seconds, begin bag-and-mask ventilation (Kattwinkel, 2011).

Newborns requiring no resuscitation or brief free-flow oxygen can usually stay with their mothers under close nursing supervision. If all appears well after assignment of the 5-minute Apgar score, the nurse can leave the newborn on the mother's chest, covered with a warm dry blanket, and maintain vigilance from a short distance. The nurse continues to assess the newborn's vital signs and temperature as appropriate and remains alert to the newborn's needs while the family enjoys a few minutes of privacy with the baby (Fig. 20.6).

Evaluation

The healthy newborn is term, pink, and active and has minimal signs of respiratory distress soon after birth.

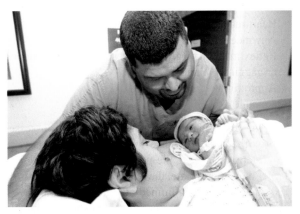

FIGURE 20.6 A family is bonding following labour and birth. (Photo courtesy of Joe Mitchell.)

EARLY NEWBORN CARE PROCEDURES

The first hours after a baby's birth are busy for perinatal and neonatal staff. The timing of procedures varies with institutional protocols and family preferences.

Identification

Identical identification bands are completed for the mother and newborn with information including the mother's hospital number, the baby's sex, and the date and time of birth. For multiple births, each baby's band denotes birth order; for example, "Twin A" signifies the firstborn of twins. Another team member present in the delivery room verifies the accuracy of information printed on the bands. The nurse places one band on the mother's wrist and usually one or two on the newborn's wrist and/or ankle. Banding the mother and newborn must occur before separating them for any reason. If at any time the newborn is separated from the mother, the nurse compares the identification bands when they are reunited to ensure a match (Fig. 20.7). This is important to avoid inadvertently giving a mother an infant who does not belong to her.

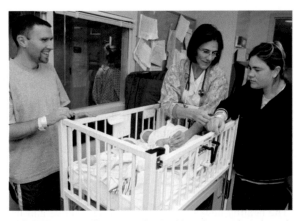

FIGURE 20.7 The nurse is checking the newborn's and mother's identification bands to ensure a match.

Weight

Parents and family members are usually eager to learn the newborn's weight. The nurse takes care to obtain an accurate weight while protecting the newborn from cold and undue stress (Nursing Procedure 20.1). He or she records the weight shortly after birth (the infant may breastfeed first, if desired). The frequency of weighing newborns varies among facilities; some may regularly weigh the newborn every day while others may only weigh on discharge.

Measurements

Measurement of length and **occipital–frontal circumference** is necessary to assess appropriateness of size for gestational age. Using a non-stretchable measuring tape, the nurse measures length by either of the following methods (Tappero, 2009):

- Place the infant supine, with the legs extended and the infant looking straight up. Place a mark on the bed to indicate the crown of the head and the infant's heel. Measure the distance between the two marks (Fig. 20.8).

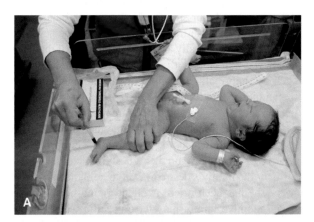

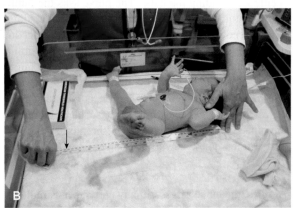

FIGURE 20.8 To measure the newborn's length, the nurse extends the baby's leg and marks the pad at the heel (**A**) and measures from the newborn's head to the heel mark (**B**).

NURSING PROCEDURE 20.1

Weighing the Newborn

PURPOSE

To measure the newborn to help determine gestational age and to establish a baseline for use in evaluating growth and development

ASSESSMENT AND PLANNING

- Assess the newborn's Apgar scores at 1 and 5 minutes *to determine newborn's transition to extrauterine life.*
- Assess the newborn's temperature and determine whether he or she is experiencing cold stress; if so, delay the procedure until temperature stabilizes.
- Calibrate the scale if necessary.
- Explain the procedure to the parents.
- Gather the necessary equipment:
    - Calibrated scale
    - Prewarmed blanket or disposable scale covering
    - Clean gloves

IMPLEMENTATION

1. Wash hands and put on gloves.
2. Place prewarmed blanket or covering on scale *to minimize risk for heat loss from conduction.*
3. Reset the scale to zero *to ensure accuracy of measurement.*
4. Place naked newborn on the covering. Position the newborn on the scale *to minimize stress;* keep one hand over the newborn body without touching the newborn *to ensure safety.*
5. Quickly note the weight.
6. Remove the newborn from the scale, and continue with care, removing gloves and washing hands when care is completed.
7. Document the weight in the newborn's medical record.

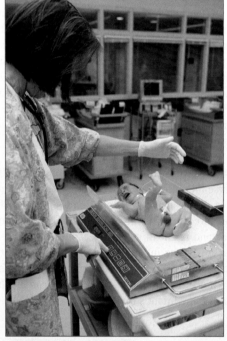

Step 4. Weighing the newborn while carefully guarding with the other hand.

EVALUATION

- Newborn is weighed without difficulty.
- Newborn experiences no evidence of cold stress.

AREAS FOR CONSIDERATION AND ADAPTATION

Lifespan Considerations

- Keep in mind that while the newborn remains at the facility, weights may be obtained daily or only at discharge obtained daily.
- Avoid placing the naked newborn directly on the scale's cold surface in the supine position. The newborn is more likely to be startled, to cry and move about, interfering with obtaining an accurate weight. Additionally, placing the naked newborn on a cold surface facilitates heat loss.

Community-Based Considerations

Obtain newborn weights at each visit. Typically, parents do not have a baby scale in their home. The home visiting nurse needs to bring a scale to the visit.

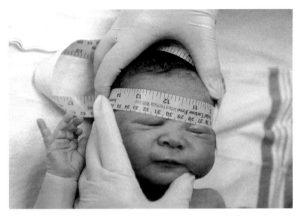

FIGURE 20.9 Measuring head circumference.

• Position the infant as described in Figure 20.8. Place the zero point of the tape measure at the heel and run it alongside the infant to the head. Mark the end spot on the tape with a finger and read the measurement.

The nurse measures occipital–frontal circumference by wrapping the tape around the infant's head, over the occipital, parietal, and frontal prominences, avoiding the ears (Tappero, 2009). He or she measures three times and records the largest finding (Fig. 20.9). Cranial moulding or scalp edema may affect the measurement (Fabris & Coscia, 2012). Because of this, the head circumference may be assessed only on discharge in some facilities.

Chest circumference measurement is optional, but is performed in many institutions (Fig. 20.10). The nurse measures the chest circumference around the nipples during newborn expiration (Tappero, 2009), making sure that, if using a paper tape, it does not stick or tear and result in an incorrect measurement. Also, the nurse lifts the infant's torso off the mattress to remove the tape measure from the back; pulling the tape measure out from under the supine infant can result in paper cuts on the infant's torso.

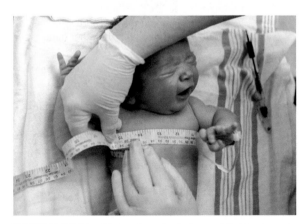

FIGURE 20.10 Measuring chest circumference.

Gestational Age Assessment

Gestational age assessment is performed to estimate a newborn's postconceptual age (Trotter, 2009). The gestational age and the appropriate growth parameters are important considerations, because neonatal risks for each classification are different. A newborn's gestational age is not evident by assessing weight alone. An infant who weighs 1,800 g at 39 weeks' gestation has a different set of risk factors and management interventions than an infant who weighs 1,800 g at 35 weeks' gestation.

Gestational age can be assessed in four ways:

1. **Maternal menstrual history:** An average term pregnancy is 266 days (38 weeks after ovulation) or 280 days (40 weeks from the first day of the last menstrual period) (Blackburn, 2013). Assessing gestational age by using the date of the last ovulation or menstrual period depends on the regularity of maternal menstrual cycles. Irregular cycles, failed contraception, and inaccurate recall by the woman can affect this method (Levine, 2008).
2. **Ultrasound examination:** Fetal measurements are taken during pregnancy and, using standard formulae, are compared with age-specific references. Using data derived from in vitro fertilization, researchers determined that in 95% of pregnancies, ultrasound was accurate to within 5 days, if done in the first trimester, and to within 7 days, if done in the second trimester (Kalish, 2008). The main criticism of ultrasound-based dating is that it does not account for normal variability (Gaillard et al., 2011).
3. **Ballard assessment:** The **Ballard Gestational Age Assessment Tool** originated from the Dubowitz Assessment of Gestational Age (Dubowitz et al., 1970). The Dubowitz scale consists of 11 external physical characteristics and 10 neurologic signs. Ballard et al. (1979) simplified the Dubowitz tool using six physical and six neuromuscular criteria. Studies have shown that, in general, these scales overestimate the gestation of infants born at less than 40 weeks, with a range of 2 weeks (Dubowitz) to 2 to 4 days (Ballard et al., 1991), and underestimate the gestation when the infant is born at or past 40 weeks (Trotter, 2009).
4. **Lens vascularity:** Used to a limited extent, this method can help determine gestational age when differences among other methods are significant. The developing lens of the eye has a vascular system that invades and nourishes the eye during fetal growth. The vascular system appears at approximately 27 weeks' gestation and disappears after 34 weeks' gestation. The stages of atrophy are divided into four grades according to the pattern and presence of blood vessels visualized on the eye lens with an ophthalmoscope. The grading system must be performed between 24 to 48 hours of age (Trotter, 2009).

Infant Classification

To determine infant gestational age following the birth of the baby, the health care provider can use the Ballard Gestational Age Assessment Tool (1991) according to the directions and descriptors. After examining the newborn and scoring each criterion, the nurse adds the two scores for neuromuscular category and the physical category to obtain the total and matches the final maturity rating with the "weeks" on the same line. Instructions are unclear as to which gestational age score to assign when the total falls between those listed. It has been suggested that the gestational age that most closely approximates the maturity rating should be chosen. For example, if the maturity rating score is 23, a gestational age of 33 weeks is assigned (Trotter, 2009).

Gestational age is based on the following definitions:

* A **preterm or premature** infant is less than 37 *completed* weeks' gestation.
* A **term** infant is 38 to 41 weeks' gestation.
* A **postterm** infant is more than 41 weeks' gestation.
* A **low birth weight (LBW) infant** weighs less than 2,500 g and can be preterm, term, or postterm.

Chapter 22 provides an illustrated comparison of the differences in preterm and term infants.

Next, the nurse plots the infant's weight on the growth curve chart. Weight is on the vertical axis; gestational age is on the horizontal axis. The nurse notes whether the plot point falls into the shaded area denoting less than the 10th percentile (**small for gestational age [SGA]**), between the 10th and 90th percentiles (**appropriate for gestational age [AGA]**), or above the 90th percentile (**large for gestational age [LGA]**). For example, if the infant is 37 weeks' gestation and weighs 1,800 g, the infant is preterm and SGA. Any newborn whose plot point falls into the SGA shading is below the 10th percentile for growth, which means that the newborn is smaller than 90% of all other babies of the same gestational age. The World Health Organization (WHO) growth charts have been adapted for use in Canada (http://www.dietitians.ca/secondary-pages/public/who-growth-charts.aspx).

Weight and gestational age combine to describe an infant who is:

* Preterm and SGA, AGA, or LGA
* Term and SGA, AGA, or LGA
* Postterm and SGA, AGA, or LGA

After plotting the weight, the nurse marks the length and head circumference on the corresponding charts and notes if an SGA infant has not grown at the expected rate for one, two, or all three growth parameters. The SGA newborn who experienced growth restriction late in gestation is usually SGA for weight only. This is termed *asymmetric growth restriction*. The infant less than the 10th percentile for weight and length experienced limited growth earlier in gestation than the newborn lacking in weight only. If all three parameters are in the 10th percentile, the infant is referred to as having *symmetric* or *proportionate growth restriction*. This type of growth restriction has a poor prognosis, given the factors that may have caused diminished growth early in gestation, such as viral infections, single-gene defects, and chromosome disorders (Trotter, 2009). However, asymmetric growth restriction has a more optimistic prognosis (Nardozza et al., 2012).

An infant at 36 weeks' gestation who weighs 3,200 g is LGA and preterm, likely to be the infant of a mother with diabetes and at risk for hypoglycemia, respiratory distress syndrome (RDS), and slow feeding. An infant of 40 weeks' gestation weighing 1,200 g is term and SGA and at risk for fetal distress, hypoglycemia, congenital anomalies, congenital infection, and polycythemia.

The experienced neonatal nurse quickly and accurately assesses gestational age during the initial newborn assessment. If the estimated date of delivery is based on the last menstrual period, ultrasound examination, or both, the nurse uses the initial assessment results to confirm the obstetrical estimation. If estimated gestational age is unclear, the nurse can quickly assess four physical parameters: ear, nipples, genitalia, and plantar creases. These findings provide enough information to develop an initial assessment and management plan. From these four criteria, the nurse can determine whether the newborn appears preterm, term, or postterm. Using an experienced eye for estimating weight, the nurse then can link the gestational age assessment to estimated weight to decide if the newborn is AGA, SGA, or LGA. This information is critical for assessing medical risks, preventing complications, assessing developmental capabilities, and implementing nursing care. Therefore, by the time the nurse has ensured that the newborn's airway is clear, wiped the baby dry, assigned the first Apgar score, and done a quick visual assessment to rule out major anomalies, he or she has also estimated gestational age and size for age and begun to formulate a plan of care based on this initial assessment.

The First Bath

The first bath is an additional opportunity to examine newborn skin and responses to stimuli. Parents often assist with the first bath and gain important information about their newborn and caregiving skills; it can also provide an opportunity for bonding. In addition, a bath can improve the newborn's appearance, provide tactile stimulation, and is important for infection control (American Academy of Pediatrics & American College of Obstetricians and Gynecologists [AAP & ACOG], 2012; Association of Women's Health, Obstetric, and Neonatal Nurses [AWHONN], 2013).

Bathing the full-term neonate immediately following birth has the potential to compromise thermal and/or cardiorespiratory adaptation during the transition period (AWHONN, 2013). Therefore, the initial bath is delayed a minimum of 1 hour (ideally 2 hours if possible) and done only if the infant has achieved thermal and cardiorespiratory stability (AWHONN, 2013). Until the initial bath is completed, health care providers use standard precautions when handling the newborn (AAP & ACOG, 2012). This includes wearing gloves whenever touching the newborn; maternal blood and blood-stained amniotic fluid may present a risk to health care providers (AWHONN, 2013).

Because bathing can be stressful, providers delay the first bath for any baby exhibiting distress during transition, such as respiratory distress, temperature instability, or hypoglycemia. Research has demonstrated no negative effects of a bath given as early as 60 minutes of age to a healthy term newborn with an axillary temperature of at least 36.8°C (AWHONN, 2013; Lund & Durand, 2011).

The first bath may take place at the bedside or in a nursery; as long as appropriate environmental controls are in place, there is no difference in heat loss (AWHONN, 2013). Limiting the bath to a short time helps maintain thermal regulation. Warm tap water and a minimal amount of pH-neutral or slightly acidic cleanser will assist with removal of blood and amniotic fluid (AWHONN, 2013). Alkaline soap destroys the skin's **acid mantle** by neutralizing the pH, which disturbs the balance of protective skin flora (Blackburn, 2013). Any soap used should be thoroughly rinsed from the infant's body (Blackburn, 2013).

Vernix should not be removed (AWHONN, 2013). If vernix is contaminated with blood, meconium, or any other uterine debris, gentle removal of the contaminant is accomplished while leaving the vernix on the skin (AWHONN, 2013). Leaving the vernix on the skin helps with early acidification of the newborn skin; attempts to remove the vernix can result in skin damage (AWHONN, 2013).

 Remember Thomas, the newborn from the beginning of the chapter. Imagine that he is 2 hours old and is to receive his first bath. The nurse is demonstrating the bath to his mother, who says, "I found a really nice fragrant soap at the bath shop that I'm going to use when I bathe him at home." How should the nurse respond?

The bathing procedure exposes the newborn to cooling and stress. Nurses take every precaution to limit adverse reactions. An efficient and organized procedure ensures that the bath, including hair washing, is completed in less than 10 minutes.

Illustrated guidelines for the initial bath appear in Nursing Procedure 20.2. The newborn may be bathed under the protection of a radiant warmer. In this

NURSING PROCEDURE 20.2
Initial Bathing of the Newborn

PURPOSE

To clean the newborn and remove any blood and secretions remaining from the birth process

ASSESSMENT AND PLANNING

- Organize supplies for bathing:
  - Basin of warm water
  - Several washcloths
  - Several towels at one end of the radiant warmer
  - Soap (optional)
  - Comb
  - Small cup for pouring water at or very near to the sink

IMPLEMENTATION

1. Wash hands and put on gloves. Keep gloves on until you have dried the baby.
2. Lay the infant under the prewarmed radiant warmer; unwrap and unclothe him or her. Change the wet or soiled diaper, if necessary. Rediaper and swaddle the newborn in a warm blanket, leaving only the head exposed.

(continued)

NURSING PROCEDURE 20.2 (CONTINUED)
Initial Bathing of the Newborn

3. Take the infant to the sink and regulate the running water temperature.
4. Use a clean washcloth to gently wash the face without soap. Include behind and inside the ears. Gently pat the face dry.
5. Wash the head and hair. Because of the possibility of fluctuating water temperature and pressure, do not hold the head directly under the running water. It is safer to collect the water in a cup or small pitcher and slowly pour it onto the infant's head over the sink. If the parent is uneasy about pouring, thoroughly soak a washcloth in running water and use it to wet the hair.
6. If using soap, use a small amount and massage it gently into the scalp. Do not rub vigorously to remove tenacious **vernix**. (Some vernix may remain firmly attached to the baby's skin.) Comb soap through the hair to loosen and remove blood, if necessary.
7. Rinse the hair thoroughly and gently dry the head with a towel. Cover the baby's head with the towel and return the infant to the radiant warmer.

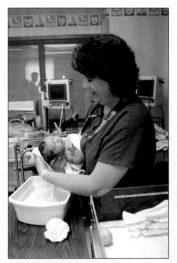

Step 5. Using a washcloth to wet the baby's hair.

8. Wash the body:
   a. Lay the infant under the radiant warmer. Positioning the infant with the head and feet across the width of the warmer provides room for a basin of clean water and supplies at the head of the warmer. Remove the baby's blanket and diaper. Expose the head to the radiant heat to help ensure drying by the end of the bath.
   b. Quickly moisten the infant's body with a wet washcloth. Do not worry about wetting the blanket underneath the baby. Work quickly and finish washing the baby's body within 1 or 2 minutes.
   c. Rub the soap into a lather with your gloved hands. Quickly massage the soap over the infant's body with your gloved hands (hands reach into infant folds faster and more efficiently than a bulky washcloth), starting at the neck creases and working down. Wash the arms, armpits, and fingers. Wash the chest. Roll the infant onto the side to wash the back. Then wash the legs and feet. Do not wash the buttocks or genitals yet.

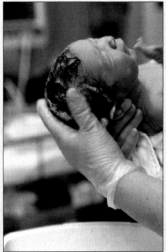

Step 6. Massaging the soap into the baby's scalp.

   d. Thoroughly wet a clean washcloth and rinse the infant, ensuring that you rinse soap from neck and armpit creases. If the infant is lying on top of soaked towels at this time, remove those towels and place the baby on a dry towel.
   e. Now use this clean wet washcloth to wash the genital area. Wipe vernix and secretions out of thigh creases. For girls, separate the labia and wipe front to back to remove secretions. Always use a clean portion of the washcloth for a front-to-back manoeuvre. Do not attempt to retract the foreskin for boys. Gently and quickly move around the genital area, remembering to lift the scrotal sac and clean the skin underneath.
   f. Clean the bottom last. Rinse any soap remaining in this area.
9. Lift the newborn off the radiant warmer to remove the waterproof pad (and with it, the wet linen on top); lay it aside or place it inside a nearby linen receptacle. Do not throw linen on the floor.

(continued)

NURSING PROCEDURE 20.2 CONTINUED
Initial Bathing of the Newborn

10. Lay the baby down on the dry towel underneath the radiant warmer. Finish drying the baby gently and thoroughly. Do not vigorously rub the skin. Discard the towel.
11. Diaper the infant.
12. Complete any necessary admission procedures, such as the vitamin K injection and cord care, if prescribed.
13. Place the newborn skin to skin with the mother or her partner if desired, with a head covering and a warm blanket over the baby. Or attach a thermistor probe to the newborn for rewarming on the radiant warmer for 10 to 15 minutes.
14. Check the baby's temperature 15 to 30 minutes after the bathing procedure is complete to monitor thermal recovery.

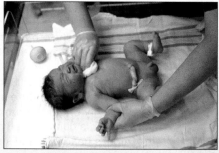

Step 8b. Bathing under the newborn's neck.

EVALUATION

• Newborn is bathed without difficulty.
• Newborn experiences no evidence of cold stress.

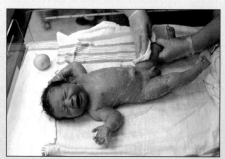

Step 8e. Cleaning the thighs and leg creases.

procedure, the infant's temperature has been taken to ensure stability within normal limits, and no transitional distress is present (Teaching Tips 20.1).

Medication Administration

Canadian newborns routinely receive two medications at birth: intramuscular vitamin K and an antibiotic agent for eye prophylaxis. In some jurisdictions, the law requires that infants receive eye prophylaxis. Parents may refuse either or both; however, it is important to document the reasons for refusal as well as information given to parents about the risks of foregoing recommended treatment. Some facilities have specific forms for parents to sign should they refuse standard procedures recommended/required for newborn care.

Vitamin K

The nurse administers vitamin K within 6 hours of birth, once the newborn is stable and there has been appropriate opportunity for interaction with the newborn (Lippi & Franchini, 2011; McMillan, 2013) (Nursing Procedure 20.3). Canadian guidelines recommend vitamin K 1 mg be given as a single intramuscular injection to all newborns with a birth weight above 1,500 g; infants who weigh 1,500 g or less should receive 0.5 mg (McMillan,

2013). If parents refuse intramuscular vitamin K, an oral dose of 2 mg is recommended at the first feeding, with follow-up oral doses given at 2 to 4 weeks of age and 6 to 8 weeks of age. Parents electing to have their newborn receive oral vitamin K should be advised that there is an increased risk of late hemorrhagic disease (including intracranial hemorrhage) with this regimen (Johnson, 2013; McMillan, 2013).

Administration of vitamin K following birth prevents hemorrhagic disease of the newborn, also known as vitamin K–deficiency bleeding (VKDB) (Blackburn, 2013; McMillan, 2013). The prevalence of VKDB is 0.4 to 1.7 per 100 infants if no vitamin K is given (Blackburn, 2013). Vitamin K is not actually required to make clotting factors. It is required to convert precursor proteins made in the liver into activated proteins with coagulant properties. Fetal vitamin K levels are low because of poor placental transport and because the fetus lacks intestinal flora that synthesize vitamin K. Infants who are exclusively breastfed have limited intake of vitamin K and may benefit from administration of vitamin K to the mother (Blackburn, 2013; McMillan, 2013). Infants with intestinal malabsorption defects, liver disease, or failure to thrive are also at risk. Without administration of vitamin K at birth,

● TEACHING TIPS 20.1 Newborn Nursing Care

- Practice newborn resuscitation skills before you need them! Palpate the umbilical pulse at the base of the umbilicus at every birth, even if the baby is pink, active, and crying. Estimate the heart rate by palpating the pulse for 3 or 4 seconds. Then double-check your estimation by counting the pulse rate for 6 seconds and multiplying by 10. Competence at palpating the umbilical pulse and quickly estimating a heart rate is important during assessment of a depressed newborn in need of resuscitative measures.
- When using the bulb syringe, suction the Mouth first, then the Nose to prevent aspiration. Remember to suction the mouth first because M comes alphabetically before N.
- Parents may wish to take a photograph of the baby being weighed at admission, with the digital readout of pounds and ounces showing on the scale. The baby will be warm and comfortable for this photograph if he or she is on a warm blanket and placed prone on the scale for this procedure.
- "Dress" the radiant warmer in layers that facilitate the admission and bathing process. Layering your linen on the radiant warmer prevents multiple errands to obtain linen during this busy time.
- Radiant warmer "dressing"
  - Layer 1: A baby blanket covers the mattress.
  - Layer 2: Two baby blankets are spread out and ready to wrap the newborn.
- Layer 3: Two towels are spread out and ready to dry the newborn after bathing.
- Layer 4: Waterproof pad
- Layer 5: Two baby blankets ready to wrap the newborn after birth.
- Top layer: Two towels ready to dry the newborn at birth.
- A clean T-shirt and two blankets are folded and set to the side on the warmer, ready to dress the infant after bathing.
- Admission and bathing supplies are within easy reach or kept in the supply drawer of the warmer.
- Perform the physical assessment in front of parents and talk through what you are seeing, hearing, and touching. Although parents may not understand everything you are doing, they will learn about things they would not have asked about, and many of their other questions will be answered as they listen. Sharing your knowledge increases parental confidence in your ability to care for their baby.
- If the physical assessment reveals a defect or variance in the midline of the body, look carefully for additional midline defects. For example, if a cleft palate is present, look closely for accompanying defects such as a two-vessel umbilical cord, hypospadias, or an imperforate anus.

---

intracranial bleeding can occur in some newborns as well as bleeding from the gastrointestinal (GI) tract, umbilicus, or any puncture or operative site (ie, circumcision) (Blackburn, 2013; McMillan, 2013).

Vitamin K prophylaxis has generated controversy since 1961 when the American Academy of Pediatrics first recommended it. Researchers have investigated its effectiveness, possible complications, and use of oral versus parenteral forms (Johnson, 2013; Lippi & Franchini, 2011). Even though it is possible that not all newborns require vitamin K, it is difficult to identify which infants require prophylaxis and which do not. Clinical decisions must be made on the best available evidence, despite controversy and a lack of definitive answers to many clinical questions.

Eye Prophylaxis

Although three topical medications, tetracycline (1%), erythromycin (0.5%), and 1% silver nitrate, are acceptable for prevention of ophthalmia neonatorum, erythromycin ointment is the prophylaxis of choice in Canada (Department of Midwifery, BC Women's, 2007). In some provinces, neonatal eye prophylaxis is mandatory; par-

ents do not have the right to consent to, or refuse, administration of the medication. This may create conflicts for health care personnel when this requirement is not consistent with patient autonomy or current evidence that questions the efficacy of the prophylaxis (Association of Ontario Midwives, ND; Darling & McDonald, 2010).

Ophthalmia neonatorum occurs when the infant is exposed to chlamydia or gonorrhea during birth. When eye prophylaxis was first introduced in the late 1800s, a dramatic decrease in the incidence of gonococcal ophthalmia neonatorum and subsequent childhood blindness resulted (Darling & McDonald, 2010). However, limitations of eye prophylaxis in the current environment have been identified (Association of Ontario Midwives, ND; Darling & MacDonald, 2010). Maternal prenatal detection and treatment or systemic antibiotics administered to the newborn in the presence of infection at the time of birth may be more effective (Association of Ontario Midwives, ND; Darling & MacDonald, 2010). The risks of long-term sequelae of ophthalmia neonatorum caused by chlamydia or gonorrhea are minimal in the presence of adequate postpartum follow-up and rapid access to antibiotic therapy on diagnosis (Association of Ontario

NURSING PROCEDURE 20.3
Administering Vitamin K to a Newborn

PURPOSE

To prevent vitamin K deficiency bleeding in the newborn

ASSESSMENT AND PLANNING

- Assess the newborn for time of birth to ensure that medication is given within 6 hours of birth.
- Check the medical record for the medication and dose ordered.
- Prepare the prescribed dose of medication in the syringe using the appropriate size needle.
- Ensure the environment is well lit.
- Explain the reason for the procedure to the parents.
- Assess the newborn's thigh to determine an appropriate injection site.
- Gather the necessary equipment:
    - Syringe with appropriate size needle attached containing prescribed dose of vitamin K (25-gauge needle recommended)
    - Alcohol wipes
    - Clean gloves
    - Clean cotton balls, gauze pads, or washcloth

IMPLEMENTATION

1. Wash hands and put on clean gloves.
2. Confirm the newborn's identity.
3. Clean the skin of the newborn's thigh with warm water, if baby has not yet been bathed, *to reduce maternal body fluids on the skin.*
4. Swaddle the newborn's upper body *to minimize movement and possible injury during injection.*
5. Locate the vastus lateralis muscle and select the injection site.
6. Clean the area with an alcohol wipe working from the centre outward in a circular pattern and allow to air dry.
7. Using the nondominant hand, grasp the newborn's thigh *to stabilize it.*
8. Remove the cap from the syringe and quickly insert the needle using a dart-like motion into the selected site at a 90-degree angle.
9. Stabilize the syringe with the nondominant hand and pull back on the plunger *to aspirate for blood.*
10. If no blood appears in the syringe, slowly inject the medication; if blood appears, quickly remove the syringe and discard; prepare a new syringe and restart the procedure.
11. When all of the medication has been injected, remove the syringe and cover the site with a gauze pad. Apply pressure and massage the site *to promote distribution of the drug into the muscle.*
12. Inspect the injection site *to check for any signs of bleeding or bruising.*
13. Discard syringe and used equipment appropriately.
14. Document administration on the newborn's medical record.

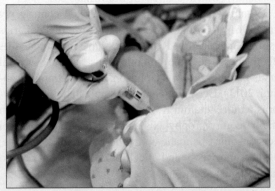

Step 8. Injecting vitamin K IM.

(continued)

NURSING PROCEDURE 20.3 (CONTINUED)
Administering Vitamin K to a Newborn

EVALUATION

- The newborn receives the prescribed vitamin K injection without difficulty.
- Injection site is free of any redness, bruising, or hematoma.
- Newborn tolerates procedure well.

AREAS FOR CONSIDERATION AND ADAPTATION

Lifespan Considerations

- If appropriate, enlist the aid of an additional person, such as support person, parent, or other health care team member *to help contain the newborn and prevent movement that could result in injury during the injection.*
- Keep in mind that a 2.5-cm needle may be necessary to reach the muscle tissue, depending on the newborn's size.
- Always double-check the dosage to be administered.
- Assess the newborn for signs and symptoms of bleeding, such as tarry stools, hematuria, blood oozing from sites such as the umbilical cord base, and decreased hemoglobin and hematocrit levels. This may indicate the need for additional vitamin K.

Community-Based Considerations

- At the follow-up home visit, question the parents about any possible signs and symptoms of bleeding and notify the health care provider if any occur.
- If the newborn was delivered at home, expect to administer vitamin K as soon as possible after the home birth.

Midwives, ND; Darling & MacDonald, 2010). As a result, some providers are calling for a re-examination of the policy on mandatory eye prophylaxis for the newborn (Association of Ontario Midwives, ND; Darling & MacDonald, 2010).

Within 1 hour of birth, the nurse deposits a 1- to 2-cm ribbon of sterile ophthalmic ointment or two drops of silver nitrate solution into the lower conjunctival sac and, after 1 minute, wipes away excess ointment with sterile cotton (Nursing Procedure 20.4).

Administration of eye prophylaxis is often challenging. It is nearly impossible to force open the eyelids of a newborn who is crying or lying under bright lights; therefore, the infant should be in a quiet, alert state.

This state is most likely if the baby is in a somewhat upright position and under dimmed lights.

Think back to William, the newborn with jaundice. When the nurse checks his medical record, which medications would William have received?

Full Physical Examination

Physical examination begins at birth and continues throughout the hospital stay. Table 20.1 summarizes the complete newborn physical examination. Table 20.2

(text continues on page 807)

NURSING PROCEDURE 20.4
Performing Eye Prophylaxis

PURPOSE

To prevent the development of severe eye infections (ophthalmia neonatorum) from gonorrhea or chlamydia that may have been transmitted to the newborn

(continued)

NURSING PROCEDURE 20.4 (CONTINUED)
Performing Eye Prophylaxis

ASSESSMENT AND PLANNING

- Check the newborn's medical record for maternal history of sexually transmitted infections.
- Review the order for prescribed agent and check to ensure that the agent is for ophthalmic use only.
- Assess the newborn's state of reactivity, ensuring that the newborn is in a quiet alert state.
- Explain the rationale for the procedure to the parents.
- Gather equipment.
  - Prescribed sterile ophthalmic ointment
  - Sterile cotton balls or dry sterile gauze pads
  - Clean gloves

IMPLEMENTATION

1. Wash hands and put on gloves.
2. Gently wipe the newborn's face with a soft gauze pad or cotton ball *to dry the face and prevent the hand from slipping.*
3. Open the prescribed ointment, making sure to keep the tip of the tube sterile.
4. Open one eye by gently separating the upper and lower lids, exposing the conjunctiva of the lower lid *to allow placement of the ointment.*
5. Lay a thin ribbon of ointment, approximately 1 to 2 cm in length, along the conjunctival sac, from the inner to outer canthus.
6. Release the eyelids and allow the newborn to close his or her eyes *to permit the ointment to be dispersed within the eye.*
7. After 1 minute, wipe away excess ointment with a sterile cotton ball or gauze.
8. Repeat the steps with the other eye *to ensure complete prevention.*
9. Document the procedure in the newborn's medical record according to agency policy.

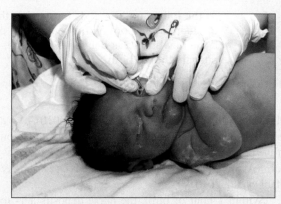

Step 5. Administering antibiotic ointment to the newborn's eye.

EVALUATION

- Ophthalmic ointment was applied to both eyes without difficulty.
- Newborn tolerated procedure without any problems.

AREAS FOR CONSIDERATION AND ADAPTATION

Lifespan Considerations

- Check the specific agency policy for the timing of eye prophylaxis. In some agencies, eye prophylaxis is performed immediately after birth. In other agencies, it may be postponed for about 1 hour to allow the parents to bond with their newborn immediately after birth without interference from the ointment, which could blur the newborn's vision.
- If necessary, dim the lights to prevent the newborn from experiencing undue discomfort and upset due to the glare of the lights.
- After instilling the ointment, do not irrigate with eyes with sterile water or saline.

Community-Based Considerations

- When making the first home visit, check with the parents to ensure that the newborn received eye prophylaxis before he or she was discharged.

● TABLE 20.1   **Physical Examination of the Newborn**

Assessment Areas and Techniques	Normal Findings	Normal Variations	Significant Deviations[a]
General Appearance			
Colour	Consistent with genetic background; pink mucous membranes Mottled with cooling Bruises over presenting part	Pigmentation: pink, ruddy, especially over face; olive; yellowish-pink; black **Acrocyanosis** (blue palms and soles) **Circumoral cyanosis** (blue around mouth): normal for first 24 hours, then evaluate **Jaundice** (yellow skin colour): mild jaundice normal after day 1 of life **Harlequin colour change** (in side-lying position, red colour demarcated on dependent side, pale colour on upper half; persists 1–30 min; colour reverses if infant is rotated to other side)	**Pallor** (grey colour could indicate hypotension) **Plethora** (deep red colour could denote polycythemia) **Central cyanosis** (blue trunk, lips, mucous membranes denote hypoxia) **Jaundice,** especially in first 24 hours of life
Respiratory effort	Diaphragmatic and abdominal breathing Rate: 40–60 breaths/min; may decrease in deep sleep and increase after crying Periodic breathing: pauses in breathing up to 20 seconds without bradycardia or colour change	Expiratory **grunting, nasal flaring,** and mild **retracting** in initial part of transition (with rapid resolution)	**Grunting, flaring, retracting** that worsens or does not resolve quickly in transition **Apnea** (cessation of breathing >20 seconds with decreased heart rate and colour change to pale or dusky) **Gasping** (intermittent rapid inhalation) **Stridor** (high-pitched sound during breathing indicates obstruction)
Tone/neuromuscular	Term infant flexed, fists clenched Term infant with healthy tone can be pulled up to sitting position using elicited palmar grasp reflex Head moves side to side Moves all extremities Moves smoothly between behavioural states (term infant)	Mild tremors with startling Frank breech: extended legs for brief time	Marked jitteriness (could indicate low blood glucose level) Tremors that continue when care provider touches or holds area (suspect seizure activity); marked hypertonia or extension Marked hypotonia
Gestational Age (see gestational assessment information on page 786)			
VITAL SIGNS: **Temperature** (broad range of normal; standard varies regionally)			
• Axillary (preferred) • Skin (usually used for special care infant) • Tympanic (not recommended)	36.5°–37.3°C 36°–36.5°C (term) 36.5°–37.0°C (preterm)		Fever is rare sign of infection; unstable temperature in stable environment is more worrisome. **Hyperthermia** or **hypothermia** is stressful and dangerous; requires evaluation of etiology such as environmental threat, sepsis, or neurologic abnormality
Heart rate (apical)	110–160 beats/min; increases with and after crying	Term infant's heart rate may increase to 180 beats/min during crying and decrease to 80–100 beats/min during deep sleep.	**Bradycardia** (persistent resting rate <100 beats/min, unless term in deep sleep without distress) **Tachycardia** (resting rate 180–200 beats/min) Persistent irregular rhythm

(table continues on page 800)

● TABLE 20.1   **Physical Examination of the Newborn** (continued)

Assessment Areas and Techniques	Normal Findings	Normal Variations	Significant Deviations[a]
Respiratory rate	Shallow, irregular 40–60 breaths/min; may decrease when in deep sleep and increase after crying **Periodic breathing** (a series of respirations followed by a pause of up to 20 seconds)	Transient **tachypnea** (fast rate) after stress or crying Rate may slow when sleeping	**Tachypnea** (resting respiratory rate >60 breaths/min) **Bradypnea** (respiratory rate <25–30 breaths/min) **Apnea** (cessation of breathing >20 seconds without respiratory effort or shorter duration accompanied by decreased heart rate and colour change to pale or dusky) **Gasping** (intermittent rapid inhalation)
Blood pressure not routinely required; oscillometric measurement preferred	Varies with weight, gestational age, and infant state; approximately 78/42 mm Hg		**Capillary refill time** >3 seconds: press on skin of trunk until it blanches and count seconds until colour returns Weak pulses Pallor, grey colour Mottling Cool skin
Measurements: **Weight**	Varies with genetic composition 2,500–3,800 g	Weight, length, and OFC must be assessed with gestational age to determine whether the newborn is SGA, AGA, or LGA. An infant is classified as SGA, AGA, or LGA *and* preterm, term, or postterm.	
Length	45–52 cm		
OFC (occipital-frontal circumference)	32–37 cm		
Chest circumference (not routinely required)	30–35 cm	Usually 2 cm smaller than the OFC; however, cranial moulding can influence OFC and chest measurements.	
Skin	Soft, smooth, elastic Hydrated skin springs back into shape if pinched Initially edematous Flaky and dry by day 2–3 **Vernix caseosa** (greasy yellow-white substance) **Lanugo** (fine hair on cheeks, shoulders, forehead, pinna of ears) **Milia** (tiny white papules on brow, cheeks, nose) **Erythema toxicum** or "newborn rash" (small white or yellow papules on a red base; lasts several hours to several days) **Sucking blisters** (vesicles on lips, hands from in utero or postnatal sucking) **Stork bite or nevus simplex** (pink macule on nape of neck, upper eyelids, bridge of nose or upper lip that usually fades)	**Meconium staining** (cord, nails, skin may be stained greenish-brown from meconium in the amniotic fluid) **Forceps marks** on cheek(s) Petechiae over presenting part **Port wine nevus** (flat pink or purple lesion on white skin and solid black on black skin, usually on face; does not blanch, grow, or fade) **Mongolian spots or hyperpigmented macule** (bluish or grey-blue areas of pigmentation on dorsum and buttocks) commonly found on non-Caucasian babies **Café-au-lait patches** (less than six) Pigmented nevus (dark brown or black macule) **Strawberry hemangioma** (bright red, raised, soft, grows then regresses over years; most appear by 6 months of age)	Loose, wrinkled skin may indicate growth aberration or dehydration. Widespread **petechiae** not associated with presenting part Rash, especially if vesicular **Skin tags** (depending on positioning and associated physical findings) **Webbing** of hands, feet **Laceration** infrequently occurs during cesarean birth. More than 6 **café-au-lait** patches may indicate **neurofibromatosis**.

(continued)

● TABLE 20.1   **Physical Examination of the Newborn** (continued)

Assessment Areas and Techniques	Normal Findings	Normal Variations	Significant Deviations[a]
Head	Fontanels: Anterior palpated as 5-cm diamond Posterior palpated as smaller triangle Palpate sutures; should be unjoined Generally symmetric shape Full range of motion	Cranial **moulding and asymmetry,** difficulty palpating fontanels and suture lines because of moulding **Scalp lesion or abrasion** (from scalp electrode, vacuum extractor) **Cephalhematoma** (hematoma between periosteum and skull bone; raised lump does not cross suture lines and resolves in months) **Caput succedaneum** (tissue swelling may cross suture lines and resolves quickly) **Petechiae** (if breech birth or cord around neck) **Torticollis** (head held immobile at angle)	Severe moulding, especially if accompanied by abnormal transition Indentation on cranium (fracture) Full, bulging fontanels Remarkable pulsation of fontanels Unusually large or small head in relation to body size Unusual hair pattern or texture Fused suture lines Significantly smaller or missing fontanelles
Eyes	Eyes placed at same level Eyelids above pupils but within iris Edema in first days of life Lashes and eyebrows present Eyes open and eyeballs present Eyes move freely, fix, and follow Eyes close in response to bright light Blinking present Occasional **strabismus** (crossed eyes) Slight **nystagmus** (involuntary eye movements) Blue colour in light-skinned baby and brown colour in dark-skinned baby (eye colour established at approximately 3 mo)	**Subconjunctival hemorrhage** (red spot on sclera; resolves) Slightly blue sclera No tears when crying	Unusually wide set eyes Eyes never seen open, even in dim light Constant strabismus, nystagmus, or both Purulent drainage Ulceration Unusual lashes (absent, bushy, unusually long) Upward slant in non-Asian (may indicate Down syndrome) Jaundiced sclera (hyperbilirubinemia)
Ears	Well-formed cartilage Visibly open auditory canal Placement: line drawn through inner and outer canthi of eye lines up with top notch of ear Responds to voices, loud noises when awake	**Darwinian tubercle** (nodule on posterior helix)	**Preauricular skin tag,** especially if accompanied by other variances **Sinus tract** near ear Low-set ears (may require assessment after cranial moulding has resolved) Abnormal ear attachment to head
Nose	Midline placement Normal breathing when mouth is closed Frequent sneezing	Asymmetric appearance because of birth trauma	Cyanosis or respiratory distress when mouth is closed (**choanal atresia**) **Nasal flaring** (respiratory distress) Persistent or marked nasal drainage Unusual nose, such as pointed or upturned

(table continues on page 802)

● TABLE 20.1   **Physical Examination of the Newborn** (continued)

Assessment Areas and Techniques	Normal Findings	Normal Variations	Significant Deviations[a]
Mouth and Throat	Symmetric movement of mouth Coordinated breathing, sucking, and swallowing during feeding Pink gums Free-moving tongue Sucking pads inside cheeks Dome-shaped hard palate Midline, single uvula Lusty cry of moderate pitch and tone	Sucking blisters on lips **Epstein's pearls** (small white epithelial cysts) on hard palate	Mouth pulls to one side (asymmetric strength or movement) **Cleft palate** (hard or soft palate) Large and/or deeply ridged tongue Excessive drooling; frequent choking (evaluate for esophageal atresia or tracheoesophageal fistula) Shrill, weak, or absent cry Cheesy coating on tongue that does not wipe off or bleeds when wiped (indicative of oral thrush—*Candida albicans*) Teeth (may be predeciduous or deciduous): aspiration risk if loose Small jaw and recessive chin, especially if accompanied by respiratory distress (Robin syndrome)
Neck	Short, straight Creased anterior Clavicles intact Head held in midline with free range of motion	Fractured clavicle(s) from difficult birth: popping or crackling felt or heard when palpated	Abnormally short neck Hyperextended or arched neck Webbing (Turner syndrome) Excessive skin folds Hypotonia (no head control)
Chest	Circular, barrel shape Symmetric respiratory movement Well-formed, symmetric nipples Clear, bilateral breath sounds	Xiphoid cartilage (lower end of sternum) may protrude Supernumerary (extra) nipples Breast enlargement (from maternal hormones) **"Witch's milk"** (milky substance from breast) Rales normal during first few hours of life	**Intercostal and/or sternal retractions** (ribs and/or sternum suck inward with inhalation due to use of accessory muscles during respiratory distress) Decreased or asymmetric breath sounds, especially with respiratory distress
Heart **(see also Vital Signs section)**	**PMI** (point of maximal impulse) heard lateral to midclavicular line at third or fourth intercostal space **Regular rate and rhythm**	Heart murmur without accompanying symptoms	PMI shifted to right or left, especially if accompanied by respiratory distress (**pneumothorax**) Distant heart sounds Extra heart sound(s) PMI on right side of chest (**pneumothorax** or **dextrocardia**) Dysrhythmia (irregular rate), tachycardia, bradycardia Heart murmur with accompanying symptoms such as edema, irregular rate/rhythm, pallor or duskiness, respiratory distress, other anomalies **Audible bowel sounds in chest, especially if accompanied by respiratory distress** (diaphragmatic hernia)

(continued)

● TABLE 20.1   **Physical Examination of the Newborn** (continued)

Assessment Areas and Techniques	Normal Findings	Normal Variations	Significant Deviations[a]
Abdomen	Cylindrical and protruding Abdominal skin colour congruent with genetic background Soft bowel sounds present 1 to 2 hours after birth No protrusion of umbilicus (*Note: palpation of liver and kidneys is not considered a nursing assessment activity in some settings.*) Liver palpable 1–2 cm below right costal margin at midclavicular line (use caution) A healthy spleen is not normally palpable. Kidneys are difficult to palpate; left more evident than right. Femoral pulses palpable, equal, bilateral Two arteries and one vein visible in umbilical cord at birth		**Scaphoid** (sunken) abdomen (diaphragmatic hernia) Bowel sounds in chest (diaphragmatic hernia) Palpable masses or bulges front or back Marked distention, shiny appearance, or visible bowel loops Inaudible bowel sounds Projectile vomiting Bilious (greenish) vomit Failure to pass meconium in 48 hours Hyperperistalsis or visible peristalsis (bowel obstruction) Absent or diminished femoral pulses (coarctation of aorta). Suspect coarctation if four-limb blood pressure demonstrates upper extremities systolic pressure is >20 points higher than systolic of lower extremities
Umbilicus	No intestinal structures visible inside cord Drying without bleeding, odour	Yellow-green staining of cord (from meconium in the amniotic fluid)	Two-vessel umbilical cord (single artery) Bleeding around cord Red or swollen umbilical area Purulent drainage from umbilical area **Omphalocele** (abdominal contents herniated into area of cord) **Gastroschisis** (abdominal contents herniated through abdominal wall)
Extremities	Term baby assumes in utero flexed positioning Symmetric full range of motion Extension limited Muscle tone congruent with gestational age Ten fingers, ten toes appropriately spaced Dry flaky hands and feet Flat sole of foot Fingernails and toenails present Fists clenched	Positional deformities (usually resolve) Polydactyly (extra digits) may be familial. **Simian crease** (single horizontal crease across palm) sometimes found in normal infants; also related to Down syndrome	Absent movement Asymmetric movement, strength, or range of motion Hypotonia Hyperflexion Limited range of motion Hypermobility of joints Polydactyly (extra digits) or syndactyly (webbed digits), especially if accompanied by additional anomalies Short fingers, incurved little finger, low-set thumb, and a simian crease (suggests Down syndrome) Persistent cyanotic nail beds Suspect dislocated or **subluxated hip:** Limited hip abduction, Unequal gluteal or leg folds, Unequal knee height, Positive Ortolani and/or Barlow sign (audible clunk on hip abduction)

(table continues on page 804)

● TABLE 20.1 Physical Examination of the Newborn (continued)

Assessment Areas and Techniques	Normal Findings	Normal Variations	Significant Deviations[a]
Genitalia	First void within 24 hours (most babies) to 48 hours (all babies) of birth Urine has mild odour	Rust-stained urine (uric acid crystals)	**Ambiguous genitalia** (sex not clearly discernible from visible anatomy) Failure to void within 48 hours of birth Foul-smelling or bloody urine
MALE	Slender penis, 2.5 cm long Urethral meatus at tip of penis Voids within 24 hours with adequate stream and volume Foreskin adheres to glans and tight 2–3 months Erection possible because of erectile tissue Scrotal skin can be loose or tight Rugae consistent with gestation Two palpable testes Testes descended but not consistently in scrotum Smegma	Scrotal bruising and edema if breech birth **Epithelial pearls** (small, firm, white lesion at tip of penis)	Undescended testes (may be in inguinal, femoral, perineal, or abdominal areas) **Hydrocele** (enlarged scrotum due to fluid) Discoloured testes **Hypospadias** (urinary meatus on ventral surface of penis) **Epispadias** (urinary meatus on dorsal surface of penis) Fecal discharge from penis
FEMALE	Edema common Development of labia consistent with gestational age Clitoris usually large Area pigment consistent with genetic background Smegma, vernix present Open vaginal orifice Urinary meatus difficult to see Mucoid discharge Bloody discharge (**pseudomenses** from maternal hormones)	Area bruised if breech birth Vaginal tag (usually disappears in first month of life)	Absent vaginal orifice Fecal discharge from vagina
Back	Spine straight, no openings, masses Term infant can raise and support head for a moment when prone Symmetric buttocks Patent single anus Meconium stool followed by transitional, then soft, yellow stool		Limited movement or flexion Nevus with tuft of hair along spine (associated with **spina bifida**) Sinus anywhere along spine **Meningocele** (lesion associated with spina bifida where meninges protrude through vertebral defect, covered by thin atrophic skin) **Myelomeningocele** (lesion associated with spina bifida, most often in the lumbar spine, characterized by protrusion of meninges, spinal roots, and nerves, remnants of spinal cord fusion and exposed neural tube) No meconium passage in first 48 hours No anus **Imperforate** anus Anal fissures or fistulas

[a]Conditions noted in this column require further assessment and evaluation. Some conditions, such as central cyanosis or gastroschisis, require immediate life-saving interventions, including support of ventilation and oxygenation, thermoregulation, perfusion, and metabolic needs. Other conditions listed in this column are less urgent, but still require evaluation and special care. See Chapter 22 for a more complete discussion of selected high-risk neonatal topics.

● TABLE 20.2   **Developmental Reflexes in the Newborn**

Name of Reflex	Figure	To Elicit Reflex	Expected Neonatal Response	Disappearance (months)
Moro		Hold the infant supine with the head a few inches above the mattress. Remove the hand supporting the infant's head and allow the head to fall back onto mattress.	Infant first extends and abducts the arms and opens the hands. Then the arms adduct with some flexion and closing of the fists. The infant may cry.	12
Palmar grasp		Press the palmar surface of the infant's hand with a finger.	Infant grasps the finger and holds tighter with attempts to withdraw. Full-term neonate can support full body weight if lifted slightly.	2
Rooting		Stroke the infant's cheek and corner of the mouth.	The infant's head turns toward the stimulus and the mouth opens.	3–4
Stepping (dance)		Hold the infant upright and touch the soles of the feet to a flat surface.	Infant makes alternating stepping movements.	3–4
Sucking		Touch or stroke the baby's lips.	Mouth opens and sucking movements begin.	12
Tonic neck		Place infant supine and turn his or her head to one side.	Infant extends the arm on the side in which the head is turned and flexes the upper extremity on the opposite side (fencing position).	7
Truncal incurvation (Galant)		Hold infant prone, in suspended position, with palm of hand against infant's chest. Apply firm pressure with the thumb or cotton swab parallel to the spine in the thoracic region.	The infant flexes the pelvis toward the side of the stimulus.	3–4

This box describes one method of organizing the newborn physical examination reviewed in Table 20.1 as a guide for inexperienced examiners. With practice, each examiner develops a personal style. It is assumed that the infant is unclothed and supine under a radiant warmer.

Observation

It can be very difficult for a practitioner to just stand at the crib and observe an infant. The immediate inclination is to touch and talk to the infant. The practitioner must delay this natural response until later in the examination, however, because observation alone produces important information about every organ system. These initial observations allow the practitioner to develop a visual differential diagnosis before employing other assessment techniques.

If these multiple observations prove normal, the examiner is less likely to find a significant abnormality upon auscultation and palpation. Each observation of normality serves to reassure the examiner—just as an observation of abnormality should heighten the examiner's suspicion that further inspection is necessary.

Observation is not an isolated technique for use only at the outset of the examination. Although spending a moment or two observing the infant at the bedside before touching him or her is important, observation of the infant's responses takes place throughout the assessment. The examiner must learn to take advantage of every opportunity the infant's behaviour offers for observation. If, for example, the infant awakens spontaneously during the examination, the practitioner should use that opportunity to examine the baby's eyes.

Hands-on inspection includes measurements and tactile inspection of the skin. It also includes manoeuvres to assess symmetry and reflexes.

Auscultation

After observing the infant closely, many examiners next auscultate the chest, heart, and abdomen. To separate the sounds of the heart from those of the lungs, concentration is important. Listen first to one type of sound, then to the other. For example, listen first to the heart—its rate, rhythm, regularity, and any added sounds. Then listen to breath sounds, ignoring the cardiac sounds.

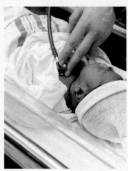

Auscultating the newborn's lungs.

Palpation

Continue with palpation. Palpating certain parts of the body disturbs the infant more than others. An ordered approach keeps the infant calm through much of the process.

Because femoral pulses are difficult to assess in a crying infant, palpate them first. Then palpate the brachial pulses. Next palpate the abdomen, beginning with the more superficial liver and spleen. (Learning to palpate the liver and spleen with the tips of the fingers as well as the lateral edges of the index fingers facilitates examination from either side of the bassinette.) Palpate for abdominal masses; then use deeper palpation for the kidneys. At this point, the infant may be disturbed and crying, but this will not impede the remainder of the examination.

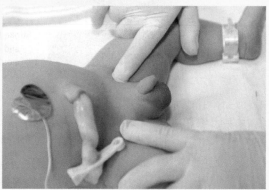

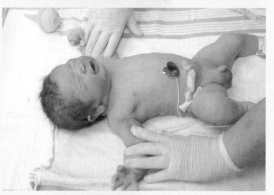

Top: Palpating the femoral pulse. **Bottom:** Palpating the brachial pulse.

The Integrated Examination

The skilled examiner integrates examination tasks. For example, after palpating the head, neck, clavicles, arms, and hands, he or she can perform the pull-to-sit manoeuvre to assess palmar grasp, arm strength, and tone. At that point, the clinician is holding the infant in an appropriate position to elicit the Moro reflex. The practitioner can examine the genitalia next, before progressing to the lower extremities. While positioning the infant prone on the practitioner's hand to assess truncal tone and the truncal incurvation reflex, the examiner also can check the baby's back. These shortcuts facilitate multiple inspections and save time.

(continues)

● **BOX 20.1 A Sample Approach to Newborn Physical Examination** (continued)

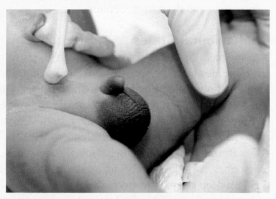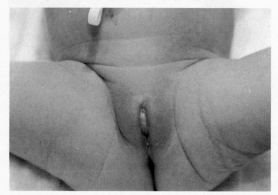

Left: Male newborn genitalia. **Right:** Female newborn genitalia.

Examination of the hips should be last because this procedure causes the most stress to the infant.

It is usually not necessary to assess reflexes separately. The examiner will most likely have observed root and suck by this point. He or she can incorporate Moro and palmar grasp into the upper extremity examination, as just explained.

Although an extremely cooperative infant may sleep through the entire process, the assessment is not complete until the infant has been observed through the various behavioural states. Facial asymmetry, for example, cannot be seen until the infant cries.

Ideally, the parents should observe the first complete examination. They appreciate demonstration of their infant's normality and uniqueness as well as early identification of unusual or abnormal findings.

Adapted from Tappero, E. P., & Honeyfield, M. E. (2009). *Physical assessment of the newborn: A comprehensive approach to the art of physical examination* (4th ed.). Santa Rosa, CA: NICU INK Book Publishers.

reviews newborn reflexes, and Box 20.1 summarizes an approach to newborn assessment. The astute nurse quickly recognizes signs of abnormalities and intervenes before further compromise develops.

When preparing to participate in the physical examination, the nurse proceeds as follows (Honeyfield, 2009):

- Wash hands before beginning. If parents are present, teach the importance of proper hand washing. If the examination takes place before the initial bath, standard precautions mandate that the nurse wear gloves (AWHONN, 2013).
- Gather necessary equipment before beginning.
- Keep the newborn warm. A radiant warmer provides a thermally safe environment and easy access to the exposed newborn. Warm hands and a warm stethoscope help decrease newborn stress.
- Look and listen before touching or handling the infant. Observe posture, muscle tone, colour, respiratory efforts, and behavioural state. Listen for expiratory **grunting,** stridor, or other audible signs of respiratory distress before disturbing the infant.
- Keep the newborn as calm as possible. Start with the least invasive and intrusive manoeuvres (observation, auscultation); finish with those assessments that may be more upsetting (assessment of Moro reflex).

Handle the newborn gently. If parents are present, use teachable moments to point out newborn developmental capabilities.
- Choose a quiet environment for auscultation.
- Establish a routine. Performing the physical assessment approximately the same way each time decreases the risk for forgetting any aspect of the examination.

THE NEWBORN TRANSITIONAL PERIOD

Full-term healthy newborns demonstrate a predictable pattern of behavioural changes, behavioural states and cues, sensory abilities, and physiologic adaptations during the first 6 to 8 hours of life. This time frame is referred to as the *transitional period* (Blackburn, 2013).

Behavioural Changes

The transitional period is divided into an initial period of reactivity and inactivity and a second period of reactivity.

Initial Period of Reactivity

The initial period of reactivity occurs in the first 30 to 60 minutes of life and is characterized by an alert, intensely exploratory newborn. At this time, the healthy,

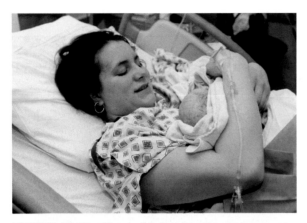

FIGURE 20.11 Maternal–infant bonding during a period of reactivity.

term newborn is fully alert and active and has a strong desire to suck. This is the optimal time for the first breastfeeding. It also is good for interaction (Fig. 20.11). The nurse can facilitate parent–child eye contact by minimizing unnecessary bright lights and delaying instillation of prophylactic eye medication. Skin to skin contact may facilitate bonding and breastfeeding.

Adaptation to extrauterine life allows for wide swings in normal parameters. The newborn may be tachypneic (up to 80 breaths/min) and tachycardic (up to 180 beats/min). The nurse may observe mild-to-moderate chest wall retractions, nasal flaring, and expiratory grunting and may hear crackles. The nurse may note **periodic breathing** (pauses in breathing of less than 15 seconds). **Acrocyanosis** (bluish hands and feet) is also normal (see Table 20.4). Bowel sounds are active.

Abnormal transition may be manifested by any signs of increasing distress instead of steady resolution. Signs that require immediate intervention include central cyanosis; apnea greater than 15 seconds, especially if accompanied by pallor, cyanosis, or bradycardia; asymmetric chest wall movement; unequal breath sounds; excessive salivation or mucus; and hypotonia or lethargy.

Period of Relative Inactivity

This period occurs 2 to 3 hours after birth. The newborn becomes less interested in external stimuli and falls asleep for a few minutes to several hours. The baby becomes less responsive. During deep sleep, the baby is difficult to arouse. Feeding is difficult, if not impossible. Heart rate stabilizes at 110 to 160 beats/min; respiratory rate decreases to 40 to 60 breaths/min. The newborn should be centrally pink with clear breath sounds and show no signs of respiratory distress. The temperature may fall.

Second Period of Reactivity

The second period of reactivity lasts approximately 4 to 6 hours and begins when the newborn fully awakens from the first sleep and is alert and responsive once again. Heart and respiratory rates may increase, but should remain within normal limits. The newborn may pass urine and the first meconium.

Behavioural States

Assessment of infant state enables caregivers to measure the newborn's response to external stimuli and to interpret physiologic and behavioural changes. The caregiver assesses infant state to evaluate the newborn's ability to control it, move smoothly from one state to another and maintain alertness (Heaberlin, 2009).

Brazelton's Neonatal Behavioural Assessment Scale describes two sleep and four awake states (Brazelton, 1978): deep sleep, light sleep, drowsy, quiet alert, active alert, and crying. Table 20.3 describes characteristics of each state and the implications for caregiving and interaction. Full-term, healthy newborns should move easily from one state to another and eventually demonstrate a unique and organized pattern of control. The nurse assesses the state as an indicator of overall well-being and central nervous system integrity (Heaberlin, 2009).

The nurse teaches parents these infant states to help them identify their newborn's unique characteristics and to facilitate optimal interactions. For example, the parent should be able to recognize the light sleep state as one in which the newborn is asleep, but may make brief fussy sounds. The parent who recognizes this state knows to wait until the infant is more fully awake before interpreting these sounds as meaning that the baby is ready to interact or feed. The parent who does not recognize light sleep may awaken the newborn prematurely and try to feed the child when he or she is not ready.

Behavioural Cues

Full-term newborns respond physiologically and emotionally to environmental stimuli. In this way, they learn to control the effects of their surroundings. They begin to display various cues to meet their needs. Caregivers who respond appropriately reinforce behavioural organization (McGrath, 2009).

Behavioural cues consist of approach and avoidance cues. **Approach cues** such as hand to mouth movements, reaching or grasping, and rhythmic sucking indicate a readiness to interact with the environment (Tappero & Honeyfield, 2009). **Avoidance cues** (time-out signals) such as frowning, fussing, stiffening, and gaze aversion indicate that the newborn is tired or overstimulated and needs a break from interaction (Tappero & Honeyfield, 2009). The caregiver who proceeds with interaction may exceed the infant's sensory threshold, meaning that the infant cannot respond appropriately and displays signs of stress and fatigue (McGrath, 2009).

Parents who learn how to interpret their infant's behaviour have stronger parent–infant interaction during the first year of life. The newborn whose parents respond

● TABLE 20.3   Infant States and Implications for Caregiving

State	Body Activity	Eye Movements	Facial Movements	Breathing Pattern	Level of Response	Implications for Caregiving
Sleep States						
Quiet (deep) sleep	Nearly still, except for occasional startle or twitch	None	Without facial movements, except for occasional sucking movement at regular intervals	Smooth and regular	Threshold to stimuli very high so that only very intense and disturbing stimuli will arouse	Caregivers trying to feed infants in quiet sleep will probably find the experience frustrating. Infants will be unresponsive, even if caregivers use disturbing stimuli to arouse infants. Infants may arouse only briefly and then become unresponsive as they return to quiet sleep. If caregivers wait until infants move to a higher, more responsive state, feeding or caregiving will be much more pleasant.
Active (light) sleep	Some body movements	Rapid eye movement (REM); fluttering of eyes beneath closed eyelids	May smile and make brief fussy or crying sounds	Irregular	More responsive to internal and external stimuli; when these stimuli occur, infants may remain in active sleep, return to quiet sleep, or arouse to drowsy	Active sleep makes up the highest proportion of newborn sleep and usually precedes awakening. Because of brief fussy or crying sounds made during this state, caregivers who are not aware that these sounds occur normally may think it is time for feeding and may try to feed infants before they are ready to eat.
Awake States						
Drowsy	Activity level variable, with mild startles interspersed from time to time; movements usually smooth	Eyes open and close occasionally; are heavy lidded with dull, glazed appearance	May have some facial movements but often there are none and the face appears still	Irregular	Infants react to sensory stimuli, although responses are delayed; state change after stimulation frequently noted	From the drowsy state, infants may return to sleep or awaken further. To awaken, caregivers can provide something for infants to see, hear, or suck, as this may arouse them to a quiet alert state, a more responsive state. Infants who are left alone without stimuli may return to a sleep state.
Quiet alert	Minimal	Brightening and widening of eyes	Faces have bright, shining, sparkling looks	Regular	Infants attend most to the environment, focusing attention on any stimuli that are present	Infants in this state provide much pleasure and positive feedback for caregivers. Providing something for infants to see, hear, or suck will often maintain a quiet alert state. In the first few hours after birth, most newborns commonly experience a period of intense alertness before going into a long sleep period.
Active alert	Much body activity; may have periods of fussiness	Eyes open with less brightening	Much facial movement; faces not as bright as in quiet alert state.	Irregular	Increasingly sensitive to disturbing stimuli (hunger, fatigue, noise, excessive handling)	Crying is the infant's communication signal. It is a response to unpleasant stimuli from the environment or within infants (eg, fatigue, hunger, discomfort). Crying says that infants' limits have been reached. Sometimes infants can console themselves and return to lower states. At other times, they need help from caregivers.
Crying	Increased motor activity with colour changes	Eyes may be tightly closed or open	Grimaces	Irregular	Extremely responsive to unpleasant external or internal stimuli	Caregivers may need to intervene at this state to console and bring the infant to a lower state.

From Blackburn, S. T. (2013). *Maternal, fetal, & neonatal physiology: A clinical perspective* (4th ed.). St. Louis, MO: Saunders Elsevier.

● TABLE 20.4   **Common Skin Manifestations of the Normal Newborn**

Skin Manifestation	Family Teaching Tips
Acrocyanosis	A bluish colour to the hands and feet of the newborn is normal in the first 6 to 12 hours after birth. Acrocyanosis results from slow circulation in the extremities.
Milia 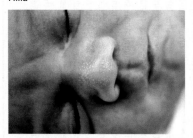	Small white spots on the newborn's face, nose, and chin that resemble pimples are an expected observation. Do not attempt to pick or squeeze them. They will subside spontaneously in a few days.
Erythema toxicum 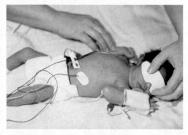	The so-called newborn rash commonly appears on the chest, abdomen, back, and buttocks of the newborn. It is harmless and will disappear.
Mongolian spot 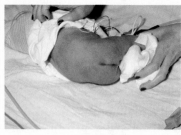	These bluish black areas of discolouration are commonly seen on the back, buttocks, or extremities of non-Caucasian newborns. These spots should not be mistaken for bruises or mistreatment; they gradually fade during the first or second year of life. Parents may require teaching about the significance of Mongolian spots because they may not be aware of this common alteration.
Telangiectatic nevi 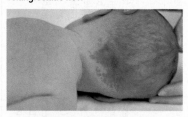	These pale pink or red marks ("stork bites") are sometimes found on the nape of the neck, eyelids, or nose of fair-skinned newborns. Stork bites blanch when pressed and generally fade as the child grows.
Nevus flammeus or port-wine stain 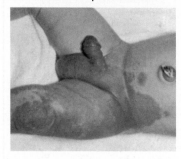	A port-wine stain is a dark reddish purple birthmark that most commonly appears on the face. It is caused by a group of dilated blood vessels. It does not blanch with pressure or fade with time. There are cosmetics available that help cover the stain if it is disfiguring. Laser therapy has been successfully used to fade port-wine stains.

to behavioural cues can better control and respond to the environment (McGrath, 2009).

Neonatal Sensory Abilities

Vision

Healthy term newborns have adequate visual abilities at birth, but eye structures continue to mature over the first 6 months. At birth, newborns can fix on an object and track its movement. They can see objects up to 5 cm away but prefer high-contrast or highly contoured objects 20 to 30 cm away (Blackburn, 2013). It is interesting to note that the traditional cradle hold positions a newborn perfectly for focusing on the adult's face.

Hearing

Healthy term newborns hear best in the low- and mid-range frequencies, but prefer high intonation and rhythmic vocalizations. They can recognize and will turn the head in response to the mother's voice. They react negatively to loud or offensive noises (Blackburn, 2013).

Newborn hearing loss is one of the most common diagnosable defects at birth (Johnson, 2009). Auditory screening before hospital discharge is discussed later.

Smell

Sense of smell is fairly well developed in healthy term newborns, enabling them to detect and identify various odours. Breastfed newborns can differentiate the odour of their mother's breast pad from pads soaked in water or other substances (Blackburn, 2013; Heaberlin, 2009). Newborns grimace, sniff, or startle in response to strong odours (eg, anise, mint) (Heaberlin, 2009).

Touch

The fetus responds to touch as early as 2 months' gestational age; by birth, the sense of touch is well developed (Kadic & Predojevic, 2012). Tactile stimulation, such as rubbing the baby's back, trunk, or extremities with a towel or flicking the soles of the feet, helps initiate respirations at birth (Kattwinkel, 2011).

Physiologic Adaptations

During the transition period, the newborn makes dramatic adaptations to extrauterine life. Thorough assessment is required to monitor progress and identify abnormalities. In this section, we present the adaptations made in several body systems and an explanation of collaborative care.

Thermoregulation

The uterine environment maintains fetal body temperature approximately 0.5°C higher than maternal body temperature. At birth, the newborn may lose heat through evaporation at a rate of 0.2° to 1°C per minute (skin temperature) (Blackburn, 2013). Maintenance of normal body temperature is critical to survival. A large ratio of surface area to body mass and decreased insulating subcutaneous fat make newborns more vulnerable to temperature variations than adults. This vulnerability is increased with decreasing gestational age (Blackburn, 2013).

The nurse strives to maintain a **neutral thermal environment** for every newborn, that is, the ambient temperature at which oxygen consumption and energy expenditure are at the minimum to sustain vital activities (Blackburn, 2013).

Range of Normal Temperature. Neonatal body temperature has a fairly broad range of normal (Sinha et al., 2012):

- Axillary: 36.7° to 37.3°C
- Skin:
    Full-term infant: 35.5° to 36.5°C
    Preterm infant: 36.2° to 37.2°C

Methods of Taking Newborn Temperatures. The nurse can assess newborn temperature as follows (Blackburn, 2013; Smith et al., 2013):

- **Axillary:** This method is safe and approximates core temperature.
- **Skin:** This method may be used for continuous assessment of the skin temperature of preterm infants or those at risk for temperature instability. Healthy newborn skin temperature is displayed when the radiant warmer is used anytime the infant must be unclothed and exposed for more than a short period. A thermistor probe is placed on the surface of the skin and displays temperature electronically. The optimal location for the thermistor probe is not known (Brown & Landers, 2011). It is usually recommended to place the probe over the liver or abdomen, or on the back of a prone infant. The nurse should make sure that the probe is in full contact with the skin and covered with a foil reflector to avoid radiant or convective cooling of the thermistor probe (see Chapter 22).
- **Tympanic:** Infrared tympanic thermometry is safe and non-invasive. However, because of unproven accuracy in newborns, it is not yet recommended for use (Duru et al., 2012).
- **Rectal:** This method is no longer recommended because of the risk of trauma, perforation, and cross-contamination (Brown & Landers, 2011).

How Newborns Lose and Gain Heat. Newborns transfer heat to and from the body surface in four ways (Blackburn, 2013; Brown & Landers, 2011) (Fig. 20.12).

- **Evaporation**
    Heat is lost when moisture from the skin and respiratory tract converts to vapor. *Example: A warm, wet newborn is exposed to cool air in the delivery room.*

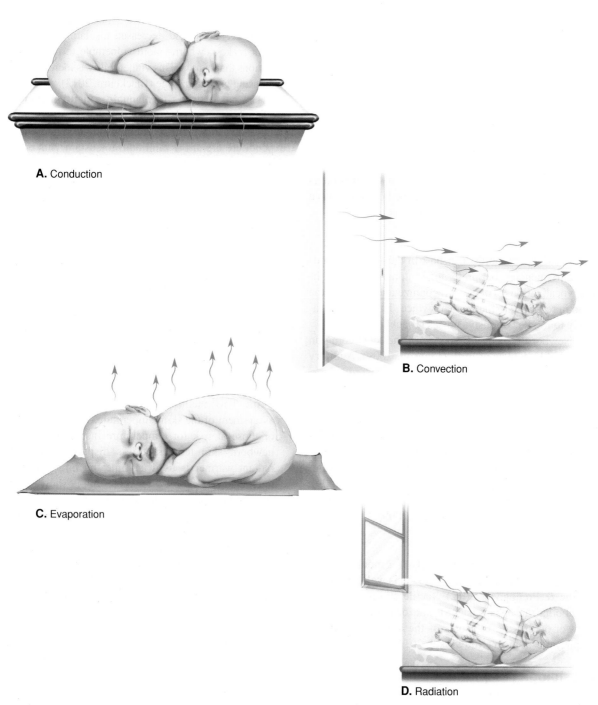

A. Conduction

B. Convection

C. Evaporation

D. Radiation

FIGURE 20.12 Heat loss in newborns occurs in four ways: (**A**) conduction, (**B**) convection, (**C**) evaporation, (**D**) radiation.

- **Conduction**

   Heat is lost from the body surface to a cooler solid surface touching the newborn. *Example: Newborn is placed on the surface of a cold scale for weighing.*

   Heat is gained from a surface warmer than the infant. *Example: Newborn is placed on a warm blanket or chemical thermal mattress.*

- **Convection**

   Heat is lost from the body surface to the surrounding air. *Example: An exposed newborn is placed in a bassinette near a door that is opened and closed frequently.*

   Heat is gained if the surrounding air temperature is higher than the infant's skin temperature.

Example: An infant is placed in an incubator with circulating air at a temperature higher than the temperature of the infant's skin.

- **Radiation**

  Heat is lost from the body surface to a cooler solid surface not touching the newborn. *Example: A newborn is placed near a cold window on an exterior wall.*

  Heat is gained when the solid surface is warmer than the infant's skin temperature. *Example: A cool infant is placed under an infant warmer (radiant heat source).*

Thomas is lying on the mother's bed, clothed in a shirt and diaper. How might he be losing heat?

Newborns produce heat in four ways (Blackburn, 2013):

- *Metabolic processes:* The amount of heat produced through this method varies with activity, state, health status, and environmental temperature. The brain, heart, and liver produce the most metabolic energy by oxidative metabolism of glucose, fat, and protein (Blackburn, 2013).
- *Voluntary muscle activity:* Increased muscle activity during restlessness and crying generates some heat. In addition, the newborn may attempt to conserve heat by assuming a flexed position to decrease surface area. Shivering, the most important method to generate heat in adults, is less important in newborns. Most likely, this is because the shivering threshold is lower in newborns than in adults and occurs as a very late response associated with decreased spinal cord temperature after prolonged exposure (Blackburn, 2013).
- *Peripheral vasoconstriction:* In response to cooling, peripheral vasoconstriction reduces blood flow to the skin and therefore decreases loss of heat from the skin's surface (Blackburn, 2013).
- ***Nonshivering thermogenesis:*** This mechanism is the main source of heat production in the newborn triggered at a mean skin temperature of 35° to 36°C (Blackburn, 2013). Thermal receptors transmit impulses to the hypothalamus, which stimulates the sympathetic nervous system and causes norepinephrine release in **brown adipose tissue**, or brown fat. Found around the scapulae, kidneys, adrenal glands, head, neck, heart, great vessels, and axillary regions, brown fat is highly vascular and accounts for 2% to 7% of the newborn's weight. It generates more energy than any other body tissue (Blackburn, 2013). Norepinephrine in brown fat activates lipase, which results in lipolysis and fatty acid oxidation. This chemical process generates heat, which is transferred to the perfusing blood and tissues near the brown fat. This increases local temperature and eventually results in increased axillary temperature.

Cold Stress. When heat loss overwhelms the newborn's ability to compensate, cold stress occurs (Fig. 20.13). Clinical signs include peripheral vasoconstriction, resulting in acrocyanosis and cool, mottled, or pale skin. The term newborn may become restless, agitated, or hypoglycemic. Signs of increased oxygen consumption include clinical signs of respiratory distress such as **tachypnea**, grunting, or lethargy (Brown & Landers, 2011). The compensatory mechanisms of the newborn with cold stress initiate a chain of metabolic events that can result in **hypoxemia**, metabolic acidosis, glycogen depletion, hypoglycemia, and altered surfactant production.

Heat Stress. The newborn is equally vulnerable to overheating. Hyperthermia (temperature above 37.5°C) can result from overheating (Blackburn, 2013). Consequences include increased heart, respiratory, and metabolic rates (increased oxygen consumption); dehydration from insensible water loss; and peripheral vasodilation that may cause hypotension (Blackburn, 2013). Clinical signs may include warm extremities, increased activity, flushing, irritability, and sweating (in term and older preterm newborns) (Blackburn, 2013).

Glucose Metabolism

Maintenance of normal blood glucose concentration can be a major problem for sick or LBW infants; however, the nurse caring for healthy, full-term newborns is aware that hypoglycemia is always possible. Because untreated hypoglycemia may result in long-term neurologic complications, immediate identification of and intervention for it are essential.

Definitions of neonatal **hypoglycemia** have been controversial over the years; no uniform standard exists. At present, a plasma glucose concentration less than 2.5 mmol/L appears to be abnormal for term and preterm infants and requires intervention (Wilson, 2011). Newborns at risk for hypoglycemia include those who are SGA, born to mothers with diabetes, premature, or stressed by sepsis, shock, hypoxia, or hypothermia (Karlsen, 2013).

At birth, the steady glucose supply from maternal circulation terminates. Plasma glucose declines to its lowest levels by 1 hour after a term, uncomplicated birth from 60% to 80% of maternal serum glucose concentration to approximately 2.5 mmol/L (Uhing & Kliegman, 2012). Liver glycogen stores, the source of the most immediately available glucose during newborn transition, are usually depleted in 3 to 12 hours. The lowest point occurs at 60 to 180 minutes of age (Uhing & Kliegman, 2012).

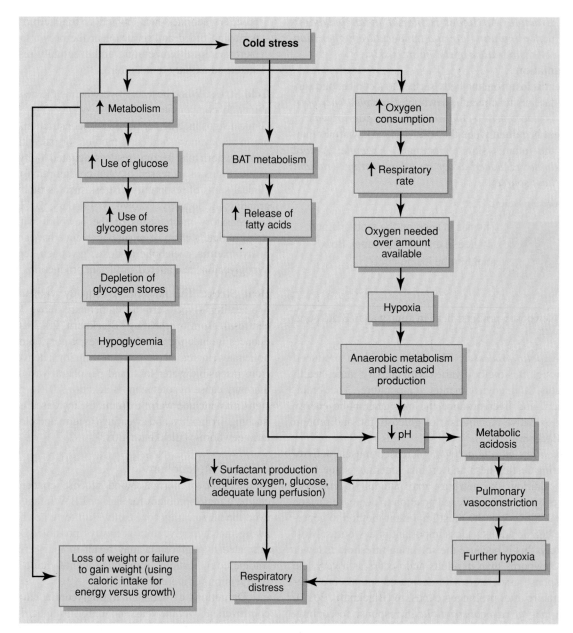

FIGURE 20.13 Physiologic consequences of cold stress. BAT, brown adipose tissue. (From Blackburn, S. T. (2013). *Maternal, fetal, & neonatal physiology: A clinical perspective* (4th ed.). St. Louis: Saunders Elsevier.)

Diminished hepatic glucose production causes most neonatal hypoglycemia. In these infants, hypoglycemia is associated with decreased availability of glycogen, lactate, glycerol, and amino acids—the substrates necessary to make glucose available to cells. In addition, the hypoglycemic newborn may have altered responses to neural or hormonal factors and immature or altered enzymatic pathways (McGowan et al., 2011).

Symptoms of hypoglycemia are not unique to that condition. For example, hypothermia, lethargy, and respiratory distress are also symptoms of neonatal sepsis. In addition, some infants with hypoglycemia are totally asymptomatic. Thus, identifying risk factors and screening those newborns most likely to develop hypoglycemia are important. Signs of hypoglycemia include jitteriness, hypothermia, lethargy, hypotonia, high-pitched or weak cry, apnea, respiratory distress, poor feeding, sweating, cyanosis, and seizures (Karlsen, 2013).

A bedside screening test (a laboratory-type test, usually involving body fluids such as blood, urine, or stool and done at the client's bedside, not sent to the laboratory) is the usual method of initial evaluation of blood glucose level. Accuracy of the initial screen depends on correct use of the evaluation method, so the nurse must be educated and proficient in the procedure. If the bedside screening reveals a low blood glucose value, the nurse usually draws a blood sample by heelstick or venipuncture for laboratory confirmation. Providers do not delay treatment of suspected hypoglycemia while waiting for test results. Interventions can include oral feeding for relatively healthy babies or intravenous (IV) therapy for more compromised or severely hypoglycemic newborns.

Prevention of hypoglycemia in term newborns is essential. Successful transition, including normal blood glucose homeostasis, is facilitated by minimizing stress, maintaining normal body temperature, and initiating feeding as soon as the newborn is stable.

Hematopoietic System

Timing of Cord Clamping. Studies in which cord clamping in full-term infants was delayed for a minimum of 2 minutes following birth demonstrated greater iron stores and a lower incidence of anemia, with the benefit extending into infancy. Although there was an increase in the need for phototherapy among infants where cord clamping was delayed, the benefits are thought to outweigh the risk of hyperbilirubinemia, providing monitoring and phototherapy is available (Garofalo & Abenhaim, 2012; McDonald et al., 2013). See Research Highlight 20.2.

Blood Components. Blood components begin to form as early as 2 to 3 weeks' gestation. By term, blood volume averages 80 to 100 mL/kg of fetal weight (Blackburn, 2013). The transition from fetal to neonatal hematologic system involves numerous changes in the structure and function of blood components, particularly those of the red blood cells (RBCs).

Red Blood Cells. Hemoglobin molecules have binding sites for oxygen molecules. When oxygen fills all the binding sites, the hemoglobin is said to be 100% saturated.

Fetal hemoglobin (HbF) differs from adult hemoglobin (HbA). HbF is saturated more readily with oxygen molecules than HbA, which is essential to fetal survival because of the low-oxygen intrauterine environment. This high affinity for oxygen molecules exists because HbF does not have binding sites for a substance called 2,3-DPG, which enables HbF to attract and hold oxygen molecules more readily than HbA. The increased affinity for oxygen molecules facilitates oxygen transfer across the placenta but reduces oxygen release to the tissues. Thus, at any given oxygen content, the oxygen saturation of the hemoglobin molecule is greater with HbF than with HbA (Blackburn, 2013).

At term, newborn cord blood contains 60% to 80% HbF and 15% to 40% HbA (Blackburn, 2013). The more preterm the newborn, the more HbF remains. This works against preterm infants, whose HbF results in a diminished ability to respond to hypoxia by releasing oxygen molecules into the tissues. The higher proportion of HbA in term newborns compared with preterm newborns makes an efficient response to oxygen needs a less significant problem. Conversion from HbF to HbA continues over the first 6 months of life, as HbA production takes over and reaches 90% (Blackburn, 2013).

Because intrauterine oxygen exchange is less efficient than extrauterine oxygen exchange through the lungs, fetuses and newborns have a higher RBC count and hemoglobin level than children and adults. Hemoglobin levels average approximately 166 to 175 g/L; the RBC count is 4.6 to 5.2 million/mm^3 (Blackburn, 2013).

● RESEARCH HIGHLIGHT 20.2   Delayed Cord Clamping

OBJECTIVE

To compare the effects of delayed versus early cord clamping on infant iron status at 4 months of age.

PARTICIPANTS AND SETTING

Four hundred full-term infants with a low-risk pregnancy were randomized to early cord clamping (<10 seconds after delivery) or delayed cord clamping (>180 seconds after delivery).

RESULTS

At 4 months of age, the infants in both groups had similar hemoglobin levels, but the infants in the delayed cord clamping group had 45% higher serum ferritin levels, a measure of iron storage. There were no differences between the groups in postnatal respiratory distress, the incidence of polycythemia, or the number of infants requiring phototherapy.

CONCLUSION

In this study, delayed cord clamping resulted in higher serum ferritin concentrations and a lower frequency of iron deficiency at 4 months of age without an increase in adverse effects.

From Andersson, O., Hellström-Westas, L., Andersson, D., & Domellöf, M. (2011) Effect of delayed versus early umbilical cord clamping on neonatal outcomes and iron status at 4 months: a randomised controlled trial. *BMJ.* 15(343), d7157.

Hemoglobin can increase up to 60 g/L in the first hours of life, resulting from the decrease in plasma volume and the net increase in RBCs. Hematocrit ranges from 0.51 to 0.56, with the aforementioned increase in the first few hours of life. Hemoglobin and hematocrit fall again to levels near the cord blood values by the end of the first week (Blackburn, 2013).

White Blood Cells. The white blood cell (WBC) count is approximately 10,000 to 26,000/mm^3 in term infants and less in preterm infants (Blackburn, 2013). It increases on the first day of life, perhaps as a result of the stress of birth, and decreases to approximately 12,000/mm^3 by 4 or 5 days in both term and preterm newborns (Blackburn, 2013). Immature forms of WBCs (eg, neutrophils, eosinophils) can be elevated in the first 3 to 4 days of life (Blackburn, 2013). Intense crying may increase the WBC count by 146% and result in a left shift in the differential (more immature cells present, which indicates mobilization of WBCs to fight infection) (Blackburn, 2013). A complete blood count (CBC) with differential is not routine for a healthy newborn, so additional diagnostic procedures, such as chest radiography, and initiation of IV therapy may occur in the same period. The infant's behavioural state just before and during a CBC with differential is helpful to note on the medical record, especially if drawing the blood was difficult, stressful, or prolonged. Personnel performing neonatal laboratory tests should be proficient and comfort newborns as much as possible during procedures by holding or swaddling them. Oral administration of 2 mL of 30% glucose to newborns 2 minutes prior to venipuncture has also been found to decrease pain (Dilen & Elseviers, 2010).

Platelets. Platelet count ranges from 150,000 to 450,000/mm^3, which is similar to that in adults. Platelet count below 150,000/mm^3 is abnormal in newborns (Blackburn, 2013). Platelet function may be hypoactive in the first few days of life, which is protective because of increased risk for thrombosis; however, this increases the risk of bleeding and bleeding disorders in preterm and compromised newborns (Blackburn, 2013). Platelet count also may be used to look for infection.

Blood Sampling. Venous sampling (blood drawn from a vein) will yield lower hemoglobin, hematocrit, and RBC values than a capillary (heelstick) sample (Blackburn, 2013). The nurse can minimize differences between capillary and venous results by prewarming the heel before drawing a capillary sample, obtaining a brisk blood flow, and discarding the first few drops of blood (Manco-Johnson et al., 2011; White, 2012). The nurse documents the site of the sample.

Hepatic System

The liver accounts for 5% of the newborn's weight (Blackburn, 2013). The maternal liver handles fetal metabolic functions, but after birth, liver function becomes essential to neonatal survival (Blackburn, 2013).

Functions of the Liver. In late gestation, the fetal liver increases glycogen storage in preparation for the newborn transition. Glycogen maintains glucose homeostasis immediately after birth. With the loss of the maternal glucose supply at birth, neonatal blood glucose level falls. The baby uses approximately 90% of liver glycogen stores in the first 24 hours as a result of rapid *glycogenolysis* (the release of glucose from glycogen). Neonatal blood glucose usually reaches its lowest level 60 to 180 minutes after birth. Steady hepatic release of glucose occurs by 3 to 4 hours of life. As glycogen levels fall, the healthy term infant mobilizes free fatty acids and ketones to stabilize blood glucose. In the first several days, blood glucose homeostasis is glucose dominant; thereafter, it becomes insulin dominant, as in adults (Blackburn, 2013).

Bilirubin Metabolism. In newborns, the liver plays a major role in the metabolism of **bilirubin,** a yellow pigment formed from hemoglobin as a by-product of RBC breakdown. In high concentrations, bilirubin is toxic to the brain (Wilson, 2011). Bilirubin production is more than twice as much in newborns as in adults because of the high volume of circulating RBCs and their shorter life span (Blackburn, 2013). These factors place newborns at risk for hyperbilirubinemia.

Cord blood bilirubin levels are approximately 24 to 33 µmol/L (Blackburn, 2013). Clamping of the umbilical cord decreases circulation to the liver. Preterm or sick newborns also may experience intermittent patency of the ductus venosus, resulting in shunting of the blood past the liver sinusoids, which interferes with bilirubin removal from the plasma (Blackburn, 2013).

Unconjugated bilirubin, also called **indirect bilirubin,** is bound to circulating albumin in the bloodstream and has not yet been metabolized by the liver. Each gram of albumin binds approximately 8.5 to 10 mg of bilirubin. As bilirubin production increases, all the albumin sites may be taken up, and the free (unbound) bilirubin can move into fatty tissue, such as the skin, where it causes **jaundice,** or into the brain, where it can cause neurologic damage (Blackburn, 2013).

The liver removes unconjugated (indirect) bilirubin from the albumin and "conjugates" it. The conversion of indirect bilirubin to **conjugated bilirubin** depends on glucose and oxygen. This process involves an important enzyme called glucuronyl transferase, in which unconjugated (indirect) bilirubin interacts with glucose and glucuronic acid to produce direct bilirubin, which is water soluble. Next, direct bilirubin is excreted into the small intestine, which processes bilirubin into urobilinogen. When oxidized, urobilinogen forms orange urobilin, giving the stool its characteristic colour.

Most urobilinogen is excreted in stool, whereas some is reabsorbed in the colon and excreted in urine (Wilson, 2011).

It is possible for urobilinogen to be converted back into indirect bilirubin, a process known as *enterohepatic shunting*. In this process, unconjugated (indirect) bilirubin is absorbed across the intestinal mucosa, re-enters the circulation, and ends up back in the liver. Any delay in intestinal movement or decrease in intestinal flora increases the risk of conversion of direct bilirubin to indirect bilirubin, thus necessitating re-entry to the liver to begin the excretion process again (Blackburn, 2013). Serum bilirubin levels are expressed as three values: total, indirect, and direct. **Total bilirubin** is simply the sum of the indirect and direct values.

Newborn jaundice progresses from head to toe. In babies with light skin, jaundice is easily seen, whereas in babies with dark skin, it can be made more evident by pressing a finger on the skin and seeing the yellow colour before capillary refill occurs. A newborn becomes visibly jaundiced as blood levels reach a total serum bilirubin (direct plus indirect) value of 85 to 120 μmol/L in the first few days after birth. This normal event is called **physiologic jaundice** and occurs in approximately 50% to 60% of term newborns, peaking at 3 to 5 days, after most newborns have been discharged from hospital (Blackburn, 2013). Visual assessment of jaundice is inadequate for diagnosing hyperbilirubinemia, since the level of bilirubin at which jaundice is evident varies considerably (Bhutani et al., 2010). See Chapters 21 and 22 for detailed discussions of other types of jaundice and their treatment.

Return to William, the newborn being screened for hyperbilirubinemia. His serum bilirubin was only mildly elevated and he did not require phototherapy. What can the nurse tell William's parents about his risk for bilirubin-related brain damage? What should William's parents be instructed to watch for after discharge?

Gastrointestinal System

Oral Feeding. The beginning of oral feeding is critical to the development of immature GI function, because it causes surges in plasma concentrations of gastric hormones and enteric neuropeptides. Human milk is rich in these factors, as well as being the preferred source of energy and fluid (Blackburn, 2013). Healthy term babies may be breastfed as soon as possible after birth and 8 to 12 times per day thereafter (Riordan & Hoover, 2010). Formula-fed babies should eat within 6 to 8 hours of birth or sooner if indicated by hunger cues or risk for hypoglycemia (see Chapter 21). The term newborn's gastric capacity is approximately 6 mL/kg body weight, which means that a newborn weighing 3,400 g has a gastric capacity of approximately 20 mL of fluid (Murray et al., 2012) (see Chapter 21).

Meconium. Meconium, the newborn's first stool, begins to form at approximately 16 weeks' gestation (Elizabeth & Jacob, 2012). This black, sticky substance consists of vernix caseosa, **lanugo,** squamous epithelial cells, occult blood, bile, and other intestinal secretions. Bacteria appear in meconium by 24 hours of life. Almost all newborns pass meconium by 24 to 48 hours. Failure to pass meconium is a sign of intestinal obstruction and places the newborn at high risk for hyperbilirubinemia (Blackburn, 2013).

Immunologic System

Susceptibility to Infection. Immature immunologic responses make the newborn susceptible to infection. In addition, lack of exposure to common organisms results in a delayed or decreased immune response. Preterm infants are especially susceptible to infection because of a markedly immature immune response (Blackburn, 2013).

Newborns can develop an infection while in utero (through transplacental passage of an organism from mother to fetus), during labour (through contact or aspiration of organisms in the birth canal), or after birth (from organisms in the environment or, less commonly, breast milk) (Venkatesh et al., 2011). The nurse is aware of prenatal, intrapartal, and neonatal risk factors for infection, uses standard precautions and thorough hand washing technique, and teaches parents basic preventive hygiene procedures.

Departure from the sterile uterine environment exposes the newborn to a host of potential pathogens. The birth process, hospital environment, and ingested and inhaled substances expose the skin, respiratory system, and GI tract. Skin flora increase immediately after birth; in term healthy newborns, the skin achieves a balance of colonized bacteria that protects them from invading pathogens. Gastric acidity initially protects the gut from gram-positive and gram-negative bacteria; breastfeeding infants receive the added benefit of antimicrobial substances in human milk (Blackburn, 2013).

Term newborns have temporary passive immunity from transplacental transfer of maternal immunoglobulins, especially immunoglobulin G (IgG). IgA levels are decreased, however, and place them at risk for viral and gram-negative bacteria (Blackburn, 2013). The inexperienced immune system fails to produce detectable type-specific antibodies. Newborns cannot localize infection because of their inability to produce adequate neutrophils and other phagocytes and transport them to infection sites. For this reason, signs of sepsis can be diffuse and nonspecific instead of localized; for example, temperature instability is a more common sign of neonatal sepsis than is fever (Blackburn, 2013) (see Chapter 22).

Infection Prevention Strategies. The best strategy for preventing nosocomial infections is thorough hand washing. The nurse's work shift may begin with a 3-minute scrub of the hands and arms above the elbow with an antiseptic soap and brush or pre-packaged antiseptic sponge. Thereafter, the nurse washes his or her hands for at least 10 seconds with bactericidal soap before and after contact with the infant and after touching objects. This rule applies regardless of whether the nurse wears gloves. The nurse removes rings, watches, and bracelets and trims fingernails short. No false or gel fingernails should be permitted, because they increase the likelihood of inadequate cleansing. Alcohol-based foams or gels, although not appropriate when hands are soiled, kill bacteria when applied to clean hands and given sufficient contact time (follow manufacturer's guidelines) (AAP & ACOG, 2012; Larson et al., 2012).

Nursery personnel managing healthy term newborns do not need to wear cover gowns as long as hand washing is strictly enforced. People with respiratory, GI, or skin infections should *not* have contact with newborns. In addition, any staff member with a skin condition or appliance that prevents or impairs hand washing should not have contact with newborns (AAP & ACOG, 2012).

Hospitals vary in their approach to staff members with herpes simplex virus. Transmission from infected personnel to infants is rare. If an infected staff member is allowed to work with newborns, he or she should cover lesions and perform meticulous hand washing. Nevertheless, any staff member with herpetic hand infections (herpes whitlow) may not have contact with any client until the infection has resolved (Sinha et al., 2012).

Ideally, each newborn has individual supplies, such as a digital thermometer and stethoscope, in his or her bassinette. If these supplies travel from baby to baby, staff members follow strict procedures for cleaning after each use to prevent infection (AAP & ACOG, 2012).

Parents also share responsibility for protecting infants. They wash their hands thoroughly before providing newborn care, before preparing for feeding, and, of course, after using the bathroom. Siblings with fever, symptoms of acute illness, or recent exposure to a known communicable disease (eg, chickenpox) should not be allowed to visit the newborn in the hospital (AAP & ACOG, 2012).

Integumentary System

Skin Functions. Newborn skin has three functions: to limit transepidermal water loss, to prevent absorption of chemicals, and to protect against pathogens (Blackburn, 2013). The epidermal thickness of the term newborn is as well developed as in an adult, although the stratum corneum does not function as well as adult skin throughout the first year of life (AWHONN, 2013; Blackburn, 2013). The more preterm the infant, the more immature the barrier (Blackburn, 2013; Dyer, 2013).

Transepidermal water loss is not a significant risk factor for healthy term infants. Term infants lose 5 to 10 $g/m^2/h$, slightly lower than in adults (Hoath, 2011). Transepidermal water loss in term infants requires consideration when their care requires a radiant warmer, an incubator, or phototherapy (Blackburn, 2013).

Skin Characteristics. Adaptation of newborn skin to the extrauterine environment occurs over the first year of life (Dyer, 2013). A newborn's skin is more permeable than an adult's to substances such as drugs and chemicals. Skin permeability is increased proportionately with decreasing gestational age.

The skin's acid mantle has a surface pH of 6.0 at birth but within 96 hours of birth, typically lowers to less than 5 and acts as a bacteriostatic barrier (AWHONN, 2013). After birth, colonization of the skin begins and "friendly" bacteria grow in balance to protect against infectious pathogens. There is a difference in skin colonization between those newborns born by vaginal birth and those born by cesarean section birth. Neonates born vaginally harbour bacterial communities most similar to the maternal vaginal community; those born by caesarian section harbour communities most similar to maternal skin communities (Dominguez-Bello et al., 2010). The relevance of this difference is not clearly understood at this time (AWHONN, 2013).

If the skin pH shifts toward alkaline, for example following bathing with an alkaline soap, there may be interference with the development and function of the acid mantle and an increase in bacteria and changes in skin permeability leading to increased transepidermal water loss (Dyer, 2013; Lund & Durand, 2011). The use of mild liquid cleansers appears similar to the use of plain water and allows more rapid acidification of the stratum corneum. Bathing normal term newborns after birth does not appear to affect either the type or amount of microbes present on the infant's skin (Dyer, 2013). Furthermore, research using a wash product specifically formulated for newborns, with a pH of about 5.5 and some buffering capacity to maintain skin pH at about the same level, found no differences between the use of the newborn wash product and plain water (Lavender et al., 2013). Bathing more frequently than every other day may lead to a drier skin surface, because bathing introduces unexpected changes in the stratum corneum (AWHONN, 2013). However, studies have shown that bathing every fourth day did not result in a significant increase in the number of skin flora, colony counts, or development of infection when compared with bathing every other day (AWHONN, 2013).

Obviously, skin disease and injury increase the risk for permeability. The historical practice of bathing newborns with hexachlorophene to prevent colonization with staphylococci was found to increase the risk for neurologic damage (Witt, 2009). Side effects from absorption and toxicity of chemicals from topical compounds can be devastating. Povidone iodine may cause hypothyroidism, and neomycin can lead to neural deafness (Thappa, 2009). Isopropyl alcohol, depending on its concentration, duration of exposure, condition of the skin, pressure on the skin, and quality of skin perfusion, can cause drying, irritation, and burns (Blackburn, 2013). Any topical preparations should be used with care and should be removed from the skin as soon as possible (Lund & Durand, 2011). Table 20.4 depicts various skin findings in newborns.

Renal System

Fetal Development. At birth, the kidneys take over fluid and electrolyte balance, metabolic excretion, and other functions from the placenta. Although the newborn has the same number of nephrons by 34 to 35 weeks' gestation as an adult, the kidneys are less functional and immature (Blackburn, 2013).

Newborn Kidney Function. Glomerular filtration rate is low in comparison to an adult's. This means that the newborn's kidneys favour resorption of sodium and cannot dispose of water rapidly when necessary. The newborn is therefore at risk for water retention and edema (Blackburn, 2013).

Tubular function is altered, so that the kidneys have less ability to concentrate urine, putting newborns at risk for dehydration. Limited ability to concentrate urine also puts the newborn at risk for acid–base abnormalities, hyperkalemia, hypocalcemia, and hypoglycemia (Blackburn, 2013).

With advancing gestational age, extracellular water and total body water decrease and intracellular water increases. Diuresis occurs shortly after birth and contributes to the loss of 5% to 10% of birth weight in the term infant's first week of life (Blackburn, 2013).

Urine. Healthy term infants urinate 15 to 60 mL/kg/day (Blackburn, 2013). The initial void occurs in the delivery room for 13% to 21% of newborns; 95% of all newborns void in the first 24 hours, and all newborns should have voided by 48 hours (Blackburn, 2013). A newborn who has not voided by 24 to 48 hours requires further evaluation (Jackman & Viessman, 2009).

The urine is usually straw coloured, but may be cloudy with mucus. Specific gravity is low (1.008 to 1.012) (Blackburn, 2013). Female infants sometimes have small amounts of bloody mucus from **pseudomenses/pseudomenstruation**, resulting from the withdrawal of maternal hormones (Cavaliere, 2009). Pink stains (**brick dust spots**) may appear in the urine of both males and females; they result from uric acid crystals and are not a cause for concern (Blackburn, 2013).

Promoting Normal Transition

No one knows exactly what the experience of birth is like for the baby. He or she likely feels the mother's muscular uterine contractions. Each contraction may lead to mild hypoxia and a transient drop in blood pressure (Blackburn, 2013). During vaginal birth, contractions and maternal pushing efforts propel the baby through the narrow birth canal and out the vaginal opening. Cesarean birth abruptly exposes the newborn to handling and light as the baby is pulled from the uterus into the extrauterine environment. For the first time, the newborn experiences cool room temperature, tactile stimulation, bright light, loud noises, and new feelings of gravity and proprioception. He or she discovers what may be a surprising ability to extend the head, arms, and legs, and reacts to this startling lack of containment around the body.

The incredible forces of the birth process may be evident during physical examination. The newborn's eyes may be puffy and bruised and the skull moulded into an elongated shape. Boggy areas of fluid may be palpable under the scalp. In some instances, the nose is flattened or pushed to one side. A large baby may even suffer a fractured clavicle as the shoulders make the tight fit through the vaginal opening, especially in the presence of shoulder dystocia.

Experienced and thoughtful neonatal nurses recognize that transition is more likely to be successful if unnecessary stressors are eliminated. Nurses who handle the newborn gently, protect the baby from unnecessary and invasive procedures, and treat him or her in accordance with developmental abilities promote successful extrauterine transitions, model excellent caregiving skills to parents, and promote parent–infant attachment. Strategies for a "gentle" newborn transition include the following:

- *Gentle handling:* Move newborns calmly and gently. Do not twist the extremities or change resting position abruptly. Speak to babies before touching them, and while providing care.
- *Use of containment:* Newborns are accustomed to containment within the uterus and are comforted by boundaries on the extremities, top of the head, and feet and legs. Swaddling is an example of containment; however, newborns can be comforted in other ways, if swaddling is not feasible. Examples include "nesting" the newborn if radiant warmer use is required, asking the mother's partner or support person to gently hold the newborn's arms across its chest during the vitamin

K injection, and quieting a newborn who is escalating from an active alert state to a crying state.

- **Avoidance of deep suction:** Vigorous or deep suctioning, especially with a suction catheter, may elicit a vagal response, slowing heart rate and causing apnea, bradycardia, and resultant hypoxia. Nurses can remove secretions at birth with a towel, bulb syringe, or suction catheter. Thereafter, in a healthy newborn, the bulb syringe is usually the only suction device needed to clear the mouth or nares, and then only to remove visible vomitus or mucus. Sick newborns may require gastric suctioning to remove gastric contents to facilitate assisted ventilation and prevent aspiration; however, routine gastric suctioning for healthy newborns is unnecessary and invasive (Gardner & Hernandez, 2011).

- **Use of ambient or dim light:** Newborns are accustomed to a dark intrauterine environment. Physical examination is best performed when newborns are in a quiet alert state. A bright overhead light causes infants to close the eyes, grimace, and become uncomfortable. Transient bright light may be required to check a blink reflex or to better visualize an aspect of anatomy. The nurse should prevent continuous bright light from shining in the baby's face.

- **Use of axillary temperature:** Routine rectal temperature measurement is now rare and not normally recommended. Axillary temperature measurement is non-invasive and approximates core temperature (Blackburn, 2013). Placement of a thermometer in the newborn's rectum does not prove rectal patency, because anal stenosis or atresia may occur at any point along the anorectal canal (Goodwin, 2009). Rectal temperature can be uncomfortable and requires removal of blankets and the diaper, exposing the newborn to chilling. Most importantly, rectal temperatures place newborns at risk for trauma, perforation, and cross-contamination (Blackburn, 2013).

If the baby is term, stable, and in good condition, and in accordance with the mother's birth plan, health care providers separate the mother and the baby as little as possible. The nurse may take the baby's axillary temperature while the mother or partner is holding the child. The nurse also can assess heart rate and breath sounds easily while parents hold the baby. Some nurses instill prophylactic eye medication and give the IM injection of vitamin K with the baby in a parent's arms.

COLLABORATIVE CARE: THE TRANSITIONAL PERIOD

Transition goes well for 85% to 90% of newborns, and these infants emerge from the first 4 to 6 hours of life healthy and ready to interact with the environ-ment. The remaining 10% to 15% develop potentially life-threatening complications that require immediate identification and intervention (Gardner & Hernandez, 2011). The nurse caring for the infant in transition must be alert for signs of abnormal transition, and the experienced nurse can assess the differences between an infant experiencing a "rocky" transition and an infant who is truly ill.

The newborn can be classified as healthy, at risk, or ill:

- The *healthy newborn* is term and AGA with no history of prenatal or intrapartal risk factors. The nurse can anticipate a smooth transition for this infant.
- The *at-risk newborn* is near term or term and has one or more risk factors relating to size for gestation, prenatal and intrapartum risk factors, or both. The nurse is alert for problems that may develop in transition. With appropriate nursing support and minimal interventions, the at-risk newborn may overcome initial challenges and become a well newborn. Conversely, the at-risk newborn may develop problems that require special care for a sick newborn.
- The *ill newborn* has clear risk factors relating to gestational age, size for gestation, and prenatal or intrapartal history. The nurse anticipates care of a sick newborn who will require evaluation and support in a special care nursery environment.

Because of the incredible complexity of adaptation necessary for the transition to extrauterine life, the term healthy newborn is allowed a short period to resolve initial challenges during transition. The nurse is aware of the prenatal and intrapartum risk factors that could place the newborn at risk. If such factors are present, the nurse anticipates potential neonatal implications and prepares to intervene during transition, as necessary. For the at-risk newborn, the nurse delays stressful procedures such as bathing until the newborn is stable. For a sick newborn, the nurse delays both bathing and feeding (see Chapter 22).

Duration and severity of symptoms differentiate normal from abnormal transition. Respiratory distress is the most common manifestation of abnormal transition (Gardner & Hernandez, 2011). If present, signs of respiratory distress (expiratory grunting, nasal flaring, and retracting) should be mild and intermittent, unaccompanied by additional problems (eg, pallor, heart murmur, lethargy), and steadily resolve in the first 15 to 20 minutes of life (Smith, 2012). It is not uncommon for near-term newborns or those born by cesarean to exhibit mild to moderate respiratory distress for several hours after birth (Gardner & Hernandez, 2011). Any newborn with moderate or severe respiratory distress requires immediate evaluation in a setting prepared to support his or

● **BOX 20.2** **Signs of Abnormal Transition**

- Abdominal distention
- Central cyanosis or duskiness requiring continuous or intermittent supplemental oxygen
- Frequent choking or drooling, especially if accompanied by apnea or cyanosis
- Hypotonia or lethargy
- Marked jitteriness or tremors
- Pale, grey, or mottled appearance, which indicates poor perfusion
- Respiratory distress that does not steadily resolve in the first 30 to 60 minutes of life or increases over time, with expiratory grunting, nasal flaring, retractions tachypnea, gasping, or apnea
- Unstable temperature in a stable thermal environment
- Unusual neurologic activity
- Vomiting of bilious material
- Weak or high-pitched cry

her thermal, pulmonary, cardiovascular, and metabolic requirements (see Chapter 22). See Box 20.2.

Assessment

The nurse assesses axillary temperature every 30 minutes after birth until the newborn's condition has remained stable for 2 hours (Brown & Landers, 2011). Thereafter, the temperature is taken during routine assessments every 3 to 4 hours, preferably when the newborn is awake for care and feeding. The nurse assesses temperature more often if the newborn is at an increased risk for heat loss from prematurity or a central nervous system anomaly; if temperature is unstable; or if the newborn shows other signs of distress related to temperature instability, such as cool or mottled skin, respiratory distress, jitteriness, or sweating (in term and postterm babies).

The nurse caring for the infant checks the prenatal and intrapartal history to identify risk factors for hypoglycemia and follows the hospital's screening protocol. Blood glucose screening is part of the assessment for any infant showing signs of hypoglycemia or respiratory or central nervous system distress. Bedside glucose monitoring is not a routine part of admission for healthy newborns with no known risk factors or symptoms (Wilson, 2011).

Inspection of colour is part of routine newborn assessment and provides information about blood volume and perfusion. Colour variations should be congruent with the newborn's genetic makeup; however, a newborn with persistently pale mucous membranes or one who is **plethoric,** that is, a deep-red colour, requires

further evaluation. Heelstick or venous blood sampling of the hemoglobin and hematocrit is indicated for these newborns to rule out anemia or polycythemia.

The nurse assesses for jaundice by pressing the newborn's skin firmly with a finger and evaluating how much jaundice appears where the skin blanches. Note that visual assessment alone is inadequate in determining the degree of jaundice present. Many settings use a transcutaneous bilirubin meter for screening. Bilirubin advances from head to foot, so a baby with jaundice to the knees has a higher bilirubin level than a baby with jaundice to the nipples. The newborn who appears slightly jaundiced by day 2 or 3 may require a laboratory evaluation of bilirubin, especially if being discharged. Follow-up examination and/or laboratory testing are indicated; the nurse may make necessary arrangements before discharge. The newborn with jaundice in the first 24 hours requires immediate evaluation by a pediatric provider. The newborn at risk for pathologic jaundice requires more intensive blood work, such as blood typing and Coombs testing (see Chapter 22). A baby whose bilirubin level rises faster than his or her capacity to metabolize it may require **phototherapy** (see Chapter 22).

The newborn has audible bowel sounds in the first few hours of life. The nurse observes and assesses ability to suck, swallow, and breathe to ensure effective feeding every 2 to 4 hours and adequate fluid intake. The newborn should pass stool by 48 hours.

The nurse routinely and periodically assesses vital signs, appearance, feeding, and activity. Signs of infection may be nonspecific and subtle. If the nurse suspects signs of developing infection, he or she performs more frequent assessments.

The healthy newborn voids by 24 hours. The nurse documents assessment of urine output and instructs parents to report the number of wet diapers they change. The nurse notifies the pediatric provider of delayed or abnormal urination (AAP & ACOG, 2012).

Potential Nursing Diagnoses

The following nursing diagnoses may be appropriate:

- **Risk for Imbalanced Body Temperature** related to large body surface in relationship to mass and decreased subcutaneous fat
- **Risk for Injury** related to hypoglycemia
- **Risk for Injury** related to blood volume excess or deficit
- **Risk for Injury** related to excess by-products of RBC breakdown and concurrent hepatic immaturity
- **Risk for Injury** related to delayed or abnormal GI function secondary to immaturity or pathology
- **Risk for Infection** related to immature immunologic defenses and environmental exposure

- **Risk for Impaired Skin Integrity** related to immature skin structure and environmental exposure
- **Risk for Deficient/Excess Fluid Volume** related to immature renal physiology

Planning/Intervention

No health care team member should ever leave a newborn exposed after unwrapping or undressing the baby for a physical examination or procedure, such as drawing blood. Parents who naturally unwrap the newborn to count the fingers and toes, to look for familial characteristics, or to make sure that "everything is there" should be allowed this important examination, but encouraged to make it brief. One strategy that helps to decrease (or correct) the risk of hypothermia is to have the mother or significant other hold the infant in what is called "skin-to-skin" or "kangaroo" care. This strategy involves holding the undressed infant against the bare chest, covered with a blanket. This has been shown to promote temperature stabilization in the newborn and to increase the infant's temperature (Chiu et al., 2005). In addition, it has also been shown to have other benefits including reduced infant crying, improved mother–infant interaction, improved breastfeeding, and increased maternal gentleness when handling the infant (Dumas et al., 2013; Haxton et al., 2012).

To avoid hyperthermia when other interventions are used to warm the infant, staff are educated in the correct use of interventions such as radiant warmers, chemical warmers, heat lamps, and incubators. Strategies to promote thermoregulation include drying the newborn immediately after birth; dressing the newborn in clothing, blankets, and a hat to conserve body temperature; ensuring that linen, blankets, and clothing are dry; placing the newborn in a draft-free area; and using necessary warming interventions, such as skin-to-skin care or the radiant warmer, appropriately and safely.

Clear and complete communication among team members is essential to identify newborns at risk for hypoglycemia. The nurse caring for the mother notifies nursery personnel, the pediatric care provider, or both when she admits a labouring woman at risk for giving birth to a baby predisposed to blood glucose instability. Risk factors include prematurity, maternal diabetes, SGA newborn, or intrapartal fetal stress. Laboratory confirmation of aberrant bedside glucose screening test results should occur quickly (see Chapter 22). Interventions vary depending on the etiology and degree of hypoglycemia. Feeding by breast, nipple, or gavage is effective in most cases. Newborns in distress and those with acute hypoglycemia are managed with IV therapy. Thermal and oxygen support are important adjuncts, because thermal stress and respiratory distress increase glucose metabolism (Brown & Landers, 2011).

The nurse caring for the newborn is aware of risk factors for anemia or polycythemia and communicates them to the pediatric provider. Communication with labour and delivery staff is important to obtain late intrapartum information, such as suspected partial placental abruption, which places the newborn at risk for decreased blood volume and anemia. Evidence of discordant placental circulation may explain anemia or polycythemia in twins. Laboratory blood work to ascertain the newborn's hemoglobin, hematocrit, or CBC and differential is not required routinely; however, any infant at risk for or showing evidence of anemia, polycythemia, or infection requires evaluation. The pale or plethoric newborn also requires support to ensure thermal stability and adequate perfusion and oxygenation.

Because healthy newborns and mothers are usually discharged by day 1 or 2, collaborative efforts are necessary to identify those babies who require treatment for hyperbilirubinemia. The nurse teaches parents when to call the health care provider, that is, when the baby is visibly more jaundiced than the previous day, or when lethargy, poor feeding, or both accompany jaundice. The nurse recommends a system of follow-up examination, either in the home or clinic, within 3 to 4 days of discharge, especially for those infants discharged before 48 hours of age (Wilson, 2011). Early and effective feeding promotes excretion of bilirubin; therefore, the baby should stay with the mother as much as possible so that feeding can occur at the first opportunity.

The nurse documents bowel sounds, feeding activity, feeding tolerance, and bowel activities and instructs parents about observing and documenting infant feeding and bowel movements. The nurse notifies the pediatric provider of delayed or abnormal bowel movements, abdominal distention, or bilious vomiting. Early and effective feeding helps promote intestinal motility. The nurse alerts the pediatric provider of abnormalities, and, when appropriate, stops feeding until medical evaluation is complete.

The infant's medical records should be complete and identify all factors that could lead to infection. Examples include prolonged rupture of membranes or maternal fever late in labour. The nurse communicates such information verbally and in the infant's care record. All team members, including the baby's parents, practise meticulous hand washing and protect the newborn from exposure to pathogens. A newborn with developing sepsis can become critically ill within hours. A CBC with differential and a blood culture is necessary for those at high risk or with abnormal transition or clinical signs of infection (see Chapter 22). In addition, the plan of care usually includes IV antibiotics and support of thermoregulation, oxygenation, perfusion, and glucose metabolism. Parents of a sick newborn require information and support during this stressful time (see Chapter 22).

Every team member works to protect the newborn's skin from damage and chemical exposure. The nurse reports skin abnormalities or breaks to the pediatric care provider in a timely manner and points out skin characteristics to parents. The nurse washes off any soap used for bathing to prevent absorption of chemicals through the skin and discourages use of perfumed baby products. If any skin dryness or cracking is present, application of an emollient to protect the integrity of the skin barrier may be indicated (AWHONN, 2013). Petrolatum or petrolatum-based ointments protect the perineal skin from moisture.

Early and effective feeding helps promote adequate voiding. Accurate documentation ensures adequate assessment of renal activity and prevents unnecessary interventions and diagnostic tests. The nurse notifies the pediatric provider of delayed or abnormal voiding.

Evaluation

Standards for normal newborn temperature vary regionally; however, axillary temperature should be stable and between 36.5° and 37.3°C. The newborn should be wrapped in dry clothing and blankets in a warm, draft-free environment. The nurse documents temperature and any interventions to adjust it and periodically re-evaluates the temperature to ensure stability or to identify instability that requires additional assessment and intervention.

Blood glucose level should be at least 2.2 to 2.7 mmol/L while weaning IV fluids or advancing oral feedings (Adamkin & Committee of the Fetus and Newborn, 2011). The nurse documents results of bedside screening and laboratory tests and symptoms of hypoglycemia, such as jitteriness or lethargy.

The healthy term newborn has no apparent risk factors for alterations in quantity or function of blood components, is pink and well perfused, and shows no signs of sepsis. RBC (including hemoglobin and hematocrit), WBC, and platelet counts vary considerably among newborns, depending on gestational age and environmental factors; however, laboratory values should be within normal limits.

Physiologic jaundice should resolve in the first week of life. Evidence of resolution includes disappearance of visible jaundice and serum bilirubin levels decreasing to normal limits.

The healthy term infant can coordinate sucking, swallowing, and breathing to feed effectively 8 to 12 times per day. He or she has audible bowel sounds, a soft protruding abdomen, no bilious vomiting, and passes meconium by 24 to 48 hours after birth.

The nurse evaluates blood work for diagnostic confirmation of infection. An infant responding positively to interventions has stable vital signs within normal limits, adequate oxygenation and perfusion, normal laboratory blood test results, and normal voiding and bowel movements. He or she also tolerates feedings when appropriate.

The newborn should void straw-coloured urine. Female infants may have small amounts of bloody mucus from pseudomenses. The nurse documents each wet diaper and may weigh the newborn daily. A loss of 5% to 10% of birth weight is expected in the first week of life from normal diuresis and passage of meconium.

ONGOING ASSESSMENTS

The nurse's vigilance does not end when the newborn transition period is over. Although this chapter focuses on a thorough newborn physical assessment, it is important that the nurse observes and assesses the newborn to some degree *every* time he or she sees the baby. Even when the nurse simply passes by the bassinette, the nurse glances at and assesses the newborn's resting position, respiratory status, colour, and state to ensure ongoing safety and well-being.

The nurse records assessments of vital signs and indicators of well-being such as colour, activity, feeding, and elimination. The nurse notes any deviations from normal, which may necessitate a narrative note for further explanation, and describes interventions and their associated outcomes.

Infant safety parameters are also part of periodic assessment. The nurse checks that newborn identification bands are secure and that mother and baby bands match. Most hospitals have flow sheets for recording specific aspects of newborn assessment and care and may include items such as a space to record the infant's position (eg, supine) and that the bulb syringe is present in the bassinette.

BASIC CARE OF THE HEALTHY NEWBORN

Basic nursing care of the healthy newborn usually differs little from care that parents render after discharge. In most cases, the healthy mother and newborn are separated as little as possible during the hospital stay; therefore, basic newborn care that the nurse performs is an opportunity to teach parents these skills (Nursing Care Plan 20.1). Hospital length of stay is typically less than 48 hours with a vaginal birth, so it is important for the mother and her partner or support person to provide newborn care, calling on the nurse to answer questions and assist as necessary. (For newborn feeding and nutrition information, see Chapter 21.)

(text continues on page 827)

NURSING CARE PLAN 20.1

●

The Healthy Newborn and Family

Recall Thomas, the 8-hour-old newborn from the beginning of this chapter. Further assessment reveals the following: weight, 3,700 g; pink colour; alert and active; axillary temperature, 36.5°C; heart rate, 148 beats/min and steady with appropriate PMI and no audible murmur; respiratory rate, 52 breaths/min, with no grunting, nasal flaring, or retractions; clear and equal bilateral breath sounds. Bowel sounds are present. Thomas voided at birth and has passed his first meconium stool. The nurse notes a small red puncture mark on the occipital part of the scalp from a fetal monitor electrode. He was lying on the bed when the nurse arrived.

NURSING DIAGNOSES

- **Ineffective Airway Clearance** related to excess mucus, gagging, and choking
- **Deficient Knowledge (Maternal)** related to newborn care and airway maintenance

EXPECTED OUTCOMES

1. The newborn will maintain a patent airway.
2. The newborn will exhibit no signs of continuing respiratory distress.
3. The mother will demonstrate beginning skill with use of the bulb syringe.

INTERVENTIONS	RATIONALES
Turn the newborn on his side.	This position promotes fluid drainage from the nose and mouth to prevent aspiration.
Suction the mouth first, then the nares with the bulb syringe.	Gentle suctioning promotes a patent airway. The baby may gasp upon placement of the bulb syringe in the nares; therefore, suctioning the mouth first prevents aspiration.
Assess for signs and symptoms of respiratory distress, such as nasal flaring or grunting respirations. Auscultate the lungs after any choking episode.	Assessment provides information to determine the effect of and recovery from choking episodes.
Replace the bulb syringe in the bassinette where it is visible.	The syringe should be available for immediate use as necessary.
Continue to assess the newborn's respiratory status frequently.	Continued assessment is necessary to allow for early identification of and prompt intervention for any additional problems.
Instruct the mother in how to use the bulb syringe; have her identify situations in which she may need the bulb syringe; have her return-demonstrate the procedure; offer praise and positive reinforcement.	Teaching assists the mother to gain necessary skills to care for her son. Return demonstration indicates the effectiveness of teaching. Positive reinforcement and praise promote feelings of confidence.

EVALUATION

1. The newborn experiences full recovery.
2. The newborn maintains a patent airway with minimal to no mucus present.
3. The mother demonstrates the ability to use the bulb syringe appropriately and correctly.

(continued)

NURSING CARE PLAN 20.1 ● The Healthy Newborn and Family *(Continued)*

NURSING DIAGNOSIS

Risk for Imbalanced Body Temperature related to immature temperature control, change in environmental temperature, and large body surface in relation to mass.

EXPECTED OUTCOME

The newborn will maintain an axillary temperature of 36.5° to 37.0°C clothed in a shirt, diaper, and two blankets.

INTERVENTIONS	RATIONALES
Assess the newborn's temperature as per agency policy.	Assessment provides a baseline from which to make future comparisons. Thomas's current axillary temperature is at the low end of the normal range.
Institute measures to conserve the newborn's heat; use warmed blankets, skin-to-skin contact with mother, and/or the overhead radiant warmer. Double-wrap the infant in a blanket and place a thermally insulated hat on his head.	Newborns need additional measures to conserve heat because of their immature ability to regulate body temperature.
Avoid situations that may promote heat loss; dry skin thoroughly, avoid placing bassinette near doorways or drafts, and avoid placing newborn on cold surfaces. Delay routine bathing until the newborn's temperature is stable.	Heat is lost through conduction, convection, radiation, and evaporation.
Continue to monitor temperature as indicated; recheck temperature 30 min after instituting warming measures.	Temperature should respond to warming measures and stabilize.

EVALUATION

The newborn maintains an axillary temperature within expected parameters.

NURSING DIAGNOSIS

Deficient Knowledge (Maternal) related to care of healthy newborn

EXPECTED OUTCOMES

1. The mother will demonstrate safe caregiving practices for her newborn.
2. The mother will demonstrate how to use the bulb syringe during choking episodes.
3. The mother will identify strategies to protect the infant from infection and injury.
4. The mother will demonstrate beginning confidence in caring for her newborn.

(continued)

NURSING CARE PLAN 20.1 ● The Healthy Newborn and Family *(Continued)*

INTERVENTIONS	RATIONALES
Assess maternal knowledge of newborn care. Provide facts; clarify misconceptions.	Assessment provides a baseline from which to develop an individualized teaching plan.
Use written, verbal, and audiovisual information to teach the mother about safe care-giving practices, such as keeping the infant in the bassinette or in her arms instead of on the bed.	Providing non-judgmental supportive information about infant safety helps ensure that the mother will listen and learn about strategies to prevent injury to her infant.
Reassure the mother that infants are competent at clearing their airways. Explain that the bulb syringe is necessary when fluids coming from the baby's mouth or nose accompany choking.	Helping the mother to perceive her infant as competent will minimize undue fear and anxiety. Additional teaching about the bulb syringe helps to promote confidence when using it.
Demonstrate the use of the bulb syringe to her. Ask for a return demonstration by placing the syringe gently inside the infant's cheek and near the nares, using correct technique to aspirate fluids.	Asking for a return demonstration during a calm moment will increase the mother's feelings of competence.
Explain that infants are vulnerable to infection. Demonstrate handwashing technique to the mother after infant caregiving, and remind the mother to wash her hands regularly before giving newborn care. Show the small scalp abrasion to the mother and explain signs to report that would indicate infection (redness, drainage, swelling, signs of illness in the newborn).	Teaching the mother about the infant's vulnerability to infection facilitates her involvement in protecting the infant from infection.
Reinforce additional measures for newborn care including bathing, diapering, clothing, using car seats, comforting, and sleeping position.	Adequate knowledge related to care measures helps to promote their use.
Review the signs and symptoms of newborn illness; encourage the mother to notify the health care provider should any occur.	Signs and symptoms of newborn illness can be vague; knowledge of when to notify the health care provider promotes early detection and prompt intervention.
Arrange for possible referral to social services and home care if indicated.	Support from additional sources helps to ease the transition and provides opportunities for additional follow-up and teaching.

EVALUATION

1. The mother demonstrates measures to provide safe newborn care.
2. The mother demonstrates calm and efficient use of the bulb syringe, identifying situations when use is necessary.
3. The mother implements appropriate measures to protect the newborn from infection and injury.
4. The mother states that she feels more confident when providing care to her newborn.

Cultural Aspects

The nurse considers cultural aspects of newborn care while teaching parents relevant skills. It is helpful to know how ethnic practices may differ from standard hospital practices. It is not safe to assume that the hospital protocol or pediatric provider's orders will be congruent with the family's cultural practices. Neither is it appropriate to stereotype the behaviour of ethnic groups by assuming that literature about cultural practices applies to everyone within each culture. The nurse observes parental responses to teaching and asks if they have a different preference. For example, the nurse who teaches umbilical cord care to a woman who has emigrated from another country may approach the situation by saying, "The way I just showed you is how many mothers in Canada do this. Is this what you expected? Would you like to talk about other methods?"

No health care professional can assume that information related to culture or ethnicity applies to each specific client just because she comes from that background. For more information about caring for clients of different cultures and ethnicities, a good place to begin is with the article by L. C. Callister on global and cultural perinatal nursing research (Callister, 2011).

Care of the Newborn Following Home Birth

Newborn care for an infant born at home follows the same principles applied to care provided in the hospital. A multidisciplinary team provides care; the nurse may coordinate the plan. Concepts important to home care of the newborn include the following:

- Women and newborns receive the same level of nursing care and expertise in the home as would be expected in a licensed birth setting.
- The nurse, health care provider, and family members develop the plan of care collaboratively with the client, with consideration of various aspects of the home life.
- Nursing practice in a home care setting is consistent with regulations that direct practice. Standards of newborn care are the same in the home setting as in the hospital setting. For example, vitamin K administration, eye prophylaxis, and newborn metabolic screening should be offered to parents in the home birth setting. The nurse documents timely assessments, the plan of care, interventions, evaluation, and outcomes.

The primary focus of home care is safety. Appropriate client selection, sound clinical judgment, and prompt transfer to a receptive environment when necessary, help ensure good perinatal outcomes (American College of Nurse-Midwives [ACNM], 2011; College of Midwives of Ontario, ND).

Infant Security

Infant abduction from hospital settings is uncommon but not outside the realm of possibility (Dalley, 2008). Hospital personnel need education regarding abductor profiles (Box 20.3), abductor behaviour, means of abduction, and their facility's emergency plan in the event of abduction. Obstetric units should have policies and procedures in place to reduce the risk for abduction (Vincent, 2009). Policies may include:

- Only those family members or support people who bear an identification bracelet matching the newborn's may transport the newborn.
- The newborn is pictured in the newborn record.
- All hospital personnel wear photo identification above the waist.

● **BOX 20.3** **Abductor Profile Characteristics**

- Female between the ages of 12 and 50 years
- Large build or overweight for height
- Married or involved in a failing relationship
- May have experienced a pregnancy loss (miscarriage, stillbirth, adoption)
- Lives in the community where the abduction takes place
- Often emotionally immature, compulsive, with low self-esteem
- May be feigning a pregnancy and have told acquaintances that she is pregnant

Typical Abduction Strategies

- Visits birthing centres asking detailed questions about procedures and unit layout
- Plans the abduction and then acts quickly when opportunity arises
- Impersonates medical, nursing, laboratory, volunteer, social work, or photography personnel
- With an accomplice or alone, may create a disturbance, such as pulling fire alarm or starting a fire, to distract staff
- Calls mother by her first name, learned from crib card or unsecured medical record
- Befriends the mother and stays for several hours to establish her trust
- Removes the newborn from the baby mother's room by saying the baby needs laboratory tests, vital signs, photographs, weight, etc.
- Removes the baby from the unit in a sport bag or under a coat
- Once the abduction has occurred, considers the baby to be her own

From Rabun, J. (Ed.). (2009). *For healthcare professionals: Guidelines on prevention of and response to infant abductions* (9th ed.). Alexandria, VA: National Center for Missing and Exploited Children. Retrieved from http://www.missingkids.com/en_US/publications/NC05.pdf

● TEACHING TIPS 20.2 Instructions for Keeping Your Baby Safe in the Hospital

- Give the baby only to hospital personnel wearing a hospital photo name tag.
- Go with any staff person who takes the baby from your room, if you wish.
- Never let the baby out of sight or leave him or her alone. Call the staff to take the baby when you shower, need to close the bathroom door, or plan to nap.
- Keep the baby on the far side of the room away from the door. This will help prevent people from moving the baby without your notice.

- Question any stranger who enters the room if the reason for the visit is unclear or strange.
- Call the nurse's station immediately to report a stranger or to check the identity of anyone who claims to work at the hospital.

Adapted from Shogan, M. G. (2002). Emergency management plan for newborn abduction. *Journal of Obstetric, Gynecologic, and Neonatal Nursing, 31*(3), 340–346.

- Infants wear security or RFID tags when practical to guard against unauthorized removal.
- All newborns are transported in their cribs. Anyone walking with a newborn in their arms is stopped and questioned.
- Unit access is controlled, unit exits have alarms, and video cameras record the faces of people leaving the unit (Vincent, 2009).

Parents play a major role in ensuring their infant's security. They must learn the basics of hospital security for their infant to help prevent abduction. See Teaching Tips 20.2 for a sample instruction sheet.

Temperature Assessment

Once the term newborn has been discharged, parents will have no reason to take his or her temperature at home unless they suspect illness. Because the nurse models the axillary method of temperature assessment, the parent usually learns this procedure. To reduce the potential for trauma and injury to the newborn during rectal assessment, nurses may advise parents to use the axillary method as their initial screen.

The nurse takes the axillary temperature by placing the thermometer deep into the baby's axilla and holding the arm down gently against the baby's chest (Fig. 20.14). The reading will be inaccurate if the thermometer tip extends past the axilla (exposed to air) or if the thermometer touches clothing instead of skin.

Use of the Bulb Syringe

The bulb syringe clears the upper airways of mucus and gastric secretions. Personnel first use it at birth to clear the mouth and nose to facilitate initial respirations. The bulb syringe then stays in the bassinette for use in the event of emesis. Healthy newborns have an active gag reflex and are adept at clearing their upper airways, however, and the bulb syringe may not be needed after the transitional period.

The nurse teaches parents to use the bulb syringe when secretions are visible in the baby's nose or mouth

or if the newborn is gagging or gurgling through oral fluids. Because the baby is likely to gasp when the syringe is placed into the nares, parents should suction the mouth before the nose to prevent aspiration (Kattwinkel, 2011). See Nursing Procedure 20.5.

During a gagging or choking episode, a calm but swift response is required. Parents gain confidence in their ability to handle this situation if the nurse can talk them through the skill, or, if necessary for a more timely intervention, demonstrate efficient use of the syringe. After the baby has recovered, the entire family may require comforting and reassurance.

Thomas, the 8-hour-old term newborn, started gagging and choking after vomiting some breast milk. His mother was visibly upset. How would the nurse calm her?

Urine and Stool

Urine output may be low for the first 2 days of life. The baby should void by 24 hours of age. By the third or

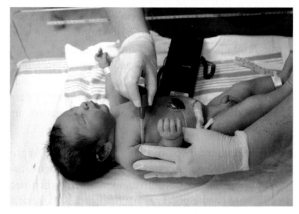

FIGURE 20.14 Taking axillary temperature in a newborn.

NURSING PROCEDURE 20.5
Suctioning With a Bulb Syringe

PURPOSE

To remove visible mucus, secretions, and vomitus from the newborn's mouth and/or nares

ASSESSMENT AND PLANNING

- Review the newborn's medical record for a history of antepartal or intrapartal problems.
- Assess the newborn's gag reflex; assess for gagging and gurgling with oral feedings.
- Auscultate the newborn's lungs *to evaluate for evidence of crackles and wheezes.*
- Inspect the newborn's mouth and nose for visible secretions or vomitus.
- Explain the procedure and its rationale to the parents.
- Gather the necessary equipment:
    - Bulb syringe (in newborn's bassinette)
    - Receptacle or tissue for discarding secretions
    - Clean gloves

IMPLEMENTATION

1. Wash hands and put on gloves.
2. Position the newborn on the side with the head slightly lower than the rest of the body *to facilitate drainage by gravity.*
3. Compress the bulb before insertion *to prevent injury to the newborn's oral mucosa.*
4. Gently insert the tip of the bulb syringe into the dependent side of the newborn's mouth *to collect drainage.*
5. Release the compression on the bulb *to allow for re-expansion and the collection of secretions.*
6. Remove the bulb syringe from the newborn's mouth and gently squeeze the bulb *to release the collected drainage into the appropriate receptacle or onto a tissue.*
7. Turn the newborn to the other side and repeat the steps to suction the other side of the newborn's mouth; if necessary, repeat the steps to suction each nares.
8. Discard the collected secretions and clean the receptacle as necessary.
9. Wash the bulb syringe in warm soapy water and rinse. Place the bulb syringe back in the newborn's bassinette for future use. Remove gloves and wash hands.
10. Reassess the newborn's lungs; provide reassurance and comforting to the parents and the newborn.

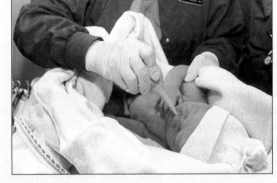

Step 7. Suctioning the newborn with a bulb syringe.

EVALUATION

- Newborn tolerated the procedure without difficulty.
- Excess secretions are removed and no longer evident.
- Lungs remained clear on auscultation.

(continued)

NURSING PROCEDURE 20.5 (CONTINUED)
Suctioning With a Bulb Syringe

AREAS FOR CONSIDERATION AND ADAPTATION

Lifespan Considerations

- As an alternative to positioning the newborn on the side in the bassinette, use the football hold with the newborn positioned on the side.
- Always suction the newborn's mouth before the nose to prevent possible aspiration of secretions as the newborn gasps when the nostril is touched.
- Never insert the bulb syringe into the middle of the newborn's mouth, toward the back of the mouth, or toward the roof of the mouth to prevent stimulating the gag reflex.
- Teach the parents how to perform suctioning with bulb syringe and signs and symptoms observed that indicate the need for suctioning; have the parents return demonstrate the procedure.
- If suctioning with bulb syringe is ineffective, anticipate the need for additional suction measures.
- Keep in mind that use of the bulb syringe is typically not necessary after the newborn's transitional period.

Community-Based Considerations

- Have the parents return-demonstrate the procedure for using the bulb syringe.
- If the infant has copious or tenacious nasal secretions, teach the parents how to instill normal saline to help loosen the secretions and aid in their removal.
- If the parents are using a humidifier in the home, review the procedure for cleaning the device to prevent growth of microorganisms.

---

fourth day, parents should note a wet diaper with every feeding—about 6 to 8 wet diapers per day.

The appearance of the first stool, called meconium, may surprise parents. This sticky black substance usually passes in the first 24 hours, although some infants do not pass meconium until 48 hours. Meconium stools persist for up to 3 days, then gradually change to the seedy yellowish colour of normal newborn stool (Fig. 20.15). Breastfed babies have softer, more liquid stools than formula-fed infants. Breastfed babies' stools are also less malodorous than stools from formula-fed babies.

Bowel movement patterns vary depending on whether the infant is breastfed or formula fed. Some breastfed infants pass stool at every feeding. Parents need to be concerned only if their baby's stool is malodorous and liquid (diarrhea stool) or if it contains mucus or blood. Newborns are rarely constipated, but parents should consult their care provider if the newborn seems to strain or cry during bowel movements or produces hard, pellet-like stools.

Diapering

Cloth or disposable diapers may be used for newborn care. Parents check the diaper when the infant awakens for a feeding. Bowel movements may occur during feeding, especially in the breastfeeding baby, which may necessitate a diaper change after feeding as well. Parents can prevent diaper rash by keeping the diaper area clean and dry. Petrolatum or petrolatum-based products will protect the perineal area from moisture (AWHONN, 2013). The buttocks and perianal region should be washed with plain or soapy water as necessary; plain water alone may not remove all feces. Stool and skin secretions can hide in vaginal folds and under the scrotum, so nurses should teach parents to wipe the vaginal area from front to back with a clean cloth, or to clean under and around the scrotal sac. Commercial diaper wipes—without alcohol or added fragrance—can be an unnecessary added expense, although they may be more comfortable than a washcloth for the infant with atopic dermatitis (AWHONN, 2013). If the diaper area is compromised with contact dermatitis, a thick application of a barrier cream or paste such as zinc oxide covers all skin that may be exposed to irritating agents. Any residual cream is not removed with a diaper change; the area should be cleaned and barrier cream reapplied (AWHONN, 2013). Parents fold the diaper down to keep the umbilicus exposed to air until after the cord falls off and the umbilical site heals (Fig. 20.16). With practice, they will be able to secure a diaper that is

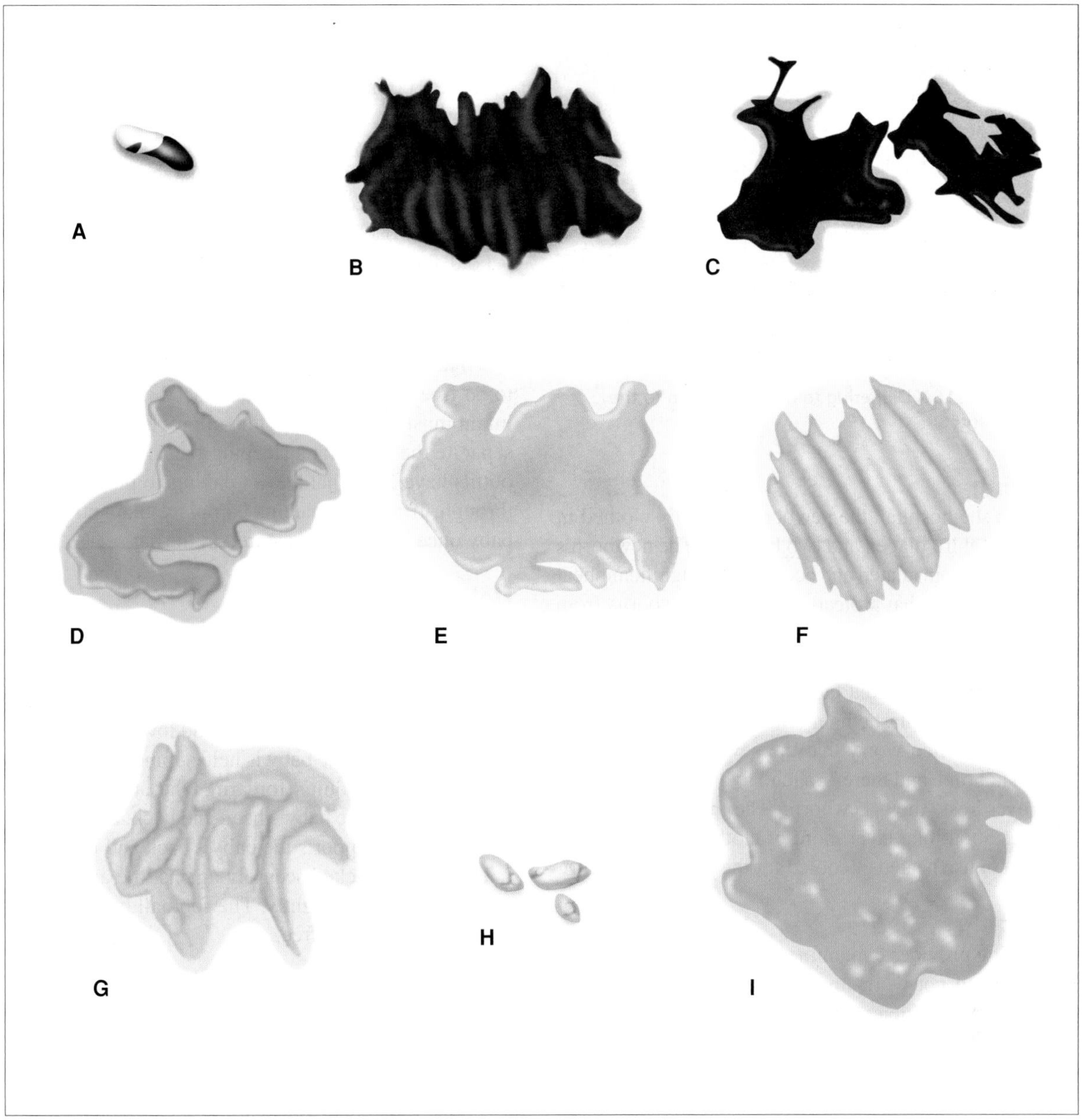

FIGURE 20.15 Characteristics of newborn stool: (**A**) meconium plug, (**B**) first meconium stool, (**C**) meconium after breastfeeding, (**D**) first transitional breastfed stool, (**E**) second transitional breastfed stool, (**F**) normal breastfed stool, (**G**) cow-milk stool, (**H**) constipated stool, (**I**) diarrheal stool.

not so tight as to press into the baby's abdomen, and not so loose as to allow the diaper to leak or fall off during handling.

Cord Care

The umbilical area is cleaned with tap water to remove any debris (AWHONN, 2013). The use of antimicrobial agents such as isopropyl alcohol, triple dye, or other agents is discouraged. Isopropyl alcohol does not decrease infection rates or bacterial colonization and increases the time for cord separation. Triple dye

can cause skin necrosis if applied to the skin and also increases the time for cord separation. Other antimicrobial agents can be absorbed into the skin because of developmental immaturity and have been associated with contact dermatitis (AWHONN, 2013). The nurse informs parents that the cord may become gooey before separation and advises parents to call the health care provider if the umbilical site becomes red or swollen, or has purulent or malodorous discharge. The parents can also be told that the stump usually drops off sometime between 5 to 13 days after birth (AWHONN, 2013).

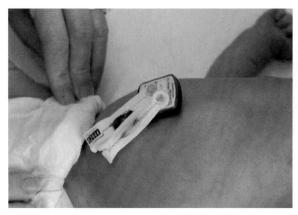

FIGURE 20.16 Diapering to avoid irritation to the umbilical area.

Clothing

While in the hospital, the newborn is usually clothed in a cotton T-shirt, diaper, and two blankets. The newborn's head is poorly insulated and accounts for significant heat loss; therefore, a hat protects vulnerable newborns from heat loss (Blackburn, 2013). The stockinette hats commonly used in hospitals are poor insulators. Preferred fabrics include insulated fabrics, wool, or polyolefin, or hats lined with a plastic liner (Blackburn, 2013).

Parents often worry that the newborn will become chilled at home and therefore tend to overheat the house and overdress their newborn. The healthy newborn requires about one layer more of clothing than the parent, in a house heated or cooled for the parent's comfort.

Wrapping

Swaddling provides containment, security, and warmth. Parents need not worry that their swaddling technique is less neat or efficient than that of the hospital staff. The nurse teaches parents how to swaddle, allowing the newborn's hands to be in close proximity to the mouth (Fig. 20.17). Hand-to-mouth behaviour is calming and an important developmental activity.

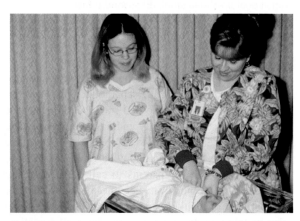

FIGURE 20.17 This nurse is teaching swaddling of a newborn to a mother.

Parents can swaddle by following these steps:

- Place a blanket on a flat surface with one corner of the blanket pointing away. Fold that corner down a few inches.
- Place the baby face up on the blanket, with the neck on the top folded edge of the blanket.
- Fold the left corner over the baby's body and tuck it under the back.
- Fold the bottom corner up over the feet and chest. Fold down any excess over the chest.
- Fold the right corner around the infant's body.

The nurse reminds parents that the baby's legs need to be free of swaddling when placed in a car seat. The infant must wear an outfit that allows the crotch strap to separate the legs (not a sleeping-bag style outfit). Some outfits have a slit that allows parents to push the buckle through. If needed, parents can place blankets over the baby once he or she is secured in the car seat.

Holding

There are two basic ways to hold a baby:

- *Cradle hold:* The baby is held supine across the adult's chest, with one arm supporting the head and neck, and the other supporting the back and lower body.
- *Football hold:* The baby is held supine along the inner aspect of the adult's forearm. The adult's hand and wrist support the baby's head and neck, and the rest of the forearm supports the baby's back and lower body. The baby is tucked securely against the adult's body, but not squeezed tightly. The football hold leaves the adult's other hand free.

Variations on these holds include the following:

- *The one-handed cradle hold:* The baby is held prone on the adult's arm, cradled against the adult's body.
- *Against the shoulder:* The baby is held upright, prone against the adult's chest, while the adult supports the baby's head and bottom.

The nurse can reassure parents that any holding position that supports the infant's head, neck, and back and prevents dangling or dropping the infant is acceptable.

Comforting

A baby's cry is a communicative signal to elicit caregiving (Zeskind, 2013). Acoustical spectrometry reveals distinct signature cries for hunger, pain, and other impetuses (Zeskind, 2013). Most parents can learn to distinguish these different cries (Lauwers & Swisher, 2010).

There is a longstanding debate about parenting practices in response to a baby's cry. Some parents practise "infant-demand" care, that is, high levels of responsiveness, breastfeeding on demand, "co-sleeping," and holding the baby. Other parents believe in routine-based or structured care. The best research evidence that has emerged from comparative studies and randomized trials is that neither of these parenting approaches is better overall; rather, there are different benefits and costs to each approach. Structured care results in babies who develop the ability to remain settled at night by 3 weeks of age. "Infant-demand" care leads to a substantial reduction in crying in the first 2 months, but to nighttime wakefulness beyond 3 months of age (St. James-Roberts, 2009).

In the "infant-demand" approach, parents can be encouraged to incorporate touching, holding, talking, and being within the newborn's field of vision when answering the cry. Skin-to-skin holding (kangaroo care) is effective (Gardner & Hernandez, 2011). Many books have been written to help parents soothe a crying baby. Suggestions include speaking softly, massaging the baby, singing, walking, or rocking (Ricci & Kyle, 2009).

The newborn who is especially sensitive to environmental stimuli may escalate crying in response to too many simultaneous quieting attempts. He or she may be overwhelmed when confronted all at once by the visual stimulation of the mother's face, as well as her voice, touch, and rocking and patting. For these newborns, the parent can experiment with a softer approach, such as briefly looking at and speaking to the newborn, then swaddling the infant or holding him or her skin to skin against her shoulder in a quiet environment. Avoiding simultaneous talking, rocking, and patting may help the newborn regain control.

Current evidence suggests (but does not confirm) that unsoothable crying bouts are common and specific to early infancy and may be the result of neurodevelopmental changes that are a normal part of development. In a small number of cases, prolonged crying in the first 3 months may be caused by food intolerance and other organic disturbances (Burns et al., 2012).

Parental Stress

Parents should know that a baby's constant demands will be stressful for them. Sometimes parents may feel angry and at risk for losing their temper. The nurse acknowledges that these feelings are normal on a tough day and a signal that the parent requires some time away. He or she helps parents plan for these times by encouraging them to arrange for a trusted friend or family member to take over baby care for a few hours, as needed. A walk around the block, warm bath, or nap can be restorative.

If no such respite care is available when the parent is losing control, the nurse can teach the parent to put the infant safely in the crib and move to another room. It is better to allow the infant to cry in the crib than to strike or shake the baby, which can cause fatalities. A parent with a fussy baby and few support systems is at risk for neglecting or abusing the newborn. The nurse is responsible for providing the parent with information about community resources to assist after discharge, such as parent support groups, parenting classes, and mother-to-mother mentoring programs.

Sleep Positioning and Sudden Infant Death Syndrome

Sudden infant death syndrome (SIDS) is defined by the Public Health Agency of Canada as "the sudden death of an infant less than one year of age which remains unexplained after a thorough case examination, including a complete autopsy, examination of the death scene, and review of the clinical history" (Public Health Agency of Canada, 2012). Although the rate of SIDS in Canada, the United States, and many other countries has declined by more than 50% over the past two decades, SIDS continues to be the leading cause of infant death, accounting for about 20% to 25% of all deaths between 1 month and 1 year of age (Kinney & Thach, 2009; Peiper & Strayer, 2013). The cause is unknown. Risk factors for SIDS include prone sleep position, sleeping on a soft surface, maternal smoking during pregnancy, overheating, late or no prenatal care, young maternal age, prematurity or LBW, and male sex. First Nations infants have a higher rate of infant mortality than non-First Nations infants, with the higher mortality rate related to causes including SIDS, infection, and other external causes (Smylie et al., 2010).

In 1992, the AAP recommended that infants be placed supine for sleeping to reduce the risk for SIDS (Fig. 20.18). Because prone sleep positioning was a modifiable risk factor, the Back to Sleep campaign was

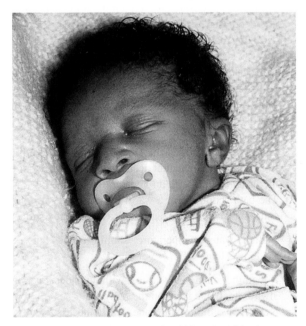

FIGURE 20.18 Newborns should be placed in the supine position when sleeping to help reduce risk of SIDS.

initiated in Canada and the United States in 1994. The campaign disseminates information to hospital nurseries and physicians, to child care education programs, and through public media campaigns.

Recommendations for parents to reduce risk of SIDS include the following (Public Health Agency of Canada, 2012):

- *Sleeping:* Put your baby to sleep on his or her back on a firm, flat surface designed for infants. Avoid soft mattresses, fluffy pillows, comforters, stuffed toys, and bumper pads in the baby's crib, as these could prevent proper air circulation around your baby's face. Plastics, such as the manufacturer's mattress wrapping, may also prevent air circulation, and should be removed to reduce the risk of SIDS. Room sharing with parent or caregiver in the first 6 months reduces the risk of SIDS. Bed sharing increases the risk of SIDS or accidental death.
- *A Smoke- and Drug-Free Environment:* Create a smoke- and drug-free environment for the baby before and after birth.
- *Dressing Baby for Sleep:* Keep your baby warm—not hot. A fitted one-piece sleep outfit that is comfortable at room temperature is recommended.
- *Breastfeeding:* Breastfeeding for any duration is protective from SIDS. Exclusive breastfeeding for the first 6 months may reduce the risk of SIDS up to 50%.

Bathing the Newborn

Only a few rules are important for infant bathing:

- Current practices range from sponge bathing to tub baths. Tub baths where the water covers the entire body helps to ensure an even temperature distribution and decreases heat loss (AWHONN, 2013).
- The baby requires a bath only once or twice a week. Parents can keep the baby's face, neck creases, and perianal area clean between baths by washing them with a cloth and plain water. Mild soap may be required to remove feces completely (AWHONN, 2013). Shampooing the hair once or twice a week is usually sufficient.
- Organize supplies before starting baths with everything within arm's reach. An extra towel is helpful to keep nearby if the parent needs to take the baby out of the water to deal with an interruption.
- The bath should be in a warm location, free of drafts, and should be in a safe place such as on a sturdy surface.

Bath water temperature should range between 38°C to less than 40°C.

- If bathing on a flat surface without sides or rails, always keep one hand on the baby.
- Never leave the infant alone. If it is necessary to get the phone or retrieve a towel from the linen closet, take the infant with you.

- Bathing products should be mild and nonirritating to the skin and eyes. Antimicrobial soaps should be avoided.
- Emollients may be used for dryness, fissures, or flaking skin (AWHONN, 2013).
- Fingernails grow quickly. Parents can file them with a soft emery board or cut them straight across with baby nail clippers or blunt-edged scissors. *Never* bite off the baby's nails—doing so can cause injury and infection. Nail care is easiest when the baby is asleep.

ADDITIONAL PARENT EDUCATION

Circumcision
Circumcision is the surgical removal of the foreskin from the end of the penis. Since ancient times in Egypt, a rationale for circumcision has been maintenance of penile hygiene; however, data fail to consistently support this association. Jewish circumcision traditionally takes place on the eighth day of the male child's life and is practised as a religious ritual, not for health (Ahmad et al., 2013). Religious circumcision is also performed for Islamic boys.

The circumcision of male infants has been a subject of debate for many years, with different benefits and risks quoted in the literature. The average complication rate is estimated to be 1.5% (Weiss et al., 2010). Most complications are minor, such as bleeding and infection, but occasionally serious complications occur (Ahmad et al., 2013).

Although circumcision remains common in the United States, it is less common in Canada and uncommon in Asia, South America, Central America, and northern Europe (WHO, 2007). In 2007, the rate of newborn circumcision in Canada was 31.9%, with wide variations across the country, for example, a high of 44.9% in Alberta to a low of 0% in Newfoundland and Labrador (Public Health Agency of Canada, 2009). Today most circumcisions are performed as an outpatient procedure.

Immunizations
Immunizations saved millions of lives in the 20th century and are an important health practice today. Without immunizations, now rare diseases are beginning to return and infect infants and children (Atkinson & Wolfe, 2012). Immunizations are safe, but not risk-free. Most side effects are mild, such as pain or soreness at the injection site. Anaphylaxis is rare, occurring on average once in every 500,000 doses, depending on the vaccine (Erlewyn-Lajeunesse et al., 2012).

In Canada the schedule of immunizations is determined by each province. While there are national recommendations and ongoing efforts to harmonize both timing

Age at vaccination	Diphtheria Tetanus Pertussis Poliomyelitis	Hib[1]	Mumps Measles Rubella	Tetanus, Diphtheria pertussis	Hepatitis B[2]	Chickenpox (Varicella)	Pneumococcal	Meningococcal conjugate	Flu	HPV[4]
Birth										
2 months	✗	✗					✗			
4 months	✗	✗					✗	Infancy 1, 2 or 3 shots depending on age or adolescence[5]	6-23 months 1-2 doses	
6 months	✗	✗			Infancy or		✗			
12 months			✗			✗	✗			
18 months	✗	✗	✗[3]							
4-6 years	✗		or ✗[3]							
9-13 years					✗					✗
14-16 years				✗						

Notes:
1. *Haemophilus influenzae* type b (Hib) requires a series of immunizations. The exact number and timing of each may vary with the type of vaccine used.
2. Hepatis B requires a series of immunizations. In some jurisdictions, they may be administered at a younger age.
3. Two-dose programs for MMR are given in all territories and provinces. Second dose MMR is given either at 18 months or 4-6 years of age.
   If the child is past the age at which the second MMR is recommended, the second dose can be given 1-2 months after the first.
4. The cost of this vaccine is not covered by all provincial/territorial health plans. You may have to pay for it yourself.
5. Recommended schedule and number of doses of meningococcal vaccine depends on the age of the child.

FIGURE 20.19 Sample Childhood immunization schedule for Ontario. For more information contact Public Health Agency of Canada. Source: Public Health Agency of Canada, http://www.phac-aspc.gc.ca/im/iyc-vve/immunizationresults-eng.php?P%2FT=9&months=7&days=5&years=2013#scheduler-frm

and financial coverage for vaccines, differences between provinces still exist (Fig. 20.19). Up-to-date information is published in the Canadian Immunization Guide, available from the Government of Canada's website (http://www.phac-aspc.gc.ca/im/ptimprog-progimpt/table-1_e.html). The Canadian Paediatric Society publishes a parent guide to immunizations entitled "Your Child's Best Shot" which can be ordered at https://bookstore.cps.ca. In addition, a free app has been developed for smart phones and other mobile devices by the Canadian Public Health Association, Immunize Canada, and the Ottawa Hospital Research Institute. This app records and stores vaccine information; provides access to vaccination schedules; manages vaccination appointments; provides access to evidence-based and expert reviews and information about recommended and routine vaccinations; and provides alerts about disease outbreaks. It is available at http://www.immunize.ca/en/app.aspx.

Prenatal blood testing for hepatitis B status is the obstetrical standard of care (Schiff et al., 2011). Women who are negative for hepatitis B surface antigen (HBsAg) may be immunized safely during pregnancy. Women not tested during pregnancy, those at high risk for infection, and those with clinical hepatitis should be tested on hospital admission (AAP & ACOG, 2012). Transmission of hepatitis B virus (HBV) from an HBsAg-positive mother to her newborn occurs primarily during childbirth. Approximately 70% to 90% of babies who become infected become chronic carriers of HBV. Preventing transmission from mother to infant, however, is possible. Perinatal HBV infection can be prevented in approximately 95% of exposed newborns who receive hepatitis B immune globulin (HBIG) within 12 hours of birth. HBIG is made of antibodies that protect against HBV, therefore providing passive immunity and immediate, although not long-term, protection. For lasting protection against HBV, the newborn must complete the three-dose immunization series (Atkinson & Wolfe, 2012). The baby may receive HBIG and HBV vaccines at the same time but at different sites (eg, in the anterolateral thigh muscle of the right and left leg). Maternal blood should be removed from the infant's skin before injection to prevent inoculation of the virus on the skin.

Parental informed consent is required before administration of HBIG or hepatitis B vaccine. Like any vaccine or medication, an adverse or allergic reaction may result. Nevertheless, HBIG and hepatitis B vaccines are very safe. Contraindications for administration include:

• The child or family has a severe allergy to baker's yeast.
• The child has had a life-threatening reaction in response to a previous dose.
• The child has a moderate or severe illness on the day the vaccination is scheduled.

Parents are provided with information on immunizations and their consent obtained prior to the administration of any immunization. Parents have the right to refuse immunization and may do so based on religious objections, a belief in homeopathy (natural health), or a belief that immunizations are ineffective or may cause harm. A study of parents' attitudes toward childhood immunizations revealed that parents want written information on immunizations and want health care providers to be aware of, and discuss, vaccine issues (Vannice et al., 2011).

Parents may voice specific concerns that vaccinations cause *autism,* a chronic developmental disorder usually identified between 18 and 30 months. This concern resulted from information in the media in the late 1990s regarding a possible link between the measles, mumps, rubella (MMR) vaccine and autism. Because vaccines, including MMR vaccine, are administered just before the peak age of onset for autism, a temporal relationship between diagnosis of autism and vaccination may be seen. At this point, health care professionals can assure parents that no convincing evidence has been found that any vaccine causes autism. This genetically based disorder has not been linked to vaccinations (Landrigan, 2011).

Signs of Newborn Illness

Many pediatric providers give parents a list of circumstances that merit a phone call or office visit. Parents need to recognize and evaluate signs of illness in a newborn immediately because newborns can develop life-threatening complications quickly. The nurse instructs parents to call their pediatric provider immediately if their baby exhibits:

- Respiratory distress, including tachypnea (more than 60 breaths/min), grunting, nasal flaring, retractions, or cyanosis
- Abdominal distention, especially if the belly is hard, or if distention is accompanied by vomiting, or there is no bowel movement for more than 1 day
- Forceful vomiting that is projectile
- Diarrhea (watery stools up to eight times per day)
- Fever (more than 37.8°C by axilla)
- Lethargy and poor feeding
- Muscle weakness
- Jitters of the whole body
- Blue colour of the face, tongue, and lips
- Persistent coughing or choking during feedings
- Excessive crying
- Watery, white, or mucous discharge from the eyes; sticky eyelashes from eye discharge
- Head-to-foot jaundice
- Umbilical cord that is red or exuding pus at the base, or that elicits a cry from the baby when touched
- Umbilicus that swells and does not dry after the umbilical cord has fallen off

Car Seats

All provinces and territories require use of a car seat or infant safety seat (Transport Canada, 2012) during any motor vehicle trip with a baby. Unfortunately, it is estimated that four out of five children are not correctly restrained in motor vehicles (Infant & Toddler Safety Association, 2012).

The nurse should become familiar with his or her institution's policy regarding the role of staff members in car seat safety. Some facilities require that nurses play an active role in placing infants in car seats and placing car seats in vehicles. Others take a "hands-off" approach—the nurse may provide verbal instructions and printed pamphlets, but parents are responsible for securing children and seats into cars. In any case, the nurse's role is to offer advice that he or she is qualified to give, and to serve as a resource for additional information.

Basic rules for car seat use apply in every case. See Figure 20.20 for correct car seat use and Teaching Tips 20.3 for written information for parents about car safety seat basics. Comprehensive information about car seats and their correct use can be found on the Transport Canada's website http://www.tc.gc.ca/eng/roadsafety/safedrivers-childsafety-index-53.htm and on the Canadian Pediatric Society's website http://www.caring forkids.cps.ca/handouts/car_seat_safety.

Siblings

Reactions of siblings to a new baby depend on age and development level (Bowden & Greenberg, 2010):

- Toddlers are likely to be upset by the change in their routine when their mother is hospitalized. They may be frightened by the unfamiliarity of the hospital environment and confused at seeing their mother in a hospital bed. Toddlers will probably be jealous of and feel displaced by the new baby. They may seek attention by misbehaving or displaying regressive behaviours, such as soiling themselves after having been successfully toilet-trained or sucking the baby's

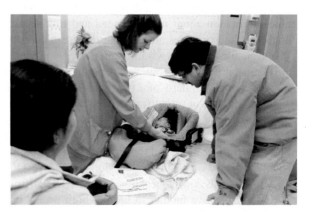

FIGURE 20.20 This nurse is checking to make sure the newborn is secured in the car seat correctly.

● TEACHING TIPS 20.3 Car Safety Seats Basics

- Use of a car safety seat may be mandatory by law. It should meet the car safety regulations from Transport Canada.
- Read the car safety seat manufacturer's instructions and always keep them in the car.
- Read your vehicle owner's manual for important information on how to install the car safety seat correctly in your vehicle, including the seating positions that can be used with the type of anchor system in the vehicle.
  - The seat should be positioned at a 45-degree angle.
  - The car seat should move no more than 2.5 cm forward or side to side when installed.
- Infants should be in rear-facing car seats until they are at least 1 year of age and weigh 10 kg.
- All children under the age of 13 years should be in the back seat; car seats should be in the middle.
- The harness straps must be snug and at or just below the baby's shoulders; the chest clip should be at the armpit level.
  - No more than one finger should fit between the shoulder harness and baby's collarbone.
  - The seat handle should be in the position recommended by the manufacturer.

- Car seats should be purchased new; a used car seat may have been in a collision.
- Replace the car seat when it has reached the expiry date. If there is no expiry date, it should be replaced when it is 10 years old, or shows any cracks or damage in the plastic.
- Do not use a car seat that has been involved in any car crash, including a minor one.
- Do not use any add-on features not provided by the manufacturer; they can affect the safety of the seat. This may include bunting bag, head-hugger, or comfort strap.
- If it is cold, tuck a blanket over the infant. Do not put anything under or behind the infant's body.
- Fill out and mail in the registration card so you can be contacted if there is any recall.

From BabyCenter. (2014). *Car seat basics in Canada.* Retrieved from http://www.babycenter.ca/a1005203/car-seat-basics-in-canada; Canadian Pediatric Society. (2011). *Car seat safety.* Retrieved from http://www.caringforkids.cps.ca/handouts/car_seat_safety

pacifier. Toddlers need extra loving attention and reassurance that they maintain their special place in the family.

- Preschoolers may feel jealousy and resentment, but discussion before the baby is born may help assuage these feelings. Parents can include preschoolers in preparations for the newborn, such as readying the crib and helping choose an outfit for the baby to wear home. If preschoolers are reassured that their status as "big sister or brother" benefits the entire family, and if they receive some special alone time with parents, they will cope more readily with changes.
- School-age children and adolescents should not feel overly threatened by the new baby. Many older children and teens are interested in the processes of pregnancy and birth and may enjoy assuming the role of older sibling. They probably will like helping with caregiving by feeding, holding, and playing with the newborn (Fig. 20.21). Parents can ensure special time alone with older siblings, and reassure them that plenty of love and attention is available for everyone.

Pet Safety

Parents can attempt to prepare pets for a new baby's arrival, although knowing whether such preparation actually works is impossible. Every pet's reaction to a new baby is unique, although knowing the pet's temperament (eg, high-strung, demanding, easy-going, moody) before the baby comes home yields many clues as to how the pet may react. Parents can bring a blanket to the hospital and use it to wrap the newborn for a period, then bring the blanket home to the pet and "introduce" the baby's scent to the animal. In any event, if the pet is used to being the centre of attention in the household, the pet may feel jealous and misbehave or

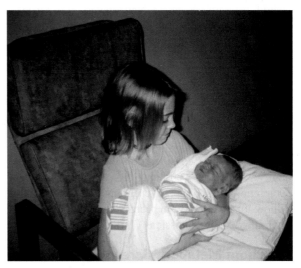

FIGURE 20.21 This older school-age child is enjoying holding her new baby sibling.

act aggressively toward other pets, family members, or the newborn.

Parents are usually eager to introduce the new baby to the family pet. This process should be gradual, and adults must closely supervise the behaviour of a pet that could potentially bite or injure the baby. They should never leave the animal alone with the baby. The animal usually grows accustomed to the newborn in 2 to 3 weeks; however, parents must be observant and cautious whenever the animal is around the baby.

Dangers of Secondhand Smoke

Passive smoking is harmful to children's respiratory health. Children exposed to secondhand tobacco smoke have increased rates of respiratory infections, middle ear effusion, asthma, and SIDS (Health Canada, 2011).

If the baby is in an environment with smokers, certain precautions can help protect the baby's health:

- No one should smoke in any area where the baby is living. The smoker must smoke outside the baby's living environment.
- If the smoker takes care of the baby, the smoker can cover his or her clothing while smoking. The smoker may use a designated shirt or jacket, which he or she wears only while outside smoking.
- No one should smoke in a car that the baby rides in, even when the baby is not in the car. As of 2013, all provinces except Quebec have made it illegal to smoke in a car in which a child is riding (CTV.ca, 2013).

The nurse caring for infants or new mothers plays a vital role in identifying families at risk from tobacco exposure. His or her role is to motivate, advise, and assist parents in starting a smoking cessation program.

Household Safety

The parent of a newborn may not be thinking yet of "child-proofing" the home. Nevertheless, it is never too early to begin to identify potential safety hazards. Even a young infant can grasp a dangerous object or roll off a bed or changing table.

READINESS FOR HOSPITAL DISCHARGE

When planning for discharge from hospital, it is important to take into consideration the physical, psychological, and social well-being of both mother and baby. Community-based support programs and post-discharge follow-up are effective in decreasing neonatal mortality, morbidity, and readmissions (Farhat & Rajab, 2011).

Newborn Metabolic Screening

Each province regulates newborn metabolic screening tests. The purpose of a metabolic screening program is to prevent complications of genetic diseases through early identification and treatment. Metabolic and genetic testing in Canada is not mandated by law, and the number of diseases included in screening programs varies (Canadian Organization for Rare Disorders, 2010). With evolving technology, the number of genetic metabolic illnesses for which screening can be done is growing constantly, and new variants of disease conditions continue to be found. Table 20.5 outlines the common metabolic diseases that are screened for in Canada.

Nurses understand that metabolic screening tests simply identify infants whose results indicate a need for further testing and diagnostic evaluation (Prows, 2011). Each hospital will have established procedures to ensure that newborn metabolic screening tests are performed before hospital discharge.

Umbilical cord blood is not adequate for testing disorders that exhibit metabolite accumulation after birth or after feeding (Prows, 2011). Ideally, the blood sample is collected between 48 and 72 hours of age; however, some healthy term newborns are discharged from the hospital before this time. Babies tested earlier than 24 hours of age (and, in some provinces, all babies) are usually retested by a pediatric care provider by 2 weeks of age to ensure detection of phenylketonuria (PKU) and congenital hypothyroidism. A heelstick sample is usually obtained. See Nursing Procedure 20.6 for an example of the heelstick collection technique.

Auditory Screening

Permanent childhood hearing loss occurs in 1.4 per 1,000 healthy newborns (CDC, 2012); 1% to 10% of premature, LBW infants have hearing impairment (Daily et al., 2011). If hearing loss is detected and appropriate interventions are made by 6 months of age, normal development can be expected. If diagnosis or treatment is delayed for longer than 6 months, however, permanent developmental delays can occur in otherwise normal babies (Wheeler, 2011).

Although in the United States newborn hearing screening is becoming the hospital standard of care, in Canada the implementation of hearing screening is variable. Some hospitals screen all newborns, while others have developed a risk-based screening program. Nurses should be familiar with the risks of congenital hearing loss and the hearing screening policies in their institution.

Hearing loss detected in the neonatal period results from various causes:

- Heredity
- Perinatal factors, such as congenital malformations of the head and neck
- Very low birth weight (VLBW) (below 1,500 g)
- Congenital infections (eg, cytomegalovirus, rubella, herpes, syphilis, toxoplasmosis)

● TABLE 20.5 **Common Newborn Screening Tests**

Test/Disorder Screened	Incidence	Characteristics	Treatment
Medium-chain acyl-CoA dehydrogenase (MCAD) deficiency	1 in 12,000	An inherited disorder of fatty acid metabolism caused by lack of an enzyme required to convert fat to energy. Seemingly well infants or children can suddenly develop seizures, respiratory failure, cardiac arrest, coma, and death. Identifying affected children before they become ill is vital to preventing a crisis and averting these consequences.	Frequent feeding or glucose intake and avoidance of fasting
Phenylketonuria (PKU)	1 in 12,000	An inability to properly process the essential amino acid phenylalanine, which then accumulates and damages the brain. PKU can cause severe intellectual disability unless detected soon after birth and treated with a special formula.	A low phenylalanine diet at least throughout childhood and adolescence and, for females, during pregnancy
Congenital hypothyroidism	1 in 4,000	Thyroid hormone deficiency that severely compromises both growth and brain development.	Oral doses of thyroid hormone
Congenital adrenal hyperplasia	1 in 16,000	A set of inherited disorders resulting from defects in the synthesis of hormones produced by the adrenal gland. Certain severe forms can cause life-threatening salt loss from the body.	Salt and hormone replacement
Glutaric aciduria type 1	Rare in general population. More common in certain ethnic groups	Deficiency of glutaryl-CoA dehydrogenase enzyme, an enzyme that breaks down amino acids. Infants with severe GA1 develop metabolic crisis triggered by illness or fever resulting in encephalopathy, coma, and, sometimes, death.	Frequent feeding or glucose especially during illness. Low-protein diet.
Maple syrup urine disease	1 in 185,000	Rare inborn error of metabolism that ranges from mild to severe. Severely affected babies rarely survive for more than 1 mo; those who do survive usually have irreversible intellectual disability. Early detection and treatment are vital for normal outcomes.	A special diet that requires frequent monitoring and must be continued indefinitely
Galactosemia	1 in 40,000	Lack of the liver enzyme needed to convert galactose into glucose. Galactose accumulates in and damages vital organs, leading to blindness, intellectual disability, infection, and death.	Elimination of milk and other dairy products from diet
Homocystinuria	1 in 200,000	Deficiency of the enzyme that converts homocysteine into cystathionine, needed by the brain for normal development. Can lead to intellectual disability, eye problems, skeletal abnormalities, and stroke.	Special diet with high doses of vitamin B_6 or B_{12}
Sickle-cell anemia	As high as 1:400 in individuals from the Caribbeans and parts of Africa	Blood disease that can cause severe pain, damage to vital organs, stroke, and early death.	Vigilant medical care, treatment with penicillin
Cystic fibrosis	1 in 3,600	Defect in chloride channel protein resulting in thick mucous secretions which damage the lung and pancreas	Breathing exercises, physical therapy, supplementation of digestive enzymes

From Perinatal Services BC: British Columbia Newborn Screening Program. Retrieved from http://www.perinatalservicesbc.ca/ScreeningPrograms/NewbornScreening/healthcare-providers/disorders-screened.htm

NURSING PROCEDURE 20.6

Performing a Heelstick on a Newborn

PURPOSE

To obtain a blood specimen for analysis

ASSESSMENT AND PLANNING

- Check the medical record to ensure that the newborn has received vitamin K.
- Assess the lower extremities for colour and warmth; if necessary, apply a warm moist pack or compress to the heel area for several minutes *to promote vasodilation.*
- Review the order for type of testing to be performed; ensure that an appropriate laboratory request form has been completed.
- Explain the reason for the procedure to the parents if appropriate.
- Gather the necessary equipment:
  - Alcohol wipes
  - Clean gloves
  - Specimen container
  - Skin puncturing device
  - Sterile gauze pads
  - Tape

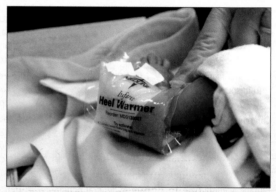

Application of a warming pad to the newborn's heel.

IMPLEMENTATION

1. Wash hands and put on clean gloves.
2. Remove the warm moist pack if applied.
3. Inspect the lateral aspects of the newborn's foot *to select a site that is free of nerves and major arteries.*
4. Support the foot with one hand covering the palmar aspect *to prevent inadvertent puncture to an area rich in nerves and major blood vessels.*
5. Palpate the selected site *to ensure that adequate padding is over the bone.*
6. Clean the site with an alcohol wipe or according to agency policy; allow to air dry.
7. Use an automated lancet device according to the manufacturer's instructions. Discard the sharp in the sharps container.
8. Obtain the first drop of blood and wipe away with a dry gauze pad *to prevent contaminating or diluting the specimen.* Obtain a second drop of blood and, if necessary, gently milk the foot instead of squeezing to obtain this drop of blood *to ensure accuracy of the results.*
9. Collect the specimen as indicated and send to the laboratory or process the specimen at the bedside, depending on agency policy.

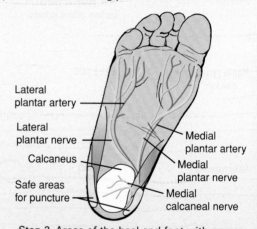

Step 3. Areas of the heel and foot with nerves and arteries.

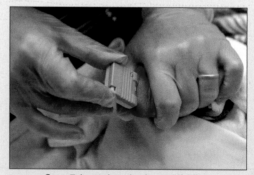

Step 7. Inserting the lancet device.

(continued)

NURSING PROCEDURE 20.6 (CONTINUED)
Performing a Heelstick on a Newborn

10. Apply a pressure dressing of gauze and tape to the puncture site *to ensure hemostasis.*
11. Remove gloves and wash hands; document procedure and disposition of the specimen.
12. Provide comfort to the newborn after the procedure.

EVALUATION

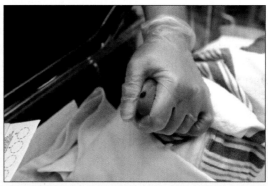

Step 8. Obtaining the first drop of blood for testing.

* Specimen is obtained without undue pain or discomfort to the newborn and sent to the laboratory.
* Newborn tolerates the procedure well.

AREAS FOR CONSIDERATION AND ADAPTATION

Lifespan Considerations

* If a pressure dressing is unavailable, use an alternate means of ensuring hemostasis by applying direct pressure to the site for several minutes until the bleeding has ceased; then apply an adhesive bandage to the site.
* When applying a warm moist pack to the newborn's heel area, check the temperature of the pack to prevent thermal injury.
* Substitute a warm washcloth, towel, or diaper for the warm moist pack if a commercial pack is unavailable. However, it is important to ensure that the cloth not be warmed in the microwave and that there are not hotspots that could result in burns to the skin.
* If the infant is somewhat older, anticipate the need to gently immobilize the lower leg temporarily to prevent sudden movements during the procedure, which may cause injury.

Community-Based Considerations

* Heelsticks may be used in the home setting to obtain blood specimens in newborns and infants. Always check with the laboratory for any specific requirements or modifications that may be necessary.
* Instruct the parents to apply topical anesthetic if ordered at the specified time before the procedure to minimize pain.

---

* Hyperbilirubinemia requiring exchange transfusion
* Apgar score of 0 to 4 at 1 minute, or 0 to 6 at 5 minutes
* Mechanical ventilation lasting 5 days or longer
* Any syndrome known to include hearing loss
* Bacterial meningitis
* Ototoxic drugs (eg, gentamicin, furosemide)

Hearing loss ranges in degree from minimal to profound. Two types are possible. If a problem lies in the outer or middle ear, the hearing loss is termed *conductive,* which can be corrected medically or surgically. If the problem is detected in the cochlea, the hearing loss is called *sensorineural.* To date, sensorineural hearing loss cannot be reversed, but it may be possible to enhance hearing through amplification. Hearing loss may also be a mix of the two types (American Speech-Language-Hearing Association, 2013).

Hospital-based screening is not diagnostic and should be followed up with re-evaluation and referral to specialists.

Post-Discharge Follow-Up

Any newborn discharged before 48 hours of age is ideally examined again within 48 hours of discharge. For healthy term newborns, the frequency of subsequent visits varies by region but should follow the Canadian Task Force on Preventive Health Care guidelines (http://canadiantaskforce.ca). Early visits include important assessments of growth (weight gain, occipital-frontal circumference, and length), general health, and attainment of developmental milestones. Immunizations should be administered according to the childhood immunization schedule. Pediatric visits also give providers an opportunity to assess parent–infant attachment; parenting skills, including breastfeeding; any remarkable stressors such as postpartum depression, intimate partner violence, or substance use; and any evidence of child neglect or abuse. Every province mandates health care professionals to report cases of suspected child abuse.

SUMMARY

- Fetal lungs are filled with fluid, not with air.
- Fetal circulation involves two important cardiac shunts, the ductus arteriosus and the foramen ovale. These shunts divert oxygenated blood to the brain and other vital organs, away from fetal lungs.
- Blood vessels in the fetal lungs are tightly constricted, and blood pressure is high (high pulmonary vascular resistance). The systemic blood pressure in the fetus is low (low systemic vascular resistance). With the newborn's first strong breaths, oxygen entering the lungs causes the vessels in the lungs to relax and allows blood to perfuse the newborn's lungs, and blood pressure in the baby's body increases. This rise in systemic vascular resistance closes the cardiac shunts and establishes newborn circulation.
- Pulmonary alveolar surfactant is a fatty substance produced by cells in the lungs. Surfactant is essential to lung function because it allows the alveoli to remain open, instead of collapsing during exhalation. Surfactant production peaks at about 35 weeks' gestation, which is why babies born before this time are likely to have surfactant deficiency, resulting in respiratory distress syndrome.
- A baby at birth who breathes or cries, demonstrates good muscle tone, and appears to be at term gestation requires little resuscitative assistance. The nurse need only provide warmth, clear the airway with a bulb syringe if necessary, and dry the baby to prevent cold stress.
- The Apgar score is a system used to evaluate the newborn at 1 and 5 minutes of age by assigning 0 to 2 points to each of five components: colour, heart rate, reflex irritability, muscle tone, and respiratory effort. Most healthy, term newborns receive a score between 7 and 9.
- The Apgar score reflects the newborn's response to extrauterine transition and resuscitative efforts, but is not used to determine the need for resuscitation. The Apgar score is not predictive of neurologic outcome.

- A newborn is term, preterm, or postterm, depending on gestational age. In addition, the newborn is SGA, AGA, or LGA, depending on weight, head circumference, and length in relation to the gestational age.
- A physical assessment should proceed with observation, auscultation, and palpation, in that order.
- The nurse can quickly approximate gestational age by assessing maturational characteristics of the infant's ear pinna, nipples, genitalia, and sole creases.
- The newborn has two sleep and four awake states: deep sleep, light sleep, drowsy, quiet alert, active alert, and crying. Each state has implications for caregiving.
- The newborn learns to control his or her environment by displaying approach cues, indicating a readiness to interact, and avoidance cues, indicating the need to disengage from interaction.
- Some newborns exhibit signs of respiratory distress immediately after birth, but a healthy newborn steadily improves and stabilizes over a short time.
- A newborn with abnormal transition shows signs of distress and does not improve or deteriorates. Signs of abnormal transition include respiratory distress, poor perfusion, hypotonia, marked jitteriness, temperature instability, abdominal distention, vomiting of bilious material, and frequent choking accompanied by apnea or cyanosis.
- The newborn transfers heat to and from the body surface in four ways: evaporation, conduction, convection, and radiation.
- The ill or the LBW newborn is at risk for hypoglycemia.
- Signs of neonatal hypoglycemia include jitteriness, hypothermia, lethargy, hypotonia, high-pitched or weak cry, apnea, respiratory distress, poor suck, vomiting, cyanosis, and seizures. A hypoglycemic newborn may be asymptomatic.
- Forty-five to sixty percent of term newborns become jaundiced in the first week of life owing to RBC hemolysis and immature liver function. Jaundice in the first 24 hours of life is never normal.
- The newborn is susceptible to infection due to immature immunologic responses to infection and because of delayed or decreased immune response due to the newborn's lack of exposure to common organisms.
- The best infection prevention strategy is thorough hand washing.
- The nurse promotes normal transition by avoiding mother–infant separation, handling the newborn gently, using containment, avoiding frequent and deep suction, avoiding bright light in the infant's face, and avoiding rectal temperature assessment.
- Acrocyanosis is normal in the few days of life, especially if the baby is exposed to cool temperatures; central cyanosis indicates hypoxia and an emergent need for supplemental oxygen.

- A healthy newborn has pink lips and mucous membranes, an axillary temperature in the range of 36.5° to 37.3°C, a heart rate of 110 to 160 beats/min, and a respiratory rate of 40 to 60 breaths/min. The healthy newborn urinates by 24 hours of age and passes meconium by 48 hours of age.
- The cause of SIDS is unknown. Risk factors for SIDS include prone sleep position, sleeping on a soft surface, maternal smoking during pregnancy, overheating, late or no prenatal care, young maternal age, prematurity or LBW, and male sex.
- The health care provider must assess the cultural and spiritual beliefs of the client. It is not safe to stereotype the behaviour or beliefs of a person from a designated ethnic group by assuming that literature about cultural practices applies to everyone within the specified ethnic group.
- Parent education before discharge includes temperature taking, use of the bulb syringe, normal amounts of urine and stool, diapering, dressing, and bathing, cord care, sleep position, car seat use, dangers of secondhand smoke, circumcision care, and signs of newborn illness.

Questions to Ponder

1. Laurie was born by scheduled repeat cesarean section to a 32-year-old woman. The mother had a healthy, uneventful pregnancy of 38 weeks' gestation by ultrasound. Apgar scores were 7 at 1 minute and 8 at 5 minutes. Laurie required less than 1 minute of free-flow oxygen for central cyanosis after delivery. Free-flow oxygen was gradually withdrawn, and her lips and mucous membranes remained pink in room air. Laurie appeared to be in good condition and was wrapped in a warm blanket, given to her father to hold in the operating room, and viewed and touched by her mother.

    Laurie is now 15 minutes old. She is lying supine on the radiant warmer with the thermistor probe in place. Her axillary temperature is 36.5°C, heart rate is 152 beats/min without murmur, and respiratory rate is 80 breaths/min with mild intermittent expiratory grunting, nasal flaring, and intercostal retracting. She has bilateral breath sounds and crackles. She has active bowel sounds. She is active and alert, with symmetric movement and good muscle tone.
    - Would you expect Laurie to be a healthy, at-risk, or ill baby?
    - Are any assessment findings of concern at this time?
    - Would any further assessment information be helpful in determining Laurie's status?

2. Ms. Chung comes to the nurses' station with her baby in her arms. You are not familiar with the Chung family. Ms. Chung asks for a warm blanket for her baby, because he is shivering. You accompany Ms. Chung back to her room and assess the infant. The baby is mottled, cool to the touch, and jittery. His cry is high-pitched. His T-shirt is wet in a large area on the front. He appears to weigh about 2,500 g.
    - How do you explain Baby Chung's "shivering" to his mother?
    - What are Baby Chung's possible problems?
    - What further information do you want to know about Baby Chung?
    - What are immediate nursing interventions for Baby Chung?

3. Ms. Taylor is 19 years old, a single woman with an uncomplicated pregnancy and delivery of her first baby. Her mother is with her. Sierra is a 2-day-old, 38-week, AGA healthy girl. You walk into Ms. Taylor's room just as Sierra begins to stir and cry. Ms. Taylor picks her up immediately and holds her under the armpits. Sierra dangles, without a blanket around her, about 25 cm away from her mother's face. "Why are you crying now?" she asks loudly, peering at Sierra intensely. The baby turns her head and cries louder and harder. Ms. Taylor rearranges her, holding her head in one hand, and supporting her bottom in the other. She bounces Sierra up and down rapidly and repeatedly speaks her name into her face. The baby arches away from her and cries louder. Grandmother Taylor then takes the baby from her daughter and begins her own bouncing, up and down and sideways in a face-to-face position, just as her daughter had done. Then she begins to walk quickly back and forth across the room as she bounces and speaks directly into her face.

    Sierra is screaming frantically now, waving her arms and legs. Ms. Taylor and her mother glare at each other, then turn and look at you.
    - What is your assessment of Sierra's behavioural state and cues?
    - What are your observations about how Sierra, her mother, and her grandmother are interacting?
    - What is your approach to supportive teaching in this situation? What interventions might help Sierra regain state control?

4. Think back to Thomas, the 40-week gestation infant from the opening scenario experiencing emesis following breastfeeding. By the second day of life Thomas is feeding 3 to 3½ hours. He continues to have a small emesis after a number of his feeds, and his mother is worried about whether or not he is taking enough milk.
    - What teaching would you provide regarding assessing the adequacy of breast milk intake?

- What suggestions can you make that might decrease the amount of emesis that Thomas has?
- How would you assess whether or not Thomas's mother is comfortable in dealing with a choking episode at home?

5. Think back to William, the 2-day-old, 37-week gestation newborn with mild jaundice.
   - What risk factors might William have that would make you more concerned about pathologic rather than physiologic jaundice?
   - What might you tell William's father about where to find reliable information about baby care on the Internet?

REVIEW QUESTIONS

1. The nurse educator is teaching a group of student nurses the differences between fetal and newborn circulation. Which of the following statements about fetal circulation would indicate that the educator's teaching plan has been successful?
   A. Fetal circulation is characterized by high pulmonary vascular resistance and high systemic vascular resistance.
   B. Fetal circulation is characterized by low pulmonary vascular resistance and low systemic vascular resistance.
   C. Fetal circulation is characterized by high pulmonary vascular resistance and low systemic vascular resistance.
   D. Fetal circulation is characterized by low pulmonary vascular resistance and high systemic vascular resistance.

2. When performing an initial newborn assessment, which of the following parameters would be most important to assess in the first minute of life?
   A. Colour, respirations, heart rate
   B. Gestational age, sex, muscle tone
   C. Weight, length, head circumference
   D. Colour, respirations, temperature

3. Oxygen administration would most likely be required 90 seconds after birth in a newborn with:
   A. Acrocyanosis
   B. Jaundice
   C. Central cyanosis
   D. Circumoral cyanosis

4. The nurse is reporting a newborn's Apgar scores to the baby's parents. The father asks what the information means. Which of the following responses, if made by the nurse, would be most appropriate?
   A. Apgar scores help determine which steps of resuscitation are required.
   B. Apgar scores reflect the newborn's response to extrauterine transition and resuscitation efforts.
   C. Apgar scores are assessed at 1, 3, and 5 minutes of age.
   D. Apgar scores are the best predictor of neurologic outcome.

5. A nurse is collecting data for a baby with suspected neonatal hypoglycemia. Which of the following sets of findings would support this diagnosis?
   A. Jitteriness, high-pitched cry, lethargy
   B. Plethoric, excess mucus production, dysrhythmia
   C. Blood glucose level of 2.7 mmol/L, no crying, fever
   D. Apnea, bradycardia, fever

6. Which of the following scenarios most clearly depicts abnormal newborn transition?
   A. Term baby; vaginal birth; Apgar scores 5 (1 minute), 8 (5 minutes); required brief free-flow oxygen for central cyanosis after birth; now 20 minutes old and pink in room air; respiratory rate 68 breaths/min; bilateral crackles heard with auscultation.
   B. Term baby; vaginal birth; Apgar scores 8 (1 minute), 9 (5 minutes); now 10 minutes old; pink when active and crying; dusky when quiet.
   C. Term baby; scheduled repeat cesarean birth; now 15 minutes old; pink with marked acrocyanosis; respiratory rate 72 breaths/min; intermittent expiratory grunting and nasal flaring.
   D. Term baby; emergency cesarean birth for fetal distress; Apgar scores 6 (1 minute), 8 (5 minutes); required free flow oxygen until 3 minutes of age, now 25 minutes old; pale pink and quiet alert; respiratory rate 68 breaths/min with periodic breathing noted.

7. When educating parents of a newborn regarding when to contact the newborn's care provider, the best statement by the nurse would be:
   A. Contact the provider if the newborn has not voided within 24 hours and passed meconium within 48 hours of birth.
   B. Contact the provider if the newborn has not voided within 12 hours and passed meconium within 24 hours of birth.
   C. Contact the provider if the newborn has not voided and passed meconium within 4 hours after the first feeding.
   D. Contact the provider if the newborn has not voided and passed meconium at least once every 8 hours times three.

8. Which of the following statements by the father of a newborn diagnosed with physiologic jaundice indicates that teaching has been effective?
   A. Physiologic jaundice is a normal result of immature liver function.
   B. Physiologic jaundice is uncommon in term infants like my baby.

C. I should have noticed the jaundice in the baby's first 24 hours.

D. The baby will have ongoing problems with his skin colouring.

9. When providing anticipatory guidance to a group of expectant parents, the nurse correctly identifies the preferred sleeping position for a term, healthy newborn as:

A. Prone

B. Supine

C. Dorsal recumbent

D. Side-lying with a blanket roll for support

10. The nurse is teaching a new mother about common signs of newborn illness. Which of the following sets of findings would the nurse alert the mother to look for and to report?

A. Respiratory distress and temperature instability

B. Fever and soft frequent stools

C. Sweating and shivering

D. Periodic breathing and nevus simplex

REFERENCES

Adamkin, D. H., & Committee on Fetus and Newborn. (2011). Postnatal glucose homeostasis in late-preterm and term infants. *Pediatrics, 127*(3), 575–579. doi:10.1542/peds.2010–3851

Ahmad, S., Goel, K., Pandey, S., Goel, P., Parashar, P., & Bhatnagar, A. (2013). Male circumcision: A modern surgical procedure and a solution to the problem. *International Journal of Contemporary Surgery, 1*(1), 15–18.

American Academy of Pediatrics, & American College of Obstetricians and Gynecologists. (2012). *Guidelines for perinatal care* (7th ed.). Elk Grove Village, IL: American Academy of Pediatrics.

American College of Nurse-Midwives. (2011). *Position statement: Home birth.* Retrieved from http://www.midwife.org/ACNM/files/ACNMLibraryData/UPLOADFILENAME/000000000251/Home%20Birth%20Aug%202011.pdf

American Speech-Language-Hearing Association. (2013). *Types of hearing loss.* Retrieved from http://www.asha.org/public/hearing/disorders/types.htm

Apgar, V. (1953). A proposal for a new method of evaluation of the newborn infant. *Anesthesia and Analgesia, 32*, 260.

Apgar, V. (1966). The newborn (Apgar) scoring system: Reflections and advice. *Pediatric Clinics of North America, 113*, 645–650.

Association of Ontario Midwives. (ND). *Neonatal eye prophylaxis.* Retrieved from http://www.aom.on.ca/Communications/Position_Statements/Neonatal_Eye_Prophylaxis.aspx

Association of Women's Health, Obstetric, and Neonatal Nurses (AWHONN). (2013). *Neonatal skin care: Evidence based clinical practice guideline* (3rd ed.). Washington, DC: Author.

Atkinson, W., & Wolfe, C. (2012). *Epidemiology and prevention of vaccine-preventable diseases* (12th ed.). Atlanta, GA: Centers for Disease Control.

Ballard, J. L., Novak, K. K., & Driver, M. (1979). A simplified score for assessment of fetal maturation of newly born infants. *Journal of Pediatrics, 95*(5), 769–774.

Ballard, J. L., Khoury, J. C., Wedig, I. K., Wang, L., Eilers-Walsman, B. L., & Lipp, R. (1991). New Ballard score, expanded to include extremely premature infants. *Journal of Pediatrics, 119*(3), 417–423.

Bhutani, V. K., Vilms, R. J., & Hamerman-Johnson, L. (2010). Universal bilirubin screening for severe neonatal hyperbilirubinemia. *Journal of Perinatology, 30*, S6–S15.

Blackburn, S. T. (2013). *Maternal, fetal, & neonatal physiology: A clinical perspective* (4th ed.). St. Louis, MO: Saunders Elsevier.

Bowden, V. & Greenberg, C. *Children and their families: The continuum of care* (2nd ed.). Philadelphia, PA: Lippincott Williams & Wilkins.

Brazelton, T. B. (1978). The Brazelton Neonatal Behavior Assessment Scale. Introduction. *Monographs of the Society for Research in Child Development, 43*(5–6), 1–13.

Brown, V., & Landers, S. (2011). Heat balance. In S. Gardner, B. Carter, M. Enzman-Hines, & J. Hernandez (Eds.), *Merenstein & Gardner's handbook of neonatal intensive care* (7th ed., pp. 113–133). St. Louis, MO: Mosby.

Burns, C. E., Dunn, A. M., Brady, M. A., Starr, N. B., & Blosser, C. (2012). *Pediatric primary care* (5th ed.). St. Louis, MO: Elsevier.

Butterfield, L. J. (1962). Practical epigram of the Apgar score. *Journal of the American Medical Association, 208*, 353.

Callister, L. C. (2011). Global and cultural perinatal nursing research: Improving clinical practice. *Journal of Perinatal and Neonatal Nursing, 25*(2), 139–143.

Canadian Organization for Rare Disorders. (2010). *Newborn Screening in Canada Status Report.* Retrieved from http://raredisorders.ca/documents/CanadaNBSstatusupdatedNov.112010.pdf

Canadian Paediatric Society. (2011). Addendum to the NRP provider textbook 6th Edition: Recommendation for specific modifications in the Canadian context. Retrieved from http://www.cps.ca/nrp/2011-NRP-Cdn-Addendum-en-Jan-2013.pdf

Canadian Paediatric Society. (2012). *Clinical and educational frequently asked questions* (FAQs). Retrieved from https://cps.ca/nrp/FAQClinicalEdu.htm

Cavaliere, T. (2009). Genitourinary assessment. In E. P. Tappero & M. E. Honeyfield (Eds), *Physical assessment of the newborn: A comprehensive approach to the art of physical examination* (4th ed., pp. 115–132). Santa Rosa, CA: NICU Ink Book Publishers.

Centers for Disease Control and Prevention. (2012). *Summary of 2009 National CDC EHDI Data.* Retrieved from http://www.cdc.gov/ncbddd/hearingloss/2009-data/2009_ehdi_hsfs_summary_508_ok.pdf

Chiu, S. H., Anderson, G. C., & Burkhammer, M. D. (2005). Newborn temperature during skin-to-skin breastfeeding in couples having breastfeeding difficulties. *Birth Issues in Perinatal Care, 32*(2), 115–121.

College of Midwives of Ontario. (ND). *The facts about home birth in Ontario.* Accessed from http://www.cmo.on.ca/documents/home-birth-sheet-FINAL.pdf

CTV.ca. (2013). *Cancer Society wants to ban smoking in cars with child passengers.* Retrieved from http://montreal.ctvnews.ca/cancer-society-wants-to-ban-smoking-in-cars-with-child-passengers-1.1301215

Daily, D., Carter, A., & Carter, B. (2011). Discharge planning and follow-up of the neonatal intensive care unit infant. In S. Gardner, B. Carter, M. Enzman-Hines, & J. Hernandez (Eds.), *Merenstein & Gardner's handbook of neonatal intensive care* (7th ed., pp. 938–961). St. Louis, MO: Mosby.

Dalley, M. L. (2008). *Infant abduction from Canadian hospitals.* Retrieved from http://cpc.phippsinc.com/cpclib/pdf/74193e.pdf

Darling, E. K., & McDonald, H. (2010). A meta-analysis of the efficacy of ocular prophylactic agents used for the prevention of Gonococcal and Chlamydial ophthalmia neonatorum. *Journal of Midwifery & Women's Health, 55*(4), 319–327.

Department of Midwifery, BC Women's. (2007). *Newborn eye prophylaxis.* Retrieved from http://www.midwivesinvancouver.ca/docs/Eye_Prophylaxis_Guideline.pdf

Dilen, B., & Elseviers, M. (2010). Oral glucose solution as pain relief in newborns: Results of a clinical trial. *Birth, 27*(2), 98–105.

Dominguez-Bello, M., Costello, E., Contreras, M., Magis, M., Hidalgo, G., Fierer, M., et al. (2010). Delivery mode shapes the acquisition and structure of the initial microbiota across multiple body habitats in newborns. *Proceedings of the National Academy of Sciences of the United States of America, 26*, 11971–11975.

Dubowitz, L., Dubowitz, V., & Goldberg, C. (1970). Clinical assessment of gestational age in the newborn infant. *Journal of Pediatrics, 77*(1), 1–10.

Dumas, L., Lepage, M., Bystrova, K., Matthiesen, A. S., Welles-Nystrom, B., & Widstrom, A. M. (2013). Influence of skin-to-skin contact and rooming-in on early mother-infant interaction: A randomized controlled trial. *Clinical Nursing Research, 22*(3), 310–336.

Duru, C. O., Akinbami, F. O., & Orimadegun, A. (2012). A comparison of tympanic and rectal temperatures in term Nigerian neonates. *BioMed Central Pediatrics, 12*, 86.

Dyer, J. A. (2013). Newborn skin care. *Seminars in Perinatology, 37*(1), 3–7.

Elizabeth, K. E., & Jacob, A. M. (2012). *Pedibloom: Pediatric cases and summaries.* London: JP Medical.

Erlewyn-Lajeunesse, M., Hunt, L., Heath, P., & Finn, A. (2012). Anaphylaxis as an adverse event following immunization in the UK and Ireland. *Archives of Disease in Childhood, 97*(6), 487–490.

Fabris, C., & Coscia, A. (2012). Physical examination of the newborn. In G. Buonocore, R. Bracci, & M. Weindling (Eds.), *Neonatology: A practical approach to neonatal diseases* (pp. 232–241). New York: Springer.

Farhat, R., & Rajab, M. (2011). Length of postnatal hospital stay in healthy newborns and re-hospitalization following early discharge. *North American Journal of Medical Sciences, 3*(3), 146–151.

Gaillard, R., de Ridder, M., Verburg, B., Witteman, J., Mackenbach, J., Moll, H., et al. (2011). Individually customized fetal weight charts derived from ultrasound measurements: The Generation R study. *European Journal of Epidemiology, 26*(12), 919–926.

Gardner, S., & Hernandez, J. (2011). Initial nursery care. In S. Gardner, B. Carter, M. Enzman-Hines, & J. Hernandez (Eds.), *Merenstein & Gardner's Handbook of Neonatal Intensive Care* (7th ed., pp. 78–112). St. Louis, MO: Mosby.

Garofalo, M. & Abenhaim, H. A. (2012). Early versus delayed cord clamping in term and preterm births: A review. *Journal of Obstetrics and Gynecology Canada, 34*(6), 525–531.

Goodwin, M. (2009). Abdomen assessment. In E. P. Tappero & M. E. Honeyfield (Eds.), *Physical assessment of the newborn: A comprehensive approach to the art of physical examination* (4th ed., pp. 105–114). Santa Rosa, CA: NICU Ink Book Publishers.

Haxton, D., Doering, J., Gingras, L., & Kelly, L. (2012). Implementing skin-to-skin contact at birth using the Iowa model: Applying evidence to practice. *Nursing for Women's Health, 16*(3), S6–S16.

Heaberlin, P. (2009). Neurologic assessment. In E. P. Tappero & M. E. Honeyfield (Eds.), *Physical assessment of the newborn: A comprehensive approach to the art of physical examination* (4th ed., pp. 159–184). Santa Rosa, CA: NICU Ink Book Publishers.

Health Canada. (2011). *Second-hand smoke.* Retrieved from http://www.hc-sc.gc.ca/hc-ps/tobac-tabac/legislation/label-etiquette/second-eng.php

Hoath, S. B. (2011). Physiologic development of the skin. In R. Polin, W. Fox, & S. Abman (Eds.), *Fetal and neonatal physiology* (4th ed., pp. 679–695). Philadelphia, PA: Saunders.

Honeyfield, M. E. (2009). Principles of physical assessment. In E. P. Tappero & M. E. Honeyfield (Eds.), *Physical assessment of the newborn: A comprehensive approach to the art of physical examination* (4th ed., pp. 1–8). Santa Rosa, CA: NICU Ink Book Publishers.

Infant & Toddler Safety Association. (2012). *Before you turn the key: Everything you wanted to know about transporting young children, but didn't know you needed to ask.* Kitchener, ON: The Association.

Jackman, M., & Viessman, S. (2009). *LANGE Q & A Pediatrics* (7th ed.). Toronto, ON: McGraw Hill.

Johnson, P. (2009). Head, eyes, ears, nose, mouth, and neck assessment. In E. P. Tappero & M. E. Honeyfield (Eds.), *Physical assessment of the newborn: A comprehensive approach to the art of physical examination* (4th ed., pp. 57–74). Santa Rosa, CA: NICU Ink Book Publishers.

Johnson, P. J. (2013). Vitamin K prophylaxis in the newborn: Indications and controversies. *Neonatal Network, 32*(3):193–199.

Kadic, A., & Predojevic, M. (2012). Fetal neurophysiology according to gestational age. *Seminars in Fetal and Neonatal Medicine, 17*(5), 256–260.

Kalish, R. (2008). Sonographic determination of gestational age. In A. Kurjak (Ed.): *Donald school textbook of ultrasound in obstetrics and gynecology* (2nd ed., pp. 165–173). London: JP Medical.

Karlsen, K. A. (2013). *The S.T.A.B.L.E. program: Pre-transport/post-resuscitation stabilization care of sick infants guidelines for neonatal healthcare providers* (6th ed.). Salt Lake City, UT: S.T.A.B.L.E. Inc.

Katakam, L. I., Trickey, A. W., & Thomas, E. J. (2012). Speaking up and sharing information improves trainee neonatal resuscitations. *Journal of Patient Safety. 8*(4):202–209.

Kattwinkel, J. (Ed.). (2011). *Neonatal resuscitation textbook* (6th ed.). Elk Grove Village, IL: American Academy of Pediatrics/American Heart Association.

Kinney, H. C., & Thach, B. T. (2009). The sudden infant death syndrome. *New England Journal of Medicine, 361*, 795–805.

Landrigan, P. (2011). Environment and autism. In E. Hollander, A. Kolevzon, & J. Coyle (Eds.), *Textbook of autism spectrum disorders* (pp. 247–264). Washington, DC: American Psychiatric Publishing.

Larson, E. L., Cohen, B., & Baxter, K. A. (2012). Analysis of alcohol-based hand sanitizer delivery systems: Efficacy of foam, gel, and wipes against influenza A (H1N1) virus on hands. *American Journal of Infection Control, 40*, 806–809.

Lauwers, J., & Swisher, A. (2010). *Counseling the nursing mother* (5th ed.). Burlington, MA: Jones & Bartlett Learning.

Lavender, T., Bedwell, C., Roberts, S. A., Hart, A., Turner, M. A., Carter, L. A., et al. (2013). Randomized, controlled trial evaluating a baby wash product on skin barrier function in healthy, term neonates. *Journal of Obstetric, Gynecologic, & Neonatal Nursing, 42*(2), 203–214.

Levine, D. (2008). Obstetrics. In R. L. Eisenberg & A. R. Margulis (Eds.), *The right imaging study: A guide for physicians* (pp. 564–580). New York: Springer.

Lippi, G., & Franchini, M. (2011). Vitamin K in neonates. *Blood Transfusion, 9*(1), 4–9.

Lund, C., & Durand, D. (2011). Skin and skin care. In S. Gardner, B. Carter, M. Enzman-Hines, & J. Hernandez (Eds.), *Merenstein & Gardner's handbook of neonatal intensive care* (7th ed., pp. 482–502). St. Louis, MO: Mosby.

Manco-Johnson, M., Rodden, D., & Hays, T. (2011). Newborn hematology. In S. Gardner, B. Carter, M. Enzman-Hines, & J. Hernandez (Eds.), *Merenstein & Gardner's handbook of neonatal intensive care* (7th ed., pp. 503–530). St. Louis, MO: Mosby.

McDonald, S. J., Middleton, P., Dowswell, T., & Morris, P. S. (2013). Effect of timing of umbilical cord clamping of term infants on maternal and neonatal outcomes. *Cochrane Database of Systematic Reviews, 7*, CD004074.

McGowan, J., Rozance, P., Price-Douglas, W., & Hay, W. (2011). Glucose homeostasis. In S. Gardner, B. Carter, M. Enzman-Hines, & J. Hernandez (Eds.), *Merenstein & Gardner's handbook of neonatal intensive care* (7th ed., pp. 185–200). St. Louis, MO: Mosby.

McGrath, J. (2009). Behavioral assessment. In E. P. Tappero & M. E. Honeyfield (Eds.), *Physical assessment of the newborn: A comprehensive approach to the art of physical examination* (4th ed., pp. 133–158). Santa Rosa, CA: NICU Ink Book Publishers.

McMillan, D. (2013). *Position Statement: Routine administration of vitamin K to newborns.* Retrieved from http://www.cps.ca/documents/position/administration-vitamin-K-newborns

Murray, S., James, S., & Nelson, K. (2012). *Maternal-Child Nursing* (4th ed.). St Louis, MO: Elsevier.

Nardozza, L., Araujo, E., Barbosa, M., Caetano, A., Lee, D., & Moron, A. F. (2012). Fetal growth restriction: Current knowledge to the general obs/gyn. *Archives of Gynecology and Obstetrics, 286*(1), 1–13.

Peiper, S., & Strayer, D. (2013). Developmental and genetic diseases. In H. Reisner (Ed.), *Essentials of Rubin's pathology* (6th ed., pp. 123–154). Philadelphia, PA: Lippincott Williams & Wilkins.

Polin, R. A., & Fox, W. W. (2011). *Fetal and neonatal physiology* (4th ed.). Philadelphia, PA: W. B. Saunders.

Prows, C. A. (2011). Hereditary influences on health promotion of the child and family. In M. J. Hockenberry & D. Wilson (Eds.), *Wong's nursing care of infants and children* (pp. 78–116). St. Louis, MO: Elsevier.

Public Health Agency of Canada. (2009). *What mothers say: The Canadian maternity experiences survey.* Retrieved from http://www.phac-aspc.gc.ca/rhs-ssg/pdf/survey-eng.pdf

Public Health Agency of Canada. (2012). *Preventing sudden infant deaths in Canada.* Retrieved from http://www.phac-aspc.gc.ca/hp-ps/dca-dea/stages-etapes/childhood-enfance_0-2/sids/jsss-ecss-eng.php

Ricci, S., & Kyle, T. (2009). *Maternity and pediatric nursing.* Philadelphia, PA: Lippincott Williams & Wilkins.

Riordan, J. & Hoover, K. (2010). Perinatal and intrapartum care. In J. Riordan & K. Wambach (Eds.), *Breastfeeding and human lactation* (pp. 215–251). Sudbury, MA: Jones and Bartlett Publishers.

Saugstad, O. D. (2012). Resuscitation of the newborn. In G. Buonocore, R. Bracci, & M. Weindling (Eds.), *Neonatology: A practical approach to neonatal diseases* (pp. 232–241). New York: Springer.

Schiff, E., Maddrey, W., & Sorrell, M. (2011). *Schiff's Diseases of the Liver* (11th ed.). Hoboken, NJ: Wiley & Sons.

Sinha, S., Miall, L., & Jardine, L. (2012). *Essential neonatal medicine* (5th ed.). Hoboken, NJ: Wiley & Sons.

Smith, J. (2012). Initial evaluation: History and physical examination of the newborn. In C. Gleason & S. Devaskar (Eds.), *Avery's diseases of the newborn* (9th ed., pp. 277–299). Philadelphia, PA: Saunders.

Smith, J., Alcock, G., & Usher, K. (2013). Temperature measurement in the preterm and term neonate: A review of the literature. *Neonatal Network, 32*(1), 16–25.

Smylie, J., Fell, D., Ohlsson, A., & The Joint Working Group on First Nations, Indian, Inuit, and Métis Infant Mortality of the Canadian Perinatal Surveillance System. (2010). A review of aboriginal infant mortality rates in Canada: Striking and persistent aboriginal/non-aboriginal inequities. *Canadian Journal of Public Health, 101*(2). Retrieved from http://journal.cpha.ca/index.php/cjph/article/viewArticle/2370

St. James-Roberts, I. (2009). *Preventing and managing infant sleeping problems.* Retrieved from http://eprints.ioe.ac.uk/3468/1/ISJR_website_article_Nov_2009.pdf

Steinhorn, R. H., & De Ungria, M. (2008). *Neonatal resuscitation. Global library of women's medicine.* Retrieved from http://www.glowm.com/section_view/heading/Neonatal%20Resuscitation/item/203

Tappero, E. P. (2009). Musculoskeletal system assessment. In E. P. Tappero & M. E. Honeyfield (Eds.), *Physical assessment of the newborn: A comprehensive approach to the art of physical examination* (4th ed., pp. 133–158). Santa Rosa, CA: NICU Ink Book Publishers.

Tappero, E. P., & Honeyfield, M. E. (2009). *Physical assessment of the newborn: A comprehensive approach to the art of physical examination* (4th ed.). Santa Rosa, CA: NICU Ink Book Publishers.

Thappa, D. (2009). *Clinical pediatric dermatology.* St. Louis, MO: Elsevier.

Transport Canada. (2012). *Child safety.* Retrieved from http://www.tc.gc.ca/eng/roadsafety/safedrivers-childsafety-index-53.htm

Trotter, C. (2009). Gestational age assessment. In E. P. Tappero & M. E. Honeyfield (Eds.), *Physical assessment of the newborn: A comprehensive approach to the art of physical examination* (4th ed., pp. 21–39). Santa Rosa, CA: NICU Ink Book Publishers.

Tutdibi, E., Gries, K., Bucheler, M., Misselwitz, B., Schlosser, R. L., & Gortner, L. (2010). Impact of labor on outcomes in transient tachypnea of the newborn: Population-based study. *Pediatrics, 125*(3), e577–e583.

Uhing, M. R., & Kliegman, R. M. (2012). Glucose, calcium, and magnesium. In J. Fanaroff & A. Fanaroff (Eds.), *Klaus & Fanaroff's care of the high-risk neonate* (6th ed., pp. 289–309). St. Louis, MO: Elsevier.

Vannice, K., Salmon, D., Shui, I., Omer, S., Kissner, J., Edwards, K., et al. (2011). Attitudes and beliefs of parents concerned about vaccines: Impact of timing of immunization information. *Pediatrics, 127*(S1), S120–S126.

Venkatesh, M., Adams, K., & Weisman, L. (2011). Infection in the neonate. In S. Gardner, B. Carter, M. Enzman-Hines, & J. Hernandez (Eds.), *Merenstein & Gardner's handbook of neonatal intensive care* (7th ed., pp. 553–580). St. Louis, MO: Mosby.

Vincent, J. L. (2009). Infant hospital abduction: Security measures to aid in prevention. *American Journal of Maternal Child Nursing, 34*(3), 179–183.

Weiss, H. A., Larke, N., Halperin, D., & Schenker, I. (2010). Complications of circumcision in male neonates, infants and children: A systematic review. *BMC Urology, 10*(2). doi:10.1186/1471-2490-10-2. Retrieved from http://www.biomedcentral.com/1471-2490/10/2/

Wheeler, B. J. (2011). Health promotion of the newborn and family. In M. J Hockenberry & D. Wilson (Eds.), *Wong's nursing care of infants and children* (pp. 227–278). St. Louis, MO: Elsevier.

White, G. (2012). *Basic clinical lab competencies for respiratory care* (5th ed.). Clifton Park, NY: Cengage.

Wilson, D. (2011). Health problems of the newborn. In M. J Hockenberry & D. Wilson (Eds.), *Wong's nursing care of infants and children* (pp. 279–313). St. Louis, MO: Elsevier.

Witt, C. L. (2009). Learning from our past, looking forward to our future. *Advances in Neonatal Care, 9*(2), 47–49.

World Health Organization. (2007). *Male circumcision: Global trends and determinants of prevalence, safety and acceptability.* Retrieved from http://www.malecircumcision.org/media/documents/MC_Global_Trends_Determinants.pdf

Zaichkin, J. (Ed.). (2011). *Neonatal resuscitation instructor manual* (5th ed.). Elk Grove Village, IL: AAP/American Heart Association.

Zeskind, D. (2013). Infant crying and the synchrony of arousal. In E. Altenmuller, S. Schmidt, & E. Zimmerman (Eds.), *The evolution of emotional communication* (pp. 155–174). Oxford: Oxford University Press.

WEB RESOURCES

Academy of Neonatal Nursing, www.academyonline.org/

American Academy of Pediatrics, www.aap.org

Association of Women's Health, Obstetric and Neonatal Nurses (AWHONN) http://www.awhonn.org/awhonn/

Canadian Association of Neonatal Nurses, www.neonatalcann.ca/

Canadian Association of Perinatal and Women's Health Nursing, www.capwhn.ca

Canadian Foundation for the Study of Infant Deaths, www.sidscanada.org

Canadian Paediatric Society, http://www.cps.ca/

Child Find Canada Inc., http://www.childfind.ca/

Transport Canada Safety in the Car, http://www.tc.gc.ca/eng/roadsafety/safedrivers-childsafety-index-53.htm

CHAPTER 21

Newborn Nutrition

Luisa Ciofani and Michelle Johnson*

Lindsay, a 35-year-old, is 6 weeks postpartum after an unplanned cesarean birth of her first baby. She is at the clinic for her scheduled follow-up appointment. The infant is thriving, but Lindsay's recovery has been slow. During discussions with the nurse, Lindsay states that she understands the benefits of breastfeeding, but that the physical demands are overwhelming her. She reports that she is debating if she should switch to formula feeding, but she feels that if she does so, she's being selfish and inadequate.

Joelle, a 24-year-old single woman, is at 25 weeks' gestation. Although she had positive results with bottlefeeding formula to her first infant, Joelle has been reading about the benefits of breast milk and the closeness provided by the breastfeeding experience, so she wants to pursue this method for the baby she is expecting. She asks the nurse for more information about breastfeeding and how to ensure a successful experience.

Nursing interactions with these clients are discussed in more detail later in this chapter. Before beginning this chapter, consider the following points related to the above scenarios:

- How will the nurse working with each of the clients tailor care to best suit the needs of the women and their families?
- What elements of teaching about newborn and infant nutrition do these women require? What issues are similar? What issues are different?
- Which points or considerations might these clients have overlooked or be unaware? What other types of information will the nurse require to assist the families to make informed decisions?
- How might the nurse involve the clients' families in care?

---

*Contributor to first U.S. edition.

Nurses are well positioned in the health care field to ensure that parents and other caregivers receive accurate information about newborn and infant feeding. They are often the first or only individuals of whom parents and families ask feeding-related questions. Nurses use anticipatory guidance with families in order to resolve any feeding problems that may occur. Nurses therefore need a thorough understanding of the various feeding techniques and strategies to ensure appropriate nutrition and to assist clients to identify and overcome feeding challenges so that they can intervene appropriately (Spatz, 2005).

In 1991, the World Health Organization (WHO) and the United Nations Children's Fund (UNICEF) launched the Baby Friendly Hospital Initiative (UNICEF, 2005). The Breastfeeding Committee for Canada (www.breastfeedingcanada.ca) is the national authority for this initiative and, in Canada, has renamed it the Baby Friendly Initiative in order to reflect the continuum of care that includes outside-the-hospital setting (Registered Nurses' Association of Ontario [RNAO], 2007). Promoting and supporting breastfeeding has become more critical as evidence shows its positive impact on addressing childhood obesity and diabetes. The Baby Friendly Initiative provides a framework to guide health care professionals in promoting, supporting, and protecting breastfeeding (Box 21.1). Several research studies have reported that hospitals that adopt these practices have higher initiation, duration, and exclusivity of breastfeeding (Ingram, Johnson & Condon, 2011).

DECISIONS ABOUT INFANT FEEDING

Determining a method of feeding is one of the most important choices parents or other caregivers must make for their newborn. Many factors influence the decision about infant nutrition, including the attitudes of the primary caregivers and significant others, as well as messages from health care professionals, the media, and personal values and choices (Kong & Lee, 2004; Labarere et al., 2005). See Research Highlight 21.1.

Maternal breast milk has unique nutritional, immunologic, developmental, and economic advantages for infants; women who breastfeed their children also experience unique health benefits for themselves (Godfrey & Lawrence, 2010). Factors that may influence a woman's decision to breastfeed include higher socioeconomic levels, higher education levels, age, occupation, and care by a midwife (Kong & Lee, 2004; Li et al., 2005;

● **BOX 21.1** Breastfeeding Committee for Canada: The 10 Steps to Successful Breastfeeding

Step 1

Have a written breastfeeding policy that is routinely communicated to all health care providers and volunteers.

Step 2

Ensure all health care providers have the knowledge and skills necessary to implement the breastfeeding policy.

Step 3

Inform pregnant women and their families about the importance and process of breastfeeding.

Step 4

Place babies in uninterrupted skin-to-skin contact with their mothers immediately following birth for at least an hour or until completion of the first feeding or as long as the mother wishes: encourage mothers to recognize when their babies are ready to feed, offering help as needed.

Step 5

Assist mothers to breastfeed and maintain lactation should they face challenges including separation from their infants.

Step 6

Support mothers to exclusively breastfeed for the first 6 months, unless supplements are medically indicated.

Step 7

Facilitate 24-hour rooming-in for all mother–infant dyads: mothers and infants remain together.

Step 8

Encourage baby-led or cue-based breastfeeding.

Encourage sustained breastfeeding beyond 6 months with appropriate introduction of complementary foods.

Step 9

Support mothers to feed and care for their breastfeeding babies without the use of artificial teats or pacifiers (dummies or soothers).

Step 10

Provide a seamless transition between the services provided by the hospital, community health services, and peer support programs.

Apply principles of Primary Health Care and Population Health to support the continuum of care and implement strategies that affect the broad determinants that will improve breastfeeding outcomes.

Source: Breastfeeding Committee for Canada 2011 http://www.breastfeedingcanada.ca/documents/2012-05-14 BCC BFI Ten Steps Integrated Indicators Summary pdf
Source: Registered Nurses' Association of Ontario (2012). Breastfeeding: Fundamental Concepts. A Self Learning Package. Toronto, Canada: Registered Nurses' Association of Ontario.

Lutsiv et al., 2013). When the use of maternal milk is contraindicated or the volume of maternal milk is insufficient to meet the newborn's needs, donor human milk is a viable alternative (Tully et al., 2004).

Commercially prepared formula is another feeding option that provides sole-source nutrition to meet the newborn's demands. These formulas have adequate nutrient composition and are appropriate for infants up to 12 months old. Some women choose to make their own, noncommercial formulas. In such instances, it is important for nutritional experts to discuss the materials being used and amounts being given, to ensure adequate nutrition for these infants.

Women who choose formula for their babies do so for a variety of reasons, some of which may be based on inaccurate information. Some of the reasons identified are as follows (Bonia et al., 2013):

• Desire to involve partners in infant feeding
• Perceived convenience of formulafeeding
• Desire to maintain a sense of "independence"

• Illness in newborns
• Problems trying to maintain milk production
• Time constraints or return to work
• Embarrassment at breastfeeding in public
• Viewing the breasts as sexual organs

It is important for clients to consider all factors that may influence their decision about choosing a method to feed their newborn. In the next sections we explore such factors in more detail and provide the information needed for nurses to address concerns, correct misperceptions, and support clients in making informed choices. See Figure 21.1 for an algorithm for assisting clients in decision making for newborn and infant feeding.

Factors to Highlight
Feeding Frequency

Breast milk, formula, or a combination of these can meet newborn nutritional needs. Breast milk is convenient, requires no special preparation, and is the nutritional

● RESEARCH HIGHLIGHT 21.1   Why do Women Stop Breastfeeding? Findings from the Pregnancy Risk Assessment and Monitoring System

OBJECTIVE

To evaluate contributing factors to breastfeeding cessation and associations between prenatal feeding intentions and actual breastfeeding results.

DESIGN

The researchers assessed 2 years of data from the Pregnancy Risk Assessment and Monitoring System for the percentage of women who began breastfeeding, continued for less than 1 week, continued for 1 to 4 weeks, and continued for more than 4 weeks. They also examined the reasons reported by the women for not beginning or stopping, as well as the clients' breastfeeding intentions before birth and subsequent outcomes.

RESULTS

Findings showed that 32% of women never started breastfeeding, 4% started but stopped within 1 week, 13% stopped within 1 month, and 51% continued for more than 1 month. Younger clients and those with limited socioeconomic resources were most likely to stop or never start breastfeeding. Participants cited sore nipples, newborn difficulties, inadequate milk supply, and hungry infant as reasons for stopping. Those clients who planned to breastfeed were more likely to initiate and continue with nursing.

CONCLUSIONS

Almost 50% of women chose not to initiate or were unable to breastfeed for longer than 4 weeks. For breastfeeding to be successful, clients need awareness and understanding of breastfeeding prenatally, as well as extensive support after birth, particularly for those with characteristics that put them in groups at risk for not breastfeeding as per recommended guidelines (6 months exclusive breastfeeding).

From Ahluwalia, I. B., Morrow, B., & Hsia, J. (2005). Why do women stop breastfeeding? Findings from the Pregnancy Risk Assessment and Monitoring System. *Pediatrics, 116*(6), 1408–1412.

substance most suited for human newborns. In addition, it comes in a relatively easy-to-use "package," although it may take a few weeks for clients to become comfortable and skilled with the process of breastfeeding. Health Canada, as well as many other professional groups and associations, recommend exclusive breastfeeding for the first 6 months of life, as breast milk is the best food for optimal growth. Breastfeeding may then continue (with gradual introduction of solid foods) for up to 2 years and beyond (Canadian Paediatric Society [CPS], 2013b; Health Canada, 2012c; Public Health Agency of Canada, 2013a ; World Health Organization (WHO), 2014).

A mother who wants to breastfeed exclusively needs to be prepared to do so regularly, every 2 to 3 hours, including through the night, for several weeks to months. In the early newborn period, 8 to 12 feedings at the breast in 24 hours are recommended, with the mother offering her breast whenever the infant shows any signs of hunger (e.g., increased alertness or activity, mouthing, rooting) (RNAO, 2007). The number of feedings needed when breastfeeding is greater than the number when formulafeeding because of the ease with which breast milk is digested.

Some women wish to breastfeed, but worry that they will not be able to meet the physical or time demands. They may also anticipate being separated from their infant or may want to involve other family members in

newborn feeding. In these situations, the nurse might suggest supplementing breastfeeding with expressed breast milk provided by an alternative method, such as a bottle or special cup. It is suggested that this occur once breastfeeding and milk supply have been well established, usually at about 4 to 6 weeks postpartum (American Academy of Pediatrics [AAP], 2012).

 Recall Lindsay, the woman at the beginning of the chapter who is having difficulty maintaining the breastfeeding of her newborn. What issues and strategies might the nurse want to investigate?

Family Involvement

The attitudes of family and friends to newborn feeding can play a major role in feeding choices. Just as some people feel pressure not to bottlefeed, others may experience similar pressures related to breastfeeding. Studies have revealed positive correlations between partner support, family knowledge about breastfeeding, and positive family attitudes about breastfeeding with a successful breastfeeding experience (Mannion et al., 2013; Meedya et al., 2010). Both breastfeeding and formulafeeding can involve multiple individuals in the feeding experience. All interested parties can easily accomplish

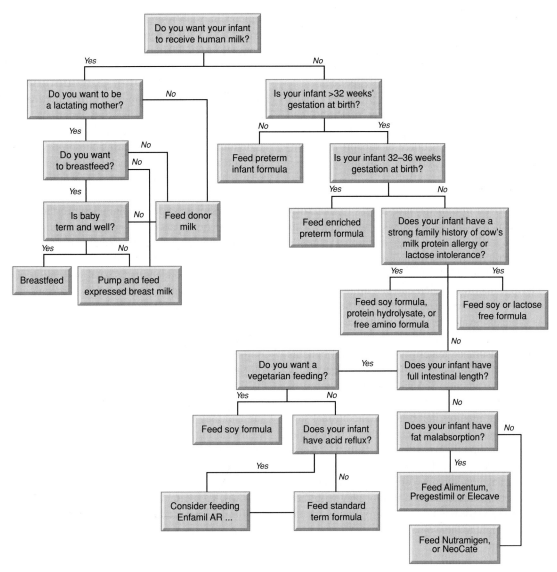

FIGURE 21.1 An algorithm for assisting clients with newborn feeding options.

formula feeding, which is simple to learn and easy to maintain. Some fathers who wish to participate in feeding their babies may be concerned that they will be unable to do so if the woman chooses to nurse. Despite this fear, individuals other than the biologic mother can be involved in caring for and giving breast milk to newborns. This requires some additional work or may become a part of a mother's routine. The mother will need to express the milk and store it in either the refrigerator or freezer.

The breasts of the breastfeeding woman should be stimulated every 2 to 3 hours as per her child's demand for the first 4 to 6 weeks after birth (AAP, 2012). This may include direct breastfeeding or expressing the breast milk. This regular stimulation of the breast helps to ensure breast milk production. Regardless of the type of feeding chosen, family members can also participate

in the many nonnutritional activities required in caring for an infant, such as preparing the newborn for feeding, changing the diaper or clothes as needed, burping, and most importantly, cuddling.

Discreet Nursing and Personal Comfort Level

Inherent in breastfeeding is the challenge of potentially exposing a part of the body that is usually covered with clothing. Although societal mores—and laws—are changing, a number of societal issues continue to be related to breastfeeding in public (Li et al., 2004). In addition, some women are uncomfortable breastfeeding in front of other people. They may be concerned about perceptions of indecency, restrictive attitudes toward exposure to the breast, or they simply might feel embarrassed (Riordan & Wambach, 2010; Spurles

& Babineau, 2011). Nurses may suggest that the client wear clothes that minimize skin exposure during nursing. Alternatively, a variety of cover ups designed specifically for breastfeeding are available that the woman may choose to use. (e.g., www.boobytrapper.ca).

Breastfeeding in Canada is protected under the umbrella of the Canadian Charter of Rights and Freedoms. Human Rights Commissions are available in all provinces and can be a source of support if a woman's right to breastfeed in public is challenged.

Returning to Work Outside the Home

Women employed in Canada have access to maternity leaves, of which many families take advantage. This may also be supplemented with additional parental leaves. Maternity leave is available to women who are pregnant, have given birth or are taking care of a newborn. During this time, which can last up to 17 weeks, the employer is required to hold her job for her. Parental leave is typically available for an additional 37 weeks, although there may be variations in some provinces. Employment Insurance maternity and parental benefits are available to those who qualify. Parental leave may be shared by two parents (Service Canada, 2014).

Breastfeeding following the return to work can be successful, but it requires flexibility and additional support from the mother's significant others. If feasible, the mother can directly breastfeed her infant at some time during the work day. For example, some places of employment have on-site day care facilities where parents are encouraged to come and feed or play with their children during work breaks. Another option is for the child to be brought to the woman at work so that she can breastfeed during breaks.

Using a breast pump at work is a viable option for many women because it fosters continued breast milk production, provides breast milk to use in bottles for future feedings, and is practical for women who do not have the flexibility or caregiving arrangements to facilitate direct breastfeeding of their newborns while working. The availability of a private place and time to pump sometimes presents a challenge in work environments. Breastfeeding support from employers (flexible work options, lactation breaks, access to private space) is essential, or the pumping, and subsequently breastfeeding, process may deteriorate (Weber et al., 2011). Fatigue, as well as high stress over job-related or other issues also may affect the woman's milk supply once she resumes employment.

Nurses who encounter women with questions about the best ways to pump milk at work and other places outside the home can encourage clients to lobby their employers for written policies regarding breastfeeding and pumping in the workplace. They can also assist clients to devise ways to approach employers for support in establishing a comfortable place and time to breastfeed, with adequate privacy and minimal disruptions (RNAO, 2007; Tsai, 2013).

Sexual and Emotional Considerations

Some women choose one type of feeding method over another because of sexual and emotional concerns. Women who breastfeed their babies have different, individualized reactions during the process. Some feel an increased emotional attachment (either immediately or eventually) with the infant as a result of breastfeeding. Other women find the sensations that accompany breastfeeding unexpected and uncomfortable. A history of sexual or physical violence where the breasts were targeted may also affect a woman's desire to breastfeed (Riordan & Wambach, 2010).

Studies have identified sexual perception of breasts and breastfeeding as constraints in women's choice to breastfeed (Hurst, 2013). They may feel awkward sharing their breasts with their baby or become uncomfortable and conflicted when attention is given to the breasts during sexual stimulation. Some women become sexually aroused during the physical act of infant suckling and have varying responses to this experience. These highly personal reactions affect a woman's attitude about feeding and may influence her decision. Nurses listen when women bring up such concerns and provide reassurance and support to help clients deal with their feelings and reach decisions appropriate for their situation.

Racial, Ethnic, and Cultural Influences

Cultural values and attitudes contribute to a woman's choice of feeding method. A woman's culture influences the initiation, frequency, and duration of breastfeeding (Kelly, 2006; Lawrence & Lawrence, 2005). Women may feel ostracized if they choose to break social or cultural normative behaviours regarding infant feeding practices. Populations differ by ethnicity in their feeding practices. In Canada, rates of breastfeeding initiation and duration are increasing. From 2009 to 2010, 87.3% of Canadian women initiated breastfeeding with their last child, increased from 84.5% reported in 2003 (Health Canada, 2012a). Furthermore, from 2009 to 2010, 25.9% of mothers exclusively breastfed their last child for the recommended 6 months (17.6%) or more (8.3%), increased from the 20.3% rate reported in 2005. Research has shown that women of Asian or other cultural backgrounds are more likely to initiate and breastfeed exclusively for the recommended 6 months or more than are women of White cultural backgrounds (Health Canada, 2012b).

Nurses consider cultural influences on feeding choices. They ask questions about beliefs and explore sources of information and knowledge. Nurses ensure that parents make informed decisions, so should strive to correct misperceptions and provide alternatives. Providing some breast milk to newborns in combination with formula or for a shorter duration than recommended will also provide benefits and can be encouraged, if a woman does not desire to exclusively breastfeed for 6 months. Ultimately, women and families are treated with respect for their decisions, and for those cultural components that influence their options.

Client Teaching and Collaborative Interventions

Women are assessed prenatally for their intent to breastfeed, attitudes about breastfeeding (including those of significant others), access to support for breastfeeding, and any physical factors that may influence their ability to breastfeed (RNAO, 2007). Interventions can then be implemented to promote breastfeeding. Information about infant feeding practices is most influential in the prenatal period before a pregnant woman has made her decision and, more specifically, before she has experienced fetal movements (Riordan & Wambach, 2010). Frequent, short discussions with health care providers regarding infant feeding choices are preferable to lengthy discussions in ensuring that women have the necessary information to make an informed decision (Taveras et al., 2004).

Women may have issues related to breastfeeding, including convenience, modesty, fear of a change in lifestyle, paternal involvement, returning to work, and their own and others' negative experiences with breastfeeding. Some women may be concerned that they may be choosing bottlefeeding for selfish reasons, rather than making a decision based on the child's best interests. Health care professionals, including nurses, are well positioned to listen to women and to address their concerns during each office visit or telephone call. An important health promotion activity for nurses is to educate the mother and family about the nutritional, immunologic, psychological, health, and developmental benefits of the different feeding strategies (Fig. 21.2). Nurses use the best evidence and resources available to provide information regarding types of feeding methods. Sharing of personal opinions may not be appropriate and should be kept to a minimum. Evidence-based guidelines to assist in decision making are available to professions and provide current information for practice (Janke et al., 2007; RNAO, 2007). The family are encouraged to consider all options.

Support for women is necessary to ensure adequate nutritional intake for the newborn. Resources providing support for different feeding methods are available, which may include formal classes, written information, internet sources, and access to health care providers. Women who choose to breastfeed may be referred to certified lactation consultants for expert assistance. These

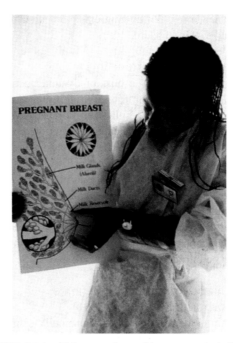

FIGURE 21.2 This nurse is teaching a group of clients about the physiology of lactation and the unique benefits of breastfeeding.

consultants are health care providers who have successfully completed additional education and achieved certification in the specialty (IBLCE, 2014). There are many resources to help health care professionals in their pursuit of breastfeeding education and increased community awareness such as the World Health Organization Baby Friendly Initiative, the Breastfeeding Committee for Canada, Breastfeeding Best Practice Guidelines for Nurses by the Registered Nurses' Association of Ontario, the Bright Future Lactation Resource Center, and Breastfeeding Inc (see Web Resources).

Women might attend nutrition classes during or after pregnancy. Classes may focus on all feeding options or on one specific method. Most classes centre on strategies for successful breastfeeding. Techniques such as positioning; objective measures to evaluate breastfeeding effectiveness, including both milk production and milk transfer assessment; management of sore nipples; returning to work or school; and feeding in public may be discussed (see later sections). Classes that include bottlefeeding may explore the differences among formulas, preparing and storing infant formula, bottle hygiene, as well as holding and positioning techniques for bottlefeeding.

BREASTFEEDING

The unique and evolving composition of breast milk is well suited to meet the nutrient and growth of all except a few newborns. All commercially prepared formulas are held to this standard.

Benefits of Breastfeeding

Human milk contains a host of dynamic and unique feeding properties not found in formula (Lawrence & Lawrence, 2005). Results from a recent systematic review revealed that the health benefits of breast milk are associated with the duration of exclusive breastfeeding (Kramer & Kakuma, 2012). Exclusive breastfeeding for 6 months and up to 2 years and beyond is recommended by Health Canada, Canadian Pediatric Society, Dietitians of Canada, and the Breastfeeding Committee for Canada (Health Canada, 2014). Nutrient-rich complementary foods, with particular attention to iron, should be introduced at 6 months of age.

Health and Immunologic Benefits to Newborns

Specific elements present in human milk enhance the normal newborn's immune system and are particularly critical for the vulnerable newborn. Prebiotics (oligosaccharides and lactoferrin) stimulate the growth and activity of the microflora in the newborn's colon. Lactoferrin binds with iron, removing it from the gut and preventing some pathogenic bacteria from growing (Kim & Froh, 2012). Human milk also contains bioactive factors such as immune cells, long chain polyunsaturated fatty acids, nucleotides, hormones, and bioactive peptides, all of which are active against pathogens including *Escherichia coli (E. coli), Vibrio cholerae, Campylobacter, Shigella, Giardia,* pneumococcus, rotavirus, cytomegalovirus (CMV), influenza virus, and respiratory syncytial virus (Kim & Froh, 2012; Nishimura et al., 2009). Therefore, human breast milk protects the newborn against gastroenteritis, respiratory infections, urinary tract infections, septicemia, necrotizing enterocolitis, and acute otitis media. Five immunoglobulins are also present in breast milk. These proteins are produced by plasma cells in response to a foreign particle and have the ability to neutralize particular antigens. Secretory immunoglobulin (IgA), the most important, is synthesized and stored in the maternal breast and is a major defense in the newborn's intestines. Lysozyme, in tandem with lactoferrin, destroys pathogenic bacteria, including *E. coli* and *Salmonella* (Kim & Froh, 2012). Human milk also contains phagocytic white blood cells, particularly macrophages and neutrophils, which protect the intestinal immune system. Recently identified is pancreatic secretory trypsin inhibitor (PSTI), which contributes to the integrity of the mucus layers of the intestinal wall (Kim & Froh, 2012).

Several studies have shown the long-range enhancements that these elements of breast milk give to children (RNAO, 2007). Infants show decreased upper and lower respiratory tract infections and cases of otitis media when fed breast milk exclusively for up to 6 months (Lawrence & Lawrence, 2005). In addition, exclusive breastfeeding for up to 6 months of age is shown to reduce asthma-related symptoms such as wheezing, shortness of breath, dry cough, and persistent phlegm (Sonnenschein-van der Voort et al., 2012). Infants breastfed beyond 6 months of age benefit from ongoing continued protection from otitis media, diarrhea, and colds (Chantry et al., 2006; Morrow & Rangel, 2004). It is recognized that additional immune-enhancing benefits of breast milk to include reduced incidence and severity of bacteremia, bacterial meningitis, botulism, urinary tract infection, and necrotizing enterocolitis (CPS, 2013b; Health Canada, 2014). Other potential benefits, for which there is no conclusive evidence, include enhanced cognitive development and reduced cases of sudden infant death syndrome (SIDS), insulin-dependent diabetes mellitus, Crohn disease, ulcerative colitis, lymphoma, and other chronic digestive diseases as well as hypertension and elevated serum cholesterol levels. (AAP, 2012; RNAO, 2007; Schack-Nielsen et al., 2005; Singhal et al., 2004).

Research findings are inconclusive whether restricting the maternal diet while breastfeeding prevents allergic conditions in infants, with the possible exception of atopic eczema. Based on recent evidence that avoiding milk, egg, peanut, or other potential allergens during pregnancy does not help prevent allergy, the Canadian Paediatric Society (CPS) and the Canadian Society of Allergy and Clinical Immunology recommend that the maternal diet during pregnancy or lactation not be restricted (CPS, 2013a).

Developmental Benefits

Benefits to cognitive development and visual acuity are attributable to the fatty acids inherent in breast milk. Premature infants fed with breast milk demonstrate improved neurodevelopment than preterm infants fed with preterm formula (Roze et al., 2012). Children who were breastfed as infants showed significantly greater IQs and better academic performance (McGill University, 2008). In addition, low–birth weight infants fed with breast milk have shown greater differences in cognitive development scores than normal–birth weight infants fed with breast milk when both were compared with formula-fed infants (Slykerman et al., 2005; WHO, 2013).

The ingestion of human milk enhances physical development. Epidermal growth factor has been shown to contribute to the growth of intestinal cells in vitro. It is thought that epidermal growth factor also promotes intestinal cell growth in living infants.

Nutritional Benefits

In comparison to cow's milk and infant formula, human milk is more easily digested and absorbed because of the bioavailability of the minerals and the unique pattern and quantity of amino acids needed for adequate growth and development. Compared with commercial infant formulas, the lower values of these nutrients in human milk give breast milk the distinction of having the lowest potential renal solute load (Lawson, 2007). This is particularly important for infants with renal impairment or immature kidneys (e.g., preterm babies).

Breast milk is also superior because it is a species-specific formulation: its nutrients are uniquely suited to support growth and development for healthy human infants. The protein in human milk is whey dominant, which forms soft, easily digested curds. Enzymes in breast milk aid digestion, enhance development of beneficial intestinal flora, and destroy harmful bacteria. Growth factors and hormones, including serotonin, insulin, prolactin, thyroid hormones, corticosteroids, ACTH, oxytocin, calcitonin, parathyroid hormone, erythropoietin, progesterone, and estrogen, are all found in human breast milk (Kim & Froh, 2012).

Another advantage of breastfeeding is that the infant leads the decision to stop breastfeeding, which assists in learning about satiety and may prevent obesity in the long term. It appears that the protection against childhood obesity is related to exclusive breastfeeding for at least 6 months (Yipu, et al., 2013).

Health Benefits to Mothers
The health advantages of breastfeeding to mothers include enhanced uterine involution. Oxytocin, a maternal hormone, triggers the milk ejection reflex in response to the baby suckling at the breast. Oxytocin also increases the rate of uterine contractions; thus, breastfeeding decreases the risk for maternal postpartum hemorrhage (RNAO, 2007).

In general, lactating women lose more weight postpartum than women not breastfeeding and are able to better maintain the weight loss (Stuebe, 2009). Heneghen (2011), in a literature review from 1926 to 2010, found that although research results were inconsistent, there was some evidence of a protective effect of breastfeeding against development of breast cancer in premenopausal women. The effect appeared to be stronger with increasing breastfeeding duration, increasing number of children, and initiating breastfeeding at a young age. Although current research has yielded conflicting results, women who breastfeed their infants may be at decreased risk for osteoporosis, diabetes, and ovarian cancer (Luan et al., 2013; Stuebe, 2009; Ziegler et al., 2012).

Economic Benefits
Breast milk undoubtedly is the most economical choice for families of all cultures. Families do not incur the costs of purchasing commercially prepared formulas and bottles. Society benefits from increased breastfeeding rates through the improved health of both mothers and infants and decreased loss of productivity due to illness (CPS, 2012b). Prolonged breast milk feedings can also potentially decrease environmental waste caused by disposal of formula containers, bottles, bags, and nipples.

Psychological Benefits
Breastfeeding offers the mother–infant dyad a unique opportunity for skin-to-skin contact 8 to 12 times each day, which contributes to emotional bonding and building trust. Skin-to-skin contact has been found to enhance mother–baby interactions, and help women to breastfeed longer (Moore et al., 2007). In addition, breastfeeding duration is increased with mother–baby contact in the immediate postnatal period (Moore et al., 2007).

Breastfeeding increases both the quality and quantity of early infant contact in the postpartum period. This, in combination with the effects of oxytocin, which is believed to contribute to maternal care-taking behaviours, is believed to lead to enhanced maternal–infant attachment. Maternal sensitivity to infants' behaviour is shown to be associated with duration of breastfeeding and attachment security (Tharner et al., 2012). In contrast, women who wean earlier than planned report experiencing feelings of loss, grief, and depression (Stuebe et al., 2012).

Contraindications to Breastfeeding and Conditions Requiring Adjustments
Earlier discussions explored the many factors that influence the newborn feeding decision. Although nurses encourage and support breastfeeding, they also treat families that choose formula feeding for reasons other than contraindications with understanding, respect, and a nonjudgmental manner (Wirihana & Barnard, 2011). Despite the advantages of feeding breast milk to infants, a handful of situations exist in which either a mother's or infant's medical condition warrants review of the risks versus benefits of feeding mother's own milk.

Medical Contraindications
- A significant challenge to universal breastfeeding practices is the increase in HIV. Approximately 10% of infants will acquire HIV from breastfeeding, if no antiretroviral treatment is used (Bode et al., 2012). With maternal use of antiretrovirals, the risk of transmission drops to 1% to 2% (WHO, 2014). Breastfeeding by HIV positive mothers poses a dilemma, because even though the rate of transmission is a risk, breastfeeding is important to child survival, the ideal way to feed an infant, and a unique bonding opportunity for child development (Jhaveri, 2013). In addition, in low and middle income countries with populations at risk for other infections and nutritional problems contributing to increased infant mortality, the risks of relying on formula feeding may outweigh the risk of transmitting

HIV (Lockman, 2011). Under these circumstances, the WHO (2014) recommends that HIV-infected mothers take antiretroviral therapy and exclusively breastfeed their babies for 6 months, then introduce solids and continue breastfeeding until the child is 1 year old. If antiretrovirals are not available, women should exclusively breastfeed for 6 months, introduce solids, and continue breastfeeding until circumstances are such that using infant formula is safe and feasible. In Canada, where a safe and culturally acceptable replacement is available to feed infants, breastfeeding is contraindicated in HIV positive women (CPS, 2012a).

- Human T-cell lymphotropic virus is transmitted through breast milk. Health care providers should advise mothers with human T-lymphotropic virus type 1 or 2 infection not to breastfeed (CPS, 2012a).
- If cytomegalovirus (CMV) is in the breast milk of CMV-positive mothers, infants who acquire CMV after birth exhibit few, if any, complications (Centers for Disease Control, 2010). Breast milk transmission of CMV has potentially the most serious consequences for CMV-seronegative or preterm infants. For premature infants, especially those less than 32 weeks' gestation, breastfeeding by a CMV-positive mother remains controversial. At present, there is support for fresh breast milk feeding even if the mother is CMV positive (CPS, 2012a).
- Mothers with active herpes simplex virus lesions on the breast should temporarily pump and discard their breast milk until lesions are healed (crusted) (CPS, 2012a). Breastfeeding is otherwise encouraged.
- Maternal varicella zoster virus infection requires temporary isolation of mother and baby until the mother is no longer infectious, there are no new lesions in 72 hours, and existing lesions have crusted over. During this time, the infant having received varicella zoster immunoglobulin may consume breast milk (CPS, 2012a).
- Breastfeeding mothers with measles should be isolated from their infants for 72 hours after appearance of the rash. As a precaution, expressed breast milk may be fed to infants who have received immunoglobulin (Lawrence & Lawrence, 2005). Although the measles vaccine virus itself passes into breast milk, it has not been reported to cause problems for the breastfed infant (Public Health Agency of Canada, 2013b).
- Maternal tuberculosis is compatible with breastfeeding, if the mother is noncontagious or has received 2 weeks of active treatment (CPS, 2012a). Active lesions on the breast must be treated on a case-by-case basis.

Nutrition- and Drug-Related Contraindications

Nutritional causes that warrant discontinuation of breast milk feedings include infantile disorders of metabolic origin. Provision of some breast milk is possible with infantile phenylketonuria, maple syrup urine disease, and mild galactosemia. Infants who present with the classic variant of galactosemia are lactose intolerant and must receive a lactose-free formula (AAP, 2012). Maternal Wilson disease is a contraindication to breastfeeding because treatment therapy is with penicillamine, which adversely alters the infant's mineral status (Roberts & Schilsky, 2008).

When a mother's treatment includes medication, the nature of the drug will determine its solubility in breast milk and the amount that will subsequently be transferred to the infant. Women for whom a prescription drug is indicated should discuss options with their health care provider so that a therapeutic regimen can be selected that will preserve the breastfeeding relationship. This may include delaying treatment or choosing alternative forms of treatment. The gestational and chronologic age of the infant, body weight, and breastfeeding pattern should also be considered (Lawrence & Lawrence, 2005). Excellent resources are available in order to facilitate selection of a drug for which the effect on infants is known, or to investigate an alternative treatment (e.g., Motherisk Program at www.motherisk.org). Illegal drugs are transferred to breast milk in sufficient concentrations to discourage breastfeeding (AAP, 2012; Lawrence & Lawrence, 2005).

Women who require chemotherapy for cancer should not breastfeed. Antineoplastic agents are toxic to the infant, suppress bone marrow, and may cause epithelial cell damage (AAP, 2012). Tamoxifen therapy is presently a contraindication to breastfeeding because of the lack of information about its transfer into human milk and effects on infants (AAP Committee on Drugs, 2001; Hale, 2006). Breastfeeding is not contraindicated for routine recommended vaccines for the mother or infant (CPS, 2012b).

Think back to Joelle, the pregnant woman who is deciding whether to breastfeed. Suppose that the nurse, when reviewing Joelle's medical record, determines that Joelle has a history of herpes simplex virus infection. Would breastfeeding be contraindicated for Joelle?

Physiology of Milk Production

In the first trimester of pregnancy, estrogen and progesterone cause the duct system in breast tissue to multiply. The Montgomery glands (on the areola and around the nipple) enlarge and begin an oily secretion that helps protect the nipple and areola (Lauwers & Shinskie, 2005). By 6 to 7 months' gestation, the pregnant woman's breasts increase in secretory activity, and the acini and

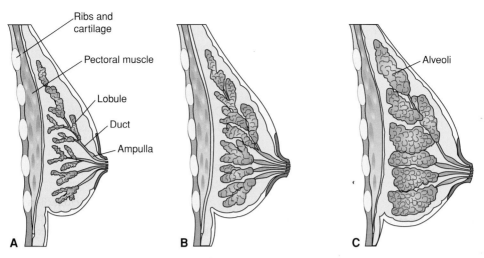

FIGURE 21.3 Comparison of the nonpregnant, nonlactating, adult breast **(A)**; pregnant breast **(B)**; and lactating breast **(C)**. In part **C**, note the increased size of the overall breast, as well as its ducts and lobules.

alveoli within the mammary tissue swell with colostrum (Cahill & Wagner, 2002a). It is not unusual for women to describe seeing drops of colostrum on their nipples in the third trimester (Wagner, 2012). The increased number of alveoli and body fluids that support lactation may increase the weight of the breast by as much as 454 to 680 g (Lauwers & Shinskie, 2005). See Figure 21.3. The expulsion of the placenta following childbirth enables reversal of the inhibitory effect of estrogen and progesterone on lactation, and prolactin levels increase (Cahill & Wagner, 2002a). A mother's breasts then continue the process that allows her to provide her newborn with human milk.

Suckling by the infant sends nerve impulses that ascend the spinal cord and stimulates the hypothalamus. In response, the anterior pituitary gland releases prolactin, which is the primary hormone responsible for milk production (Fig. 21.4). In addition, the posterior pituitary gland releases oxytocin, which causes the cells in the alveoli to contract, initiating the milk ejection reflex (Wagner, 2012). The alveoli actively produce milk during the breastfeeding or pumping session and, when active suckling ceases, the alveoli in the breasts continue the process of refilling the ductal system with milk in preparation for the next breastfeeding or breast milk pumping session. When emptying of accumulated milk from the breast is inadequate, the levels of prolactin and oxytocin decrease, causing milk production to decrease as well (Cahill & Wagner, 2002a).

The early production of breast milk is in response to the endocrine system. The hormonal shifts initiate the production of colostrum. Beyond the first 2 to 3 days, the shift is made to an autocrine system, and milk removal ensures further production. This phase signals the beginning of a new phase of lactogenesis and

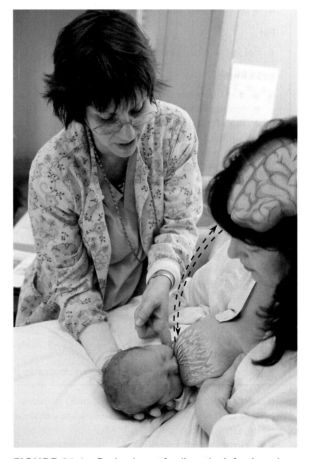

FIGURE 21.4 During breastfeeding, the infant's suckling stimulates the anterior pituitary gland to secrete prolactin, which in turn stimulates the breasts to secrete milk. Suckling also causes the posterior pituitary gland to secrete oxytocin, which in turn stimulates the breasts to eject milk into the ducts for removal by the newborn.

is accompanied by primary engorgement. The mother's breasts will feel warm, fuller, and heavier. Decreasing the amount of milk removal will signal a desire to decrease milk production.

Composition

Box 21.2 provides an overview of the components of human milk.

This section describes the evolution of breast milk both throughout the breastfeeding session as well as throughout the breastfeeding experience.

Evolution of Breast Milk During Stages of Lactation

During pregnancy, the breasts prepare to produce milk during the phase known as lactogenesis I. In the first

---

● **BOX 21.2** **Components of Human Milk and Their Benefits**

Protein

- The amount of protein in breast milk is perfect for infant growth and brain development.
- Protein in breast milk is easily digested and well-absorbed.
- Whey:casein ratio of breast milk is 60:40.
- Whey is more easily digested than casein.
- Whey is predominant in breast milk.
- Casein is predominant in cow's milk and infant formulas, making the protein in cow's milk formula harder to digest.
- 8 of 20 amino acids in breast milk are essential.

Fat

- Fat is the most variable component in breast milk.

It Changes

- During the feeding
  - low-fat foremilk at the beginning
  - high-fat hindmilk at the end
- Throughout the day
  - high milk volume/low fat content in morning (fat content lowest at 6 AM)
  - low milk volume/high fat content later in the day (fat content peaks at midafternoon)
- With age of infant
  - preterm breast milk has 30% higher fat concentration for some time
- Lipase enzyme (found in the infant's intestine and in the breast milk itself) breaks down fat so that it is more easily digested and utilized.
- Half of breast milk calories come from fat.
- Fat is found mostly in the hindmilk.
- Breast milk contains 20 calories/oz.

Carbohydrate

- Lactose accounts for most of the carbohydrates in human milk.
- Lactase enzyme (present in breast milk) is necessary to convert lactose into simple sugars that can be easily used.
- Lactose is metabolized easily.
  - Provides energy to the growing brain
  - Enhances calcium absorption, helping to prevent rickets

- Promotes growth of lactobacillus bifidus and lowers harmful organisms in the gut
- Is an available source of galactose

Vitamins and Minerals

- Complete, but lower levels found in breast milk than in formula
- More easily absorbed from breast milk
- Higher levels in formula, but more are excreted

Renal Solute Load (RSL)

- Renal solute load of breast milk is a third of that in formula, placing less stress on the kidneys.

Vitamin D

- Breastmilk contains small amounts (15 to 40 IU/litre) of vitamin D.
- Those most at risk for vitamin D deficiency are preterm babies, and dark-skinned babies in northern climates.
- The need for vitamin D supplementation for healthy full-term infants is controversial; however, it is recommended that all healthy, full-term breast-fed infants receive a supplement of 400 IU/day from birth, continuing until the infant's diet includes at least 400 IU/day of Vitamin D from other dietary sources, or until the breastfed infant reaches 1 year of age. (Health Canada, 2012c)

Iron

- Iron is found in smaller amounts in breast milk (0.5 to 1 mg/L), but iron absorption is increased due to high lactose and vitamin C content.

Enzymes

- There are 20 active enzymes in human milk. There are none or limited amounts in cow's milk.
- Help to digest fat
- Increase bio-availability of other components

Source: Registered Nurses' Association of Ontario. (2006). *Breastfeeding: Fundamental concepts. A self-learning package.* Toronto: Registered Nurses' Association of Ontario 15–16. Reproduced with permission.

few weeks postpartum, the type and composition of milk the woman produces changes. **Colostrum**, the milk produced in the first 1 to 4 days of lactation, is clear to yellowish in colour. It is present in small amounts of 5 to 10 mL per feed; the infant's kidneys are not able to handle large volumes of fluid initially (RNAO, 2006). Colostrum contains increased amounts of protein and minerals and is lower in fat, carbohydrates, and some vitamins than mature milk (RNAO, 2006). It contains large amounts of antibodies and immunoglobulins, which help boost the newborn's immature immune system. It is easily digested and acts as a laxative to assist in the elimination of meconium (RNAO, 2006).

Transitional human milk, produced at approximately 5 to 10 days of lactation, is a mixture of colostrum and mature breast milk (RNAO, 2006). It has increased concentrations of lactose, fat, and calories, but a lower concentration of immunoglobulins and total proteins, than colostrum. Its production signals the beginning of lactogenesis II and is accompanied by changes to the breasts, including warmth, heaviness, and some engorgement.

Mature human milk contains more lactose and fat than does colostrum. It begins approximately 2 weeks postpartum and lasts until 7 to 8 months of lactation. Milk produced after this time has reduced amounts of some vitamins and minerals.

Evolution of Breast Milk During a Feed

Not only does breast milk vary in nutrient content by stage of lactation, but it also varies for each woman according to the time of day, volume of milk available, and whether the infant feeds from one breast or both breasts at a feeding. For example, breast milk fat content is higher in the day and evening than in the morning and night (Kent et al., 2006). It is important to note, however, that fat intake of infants is not related to breastfeeding frequency, and infants have the same fat intake whether they take small frequent feedings or large, infrequent feedings (Kent et al., 2006). Mothers of premature infants produce breast milk that is higher in iron, sodium, and energy as a result of increased levels of protein and fat.

Mature milk is composed of foremilk and hindmilk. **Foremilk**, breast milk delivered during the first 5 to 10 minutes of a feeding, is lower in calories and fat than is breast milk produced in the latter part of the feed. **Hindmilk**, breast milk at the end of a feeding session, is higher in fat and energy. Because of the different properties of the milk found throughout a feeding session, it is important to allow the infant to nurse effectively at one breast prior to switching to the opposite breast (Kent et al., 2006).

 Recall Lindsay, the young woman returning for her 6-week clinic appointment. What type of breast milk is her newborn receiving?

Medicinal Supplementation for Breastfed Infants

Vitamin D

Health Canada (2012c) as well as the CPS (2013d) recommends 10 μg (400 IU) of vitamin D supplement daily for all breastfed infants. This supplementation should start at birth and continue until the diet includes at least 10 μg (400 IU) per day of vitamin D from other dietary sources, or until the breastfed infant reaches 1 year of age. For those infants who live in a Northern community, that is, north of the 55th parallel (approximate latitude of Edmonton), intake of vitamin D should be increased to 800 IU/day from all sources during the winter months, when there is less sunlight. Premature infants should receive 200 IU/kg/day to a maximum of 400 IU/day.

Iron

According to Health Canada (2012c), caregivers should introduce breastfed infants to iron-rich complementary foods gradually beginning around 6 months of age. Preterm infants, low–birth weight infants, infants with hematologic disorders, and infants with inadequate iron stores at birth generally require iron supplementation before 6 months of age. Iron may be administered while continuing exclusive breastfeeding.

Donor Human Milk

For a small minority of women who are not able to supply their own breast milk to their infant (e.g., a mother who cannot pump sufficient milk for her immunocompromised newborn), donor human milk is a more readily available alternative to commercial formula (Tully et al., 2004). Indications for the use of donor human milk include prematurity, feeding intolerance, burns, gastrointestinal surgery, immunodeficiency diseases, and prevention or treatment of allergies. Immunologic benefits, enhanced nutrient absorption, low allergenicity, growth factors, and maturation of organ systems contribute to the development of the infants who receive donor human milk (Tully et al., 2004).

A **human milk bank** is an agency that operates to collect donor human milk, verify its safety for use, and distribute it to those who request it. The Human Milk Banking Association of North America (HMBANA) was established in 1985 to develop standards for the operation of donor milk banks in cooperation with the U.S. Food and Drug Administration and the Centers for Disease Control and Prevention. The HMBANA also serves to enhance information sharing among milk banks and to improve societal awareness of the benefits of donor human milk for ill infants and children.

As of this writing, three human milk banks are operating in Canada, namely in Vancouver, Calgary, and Toronto (HMBANA, 2013), with a fourth opening in Quebec in 2014. Donors complete a verbal and written questionnaire and are screened serologically for infectious diseases, including HIV, syphilis, hepatitis B, and hepatitis C (BC Women's Hospital & Health Centre, 2008). Donors must follow specific procedures during pumping, storing, and transit to ensure the quality of the donated milk. Once the frozen milk is at the milk bank, a number of donations may be pooled to promote a more homogeneous mixture, as each woman's breast milk differs slightly in composition. The milk is pasteurized, then repackaged and refrozen until distribution. Pasteurization and freezing affect several vitamins, minerals, immunoglobulins, enzymes, and lipids (Lawrence & Lawrence, 2005); however, the risk for viral or bacterial contamination outweighs the benefit of preservation of these human milk components. The milk is shipped in an insulated box that may contain dry ice when moved over long distances. Human milk from the BC Women's Milk Bank is available by prescription. A processing fee is charged for recipients outside of BC Women's and BC Children's Hospitals (BC Women's Hospital & Health Centre, 2008). Dilemmas concerning wet-nursing practices still have implications in today's society. Women who wish to directly donate milk to the infant of a friend or family member must consider the legal ramifications if such milk contains harmful bacteria or viruses. The CPS and the American Society of Paediatrics do not support the sharing of unprocessed human milk.

COLLABORATIVE CARE: BREASTFEEDING

Breastfeeding classes taken before a baby's birth introduce parents to techniques that help ensure breastfeeding success. Involvement of the woman's partner in breastfeeding education helps to build a supportive environment for the mother contemplating lactation (Pisacane et al., 2005). Peer counselling from mothers, sisters, aunts, or close friends with lactating experience can help the woman as she encounters situations that are new and different to her. Mothers in particular situations can act as peer counsellors to new mothers (e.g., breastfeeding twins or triplets). The lactation consultant is an invaluable professional resource to the breastfeeding dyad (IBCLE, 2014).

Professional organizations exist in support of breastfeeding, such as La Leche League Canada (www.lllc.ca), and Infact Canada (http://www.infactcanada.ca/index.htm). For example, La Leche League Canada's Web site has breastfeeding information, and information about groups throughout Canada, including maps of their locations. The Breastfeeding Committee for Canada (BCC) (www.breastfeedingcanada.ca) is useful to professionals who want to work with the BCC to establish breastfeeding as the infant norm for Canada.

Assessment

Welcoming a new baby into the home requires lifestyle considerations. A mother who is breastfeeding will require additional support in the early weeks to facilitate optimal results for both her and her baby. Exploring areas such as rest, nutrition, and hydration can identify potential problems or concerns and may provide a good opportunity for nurses to involve the baby's father or other family members in facilitating an optimal environment. Encouraging the infant's siblings to participate in feeding sessions by sitting close to the nursing dyad, asking questions, and even holding the infant's hand may help them become more comfortable with a new feeding process in the home. Assessment Tool 21.1 provides a foundation for obtaining information about the woman's knowledge and understanding of breastfeeding that the nurse can use to shape education and interventions.

Rest and Environment

Nurses evaluate the woman's patterns of rest to ensure that she is getting sufficient sleep to prevent excessive fatigue, which might interfere with milk production. This can be difficult because the woman is adjusting to the unpredictable sleep–wake cycles of the newborn. Nurses remind breastfeeding mothers to get appropriate rest, which often means sleeping when the infant is sleeping. Nurses encourage family members to assist the new mother with household chores so that she can focus on caring and feeding her infant. This becomes especially important in the first few weeks of breastfeeding twins or triplets.

Nutrition

The nutritional status of a woman in the postpartum period will depend on her nutritional status prior to the pregnancy and the number of pregnancies she has carried. Some of a pregnant woman's nutrient reserves may be tapped during pregnancy. A lactating mother who is in generally good health and consumes a variety of nutritious foods to satisfy hunger can replenish the nutrient stores that she used to support her pregnancy.

The nurse performs a detailed nutritional history and review of the client's dietary behaviours to ensure

● **ASSESSMENT TOOL 21.1 Breastfeeding**

BREASTFEEDING—INITIAL ASSESSMENT

- Has the client ever breastfed before?
  - If yes, what was her experience like?
  - If no, has she had close contact with anyone who has breastfed?
  - What was the feeding intention prior to the birth of the baby?
- Has the client taken prenatal classes?
- Has she attended any specific breastfeeding classes?
- What books, Websites, or other materials has she read about breastfeeding?
- How long ago did the client give birth?
- What kind of birth did the client have?
- What is the client's mood, physical condition, and overall state of health?
- What is the client's support system?
- What are the client's breasts like?
- What are the client's nipples like?
- What is the infant's physical condition and overall state of health?

- Does the mother seem confident in handling the newborn?

BREASTFEEDING—ONGOING ASSESSMENT

- Has the mother assumed a comfortable position for herself and her infant?
- Is the mother holding the newborn correctly?
- Does the mother bring the infant to her breast?
- Does the mother feed the newborn every 2 to 3 hours?
- Is there any evidence of milk production? Are the mother's breasts engorged?
- Do the nipples show any signs of bruises, cracks, or abrasions?
- Does the mother report any signs of pain or discomfort?
- Is the infant opening the mouth wide?
- Is there any evidence of milk transfer?
- What are the urine and stool outputs of the infant?

adequate intake and to correct any identified problems. During the first 6 months of lactation, women aged 14 to 50 years require approximately 330 calories/day more than nonlactating women of the same age (see Chapter 3). Estimated energy requirements for a lactating woman are 400 to 500 kcal/day more than for a nonlactating woman (Yon & Johnson, 2005). A lactating woman's Recommended Dietary Allowances (RDA) for protein is that of a nonpregnant, nonlactating woman plus 25 g/day of protein. This equates to approximately 71 g/day of protein (Health Canada, 2006a).

A lactating woman should follow Canada's food guide and consume nutritious foods she enjoys. Calcium needs are the same as for the nonpregnant, nonlactating woman: 1300 mg/day for those 18 years or younger, and 1000 mg/day for those 19 to 50 years. Iron needs are actually less during lactation than for nonpregnant, nonlactating women and pregnant women: 10 mg/day for women 18 years or younger, and 9 mg/day for women 19 to 50 years (Health Canada, 2005). The lactating woman's dietary intake influences the amounts of some nutrients in her breast milk (Box 21.3). **Fluid Intake.** The nurse should discuss the client's fluid intake. Breastfeeding mothers do not need to drink milk to make milk. Breastfeeding mothers should drink to satisfy thirst (RNAO, 2006). One of the body's chemical responses to breastfeeding is thirst. A woman who is

nursing will likely find it essential to have something to drink available while breastfeeding.

Allergens, Potentially Offending Foods, and Substances to Avoid. A lactating woman may notice changes

● **BOX 21.3 Vitamins and Minerals in Breast Milk Influenced by Maternal Diet**

Vitamins

Vitamin A
Vitamin D
Vitamin C
Thiamin
Riboflavin
Niacin
Vitamin E
Pyridoxine
Biotin
Pantothenic acid
Cyanocobalamin

Minerals

Manganese
Iodine
Fluoride
Selenium

in her infant's behaviour after her consumption of a particular food and subsequent provision of breast milk to her infant. Foods such as chocolate, peanuts, milk or milk products, chocolate, and cruciferous vegetables (broccoli, cabbage, cauliflower, onion), cherries, and prunes have been reported by mothers to be associated with infantile fussy behaviour (Pryor & Pryor, 2014). The lactating woman does not need to eliminate all these foods from her diet simply because of the potential for changes in the behaviour of her infant. The nurse would advise her to eliminate one food at a time from her diet to determine which food, if any, seems to be causing irritability in the newborn. Once identified, the woman can eliminate or replace that food with another that is less offending and offers the same nutrients. A recent systematic review revealed that there is little evidence to support restricting a breastfeeding woman's diet to prevent infant allergies, with the exception of atopic eczema (Kramer & Kakuma, 2012). There are currently two studies under way in the United Kingdom—the Learning Early About Peanut (LEAP) allergy study and the Enquiring About Tolerance (EAT) study—to explore whether introducing solids before 6 months decreases the risk of childhood food allergies.

Caffeine. Women secrete peak levels of caffeine into breast milk 60 to 120 minutes after consumption; the infant excretes the caffeine it receives slowly (Hale, 2006). Maternal caffeine intake greater than three cups per day can result in an irritable infant and an altered sleeping pattern (AAP Committee on Drugs, 2001). Caffeinated coffee, soft drinks, tea, and chocolate contribute to daily caffeine intake.

Alcohol. Alcohol secreted into breast milk can be harmful to the breastfed infant, causing symptoms in the baby such as drowsiness, weakness, diaphoresis, and decreased weight and length gain. Alcohol is transferred into breast milk in a similar concentration to that present in maternal serum. Alcohol can impede the let-down reflex, and excessive alcohol may impair milk production. Maternal consumption of 1 g/kg body weight per day of alcohol decreases milk production (Riordan & Wambach, 2010). This equates to four 12-oz beers, 16 oz of table wine, or 4 to 5 oz of liquor per day for a woman who weighs 60 kg. Breastfeeding mothers are advised to limit alcoholic beverages because alcohol readily passes into breastmilk and is ingested by the infant, causing sedation and impairing motor skills (Motherisk, 2013). Heavy alcohol intake should be avoided; occasional, moderate alcohol consumption is unlikely to create issues for the infant. Peak alcohol concentrations in breast milk occur approximately 30 to 60 minutes after ingestion. Lactating women who want to consume an alcohol-containing beverage may drink it shortly after nursing to allow peak concentration to rise and fall before the next breastfeeding. The woman should ideally refrain from breastfeeding for a minimum of 2 hours per drink following consumption (Motherisk, 2013).

Nicotine. Nicotine and its primary metabolite, cotinine, are present in human milk of lactating women who smoke. It has not been determined whether nicotine, other compounds in tobacco, or environmental exposure to tobacco smoke are responsible for increased infant respiratory illness, decreased infant weight gain, or decreased maternal milk production (AAP, 2001). One Canadian study found that fetal exposure to household second-hand smoke during pregnancy is associated with increased childhood asthma (Simons et al., 2012). Although there is not enough evidence that nicotine itself causes health risks for breastfeeding infants, health care providers should consider pregnancy and lactation as opportune times to encourage cessation of smoking (AAP, 2012; Motherisk, 2013).

Contraceptives. Research evidence on the safety of combined oral contraceptives during lactation is of variable quality, and there is little information about the low-dose estrogen combinations. It is also believed that combination oral contraceptives do not affect the composition of breast milk in women who are healthy and well nourished (Drugs.com, 2014a). Injectable depot medroxyprogesterone acetate (Depo-Provera) has not been shown to adversely affect the composition, quality, or amount of breast milk. It can be given immediately postpartum regardless of breastfeeding (SOGC, 2012). The long-term effects of vaginal rings that contain some progesterone are currently unknown (see Chapter 8). The vaginal ring may be started 3 weeks postpartum if not breastfeeding; if breastfeeding, it is recommended to be started after 6 weeks postpartum (SOGC, 2012). After 6 months postpartum, combination oral contraceptives, including the vaginal ring and transdermal patch, can be used, but it is preferable to use progestin-only methods (Drugs.com, 2014a). Barrier methods such as diaphragms, cervical caps, condoms, or sponges may be used to avoid exposure to hormones, as desired by the couple. The Lactational amenorrhea method (LAM) is highly effective if certain conditions are met (Black et al., 2004).

Herbs and Galactagogues. Certain substances have been identified as increasing milk production by increasing prolactin levels. These substances are known as *galactagogues* and include herbs, typically in the form of pills or teas. Little research exists to support their efficacy, safety, mechanism of action, or potential side effects. As well, currently no regulations enforce herbal

● COMPLEMENTARY/ALTERNATIVE MEDICINE 21.1
Galactogogues

Lactating mothers should discuss the intake of herbal teas with their health care providers because some herbs may be transferred to their infants or affect milk production (Hale, 2006). Herbs purported to enhance milk production include fenugreek, goat's rue, milk thistle, and fennel. Medicinal galactogogues such as metoclopramide and domperidone are also believed to increase the rate of milk synthesis (Drugs.com, 2013, 2014b). Oxytocin nasal spray enhances the milk ejection reflex, but is not available in Canada (Hale, 2006). Health Canada has not

approved any prescription drug or herbal remedies for use in increasing milk production (Saskatchewan Drug Information Services, 2012). Consultation with a lactation consultant can help identify causes of insufficient milk production or impaired milk ejection reflex. The solution to a particular woman's problem may be rectified by a change of position, environment, or other behaviours unrelated to the need for a galactogogue.

---

labelling or dosing. See Complementary/Alternative Medicine 21.1 for further discussion.

Select Potential Nursing Diagnoses
The following nursing diagnoses may apply to the care of the breastfeeding woman and newborn:

- **Lack of Knowledge** related to breastfeeding techniques and the process of lactation
- **Anxiety** related to concerns about infant feeding patterns
- **Effective Breastfeeding** as evidenced by correct technique, content infant, and mother's reports of satisfaction
- **Effective Breastfeeding** as evidenced by appropriate milk production and milk transfer (ability of the baby to access the milk that is produced)
- **Pain** related to engorged breasts and/or sore nipples
- **Ineffective Breastfeeding** related to poor infant sucking reflex or inappropriate latch

Planning and Intervention
Nursing Care Plan 21.1 highlights the care of a pregnant woman who is deciding to breastfeed. Although the nurse should always tailor care to be appropriate for the specific client's and her infant's circumstances, there are general interventions which may be used for various stages and issues related to breastfeeding.

Supporting the First Breastfeed
Newborns are placed on the mother's chest in skin to skin contact within the first half hour of life; during this time, some infants have actually started to "crawl" towards the mother's nipple to latch on and breastfeed. When a woman puts her newborn to breast shortly after birth, the posterior pituitary gland releases oxytocin, which causes myoepithelial cells of the uterus and ductal system of the breast to contract. Uterine contractions, in response to infant suckling following birth,

promote the expulsion of the placenta and decrease the risk for maternal hemorrhage. The delivery of the placenta promotes a hormonal milieu that is low in estrogen and progesterone and high in prolactin levels. The infant suckling at the breast also stimulates the release of prolactin, which is essential for milk production.

Newborns may lick or explore the nipple without nutritive sucking during the first encounter at the breast. The nurse helps mothers to interpret this experience as positive and as a way for mother and baby to begin bonding.

The nurse assists with breastfeeding by helping secure privacy for the family. He or she assists the woman to find a comfortable breastfeeding position. Pillows are helpful in offering adequate physical support for the mother and baby. The nurse may place a pillow where the mother's body does not support the baby's body. Common bed pillows can be manipulated to accommodate positioning. Some companies manufacture pillows that are curved much like a C-shape: the mother places the pillow around her abdomen and uses it to support her arms, which are supporting the infant. Pillows may also be useful to support the arms, feet, or legs of the mother who is upright in bed. The father can be recruited to become involved and can assist the mother in positioning their infant.

Support of Ongoing Breastfeeds
Positions. Several holds are used for successful breastfeeding (Fig. 21.5). In most positions, the mother supports her breast with one hand while supporting the newborn's head and back with the other hand.

- The *cradle hold* may be most intuitive for new mothers; however, it offers minimal control of the baby's head (Fig. 21.5A). The *cross-cradle hold* works better because it allows the mother to support the baby's head with one hand and offer the breast with the other

(text continues on page 868)

NURSING CARE PLAN 21.1

●

The Client Who is Deciding to Breastfeed

 Recall Joelle from the start of this chapter. Further conversation reveals that she will be taking a leave of absence from work for approximately 6 months. She states, "I really would like to try breastfeeding, and my husband is supportive and thinks we should try it, too. But I'm a bit nervous. This is all so new to me."

NURSING DIAGNOSIS

Deficient Knowledge related to lack of experience with breastfeeding.

EXPECTED OUTCOMES

1. The client will identify advantages and disadvantages of breastfeeding.
2. The client will state appropriate information related to measures to promote effective breastfeeding.

INTERVENTIONS	RATIONALES
Assess the client's and her partner's level of understanding about breastfeeding.	Assessment provides a baseline to identify specific client needs and develop an individualized teaching plan.
Explore the client's and her partner's exposure to breastfeeding. If previous pregnancies, explore methods of feeding and rationale for choice. Correct any misconceptions or myths. Allow time for questions.	Information about previous exposure helps to identify possible reasons for her choice and provides opportunities to clarify or correct misinformation and teach new information.
Describe the advantages and disadvantages of breastfeeding.	This information provides additional knowledge from which clients can make an informed effective choice.
Teach the client about the need for proper nutrition. Inform the client and her partner about the need for support for breastfeeding mothers. Demonstrate breast care techniques.	Proper nutrition is recommended to ensure an adequate milk supply and to promote well-being. Preparation for breastfeeding helps the client to become comfortable with handling her breasts; teaching about breast care techniques reduces the risk for future problems.
Demonstrate positions for breastfeeding and review measures for stimulating the neonate to suck and latch on, and for alternating breasts for feedings; allow the client time to practice.	Practice promotes understanding and opportunities to troubleshoot any problems that may arise; practice also helps to increase self-confidence.
Include the client's partner in teaching sessions.	Participation of the client's partner provides support and enhances the chances for a successful experience.
Arrange for the client to meet with a lactation consultant.	This referral provides additional opportunities for teaching and learning and allows for feedback and positive reinforcement, thus promoting a positive experience. The lactation consultant can also be a source of support in the postpartum period.

(continued)

NURSING CARE PLAN 21.1 ● The Client Who is Deciding to Breastfeed *(Continued)*

EVALUATION

1. The client states rationale for choosing breastfeeding.
2. The client demonstrates measures to prepare for breastfeeding.
3. The client demonstrates an understanding for support needs in the postpartum period.

NURSING DIAGNOSIS

Anxiety related to inexperience with breastfeeding.

EXPECTED OUTCOMES

1. The client will express concerns related to breastfeeding.
2. The client will identify strategies to cope with the new experience of breastfeeding.

INTERVENTIONS	RATIONALES
Assess the client's current understanding about breastfeeding; communicate accurate facts and answer questions honestly.	Assessment of current understanding provides direction for individualized care targeted to the client's needs; honest communication promotes trust.
Discuss with the client and her partner their concerns related to breastfeeding; encourage clients to verbalize their feelings, concerns, and perceptions.	Discussion provides opportunities to emphasize positive aspects and correct any misconceptions or misinformation; verbalization of fears and concerns aids in establishing sources of stress and problem areas that need to be addressed.
Include the client and her partner in discussion about breastfeeding.	Client participation increases feelings of control over the situation and promotes support and sharing.
Evaluate the client's past coping strategies to determine which strategies have been most effective.	Use of appropriate coping strategies aids in reducing anxiety.
Ask the client about available support systems, such as family, friends, community.	Additional sources of support are helpful in alleviating anxiety.
Provide the client with information about support groups, Web sites, and other sources of information related to breastfeeding.	Shared experiences and knowledge of similar situations can aid in preparing the client and her partner for what to expect with breastfeeding.

EVALUATION

1. The client and her partner state they are comfortable with the decision to breastfeed.
2. The client verbalizes decreased anxiety when discussing breastfeeding.
3. The client uses appropriate resources for support.

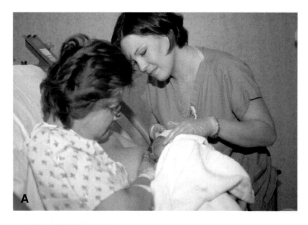

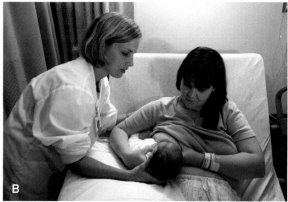

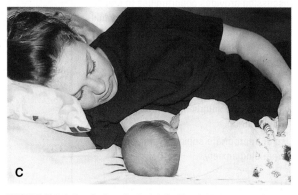

FIGURE 21.5   **A:** Cradle hold. **B:** Football hold. **C:** Side-lying hold.

hand. In the cross-cradle hold, the breast is supported from underneath with the hand leaning against the chest wall. The infant will be tummy-to-tummy in the cross-cradle hold.

- The mother who has had a cesarean birth may find the football (Fig. 21.5B) or side-lying (Fig. 21.5C) positions comfortable. Side-lying also may be a convenient position for feeding during periods of rest for the mother and infant.
- The C-hold refers to supporting the breast by the mother's thumb resting above the areola with the other fingers under the breast and away from the are-

ola. In this way she can lift the breast and help the baby take as much of the areola into the mouth as possible (Lauwers & Shinskie, 2005).
- The scissor grasp allows for some compression of the areola, although it is less effective if the mother's breast is small or her hand is large. The woman places her thumb on top of the breast, close to the thorax, with her index finger above the areola, and places the other fingers beneath the breast for support. This position may limit access to the areola, and so is discouraged if the baby does not latch on easily.

The infant should be well aligned and turned toward the mother, tummy to tummy, in all positions. The nurse instructs the woman that, once the baby is sucking, the mother should continue to support the breast until she and the baby are comfortably positioned. She can then wrap both arms around her infant to keep the infant close and well-positioned. A mother with large breasts may need to support the breast so that its weight does not break the seal that the baby's mouth has made.

Lindsay reports discomfort with breastfeeding. Which positions might the nurse suggest to enhance Lindsay's comfort during feeding sessions?

Infant Feeding Cues. With the **rooting reflex**, infants open their mouths and turn their heads toward the stimulus in search of a nipple. Infants will spontaneously exhibit this behaviour when a stimulus touches the cheek and this may be an indication that the infant is preparing for feeding. Infants may also wake spontaneously and start to stir, or they may suck on their fingers or hands to indicate they are preparing for a feeding (see Table 20.3 in Chapter 20). Inducing the rooting reflex can facilitate latching. This may include stroking the baby's cheek with the nipple or a finger to get the baby to turn toward the breast. Getting the baby to open the mouth to accept the breast may also include stroking the baby's lower lip with the nipple until the mouth opens wide. Another technique is to express a little colostrum from the nipple and allow the baby to lick it, or to place it on the baby's lips to elicit interest.

A hungrier baby may present with clenched fists, flexed arms, and moving legs as though riding a bicycle. Crying is a late sign of hunger (AAP, 2012; RNAO, 2006).

Latching. In the early days, arousing a sleeping baby to feed can be a challenge. The nurse can suggest unwrapping the baby from blankets, or even removing some of his or her clothing and positioning the baby skin-to-skin. Stroking the baby's feet, changing his or her diaper, or applying a warm, moist washcloth may help stimulate the baby as well. The father or other family members eager for involvement in feeding may be good candidates for helping to ready a baby for feeding.

Once the infant is awake, the mother can facilitate latching by holding the infant close and in good alignment, supporting the infant's nape and back, as the infant's head is slightly extended and tilted back. The mother then brings the infant to her with the mouth opposite the nipple. When the baby opens his or her mouth wide, the nurse advises the mother to quickly bring the baby onto the areola (the nipple may be off centre so that the baby takes a larger part of the breast in the lower jaw), without pushing the baby's head, which will cause the baby to arch away from the breast. Approximately 3.8 cm of areolar tissue should be centred in the infant's mouth. When an infant is latched correctly, his or her lips are flanged out over the areola, with the nose and chin touching the breast (Fig. 21.6). Most infants suck rapidly for 30 to 90 seconds (Cahill & Wagner, 2002b) until the mother experiences the milk ejection reflex, also known as the let-down reflex.

The nurse advises the mother that she will feel as though the baby is tugging on her breast tissue, but that a good latch is not painful; some sensitivity may be experienced in the first week. Audible assessment of swallowing in the first 24 to 48 hours is likely after three to four high-powered sucks and may sound like small puffs of air (Lauwers & Shinskie, 2005). After the mother's milk supply is established, the baby will develop a series of deeper and more rhythmic sucks followed by a pause, for swallowing and breathing. This series is often referred to as the *suck-swallow-breathe sequence.*

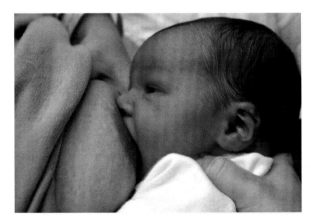

FIGURE 21.6 With correct latching, the newborn's lips flange out over the mother's areola, and the baby's nose and chin touch the mother's breast.

Infant Satiety Cues. Once the baby is latched onto the breast correctly, the mother allows the infant to suckle until he or she spontaneously comes off the breast, pushes the nipple from the mouth, or stops sucking entirely. These behaviours are *satiety cues.* The nurse instructs the mother to watch for the infant's satiety cues to determine when to stop the nursing session, rather than concentrating on how long the baby has been breastfeeding. Signs of effective milk transfer that can support the assessment of satiety include having seen the infant's lower jaw moving deeply and rhythmically, hearing swallows, seeing breast milk in the mouth, and soft maternal breast tissue after a feed. A satisfied postprandial baby has relaxed the arms and legs, appears drowsy, or falls asleep. During the first 2 months of life, a breastfed infant should nurse 8 to 12 times in a 24-hour period (AAP, 2012).

When a mother requests a general timeframe to gauge the length of a breastfeeding session, the nurse can suggest 20 to 30 minutes on the first breast, or as long as the infant continues to transfer milk, or until the baby spontaneously releases from the breast. The second breast can then be offered (Riordan & Wambach, 2010; RNAO, 2006). The nurse encourages the mother to offer both breasts during each early feeding session to stimulate milk production. Breast compression while the baby is at the breast can also enhance infant intake and milk production.

The nurse reminds the client to allow the baby to effectively feed on one breast during a feeding session, and then to offer the other breast if the baby desires. He or she instructs the client to alternate the breast offered first so that each breast is equally stimulated. Another technique is to offer just one breast during each feeding, and to alternate breasts with each feeding. If the client must break the suction during a feeding, the nurse instructs her to insert her finger into the corner of the baby's mouth between the gums to break the seal so that nipple trauma is minimized.

Burping. The primary reason to burp an infant is to help the baby expel air ingested during feeding or crying. Breastfed infants create a seal on the breast so that a correct latch does not allow for ingestion of air during suckling. Some breastfed infants, however, may benefit from burping during feedings if air was swallowed during crying prior to breastfeeding.

Use of Artificial Nipples. The use of pacifiers remains controversial and further research is needed to better understand the relationship between pacifiers and breastfeeding duration and exclusivity (O'Connor et al., 2009). Recent evidence regarding pacifier use suggests that families be advised to delay the introduction of artificial nipples from pacifiers and bottles until breastfeeding is well established, usually about 3 to 6 weeks; however, nurses need to recognize that pacifier use is a parental choice (CPS, 2013c). Newborns begin to recognize their mothers through touch, taste, and smell. They are forming both a nipple preference and comfort with sucking during this time; introduction of more than one type of nipple may impede breastfeeding. The sucking mechanism for breastfeeding differs from that of bottlefeeding. The breastfed infant's mouth must open wide to take in breast tissue, while the tongue protrudes over the lower lip as it flanges outward. Bottle-fed infants have a partially closed mouth, and the tongue does not protrude quite so far.

Pumping. Most lactating women can anticipate occasions when they will need to express breast milk to be fed to their babies during their absence. Breastfeeding mothers do not need to be present for every infant feeding. *Breast pumping* allows lactating women to express breast milk through manual stimulation or a mechanical device, so that they can store and subsequently feed the milk to their infants. Breast pumping is useful for women who return to work or school. Expressing breast milk affords other caregivers the opportunity to feed the infants without interrupting breastfeeding or exposing the infant to formula. Pumping can also be used in special circumstances to supplement infants who have inadequate intake at the breast, for example, a sleepy baby with hyperbilirubinemia, or when mothers are separated from their infant for maternal or infant illness. A mother could produce an excessive milk supply and so should be discouraged from pumping routinely in addition to breastfeeding if the baby is nursing well and she does not need the expressed breast milk. Mothers of multiples may choose a combination of breastfeeding and pumping in order to meet the demands of caring for twins or triplets.

If a mother gives birth to a newborn who cannot be put to the breast (e.g., due to prematurity), a pumping regimen should be initiated within 6 to 24 hours after birth (Bonyata, 2011). A hospital-grade, electric pump is most efficient at extracting milk from the breasts (Fig. 21.7). Maternal comfort and effectiveness of milk expression are enhanced when breast pump features include hospital-grade electric capability, double breast shields that enable pumping both breasts at the same time, and the ability to adjust for suction and the number of cycles per minute. Other pumps available, including manual pumps, battery-powered pumps, and mini-electric pumps may not have enough power for adequate suction or adjustment of suction or cycles. Nurses consider the indication for pumping and ensure that mothers use an appropriate breast pump for the circumstance.

Some insurance plans reimburse the cost of a breast pump when infants are born prematurely. In these cases, the nurse encourages the client to inquire about insur-

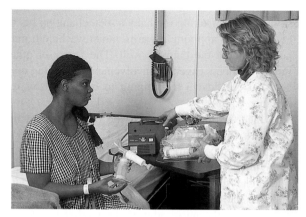

FIGURE 21.7 This nurse is teaching a client about the differences between a hand-held breast pump and an electric breast pump (shown on the table).

ance coverage for a breast pump and the documentation required for reimbursement. Breast pumps are often available where other baby supplies are sold, with a large variety of pumps found at stores dedicated to baby supplies. The internet is another resource for mothers who wish to purchase a breast pump. Caution should be exercised when sharing breast pumps with different mothers.

Pumping both breasts simultaneously helps increase milk volume and decreases time spent pumping each breast consecutively (Fig. 21.8). Mothers should set the level of suction on low and increase suction throughout the session as comfort allows. The breast pump should provide cycles of suction and release as many times as the infant would suckle.

Milk supply is stimulated by demand. Increasing pumping frequency increases supply. The stress of needing to pump and having a baby who is not well can adversely affect milk production, milk release, or both. Teaching Tips 21.1 provide suggestions to improve the volume of milk expression.

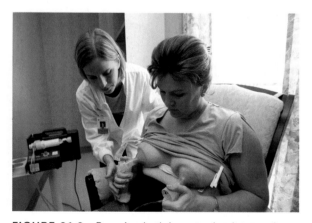

FIGURE 21.8 Pumping both breasts simultaneously will provide the most milk volume and minimize the time the client must spend performing the activity.

● TEACHING TIPS 21.1   Improving Milk Volume and Expression

- Use an electric, double pump. Single pumping accompanied by massage of the breast can also be effective.
- Pump 8 times in a 24-hour period, allowing for 4 to 5 hours of continuous sleep through the night.
- Provide a comfortable and private environment.
- Play soft music.
- Use imagery to imagine your baby successfully breast-feeding.
- Use imagery to imagine milk flowing from your breasts.
- Apply clean, warm, and moist compresses to breasts before pumping.

- Maintain adequate fluid and nutrient intake.
- Maintain adequate rest.
- Massage shoulders.
- Promote skin-to-skin contact with the baby before pumping ("kangaroo care").
- Place a picture of the baby or an article that belongs to him or her within sight.
- Accept support to free up time for meeting pumping and rest regimens.

An appropriate pumping regimen for a mother who is separated from her infant includes encouragement to pump every 2 to 3 hours during the day, and at least once or twice during the night (much the same timing as if the baby were nursing). Pumping sessions should last 12 to 15 minutes. The frequency of pumping sessions is more important to stimulating milk production than is extending the length of pumping sessions. Personal hygiene and pump equipment cleanliness are important to avoid contamination of expressed breast milk. See Teaching Tips 21.2 for details.

Milk Storage. The duration for which breast milk can be stored for use depends on the storage conditions. Mothers should feed freshly expressed breast milk to the infant or chill it as soon as possible to retain maximum immunologic and nutritional benefits and to decrease the possibility of bacterial contamination. Expressed breast milk may be refrigerated before use

for a maximum of 48 hours. Breast milk should be frozen within 24 hours of pumping and may be stored in the freezer of a two-door refrigerator–freezer combination unit for a maximum of 3 months (The Hospital for Sick Children, 2008). Breast milk stored in a deep freezer may be used within 6 to 12 months (Lauwers & Shinskie, 2005; The Hospital for Sick Children, 2008). Refrigerated and frozen human milk should be placed toward the back of the cooling unit to avoid partial warming with repeated opening of the unit's door. Once thawing begins, breast milk should be used within 24 hours and should not be refrozen (The Hospital for Sick Children, 2008).

Optimal storage containers for breast milk include specialized disposable breast milk storage bags or glass containers. Glass containers are the least destructive of milk components (Rasmussen & Geraghty, 2011). Glass has a durable, smooth surface for cleaning and is reusable, making it economical. The interior of soft

● TEACHING TIPS 21.2   Maintaining Breast and Equipment Hygiene

- Cleanse the breast area every day with warm water only; avoid soap on the breast because it can dry the skin.
- Wear a clean bra daily.
- Change breast pads as they become damp.
- Wash hands with warm water and soap just before pumping.
- Express milk into a sterile bottle or container.
- Maintain a "clean" area for equipment. Do not place equipment into sink for cleaning.
- Wash flange and one-way valve with hot water and dish soap (not antibacterial); rinse well with hot water.
- Allow equipment to air-dry.
- Once daily, sterilize equipment that comes in contact with milk by boiling for 3 to 5 minutes in a covered pan or washing in the top rack of a dishwasher.

- Take care not to allow backflow of milk into tubing.
- Label container with baby's name, date, and time of expression.
- Store expressed milk in the refrigerator toward the back for use within 48 hours.
- Store expressed milk in the freezer within 24 hours of pumping. Cool milk in refrigerator first.
- Thaw frozen expressed milk in a warm water bath, taking care not to allow water to spill into the container.
- Use previously frozen expressed milk within 24 hours. Do not refreeze if any thawing has occurred.

plastic (polypropylene) bottles is prone to scratches during the cleaning process, making adequate cleaning difficult. Bacteria thrive in scratches. Hard plastic (polycarbonate) bottles should not be used because of recent concerns about the release of the potentially harmful chemical bisphenol A (Health Canada, 2008). Soft, plastic bottle liners (polyethylene bags), such as those used inside hard plastic bottles, are prone to leaking breast milk during freezing and thawing. Use of bottle liner bags also reduces antibody retention. In addition, these bags may alter the smell and taste of human milk, causing the infant to refuse it (Lauwers & Shinskie, 2005).

Management of Problems Related to Breastfeeding
Nipple Protractility. A nipple that everts easily helps to provide the infant with a stimulus on the hard palate, which will stimulate the sucking reflex and promote effective milk extraction. The nurse can perform a simple pinch test, which consists of applying pressure and pinching on the areola at the base of the nipple with the forefinger and at the top of the nipple with the thumb. A protracting nipple moves outward; an inverted nipple moves inward. Women with nipples that remain inverted into the third trimester can do several things to evert their nipples. They should consult with their practitioner about the safety of such techniques because nipple stimulation can cause preterm labour in some women by liberating oxytocin from the posterior pituitary gland.

One technique is to cut a small hole in the bra at the place of the nipple and allow the pressure around the nipple to push it forward (Lauwers & Shinskie, 2005). This acts in a similar fashion to wearing breast shells which, though not proven to be an effective means of everting nipples prenatally (Lauwers & Shinskie, 2005), some women will opt to try. The niplette, an instrument that applies continuous suction, may be worn for increasing periods of time after the third trimester (Avent, 2008). In the postpartum period, a mother may manually form the nipple or apply ice to the nipple before each feed to promote protractility (Lauwers & Shinskie, 2005). She may also use a breast pump to assist with stretching the nipple and she can offer the breast to the newborn, who may be able to latch if the surrounding tissue is soft and malleable in the infant mouth.

Plugged Ducts. A **plugged milk duct** is a localized blockage of milk that results from stasis of milk. The affected breast may present with a tender lump that feels hot to the touch. The lactating woman remains afebrile and does not have signs of infection (Walters, 2007).

The nurse instructs the client that offering the breast with the plugged duct first may help remove the blockage, as a result of the infant's vigorous sucking at the beginning of a feed. Maximizing suction by changing the infant's feeding position to point his or her nose in the direction of the plugged duct may be beneficial (Riordan & Wambach, 2010). Other helpful measures include massaging the affected area during a warm shower or after applying heat from a hot water bottle (Walters, 2007). If the baby cannot directly breastfeed, the nurse can suggest hand expression while leaning over a container of warm water. Alternatively, the woman may apply warm, moist compresses followed by hand expression to release the blockage (Lauwers & Shinskie, 2005). In order to prevent recurrence, the nurse advises the woman to allow the baby to lead the breastfeeding (paying attention to her infant's cues), to ensure a good latch, and to recognize effective emptying of her breasts. She should also be advised to avoid wearing constrictive clothing (e.g., underwire bras) and baby carriers.

Mastitis. Mastitis means inflammation of the mammary gland (usually unilateral); it may involve bacterial infection. Infection may be detected through cultures of breast milk, although it is difficult to obtain a sample not contaminated by skin flora. Causative organisms vary and may include common nasal and skin flora such as *Staphylococcus aureus.* Organisms that are also implicated in mastitis are Streptococcus A and Streptococcus B which should always be considered in the case of a bilateral mastitis. Mastitis may be associated with an unresolved plugged milk duct, inadequate milk removal or oversupply, and maternal fatigue and stress. It is characterized by maternal flu-like symptoms (e.g., fever, malaise). The breast tissue appears red and inflamed and is tender (Walters, 2007).

Mastitis occurs most frequently after the breastfeeding dyad has been discharged from the hospital. Nurses advise mothers to continue to breastfeed and use the same techniques as for a plugged duct. In addition, treatment includes analgesics and plenty of maternal rest and fluids. If a fever persists or the mother continues to feel ill, she should contact her primary health care provider, who will probably prescribe antibiotics. Mothers who require antibiotic therapy should complete the entire course of medication while continuing to breastfeed. Untreated mastitis or discontinuing breastfeeding in the acute phase may lead to an abscess, in which needle aspiration or drain placement is necessary to remove the accumulated pus.

Evaluation
Expected outcomes for a breastfeeding dyad are a satisfying, comfortable, feeding relationship for mother and child, where the mother is producing an appropriate milk supply and the infant is growing and thriving.

FORMULA FEEDING

Infant formula is patterned after the composition of breast milk or the outcomes of the postprandial breastfed infant. In Canada, Good Manufacturing Practices for infant formulas establish general requirements for the effective control of ingredients, formulations, processes, facilities, and equipment used for production of infant formula products. This is particularly important, as infant formulas may constitute the sole or major source of nutrition of an infant for up to a year after birth (Health Canada, 2006b). This is a period of rapid growth and development that affects a child's long-term health status and well-being (Health Canada, 2006b). Many nutrient levels in infant formulas are higher than in breast milk because of the lower bioavailability of the formulas. Infant formulas fall into several main classes: standard term, soy, protein hydrolysate, free amino acid-based, metabolic, and preterm. Table 21.1 contains indications for the different formulas.

Composition

Standard formulas for term infants over 2 kg contain 68 kcal/100 mL and are made from cow's milk protein and contain lactose and a blend of fats. Infant soy formulas are made using a soy protein isolate and are lactose free.

Preterm infant formulas are made with intact cow's milk protein and dual sources of carbohydrates and fats to increase absorption. Commercially prepared preterm infant formulas are available in 68 and 80 kcal/100 mL. The main features of preterm formulas are higher levels of protein, vitamins, minerals, and electrolytes than formulas designed for term infants. In addition, there are breast milk fortifiers that enhance the composition of expressed breast milk and better meet the high nutrient needs of premature newborns. They are available in liquid or powdered form, and are added to breast milk; the liquid form may be fed alternately with breast milk.

Considerations Related to Formula Type

Most healthy, full-term infants who are bottlefed can be fed a standard cow's milk-based, iron-containing infant formula. Formulas sold in Canada adhere to the Food Manufacturing Practices regulations regarding manufacturing of infant formulas. The use of specialized

● TABLE 21.1 **Indications for Various Feeding Types**

Feeding Type	Brand Name	Indications for Use
Human milk		Healthy, full-term infants; most sick-term infants; most healthy and sick preterm infants, with supplementation
Human milk fortifier as a supplement to human milk	Similac Human Milk Fortifier (powder), Enfamil Human Milk Fortifier (powder), Similac Natural Care (liquid)	Preterm infants fed human milk in the hospital
Standard cow's milk-based formula	Similac With Iron Enfamil With Iron Carnation Good Start Similac Lactose Free Lacto-Free	Healthy, full-term infants Same as above, with family history of atopy Healthy, full-term infants with lactose intolerance Same as above
Soy	Isomil ProSobee Isomil DF	Family history of allergy to cow milk protein, lactose intolerance, galactosemia, vegetarianism Same as above, and with sucrose intolerance Decreases duration of loose stools
Protein hydrolysate	Nutramigen Alimentum, Pregestimil	Family history of allergy to cow milk protein, multiple food allergies, idiopathic defects of protein digestion or absorption Same as above, and fat malabsorption
Free amino acid	Neocate	Infants sensitive to intact proteins, multiple food allergies, severe gastroesophageal reflux, Kosher feeding
Metabolic	RCF 3232 A 80056 Pro-Phree ProViMin	Used under the precise direction of a physician and dietitian for malabsorptive syndromes requiring protein, carbohydrate, or fat manipulations
Preterm	Similac Special Care With Iron Enfamil Premature With Iron Similac NeoSure Enfamil EnfaCare	Preterm infants, until a weight of ~2500–3600 g Preterm infants ready for hospital discharge who weigh ~1800 g; to be fed until 9 to 12 mos corrected gestational age

formulas is not indicated for routine use. An evaluation of the infant's health status and nutritional needs must be performed prior to the use of such products.

Soy formulas are appropriate for infants with galactosemia or primary lactase deficiency, an allergy to cow's milk proteins, or whose caregivers desire a vegetarian formula (Seppo et al., 2005; The Hospital for Sick Children, 2008). Cow's milk protein formulas that contain no lactose are appropriate for infants with primary lactose intolerance. Formula with added rice starch may be helpful for infants who require thickened feedings, such as those with gastroesophageal reflux (Health Canada, 2012c). The formula is only slightly thicker than regular formula during feeding, but upon entering the acidic environment of the stomach, it becomes more viscous, thus decreasing the amount of emesis (Arguin & Swartz, 2004).

Protein hydrolysate formulas are appropriate for infants at risk for allergy to cow's milk or soy protein, or impaired protein metabolism (Hays & Wood, 2005; The Hospital for Sick Children, 2008). Soy formulas may be suitable for allergic infants in select cases, depending on the type of allergy manifested (Seppo et al., 2005). Some infants who are allergic to cow's milk protein may also become sensitized to the soy protein because there is a 40% cross sensitivity (The Hospital for Sick Children, 2008). In the case of fat malabsorption, specialized formulas will provide alternative pathways for metabolism of fat and increase absorption. Preterm formulas were designed to meet high nutrient needs of the preterm infant weighing less than 2,000 g. See Figure 21.1 for guidance on choosing a feeding type.

The Canadian Paediatric Society, Dieticians of Canada, and Health Canada do not recommend homemade formula made with canned evaporated milk as an alternative to breast milk or commercial infant formula because it is nutritionally incomplete. Formula based on evaporated milk has low iron content, is low in essential fatty acids, and delivers a high renal solute load. These feedings are not sufficient in iron and vitamins C, A, and D to promote normal growth and development. Although medicinal supplements may be provided, the fat content of evaporated milk is digested poorly, and the sodium and phosphorus contents are excessive. However, evaporated milk formulas are used in some areas of Canada because of cost, convenience, and tradition. If evaporated milk formula is used, it must be adapted to ensure proper dilution and appropriate amounts of energy, protein, and carbohydrate. Only evaporated whole milk should be used.

Infants should not receive regular cow's milk because of the possibility of excessive protein load, allergic response, microintestinal blood loss, inferior protein absorption with increased renal solute load, low iron bioavailability, and dehydration.

Additives

Health Canada (2013) has approved two fatty acids found in breast milk for inclusion in infant formulas. Literature supporting their use in infant formula shows that their symbiotic relationship can help stimulate infants' mental development and visual acuity (Clandinin et al., 2005; Innis, 2004).

Most infant formulas contain iron, which is important for cognitive development. Infants who have experienced iron deficiency have shown behaviour, motor, and developmental impairment (Akman et al., 2004; Eden, 2005). Informing caregivers of the importance of feeding iron-fortified infant formula and addressing their concerns about feeding iron-containing formulas are vital interventions. Iron-fortified infant formulas do not change the consistency or frequency of stools; they simply darken them, while medicinal iron and iron from fortified infant cereals may contribute to constipation. Since 1969, the American Academy of Pediatrics Committee on Nutrition (1999) has recommended that infants be fed iron-fortified formula, as a way of decreasing the prevalence of iron-deficiency anemia and its sequelae. However, as a result of a large, 10-year follow-up study, Lozoff, et al. (2012) suggested that the optimal level of iron in infant formula needs further study to avoid giving infants more iron than they need.

Client Teaching and Collaborative Interventions

Results from a systematic review of women's experience of formula feeding revealed that they received inadequate information and support from health providers, and many mothers expressed feelings of guilt, anger, and failure (Lakshman et al., 2009). Women who choose to bottlefeed require instruction regarding physical delivery of the feeding (Fig. 21.9). Caregivers need to develop new feeding skills and begin to understand the feeding relationship they are developing with the infant. All caregivers will benefit from support and nursing advice that feeding should be a time to enjoy the newest family member. Nurses can give assistance and reassurance regarding reading hunger and feeding cues that signal the infant's need to be fed, burped, for rest, or the end of a feeding session.

Artificial Nipples

Most infants of term gestation suck well from standard rubber nipples stocked in most well-baby nurseries and stores. Preterm infants benefit from softer nipples with smaller holes. Orthodontic nipples have a flattened appearance, and some infants show a preference for

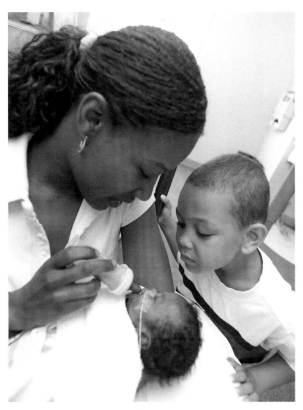

FIGURE 21.9 Nurses teach clients who bottlefeed their newborns about the importance of correct feeding position, eye contact, and appropriate hygiene measures.

them. Other nipples are marketed as being most like a breast, based on a shape similar to the human breast. Silicone nipples are available in different artificial nipple shapes. Infants with congenital anomalies that involve the tongue, palates, lips, or chin may feed successfully using feeding devices specifically designed for them. A speech pathologist or an occupational therapist is most appropriate to make recommendations for safe and effective oral feeding programs.

If an infant does not do well with the choice of artificial nipple, a different shape or material may result in more effective bottlefeeding. Once the oral cavity of the infant has grown, he or she may benefit from a nipple with a bigger overall size as well as a larger hole from which the feeding flows.

Formula Preparation

Preparation of infant formula depends on the type used. Ready-to-feed bottles and cans are the most convenient and most expensive. Concentrated liquid formulas which require dilution are also available. Powdered formula is available and is the most economical choice.

Before preparing formula, caregivers should wash their hands with warm, soapy water to decrease the risk for contamination of formula with bacteria or viruses. They should use a clean, damp cloth to wipe the top of the can and a clean punch-type can opener for puncture. Ready-to-feed and concentrated liquid formulas must be shaken before opening to suspend any particles that have settled out of solution. Concentrated liquid formulas are reconstituted by adding an equal amount of water to the formula and shaking or stirring. A glass liquid measuring cup is the best device to use because of concern about the release of bisphenol A from bottles and utensils made of polycarbonate. Bisphenol-free polycarbonate containers are also available.

When making formula from powder, caregivers should use the scoop included in the can to measure the powder. Household measures may seem like a good way to make a large volume of formula at once without losing count of the number of scoops; however, they are less accurate than scoops. Stirring the formula powder slightly will make it free flowing. Caregivers should dip the scoop into the powder, draw the scoop up the side of the can, and tap or redip the scoop to release any air pockets. The powder should be level with the side of the scoop. Caregivers should pack or unpack scoops according to label directions.

Formula may be prepared in a clean pitcher or individual bottles. Prepared formula may be kept in the refrigerator and covered for use within 48 hours. Any unused powdered formula should be discarded within 30 days of opening, according to label directions.

Sterilization

Water may be sterilized before reconstituting infant formula. Some pediatricians advise sterilization of the water and equipment used to make formula during the first 3 months of life, when the infant's immature immune system is not fully equipped to fight infection. After 3 months, it is assumed that the baby's increased activity and exploration will have already exposed him or her to the pathogens that could cause illness from bottlefeeding. Preterm infants or babies with an impaired immune system stand to benefit the most from a sterile water source. Baby or nursery waters are unnecessary and expensive. If caregivers choose nursery water, they should remember that it is not a sterile water source. If well water or pond water is used to prepare formula, it should be sterilized before use. Well water should be tested to make sure it does not contain toxic levels of lead (Health Canada, 2007).

To sterilize water or equipment, caregivers should boil it for 2 to 5 minutes, allowing the water to cool before making formula. Extremely hot temperatures may alter the nutrient composition of formula, removing or inactivating some of the nutrients. An alternative to boiling equipment for sterilization includes countertop electric steam sterilizers. Caregivers should clean the equipment used to make formula, sterilize it if they desire, and allow it to air-dry. The nurse discusses the importance of adequately cleaning away debris that may support the growth of harmful pathogens from equipment. Pathogens can survive the sterilization process if the equipment is improperly cleaned.

Warming

When warming a feeding for an infant, caregivers must allow it to come to temperature slowly under a running warm water bath. The level of the water should not be so close to the opening to allow water to seep into the container. Electric bottle warmers use steam to warm the feeding. Care must be taken to ensure even heating to avoid burning the baby with the formula that's been heated the most on the outside of the bottle. Caregivers should be reminded to avoid warming feedings in microwave ovens because the uneven heating of microwaves can cause hot spots, which can burn a baby's mouth. In addition, the buildup of steam can cause hot liquid to seep or spray out of the bottle.

Positioning and Burping

When discussing positioning for bottle-fed babies, the nurse provides the following instructions:

- Wash hands before feeding to limit the transmission of infectious microorganisms to the baby.
- Hold the infant semiupright and close to promote eye contact. Eye contact increases both the caregiver's and the infant's sense of attachment and promotes bonding. Infants who are bottlefed also benefit from skin-to-skin contact that promotes physical closeness and bonding. Wearing short-sleeved shirts or placing the diapered baby on a parent's bare chest ("kangaroo care") can accomplish this (Fig. 21.10).
- Take care to interact with the baby during feedings because feeding can evoke feelings of nurturing and attachment. As much as possible, feedings should take place in a quiet environment without distractions for the caregiver or baby. Without removing the bottle from the infant's mouth, or during times of rest, the caregiver can talk to the infant in soft, sing-song tones, which infants respond to favourably. Some infants are calmed by their mother's voice and may show interest in her singing.
- Tilt the bottle so that the nipple remains filled with formula or breast milk.
- A bottle should never be propped. It is possible for prolonged exposure to carbohydrate from infant formula or juice to damage both the exposed and unexposed teeth. For this same reason, a child should never be put to sleep with a bottle. In addition, a baby with a propped bottle or the baby left to self-feed does

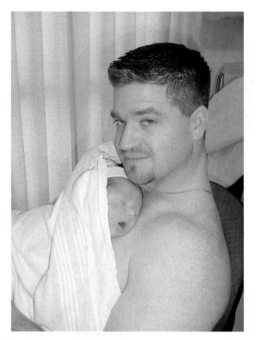

FIGURE 21.10 One measure to promote parent–infant bonding is kangaroo care, in which the newborn is held against a parent's bare chest.

not benefit from the bonding that develops during the feeding relationship.

Caregivers allow infants to pace themselves with bursts of sucking and periods of rest.

During a feeding, the infant may push the nipple out of the mouth, pull away from the bottle, or turn the head to indicate that he or she has swallowed some air before or during the feed and that a burp is appropriate.

Burping

Placing the infant over the shoulder creates abdominal pressure that helps to expel air. The infant is held upright and the back is patted to allow air to rise and to be expelled. Other positions that create the same effect are to place the prone infant over the lap, or in a sitting position on the lap, while patting the infant's back with one hand and supporting the chin and head with the other hand (Fig. 21.11).

Feeding Cues

Caregivers should never force infants to finish a bottle, unless indicated for a specific purpose, such as poor weight gain or dehydration. Caregivers watch for satiety cues (e.g., pushing the nipple from the mouth, pulling away from the bottle, and longer pauses between sucks) that the feeding is complete. In addition, if an infant does not finish a feeding and it appears that the baby wants more later, it is acceptable to give the same bottle to the baby as long as it is no longer than 90 minutes from the start of the original feeding.

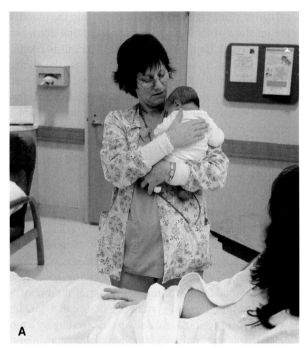
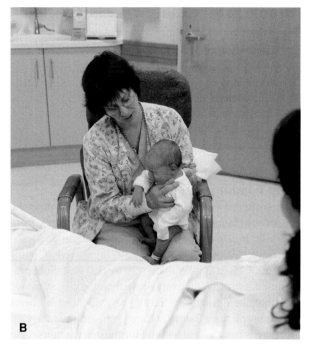

FIGURE 21.11 A: Burping over the shoulder. **B:** Burping with the newborn on the lap, while the nurse supports the head and neck.

OTHER FEEDING DELIVERY STRATEGIES

Parenteral and Enteral Nutrition

Several conditions warrant parenteral nutrition (Box 21.4). Examples include babies who are ill following birth or are premature. Preterm infants may begin to suck on their tongues, feeding tubes, or hands and fingers as early as 30 to 32 weeks' postconceptual age and have the ability to suck nutritively at approximately 33 weeks' gestational age (Breton & Steinwender, 2008). Such behaviour may not be coordinated, however, in terms of the suck-swallow-breathe pattern required for oral eating. Other indications for parenteral or enteral feedings include anatomic anomalies of the gastrointestinal tract (e.g., tracheoesophageal fistula);

● **BOX 21.4   Indications for Parenteral Nutrition**

- Gastrointestinal tract anomalies
- Inadequate enteral nutrition for 3 days or more, sooner if possible
- Intractable diarrhea of infancy
- Meconium ileus
- Necrotizing enterocolitis
- No enteral tolerance or availability
- Postoperative correction for gastrointestinal tract anomalies

cleft lip, cleft palate, or both; neurologic impairment; and short bowel syndrome.

Initially, the goals of parenteral nutrition are to minimize catabolism and to provide glucose in amounts that will prevent *glycogenolysis* (the breakdown of the body's stores of glucose) and *gluconeogenesis* (the formation of glycogen from fat and protein). Parenteral nutrition consists of carbohydrates combined with a crystalline amino acid solution. Lipid infusions are either hung separately or are part of the crystalline solution.

For newborns receiving parenteral nutrition, small-volume (enteral) feedings (less than 20 to 30 mL/kg/day) should start as soon as they are medically stable. These small-volume feeds are not nutritive; rather, they prime the gut for future success with enteral feeding. Generally, small-volume feeds are initiated as an adjunct to intravenous (IV) fluids or parenteral nutrition, and feeds are advanced while the contribution from IV fluids is decreased.

Whenever possible, enteral nutrition is preferable to parenteral nutrition. After several days without enteric stimulation, mucosal cell may be damaged. The villi of the intestinal wall become blunted and progression of feedings becomes more difficult. Secretion of sucrase and lactase decreases, absorption of amino acids declines, and bacterial translocation from increased gut permeability is possible, which may lead to necrotizing enterocolitis. Enteral nutrient needs are available as Adequate Intakes set to meet the needs of most infants up to 6 months of age. See Box 21.5.

Calculation of Fluid Intake

Volume received over 24 hours = mL/kg/day
Weight in kg
Calculation of calorie intake
Fluid intake (mL/kg/day) × Caloric density of formula (cal/mL) = cal/kg/day

Cup Feeding

Cup feeding evolved in developing countries to meet the needs of infants who could not breastfeed or suck from a bottle. It is used most often to feed preterm and low–birth-weight infants until they can breastfeed (Collins et al., 2004). At approximately 30 weeks' gestation, preterm infants can effectively move their tongue, swallow, and breathe during cup feeding as evidenced by heart rates, respiratory rates, and oxygen saturations. Cup feeding is not an ideal method for full-term infants, who tend to dribble the feeds from the cup and may show a strong preference for the cup when presented with the opportunity to again breastfeed.

During cup feeding, the infant is held in a semi-upright position. A cup specifically developed for infant feedings may be used. A small cup without a spout, such as a pliable medicine cup, shot glass, or plastic condiment cup used at fast food restaurants may also be used. The cup is placed on the infant's lower lip so that it touches the corners of the mouth. This tactile stimulation, as well as the infant's olfactory sense, provides information that feeding is about to commence. The caregiver allows the infant to lap milk with the tongue into the mouth (Lauwers & Shinskie, 2005). Cup feeding should be first attempted when the infant is quiet, alert, and not overly hungry or crying. Establishing cup feeding may require practice and patience on the part of the caregiver. As infants become more proficient at cup feeding, a sipping technique may be used. Feedings should never be poured into the mouth. The infant may hold the breast milk or formula in the mouth until ready to swallow. The infant controls the total amount fed.

A Cochrane review reported that, as a supplement to breastfeeding, cup feeding is less effective than bottlefeeding because it may result in a longer stay in hospital and does not promote maintenance of breastfeeding after hospital discharge. (Flint et al., 2008).

Finger Feeding

Another feeding method is *finger feeding*. One end of a small-bore tube extending ¼ inch beyond the tip of the finger is secured to the caregiver's finger. The other end is placed in a syringe containing the feeding, with the plunger removed (Lauwers & Shinskie, 2005). The caregiver places the finger pad side up into the mouth at the juncture of the hard and soft palates and allows the infant to suck the finger, while the feeding is running through the tube. Another variation is to use the plunger of the syringe to deliver approximately 0.5 mL of feeding with every third suck. Caregivers should maintain caution not to allow infants to become accustomed to this mode of feeding so that they begin to prefer it to the exclusion of all other feeding methods. They also must be sure to assess the integrity of the roof of the infant's mouth where the tubing is placed.

Nursing Supplemental System

When a breastfed infant requires more feeding volume than breastfeeding is providing, or for adopted babies, a nursing supplemental system may be a good option. This is an excellent means of reinforcing breastfeeding behaviour by rewarding the infant at the breast. A **nursing supplemental system** is a device that contains breast milk or formula and delivers the feeding by a tube placed near the mother's nipple and into the infant's mouth (Fig. 21.12). While the infant is breastfeeding, one end of the tube is taped to the mother's breast so that it goes into the baby's mouth. The other end of the tube is connected to a feeding container filled with additional breast milk or infant formula. The container may be pinned to the mother's shirt or hung around her neck.

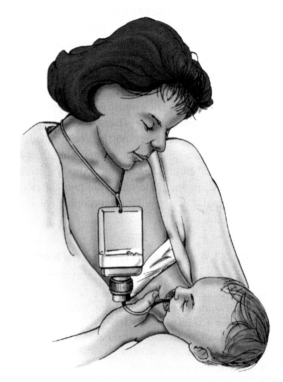

FIGURE 21.12 By using a nursing supplemental system, the client can simulate the breastfeeding experience with a formula-fed infant, or with an infant who cannot take sufficient breast milk directly from the mother's nipple.

In this way, the infant can continue to breastfeed and stimulate milk production while receiving the additional nutrients required for growth. Consultation with a lactation consultant can provide answers on how to physically manage the baby and the supplementary nursing system. A neonatal nutritionist can provide guidance on how much additional feeding to infuse.

MEASURES OF SUCCESSFUL FEEDING

Signs of a successful breastfeeding session include seeing the baby's lower jaw moving deeply, hearing the baby swallow, having a soft breast after feeding, and seeing typical behaviours of a satisfied baby. Infant weight is the gold standard for evaluating adequacy of feeding. Other ways to measure the success of feeding are discussed in the following sections.

Fluid Intake

Fluid needs in the first 24 hours of life for a full-term newborn are minimal. Mothers produce an average of 10 to 100 mL of colostrum in the first 24 hours. (Riordan & Wambach, 2010) A preterm newborn requires approximately 80 mL/kg/day in the first 24 hours of life. Fluid needs increase to 135 mL/kg/day by day 14 (Bell & Acarregui, 2014).

Wet Diapers

By the end of the first day of life, the newborn should have voided. If within the first 24 hours of life the infant has not voided, health care providers consider and investigate possible causes. By days 2 and 3 of life, the newborn should have two to three wet diapers per day. The urine should be pale and odourless. By day 4, the newborn should have six to eight voids in a 24-hour period (RNAO, 2006).

Stools

Infants develop uniquely recognizable, characteristic, and individual stool patterns. Infants may have one or more bowel movements in a day. When counselling parents on the type of stool to expect from their infants, nurses are aware of the expected characteristics. It is important to remember that when an infant changes from one type of feeding to another, stool habits may also change.

Meconium is the first stool that the newborn produces; it is black, tar-like, and sticky. Meconium consists largely of bilirubin and biliverdin, substances that accumulate during gestation. The baby eliminates meconium during the first 48 to 72 hours of life (Lauwers & Shinskie, 2005).

Many newborns have at least one to two bowel movements a day. By the end of the first week, the newborn may have as many as 5 to 10 bowel movements a day and may pass a stool with each feeding, as a result of a strong gastrocolic reflex (WebMD, 2013). The number of bowel movements per day may decrease as the baby matures.

The stools of breastfed infants change from black to greenish-brown to yellow and seedy, and may be very soft, or liquid. Infants fed breast milk are reported to have twice as many stools as formula-fed infants (Tunc et al., 2008). Stools of infants fed iron-fortified formulas may be green in colour. In addition, infants fed soy-based formulas may have harder stools more often than other feeding groups. Hard or dry stools may also be an indication that the baby is not getting enough liquid or is losing fluid because of a fever (WebMD, 2013).

 Joelle says, "When I bottlefed my first baby, I knew exactly how much milk she took. But how will I know if the baby is getting enough when I'm breastfeeding?" How would the nurse respond?

Weight Gain and Growth

Appropriate gains in weight, length, and head circumference give everyone caring for an infant the opportunity to take pride in a thriving baby with good nutritional status. Conversely, too small or too large gains can alert the health care team to genetic, metabolic, physiologic, or iatrogenic complications. Nurses are often expected to weigh infants and measure length and head circumference. Serial measurements are invaluable tools in evaluating infant growth and subsequent development. Newborns lose approximately 5% to 10% of their birth weight as interstitial fluid and stool in the first 5 to 7 days, and by 10 to 14 days of life, the infant should have regained its birth weight (MedlinePlus, 2012).

The Dietitians of Canada, Canadian Paediatric Society, The College of Family Physicians of Canada, and Community Health Nurses of Canada recommend that the growth of all full-term infants be monitored using the growth charts developed by WHO in 2007 (Dietitians of Canada and Canadian Paediatric Society, 2010). These charts represent a more ethnically diverse population than did previous charts. These percentile charts include the third and 97th percentiles for better assessment of growth at the extremes of normal distribution. Growth curves specific to breastfed infants have been developed and may be used for specific infants. When an infant's growth parameters channel upward or downward sharply by crossing percentiles for weight, length, or head circumference, the nurse suggests a consultation with a pediatric dietitian to determine a suitable course of action.

FEEDING-RELATED ISSUES

Jaundice

Breakdown of fetal red blood cells (RBCs) results in bilirubin. **Jaundice** results from accumulation of bilirubin in tissue (hyperbilirubinemia) and is characterized by yellowing of the sclera and skin (see Chapters 20 and 22). Physiologic jaundice is characterized by a natural and expected rise and fall in bilirubin levels in healthy, term infants; it peaks at approximately 3 to 5 days of life (Riordan & Wambach, 2010). Pathologic jaundice results from disease processes, such as blood abnormalities, liver impairment, metabolic disease, carrier protein deficiency, or binding site deficiencies.

Nonphysiologic Jaundice

When bilirubin levels exceed accepted norms for physiologic jaundice, and pathologic jaundice can reasonably be ruled out, nonphysiologic jaundice is the diagnosis (Lauwers & Shinskie, 2005). Nonphysiologic jaundice in breastfed infants may be compounded from inadequate intake of breast milk, not dehydration. Decreased caloric intake leads to fewer stools, which is the primary means of biliary excretion. The infant may appear lethargic and weak. The danger of high levels of circulating bilirubin is that it is not attached to carrier proteins, which would prevent its passage through the blood–brain barrier, skin, muscle tissue, and mucous membranes. Neurologic damage, known as kernicterus, can result.

Primary treatment includes unlimited access to breastfeeding; evaluation of appropriate positioning, latch, and intake; and possibly supplementary tube feeds of expressed breast milk or infant formula, while infant energy levels and successful breastfeeding are re-established. Phototherapy (artificial light) may be directed to the infant's exposed skin to convert bilirubin to a form that can be excreted without assistance from the liver (see Chapters 20 and 22).

Late-Onset Jaundice

Late-onset jaundice, also known as breast milk jaundice, is thought to result from a rare factor in some breast milk. Identification of this factor has been met with controversy and conflicting evidence. Late-onset jaundice develops slowly; peak bilirubin levels do not appear until the second or third week of life. Treatment includes increased breastfeeding and possibly increased light exposure (Riordan & Wambach, 2010).

Thrush

Thrush is an oral yeast infection, commonly caused by pathogens of the *Candida* species (Papon et al., 2013). Also known as candidiasis, thrush results from an overgrowth of, or infection with, the yeast-like fungus candida. Modes of person-to-person transmission include saliva, mucosa, breast milk, sexual contact, and stool. The characteristic manifestations of oral thrush in the infant are white patches on the mucous membranes of the mouth and a rash in the genital area with characteristic satellite lesions. Yeast infections on the diaper area, breasts, or under the arms may be red or bright pink. The rash is macular and raised. Patches of yeast appear darker on dark skin. The breastfeeding mother may experience extreme pain, described as burning or stabbing in the breast, which could lead to premature weaning (Morrill et al., 2005). Unique features of a yeast infection in the breast are the appearance of pain after a period of pain-free nursing, and pain in the breast while the mother is not breastfeeding.

When infected, both mother and infant require concurrent treatment. Nurses advise women to apply a topical antifungal cream to water-cleansed breasts after each breastfeeding (Wiener, 2006). Mothers are advised to not rinse off any residue left on the breast before the next feeding to enhance treatment. In severe cases of recurrent yeast, providers often consider a systemic antifungal medication for the mother (Wiener, 2006). Ibuprofen may be appropriate for pain relief. Breast shells may protect sore nipple areas from friction caused by clothing. Women wear clean bras daily and change breast pads at least with every feeding to deprive yeast of the moist environment which promotes growth. When breastfeeding, the infant should not be so hungry that he or she nurses ravenously. The mother offers the least sore breast first to promote let-down. Pumping the breasts may be more comfortable than breastfeeding. Women feed expressed breast milk the same day to avoid possible infant recolonization. The addition of acidophilus from yogurt or cottage cheese to the maternal diet may help replace appropriate bacteria in the intestines. Temporary maternal dietary restriction of refined sugars and dairy products may help resolve persistent infections. Some women consume additional garlic, zinc, water, and the vitamin B complex to discourage growth of yeast.

Caregivers thoroughly swab the infant's oral cavity (including the cheek and pouches) with oral nystatin suspension every 3 hours. The diaper area should be kept clean with clear water, allowing the area to air-dry several times a day. A prescription topical antifungal cream is applied when changing the diapers.

Other family members with yeast infections will receive treatment as well. All family members should wash hands before and after handling feeding and breast pump equipment, feeding the baby, changing diapers, using the restroom, or handling toys mouthed by the infant. The hands of infants are washed frequently as well. Paper towels should be used to dry hands, and bath towels used only once before laundering. Laundry must be washed in hot water (50°C or more) and dried in the sun or high heat of a clothes dryer. Each day, the infant's toys and pacifier, artificial nipples, breast pump equipment that has come in contact with breast milk, and breast shells require washing in hot soapy water, rinsing, and boiling for 5 minutes. Any medicine droppers that come in contact with the infant's mouth require washing in hot, soapy water and thorough rinsing before storing them in the bottle.

Gastroesophageal Reflux

Gastroesophageal reflux may be characterized by occasional burps, emesis, or nonregurgitant reflux. It is associated with failure to thrive, irritability with feeding, anemia, hematemesis, pneumonia, and apnea. Regurgitation, more than once a day, occurs in up to 50% of healthy infants and does not necessitate intervention, depending on the caregiver's anxiety (Craig et al., 2004).

Changes in caregiver practices can eliminate or reduce symptoms of gastroesophageal reflux. In breastfed infants, a maternal diet that excludes or restricts milk and eggs has been found to reduce episodes of reflux (Lightdale & Gremse, 2013). Small frequent feeds (every 2 to 3 hours) decrease the volume to the stomach at one time. Thickened feeds will increase viscosity to decrease episodes of reflux (Lightdale & Gremse, 2013). Small and frequent thickened formula feeds may be appropriate for infants with failure to thrive as a result of gastroesophageal reflux (Goessler, 2012). Breast milk contains the enzyme amylase, which breaks down the starch in most thickening agents. Nutritionally, extra calories from feeds thickened with absorbable carbohydrate increases the percentage of calories from carbohydrate. This decreases the percentage of calories from protein and could serve to make an infant overweight from overfeeding. This also could make it difficult to achieve age-appropriate physical milestones. The viscosity of thickened feeds may prevent it from flowing freely from the artificial nipple on a bottle, making it necessary to slit the nipple for a larger opening. Conversely, making the slit too big could cause the feeds to flow too quickly, and the infant would not be able to control the volume extracted.

One of the most traditional therapies for gastroesophageal reflux has been to change the positioning of the infant. Studies have shown that elevating the head of the bed or using upright seat positioning help to reduce gastroesophageal reflux symptoms (Goessler, 2012; Lightdale & Gremse, 2013). Pharmacologic agents may be used for infants with reflux and resultant failure to thrive, apnea, or recurrent pneumonia (Lightdale & Gremse, 2013).

Colic

The etiology of **colic** has not been determined (Mayo Clinic, 2014). Gastrointestinal symptoms include sensitivity to dietary intake, excessive flatulence, and gastric and colonic hypermotility. The infant's legs may be drawn up into the abdomen, fists may be clenched, and facial grimaces may be noted, with body stiffening. Colic appears in both breastfed and bottle-fed infants, and is characterized as irritability, fussiness, or high-pitched crying episodes lasting 3 hours or more per day at least 3 days out of a week, for a duration of 1 week or more (Mayo Clinic, 2014).

Strategies to reduce colicky behaviour include elimination of dairy products from the breastfeeding mother's diet with gradual, weekly reintroduction of specific products (Riordan & Wambach, 2010); cessation of smoking for the breastfeeding mother; and effective feeding from only one breast during a feed to allow the infant to receive high-fat hindmilk. A hypoallergenic diet for breastfeeding mothers has limited effectiveness in reducing colic and if introduced, expert nutritional consultation is recommended to ensure adequate maternal dietary intake (Iacovou et al., 2012).

Weaning a colicky breastfed infant does not improve symptoms of colic (Roberts et al., 2004). Soy protein-based formulas have not proven to provide relief from symptoms and are to be avoided as a treatment strategy (Bhatia & Greer, 2008). Relief from symptoms appears to be achieved by holding the infant over the shoulder and thereby applying some pressure on the infant's abdomen. Rocking the infant and rubbing his or her back may have a soothing effect. Bottle-fed infants may benefit from a change in the size of the nipple opening. Encouraging the bottle-fed infant to burp frequently during a feeding may decrease the amount of air that the infant swallows.

Water Intoxication

Water intoxication, which can lead to brain injury, seizures, hypothermia, and edema, can result from feeding too much water, either enterally or parenterally. Inappropriately diluting infant formula, feeding water in place of formula, or giving extra water in hot weather can have negative outcomes, especially during the first month of life, when the newborn's glomerular filtration rate and ability to excrete excess water are decreased. Nurses should mention the inappropriateness of feeding any water to a baby less than 6 months old, especially in warm climates where the practice may be more commonplace.

SUMMARY

- Feeding a baby is an opportunity for the caregiver and infant to begin developing a personal relationship of trust and affection.
- The nurse is well-positioned to assist families with making their choice of how to nourish their baby. Sharing techniques for the chosen feeding method is an important part of successful feeding and subsequent growth and development.

- The nutritional benefits of breast milk include high bioavailability and ease of digestion, low potential renal solute load, and epidermal growth factor.
- The immunologic benefits of human milk include factors that help fight infection and prevent allergic diseases.
- Developmental advantages of breastfeeding are psychological and neurologic. Breastfeeding offers the mother and infant dyad a unique opportunity to nurture a trust relationship. Neurologic benefits from feeding breast milk include cognitive development and visual acuity.
- Health advantages to the breastfeeding mother include earlier return to pregravida weight, less risk for osteoporosis and premenopausal ovarian and breast cancers, and protection against anemia and some infections.
- Economically, breast milk offers families substantial savings over the cost of purchasing infant formulas. In addition, there is no environmental waste, and caregivers lose less work time because of fewer infant illnesses.
- Only a few maternal infectious diseases, metabolic disorders, and drugs are contraindications to feeding human milk. Sometimes a short separation and breast milk substitute are indicated during maternal illness. HIV and human T-cell lymphotropic virus are known absolute contraindications to feeding mother's own milk in Canada.
- Alternatives to feeding mother's own milk include donor human milk, commercially prepared infant formulas, and parenteral nutrition. Indications for each feeding type have been established; care should be taken to choose the appropriate means of nutrition.
- Feeding methodologies include breastfeeding, bottle feeding, cup feeding, tube or gavage feeding, finger feeding, and parenteral nutrition.
- Nurses can assess the adequacy of infant feeding through infant feeding cues, assessment of intake and output, and growth and weight trends.
- Common problems in the newborn period include jaundice, gastroesophageal disease, colic, thrush, and water intoxication. The nurse can be instrumental in making recommendations to the physicians and parents that are consistent with current literature, and in providing supportive measures for infants with these complications.

Questions to Ponder

1. During an appointment with her obstetrician, a 22-year-old pregnant woman confides that she would like to breastfeed her newborn. She shares that one of her biggest obstacles is her fear of breastfeeding in public places. Specifically, her father-in-law has voiced his opinion that he does not feel it is an appropriate thing to do in public.
   - What are your personal feelings about mothers' breastfeeding in public? What are the national and provincial laws about public breastfeeding?
   - What type of dialogue might the nurse suggest for the woman to have with her father-in-law?
   - What might the nurse suggest to the woman that might make breastfeeding in a public place more comfortable?

2. During a well-baby visit, a mother shares with her nurse that her newborn has been constipated for the past 2 weeks. The mother reports that her baby strains with bowel movements, turns red in the face, and has clenched fists, and that her infant's stool is formed, soft, and brown. After talking with the baby's grandmother, the mother changed to a low-iron–containing formula and started giving the infant 60 mL of apple juice in a bottle every day. The mother reports that the baby appears happier.
   - What additional information would the nurse need to gather?
   - What guidance could the nurse give the mother regarding this problem?
   - Ideally, who would be involved in the counselling session?

REVIEW QUESTIONS

1. During a 2-week well-baby visit to the baby's primary physician, the infant's mother explains that she's not sure how often to feed her baby based on the baby's cues. The mother shares the following cues with the nurse. Which cue would the nurse correctly identify as a late sign of hunger?
   A. Crying
   B. Sucking on fingers
   C. Sleeping
   D. Licking or smacking lips

2. A woman at 29 weeks' gestation with her first pregnancy is not sure she should breastfeed her newborn. Which statement, if made by the nurse, would be most accurate in describing a benefit of breastfeeding?
   A. "You'll lose more weight than with bottlefeeding."
   B. "The baby will gain more weight more quickly with breastfeeding."
   C. "Breast milk will provide the baby with maternal antibodies."
   D. "Maternal–child bonding occurs only with breastfeeding."

3. A bottle-feeding primipara calls the nurse helpline at the primary pediatrician's office, stating that her 2-week-old is "throwing up" after every feeding. The mother states that she feeds him soy formula, 150 mL every 3 hours, and that she has to work to get him to finish each bottle. Based on the information, which of the following suggestions should the nurse make to the mother?
   A. Make an appointment with the pediatrician to explore antireflux medications.
   B. Feed the baby until he appears satisfied instead of making him finish the bottle.
   C. Consider switching to a low-iron formula.
   D. Come to the emergency department to rule out anatomic abnormalities.

4. The mother of a breastfeeding 6-week-old calls the pediatrician's office, stating that her baby is constipated. She describes the stool as sometimes hard. Which of the following actions should the nurse suggest that the mother take next?
   A. Give the baby 60 mL of water daily.
   B. Weigh urine output at home for 24 hours and call back with the results.
   C. Change to a low-iron–containing formula.
   D. Keep a list of what the baby consumes in 24 hours.

5. When teaching a new mother about warming formula for a feeding, the nurse should include that the new mother should:
   A. Run warm water over the base of the closed feeding container.
   B. Place the bottle in the microwave for 20 seconds.
   C. Pour the feeding into a saucepan and place on the stove on low heat.
   D. Allow the formula to come to room temperature on the counter.

6. The mother of a 2-day-old in the newborn intensive care unit tells the nurse that she's not getting any milk when she pumps her breasts. She shares that she is pumping four times a day for 5 to 10 minutes each pumping session. Which of the following recommendations should the nurse share with the client?
   A. Increase pumping time to 30 minutes per session.
   B. Stop pumping because her milk is not coming in quickly enough.
   C. Take 1 day off from pumping and try again the next day.
   D. Pump every 3 hours and once through the night for 12 to 15 minutes each session.

7. The mother of a newborn who is 24 hours old, states that her baby is falling asleep after just 3 to 5 minutes of breastfeeding. The baby has awakened himself to eat only once since birth. Based on this information, the nurse should advise the woman to:
   A. Wake the baby up to eat every 3 hours.
   B. Allow the baby to sleep as much as possible to regain strength.
   C. Start formulafeeds and monitor for improved hunger cues.
   D. Express human milk and try bottlefeeding.

8. A lactating mother calls the maternity nurse with complaints of right-sided breast pain with breastfeeding. The woman describes her breast as warm to the touch with a palpable lump; she is afebrile. Based on this information, the nurse should advise the client to:
   A. Stop breastfeeding immediately and take 200-mg ibuprofen every 4 hours as needed for pain.
   B. Continue to breastfeed 8 to 12 times per day to resolve a likely plugged milk duct.
   C. Schedule a mammogram immediately.
   D. See her primary care provider for an antibiotic prescription.

REFERENCES

Akman, M., Cebeci, D., Okur, V., Angin, H., Abali, O., & Akman, A. C. (2004). The effects of iron deficiency on infants' developmental test performance. *Acta Paediatrica, 93*(10), 1391–1396.

American Academy of Pediatrics (AAP). (2012). Policy statement: Breastfeeding and the use of human milk. *Pediatrics, 129*(3), e827–841.

American Academy of Pediatrics (AAP) Committee on Drugs. (2001). Transfer of drugs and other chemicals into human milk. *Pediatrics, 108*(3), 776–789.

American Academy of Pediatrics (AAP) Committee on Nutrition. (1999). Iron fortification of infant formulas. *Pediatrics, 104*(1), 119–123.

Arguin, A., & Swartz, M. (2004). Gastroesophageal reflux in infants: A primary care perspective. *Pediatric Nursing, 30*(1), 45–51, 71. Retrieved from http://www.medscape.com/viewarticle/470698_7

Avent. (2008). Avent niplette: Helping mothers breastfeed longer. Retrieved from http://aventniplette.com

BC Women's Hospital & Health Centre. (2008). *Breastfeeding.* Retrieved from http://www.bcwomens.ca/info/search.htm?query=breastfeeding

Bell, E. & Acarregui, M. (2014). Fluid therapy in the neonate. University of Iowa Children's Hospital. Retrieved from http://www.uichildrens.org/fluid-therapy-in-the-neonate

Bhatia, J., & Greer, F. (2008). American Academy of Pediatrics, Committee on Nutrition. Use of soy protein-based formulas in infant feeding. *Pediatrics, 121,*1062–1068.

Black, A., Francoeur, D., & Rowe, T. (2004). SOGC clinical practice guidelines; Canadian contraception consensus. *Journal of Obstetrics and Gynaecologists of Canada, 26*(3), 219–254.

Bode, L., Kuhn, L., Kim, H. Y., Hsiao, L., Nissan, C., Sinkala, M., et al. (2012). Human milk oligosaccharide concentration and risk of postnatal transmission of HIV through breastfeeding. *American Journal of Clinical Nutrition, 96*(4), 831–839. Retrieved from http://www.ncbi.nlm.nih.gov/pmc/articles/PMC3441110

Bonia, K., Twells, L., Halfyard, B., Ludlow, V., Newhook, L., & Murphy-Goodridge, J. (2013). A qualitative study exploring factors associated with mothers' decision to formula-feed their infants in Newfoundland and Labrador, Canada. *BMC Public Health, 13,* 645. Retrieved from http://www.biomedcentral.com/content/pdf/1471–2458–13–645.pdf

Bonyata, K. (2011). Establishing and maintaining milk supply when baby is not breastfeeding. Kellymom Parenting Breastfeeding. Retrieved from http://kellymom.com/bf/pumpingmoms/pumping/maintainsupply-pump

Breastfeeding Committee for Canada. (2014). Baby-Friendly™ hospitals, birthing centres and community health services in Canada. Retrieved from http://breastfeedingcanada.ca/Default_en.aspx

Breton, S., & Steinwender, S. (2008). Timing introduction and transition to oral feeding in preterm infants: Current trends and practice. *Newborn & Infant Nursing Reviews, 8*(3), 153–159.

Cahill, J., & Wagner, C. (2002a). Challenges in breastfeeding: Maternal considerations. *Contemporary Pediatrics, 5*, 94.

Cahill, J., & Wagner, C. (2002b). Challenges in breastfeeding: Neonatal concerns. *Contemporary Pediatrics, 5*, 113.

Canadian Paediatric Society (CPS). (2012a). Maternal infectious diseases, antimicrobial therapy or immunizations: Very few contraindications to breastfeeding. *Paediatrics & Child Health, 11*(8), 489–491.

Canadian Paediatric Society (CPS). (2012b). The Baby-Friendly Initiative: Protecting, promoting and supporting breastfeeding. *Paediatrics & Child Health, 17*(6), 317–321.

Canadian Paediatric Society (CPS). (2013a). Dietary exposures and allergy prevention in high risk infants. *Paediatrics & Child Health, 18*(10), 545–549.

Canadian Paediatric Society (CPS). (2013b). Nutrition for healthy term infants, birth to six months: An overview. *Paediatrics & Child Health, 18*(4), 206–207.

Canadian Paediatric Society (CPS). (2013c). Recommendations for the use of pacifiers. *Paediatrics & Child Health, 8*(8), 515–519.

Canadian Paediatric Society (CPS). (2013d). Vitamin D supplementation: Recommendations for Canadian mothers and infants. *Paediatrics & Child Health, 12*(7),583–589.

Centers for Disease Control and Prevention. (2010). *Cytomegalovirus and congenital CMV infection.* Atlanta, GA. Retrieved from http://www.cdc.gov/cmv/transmission.html

Chantry, C. J., Howard, C. R., & Auinger, P. (2006). Full breastfeeding duration and associated decrease in respiratory tract infection in U.S. children. *Pediatrics, 117*(2), 425–432.

Clandinin, M. T., Van Aerde, J. E., Merkel, K. L., Harris, C. L., Springer, M. A., Hansen, J. W., et al. (2005). Growth and development of preterm infants fed infant formulas containing docosahexaenoic acid and arachidonic acid. *Journal of Pediatrics, 146*(4), 461–468.

Collins, C. T., Ryan, P., Crowther, C. A., McPhee, A. J., Paterson, S., & Hiller, J. E. (2004). Effect of bottles, cups, and dummies on breast feeding in preterm infants: A randomized controlled trial. *British Medical Journal, 329*(7459), 193–198.

Craig, W. R., Hanlon-Dearman, A., Sinclair, C., Taback, S., & Moffatt, M. (2004). Metoclopramide, thickened feedings, and positioning for gastro-oesophageal reflux in children under two years. *Cochrane Database of Systematic Reviews, 4*, CD003502.

Dietitians of Canada and Canadian Paediatric Society. (2010). Promoting optimal monitoring of child growth in Canada: Using the new WHO growth charts. Retrieved from http://www.cps.ca/tools/growth-charts-statement-FULL.pdf

Drugs.com. (2013). Metoclopramide use while breastfeeding. Retrieved from http://www.drugs.com/breastfeeding/metoclopramide.html

Drugs.com. (2014a). Contraceptives, oral, combined levels and effects while breastfeeding. Retrieved from http://www.drugs.com/breastfeeding/contraceptives-oral-combined.html

Drugs.com. (2014b). Domperidone use while breastfeeding. Retrieved from http://www.drugs.com/breastfeeding/domperidone.html

Drugs.com. (2014c). Depo-Provera. Retrieved from http://www.drugs.com/pro/depo-provera.html

Eden, A. N. (2005). Iron deficiency and impaired cognition in toddlers: An underestimated and undertreated problem. *Paediatric Drugs, 7*(6), 347–352.

Flint, A., New, K., & Davies, M. (2008). Cochrane review: Cup feeding versus other forms of supplemental enteral feeding for newborn infant unable to fully breastfeed. *Evidence-Based Child Health: A Cochrane Review Journal, 3*(3), 642–664.

Godfrey, J. R., & Lawrence, R. A. (2010). Toward optimal health: The maternal benefits of breastfeeding. *Journal of Women's Health, 19*(9), 1597–1602.

Goessler, A. (2012). Gastroesophageal reflux in children-news, trends and standards. *European Surgery, 44*(4), 212–221.

Hale, T. (2006). *Medications and mothers' milk.* (10th ed.). Amarillo, TX: Pharmasoft Publishing.

Hays, T., & Wood, R. A. (2005). A systematic review of the role of hydrolyzed infant formulas in allergy prevention. *Archives of Pediatric and Adolescent Medicine, 159*(9), 810–816.

Health Canada. (2005). *Food and nutrition. Dietary Reference Intakes: Reference values for elements.* Retrieved from http://www.hc-sc.gc.ca/fn-an/nutrition/reference/table/ref_elements_tbl-eng.php

Health Canada. (2006a). *Food and nutrition. Dietary Reference Intakes.* Retrieved from http://www.hc-sc.gc.ca/fn-an/nutrition/reference/table/ref_macronutr_tbl-eng.php

Health Canada. (2006b). *Good manufacturing practices (GMPs) for infant formula.* Retrieved from http://www.hc-sc.gc.ca/fn-an/legislation/codes/infant_formula_gmp-eng.php

Health Canada. (2007). Minimizing exposure to lead from drinking water distribution systems. *Environmental and Workplace Health.* Retrieved from http://www.hc-sc.gc.ca/ewh-semt/pubs/water-eau/lead-plomb-eng.php

Health Canada. (2008). *Health risk assessment of Bisphenol A from food packaging applications.* Retrieved from http://www.hc-sc.gc.ca/fn-an/securit/packag-emball/bpa/bpa_hra-ers-eng.php

Health Canada. (2012a). Breastfeeding Initiation in Canada: Key Statistics and Graphics (2009–2010). Retrieved from http://www.hc-sc.gc.ca/fn-an/surveill/nutrition/commun/prenatal/initiation-eng.php

Health Canada. (2012b). Duration of Exclusive Breastfeeding in Canada: Key Statistics and Graphics (2009–2010). Retrieved from http://www.hc-sc.gc.ca/fn-an/surveill/nutrition/commun/prenatal/exclusive-exclusif-eng.php

Health Canada. (2012c). *Nutrition for healthy term infants: Recommendations from birth to six months.* Retrieved from http://www.hc-sc.gc.ca/fn-an/nutrition/infant-nourisson/recom/index-eng.php

Health Canada. (2013). Novel food information—DHASCO and ARASCO as sources of docosahexaenoic acid and arachidonic in infant formula. *Food and nutrition.* Retrieved from http://www.hc-sc.gc.ca/fn-an/gmf-agm/appro/dhasco_arasco-eng.php

Health Canada. (2014). *Nutrition for healthy term infants: Recommendations from birth to six months.* Retrieved from http://www.hc-sc.gc.ca/fn-an/nutrition/infant-nourisson/recom/index-eng.php

Heneghen, M. (2011). The association between breastfeeding and the incidence of premenopausal breast cancer: Modification by breast cancer hormone receptor status. *Doctoral Dissertation,* Weill Medical College of Cornell University. Abstract retrieved from http://gradworks.umi.com/14/90/1490042.html

Human Milk Banking Association of North America (HMBANA). (2013). *Milk bank locations.* Retrieved from https://www.hmbana.org/milk-bank-locations

Hurst, C. (2013). An initial validation of a measure of sexual perceptions regarding breastfeeding. *Social Work and Public Health, 28,* 21–31.

Iacovou, M., Ralston, R., Muir, J., Walker, K., & Truby, H. (2012). Dietary management of infantile colic: A systematic review. *Maternal and Child Health Journal, 16*(6),1319–1331.

Ingram, J., Johnson, D., & Condon, L. (2011). The effects of Baby Friendly Initiative training on breastfeeding rates and the breastfeeding attitudes, knowledge and self-efficacy of community health-care staff. *Primary Health Care Research & Development, 12*(3), 266–275.

Innis, S. M. (2004). Polyunsaturated fatty acids in human milk: An essential role in infant development. *Advances in Experimental Medicine and Biology, 554,* 27–43.

International Board of Lactation Consultant Examiners [IBCLE]. (2014). *About IBLCE.* Retrieved from http://iblce.org/about-iblce/

Janke, J., Ciofani, L., Creehan, P., Ekkerbee, S. M., Hill, P. D., & Johnson, T. S. (2007). *AWHONN (Association of Women's Health, Obstetric and Neonatal Nurses) breastfeeding support: Prenatal care through the first year: Evidence based clinical practice guideline* (2 nd ed.). Washington, DC: AWHONN.

Jhaveri, R. (2013). Protection against hepatitis c and other enveloped viruses? Another reason why "breast is best". *The Journal of Infectious Diseases, 208*(12), Retrieved from http://jid.oxfordjournals.org/content/early/2013/10/15/infdis.jit521.full

Kelly, Y. (2006). Racial/ethnic differences in breastfeeding initiation and continuation in the United Kingdom and comparison with findings in the United States. *Pediatrics, 118*(5), e1428–e1435.

Kent, J. C., Mitoulas, L. R., Cregan, M. D., Ramsay, D. T., Doherty, D. A., & Hartmann, P. E. (2006). Volume and frequency of breastfeedings and fat content of breast milk throughout the day. *Pediatrics, 117*(3), e387–e395.

Kim, J., & Froh, E. (2012). What nurses need to know regarding nutritional and immunological properties of human milk. *Journal of Obstetric Gynecologic & Neonatal Nursing, 41*(1), 122–137.

Kong, S. K., & Lee, D. T. (2004). Factors influencing decision to breastfeed. *Journal of Advanced Nursing, 46*(4), 369–379.

Kramer, M., & Kakuma, R. (2012). Optimal duration of exclusive breastfeeding. *Cochrane Database Systematic Review, 8*, CD003517.

Labarere, J., Gelbert-Baudino, N., Ayral, A. S., Duc, C., Berchotteau, M., Bouchon, N., et al. (2005). Efficacy of breastfeeding support provided by trained clinicians during an early, routine preventive visit: A prospective, randomized, open trial of 226 mother–infant pairs. *Pediatrics, 115*(2), e139–e146.

Lakshman, R., Ogilvie, D., & Ong, K. (2009). Mothers' experiences of bottle-feeding: A systematic review of qualitative and quantitative studies. *Archives of disease in childhood, 94*, 596–601.

Lauwers, J., & Shinskie, D. (2005). *Counseling the nursing mother: A lactation consultant's guide* (4th ed.). Sudbury, MA: Jones and Bartlett.

Lawrence, R. A., & Lawrence, R. M. (2005). *Breast-feeding: A guide for the medical profession* (6th ed.). St. Louis, MO: Mosby.

Lawson, M. (2007). Contemporary aspects of infant feeding. *Paediatric Nursing, 19*(2), 39–44.

Li, R., Darling, N., Maurice, E., Barker, L., & Grummer-Strawn, L. M. (2005). Breastfeeding rates in the United States by characteristics of the child, mother, or family: The 2002 National Immunization Survey. *Pediatrics, 115*(1), e31–e37.

Li, R., Hsia, J., Fridinger, F., Hussain, A., Benton-Davis, S., & Grummer-Strawn, L. (2004). Public beliefs about breastfeeding policies in various settings. *Journal of the American Dietetic Association, 104*(7), 1162–1168.

Lightdale, J., & Gremse, D. (2013). Gastroesophageal reflux: Management guide for the pediatrician. *Pediatrics, 131*(5), e1684–e1695.

Lockman, S. (2011). HIV and Infant Feeding: Review of Updated 2010 WHO Guidelines. *Medscape.* Retrieved from http://www.medscape.com/viewarticle/735119

Lozoff, B., Castillo, M., Clark, K., & Smith, J. (2012). Iron-fortified vs low-iron formula: Developmental outcome at 10 years. *Archives of Pediatrics and Adolescent Medicine, 166*(3), 208–215.

Luan, N., Wu, Q., Gong, T., Vogtmann, E., Wang, Y., & Lin, B. (2013). Breastfeeding and ovarian cancer risk: A meta-analysis of epidemiologic studies. *American Journal of Clinical Nutrition, 98*(4), 1020–1031.

Lutsiv, O., Pullenayegum, E., Foster, G., Vera, C., Giglia, L. Chapman, B., et al. (2013). Women's intentions to breastfeed: A population-based cohort study. *British journal of obstetrics and gynaecology, 120*, 1490–1499.

Mannion, C., Hoobs, A., McDonald, S., & Tough, S. (2013). Maternal perceptions of partner support during breastfeeding. *International Breastfeeding Journal, 8*(4), Retrieved from http://www.internationalbreastfeedingjournal.com/content/8/1/4

Mayo Clinic. (2014). Colic. *Patient Care and Health Info, Diseases and Conditions.* Retrieved from http://www.mayoclinic.org/diseases-conditions/colic/basics/definition/con-20019091

McGill University. (2008). Breastfeeding associated with increased intelligence, study suggests. *Science Daily.* Retrieved from http://www.sciencedaily.com/releases/2008/05/080505162902.htm

MedlinePlus. (2012). *Health topics: Normal growth and development.* Bethesda, MD: National Center for Biotechnology Information. Retrieved from http://www.nlm.nih.gov/medlineplus/ency/article/002456.htm

Meedya, S., Fahy, K., & Kable, A. (2010). Factor that positively influence breastfeeding duration to 6 months: A literature review. *Women and Birth, 23*(4), 135–145.

Moore, E. R., Anderson, G. C., Bergman, N. (2007). Early skin-to-skin contact for mothers and their healthy newborn infants. *Cochrane Database of Systematic Reviews, 3*, CD003519. DOI: 10.1002/14651858.CD003519.pub2.

Morrill, J. F., Heinig, M. J., Pappagianis, D., & Dewey, K. G. (2005). Risk factors for mammary candidosis among lactating women. *Journal of Obstetric Gynecologic and Neonatal Nursing, 34*(1), 37–45.

Morrow, A. L., & Rangel, J. M. (2004). Human milk protection against infectious diarrhea: Implications for prevention and clinical care. *Seminars in Pediatric Infectious Diseases, 15*(4), 221–228.

Motherisk. (2013). *Breastfeeding and drugs.* Retrieved from http://www.motherisk.org/women/breastfeeding.jsp

Nishimura, T., Suzue, J., & Kaji, H. (2009). Breastfeeding reduces the severity of respiratory syncytial virus infection among young infants: a multi-center prospective study. *Pediatrics International, 51*(6), 812–816.

O'Connor, N., Tanabe, K., Siadaty, M., & Hauck, F. (2009). Pacifiers and breastfeeding: A systematic review. *Archives of Pediatrics Adolescent Medicine, 163*(4):378–382.

Papon, N., Courdavault, V., Clastre, M., & Bennett, R. (2013). Emerging and emerged pathogenic *Candida* species: Beyond the *Candida albicans* paradigm. *PLOS Pathogens, 9*(9):e1003550. DOI: 10.1371/journal.ppat.1003550. Retrieved from http://www.plospathogens.org/article/info%3Adoi%2F10.1371%2Fjournal.ppat.1003550

Pisacane, A., Continisio, G. I., Aldinucci, M., D'Amora, S., & Continisio, P. (2005). A controlled trial of the father's role in breastfeeding promotion. *Pediatrics, 116*(4), 494–498.

Pryor, K., & Pryor, G. (2014). Are there any foods I should avoid when breastfeeding? Babycenter. Expert Advice. Retrieved from http://www.babycenter.com/404_are-there-any-foods-i-should-avoid-while-breastfeeding_8906.bc?startIndex = 10&questionId = 8906

Public Health Agency of Canada. (2013a). *Breastfeeding & infant nutrition.* Retrieved from http://www.phac-aspc.gc.ca/hp-ps/dca-dea/stages-etapes/childhood-enfance_0–2/nutrition

Public Health Agency of Canada. (2013b). Vaccination of specific populations: Immunization in pregnancy and breastfeeding. *Canadian Immunization Guide.* Retrieved from http://www.phac-aspc.gc.ca/publicat/cig-gci/p03–04-eng.php

Rasmussen, K., & Geraghty, S. (2011). The quiet revolution: Breastfeeding transformed with the use of breast pumps. *American Journal of Public Health, 101*(8), 1356–1359. Retrieved from http://europepmc.org/articles/PMC3134520

Registered Nurses' Association of Ontario. (2006). *Breastfeeding: Fundamental concepts. A self-learning package.* Toronto, Canada: Registered Nurses' Association of Ontario. Retrieved from http://rnao.ca/bpg/guidelines/resources/breastfeeding-fundamental-concepts-selflearning-package

Registered Nurses' Association of Ontario. (2007). *Breastfeeding best practice guidelines for nurses.* Toronto, Canada: Registered Nurses' Association of Ontario. Retrieved from http://rnao.ca/bpg/guidelines/breastfeeding-best-practice-guidelines-nurses

Riordan, J. & Wambach, K. (2010) *Breast-feeding and human lactation* (4th. ed.). Sudbury, MA Jones and Bartlett.

Roberts, D. M., Ostapchuk, M., & O'Brien, J. G. (2004). Infantile colic. *American Family Physician, 70*(4), 735–740.

Roberts, E., & Schilsky, M. (2008). Diagnosis and treatment of Wilson disease. *Hepatology, 47*(6), 2089–2111.

Roze, J., Darmaun, D., Boquien, C., Flament, C., Picard, J., Savagner, C., et al. (2012). The apparent breastfeeding paradox in very preterm infants: Relationship between breastfeeding, early weight gain and neurodevelopment based on results from two cohorts, EPIPAGE and LIFT. *Pediatrics BMJ, 2*(2), 1–11.

Saskatchewan Drug Information Services. (2012). Galactogogues: Effectiveness and safety. *Drug News, 29*(12). Saskatoon, SK: College of Pharmacy and Nutrition, University of Saskatchewan. Retrieved from http://medsask.usask.ca/documents/newsletters/29.2.Galactagogues.pdf

Schack-Nielsen, L., Larnkjaer, A., & Michaelsen, K. F. (2005). Long term effects of breast feeding on the infant and mother. *Advances in Experimental Medicine and Biology, 569,* 16–23.

Seppo, L., Korpela, R., Lonnerdal, B., Metsaniitty, L., Juntunen-Backman, K., Klemola, T., et al. (2005). A follow-up study of nutrient intake, nutritional status, and growth in infants with cow milk allergy fed either a soy formula or an extensively hydrolyzed whey formula. *American Journal of Clinical Nutrition, 82*(1), 140–145.

Service Canada. (2014). *Employment insurance maternity and parental benefits.* Retrieved from http://www.servicecanada.gc.ca/eng/sc/ei/benefits/maternityparental.shtml

Simons, E, Teresa, T. O., Moineddin, R., Stieb, D., & Dell, S. (2012). Associations between second-hand smoke exposure in pregnancy and age of childhood asthma development. *Allergy, Asthma & Clinical Immunology, 8*(Suppl 1):A4.

Singhal, A., Cole, T. J., Fewtrell, M., & Lucas, A. (2004). Breastmilk feeding and lipoprotein profile in adolescents born preterm: Follow up of a prospective randomized study. *Lancet, 363,* 1571–1578.

Slykerman, R. F., Thompson, J. M., Becroft, D. M., Robinson, E., Pryor, J. E., Clark, P. M., et al. (2005). Breastfeeding and intelligence of preschool children. *Acta Paediatrica, 94*(7), 827–829.

Society of Obstetricians & Gynaecologists of Canada. (2012). *What are my birth control options post partum?* Retrieved from http://www.sexualityandu.ca/sexual-health/pregnancy/what-are-my-birth-control-options-post-partum

Sonnenschein-van der Voort, A., Jaddoe, V., van der Valk, R. J., Willemsen, S., Hofman, A., Moll, H., et al. (2012) Duration and exclusiveness of breastfeeding and childhood asthma-related symptoms. *European Respiratory Journal, 39*(1), 81–89.

Spatz, D. L. (2005). The breastfeeding case study: A model for educating nursing students. *Journal of Nursing Education, 44*(9), 432–434.

Spurles, P., & Babineau, J. (2011). A qualitative study of attitude toward public breastfeeding among young Canadian men and women. *Journal of Human Lactation, 27*(2), 131–137.

Stuebe, A. (2009). The risks of not breastfeeding for mothers and infants. *Reviews in Obstetrics & Gynecology, 2*(4), 222–231.

Stuebe, A., Grewen, K., Pederson, C., Propper, C., & Meltzer-Brody, S. (2012). Failed lactation and perinatal depression: Common problems with shared neuroendocrine mechanisms? *Journal of Women's health, 21*(3), 264–272.

Taveras, E. M., Li, R., Grummer-Strawn, L., Richardson, M., Marshall, R., Rego, V. H., et al. (2004). Mothers' and clinicians' perspectives on breastfeeding counseling during routine preventive visits. *Pediatrics, 113*(5), e405–e411.

Tharner, A., Luijk, M., Raat, H., Ijzendoorn, M., Bakermans-Kranenburg, M., Moll, H., et al. (2012). Breastfeeding and its relation to maternal sensitivity and infant attachment. *Journal of Development Behavior. Pediatrics, 33*(5), 396–404.

The Hospital for Sick Children. (2008). *Feeding infants and toddlers.* Retrieved from http://www.sickkids.ca/Nursing/Education-and-learning/Nursing-Student-Orientation/module-two-clinical-care/Feeding/index.html

Tsai, S. Y. (2013). Impact of a breastfeeding-friendly workplace on an employed mothers' intention to continue breastfeeding after returning to work. *Breastfeeding Medicine, 8*(2), 210–216.

Tully, M. R., Lockhart-Borman, L., & Updegrove, K. (2004). Stories of success: The use of donor milk is increasing in North America. *Journal of Human Lactation, 20*(1), 75–77.

Tunc, V., Camurdan, A., Ilhan, M., Sahin, F., & Beyazova, U. (2008). Factors associated with defecation patterns in 0–24 month old children. *European Journal of Pediatrics, 167*(12), 1357–1362.

United Nations Children's Fund (UNICEF). (2005). *The baby friendly hospital initiative.* Retrieved from http://www.unicef.org/nutrition/index_24806.html

Wagner, C. (2012). Human milk and lactation. Retrieved from http://emedicine.medscape.com/article/1835675-overview#showall

Walters, S. (2007). Dealing with a plugged duct or mastitis. *New Beginnings, 24*(2), 76–77. LaLeche League International.

Weber, D., Janson, A., Wen, L., & Rissel, C. (2011). Female employees' perception of organisational support for breastfeeding at work: findings from an Australian health service workplace. *International Breastfeeding Journal, 6*(19) Retrieved from http://www.internationalbreastfeedingjournal.com/content/6/1/19

WebMD. (2013). Bowel movements in babies. 119502014 *Healthwise, Inc.* Retrieved from http://www.webmd.com/a-to-z-guides/bowel-movements-in-babies-topic-overview

Wiener, S. (2006). Diagnosis and management of Candida of the nipple and breast. *Journal of Midwifery and Women's Health, 51*(2), 125–128.

Wirihana, L., & Barnard A. (2011). Women's perceptions of their healthcare experience when they choose not to breastfeed. *Women & Birth, 25*(3), 135–141.doi: 10.1016/j.wombi.2011.08.005. Retrieved from http://www.infantformula.org/sites/default/files/Womens_healthcare_experience_when_choosing_not_to_breastfeed_0.pdf

World Health Organization. (2013). Long-term effects of breastfeeding: A systematic review. NLM classification: WS 125. Retrieved from http://www.who.int/maternal_child_adolescent/documents/breastfeeding_long_term_effects/en/

World Health Organization. (2014). Infant and young child feeding. *Fact Sheet No. 42.* World Health Organization. Retrieved from http://www.who.int/mediacentre/factsheets/fs342/en/

Yipu, S., deGroh, M., & Morrison, H. (2013). Perinatal and early childhood factors for overweight and obesity in young Canadian children. *Canadian Journal of Public Health, 104*(1), e69–e74.

Yon, B., & Johnson, R. (2005). US and Canadian Dietary References Intakes (RNIs) for the macronutrients, energy and physical activity. *British Nutrition Foundation Bulletin, 30,* 176–181.

Ziegler, A., Wallner, M., Kaiser, I., Rossbauer, M., Harsunen, M., Lachmann, L., et al. (2012). Long-term protective effects of lactation on the development of type-2 diabetes in women with recent gestational diabetes mellitus. *Diabetes, 61,* 3161–3171.

WEB RESOURCES

Academy of Breastfeeding Medicine Web site (www.bfmed.org)
Breastfeeding Committee for Canada (www.breastfeedingcanada.ca)
Breastfeeding Inc. (http://www.breastfeedinginc.ca)
Bright Future Lactation Resource Center (www.bflrc.com/index.htm)
Infact Canada (http://www.infactcanada.ca/InfactHome Page.htm)
La Leche League Canada (www.lllc.ca)
Motherisk Program, Sick Kids Foundation (www. motherisk.org)
Registered Nurses' Association of Ontario (http://rnao.ca)
Health Canada: Infant Feeding (http://www.hc-sc.gc.ca/fn-an/nutrition/infant-nourisson/recom/index-eng.php)

CHAPTER 22

The High-Risk Newborn

Debbie Fraser and Mary F. King*

 Baby Mitchell was born at 30 weeks' gestation 48 hours after his mother experienced premature rupture of membranes. His birth weight was 1590 g, considered appropriate for gestational age (AGA). Mitchell received one dose of surfactant and was placed on a ventilator because of difficulty establishing respirations.

 Baby Madeline was born at 39 weeks' gestation following uneventful labour and a vaginal birth. Her weight was 4100 g, considered large for gestational age (LGA); her length was 54.6 cm. Madeline's parents, Louie and Danita, learned during a routine prenatal ultrasound that Madeline had congenital cleft lip and palate. The early diagnosis provided an opportunity for the parents to research the defect and to receive counselling and teaching about it. Nevertheless, actually seeing Madeline at birth came as "a shock" to Danita. While holding Madeline, she said "Oh, my poor baby." Louie tried to comfort them both.

You will learn more about these stories later in this chapter. Nurses working with such families need to be able to manage care and address issues appropriately. Before beginning, consider the following points related to the above scenarios:

- What aspects present issues of immediate concern? What interventions are needed? Explain your answers.
- What are the priorities of care for baby Mitchell? For baby Madeline?
- How might the nurse promote parental attachment in each situation?
- What long-term effects related to each newborn's condition does the nurse need to address when teaching the parents? How might these factors affect family functioning?

---

*Contributor to first U.S. edition.

On completion of this chapter, the reader should be able to:

- Correlate small-for-gestational-age (SGA) and LGA status with precipitating factors and common complications.
- Prioritize the needs of newborns experiencing complications related to size, gestational age, or both.
- Discuss collaborative care for newborns with complications related to size, gestational age, or both.
- Identify major congenital anomalies experienced by newborns and their underlying factors and conditions.
- Analyze physiologic stressors related to congenital anomalies that may negatively affect newborn extrauterine adaptation.
- Establish immediate priorities for care and provisions for transfer to the home when congenital anomalies lead to alterations in oxygenation, nutrition, growth, and development.
- Discuss the effects that newborn complications may have on family attachment and coping.
- Describe collaborative management strategies for newborns with common congenital anomalies.

appropriate for gestational age (AGA)
bronchopulmonary dysplasia
congenital diaphragmatic hernia
developmental dysplasia of the hip
esophageal atresia
gastroschisis
hydrocephaly
hyperbilirubinemia
hypoglycemia
imperforate anus
intrauterine growth restriction (IUGR)
kernicterus
large for gestational age (LGA)
late preterm newborn

meningocele
myelomeningocele
omphalocele
oral–facial cleft
phototherapy
postterm newborn
preterm newborn
respiratory distress syndrome
retinopathy of prematurity
small for gestational age (SGA)
spina bifida
talipes equinovarus
tracheoesophageal fistula
trophic feedings

With the first cry at birth, newborns begin the transition from fetal to extrauterine life, which involves marked cardiovascular and respiratory changes (see Chapter 20). In addition, newborns require energy to consume and metabolize nutrients as well as to maintain and produce heat. Preparations for these changes begin in utero, where the maternal body normally provides an optimal environment for fetal growth. For example, during gestation, the fetus develops fat for insulation against heat loss and stores liver glycogen for energy. The fetal lungs produce surfactant to facilitate breathing. Primitive neurologic reflexes support future adaptation.

Unfortunately, not all newborns have the necessary physiologic reserves for an uneventful extrauterine transition. Certain complications can affect the newborn's ability to successfully adapt, grow, and not only survive, but also *thrive*. For example, birth asphyxia threatens oxygenation and usually requires immediate resuscitation (see Chapter 20). Congenital anomalies may interfere with the ability to make necessary adjustments. For example, cleft lip and/or palate compromise the baby's ability to feed optimally and may pose problems for parental–newborn attachment.

Antepartal and intrapartal history taking and physical examination can help nurses identify risk factors that may contribute to neonatal complications, thus forewarning the health care team attending a birth to be prepared to accommodate special needs (see Chapters 13 and 16). In some cases, however, risk factors or problems are not readily apparent at birth, and poor adaptation, complications, or congenital defects catch the health care team by surprise. Thus, vigilant ongoing newborn assessment is essential to detect any gradually evolving problems. The nurse should be alert to subtle changes in newborn behaviour, crying, and feeding and be prepared to intervene promptly and aggressively as a family care provider.

All parents hope and expect that their newborn will be perfect in every way. When a newborn has an obvious congenital anomaly, injury from birth trauma, or other complication requiring aggressive management, nurses intervene therapeutically with the entire family to facilitate grieving over the loss of what was expected and healthy coping with the real situation. Nurses also assist families to accept the outcome and to adjust psychosocially, making the necessary role adaptations to accommodate their new family member.

Occasionally, problems or deviations from normal cause no obvious symptoms or ones that manifest slowly. In such cases, family members may deny or ignore these emerging problems. Nurses are aware of individual and collective needs in order to interact effectively in such cases and develop a culturally sensitive and acceptable plan of care with families. Knowledge of available resources and community and agency contacts is crucial for collaborative long-term planning.

NEWBORN RISK IDENTIFICATION

Many different factors can influence fetal risks and lead to newborn complications. Attempts to identify such risks begin as early as possible with prenatal screening, risk assessments, and early prenatal care and testing (see Chapters 11 and 12). Ongoing nursing assessments and evaluations during the first hours of life also help identify newborns at risk (see Chapter 20). A careful and complete nursing history reviews pre-pregnancy and antepartal maternal health, labour and birth history, and the family's cultural and lifestyle practices.

With all clients, the nurse strives to establish rapport during the initial antepartum visit, regardless of timing. Rather than admonishing a client who is late seeking prenatal care, the nurse praises her current initiative and uses verbal and nonverbal communication to make the client feel that her own needs and those of the fetus are priorities. The nurse first establishes credibility; through active listening, positive attention, eye contact, and touch (when appropriate), the nurse can establish trust. During subsequent visits, a trusting relationship between nurse and client facilitates acceptance of such things as community support systems for nutrition and transportation when personal resources are limited or absent.

Nurses interact with pregnant clients in various settings and collaborate with other members of the health team to provide education and interventions for expectant parents, the fetus, the newborn, and other important parties (eg, siblings). Chapters 13 and 16 cover in detail potential problems in pregnancy, labour, and birth. See Table 22.1 for a summary of common risk factors and their possible neonatal consequences.

PROBLEMS RELATED TO SIZE AND GESTATIONAL AGE

Newborns vary in size and gestational age. Differences in size can result from genetics or be related to alterations in the quantity and quality of nutrients transferred to the fetus through the placenta during gestation. Differences in duration of gestation vary based on several factors, including whether this is a woman's first pregnancy, any complications that occurred during gestation, problems with estimating correct due date, genetics, and reasons yet unidentified. As discussed in Chapter 20, a baby born between 38 and 41 weeks' gestation is considered *term*. When gestation is less than 34 completed weeks, the newborn is considered a **preterm newborn**; when gestation is between 34 and 37 completed weeks, the newborn is considered a **late preterm newborn**; when gestation is more than 41 weeks, the newborn is considered a **postterm newborn**. Preterm, late preterm, and postterm newborns are at risk for complications.

Birth weights vary normally and can be correlated with gestational age. Soon after birth, the nurse weighs the newborn and estimates gestational age (see Chapter 20). Typical weight for a term newborn ranges from 3000 to 4000 g. Weights below this range

● TABLE 22.1 **Pregnancy Risk Factors and Potential Newborn Complications**

Problem	Possible Neonatal Consequences
Maternal Infections	
Toxoplasmosis	Cranial deformity
	Microcephaly
	Hydrocephaly
Rubella	Cataracts
	Deafness
	Cardiac anomalies
	Cognitive and motor deficits
	Cleft lip and palate
	Intrauterine growth restriction (IUGR)
Syphilis	Cognitive deficits and orthopedic deformities
	Congenital syphilis
Cytomegalovirus	Severe disability
	Cranial nerve damage
	Blindness
	Deafness
	Hepatic dysfunction
Herpes	Congenital herpes simplex virus infection
	Encephalitis
	Convulsions
	Shock
	Neurologic damage
	Death
Gonorrhea	Severe eye infection (ophthalmia neonatorum)
	Blindness (if untreated) from corneal damage
Hepatitis B virus (HBV)	Hepatitis B infection with potential for becoming a chronic carrier
Chlamydia	Severe eye infection (ophthalmia neonatorum)
Candidiasis	Thrush (oral *Monilia*)
	Systemic candida infection
Human immunodeficiency virus (HIV)	Possible HIV infection resulting from placental transmission, perinatal exposure, or breast milk
Group B streptococcus	Early onset (day of birth):
	Rapidly progressing pneumonia
	Respiratory distress
	Late onset (2–4 wk):
	Meningitis
	Intracranial pressure
	Bulging fontanels
	Neurologic deficits
Maternal Substance Use	
Alcohol use	Fetal alcohol spectrum disorder
	Spontaneous abortion
	Low birth weight
	Low Apgar scores
Cocaine use	Congenital anomalies of the brain, kidneys, and urogenital tract
	SGA
	IUGR
	Prematurity
	Necrotizing enterocolitis (NEC)
	Birth asphyxia secondary to placental abruption
	Brain infarcts
	Neurobehavioural abnormalities

(continued)

● TABLE 22.1 **Pregnancy Risk Factors and Potential Newborn Complications** (continued)

Problem	Possible Neonatal Consequences
Smoking or exposure to secondhand tobacco smoke	Spontaneous abortion SGA Low birth weight Increased risk for sudden infant death syndrome (SIDS) Birth defects including congenital urinary tract anomalies
Heroin	IUGR SGA Increased risk for SIDS Newborn withdrawal Poor feeding Dehydration and electrolyte imbalance related to vomiting and diarrhea
Marijuana	Preterm birth Decreased birth weight and length Possible delays in growth and development
Common Maternal Conditions	
Maternal–newborn blood group/Rh incompatibility	Hyperbilirubinemia Kernicterus Erythroblastosis fetalis
Hypertensive disorders	IUGR SGA Preterm birth Hypoglycemia Intrauterine hypoxia Birth asphyxia
Diabetes mellitus	Hypoglycemia Congenital anomalies Macrosomia with an increased risk for birth injury (shoulder and neck) IUGR or SGA from poor placental perfusion

indicate a problem related to size and may be categorized as follows:

- Low birth weight (LBW): The newborn weighs 1500 to 2500 g.
- Very low birth weight (VLBW): The newborn weighs 1000 to 1500 g.
- Extremely low birth weight: The newborn weighs 1000 g or less (Ives & Austin, 2009).

Major problems associated with an extremely LBW newborn include intracranial hemorrhage and pulmonary dysfunction. Neurosensory impairments in extremely LBW newborns include cerebral palsy, deafness, and blindness, which create long-term health and educational needs.

Size, gestational age, and condition are variables that help predict how well a newborn will adapt to the extrauterine environment. The newborn whose growth and development are AGA meets the normal expected size for weeks' gestation. The newborn whose growth pattern is at either extreme, either **small for gestational age (SGA)** or **LGA**, may be at risk for predictable complications. Mortality and morbidity rates are linked directly with birth weight and gestational age (Gardner & Hernandez, 2011; Miltenburg et al., 2011).

Classifications of SGA, AGA, and LGA are independent from classifications of preterm, term, and postterm newborns. For example, a baby born at 40 weeks' gestation would be considered term. If he or she also weighed less than 2500 g, the newborn would be considered SGA. Similarly, a baby born at 34 weeks' gestation who weighed 2500 g would be LGA, despite his or her preterm status.

 Consider baby Mitchell, described at the beginning of the chapter. How would the nurse classify Mitchell based on gestational age? Suppose Mitchell was born at 40 weeks' gestation, how would the nurse then classify him based on his birth weight?

Small-for-Gestational-Age Newborn

The weight of the SGA newborn is typically below the 10th percentile on the intrauterine growth chart for gestational age (see Chapter 20). SGA newborns near or at term typically weigh less than 2500 g.

Etiology

Some newborns have genetically small stature and thus are SGA. Many SGA newborns, however, experienced growth problems in utero. **Intrauterine growth restriction (IUGR)** is the term used when fetal growth is less than normal because the fetus is not receiving the nutrients and oxygen required for development. IUGR can develop at any time in pregnancy, but the point in gestation at which it occurs can have different effects. With *symmetric (early-onset) IUGR,* the fetus lags behind in growth for most of the pregnancy, resulting in a newborn that is proportionally small. This condition usually results from a long-term or chronic prenatal problem, such as placental dysfunction, maternal substance use, phenylketonuria, or chromosomal abnormalities. With *asymmetric (late-onset) IUGR,* the fetus typically grows normally until the third trimester. Subsequent growth problems cause the head to continue normal development, but body size falls behind normal parameters as a result of "brain sparing" (nutrients and oxygen are diverted away from the body to salvage the brain at the expense of other organs) (Singh, 2010).

Box 22.1 lists risk factors contributing to SGA, IUGR, or both. Some of these conditions are modifiable. For example, smoking in pregnancy has been found to triple or quadruple the incidence of IUGR (Simmons, 2012).

Newborn Characteristics

SGA newborns are similar in physical appearance to, and share some needs with, preterm newborns. Both appear scrawny and underdeveloped with little subcutaneous fat for insulation and scant brown fat for heat production, making hypothermia a common problem. With SGA babies, the head may appear large in proportion to the body; poorly developed suck pads give the head an oval appearance. The face is angular and pinched. Decreased muscle mass is most evident in the buttocks, thighs, and cheeks.

The stomachs of SGA newborns have a small capacity. Unlike preterm newborns, however, term SGA newborns with no additional complications have coordinated suck and swallow (Blackburn, 2013). This enables them to tolerate early oral feedings safely. Some SGA newborns do not demonstrate "catch-up" growth. Slow growth velocity and problems related to poor development of vital organs may persist beyond the preschool years.

Large-for-Gestational-Age Newborns

Excessive body weight is the defining criterion for the LGA newborn (also called *macrosomia*). Depending on

● **BOX 22.1** **Risk Factors Associated With IUGR, SGA, or Both**

Maternal Factors
- Anemia
- Cardiac disease
- Chronic renal disease
- Cigarette smoking
- Diabetes
- Hypertension
- Infection
- Malnutrition
- Residence at high altitude
- Respiratory disease
- Sickle cell disease
- Substance use (alcohol, drugs)

Uterine/Placental Factors
- Abruptio placentae
- Decreased blood flow in the uterus and placenta
- Infection in the tissues around the fetus
- Placenta previa

Fetal Factors
- Birth defects
- Chromosomal abnormalities
- Infection
- Multiple gestation

the assessment tool used, adjustments may be considered for gestational age and sex. Typically, newborns above the 90th percentile on growth charts (which equals approximately two standard deviations above the mean for weight) are considered LGA (Rahimian, 2013). In some cases, birth weight above 4000 g alone has been used to classify a newborn as LGA. Regardless of preterm, term, or postterm status, any birth weight exceeding 4500 g is considered excessive (Simpson, 2012). See Box 22.2 for risk factors.

Newborn Characteristics

LGA newborns typically have rounded, flushed faces and prominent chin pads. Shoulders are large and broad;

● **BOX 22.2** **Risk Factors for LGA Newborn**

- Excessive pregnancy weight gain
- Fetal exposure to high estrogen levels
- High maternal birth weight
- LGA in previous infants
- Maternal diabetes
- Maternal pregravid obesity
- Multiparity

abdomens are round and protuberant, with increased body mass. Because of their physical size, they may be mistaken at first glance for "older" infants.

LGA newborns may appear healthy and normal, pending physical appraisal for gestational age and neurologic maturity. Nevertheless, they are at risk for such complications as birth trauma, hypoglycemia, and congenital anomalies.

Associated Complications

Birth Trauma. Trauma can occur during vaginal or cesarean birth of the LGA newborn (see Chapter 16). Ecchymosis and erythema may develop from birth injuries related to cephalo-pelvic disproportion or from the use of instruments during delivery (ie, forceps, vacuum). Subcutaneous bleeding or extensive bruising can lead to jaundice. Observation and inspection of the newborn's symmetry of movement may reveal neurologic trauma or paralysis.

Head trauma may result in increased intracranial pressure (ICP). Close monitoring of the newborn's behaviour may provide clues for detecting subtle and insidious signs of increased ICP, which include altered sleep–wake cycles, crying, and pain. Later signs of increased ICP are more ominous and include bulging fontanels, high-pitched crying, and seizure activity.

Vaginal birth of the LGA newborn with very wide shoulders may lead to shoulder dystocia and result in clavicular fracture (Simpson, 2012). Supraclavicular edema and ecchymosis may be apparent on inspection; crepitus can be palpated over the fractured clavicle. Swaddling, careful handling, and gentle cuddling promote comfort for the newborn with birth trauma.

Hypoglycemia. LGA newborns are at risk for **hypoglycemia** (serum blood glucose level below normal values). In term newborns, normal blood glucose values should be above 2.6 mmol/L (Aziz et al., 2004/2013). This common complication usually develops within 2 to 6 hours of birth.

Newborn hypoglycemia is related closely to size and condition as well as to complications of labour and birth (Wilson, 2011). A close relationship between maternal and fetal glucose concentrations during both early and late gestation has been well documented (McGowan et al., 2011), so a drop in maternal glucose level affects the fetus as well.

Indications of hypoglycemia may include a change in level of consciousness (fretfulness, lethargy, stupor) and poor feeding despite previous successful efforts. The nurse is alert for a whimpering or weak cry, tremors or jitteriness, respiratory difficulties, and central cyanosis. Often, however, low blood glucose levels in newborns have no accompanying clinical signs or symptoms. Untreated hypoglycemia may result in long-term

neurologic injury (Boardman et al., 2013; McGowan et al., 2011).

Congenital Anomalies. LGA newborns are at an increased risk for skeletal deformities such as hip subluxation (Loder & Skopelja, 2011). These problems are thought to be related to mechanical factors secondary to a cramped intrauterine environment with little amniotic fluid to facilitate movement and positioning.

Preterm Newborn

A classification of preterm (premature) is used when a baby is born any time before 38 weeks' gestation, independent of birth weight. Birth before 34 completed weeks' gestation is considered "very preterm" (Arduini & Vendola, 2012). LBW typically accompanies preterm status, because the untimely birth interrupts normal growth and development. See Box 22.3 for factors associated with preterm birth.

Newborn Characteristics

Characteristics of preterm newborns are related to gestational age. The Ballard Gestational Age assessment tool correlates findings with gestational age, including in VLBW newborns (see http://www.ballardscore.com/Pages/ScoreSheet.aspx).

The appearance of preterm newborns often differs significantly from that of term babies. Generally, the preterm newborn's skin is ruddy, thin, and permeable, with visible blood vessels. Fine, downy lanugo covers the skin; vernix is present. Plantar and palmar surfaces are shiny and gelatinous, with a few creases. The head appears large in proportion to the body; the eyelids may still be fused in very preterm newborns. Eyelids may be edematous, and eye rolling may be noted, with wakefulness and spontaneous eye opening if the eyelids are not fused. Fontanelles are large; cranial suture lines are prominent and moveable. The chest is small, with little to no breast tissue. The abdomen has a "pot-belly" appearance. In females, the external genitalia appear large with widely separated labia and a large clitoris. In males, the scrotal sac is loose with a few rugae. Testes may be undescended.

● **BOX 22.3   Factors Associated With Preterm Birth**

- Previous preterm birth
- Uterine anomalies: bicornate uterus, cervical insufficiency
- Multiple gestation
- Polyhydramnios (uterine stretching)
- Trauma
- Obstetric conditions requiring pregnancy termination
- Maternal urinary tract infection

The cry of preterm newborns may be weak and whimpering. Respirations are typically rapid, irregular, possibly shallow, and diaphragmatic, with periods of apnea. Respiratory distress is evidenced by sternal, intercostal, or subcostal retractions; inspiratory lag; flared nostrils with inspiration; or grunting on expiration.

Posture is reflective of limp, weak muscles. Preterm newborns tend to stay in place when positioned. Seizure activity may be evidenced by stiffness.

Preterm newborns also demonstrate specific behavioural responses to stress. Examples include averting gaze, tremors, and splaying of fingers of one or both hands. In some cases, they may simply sigh and become flaccid. Such behaviours, in conjunction with physiologic indicators of poor tolerance to stress (eg, tachycardia), brief periods of apnea, and colour changes, are cues that the newborn is becoming overstressed and needs rest.

Figure 22.1 compares in detail typical physical examination findings and reflex characteristics in preterm versus term infants.

Associated Complications

Preterm newborns face complications related to immaturity of the central nervous system and other vital organs, making the already stressful extrauterine transition (see Chapter 20) even more challenging. Consequently, preterm newborns are at risk for numerous complications. Most of them receive care in a neonatal intensive care unit (NICU). If the birth facility does not have an NICU and preterm birth is expected, ideally the labouring woman will be transferred to a facility with an NICU, if time permits. Otherwise, the newborn will be transported to the facility immediately after birth.

Birth Asphyxia. Preterm newborns may develop birth asphyxia from inadequate oxygen transfer during labour and birth. If a preterm newborn does not breathe spontaneously, is gasping, or the heart rate is below 100 beats/min, the health care team begins positive-pressure ventilation (PPV) with room air following 30 seconds of stimulation, drying the skin (for preterm infants of at least 29 completed weeks' gestation), and provision of warmth (Kattwinkel, 2011). Preductal pulse oximetry (applied to the right hand/wrist) should be used for all infants receiving PPV, those who remain cyanotic at 5 minutes of age, or those who have laboured respirations (Canadian Pediatric Society, 2011). If the heart rate remains below 60 beats/min following 30 seconds of effective PPV, chest compressions should be started with PPV delivered via a blend of oxygen and room air based on the neonate's oxygen saturation level (SpO_2) (Kattwinkel, 2011). Development of tissues during the fetal stage takes place in a hypoxic environment; excessive amounts of oxygen can lead to oxidant injury

(Kattwinkel, 2011). Oxygen should therefore always be delivered to the preterm infant blended with room air at a concentration that achieves a targeted SpO_2 level: 60% to 65% at 1 min, increasing by 5% each minute until 80% to 85% is reached at 5 minutes; at 10 minutes the target is 85% to 95% (Kattwinkel, 2011).

Intubation may be necessary to maintain a patent airway and to deliver more effective ventilations. The size of the endotracheal tube used for intubation reflects the tiny lumen of the preterm baby's airway. An endotracheal tube of 2.5 to 3 mm is used for VLBW newborns, whereas an endotracheal tube of 3 mm is used for LBW newborns. Arterial blood gases are evaluated for oxygen and carbon dioxide concentrations and acid–base balance.

 Think back to baby Mitchell from the beginning of the chapter. Mitchell was intubated and placed on a ventilator. What size endotracheal tube would the nurse expect to be used for care?

Cold Stress. The preterm infant is susceptible to cold stress because of an inability to generate heat, increased heat loss, and impaired thermoregulation resulting from immaturity of the central nervous system. Brown fat deposits develop around vital organs late in gestation; the preterm infant lacks this protection against hypothermia (Blackburn, 2013). Excessive heat loss is also attributable to the lack of insulating subcutaneous fat, a high body-surface-area–to–body-mass ratio, and thin permeable skin, with increased insensible fluid loss (Blackburn, 2013). In term infants, positions that hold the extremities close to the body, such as full flexion, serve to prevent heat loss. The lack of flexion in preterm infants is demonstrated by a frog-like position with splayed extremities. Heat is readily lost to the environment through radiation. The ambient temperature in the delivery room should be increased to approximately 25°C to 26°C to prevent heat loss in the preterm infant. A portable warming pad may be useful under layers of towels on the resuscitation surface to prevent loss of heat by conduction. The preterm infant born at less than 29 completed weeks' gestation should not be dried at birth. Rather the infant's body should be wrapped in polyethylene or food grade plastic wrap up to the neck to maintain body temperature and prevent heat loss through evaporation (Kattwinkel, 2011).

Respiratory Distress. The preterm newborn's most crucial need is adequate oxygenation. When a woman goes into preterm labour, corticosteroids (eg, betamethasone) are administered; this is transferred via the

(text continues on page 898)

Premature Infant

Full-term Infant

A

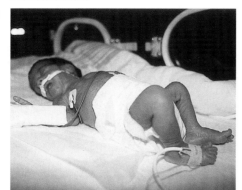
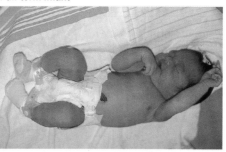

RESTING POSTURE   *The premature infant is characterized by very little, if any, flexion in the upper extremities and only partial flexion of the lower extremities. The full-term infant exhibits flexion in all four extremities.*

Premature Infant, 28–32 Weeks

Full-term Infant

B

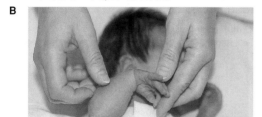
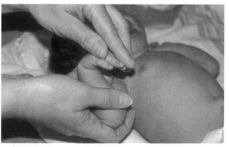

WRIST FLEXION   *The wrist is flexed, applying enough pressure to get the hand as close to the forearm as possible. The angle between the hypothenar eminence and the ventral aspect of the forearm is measured. (Care must be taken not to rotate an infant's wrist.) The premature infant at 28–32 weeks' gestation will exhibit a 90° angle. With the full-term infant it is possible to flex the hand onto the arm.*

Premature Infant

Full-term Infant

C

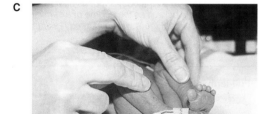
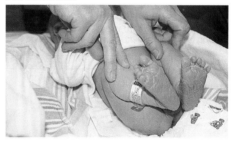

Response in Premature Infant

Response in Full-term Infant

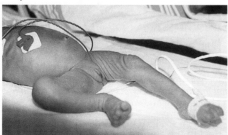
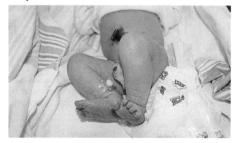

RECOIL OF EXTREMITIES   *Place an infant supine. To test recoil of the legs (1) flex the legs and knees fully and hold for 5 seconds (shown in top photos), (2) extend the legs fully by pulling on the feet, (3) release. To test the arms, flex forearms and follow same procedure. In the premature infant response is minimal or absent (bottom left); in the full-term infant extremities return briskly to full flexion (bottom right).*

FIGURE 22.1   Physical and neuromuscular maturation in preterm and term newborns.
A: Resting posture. **B:** Wrist flexion. **C:** Recoil of the extremities.   *(continued)*

D

Premature Infant   **Full-term Infant**

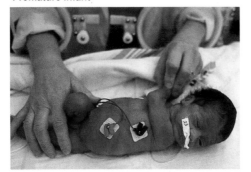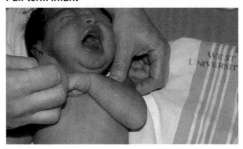

SCARF SIGN   *Hold the baby supine, take the hand, and try to place it around the neck and above the opposite shoulder as far posteriorly as possible. Assist this maneuver by lifting the elbow across the body. See how far across the chest the elbow will go. In the premature infant the elbow will reach near or across the midline. In the full-term infant the elbow will not reach the midline.*

E

Premature Infant   **Full-term Infant**

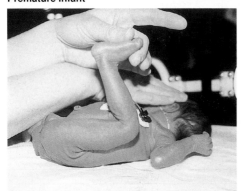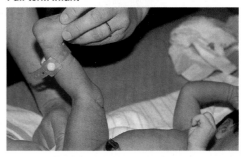

HEEL TO EAR   *With the baby supine and the hips positioned flat on the bed, draw the baby's foot as near to the ear as it will go without forcing it. Observe the distance between the foot and head as well as the degree of extension at the knee. In the premature infant very little resistance will be met. In the full-term infant there will be marked resistance; it will be impossible to draw the baby's foot to the ear.*

F

Premature Infant   **Full-term Infant**

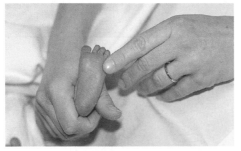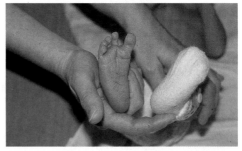

SOLE (PLANTAR) CREASES   *The sole of the premature infant has very few or no creases. With the increasing gestation age, the number and depth of sole creases multiply, so that the full-term baby has creases involving the heel. (Wrinkles that occur after 24 hours of age can sometimes be confused with true creases.)*

FIGURE 22.1   *(Continued)* **D:** Scarf sign. **E:** Heel to the ear. **F:** Sole (plantar) creases.

(continued)

G

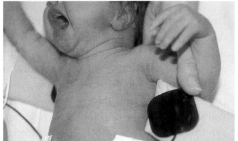 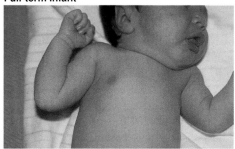

BREAST TISSUE   *In infants younger than 34 weeks' gestation the areola and nipple are barely visible. After 34 weeks the areola becomes raised. Also, an infant of less than 36 weeks' gestation has no breast tissue. Breast tissue arises with increasing gestational age due to maternal hormonal stimulation. Thus, an infant of 39 to 40 weeks will have 5 to 6 mm of breast tissue, and this amount will increase with age.*

Premature Infant, 34–36 Weeks   Full-term Infant

H

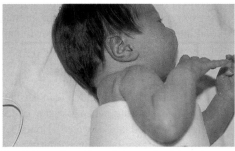 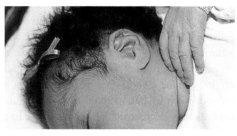

EARS   *At fewer than 34 weeks' gestation infants have very flat, relatively shapeless ears. Shape develops over time so that an infant between 34 and 36 weeks has a slight incurving of the superior part of the ear; the term infant is characterized by incurving of two thirds of the pinna; and in an infant older than 39 weeks the incurving continues to the lobe. If the extremely premature infant's ear is folded over, it will stay folded. Cartilage begins to appear at approximately 32 weeks so that the ear returns slowly to its original position. In an infant of more than 40 weeks' gestation, there is enough ear cartilage so that the ear stands erect away from the head and returns quickly when folded. (When folding the ear over during examination be certain that the surrounding area is wiped clean or the ear may adhere to the vernix.)*

Premature Male   Full-term Male

I

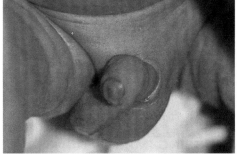 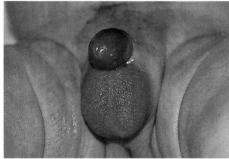

MALE GENITALIA   *In the premature male the testes are very high in the inguinal canal and there are very few rugae on the scrotum. The full-term infant's testes are lower in the scrotum and many rugae have developed.*

Premature Female   Full-term Female

J

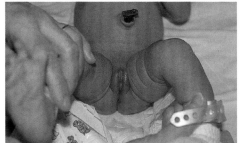 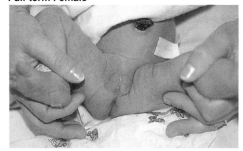

FEMALE GENITALIA   *When the premature female is positioned on her back with hips abducted, the clitoris is very prominent and the labia majora are very small and widely separated. The labia minora and the clitoris are covered by the labia majora in the full-term infant.*

FIGURE 22.1   *(Continued)* **G:** Breast tissue. **H:** Ears. **I:** Male genitalia. **J:** Female genitalia.

placenta to the fetus. Corticosteroids hasten fetal lung maturity by stimulating the production of surfactant, and thus reduce the severity of respiratory illness. In addition to its respiratory benefits, antenatal corticosteroid therapy contributes to decreased cerebroventricular hemorrhage, necrotizing enterocolitis, and mortality (Carlo et al., 2011; Dutta, 2012).

Respiratory distress may become apparent shortly after birth. Regardless of size, all preterm newborns are at risk for **respiratory distress syndrome** related to deficiency of surfactant secondary to lung immaturity. Without adequate surfactant to reduce surface tension in the lungs and to promote alveolar stability, the alveoli tend to collapse with each expiration. Consequently, each breath requires the same high pressure as the initial breath at birth to inflate the lungs. The weak preterm newborn cannot sustain the work of breathing, even with the use of accessory muscles and grunting, both of which are used in an attempt to keep the alveoli open. Administration of antenatal steroids such as betamethasone helps mature the fetal lungs, thereby decreasing the risk of severe lung disease and resultant hypoxia after delivery.

Preterm newborns may receive exogenous surfactant at birth, which requires the presence of an endotracheal tube immediately after birth (Pharmacology Box 22.1). A commercial preparation of surfactant is administered directly into the lungs through the endotracheal tube. Bovine lipid surfactant and beractant are the two surfactant preparations available in Canada. Suctioning is avoided for at least 1 hour, if possible, to prevent inadvertent removal of the surfactant before it can coat the alveoli. Auscultation of the lung fields of the newborn who has received endotracheal surfactant typically reveals coarse rhonchi and crackles until the alveoli have absorbed the medication.

Bronchopulmonary Dysplasia. Preterm infants often require continuous oxygen therapy through nasal cannula or by mechanical ventilation or continuous positive airway pressure (CPAP). **Bronchopulmonary dysplasia** is a chronic lung disease that results from immaturity of the lungs and the use of long-term mechanical ventilation after the development of respiratory distress syndrome (Gardner et al., 2011). Bronchopulmonary dysplasia predisposes the infant to respiratory infections and reactive airway disease.

Retinopathy of Prematurity. Retinopathy of prematurity (ROP) results from a combination of factors, including prematurity and the administration of oxygen. High oxygen concentrations in the premature infant's blood interfere with the normal growth patterns of retinal blood vessels, leading in some cases to structural changes to the retinal tissue, tangling of retinal vessels, retinal detachment, and blindness (Fraser, 2012).

The retinal vascular bed can sustain permanent damage and scarring when oxygen concentrations in the infant's blood are elevated. Nevertheless, oxygen administration may be required during resuscitation to ensure perfusion of the brain and vital organs. The lowest possible concentration of oxygen is used to reduce the risk for oxygen toxicity while maintaining adequate oxygenation. This is accomplished by the initial use of room air (this concentration is elevated from the intrauterine environment) and the use of preductal pulse oximetry (the probe is applied to the right hand/wrist) to determine appropriate concentrations of oxygen administration during resuscitation (Kattwinkel, 2011). The very preterm newborn may require supplemental oxygen initially rather than room air in order to maintain appropriate oxygen saturation levels (Finan et al., 2011).

● PHARMACOLOGY 22.1   Surfactant

ACTION

Exogenous surfactant coats the alveoli, decreasing surface tension and improving oxygenation and lung compliance.

PREGNANCY RISK CATEGORY

X

DOSAGE

5 mL/kg intratracheally; one to two doses given in first 48 hours of life

POSSIBLE ADVERSE EFFECTS

Transient bradycardia, pulmonary hemorrhage

NURSING IMPLICATIONS

- Suction infant before administration, if necessary.
- Assess infant's respiratory rate, rhythm, arterial blood gases, and colour before administration.
- Ensure proper endotracheal tube placement before dosing.
- Assess infant's respiratory rate, colour, and arterial blood gases after administration.
- Do not suction endotracheal tube for at least 1 hour after administration to avoid removing drug.

Oxygen saturations above 93% should be avoided when supplemental oxygen is used for preterm infants (Gardner et al., 2011). Monitoring oxygen saturation levels through evaluation of arterial blood gases and pulse oximetry is essential. In addition, referrals for eye examinations are indicated for all preterm newborns born at less than 30 weeks' gestation or with a birth weight of less than 1500 g (American Academy of Pediatrics Section on Ophthalmology et al., 2013).

Feeding Problems. For preterm newborns, oral feedings may begin when the infant is medically stable. Infants born prior to 32 to 34 weeks' gestation may have difficulty coordinating suck, swallow, and breathing and therefore are prone to aspiration (Askin & Wilson, 2011). The underdeveloped esophageal sphincter predisposes the baby to painful gastroesophageal reflux. Stomach emptying is delayed; gut motility is diminished. Bile salts and pancreatic enzymes for digestion of enteral feedings are lacking, depending on gestational age (Blackburn, 2013).

To compound the feeding difficulties faced by preterm newborns, their nutritional needs are greater because fetal growth was interrupted at its peak by the birth. Fluid needs are also greater than that of term newborns because of increased insensible losses through permeable skin surfaces and increased excretion related to inability of the renal system to concentrate urine. If the preterm newborn does not receive fluid and nutritional support from the first day of life, dehydration and catabolism begin (Blackburn, 2013).

Necrotizing Enterocolitis. Necrotizing enterocolitis (NEC) is a multifactorial bowel disorder associated with ischemia leading to bowel inflammation and necrosis. Hypoxic damage to the bowel wall allows the invasion of bacteria. When stressors such as infection, prematurity, enteral formula feeding, or other inflammatory mediators are present, gastrointestinal (GI) mucosal injury may lead to necrotizing enterocolitis (Siggers et al., 2013). The risk for necrotizing enterocolitis is increased with persistent patent ductus arteriosus following birth (Sellmer et al., 2012).

Because the premature newborn is susceptible to necrotizing enterocolitis, all efforts are made to halt preterm labour. Breast milk feedings protect the GI tract from injury and bacterial invasion, reducing the incidence and severity of necrotizing enterocolitis (Noble, 2010). Administration of probiotics to accompany feedings may be beneficial, although further research is needed prior to routine use (Caplan, 2009; Li et al., 2013). Symptoms of necrotizing enterocolitis in early stages may be somewhat vague and include abdominal distention, apnea, bradycardia, feeding intolerance, and lethargy. As the condition progresses, frank rectal bleeding and abdominal tenderness may develop. Bowel sounds may be diminished or absent.

If a newborn exhibits the onset of symptoms of necrotizing enterocolitis, the nurse withholds all oral or enteral feedings and notifies the health care provider immediately. An abdominal x-ray should be done and may confirm necrotizing enterocolitis. The nurse administers and monitors total parenteral nutrition until enteral feedings can be resumed. Surgical resection of the affected bowel segment and possible formation of an ostomy may be necessary when the intestine perforates or in the presence of peritonitis. The nurse administers broad-spectrum antibiotics and IV fluids as prescribed. He or she is vigilant and monitors continuously for changes in the newborn's condition, as necrotizing enterocolitis is potentially life-threatening.

Anemia of Prematurity. Anemia of prematurity primarily results from the physiologic immaturity of the hematologic system, leading to diminished erythropoiesis. Frequent blood specimens needed for laboratory analysis can further exacerbate this condition.

Early cord clamping in the preterm birth is defined as clamping of the umbilical cord within 15 to 30 seconds after birth. Delayed cord clamping (DCC) is defined as clamping that occurs at any time after 30 seconds. The amount of blood that is transferred from the placenta to the preterm neonate is not as well understood as in the term infant, although several studies have shown that a delay of a minimum of 30 seconds in clamping the cord increased the blood volume transferred (Garofalo & Abenhaim, 2012). DCC (or even milking the cord) in the preterm infant has been shown to decrease the need for blood transfusions for anemia, as well as decrease the risks for intraventricular hemorrhage and late-onset sepsis (Garofalo & Abenhaim, 2012). The Society for Obstetricians and Gynecologists of Canada (SOGC) recommends that cord clamping in preterm infants should be delayed by at least 60 seconds whenever possible (Leduc et al., 2009).

Persistent Patent Ductus Arteriosus. The ductus arteriosus, a fetal circulatory structure, allows blood to bypass the fetal lungs and normally closes at birth with the first cry (see Chapter 20). In preterm newborns, however, this structure may remain open (patent), especially in cases of respiratory distress syndrome (Askin & Wilson, 2011). With a patent ductus arteriosus, assessment findings reveal bounding pulses, an active precordium (the region over the heart and lower thorax), and auscultation of a long systolic murmur (Evans, 2012). An echocardiogram confirms the diagnosis. The duct is closed either pharmacologically with indomethacin or ibuprofen, or surgically with ligation. Because a secondary effect of indomethacin is vasoconstriction of the mesenteric blood vessels, this drug was thought to be implicated in bowel ischemia, contributing to necrotizing enterocolitis. Current research, however, does not support this finding.

Rather, patent ductus arteriosus independently contributes to necrotizing enterocolitis, distinct from administration of indomethacin (Sharma et al., 2010). Ibuprofen is now used more commonly because it has less impact on renal blood flow than indomethacin (Hammerman et al., 2012).

Intracranial Hemorrhage. The most common type of intracranial hemorrhage is bleeding within the brain ventricles, which may develop in 15% to 20% of preterm infants who weigh less than 1500 g (Robinson, 2012). The germinal matrix, a vascular embryonic lining of the ventricles that persists up to 35 weeks' gestation, increases susceptibility to bleeding under certain conditions. The most serious effects of intraventricular hemorrhage in this area are neurodevelopmental disability and death (Klebermass-Schrehof et al., 2012).

Preterm infants at the greatest risk for spontaneous intraventricular bleeding include those who have experienced stressors such as birth trauma, birth asphyxia, or respiratory distress syndrome in addition to prematurity. Administration of antenatal magnesium sulphate to the woman in preterm labour has been found to decrease the incidence of death, cerebral palsy, and substantial gross motor dysfunction (Magee et al., 2011). Women who are in active preterm labour or with a planned preterm birth due to maternal or fetal indications at ≤31 6/7 weeks' gestation should receive magnesium sulphate for fetal neuroprotection (Magee et al., 2011). A loading dose of 4 g IV administered over 30 minutes should be followed by a 1 g/hour infusion until birth; if birth is no longer imminent or the magnesium sulphate has been administered for a maximum of 24 hours, it should be discontinued. There is no evidence to support repeated administration of the medication for the purpose of fetal neuroprotection (Magee et al., 2011). The health care provider monitors both the woman and fetus with existing protocols and guidelines for administration of magnesium sulphate and fetal surveillance.

Infants born at less than 32 weeks' gestation should have a screening cranial ultrasound at 1 week of age and again at 4 weeks of age. More frequent ultrasounds may be necessary if the initial ultrasound demonstrates evidence of an intracranial hemorrhage.

When parents learn that their newborn has been diagnosed with intraventricular bleeding, they are likely to become alarmed and extremely fearful about this immediate threat to well-being. Once the bleeding begins to decrease and resolve, other fears may begin to surface. Parents may worry that the infant will face subsequent learning disabilities, poor school performance, and decreased quality of life. Nurses can support and remind parents that unless the neurologic defects are major and irreversible, predictions about future developmental growth and adaptation depend on many variables, including family support, home environment, and the socioeconomic availability of resources. See Teaching Tips 22.1.

The Late-Preterm Infant

A group of infants now recognized as being at significant risk for morbidity is the late-preterm infant. Originally referred to as the near-term infant, the late-preterm infant is born between 34 and 36 6/7 weeks' gestation (Forsythe & Allen, 2013; Gyamfi-Bannerman, 2012). This group of infants comprises about 76% of all preterm births in the United States (Gyamfi-Bannerman, 2012). Statistics for the incidence in Canada are not available.

In the past 20 years the incidence of preterm delivery has increased by approximately 20%, with late-preterm births accounting for the majority of the increase (Muglia & Katz, 2010). The increase in deliveries between 34 and 37 weeks' gestation has been attributed to a number of factors: improvements in prenatal diagnosis and management of complications of pregnancy; increasing maternal age and the use of fertility treatments; and the increase in elective cesarean deliveries with the increased risk of miscalculation of gestation (Muglia & Katz, 2010). These infants are at an increased risk for a number of short- and long-term problems, including respiratory distress, hyperbilirubinemia, feeding difficulties, temperature instability,

---

● **TEACHING TIPS 22.1** **Providing Developmental Stimulation for a Preterm Infant**

The nurse should review with parents and caregivers the following tips for maximizing cerebral function in the stable premature infant:

- Visual stimulation, after determining developmental readiness:
  - Present human faces in close proximity to the infant.
  - Use crib mobiles with colours, designs, and well-defined and distinctive patterns.

- Auditory stimulation
  - Regularly expose the newborn to voice interactions.
  - Play music around the infant.
- Motor stimulation
  - Assist the infant with patterning exercises to simulate crawling.

infection, learning difficulties (Forsythe & Allen, 2013; Harijan & Boyle, 2012), and increased health care costs (Bérard et al., 2012).

Newborn Characteristics

Because of their larger size and more mature appearance, late-preterm infants are often treated as term infants and cared for in the normal nursery; however, these infants are at an increased risk of experiencing complications related to prematurity.

Associated Complications

Like preterm infants, the late-preterm infant has an increased risk of developing complications such as hypothermia, hypoglycemia, respiratory distress, and hyperbilirubinemia. In a 2010 study, Kalyoncu et al. found that, compared with term infants, late-preterm infants were 11 times more likely to have respiratory distress or hypoglycemia. The late-preterm infant also has immature sucking and swallowing behaviours, which interfere with breastfeeding (Askin & Wilson, 2011).

Postterm Newborns

Postterm newborns are born after 41 completed weeks of gestation (see Chapter 16). Problems arise when the aging placenta can no longer deliver adequate oxygen and nutrients. As a result, the fetus uses nutritional reserves, potentially catabolizing proteins for energy and survival. With placental insufficiency, the fetus receives poor oxygenation (hypoxemia) and nutrient transfer (starvation), which depletes glucose reserves normally stored in the liver. Hypoxia triggers increased production of red blood cells (polycythemia), which can pose serious problems (eg, thick viscous blood) when coupled with dehydration. Consequently, the baby may be predisposed to a debilitating or possibly fatal thrombotic event, such as stroke.

Newborn Characteristics

A postterm newborn typically looks lean, with a long angular body and little subcutaneous fat. This appearance is due to depletion of the nutritional reserves developed during pregnancy, leading to metabolism of body fats and protein.

Because the newborn is gestationally mature, plantar and palmar surfaces are deeply wrinkled. Hair is coarse and abundant. Nails are long and possibly meconium-stained if there has been a history of fetal distress. The skin appears scaly and dry and also may be meconium-stained.

Associated Complications

A postterm newborn is at risk for complications resulting primarily from inadequate nutrition and hypoxemia.

Examples include meconium aspiration syndrome, polycythemia, and hypoglycemia.

Meconium Aspiration Syndrome. In the presence of distress commonly precipitated by hypoxemia, the fetus makes gasping respiratory efforts and releases meconium into the amniotic sac. Meconium in the amniotic fluid increases the risk for meconium aspiration, another serious complication. Meconium may be aspirated in utero or with the newborn's first breath. When amniotic fluid is thick with tenacious meconium, the rush of air into the lungs with the first cry also transports these waste products into the lungs, forming plugs that reduce oxygen diffusion and may lead to air trapping and rupture of the alveoli. The presence of meconium in the airways results in inflammation and a chemical pneumonitis similar to pneumonia.

Risk for meconium aspiration syndrome may be identified intrapartally when rupture of the membranes reveals green amniotic fluid. Depending on the amount of meconium, the amniotic fluid can range from being lightly stained to thick, viscous, and opaque green (similar to pea soup). The health care team can intervene to minimize complications. Based on results of a nonstress test, contraction stress test, or sonographic assessment of fetal behaviour and/or amniotic fluid volume, health care providers may determine that placental insufficiency and resultant fetal hypoxemia contraindicate the stress of labour and vaginal birth. Fetal monitoring or fetal scalp sampling may identify the fetus in need of urgent delivery. A cesarean birth may be deemed appropriate.

Health care personnel perform endotracheal intubation and suctioning in infants, born in the presence of meconium-stained amniotic fluid, who are not vigourous at birth (see Chapter 20). Newborns with poor tone and no spontaneous respiratory efforts after delivery should be intubated prior to drying and stimulation and the endotracheal tube suctioned to remove any meconium from the trachea (Kattwinkel, 2011).

Meconium aspiration syndrome results in hypoxemia, as evidenced by tachypnea, retractions, and nasal flaring. Oxygen therapy is instituted to prevent blood from shunting away from the lungs secondary to increased pulmonary pressures. Continuous monitoring of respiratory status and vital signs is essential.

Polycythemia. Dehydration and hemoconcentration in postterm newborns can result in polycythemia. Sluggish blood flow can predispose the newborn to thrombi, pulmonary emboli, and stroke. Neonatal nurses monitoring behaviour, symmetry of movement, suck, cry, and Moro reflex may be the first to detect a stroke. In such cases, after the airway is maintained, adequate hydration is the next priority; oxygen is bound to hemoglobin on the red blood cell and thick viscous blood can obstruct oxygen transport.

COLLABORATIVE CARE: COMPLICATIONS RELATED TO SIZE, GESTATIONAL AGE, OR BOTH

Newborns with complications related to size, gestational age, or both need astute assessment, early detection of problems, and prompt interventions. Typically, they require a multidisciplinary approach to meet their numerous and varied needs.

Assessment

The process of assessment for newborns with size- or age-related complications is the same as for normal newborns (see Chapter 20). Certain areas, however, require close investigation to prevent or to minimize problems.

Respiratory Status

General respiratory assessments include initial and continuing appraisal of the motion of the chest wall and abdomen to detect any inspiratory lag or asynchrony. The nurse assesses use of the nares and intercostal muscles (between the ribs) and notes any undue effort manifested by xiphoid retraction or grunting sounds, which increases intrathoracic pressure and maintains alveolar stability during exhalation.

If complications compromise the ability to exchange oxygen and carbon dioxide, the nurse assesses for manifestations of respiratory insufficiency. Respiratory instability may progress to diminished respiratory effort that is unresponsive to stimulation, with eventual deterioration to a total lack of respiratory effort. Team members promptly identify and remedy the cause of the respiratory distress before the newborn begins to decompensate and deteriorate. Using Assessment Tool 22.1, the nurse evaluates the five criteria and assigns a value of 0, 1, or 2 to each. A total of zero reflects no respiratory distress; a total of 2 to 4 indicates mild distress; a total of 5 or 6 signifies moderate distress; and totals of 7 or above indicate severe respiratory distress. The higher the number on this Silverman/Anderson tool, the greater the respiratory effort and energy expenditure, and the incidence of eventual exhaustion, respiratory acidosis, and hypoxemia.

Special Concerns for Preterm Newborns

Tactile and thermal stimuli trigger respirations at birth. Additionally, chemoreceptors respond to low oxygen tension and elevated arterial carbon dioxide tension to stimulate the brain's respiratory centre. Because preterm newborns lack the lung and neuromuscular maturity to respond to birth with stable, effective respirations, the nurse assesses respiratory rate, depth, and regularity and documents findings frequently. Rapid, irregular respirations are normal initially but should slow to 40 to 60 breaths per minute at rest. When stressed or with excessive stimulation, the newborn will respond with rapid, irregular respirations. Tachypnea, tachycardia, and central cyanosis are indicators of poor tolerance of noxious stimuli or poor extrauterine transition. Unlike the acrocyanosis (mottled, bluish discolouration of extremities) seen in normal newborns, central cyanosis is seen in the head and trunk and indicates insufficient oxygen and arterial desaturation.

Special Concerns for LGA Newborns

During labour and vaginal birth, compression of the chest squeezes lung fluid from the alveoli and air passageways. Vaginal birth stimulates chest wall recoil to facilitate the initial breath, which also draws air into the partially cleared passageways. Newborns, delivered by cesarean birth because of excessive size, miss these benefits. The nurse assesses these infants for excessive mucus, regurgitation of mucus, or gagging efforts and diminished respiratory effort.

Skin

Newborn skin may reflect various stages of fetal development and complications related to size, gestational age, or both. See Table 22.2.

Special Concerns for Postterm Newborns

Postterm newborns may have little vernix, leading to skin desquamation and peeling. Additionally, if the postterm newborn experienced intrauterine hypoxia from placental aging and deterioration, the skin may be stained greenish yellow from meconium in the amniotic fluid.

Special Concerns for LGA Newborns

When assessing an LGA newborn whose mother had diabetes, the nurse may observe opaque skin common

● TABLE 22.2 **Common Skin Assessment Findings and Associated Complications**

Finding	Associated Complication
Reddish colour	Preterm birth
Greenish tint	Meconium staining
Puffy and opaque	Infant of mother with diabetes
Bluish head/trunk	Deficient oxygen
Copious lanugo	Preterm birth
Scanty lanugo	Postterm birth
Yellow	Jaundice
Loose/wrinkled	Dehydration, postterm birth
Pallor	Hypoglycemia
Flushed face	Hyperglycemia
Bluish mottled extremities	Acrocyanosis, exposure to cold
Peeling/scaliness	Postterm birth

● ASSESSMENT TOOL 22.1   **Grading of Neonatal Respiratory Distress Based on the Silverman–Anderson Index**

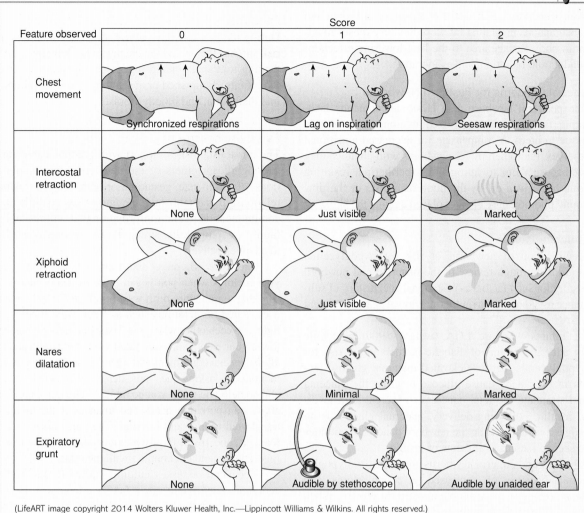

Feature observed	Score		
	0	1	2
Chest movement	Synchronized respirations	Lag on inspiration	Seesaw respirations
Intercostal retraction	None	Just visible	Marked
Xiphoid retraction	None	Just visible	Marked
Nares dilatation	None	Minimal	Marked
Expiratory grunt	None	Audible by stethoscope	Audible by unaided ear

with a full-term infant; excess body fat and fluid retention also may add a puffy edematous appearance.

Thermoregulation

Temperature control is an important goal for newborns with complications related to size, age, or both. Axilla temperature assessment and the use of skin temperature probes do not require contact with delicate, easily traumatized mucous membranes. Rectal thermometers increase the risk for trauma to the rectal mucosa and should be avoided (Blackburn, 2013).

The nurse carefully obtains an initial baseline temperature on the high-risk newborn, continuing to assess the temperature every 15 minutes until stable. Since the preterm infant can have differences in both the core and body surface temperatures, both axilla and skin probe assessments are instituted simultaneously (Brown &

Landers, 2011). Thereafter, temperature is assessed every 1 to 4 hours in stable newborns (Brown & Landers, 2011).

The nurse assesses any deviation from normal temperature (36° to 36.5°C [skin]; 36.5° to 37.3°C [axilla]), being constantly alert to all indicators of ineffective thermoregulation (Brown & Landers, 2011). Changes in feeding behaviours and tolerance and onset of lethargy or irritability are signs of ineffective regulation. Cool, mottled skin may indicate hypothermia. When the nurse assesses such signs, he or she checks for accompanying signs of respiratory distress and obtains a heelstick blood sample for blood glucose monitoring; respiratory distress, hypoglycemia, and hypoxia are often seen together (Aylott, 2006; Karlsen, 2013). Because temperature instability can indicate infection, the nurse looks for other evidence, being especially alert in a baby with invasive lines.

Special Concerns for Preterm Newborns

Preterm newborns have an immature regulatory control centre, lose heat to the environment, and cannot effectively generate heat because of a paucity of brown and subcutaneous insulating fat. Poor flexion exposes maximum body surface area to the heat-lowering effects of conduction, radiation, and evaporation.

Special Concerns for Postterm Newborns

The postterm newborn also lacks subcutaneous insulating fat, having metabolized it along with muscle tissue in utero to compensate for decreased nutritional reserves. Phototherapy for newborns with jaundice may predispose them to iatrogenic hyperthermia resulting from heat given off by the fluorescent rays or the fibreoptic phototherapy blanket placed against the skin.

Glucose Levels

Identification of newborns at risk for hypoglycemia requires thorough review of the maternal and newborn history for such factors as gestational age, history of substance use, diabetes, hypothermia, low Apgar scores, and LGA.

Infants who are LGA (weight >90th percentile for age) and infants of diabetic mothers are at risk for hypoglycemia, because elevated maternal glucose levels in pregnancy cause glucose to cross the placenta and stimulate the fetal pancreas to secrete high levels of insulin. Following delivery, maternal glucose is no longer available, while the newborn pancreas continues to secrete increased amounts of insulin.

SGA and preterm newborns are at risk for hypoglycemia because of decreased glycogen stores and decreased nutrients available in utero for growth. When glucose supplies are limited or scarce, any available glucose is used for metabolic needs, with none available for storage in the liver as glycogen.

The Canadian Paediatric Society (CPS) recommends that neonates who are asymptomatic but at risk for hypoglycemia should have an effective feeding and then have their blood glucose checked at 2 hours of age and then every 3 to 6 hours (Aziz et al., 2004/2013). If the blood glucose at 2 hours of age is less than 1.8 mmol/L after one feeding or less than 2.0 mmol/L after a subsequent feeding, then a dextrose infusion is established. Intravenous dextrose is also considered for neonates whose blood glucose levels are repeatedly below 2.6 mmol/L after subsequent feedings. Newborns who are symptomatic or unwell have their blood glucose levels checked immediately. Infants with hypoglycemia who are symptomatic or unwell require treatment with intravenous dextrose (Aziz et al., 2004/2013). The CPS algorithm for screening and immediate management of babies at risk for neonatal hypoglycemia (Aziz et al., 2004/2013) is found at www.cps.ca/documents/blood-glucose-en.pdf.

Feeding

During the first few days of life, the nurse monitors at-risk infants for behaviour changes (eg, lethargy), poor feeding tolerance, increasing gastric residuals in tube-fed infants, diminished or absent bowel sounds, abdominal distention, and bloody stools.

Family Assessment

The nurse establishes rapport with parents, caregivers, and significant others of the newborn with complications related to size, gestation, or both. Once a trusting relationship is established, the nurse uses goal-directed communication to elicit information that will reveal the family's coping skills, strengths, and resources needed to adapt effectively.

The nurse asks direct questions such as, "What were your feelings when you began preterm labour and realized that a premature birth was imminent?" Or the nurse uses shared observations such as "You were holding so tightly to each other when you first came into the nursery to see your baby. It appeared that you were frightened by all the special equipment and lines." Discharge needs are identified by asking questions such as "Who will be available to help you when you go home?" The nurse inquires about transportation needs and finances if the infant is transferred to a distant hospital. The nurse assesses any fears or concerns of family members that could compromise attachment and bonding with the infant.

The nurse assesses cultural, spiritual, and socioeconomic factors that affect family adaptation, as well as beliefs about the health care delivery system. In that way, the nurse is prepared to share a thorough but concise nursing assessment with other team members to effectively plan collaborative care that meets the unique needs of newborn and family.

The nurse works with other team members to determine special equipment, supplies, or services needed at home (eg, oxygen, special appliances for feeding). He or she directs caregivers toward specific agencies for the recommended resources and collaborates with social service personnel. Public health or home care nurses are invaluable for family members caring for newborns with complications. They provide teaching, as well as physical and emotional support, and evaluate the effectiveness of supportive, preventive, and restorative care.

Select Potential Nursing Diagnoses

Nursing diagnoses appropriate for newborns with complications related to age, size, or both can be wide-ranging. Some common examples include the following:

- **Impaired Gas Exchange** related to inadequate surfactant production
- **Ineffective Breathing Pattern** related to internal and external factors including cold stress, hypoglycemia, lack of surfactant, and birth asphyxia
- **Ineffective Thermoregulation** related to immature central nervous system, inability to generate and conserve heat, excessive heat loss to the environment, and inadequate quantities of brown fat
- **Risk for Imbalanced Nutrition, Less Than Body Requirements** related to problems with ingestion, digestion, and metabolism
- **Risk for Infection** related to poorly developed immune system and invasive procedures
- **Risk for Disorganized Infant Behaviour** related to noxious stressors required in the care of the high-risk infant (eg, frequent arterial specimen collection, arterial blood gases, intubation, mechanical ventilation)
- **Parental Anxiety** related to uncertain outcomes of a newborn with complications

- **Risk for Impaired Parenting** related to poor role transition secondary to added stressors
- **Risk for Caregiver Role Strain** related to fatigue and stress secondary to multiple needs of an ill newborn

Planning/Intervention

Sophisticated technology and equipment may be necessary for the newborn's specific circumstances and care requirements. See Nursing Care Plan 22.1.

Outcomes are highly individualized and may include the following:

- The newborn will maintain adequate oxygenation and respirations.
- The newborn will maintain a stable temperature.
- The newborn will ingest adequate nutrients.
- The newborn will remain free of infection.
- The parents will demonstrate appropriate coping behaviours related to the newborn's status.
- The parents will exhibit positive responses to their newborn.
- The parents will participate in the care of their newborn.

(text continues on page 910)

NURSING CARE PLAN 22.1
●
The Preterm Newborn

Recall Baby Mitchell, the preterm newborn described at the beginning of the chapter. Maternal history reveals two spontaneous abortions related to cervical insufficiency. With the pregnancy that produced Mitchell, cervical cerclage was performed.

Mitchell and his 34-year-old mother Alisha were febrile at Mitchell's birth. Both are now afebrile. Mitchell required ventilator support with 50% to 60% oxygen for the first 3 days of life before being weaned from the ventilator. He was extubated on day 5 and received oxygen therapy at 30%, which was gradually discontinued. Oxygen saturation levels on room air are now at 90% to 92%. He is to be weaned gradually from total parenteral nutrition (TPN) and glucose-containing IV fluids. A nasogastric tube has been inserted to begin gavage feedings with his mother's breast milk, with the ultimate goal of progressing to oral feedings. Alisha states a desire to continue pumping breast milk to increase her supply in preparation for Mitchell's anticipated discharge home in 6 to 8 weeks.

NURSING DIAGNOSIS

Risk for Imbalanced Nutrition, Less Than Body Requirements related to increased needs for nutrients, small stomach capacity, and immature gastrointestinal tract

EXPECTED OUTCOMES

1. Mitchell will demonstrate steady weight gain appropriate to developmental age (minimum 20 to 30 g/day).
2. Mitchell will demonstrate an ability to tolerate gavage feedings.

(continued)

NURSING CARE PLAN 22.1 ● The Preterm Newborn *(Continued)*

INTERVENTIONS	RATIONALES
Administer prescribed IV glucose, amino acids, and essential fatty acids (TPN), observing protocols for monitoring serum glucose, electrolytes, and urine specific gravity.	Glucose has a critical role in brain metabolism. Amino acids and proteins are required for growth. Fatty acids in the form of linoleic acid provide the major source of calories for energy. Monitoring glucose, electrolytes, and urine-specific gravity provides valuable information about the therapeutic effectiveness of TPN and allows for early identification of potential complications.
Provide opportunity for non-nutritive sucking if suck reflex is present and respiratory distress is absent.	Non-nutritive sucking helps satisfy the newborn's sucking need and promotes readiness for oral feedings. It also allows the newborn the opportunity to associate feelings of satiety and gastric fullness with the act of sucking.
Collaborate with healthcare practitioner regarding timing, volume, and frequency of breast milk gavage feedings. Anticipate the introduction of small volumes of milk (minimal enteral feeding) as soon as the infant is medically stable.	Timing and readiness are paramount to tolerance of feedings, which must be individualized to each newborn's physiologic condition. The early introduction of small volumes of milk (usually 1 mL/kg) enhances maturation of the intestine and has been shown to result in earlier achievement of full enteral feeding without increasing the risk of NEC.
	Gastrointestinal mucosal inflammation or injury also may have been mediated by infection such as that associated with premature rupture of membranes.
Confirm tube placement; once confirmed, begin gavage feedings as ordered.	A malpositioned feeding tube can lead to aspiration.
Weigh newborn at the same time each day using the same scale with the newborn wearing the same amount of clothing.	Weight is a reliable indicator of the newborn's overall condition, including nutritional status. It provides an objective measure of the effectiveness of therapy.
Assess newborn's tolerance to enteral feeding. • Check gastric residuals before each feed; measure and replace gastric contents. • Subtract the amount of the gastric residual before and after the flush of the nasogastric tube from the total prescribed volume.	Assessment of feeding tolerance helps evaluate effectiveness. Measuring gastric residuals provides information about the newborn's ability to absorb feedings; replacing residuals prevents fluid loss and electrolyte imbalances.
Assess urine output, recording the number and amount of voidings. Weigh each saturated diaper, subtracting dry weight of the diaper for output (1mL urine = 1 g). Amount of voiding depends on renal maturity and ability of the kidneys to concentrate urine).	Urine output is a reliable indicator of renal function and hydration status. Accuracy in measurements is key.
Record the number, amount, and character of stools.	Stool assessment provides important information about gastrointestinal tract function. Abdominal distention, increasing gastric residuals, and blood in the stools are classic signs of necrotizing enterocolitis.

(continued)

NURSING CARE PLAN 22.1 ● The Preterm Newborn *(Continued)*

INTERVENTIONS	RATIONALES
Collaborate with healthcare team to progressively advance enteral feeding as TPN is decreased.	Feedings are individualized and progressed as the newborn develops. The expectation is that the newborn would be able to tolerate increased feedings.
Change to reflect cue-based feeding. As tolerated and ordered, gradually introduce oral feedings with breast milk through soft premature nipple or breast milk reservoir using gravity flow through a tiny soft tube allowing milk droplets into the newborn's mouth without sucking.	Excessive energy expenditure with the work of sucking negates the benefits of oral caloric intake by using the available calories for energy rather than for weight gain.
Hold the newborn upright with the head forward and chin tucked inward.	The chin-tuck manoeuvre minimizes the risk for aspiration.
Observe carefully for fatigue; cut back oral feeding if newborn tires or feeding takes longer than 30 minutes; administer remainder of feeding by gavage.	Fatigue interferes with the newborn's ability to ingest the feeding and increases energy expenditure and oxygen demand.
Involve mother in feeding opportunities; provide teaching and support. Give praise, encouragement, and support to the mother pumping breast milk. Advise her of the value of breast milk in the infant's health and nutrition.	Pumping can be uncomfortable and requires considerable motivation to continue for a prolonged period when the newborn is too ill or weak to suckle.
Involve a lactation specialist to assist mother in obtaining a full-sized, hospital-grade breast pump and provide instructions. Initiate pumping within 6 to 8 hours postpartum. Help her double pump (both breasts) simultaneously for 15 minutes every 2 to 3 hours until a good supply of breast milk is obtained.	A lactation specialist can provide valuable information, support, and guidance to the mother about breastfeeding and maintaining her milk supply.
Encourage mother to pump once or twice during the night when prolactin levels are high.	The release of prolactin results in milk production and release in the breast.
Collaborate with a lactation specialist in teaching the mother how to store, transport, and prepare breast milk.	The woman can pump with privacy in the NICU while she provides "kangaroo care" (skin-to-skin physical contact to maintain warmth and colonize normal flora on the skin surface); however, not all feedings can be accomplished with freshly pumped breast milk because of the mother's need for rest. Breast milk must be stored in clean containers and refrigerated or frozen. Stored breast milk is warmed in a water bath rather than a microwave to prevent dangerous hot spots from causing burns.

(continued)

NURSING CARE PLAN 22.1 ● The Preterm Newborn *(Continued)*

INTERVENTIONS	RATIONALES
Advise the mother to apply warm compresses and massage breasts before pumping; suggest the use of mental imaging of her baby.	Warm compresses and massage promote the let-down reflex; mental imaging stimulates the release of oxytocin, which in turn aids in the let-down reflex.
Reinforce positive gains made by the newborn with gavage and progression to oral feedings.	Positive reinforcement promotes continued participation and enhances feelings of self-esteem, thereby enhancing the chance for success.

EVALUATION

1. The newborn demonstrates increased body weight and is AGA by discharge.
2. The newborn ingests oral feedings of breast milk through premature nipple without evidence of difficulty swallowing or aspiration.

NURSING DIAGNOSES

- **Risk for Caregiver Role Strain** related to fatigue and stress secondary to added burdens of needs of preterm infant
- **Deficient Knowledge** related to multiple ongoing needs of preterm newborn

EXPECTED OUTCOMES

1. The mother and caregivers will identify possible areas of stress.
2. The mother and caregivers will list acceptable sources of support by which to reduce stress of caring for preterm newborn.
3. The mother and caregivers will identify the specific care measures required by her newborn.
4. The mother and caregivers will demonstrate beginning skills to care for the preterm newborn.

INTERVENTIONS	RATIONALES
Assess the client's level of understanding about needs of preterm newborn and required care.	Assessment provides a baseline to identify specific client needs and develop an individualized plan.
Discuss with the client her concerns, feelings, and perceptions related to the preterm newborn and care measures during labour and birth.	Discussion provides opportunities to emphasize positive aspects of the current situation; verbalization of concerns aids in establishing sources of stress and problem areas that need to be addressed.
Communicate accurate facts and answer questions honestly. Reinforce factual information, emphasizing the uniqueness of each preterm newborn.	Open, honest communication promotes trust and helps correct any misconceptions or misinformation. Facts help dispel unfounded fears, myths, or guilt feelings.

(continued)

NURSING CARE PLAN 22.1 ● The Preterm Newborn *(Continued)*

INTERVENTIONS	RATIONALES
Initiate a supportive approach for the breast-feeding mother of a premature infant.	A supportive approach fosters a trusting relationship and enhances the chances for success.
Teach the client what to expect relative to the preterm newborn's needs and care. Review expectations for growth and development.	An understanding of what to expect aids in reducing fear of the unknown.
Instruct the client in care measures, including necessary adaptations, such as use of premie nipple and small frequent feedings; also review measures for routine newborn care. Have the client return-demonstrate measures or skills as indicated.	Teaching enhances understanding. Return demonstration provides information for evaluating the success of teaching and aids in identifying areas needing additional education.
Encourage ample rest, including an afternoon nap, extra fluids (8 to 10 glasses per day), and balanced nutrition with extra protein. Advise mother to continue taking antepartal multivitamins.	Ample fluids and high-quality proteins are required to increase the quantity and quality of breast milk produced. Fatigue and anxiety can influence the breastfeeding experience negatively, which may hinder the let-down reflex. Adequate rest aids in meeting the demands of care.
Initiate a referral for social services and home care follow-up. Investigate resources for help with household tasks. Encourage mother to use appropriate resources.	Social services can provide the family with additional resources for assistance and support. Home care follow-up provides additional opportunities for assessment and teaching as well as for determining the success of previous teaching.
Encourage participation in community support groups of parents with preterm newborns.	Participation in support groups allows for sharing and helps diminish feelings of being overwhelmed and alone.
Maintain open lines of communication, including phone contact after discharge to inquire as to adjustment to full-time care of infant; allow verbalization of feelings and offer encouragement and tips for self and infant care as needed.	Follow-up communication aids in determining the transition to home, providing opportunities for positive reinforcement and identification of any areas that may develop into potential problems. Allowing the mother to verbalize feelings helps alleviate stress and anxiety.

EVALUATION

1. The mother and caregivers identify acceptable resources by which to reduce their stress, verbalizing an intent to use these resources as needed.
2. The mother and caregivers participate in developing a plan for home care with assistance from the health care team and community.
3. The mother and caregivers demonstrate safe and effective physical and developmental care, while verbalizing an understanding of the special needs of the preterm newborn.
4. The mother and caregivers create a plan for family adaptation to added time, energy, and fiscal resources and family responsibilities.

- The parents will demonstrate confidence in their ability to provide care for their newborn.
- The parents will verbalize measures to balance demands of caring for their newborn with other aspects of their life.

Oxygenation

When an infant demonstrates respiratory compromise (apnea, gasping respirations, heart rate below 100 beats/min refractory to bag and mask ventilation with room air, persistent central cyanosis), the nurse institute ventilation with oxygen immediately.

A T-piece resuscitator is ideal for resuscitation, as it is able to control target peak inspiratory pressure and deliver positive end-expiratory pressure. A self-inflating bag with a reservoir or flow-inflating device is also acceptable for preterm infants as long as a pressure manometer is used. The pressure manometer provides visual information about airway pressure in the newborn during ventilation and allows the amount of pressure given with each breath to be controlled. Recommended initial pressures are 20 cm for a preterm infant and 30 cm for a full-term infant; however, the amount of pressure used should be the minimum amount necessary to visualize the infant's chest rising. Excessive pressure should be avoided to reduce the risk for pneumothorax.

When newborns younger than 32 weeks' gestation require resuscitation, guidelines (Kattwinkel, 2011) recommend blended oxygen (room air with 100% O_2 mix) and use of an oximeter to maintain pre-ductal oxygen saturations between 85% and 90%. The infant's heart rate is used as an indicator of effectiveness: if, during resuscitation, the heart rate does not rapidly accelerate to above 100 beats/min or there is no appreciable improvement in condition, the oxygen concentration is increased according to the pre-ductal oxygen saturation (Finan et al., 2011). A carbon dioxide detector should always be used in conjunction with endotracheal intubation to ensure tube placement. Oxygen administered by all sources must be warmed to avoid cold stress.

Effectiveness of oxygen administration with assisted ventilations result in the following outcomes:

- The newborn shows improved colour and no central cyanosis after 30 seconds of PPV.
- The limp, flaccid newborn regains visible muscle tone.
- The newborn begins spontaneous breathing with oxygen.
- Saturation remains at the appropriate level for the time elapsed since birth.
- Infants who are unable to maintain effective breathing independently and oxygen saturation levels may receive oxygen with or without assisted ventilation. Method, flow rate, and percentage of oxygen

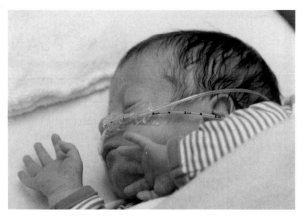

FIGURE 22.2 Delivery of oxygen therapy via nasal cannula in a preterm newborn.

administration are individualized. Examples include the following:

- Flow-by oxygen: A mask placed in close proximity to the infant's face.
- Oxygen hood: A hard, clear material with a U-shaped cut out for the infant's neck and an inlet for oxygen.
- Nasal cannula
- CPAP

As the newborn matures or as complications related to size resolve, team members wean him or her from invasive forms of oxygen administration. Lesser concentrations of oxygen are delivered by nasal cannula. The two tiny prongs must be applied with the curve pointing downward (fitting the anatomy of the nares) and may be secured with small patches of paper, or hypoallergenic tape to the cheek (Fig. 22.2).

When a newborn requires extended oxygen delivery after discharge from the health care facility, the nurse teaches parents and other caregivers how to provide oxygen at home. Usual administration is by nasal cannula. The nurse emphasizes safety precautions. For example, candles and open gas flames must be avoided to prevent combustion. Smoking around infants must always be strictly avoided.

Thermoregulation

To prevent cold stress in preterm newborns, the nurse immediately dries the newborn at birth to control a significant cause of heat loss, promptly removing any damp towels if the gestation is 29 weeks or more (Blackburn, 2013; Kattwinkel, 2011). If the gestation is less than 29 weeks, the newborn should not be dried; instead the preterm should be wrapped up to their neck in polyethylene plastic or food grade plastic wrap immediately after birth to prevent heat loss and damage to the delicate immature skin (Kattwinkel, 2011). Any surface coming into contact with the infant (eg, x-ray cassette) is covered with a warmed receiving blanket. Oxygen, if indicated, is warmed and humidified.

Keeping the newborn in an open-air, infrared radiant warmer equipped with a skin-temperature probe assists in regulating temperature and decreasing heat loss. The radiant warmer comes on when the temperature drops below a preset range, and automatically turns off if the temperature rises above the set range. A continuous digital reading is available. The nurse documents the temperature every 30 to 60 minutes initially, and then every 3 to 4 hours when the newborn is stable. Plexiglas shields surround the infant to block heat loss by convection. The nurse continually monitors the functioning of all heat control mechanisms used to maintain a neutral thermal environment as well as the ambient temperature.

Preventing cold stress and minimizing heat loss through conduction, convection, evaporation, and radiation conserve energy in LBW infants. Commercial knit caps are available, and some hospital auxiliary organizations provide hand-knit newborn caps that become keepsakes. If neither is available, the nurse fashions a newborn cap from tubular cotton material called stockinette, which may be found in most hospitals. Scalp vessels bring blood and body warmth close to the skin surface; a cap reduces the energy expenditure required for thermoregulation.

Ethical Dilemmas

Resuscitation may not be appropriate for all newborns with complications related to size, gestation, or both. Conditions that result in almost certain early death or rare survival pose ethical dilemmas for families and health care providers alike (Kattwinkel, 2011). Examples include gross immaturity (gestational age <23 weeks or birth weight <400 g) and congenital conditions with high mortality rates (anencephaly or trisomy 18). Once a decision has been made to withhold resuscitation, or if resuscitation efforts have been unsuccessful, priority nursing considerations include giving consistent, quality care to the dying newborn and showing compassion and sensitivity to the wishes and needs of the family. Communication by and among all team members reflects cultural and spiritual sensitivity.

Nurses may feel poorly prepared to deal with ethical issues arising from newborn complications related to size, gestation, or both. It is of tremendous benefit for novice nurses to volunteer to serve on hospital ethics committees and to take every opportunity for training and practice in advance of situations that require such skilled communications and sensitivity (see Chapter 1).

Nutrition

Term newborns have the necessary neuromuscular reflexes (root, suck, and swallow) and fully developed suck pads to ingest oral feedings without difficulty. The rhythm of intermittent feeding, internal feelings of hunger alternating with satiety, and a consistent caregiver provide the foundation for satisfying feeding behaviours. When newborns are medically unstable, oral feedings might need to be delayed. This is most common in SGA and preterm newborns.

Oral Feedings

When the newborn has adequate sucking and swallowing reflexes, GI functioning, and energy levels, oral feedings are preferred. Breast milk, ideally from the newborn's mother rather than from a donor or milk bank (see Chapter 21), is most desirable, especially for preterm newborns. Preterm birth greatly affects the quality of maternal breast milk, increasing the concentration of immune globulins, increasing absorption of fat, zinc, and iron, and providing increased protection against sepsis and NEC (Blackburn, 2013). In the case of LBW infants, human milk may not provide adequate calories, proteins, and minerals for growth. Human milk supplements (liquid or powder formulations) can be added to breast milk to ensure adequate growth. If human breast milk is unavailable, specialized premature infant formulas can supply needed extra calories and other nutrients (80 kcal/100 mL, rather than 68 kcal/100 mL, in term infant formulas). These specialized formulas also are fortified with calcium, phosphorus, and iron to combat anemia of prematurity.

Commercially available "premie" nipples are shorter and softer, making them easier for a preterm or weak LBW infant to compress. Frequency and amounts of feedings vary according to the newborn's size, age, and physical condition. Typically, a near-term newborn can consume 10 mL to 15 mL orally every 1 to 2 hours, whereas the very preterm newborn requires enteral feeding by orogastric or nasogastric tube because of absent or uncoordinated suck and swallow reflexes. During oral or enteral feeds, the nurse observes the infant closely to evaluate tolerance. If heart rate or respiratory effort is increased, the nurse stops the feeding to allow time for the baby to rest and recover. Oral and enteral feedings may be combined. The preterm infant who is neurologically mature enough for oral feedings may consume 8 mL of the prescribed 15 mL formula or breast milk before slowing or sleeping. He or she may take the remaining 7 mL by feeding tube. If the infant continues to tolerate oral or enteral feedings, the nurse increases the amount gradually according to metabolic needs (115 to 140 cal/kg/day of body weight), which are somewhat higher than that of full-term newborns.

Gavage Feedings

Gavage feedings are indicated for physiologically stable newborns who cannot ingest sufficient breast milk or formula orally to satisfy nutritive requirements (Nursing Procedure 22.1). Enteral feedings are withheld in cases

(text continues on page 914)

NURSING PROCEDURE 22.1
Administering a Gavage Feeding

PURPOSE

To provide nutrition to a physiologically stable newborn who cannot orally ingest sufficient breast milk or formula to satisfy normal nutritive requirements

ASSESSMENT AND PLANNING

- Check the newborn's medical record for frequency of feeding (continuous or intermittent), amount to give, and type (breast milk, formula, or specialized feeding).
- Assess the newborn's ability to suck and swallow.
- Inspect the nares and mouth for deformities that may contraindicate insertion of a tube into the mouth or nares.
- Assess parental knowledge of and previous exposure to this feeding method.
- Ensure that feeding is at room temperature. If necessary, remove feeding from refrigerator approximately 30 minutes before use; warm in a warm-water bath if indicated.
- Gather the necessary equipment:
  - 20- to 50-mL syringe or feeding solution container
  - Syringes for checking tube placement and flushing as appropriate (5 to 10 mL)
  - Appropriate-sized feeding tube depending on the size of the newborn (usually 5 or 8 French tube)
  - Feeding
  - Hypoallergenic tape
  - Stethoscope
  - pH paper
  - Water or water-soluble lubricant
  - Small rolled towel or blanket for positioning if appropriate
  - Clamp or cap for feeding tube (if tube is to remain in place)
  - Infusion pump (if a continuous feeding)

IMPLEMENTATION

1. Explain the procedure to the parents and answer any questions *to help allay their anxiety.*
2. Wash hands.
3. Position the newborn with the head slightly elevated. Measure the length of the catheter to be inserted from the tip of the nose to the earlobe and then to the midpoint of the area between the xiphoid process and umbilicus *to ensure that the tube reaches the stomach.* Mark the point with tape or indelible pen *to provide a reference point for insertion.*
4. Lubricate the feeding tube generously with sterile water *to ease passage of the tube and minimize the risk for trauma to the newborn's mucosa.*
5. Ensure that the newborn is positioned so that his or her head is slightly hyperflexed or in the "sniff" position. If necessary, use a rolled towel under the neck to help maintain this position. Insert the tube into one of the nares or through the mouth, directing the tube toward the back *to facilitate passage along the natural curvature of the area;* continue to pass the tube to the identified mark *to promote passage into the stomach.*
6. Check the position of the tube using two methods *to ensure proper placement in the stomach:*
   a. Attach a small syringe to the feeding tube and aspirate stomach contents, noting the amount, colour, and consistency and return the fluid to the stomach *to prevent possible fluid and electrolyte imbalances.* If there is any question as to whether the fluid is stomach or respiratory fluid, test the fluid with pH paper. *Stomach fluid is acidic and has a pH of 1 to 3.*
   b. Attach a syringe filled with a small amount of air (up to 5 mL); instill air into the tube while auscultating the abdomen at the same time for gurgling or growling sounds *to identify accurate placement.*

(continued)

NURSING PROCEDURE 22.1 (CONTINUED)
Administering a Gavage Feeding

7. Tape the tube in place *to secure it.* Measure and record the length of the tubing from where it exits the nose or mouth to the end of the tubing *for use as a reference to aid with future determinations of placement.*

8. Attach the syringe (with the barrel removed) or feeding solution container to the tube. Pour the specified amount of feeding into the syringe or container and allow the feeding to flow slowly into the tube by gravity. Adjust the height of the syringe or container to allow for a gentle slow flow of the feeding *to prevent too fast a flow, which could lead to regurgitation and aspiration.* Feeding time should range from 15 to 30 minutes.

9. If feeding does not flow from the syringe, reinsert the plunger and apply gentle pressure to initiate the flow and then allow the feeding to flow by gravity. Do not continue to push the entire feeding through the tube *to prevent excess pressure that could traumatize the mucosa and overdistend the stomach.*

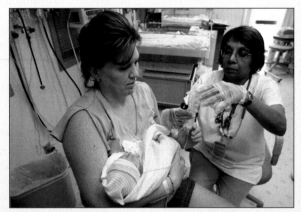

Step 8. Attaching the tube and feeding.

10. If the tube is to be removed after the feeding, when the syringe or container empties, remove the tape while pinching the feeding tube to close it off and quickly, yet gently, remove the tube *to reduce the risk for irritation to the gastrointestinal tract and potential leakage of feeding into the trachea with withdrawal.*

11. If the tube is to remain in place, as the syringe or container empties, flush the feeding tube with sterile water (approximately 1 to 5 mL) *to maintain tube patency* and then clamp or cap the tube *to prevent additional air from entering the stomach.*

12. Burp the newborn after the feeding if appropriate *to aid in air removal* or position the newborn on his or her right side with the head of the bed elevated approximately 30 degrees for 1 hour *to facilitate stomach emptying and reduce the risk for regurgitation and aspiration.*

13. Dispose of equipment and supplies as appropriate. Wash hands.

14. Record the time, amount of feeding, type of feeding, and how the newborn tolerated the feeding.

EVALUATION

- Feeding tube is inserted without injury to the newborn.
- Feeding tube is positioned in the stomach.
- The newborn received the feeding in the correct amount over 15 to 20 minutes without difficulty.
- The newborn tolerated the procedure well, without any episodes of regurgitation, vomiting, or signs and symptoms of aspiration.

AREAS FOR CONSIDERATION AND ADAPTATION

Lifespan Considerations

- Orogastric feedings are preferred for small infants because they are obligate nose breathers and insertion through the mouth is less disruptive and stressful. It also stimulates the sucking reflex. If continuous feedings are ordered, typically nasogastric feedings are used.
- If necessary, use a small rolled towel draped across the newborn's chest and secured under the shoulder *to help prevent inadvertent arm movement by the newborn.*

(continued)

NURSING PROCEDURE 22.1 (CONTINUED)
Administering a Gavage Feeding

- If appropriate, enlist the aid of an additional person, such as support person, parent, or other health care team member, *to help contain the newborn and prevent movement that could result in injury.*
- Encourage the parents to hold and swaddle their newborn during the feeding, just as if the newborn was being fed by the breast or bottle *to help promote a positive experience for the newborn.*
- Provide the newborn with non-nutritive sucking *to help satisfy the newborn's need to suck.*
- Always check gastric residuals before each intermittent feeding and reinstill the amount aspirated. Typically, the amount of residual aspirated is deducted from the prescribed amount of the planned feeding *to prevent overdistention.* Follow the agency's policy regarding residual amounts requiring notification of the health care provider.
- When administering continuous feedings, use an infusion pump *to regulate flow* and check residuals at specified intervals, such as every 4 hours *to evaluate the newborn's tolerance of the feeding.*
- Always check the placement of the tube before each intermittent feeding and at specified intervals during continuous feedings when the tubing remains in place.

Community-Based Considerations

- Keep in mind that infants are occasionally discharged home with gavage or gastrostomy feedings. Teach the parents or caregivers how to perform the feeding and have them return-demonstrate the procedure before discharge. For infants with a gastrostomy tube, parents should perform a return-demonstration of gastrostomy tube insertion. Clean tap water, instead of sterile water, may be used to lubricate the gavage tube for insertion and both gavage and gastrostomy tube flushing.
- Reinforce the need for non-nutritive sucking opportunities and for cuddling and swaddling.
- Arrange for a home care follow-up to assist with the transition to the home. Enlist the aid of social services to help arrange the necessary supplies and equipment.
- Provide the family and caregivers with telephone numbers for use should a problem or difficulty arise.

of cardiovascular compromise (eg, respiratory distress, central cyanosis, tachypnea). Gestational or neurologic immaturity and birth conditions often necessitate gavage feedings, which require the insertion of a small-bore, soft, pliable feeding tube through either the nose or the mouth and advanced into the stomach. Gavage feedings through a nasogastric or orogastric tube may be intermittent bolus or continuous. The pediatrician or neonatologist prescribes the type and volume of the formula and the frequency. When feedings are continuous, the orogastric or nasogastric tube is secured with hypoallergenic tape and changed according to unit policy. When feedings are intermittent, the tube can be left in place for bolus feedings or removed after each feeding and reinserted for the next. The preterm infant who requires intermittent bolus feedings has a poor gag reflex, and the soft tiny tube that is inserted intermittently causes less trauma than does the indwelling tube, which also can cause pressure and mucosal ischemia, especially with the nasogastric approach. Gastric residuals are aspirated and measured every 3 to 4 hours, as specified, when the feeding is continuous; the stomach contents are replaced unless there is a trend of increasing residuals, or half the total hourly feed is aspirated. Gastric residuals are measured before each intermittent bolus feed, and gastric contents are replaced and the volume of gastric residual is deducted from the prescribed bolus feed.

Trophic Feedings

Trophic feedings, also called early or minimal enteral feedings, are given to stimulate the gut and to prime the GI tract. Trophic feedings also prevent deterioration of the intestinal villi. They are not sufficient for meeting nutritional needs. Rather, they provide small-volume feedings (preferably breast milk) to nourish the gut, promote intestinal maturation, and stimulate motility (Blackburn, 2013).

Non-nutritive Sucking

During the 8 to 10 weeks of alternative feedings that some preterm newborns require, many factors can contribute to feeding aversion and difficulties. Examples include unpleasant feelings associated with intubation or suction, IV feedings without oral stimulation, and decreased physical contact during feedings. For successful oral feedings, the newborn must create suction and then compress the nipple against the hard palate with anterior–posterior tongue movements. Each of these motions requires neurologic maturity and practice, because feeding is a learned behaviour for preterm newborns. Thus, newborns with complications related to size or gestational age still need to suck, although this reflex may not be well-developed.

Preterm infants can be observed sucking on feeding tubes that have been inserted orally rather than nasogastrically. This spontaneous behaviour satisfies the need to suck and serves to increase readiness for oral feeding. An additional benefit of tube feeding is conservation of energy. However, when parents feed a preterm infant orally and see that the suck reflex is effective, it is difficult for them to understand the need for supplemental enteral feeding by tube. The nurse explains energy conservation and its relationship to weight gain. The work of sucking requires energy, and energy expenditure requires calories to support the physical effort of ingestion. The nurse explains to the parents that a preterm or LBW infant has poorly developed suck pads, a small stomach capacity, and low capacity for activity. The baby is easily stressed by the need for frequent feedings beyond the capability to adapt. Allowing the infant to suck until sufficient calories are consumed to support growth and metabolism may overtax the preterm infant and result in overstressing him or her. Weight gain is less than expected when calculating total caloric intake, because calories used for energy do not contribute to weight gain. Newborns who are too immature or sick to tolerate enteral feeding are fed parenterally but still require a pacifier for nonnutritive sucking, which satisfies a physiologic need as well as being a source of comfort (Fig. 22.3). The nurse can offer a commercial premie nipple, leaving the sterile covering over the rim that houses it. This measure prevents the newborn from sucking air and distending the abdomen. If the soft premie nipples available do not have a peel-away sterile covering on the back, the nurse can stuff the nipple with sterile gauze and occlude the nipple back with water-resistant or paper tape. The nurse offers the pacifier in conjunction with enteral feedings, so that the infant associates the feeling of a full stomach (satiety) with sucking.

Parenteral Nutrition

VLBW newborns are very physiologically immature and cannot ingest and digest breast milk or formula by the enteral route. In such cases, the parenteral route is used to provide nutrition until the infant is stable enough. In

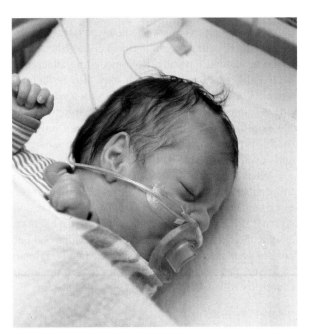

FIGURE 22.3 Non-nutritive sucking in a preterm baby.

the past, VLBW infants were not given parenteral amino acids early enough, or in sufficient amounts, to support their protein needs related to a fear of protein intolerance and development of toxicity. Evidence-based nursing, however, demonstrates no complications in the VLBW newborn receiving amino acids parenterally up to 3.5 g/kg/day (Ziegler, 2011).

Maintenance of Glucose Levels

Promotion of early and frequent oral feedings is a primary nursing intervention to maintain glucose levels. If rooming-in is not an option, nursing infants are taken to breast every 2 hours or on demand. When the newborn cannot ingest breast milk orally, the nurse encourages the mother to pump milk for gavage feedings. Infants who cannot tolerate enteral feedings may require parenteral nutrition, such as those for whom enteral feeding is contraindicated (eg, NEC).

 Baby Mitchell was placed on a ventilator. Which method(s) for providing nutrition would be most appropriate for him?

Attachment Promotion

Nurses can be instrumental in promoting family attachment when parents are separated from newborns in the NICU, the mother cannot breastfeed the baby, or both. Initially, they can give cues to promote identification.

Nurses may wish to remark about any physical likeness of the child to parents or siblings and discuss the significance of naming the baby. Role-modelling attachment behaviours while parents watch may also be helpful. Once the infant is medically stable, skin-to-skin holding, also known as kangaroo care, can be initiated. During skin-to-skin holding, the infant, clothed only in a diaper, is placed against the mother's or partner's chest and covered with a blanket.

When fetal illness or complication causes serious or irreversible disabilities, the nurse allows family members to express anger, guilt, shame, remorse, or fear. Demonstrations of respect, caring, and empathy assist clients to assume their parental roles and to find meaning and purpose in whatever the future holds for the family. Primary caregivers discuss and thoroughly understand the implications for follow-up care and ongoing monitoring.

 Think back to Madeline, the baby at the beginning of the chapter born with congenital cleft lip and palate. Madeline's mother, Danita, was visibly upset when she saw her baby. How could the nurse assist the family in promoting attachment?

Transcultural Awareness and Sensitivity

When newborn complications require intensive medical and nursing interventions, the family unit responds to the crisis based on a combination of their own experiences, their educational levels, and cultural and religious beliefs. They can derive much comfort and stability from sensitive, caring nurses who demonstrate acceptance of and respect for practices families believe to be healing. Differences in what is acceptable with regards to communication, personal space, voice tone, eye contact, and touch vary across cultural boundaries and even within cultures. Often, failure to agree to a prescribed treatment plan for a newborn experiencing a complication is related to parental cultural orientation. Culturally sensitive nurses are responsible for exploring beliefs, expectations, and desired practices.

The nursing care plan incorporates and accommodates provisions for any belief system, unless doing so may result in harm to the newborn. In this case, nurses provide explanations and determine what modifications to a particular desired practice would be acceptable to the family caregivers. For example, if it is important to the parents to tie a red string around the newborn's limb or rub the baby with oil, the nurse finds ways to accommodate such requests without jeopardizing an IV site or electrodes or temperature sensors adhered to the skin

of a newborn who requires monitoring (Thibodeaux & Mooney-Doyle, 2011).

Communication with the family is essential to learning what practices they deem important and what substitutions or adaptations they will accept. Reasonable cultural and religious provisions can be made without compromising treatment when the health care team demonstrates a willingness to accommodate special needs. For example, some First Nations groups practice "smudging" to purify the body, which involves the burning of sweet grass by an elder, a medicine man or a *shaman.* The nurse helps the family find a place within the facility to perform smudging without compromising safety. He or she promotes and respects privacy unless the newborn's condition is too unstable for him or her to be away from an oxygen source or monitoring equipment during the 30-minute healing ceremony. Some practices that are common to nursing may be inappropriate within certain beliefs. For example, prior to taking pictures of the baby or providing mementos such as a lock of hair, the nurse ensures that these well-meaning gestures do not violate the family's religious or cultural beliefs.

Discharge Planning

In preparation for discharge, nurses establish follow-up contact information with the parents, who are likely to feel anxious and overwhelmed by the total responsibility of care that they are assuming. Close relationships are common when health care providers work with preterm or ill newborns and their families for extended periods of time during long hospitalizations. Families become attached to nurses and vice versa, which requires intervention to bridge the gap between critical care and parent care.

Discharge planning for the family of the newborn with ongoing complications related to size, gestation, or both must include teaching about the use of any specialized equipment, formulas for feeding, or medications that the infant requires after discharge. Where possible, parents are instructed in newborn resuscitation, in addition to the obstructed airway manoeuvre for infants. Parents may feel safe when caring for infants under nursing supervision, but be frightened by the prospect of independent care at home. Some units provide the opportunity for parents to room-in or stay overnight with the baby in a designated hospital room prior to discharge. This provides an opportunity for parents to increase their level of confidence and comfort in their ability to care for the baby following discharge. For premature infants discharged home during the winter months, arrangements are made for respiratory syncytial virus (RSV) prophylaxis, which is normally offered to infants born at less than 32 weeks' gestation and must be administered on a monthly basis for the duration of the RSV season (usually November until April).

Follow-up visits focus on assessment of newborn weight gain and attainment of normal developmental milestones. The nurse plots weight and length in two distinct colours: one to represent the percentile for actual chronologic age from birth date, and the other to reflect the percentile based on adjusted age using the expected term gestation age.

Long-term collaborative care requires referrals for hearing and vision screenings. The organ of Corti is sensitive to oxygen deficits; thus, deafness may result from any early hypoxemia that requires resuscitation. Premature infants born at less than 32 weeks, especially those requiring supplemental oxygen, are prone to retinal bleeding and scarring, a process known as retinopathy of prematurity (ROP). Follow-up by a pediatric ophthalmologist is important to identify infants at risk for retinal scarring requiring treatment and because preterm newborns are more prone to strabismus and nearsightedness.

Evaluation

When a newborn has a complication related to size, gestational age, or both, the nurse evaluates the effectiveness of care to promote nutrition. The underweight postterm newborn should demonstrate weight gain and increased urinary output as indicators of dietary well-being and hydration. Desired blood glucose levels are 2.6 to 4.0 mmol/L.

Other indications of effective care include thermal stability and satisfactory extrauterine adaptation as evidenced by stable vital signs within normal ranges. Behaviourally, the newborn should demonstrate appropriate sleep–wake cycles and intact protective neurologic reflexes. Freedom from complications (eg, respiratory distress syndrome, sepsis) reflects successful supportive and restorative management.

HYPERBILIRUBINEMIA

Hyperbilirubinemia refers to elevated serum bilirubin levels. The normal polycythemic state of the newborn accounts for nearly 80% of serum bilirubin, which results from the breakdown of damaged, dead, or dying red blood cells and subsequent hemoglobin metabolism. Metabolism of 1 g of hemoglobin can release as much as 35 mg of unconjugated bilirubin into the bloodstream. The unconjugated (indirect) bilirubin is transported to the liver, where it is chemically changed to conjugated (direct) bilirubin. The conjugated bilirubin then combines with bile and is deposited into the GI tract for excretion in the stool. Intestinal flora act on a smaller portion of conjugated bilirubin molecules, converting them to urobilinogen for urinary excretion. The chemical conversion of indirect to direct bilirubin, however,

requires ample available glucose and serum albumin as well as adequate oxygenation (Blackburn, 2013).

The typical manifestation of hyperbilirubinemia is yellow discolouration of the skin and tissues called *jaundice*. Many newborns experience mild, self-limiting *physiologic jaundice* (see Chapter 20) after the third day of life in formula-fed babies, and later in breastfed babies. After the normal peak in breastfed newborns, the level slowly declines to normal (see Chapter 21). Some neonates are at risk for severe hyperbilirubinemia (total serum bilirubin [TSB] >340 µmol/L) leading to *acute bilirubin encephalopathy*, a clinical syndrome characterized by lethargy, hypotonia, and poor suck that may proceed to hypertonia, high-pitched cry, and fever (Sgro et al., 2011).

Excessive indirect serum bilirubin may lead to neurotoxicity because bilirubin readily crosses the blood–brain barrier. Bilirubin deposited in the newborn's brain produces a condition called **kernicterus**, which can lead to serious neurologic sequelae, including permanent damage to the central nervous system, motor abnormalities, deafness, developmental delay, and seizures (van Imhoff et al., 2012; Shapiro, 2010). Kernicterus also occasionally results in death (Kaplan et al., 2011).

Increasingly shorter postpartum hospital stays make identifying and monitoring newborns at risk for hyperbilirubinemia difficult. Jaundice and hyperbilirubinemia are responsible for most newborn readmissions to the hospital after early discharge (Buescher & Bland, 2011). The increased incidence of hyperbilirubinemia and an upward trend in cases of the less-common kernicterus prompted the CPS to issue guidelines for the detection, prevention, and management of hyperbilirubinemia in term and late-preterm infants (Barrington & Sankaran, 2007). According to the CPS, predicting which infants may develop severe hyperbilirubinemia is based on an assessment of risk factors (Assessment Tool 22.2) and also on the information collected from TSB measurements. The CPS recommends that all infants have either a TSB or a transcutaneous bilirubin measurement at the same time as the metabolic screening test; alternatively at discharge or prior to 72 hours of life. If the infant is visibly jaundiced in the first 24 hours of life, a bilirubin level test is indicated. The results of the bilirubin screening test are plotted on an hour-specific nomogram (Fig. 22.4) and follow-up determined by the infant's level of risk (Barrington & Sankaran, 2007).

COLLABORATIVE CARE: THE NEWBORN WITH HYPERBILIRUBINEMIA

Newborns require astute observation for jaundice and careful review of possible risk factors for hyperbilirubinemia. The nurse collaborates with other team

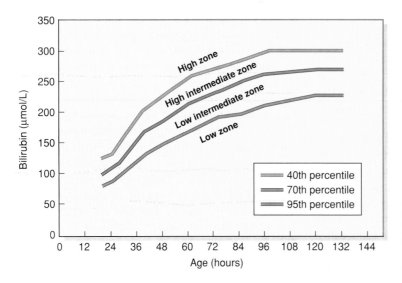

FIGURE 22.4 Hour-specific nomogram for assessing serum bilirubin (Canadian Paediatric Society, 2004/2011). Reproduced with permission from *Pediatrics, 114*(1), Pages 297–316, Copyright © 2004 by the AAP.

members to identify infants who may require follow-up after early discharge and to educate parents about jaundice and the normal time frame for its resolution. As client advocates, nurses initiate collaborative therapeutic interventions as soon as they detect jaundice.

Assessment

Some newborns are at an increased risk for hyperbilirubinemia because of prematurity, family history, ethnic background, birth trauma, and illness. Assessment Tool 22.2 provides a checklist for assessing a newborn's risk.

The nurse correlates any onset of jaundice with the baby's age (in hours and gestational age) and feeding method (breast versus bottle) to help differentiate between physiologic and pathologic jaundice. When

assessing for signs of hyperbilirubinemia, the nurse notes the location of jaundice. The nurse reports any visible jaundice and inspects the urine for a dark tea-coloured appearance, which is indicative of urobilinogen. In addition, the nurse assesses the newborn's feeding behaviour and alertness. He or she reports any feeding problems and lethargy immediately.

Select Potential Nursing Diagnoses

Many nursing diagnoses may be applicable to the newborn with hyperbilirubinemia. Common examples include the following:

- **Risk for Injury** related to increased serum bilirubin levels

---

● **ASSESSMENT TOOL 22.2** **Checklist for Evaluating Hyperbilirubinemia Risks**

- Is the baby of Asian, African, or Mediterranean descent? _____
- Did any of the baby's siblings have newborn jaundice? _____
- Was the baby born before the expected due date? _____
- Is the baby being exclusively or partially breastfed? _____
- Did the baby experience birth trauma or bruising? _____
- Did the baby fail to pass meconium within the first 24 hours? _____
- Are fewer than six diapers saturated with urine per day? _____
- Does the baby have visible jaundice? _____
- Is the baby a boy? _____
- Is the mother older than 25 years of age? _____
- Are medications given or passed through breast milk that impair bilirubin excretion
  (eg, Aspirin, acetaminophen, sulfa, alcohol, rifampin, erythromycin, corticosteroids, tetracycline)? _____
- Is there ABO or Rh mother–infant incompatibility? _____
- Does the newborn show signs of infection or sepsis? _____

A yes answer to any of these questions increases the risk for hyperbilirubinemia.

- **Risk for Impaired Skin Integrity** related to effects associated with phototherapy
- **Risk for Deficient Fluid Volume** related to increased insensible fluid losses related to phototherapy
- **Lack of Knowledge** (parental) related to use of phototherapy and necessary newborn care
- **Anxiety** (parental) related to newborn requiring treatment for hyperbilirubinemia

Planning/Intervention

Goals are individualized based on the severity of hyperbilirubinemia and proposed treatment. When planning care, prevention of common potential complications and monitoring the effectiveness of treatment are essential.

Bilirubin Level Monitoring

The newborn's bilirubin levels require close monitoring. Discharge from the facility will be delayed if an infant shows signs of significant hyperbilirubinemia. These include late passage of meconium stool, light tan–coloured stools after ingestion of milk, dark urine, poor feeding, and lethargy.

All breastfeeding mothers are assessed and provided support by knowledgeable individuals. The newborn's weight loss is monitored and any infant losing in excess of 10% of its birth weight is further evaluated for adequacy of feeding intake and signs of dehydration (Tasker et al., 2013). Supplements of water, glucose water, or both are avoided, because they reduce caloric intake and may lead to iatrogenic hyponatremia.

Monitoring of Intake and Output

The nurse monitors and records the frequency and amount of each feeding. Often, the nursing mother voices anxiety about being unable to determine the actual quantity of breast milk the baby takes and the correlation between breastfeeding and jaundice, which can persist for weeks to months. The nurse monitors the effectiveness of breastfeeding technique and reassures the mother that wet diapers are excellent indicators of a newborn's hydration status. Six to 10 wet diapers per 24 hours is acceptable. As the baby is excreting bilirubin (urobilinogen), the urine will be dark-tea coloured initially and gradually lighten. The nurse monitors and records intake and output. He or she may use a gram scale to weigh wet diapers (1 g = 1 mL).

Phototherapy

Phototherapy involves exposing as much of the newborn's skin surface as possible to blue wavelengths of light to assist with the excretion of excess bilirubin. To prevent neurotoxicity, phototherapy is instituted when the TSB level reaches the treatment threshold appropriate for the newborn's gestational age and age in hours (Wilson, 2011) (Fig. 22.5). An effective arrangement consists of four special blue bulbs with two daylight fluorescent tubes on either side (Fig. 22.6). To maximize conversion of bilirubin to the water-soluble form for excretion, the newborn may be placed on a fibreoptic pad as an additional modality for applying a light source. The fibreoptic pad may be less disturbing, because it allows interaction with the infant (Dent & McKenna, 2010).

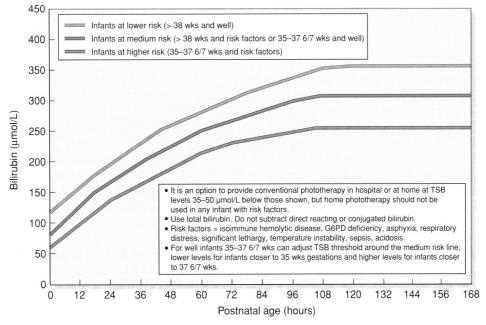

FIGURE 22.5 Phototherapy guidelines (Canadian Paediatric Society, 2004/ 2011). (Reproduced with permission from *Pediatrics,* Volume 114, Pages 297–316, Copyright © 2004 by the AAP.)

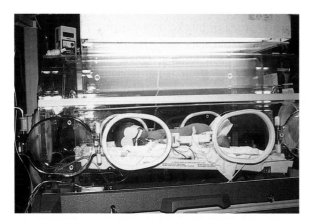

FIGURE 22.6 Newborn receiving phototherapy.

The eyes of newborns receiving phototherapy are protected from the light source. After carefully closing each of the baby's eyes, the nurse applies small patches to each eye and secures them with a Velcro band around the oval circumference of the newborn's head (above the ears). The band should be snug and stay in place at all times while the newborn is under the lights. The nurse removes the eye pads when the infant is away from the UV light source for physical care, during breastfeeding, or when the nonbreastfeeding newborn visits with parents. The nurse changes the eye pads each time he or she removes them, and discards the Velcro straps when phototherapy is discontinued.

Phototherapy can contribute to overheating and dehydration because it increases insensible fluid losses. Thus, the nurse closely monitors newborn temperature and hydration. Some newborns develop a minor transient rash that requires no intervention (Wilson, 2011). Diarrhea may necessitate oral administration of supplemental fluids. See Nursing Procedure 22.2.

Exchange Transfusion

Should jaundice fail to respond to intensive phototherapy, the team caring for the newborn may consider exchange transfusion. This may have religious or cultural implications for the family; for example, if the infant's family members are Jehovah's Witnesses, they may refuse blood and blood products. The nurse assumes a nonjudgmental and supportive role, while keeping lines of communication open and continuing other therapeutic treatment modalities acceptable to these families.

When a newborn is to undergo exchange transfusion, the nurse first positively identifies the baby and obtains verification by a second licensed health care provider who also verifies the blood product, blood type (donor and recipient), cross-match number, and expiration date. The nurse ensures patency of the venous access, which is usually a catheter inserted into the umbilical vein. The total amount of blood to be transfused as well as the volume (usually 2 to 10 mL) to withdraw and discard before the infusion of each replacement volume (2 to 10 mL) of compatible donor blood is identified. Depending on how often the blood is alternately withdrawn and replaced to administer the prescribed total volume, the entire transfusion process may take 1 to 4 hours. Fresh blood from a compatible donor is required for infant transfusion because of the risk for electrolyte imbalance (calcium in particular) from the preservative (citrates) used in stored blood. The blood for each exchange is administered at room temperature; the nurse can employ a commercial blood warmer when the remaining volume remains cold. Any blood outside of refrigeration for more than 4 hours must be discarded. The nurse monitors the baby's vital signs closely and rechecks indirect bilirubin levels after the infusion and for several subsequent days to ensure that they do not rise again.

Parental Education

Because of the increasing trend toward early discharge, nurses frequently instruct parents and caregivers in strategies to monitor the progress of their newborns with complications. The nurse teaches parents to carefully inspect for jaundice that develops, increases, or persists after discharge. If previously pale urine becomes dark or scant, the parents are taught to notify a health care provider immediately. The caregivers also monitor feeding behaviour. Other indicators that parents should report promptly are lethargy, as evidenced by a sluggish newborn who fails to nurse vigorously, and excessive sleep.

Breastfeeding mothers are urged to consume enough fluids to support milk volume and enable frequent nursing; nonbreastfeeding mothers may offer water between feedings. Parents should check stools for excreted bile pigments as bilirubin levels decrease. Stools will be greenish initially, becoming normal yellow-gold (depending on the type of liquid consumed) as bilirubin levels become normal.

Evaluation

The following outcome and discharge criteria ensure that treatment of hyperbilirubinemia has been effective:

- The newborn ingests sufficient formula or breast milk to saturate five or more diapers per day.
- The newborn demonstrates intact skin with diminishing visible bilirubin pigment on the surface and in the excreta.
- Newborn behaviour is appropriate to gestational age, with vigourous suck reflex and no irritability or lethargy.
- Parents and caregivers express confidence in their ability to monitor the newborn's health status relative to jaundice and state the intent to notify a health care provider promptly in the event of complications.

NURSING PROCEDURE 22.2

Administering Phototherapy

PURPOSE

To reduce serum bilirubin levels

ASSESSMENT AND PLANNING

- Assess parental knowledge of and previous exposure to the procedure.
- Inspect the newborn for signs and symptoms of jaundice.
- Evaluate test results of serum bilirubin levels.
- Assess overall newborn status, including vital signs, intake and output, and other parameters *to establish a baseline for future comparison.*
- Gather equipment
- Light source (bilirubin lights or fibreoptic blanket or panel with protective covering)
- Eye shields
- Check the light source for proper functioning.
- Review manufacturer's and agency's policy for light intensity and distance of lights from newborn.

IMPLEMENTATION

1. Explain the procedure to the parents; answer any questions they may have *to help alleviate fear and anxiety;* review the need for eye shields while the baby is under overhead bilirubin lights *to protect the eyes;* reinforce the need to interact with the newborn; encourage parents to hold and cuddle baby when out of the lights and especially while feeding *to promote attachment.*
2. Set up bili lights over the newborn's crib or isolette at the proper distance from the baby, according to agency policy *to ensure adequate exposure while minimizing risk for thermal injury.* If using a blanket or wrap, turn on the device.
3. Check the intensity of the lights with a photometer *to prevent injury to the newborn,* as per facility policy.
4. Apply eye shields to the newborn's eyes, checking that the eyelids are closed before application *to prevent corneal injury.* Ensure a snug fit that occludes the eyes but not the nares. (Eye shields may or may not be needed if a blanket or wrap device is used. Check the manufacturer's instruction.) Place the newborn unclothed except for a small diaper under the lights *to maximize skin exposed to the lights while protecting the external genitalia.* If using a blanket or wrap, wrap the newborn in it.
5. Turn the newborn frequently while under the lights, approximately every 2 hours *to ensure exposure of all body parts, thereby promoting breakdown of bilirubin, preventing pressure areas, and providing stimulation.*
6. Monitor vital signs at least every 4 hours *to allow for early detection of complications.*
7. Assess intake and output; weigh diapers *to ensure accurate determination of output;* assess skin turgor and mucous membranes *to evaluate for possible dehydration secondary to increased insensible fluid losses.* Provide additional fluids as ordered *to prevent dehydration.*
8. Assess stool characteristics; change diapers frequently, and inspect perianal area closely for irritation or excoriation *because stools are often loose and may be irritating to the skin.*
9. Provide meticulous skin care *to prevent irritation and breakdown;* avoid the use of oily lubricants or skin lotions *to reduce the risk for intensifying the heat of the lamps leading to thermal injury.*
10. Assess serum bilirubin levels as ordered *to evaluate effectiveness of therapy.*
11. Replace eye shields frequently to prevent the risk for infection. Ensure that they are secured in the proper position *to prevent damage to the eyes and surrounding skin.*

(continued)

NURSING PROCEDURE 22.2 (CONTINUED)
Administering Phototherapy

12. Periodically, according to agency policy and manufacturer's instructions, monitor light intensity with a photometer *to reduce the risk for injury and ensure appropriate exposure.*

13. Encourage parents to soothe and touch the newborn while under the lights; role-model soothing behaviours *to promote parental participation.* If using a blanket or wrap, encourage the parents to hold the newborn frequently *to promote bonding.*

14. Remove the newborn from the lights for feeding and periodically, but at least once every 8 hours, *to promote bonding and attachment;* remove eye shields while out of the bilirubin lights *to provide visual and sensory stimulation and allow for eye-to-eye contact between newborn and parents or caregivers.*

15. Arrange care activities *to promote comfort, reduce energy expenditure, and maximize time spent under the lights.*

16. Wash hands and document time therapy was started; type of therapy, including number of lights and type; light intensity; vital signs; use of eye shields; serum bilirubin levels; and newborn's status and response to therapy.

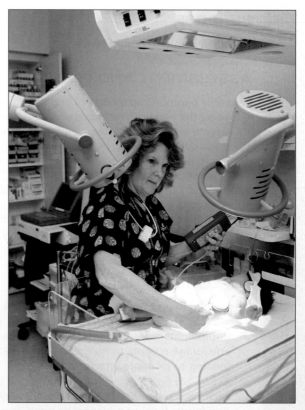

Step 12. Adjusting the lights.

EVALUATION

- Newborn tolerated therapy and remained free of complications and pain.
- Newborn's serum bilirubin levels demonstrated a gradual decrease to acceptable levels.
- Newborn and parents demonstrated positive attachment and bonding behaviours.

AREAS FOR ADAPTATION AND CONSIDERATION

Lifespan Considerations

- Bili lights may be used in conjunction with a blanket or wrap device to enhance the effect when serum bilirubin levels continue to increase or are approaching critical levels.
- Document the newborn's ongoing status, including time spent out of the lights and parents' interaction with the newborn.

Community-Based Considerations

- Phototherapy may be provided in the home with conventional bili lights or a blanket or wrap device. Often, a blanket or wrap device is chosen because of its ease of use.
- Ensure that parents understand how to administer phototherapy in the home; arrange for parents to provide a return demonstration of the procedure and care required.

(continued)

Administering Phototherapy

- Arrange for home health care follow-up to assist with initiating therapy, provide ongoing education and assessment, obtain serial serum bilirubin levels, and offer support and guidance to the parents.
- Remind parents to ensure that they use a protective covering at all times with a blanket or wrap device to reduce the risk for injury to the newborn's fragile skin.
- Demonstrate to the parents how to record the necessary information about their newborn when receiving phototherapy, such as temperature, number of stools, and number of wet diapers. If appropriate, provide the parents with forms to use to record the data.

FETAL ALCOHOL SPECTRUM DISORDER

Fetal alcohol spectrum disorder results from maternal use of alcohol during pregnancy. Fetal alcohol spectrum disorder is a term used to represent the continuum of effects seen with alcohol exposure in utero and includes several alcohol-related syndromes and disorders, including Fetal Alcohol Syndrome and alcohol-related neurodevelopmental disorder (Public Health Agency of Canada, 2012). Although the development of fetal alcohol spectrum disorder is strongly linked to levels of alcohol ingestion, no safe levels of alcohol consumption in pregnancy have been established.

The characteristic craniofacial deformities of fetal alcohol spectrum disorder that may be apparent at birth include a flat, thin upper lip; small eyes with short slits for openings (short palpebral fissures); and a flattened midface and profile with a short nose and low nasal bridge (Riley et al., 2011) (Fig. 22.7). These features result from fetal exposure to the metabolites of alcohol early in pregnancy.

Children with fetal alcohol spectrum disorder may face difficulties, including speech problems, inappropriate social interactions, developmental delays, and aggressive behaviour. Later in childhood, cognitive deficits and learning disabilities may contribute to poor school performance. The child with fetal alcohol spectrum disorder requires patience, nurturing, and special education; however, if parental substance use is ongoing, the chances that the child will receive appropriate care are not high.

Nurses direct their care toward the newborn's immediate physical and psychosocial needs. If the mother continues to ingest alcohol to the point of intoxication, newborn care will be compromised, and the parent requires referral to community resources for alcohol addiction. In this event, social services is contacted to evaluate safety issues (nurturing, feeding, risk for neglect) and possible placement of the child with foster care. Initially, the nurse assesses parent–infant attachment. Because of alcohol's effects and the characteristic appearance of the baby with fetal alcohol spectrum disorder, parents may view the newborn negatively, rather than accepting him or her as a person to be nurtured and protected. Guilt may negatively influence the parent–child relationship, especially if the mother realizes the lifelong implications of impaired cognitive function. The nurse role-models care by making eye contact with the newborn and demonstrating to the parents the baby's capabilities. He or she shows parents how to cuddle, feed and burp, diaper, and perform cord care for the baby. The nurse discusses parameters for normal growth and development and encourages parents to stimulate the baby with bright-coloured mobiles, talking, and singing. Praise for all demonstrations of nurturing care is essential. Team members encourage follow-up care, because these newborns may have ongoing special needs.

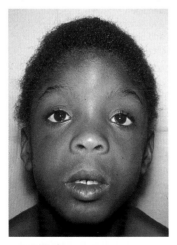

FIGURE 22.7 Facial characteristics of a child with fetal alcohol spectrum disorder include short palpebral features, a wide and flattened groove in the midline of the upper lip, and thin lips.

CONGENITAL ANOMALIES

The embryonic period refers to the time before organogenesis (formation of organs) (see Chapter 11). Three layers of primary cells (ectoderm, endoderm, and mesoderm) are the basis of all body structures and are susceptible to malformations. The ectoderm lines the amniotic cavity; the endoderm lines the yolk sac; the mesoderm arises in between.

Multiple congenital anomalies may arise from the same germ layer. When one congenital anomaly is present, other anomalies within that germ layer are also common. For example, the heart and kidneys both arise from the mesoderm; therefore, a newborn with a congenital heart defect may also have a kidney defect. The trachea and esophagus both form from the endodermic layer; thus, anomalies in both of these organs often occur together.

Genetic factors and teratogenic exposure are associated with congenital anomalies. Defects resulting from inherited traits usually involve only one germ layer. A virulent viral teratogen (eg, measles) can affect all germ layers and cause multiple anomalies. In a study of infants with congenital esophageal atresia, congenital heart disease was noted to be the most commonly associated defect (Stoll et al., 2009). Cardiac defects are also linked with omphaloceles and neural tube defects (Greer, 2010;

Morton et al., 2011). When one major congenital anomaly is present, the nurse is alert to other anomalies.

Nurses play a key role in educating women about factors associated with congenital anomalies. Because the embryonic heart begins beating only 24 days after conception, waiting until pregnancy is confirmed may be too late to begin teaching about the avoidance of teratogens. When pregnancies are planned, the nurse can influence quality of life significantly through early interventions, such as referrals to smoking cessation and alcohol abstinence programs and avoidance of workplace teratogens. If primary prevention is impossible, the nurse can be involved with early detection of congenital anomalies and begin providing information and preparing parents while the fetus is still in utero. See Chapter 11 for more discussion.

Some congenital defects require emergency stabilization, possible transport to a distant facility, or corrective or palliative surgery. For example, anomalies involving the anterior abdominal wall and diaphragm pose serious complications and require immediate therapeutic intervention to avoid further damage and preventable complications. Table 22.3 identifies some common complications associated with congenital anomalies.

Having a newborn with a congenital anomaly is stressful to parents, especially when the problem is unexpected and families are not prepared. In some cases, a

● TABLE 22.3   **Incidence of Congenital Anomalies and Associated Newborn Complications**

Anomaly	Incidence	Associated Complications
Diaphragmatic hernia	Unreported in Canada	Respiratory distress at birth Poor prognosis with extensive pulmonary hypoplasia Chronic lung disease, feeding problems, gastroesophageal reflux diseases (GERDs)
Neural tube defects	4 per 10,000 total births	Trauma, infection secondary to break in the sac Nerve damage Motor and sensory impairment below the defect Bowel and bladder complications Latex allergy
Abdominal wall defect (includes omphalocele, gastroschisis, and other unspecified abdominal wall defects)	Unreported in Canada	Mechanical trauma, infection secondary to leak in the sac Heat loss from exposure of internal organs to ambient temperature
Cleft lip with cleft palate	9.7/10,000 total births	Feeding difficulties, facial deformity
Cleft palate	6.5/10,000 total births	Feeding difficulties, frequent ear infections; impaired speech development, orthodontic problems
Esophageal atresia	Unreported in Canada	Alteration in nutrition/hydration requiring alternative route for food and fluids Aspiration from overflow of esophageal pouch
Tracheoesophageal fistula	Unreported in Canada	Aspiration with sudden coughing, choking, and cyanosis
Developmental dysplasia of the hip	Unreported in Canada	Abnormal development of the affected hip; avascular necrosis of the femoral head if arterial blood flow is disrupted with osteoarthritis later in life

From Health Canada. (2008). Canadian Perinatal Health Report. Retrieved from http://www.phac-aspc.gc.ca/publicat/2008/cphr-rspc/pdf/cphr-rspc08-eng.pdf

● **BOX 22.4** **Risk Factors for Congenital Heart Disease**

- Family history of congenital heart disease
- Maternal diabetes
- Maternal lupus erythematosus
- Living at high altitude
- First-trimester rubella exposure
- Maternal viral infections: cytomegalovirus, herpes, Coxsackie B
- Down syndrome (and other abnormal karyotypes)
- Preterm tocolysis with indomethacin (Indocin)
- Drug exposure: amphetamines, phenytoin, trimethadione, estrogen, progesterone, alcohol

congenital anomaly is diagnosed prenatally, but its full effects are not realized until birth when it is actually visible or necessitates decisions and surgical consents.

Congenital Heart Disease

Congenital heart disease (CHD) refers to a group of cardiac defects that change either the direction of blood flow or the normal structure and function of the heart chambers or great vessels. These anomalies range in severity from a single, common defect (ventricular septal defect [VSD]) to a syndrome of multiple defects. Antepartal diagnosis is possible through transvaginal four-chambered ultrasound.

Etiology

Several factors increase a newborn's risk for congenital heart disease (Box 22.4). Mortality rate depends on the severity of the lesion and newborn birth weight. Preterm and VLBW newborns are at an increased risk for adverse outcomes and higher mortality (Polito et al., 2013).

Classification

Historically, congenital heart disease has been categorized as acyanotic (oxygenated blood is shunted left to right, placing added strain on the heart) or cyanotic (deoxygenated blood is shunted right to left and pumped into the systemic circulation); these terms are still in use. This classification system, however, may lead to an erroneous belief that a newborn having only oxygenated blood pumped forward into systemic circulation cannot become cyanotic, or that the newborn with a "cyanotic" heart defect is cyanotic at all times. Visible cyanosis is related directly to the amount of circulating oxyhemoglobin.

A more explanatory classification groups defects according to abnormalities involving inflow of blood to the lungs or outflow of blood from the heart, and the mixing of oxygen-saturated with desaturated blood in the heart or great vessels (Table 22.4). VSD and atrial septal defect (ASD) and patent ductus arteriosus are examples of defects that increase pulmonary blood flow, and thus can lead to pulmonary congestion and heart failure.

When blood outflow is obstructed from the right side of the heart en route to the lungs for oxygenation, back pressure builds, and desaturated blood is shunted from right to left through the foramen ovale (the fetal structure between the right and left atria to bypass fetal lungs). Cyanosis occurs when blood leaving the heart for the systemic circulation has not been routed through the lungs for oxygenation. Pulmonary stenosis is an example of an outflow defect. Blood outflow also can be obstructed from the left side of the heart with aortic stenosis or coarctation. Again, the obstructed outflow results in back pressure, forcing blood back into the pulmonary veins, resulting in pulmonary edema.

Ventricular Septal Defect. VSD is the most common of all congenital cardiac anomalies. The defect, an abnormal opening between the right and left ventricles, can be small and relatively asymptomatic, with possible spontaneous closure. It may produce significant shunting of blood, resulting in neonatal hypoxemia and congestive heart failure.

Tetralogy of Fallot. Tetralogy of Fallot consists of four defects: (1) VSD high in the ventricular septum, which allows for (2) the overriding aorta to be dextropositioned over the right and left ventricle; (3) stenosis of the pulmonary artery arising from the right ventricle; and (4) hypertrophy of the right heart secondary to the increased cardiac effort required to pump blood to the lungs. Depending on the severity of the defects and pump dysfunction, newborn survival may depend on patency of the ductus arteriosus to support pulmonary blood flow. In this case, prostaglandin E_1 is used to keep the ductus arteriosus open (Kohr, 2012). Provisions for immediate intubation must be readily available if apnea occurs during prostaglandin infusion (Stewart et al., 2012).

Patent Ductus Arteriosus. Patent ductus arteriosus occurs when the fetal structure connecting the aorta and pulmonary trunk remains open after birth. In utero, the ductus arteriosus allows blood oxygenated from the placenta to bypass the airless collapsed fetal lungs. This structure should functionally close within 48 hours after lung expansion with ambient air as a result of hormonal changes, increased arterial oxygen levels, and pressure changes in the lungs. By 3 months of age, complete closure of the ductus arteriosus should be attained, if it is not completely closed shortly after birth (Blackburn, 2013). With patent ductus arteriosus, left-to-right shunting reroutes oxygenated blood to the pulmonary circuit, increasing workload on the heart. Congestive heart failure can develop.

(text continues on page 929)

● TABLE 22.4 Classifications of Congenital Heart Disease

Heart Defect	Cyanotic vs. Acyanotic	Blood Flow	Comments	Figure
Ventricular septal defect (VSD)	Acyanotic	Because pressure is higher in the left side of the heart, oxygenated blood will be shunted from the left to the right ventricle to be recirculated to the lungs. This left-to-right shunting does not impair oxygenation of blood, but cardiac output is decreased, and cardiac workload is increased.	Size of defect dictates hemodynamic presentation. In 30% to 40% of cases, closure is spontaneous within the first 6 months. Surgical repair is required if infant exhibits failure to thrive, pulmonary hypertension, or right-to-left shunt greater than 2 to 1.	Aorta; To left lung; Pulmonary artery; Left ventricle; Ventricular septal defect; Right ventricle; Vena cava; To right lung
Atrial septal defect (ASD)	Acyanotic	Blood flow is inefficiently divided as some blood is directed back to the right atria to return to pulmonary circulation and some is directed forward into the left ventricle to be pumped into systemic circulation. The left-to-right shunting of blood decreases cardiac output and increases preload. Cyanosis is not typical because only oxygenated blood moves forward; however, congestion in the lungs can impair oxygenation and result in cyanosis.	Often symptomatic; 87% of secundum types close by 4 years. Primary and sinus types require surgery. Late sequelae include mitral valve prolapse, atrial fibrillation or flutter, and pulmonary hypertension. Congestive heart failure may develop from the increased work load on the heart.	Aorta; Pulmonary artery; Left atrium; Right atrium; Atrial septal defect; Vena cava
Atrioventricular canal	Acyanotic	This defect allows oxygenated blood from the left atrium to flow backward into the right atrium. The abnormal tricuspid valve does not close properly to prevent backflow in the right atrium when the ventricle contracts. The ventricular septal defect produces left-to-right blood shunting, which mixes with deoxygenated blood in the right atrium.	Combination of the primum type of ASD, VSD, and common atrioventricular valve. Presentation similar to that of VSD. Palliative pulmonary artery banding in refractory congestive heart failure.	Left atrium; Fused mitral and tricuspid valve leaflets; Vena cava; Foramen ovale; Right atrium; Persistent common atrioventricular canal (atrial and ventricular septal defect)

Pulmonary stenosis	Acyanotic	Forward blood flow by way of the pulmonary artery is impeded by narrowing of the lumen of the pulmonic valve or the artery just distal to the valve. Blood distends the right ventricle, leading to hypertrophy from excessive workload.	May be asymptomatic or result in severe congestive heart failure. Prostaglandin E₁ infusion at birth may be helpful. Valvular type may require balloon valvuloplasty.	Aorta — Pulmonary artery; Pulmonary stenosis; Right atrium; Right ventricle
Patent ductus arteriosus	Acyanotic	Aortic blood is shunted back into the pulmonary artery through the fetal structure (ductus arteriosus).	In preterm infants, spontaneous closure or indomethacin-induced closure. In term infants, spontaneous closure is less likely, and indomethacin is not helpful. Recurrent pneumonia may occur. Surgical ligation is usually required. No long-term sequelae if treated adequately.	Aorta; Patent ductus arteriosus; Pulmonary artery
Aortic stenosis	Acyanotic	Narrowing or stricture of the aortic valve restricts forward blood flow from the left ventricle. Blood distends the left ventricle, leading to hypertrophy from excessive workload. Back pressure may result in distention of pulmonary veins and pulmonary edema.	May be asymptomatic. Valve replacement and anticoagulation may be required.	Aorta; Pulmonary artery; Subaortic stenosis; Left ventricle

(table continues on page 928)

● TABLE 22.4   Classifications of Congenital Heart Disease (continued)

Heart Defect	Cyanotic vs. Acyanotic	Blood Flow	Comments	Figure
Coarctation of the aorta	Acyanotic	Because of kinking of the aorta, there is high pressure, turbulent blood flow proximal to the coarctation, and low pressure with decreased blood flow distal to the coarctation.	Up to 98% of cases occur at origin of left subclavian artery. Blood pressure is higher in the arms than in the legs. Bounding pulses in the arms and decreased pulses in the legs.	
Tetralogy of Fallot	Cyanotic	Because of pulmonary stenosis that restricts blood flow from the right heart into the pulmonary artery, and the VSD that is high in the ventricles and allows the aorta to override at the top of the VSD, blood from the right heart and left heart is pumped simultaneously forward via the aorta into the systemic circulation. The defect is classed as cyanotic because blood from the right heart is pumped forward into circulation bypassing oxygenation in the lungs.	Most common CHD beyond infancy. Defects include VSD, right ventricular hypertrophy, right outflow obstruction, and overriding aorta. Intermittent episodes of hyperpnea, irritability, cyanosis with decreased intensity of murmur. Palliative shunting may be necessary. Surgical repair required before age 4 years.	
Transposition of the great arteries	Cyanotic	Deoxygenated blood from the right ventricle is pumped forward through the aorta, which arises from the right ventricle instead of the left. Blood is pumped to the lungs from the left ventricle through the pulmonary artery, which arises from the left rather than the right ventricle. The patent ductus that connects the aorta and pulmonary circulation allows some blood to be oxygenated and return to the left heart via the pulmonary veins to be shunted through the right atria through a defect in the atrial wall. This small amount of oxygenated blood can be moved forward into systemic circulation from the right ventricle and out the connecting aorta.	Transposition of the pulmonary artery and aorta. Ductus dependent. Consider palliative balloon atrial septostomy, but definitive surgical switch of the aorta and pulmonary artery required as soon as possible. Late complications include pulmonary stenosis, mitral regurgitation, aortic stenosis, coronary artery obstruction, ventricular dysfunction, and dysrhythmias.	

Text adapted from Saenz, R. B., Beebe, D. K., & Triplett, C. (1999). Caring for infants with congenital heart disease and their families. *American Family Physician, 59(7)*, 1857–1868.

Classic symptoms of patent ductus arteriosus are bounding pulses, a long systolic and an active precordium (Evans, 2012). Many newborns, however, especially those born preterm, present with only respiratory distress, tachypnea, and tachycardia, which may be confused with signs of sepsis. Echocardiography can confirm a diagnosis of patent ductus arteriosus. The conservative approach for closure is indomethacin, unless drug-related complications are considered too risky. An infant who is unresponsive to indomethacin may require surgical ligation (Kenney et al., 2011).

When the foramen ovale (a fetal structure between the right and left atria) remains open in addition to a patent ductus arteriosus, deoxygenated blood from the right atrium mixes with oxygenated blood in the left atrium.

Transposition of the Great Vessels. Oxygenated and deoxygenated blood mix when there is communication between the right and left heart chambers. The position of the great vessels can be switched, with the aorta (rather than the pulmonary artery) arising from the right side of the heart and the pulmonary artery (rather than the aorta) arising from the left side. The implication of this congenital defect is blood being moved forward into the systemic circulation without first being routed to the lungs for oxygenation. This defect is called transposition of the great vessels and is incompatible with life. Immediate stabilization and surgical intervention are necessary. The ductus arteriosus and foramen ovale must remain open to allow oxygenated blood to be pumped to the systemic circulation to sustain life until surgical correction is accomplished. Prostaglandin E_1 is administered to prevent normal closure of the ductus arteriosus, and the foramen ovale is enlarged by a balloon to create an artificial ASD.

Collaborative Management

A review of the antepartal record for factors that increase the risk for congenital heart disease is essential. The nurse is also especially aware of the newborn's gestational age, respiratory status, and feeding behaviour. In preterm newborns, patent ductus arteriosus is often manifested by respiratory distress (Kenney et al., 2011). Recent research has found no association between antenatal indomethacin and patent ductus arteriosus in the neonate (Klauser et al., 2012).

Many newborns with congenital heart disease appear normal in the first days or weeks of life and only begin to decompensate when stressed. The nurse closely monitors for signs and symptoms associated with congenital heart disease (Box 22.5). He or she also monitors bilateral pulses of the upper and lower extremities. When monitoring the newborn's response to oxygen therapy, the nurse positions the pulse oximeter sensor device on the newborn's right hand and then

● **BOX 22.5** **Signs and Symptoms Associated With Congenital Heart Disease**

- Tachycardia > 200 beats/min
- Feeding difficulties; poor feeding; feeding times longer than 30 min
- Tachypnea; respiratory distress
- Diaphoresis
- Irritability
- Murmurs
- Pallor
- Cold extremities
- Cyanosis
- Hepatomegaly
- Recurrent pneumonia

on either foot, making note of any differences in oxygen saturation.

Newborns with congenital heart disease may also experience structural anomalies or diaphragmatic hernia, predisposing them to persistent pulmonary hypertension. Risk factors include meconium aspiration, respiratory distress syndrome, heart anomalies with shunting, congenital diaphragmatic hernia, pneumonia, and sepsis. Depending on the severity of the hypoxemic respiratory failure, various treatments may be used: inhaled nitric oxide, high-frequency oscillatory ventilation, and extracorporeal membrane oxygenation. Extracorporeal membrane oxygenation may be used for respiratory failure of any origin.

Supportive nursing management for the newborn includes minimal handling to reduce energy expenditure and swaddling to provide containment and comfort. Noxious stimuli, such as obtaining blood specimens for arterial blood gases or manipulating the newborn, tend to induce respiratory distress and cyanosis. The nurse may premedicate the newborn with a prescribed sedative before activities known to precipitate agitation (Wolf & Jackman, 2011).

Feeding is a stressor and may fatigue a seriously compromised newborn. Difficulties are associated with distress in the form of tachypnea, perspiring around the forehead and hairline during feeding, subcostal retractions, and feeding lasting more than 30 minutes. Using soft, smaller preterm nipples with enlarged holes can reduce the work of sucking.

Depending on the severity of congenital heart disease, the newborn may be able to breastfeed and may demonstrate satisfactory weight gain. If weight gain is insufficient, breastfeeding should be supplemented with high-caloric formulas or enteral feedings through orogastric-nasogastric or gastrostomy-duodenal tubes. Nutritional intake is often insufficient to meet the metabolic demands of congestive heart failure: tachycardia, increased oxygen consumption, and recurrent respiratory illness. Reduced nutritional intake may also be related to fatigue and the side effects of prescribed medication such as nausea, vomiting, and anorexia.

Because a diagnosis of congenital heart disease causes much distress for families, supportive interventions involve a collaborative, culturally sensitive approach based on identified family needs. Caregiver role strain may be related to the demands of medical treatment and frequent transportation and visits to a distant facility with pediatric cardiology offices. These demands may be coupled with common stressors related to careers, care of other children, and housekeeping. The nurse is aware of community resources, parental support groups, homemaker services, and respite care, giving appropriate referrals and recommendations according to the family needs. The availability of tele-echocardiography and pediatric cardiology through telemedicine can reduce medical expenses and improve time management when the family's community does not have immediate access to pediatric sonographers, pediatric cardiologists, or both (Grant et al., 2010).

The nurse supports positive coping by encouraging members of the family unit to focus on the newborn rather than the illness. Protectiveness must be balanced with normalcy. Caregivers can become so fearful of exposing the baby to infection sources that they isolate themselves with the infant. In becoming consumed with the care that the newborn with congenital heart disease requires, parents may ignore or neglect other siblings and their own relationship.

Some defects are not always treated immediately in the newborn period. For example, sometimes surgery is delayed until an organ suitable for transplant is available. The effect that such delays can have on families may be significant. In such instances, nurses help the family cope by providing teaching about areas such as the best way to handle cyanotic episodes. Referrals to support groups, websites hosting other parents in similar situations and other mechanisms for sharing common experiences may also be helpful.

Congenital Diaphragmatic Hernia

Congenital diaphragmatic hernia refers to the protrusion of abdominal contents (eg, a portion of the stomach or intestine) through an abnormality in the diaphragm. It usually develops between 8 and 10 weeks' gestation, when the pleuroperitoneal canals are fusing. As a result, the abdominal organs rise up through the defect and occupy space in the thoracic cavity. Intestinal organs may not actually invade the thoracic cavity, however, until later in pregnancy. Depending on the degree of pulmonary compression during the time when lung tissue should be developing, potentially fatal lung hypoplasia may also result.

Assessment Findings

If prenatal ultrasound identifies a congenital diaphragmatic hernia, birth in a facility with specialized care and a pediatric surgeon is advised (Wilson et al., 2011). Fetal surgery has been possible for the past 20 years, but as of this writing, no Canadian sites and only two US sites perform it. Ten years ago at the University of California, San Francisco, fetal surgery was performed to repair a diaphragmatic hernia. After performing a maternal hysterotomy, the fetal torso was partially outside the uterus for this repair. The maternal risk at the time of surgery and future implications of possible uterine rupture coupled with the fetal outcome did not appear to be worth the risk to the mother and fetus.

Collaborative Management

At birth, after determining the adequacy of oxygen exchange and ventilation, surgery is an immediate priority and the only option. The nurse is alert to signs of respiratory distress, which may be present with the first cry at birth or develop hours or even days later, depending on the size of the herniation. Resuscitation may be necessary at birth. Assessing the newborn's respiratory effort and colour provides immediate indicators of respiratory distress. Tachypnea, grunting, and intercostal retractions may be present because of impaired ventilatory exchange, which results from herniation of the stomach (normally in the abdominal cavity) into the thorax and displacement of the lungs. Auscultation may reveal absent or decreased breath sounds and audible bowel sounds on the side of the chest with the herniation.

The nurse may detect an abnormal contour of the abdomen, chest, or both in the affected newborn. When appreciable loops of bowel are in the chest cavity rather than in the abdomen, the abdomen may appear flat or concave instead of rounded. A chest cavity filled with abdominal contents appears barrel shaped.

Endotracheal intubation is indicated immediately. Increasing intrathoracic pressure with positive pressure bag-mask resuscitation increases mediastinal shifting and can lead to pneumothorax; the intestines in the chest are filled with air, which further compromises breathing. For these reasons, bag-mask resuscitation is contraindicated (Wilson et al., 2011). An orogastric catheter should be placed, accompanied by decompression with gentle suction to prevent gastric distention and further restriction of respiratory excursion (Wilson et al., 2011).

Pulse oximetry is used as a tool to monitor adequacy of respirations and ventilation. Maintaining the oxygen saturation above 90% ensures the adequacy of oxygenation. The probe for pulse oximetry is positioned on the newborn's right hand. The umbilical cord is left long to allow for cannulation and IV access. Because the infant will be NPO, IV fluids are administered to maintain hydration. Antibiotic therapy may be prescribed preoperatively because of the newborn's altered immune response (Bruzoni & Albanese, 2012).

Parental anxiety and concern are extremely high when resuscitation is required at birth. This anxiety is further compounded when plans are made for stabilization, possible transport to a tertiary care facility, or use of extracorporeal membrane oxygenation. Family-centred care requires honest, straightforward, positive communication, providing information, and frequent updates regarding the newborn's condition and the plans for care.

Minimal handling of the newborn is indicated, because of his or her increased oxygen needs related to stress and agitation. The nurse promotes attachment, however, by providing physical contact between the newborn and family as much as possible. Because of the relationship between cold stress and the development of acidosis, the newborn is kept warm at all times. Swaddling promotes both comfort and warmth.

Neural Tube Defects

Neural tube defects refer to a group of anomalies involving the brain and spinal cord. Abnormal neural development may result in cephalic or spinal defects that range from mildly serious, to severe and disabling, to incompatible with life.

Types

Neural tube defects include anencephaly, spina bifida, and encephalocele. Newborns with anencephaly have no cerebral hemispheres (Fig. 22.8). These infants may have functioning centres for cardiac and respiratory function

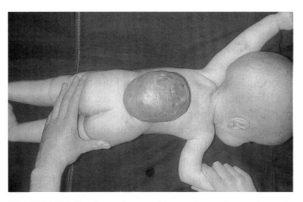
FIGURE 22.9 A newborn with myelomeningocele and hydrocephaly.

because of an intact medulla oblongata. The condition is suspected antepartally in the presence of elevated levels of alpha-fetoprotein and confirmed diagnostically by sonogram. Parents are usually presented with the option to terminate the pregnancy because the fetus with only a brain stem will likely die soon after birth.

The most common neural tube defect is **spina bifida**, which develops between 3 and 4 weeks' gestation (Blackburn, 2013). It occurs at a rate of 5.6 per 10,000 births in Canada (Wilson, 2007). The incidence of spina bifida has decreased significantly in recent years because of the introduction of folic acid supplementation. Spina bifida involves a failure of the neural tube to close because of internal and external factors (Blackburn, 2013). It is not always fatal; however, it can create significant stress for families, because the baby may have paralysis below the level of the defect and hydrocephaly that can lead to brain injury secondary to ICP. Because of quality-of-life issues, women may choose to terminate pregnancies with fetuses who have spina bifida. Others continue the pregnancy and assume care of the affected infant.

Spina bifida can be manifested in one of three forms: spina bifida occulta, meningocele, or myelomeningocele (Fig. 22.9).

* *Spina bifida occulta* is the mildest form of spina bifida. The area where one or more vertebra are malformed is covered by a layer of skin (Wilson et al., 2011). Although there is an opening in the spinal column, there is no sac and the spinal cord does not protrude ("occulta" means hidden). It results in a few sensory or motor deficits at birth. Assessment reveals a dimple, thickening of the overlying skin, and possibly hair growth at the site.
* With **meningocele**, the neural tube fails to close, leaving an opening in the vertebral column, with an external pouch containing cerebrospinal fluid. Meningocele is evident when the meninges (three-layered covering of the spinal cord) protrude through the

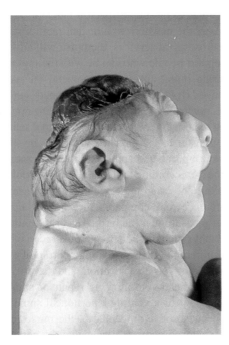
FIGURE 22.8 The newborn with anencephaly.

congenital opening into a sac on the external surface of the back. The defect can occur anywhere along the spinal column, but is most common in the lumbar area. The sac contains only cerebrospinal fluid and meninges; no spinal cord nerves are present in the sac (Blackburn, 2013). Therefore, there are a few accompanying motor or sensory deficits (Blackburn, 2013).

- The most serious and disabling form of spina bifida is **myelomeningocele.** With failure of neural tube closure, the spinal nerves protrude into the sac with the cerebrospinal fluid and meninges. Subsequently, nerve damage and severe motor and sensory disabilities can occur. **Hydrocephaly** (fluid collection in and surrounding the brain ventricles, resulting in an enlarged head) frequently accompanies myelomeningocele, because herniation of brain tissue into the foramen magna prevents drainage of cerebrospinal fluid while it is being manufactured continually in the brain (Wilson et al., 2011).

Assessment Findings

All women in Canada should be offered routine screening for neural tube defects (Chitayat et al., 2011) (see Chapter 11). When spina bifida is diagnosed prenatally, treatment options include prenatal surgery to close the sac, and cesarean birth to avoid trauma to the sac.

At birth, with the newborn prone, the nurse visually inspects the spine from the base of the skull to the sacrum. He or she documents and reports any dimpled indention or tuft of hair over any area. An external mass may be readily visible on inspection and appears as a glistening fluid-filled outpouching. The nurse takes extreme care to prevent trauma to a visible sac.

With a dressing protecting any visible sac in place (Wilson et al., 2011), the nurse assesses and documents the baby's neurologic reflexes (Babinski and leg recoil) below the defect and notes any mobility impairment or flaccidity. Assessment of bowel and bladder elimination patterns also provides clues to neurologic dysfunction. Lack of sphincter function may lead to constant leakage of urine and stool (Wilson et al., 2011).

The nurse inspects the head for signs of hydrocephalus, which includes an enlarged head with visible vessels. This enlargement, transmitted anteriorly, gives an appearance of an unusually high, wide, and protuberant forehead, which is called "bossing." The nurse documents a baseline head circumference at the level of the eyebrows to detect and evaluate the degree of bossing.

While the newborn is prone, the nurse assesses the skin for pressure areas, particularly on the knees and feet. A folded infant blanket under the groin area reduces strain on any lumbar lesion by keeping the hips slightly flexed.

Collaborative Management

Primary prevention of neural tube defects begins with optimal prepregnancy nutrition and multivitamin and folic acid (0.4 to 1.0 mg daily) supplementation, which should continue throughout the first trimester (Wilson, 2007) (see Chapters 2, 3, and 12). Newborns with spina bifida occulta typically require no treatment; however, their bowel and bladder function is assessed. For newborns with meningocele, surgery is initiated within 24 hours of birth to close and prevent any further damage or infection from a break in the sac. Preoperatively, the nurse employs protective prone positioning, careful handling, and other measures to avoid trauma to the sac. Any crack in the sac, no matter how minute, can be a portal of entry for organisms that can lead to possibly fatal meningitis. Thus, strict asepsis is a nursing priority at all times.

Fetal surgery to repair myelomeningocele is risky, although it has been performed. The most publicized of these surgeries involved a couple who refused a therapeutic abortion. The now-famous surgeon successfully performed the fetal procedure in 1999 at Vanderbilt University Hospital. At the time of the repair, Samuel was 21 weeks' gestation.

Before birth of the newborn, regardless of the type of defect, anxiety in parents and family members is common because of uncertain outcomes for both mother and baby. The nurse preparing the woman for a cesarean birth offers reassurance, information, and explanations regarding preoperative and postoperative expectations, including when she will be able to see her newborn (see Chapter 16). Ideally, transport of the newborn to surgery should occur after the mother can view and touch him or her. If the newborn's father or another relative or support person indicates a desire to accompany the newborn to a distant facility with pediatric neurosurgical services, the nurse will advocate for other support people who can be with the mother.

During initial airway management, the nurse supports the sac (if large) gently with a cupped, sterile, powder-free, nonlatex, gloved hand, lined with a nonadherent dressing material premoistened with normal saline. After careful transfer to the radiant warmer, he or she places the newborn prone and applies a protective moist dressing to the sac according to the facility's protocol.

Before and after surgery, the nurse measures head circumference and compares the finding against the baseline measurement at birth. He or she notifies the primary physician or pediatric neurosurgeon of increasing circumference or deteriorating neurologic status.

Depending on the location and severity of the defect, complications following repair of spina bifida, and placement of a ventriculoperitoneal shunt (if warranted because of hydrocephaly), the nurse reinforces health care teaching with parents and the possible need for neurology and physical therapy referrals for later

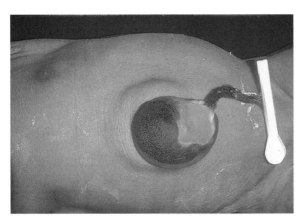

FIGURE 22.10 A newborn with the large and protruding sac characteristic of omphalocele.

mobility problems, as well as bladder and bowel training. Physical growth will require periodic shunt revisions. The nurse teaches caregivers to be alert to any behavioural changes, especially decreased level of consciousness, which could indicate increasing intracranial pressure from shunt malfunction.

Congenital Defects of the Abdominal Wall

Congenital defects of the abdominal wall typically include omphalocele and gastroschisis. **Omphalocele** results from a defect in the umbilical ring that allows abdominal contents contained within a peritoneal sac to protrude through the external abdominal surface at the base of the umbilical cord (Fig. 22.10). The less common **gastroschisis** also involves an opening in the anterior abdominal wall, usually to the right of the umbilical cord insertion (Wilson et al., 2011), through which eviscerated abdominal contents protrude. Because gastroschisis is a full-thickness defect of the abdominal wall and abdominal contents are *not* contained within a peritoneal sac, the internal abdominal contents are exposed to amniotic fluid. Amniotic fluid, composed largely of fetal urine and intestinal waste products, irritates the intestines and causes bowel thickening. When meconium is excreted into the amniotic fluid, a thick peel develops over the exposed intestines (Barseghyan et al., 2012). This is visible on prenatal ultrasound as matting of the bowel. Incidence of other associated defects is high and may involve anomalies of the heart, GI system, genitourinary system, and central nervous system.

Unlike gastroschisis, omphalocele is linked to genetic and chromosomal syndromes. Risk factors include young maternal age, lower socioeconomic status, smoking, and use of over-the-counter preparations containing vasoactive properties such as pseudoephedrine (a common nasal decongestant). Findings also implicate the use of cyclo-oxygenase inhibitors and maternal substance use in gastroschisis (Jones et al., 2009).

Assessment Findings

Omphalocele and gastroschisis are readily visible at birth. When assessing omphalocele, the nurse looks for intactness of the peritoneal sac and evidence of organs visible within the sac. Usually the sac contains only the intestines, but sometimes the liver is there as well. The nurse documents the size of the omphalocele, which can range from 2 to 12 cm.

Assessment of gastroschisis involves additional inspection (not manipulation) for twisting of intestines and changes in the colour of the exposed intestines. The nurse completes a thorough physical examination to evaluate for evidence of associated defects.

Collaborative Management

Any open abdominal defect predisposes the newborn to trauma of internal organs, infection, fluid loss, and hypothermia. Timing and method of birth are related to fetal well-being, with best outcomes after 36 weeks' gestation (Lovvorn et al., 2011). Procedures start immediately after birth to stabilize the newborn and prepare for surgery. An elective cesarean birth may be planned to allow the newborn with known problems to emerge when pediatric surgical teams and intensive care beds are available; however, research findings do not support cesarean over vaginal birth in cases of the abdominal defect alone (Lovvorn et al., 2011). The high risk of stillbirth with gastroschisis (6% to 12%) may also be an indicator for cesarean birth when the pregnant woman reports decreased fetal movements. Follow-up ultrasound may demonstrate fetal gastric distention and an abnormal nonstress test, indicating that the fetal heart does not accelerate as normal with movement felt by the pregnant woman (Kuleva et al., 2012). With smaller defects, a single surgery replaces internal contents (usually only intestines, but may include other organs as well, such as the liver) back into the abdominal cavity. When the defect is large or there is significant bowel edema, a staged repair may be undertaken. Initially a silastic pouch may be placed over the abdominal contents and then secured to the abdominal wall. In subsequent procedures the pouch is gradually reduced in size, gently forcing the abdominal contents back into the abdominal cavity.

Gentle handling is indicated to prevent trauma to the sac or exposed abdominal organs. Because newborns readily lose body heat to the environment through evaporation and radiation, the nurse places the baby in a servocontrolled open-air radiant warmer. If not readily available, the nurse obtains a sterile bowel bag (usually available where abdominal surgeries are performed). Wearing sterile, nonlatex, powder-free gloves, the nurse inserts the newborn, feet first, into the bag. A high incidence of latex allergy in infants with congenital defects with organs on the outside of the body may be related to the frequency of exposure to latex materials

(Chua et al., 2013); hence, all products in contact with the infant should be latex-free. After containing the newborn within the sterile bag, the nurse secures the drawstring tie on the bowel bag at the nipple level. This intervention helps preserve warmth and protect against microbial contamination until transport and surgery can be accomplished.

The appearance of intestines outside the abdominal cavity can be a frightening sight for parents. Nurses assess their interpretation of what they have seen and explain the defect and measures being taken to ensure stabilization of the baby. When discussing surgery, the nurse emphasizes that the abdominal organs themselves are normal, and surgery to replace them into the abdominal cavity usually corrects the problem. If kinking or constriction have interrupted blood flow to the intestines, the nonviable intestines are surgically excised with anastomosis of the bowel. A temporary ostomy may be created.

Postoperatively, the newborn is monitored for arterial hypertension. The cause of this hypertension is unknown and is more common with omphalocele (40% of cases) than with gastroschisis (10% of cases) (Cachat et al., 2006). Although such hypertension is usually transient, the newborn is observed in a critical care setting for several days before antihypertensive therapy is begun. The nurse is alert to signs of other postoperative complications such as sepsis, bowel obstruction, and necrotizing enterocolitis. Parenteral nutrition and fluids are indicated, because oral feedings must be delayed until bowel function is well-established (Wilson et al., 2011).

Cleft Lip and Cleft Palate

When embryonic structures of the upper lip, nose, and hard and soft palate fail to close and fuse, clefting results. Clefting may take many forms: complete or incomplete clefting of the lip only, which may be either unilateral or bilateral; clefting of the palate alone, which may involve only the soft or hard palate or both; or clefting of the lip in combination with complete or incomplete clefting of the palate (Fig. 22.11). **Oral–facial cleft** refers to a defect involving both the lip and palate. Typically, when a cleft lip develops, the possibility of cleft palate is also high. Infants having an isolated cleft palate (without cleft lip) are more prone to genetic syndromes accompanied by multiple other birth defects.

Etiology

The face and palate develop from embryonic cells that form the facial structures and separate the nasal passage from the oral cavity. These cells begin to coalesce, coming together from either side of the midline to the line that passes through the upper lip into each nostril. The hard palate likewise is formed by two shelves of tissue that grow from the sides and join together in the

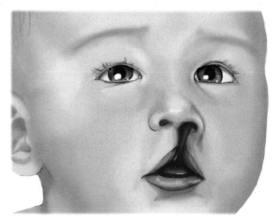

FIGURE 22.11 Cleft lip.

midline to separate the nasal and oral cavities (Nanci, 2008). Failure to fuse by the end of 7 to 8 weeks' gestation results in a congenital craniofacial defect. Cleft lip occurs in approximately 1 in 600 births and occurs more frequently in males than in females; cleft palate occurs in 1 in 2,500 births, with females affected more than males (Wilson et al., 2011).

Heredity and modifiable environmental factors have been implicated, but the exact cause of craniofacial clefting is unknown (Centers for Disease Control and Prevention, 2013). It has been suggested (Wilson et al., 2011) that maternal smoking, alcohol consumption, and folic acid deficiency may be implicated; maternal use of antiseizure medications also may increase risks for cleft lip.

Assessment Findings

Defects involving the lip are apparent at birth, with a flattened nose and profile and clefts of the lip that extend into the nostrils. Palpating the hard and soft palates with a gloved finger can easily reveal a large or a complete cleft palate. A small incomplete cleft palate may not be detected, unless visualized with a light source.

Collaborative Management

Surgery is the primary treatment. Cleft lip can be repaired any time after birth. Early closure of the lip allows the infant to be able to create suction for nursing. Advances in neonatal surgery and anaesthesia have made safe repair possible at ages younger than the 10-week age cut-off traditionally used. As the child grows, lip and nasal revisions may be necessary to improve appearance (Wilson et al., 2011; Harris et al., 2010).

Repair of a cleft palate may be delayed until 10 to 12 months of age to allow time for muscular growth. Surgery as early as possible during this time supports speech development. Later revisions to the palate may be necessary if speech is nasal (Wilson et al., 2011). See Nursing Care Plan 22.2.

NURSING CARE PLAN 22.2

●

The Newborn With Cleft Lip and Palate

Recall Baby Madeline, described at the beginning of this chapter, who was born with a congenital cleft lip and palate. When taking a nursing history, Madeline's mother Danita denies any modifiable environmental risk factors during the pregnancy such as smoking or alcohol consumption. She reports that she took 400 mg of folic acid daily for an entire year before Madeline was conceived. Family history reveals two cousins born with craniofacial clefting deformities.

Baby Madeline appears healthy in every other way. Her mother continues to request verification that she has no other congenital defects. Neither parent has achieved a level of comfort with feeding. Danita and Louis decline the hospital's newborn photography plan, stating that they will wait to take photographs after Baby Madeline's lip is "fixed."

NURSING DIAGNOSIS

Risk for Impaired Parenting related to difficulty with role transition secondary to added stressors of visible craniofacial defect

EXPECTED OUTCOMES

1. The parents will express their feelings of anger, grief, and guilt.
2. The parents will work together to nurture and protect their newborn.
3. The parents will verbalize positive remarks about the newborn and optimistic plans for repair of the craniofacial defect.
4. The parents will demonstrate progressive attachment and engrossment behaviours.

INTERVENTIONS	RATIONALES
Show before and after pictures of infants having craniofacial defects similar to Madeline's.	Photographs evoke less emotion than an actual defect and can help desensitize the real experience. Seeing "after" photographs helps the parents visualize past the defect toward the future.
Give updated reports about the newborn frequently, calling her by name and citing her positive behaviours. For example, "She likes to cuddle when you hold her close for bubbling"; "Madeline is such a good baby. She goes right to sleep after feeding!"	The newborn becomes more of a personality when behaviours are assigned to her.
Feed, diaper, and bring the newborn to visit during a quiet alert state when the baby is awake, but not hungry, wet, or crying.	The defect will look worse when the infant is red faced and upset, with eyes shut and mouth wide open and crying. Parents may face additional stressors in the urgency of comforting the infant.
Remain with the parents to hold the newborn while pointing out her positive traits. Point out positive normal characteristics such as eyes, long lashes, pretty hair, strong grasp, etc. Emphasize that the newborn is perfectly healthy in every other way.	Physical presence is a "buffer" and allows parents some space during appraisal of the newborn. Verbal encouragement and physical presence are supportive and provide reassurance.

(continued)

NURSING CARE PLAN 22.2 ● The Newborn With Cleft Lip and Palate (Continued)

INTERVENTIONS	RATIONALES
Smile while looking the newborn in the face to role-model attachment behaviours for the parents. Use the en face position and speak words of comfort and love in a soft voice. Hold and cuddle the newborn before handing her off to a parent.	Role modeling reinforces the normalcy of the newborn and affirms her value.
Encourage similar behaviours in the parents. Reinforce that it is okay to touch, stroke, or cuddle the newborn.	
Introduce parents to a support group or Internet site for contact with other parents of children with cleft lip and palate to share reactions and feelings as well as encouragement and support.	Group interactions with people who have had similar experiences can be an effective means by which to cope with similar stress reactions.

EVALUATION

1. The parents demonstrate acceptance of their newborn.
2. The parents show affection to their baby by such measures as kissing, holding, and looking directly at her.
3. The parents verbalize a realistic perception of the craniofacial defect and a plan for future care.

NURSING DIAGNOSIS

Risk for Imbalanced Nutrition: Less Than Body Requirements related to feeding difficulties associated with craniofacial defect

EXPECTED OUTCOMES

1. The parents will establish successful and satisfying feeding techniques.
2. The newborn will consume and retain 350 to 500 mL of formula or breast milk daily.
3. The newborn will produce sufficient urine to wet 6 to 10 diapers per day.

INTERVENTIONS	RATIONALES
Collaborate with the healthcare team to establish successful feeding techniques before introducing parents to the feeding behaviours.	Finding a successful feeding technique is a first step in teaching, avoiding the stress associated with trial and error.
Assist the parent to a comfortable, upright position; place the newborn in the parent's nondominant arm.	Sitting upright during feeding helps prevent aspiration in the newborn. Use of the nondominant arm keeps the dominant hand available to manipulate the bottle and nipple for feeding.

(continued)

NURSING CARE PLAN 22.2 ● The Newborn With Cleft Lip and Palate *(Continued)*

INTERVENTIONS	RATIONALES
Supply the parents with special equipment for feeding. Demonstrate how to place the elongated, soft, and easily compressed nipple into the newborn's mouth. Have the parents return-demonstrate.	Special nipples simplify feeding by closing off the cleft palate or being compressed easily by the existing portion of the palate. Demonstration is the optimal mode of teaching. Return demonstration indicates the extent of learning.
Teach the caregiver to sit the newborn upright on the lap, or to hold the newborn upright against the shoulder and to pat the back to burp or bubble the newborn after each 15 to 30 mL of liquid.	Typically, newborns swallow air with feeding, which may distend the stomach if unrelieved.
Monitor the amount of breast milk or formula ingested. Assess daily weights and evaluate the number of wet diapers produced.	Monitoring intake and output provides an indication of hydration status. Weight gain is helpful in determining whether the newborn is receiving adequate calories for growth and development.

EVALUATION

1. The parents demonstrate feeding without difficulty, expressing confidence with feeding their newborn.
2. The newborn consumes and retains 60 to 90 mL of fluid with each feeding.
3. The newborn wets the established number of diapers.

Communication and Bonding. Therapeutic communication with the parents about the defect is essential immediately after birth. Even when they know about the problem in advance and have participated in antepartal interventions (eg, education, showing photos), parents and family members may be upset when they see the actual cleft. The nurse provides explanations and the opportunity for the parents to discuss their feelings, as well as answering any questions they may have. The nurse models attachment behaviours in the presence of the parents and family unit. Looking into the newborn's face (en face position), smiling, enfolding, patting, and talking to the baby are all nurturing behaviours that may help the parents feel that others are accepting of their child.

Feeding Assistance. Before a parent's first feeding sessions with the newborn, the nurse reviews techniques known to be effective for the particular defect. A team approach and practice are helpful before the first feeding, which the mother may find difficult. Various organizations offer tips and video instructions for new parents facing the challenge of feeding an infant with an oral–facial defect. Consultations with specialists who work with children with clefting disorders may be helpful.

Feeding tips include basic guidelines of holding the infant upright, using special cleft palate nipples, and increasing the hole in a regular nipple to ensure a constant drip (Fig. 22.12). If a feeding takes longer than 30 minutes, parents can enlarge the hole by cutting an "X" into the distal end of the nipple. If the infant is receiving too much flow and appears to be struggling with the liquid, the size of the nipple hole is obviously too large and a smaller hole should be cut into a new nipple.

By visualizing the hard palate, the nurse determines the side of the oral cavity having the larger solid strip of hard palate. By offering a long, soft nipple (Lamb nipple) to the larger side directed toward the back of the oropharynx, the infant can simply compress the nipple between the flattened tongue and existing portion of hard palate to express milk without suction. The flanged nipple provides an attached covering that occludes the

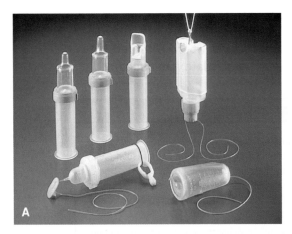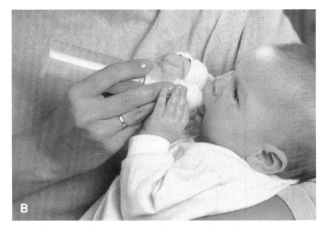

FIGURE 22.12 **A:** Special nipples and feeding devices for the newborn with congenital cleft lip or palate. **B:** Correct positioning for feeding the infant with cleft lip or palate disorders.

cleft in the hard palate and allows the infant to create suction. This device may be effective initially (although hard to use with very small infants); it must be resized as the infant grows. The nurse advises the parents to burp the newborn frequently to control problems related to excess swallowed air.

Breastfeeding is possible with cleft lip, because breast tissue can close off the cleft effectively. Breastfeeding may be difficult, however, if there is a wide separation of the palate. The nurse encourages mothers to pump breast milk and feed their babies through special nipples and appliances, if needed.

The nurse encourages new parents not to be afraid and reassures them that health care providers are committed to helping them learn how to successfully feed their baby. Expressing confidence that the parent possesses the necessary skills to meet the challenges ahead fosters self-esteem. A satisfactory feeding takes no longer than 30 minutes; the infant should consume 60 to 90 mL of fluid. Weight gain and saturated diapers offer good indicators of sufficient nutritional intake.

 Remember Madeline, who had a congenital cleft lip and palate. Would she be a candidate for breastfeeding?

Parents should express comfort and confidence with infant feeding before discharge from the acute care setting. If the primary caregiver feels insecure with feedings, referral for a home health nurse or an early visit from the public health nurse is indicated. The nurse also can be instrumental in introducing the family unit to community and on-line support groups and interactive chat sessions with other parents of infants with clefting defects. Additionally, the nurse can give the parents

contact information for various manufacturers of specialized feeding devices.

Surgical Preparation and Support. In preparation for surgical repair, the parents and family meet with members of the craniofacial team who explain, inform, and prepare them for the infant's dramatic new look and oral capabilities (Box 22.6). The nurse listens to fears and concerns and verifies that parents correctly understand preoperative and postoperative events and care. Depending on the extent of repair, the operation may last approximately 3 hours (Lee, 2010). The nurse relays frequent updates and reports from the operating room to the parents and ensures that the family has a comfortable area for waiting.

Postoperatively, the infant is likely to be somewhat fussy upon awakening from anaesthesia. He or she is quickly reunited with parents for comfort and nurturing. Feeding by breast or bottle (a primary comfort measure) is allowed immediately after surgery. Contrary to beliefs that led to previously rigid postoperative measures to protect the surgical site, feeding has not been proven to compromise the integrity of the suture line (Kim et al.,

● **BOX 22.6   Members of the Craniofacial Team**

- Nurse
- Physician
- Dentist
- Orthodontist
- Prosthodontist
- Speech therapist
- Social worker
- Child psychologist
- Otolaryngologist
- Plastic surgeon
- Pediatric anaesthesiologist

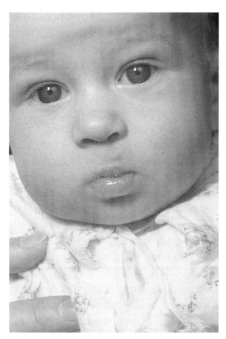

FIGURE 22.13 Appearance of the older infant who has undergone surgical correction of a cleft disorder.

2009; Wilson et al., 2011). The nurse is alert to patency of small airways that swelling or secretions could easily obstruct. A splint-like appliance is usually applied in the operating room to prevent the child from stretching the upper lip when crying. The Logan bar (also called a Logan bow) helps protect the suture line and maintains approximation until healing by primary intention is established. Usually, the infant is discharged from the facility 1 to 2 days after surgery. By that time, the infant should be consuming and retaining the usual full feeding. Once healing is complete, families often feel much more positive (Fig. 22.13).

Discharge Planning. Discharge instructions emphasize the need to monitor for signs of infection, including temperature above 38.4°C (axillary or tympanic), erythema or drainage from the surgical site, or pain uncontrolled by acetaminophen. Infection can interfere with normal healing and may result in a less-than-optimal cosmetic result.

Esophageal and Tracheal Defects

Esophageal abnormalities develop early in utero. During the 4th to 5th gestational week, the foregut normally lengthens and separates into two distinct structures that eventually become the trachea and esophagus. Several congenital anomalies may occur.

With **esophageal atresia**, the esophageal passageway to the stomach is disrupted and closed off, ending in a blind pouch. The newborn may appear normal and healthy at birth with no visible abnormalities. When secretions or initial feedings drain into the blind pouch, overflow may cause aspiration, coughing, and choking. Without surgery, the newborn has no means of ingesting fluid and receiving nutrition. Associated risks include aspiration and pneumonia.

A more immediately dangerous and potentially lethal condition, **tracheoesophageal fistula** can compromise respiratory status at birth or soon after. With this defect, an abnormal connecting passageway (fistula) exists between the trachea and esophagus, created while these two structures were developing to form two separate tubes. Because of the abnormality, fluid or food that should pass from the mouth to esophagus and onward to the stomach may instead be diverted into the lungs. Air taken in through the trachea and intended for the lungs may enter the stomach and cause gastric distention. Crying that compresses the abdominal musculature or having the head or chest in the dependent position may propel gastric contents upward into the fetal lung.

Types of Defects

Some varieties of tracheoesophageal fistula are more common than others.

1. In type A, the distal end of the esophagus is attached to the trunk of the trachea above the carina. The proximal end of the esophagus is a short stump that forms a blind pouch. Food and fluids have no route by which to enter the stomach; with each inspiration, air from the trachea enters and distends the stomach. This route also allows gastric juice to enter the lungs through the fistula.
2. Type B is esophageal atresia only (without a corresponding fistula). The proximal esophagus ends in a blind pouch, and the distal esophagus is a closed stump that is not attached to the trachea. Because the stomach is not connected to the lung, gastric distention is not possible. The two ends of the esophagus are not joined; thus, there is no passageway for fluid or nutrition to enter the stomach. The blind pouch can fill with secretions or fluid that could overflow into the back of the oropharynx and be aspirated into the lung.
3. Type C is a rare "H-type" tracheoesophageal fistula, representing about 4% of all tracheoesophageal fistulas (Mattei, 2012). It does not have accompanying esophageal atresia, but incomplete division of the esophagus and trachea is apparent. The passageway from the oropharynx through the esophagus and into the stomach is patent. The fistula, which allows concurrent flow of oral fluid or tracheal air, usually is located high, near the second thoracic vertebra. This diagnosis is commonly missed because passage of a small-bore feeding tube at birth reveals a patent esophagus and aspiration of gastric fluid. Only when

the esophagus is distended fully with diagnostic contrast media can the defect be visualized during a technique called the "pull-back" esophagram (Bruch et al., 2010). Obviously, during this procedure, care must be taken to avoid overflowing the contrast medium into the infant's lungs.

4. The type D defect can be rapidly fatal. Because the proximal esophagus is attached directly to the trachea, any oral feeding will go directly into the infant's lungs. The distal esophagus is closed off, and the stomach is flat and undistended. Gastric distention is impossible because the esophageal stump near the cardiac orifice of the stomach is not connected by way of fistula to the trachea.

5. Type E is a tracheoesophageal fistula with a connecting tracheal passageway to both the proximal and distal ends of the esophagus. Both fluid and air can enter the stomach and lung. This defect can be rapidly fatal with the initial feeding of the newborn if the defect is not suspected and detected early. See Figure 22.14.

Assessment Findings

With esophageal anomalies, the fetus cannot suck and swallow amniotic fluid. The health care practitioner monitoring antepartal measurements may notice increasing fundal height. Subsequent prenatal ultrasound may verify maternal polyhydramnios and no fetal fluid-filled stomach bubble (Wilson et al., 2011; Ojha et al., 2011). Brown and Nicolaides (2000) also described a high suspicion of esophageal atresia with tracheoesophageal fistula based on increased first-trimester fetal nuchal translucency. Antenatal recognition and in utero diagnosis of esophageal abnormalities may afford improved clinical outcomes based on measures to prevent aspiration pneumonia and early surgical correction (Czerkiewicz et al., 2011).

Symptoms at birth or shortly after vary in severity depending on the type of problem. Typically, the infant with the type A defect experiences noticeable abdominal distention because inhaled air with the birth cry goes directly into the stomach as well as the lungs. The flat stomach of the newborn before the first cry at birth immediately changes in contour, becoming rounded or convex with the first breath. With the newborn's head in a dependent position to facilitate normal drainage of oral secretions, the esophageal pouch may drain amniotic fluid and secretions that can be aspirated into the lung. Respiratory distress may develop. Conversely, the defect may not be noted until newborn nursery personnel detect indicators of tracheoesophageal atresia, fistula, or both. With esophageal atresia, an orogastric tube cannot be passed into the stomach. Rather, the tube coils into a blind esophageal pouch (Wilson et al., 2011; Lovvorn et al., 2011).

Close observation of all newborns for cardinal symptoms of tracheoesophageal atresia and fistula is essential. Coughing, choking, and cyanosis with feeding are classic findings (Wilson et al., 2011). Excessive salivation and drooling when in the side-lying position are additional indicators of esophageal atresia. Abdominal distention is apparent when the distal segment of the esophagus is connected to the trachea. Crying (which compresses abdominal musculature) may result in cyanosis, yet when the oropharynx is suctioned, no secretions are present. Based on this assessment, the astute nurse suspects aspiration of gastric contents into the lung. Because signs and symptoms may be intermittent and variable, a small trial feeding of sterile distilled water may be attempted to reproduce them under the watchful eye of the pediatrician, the pediatric gastroenterologist, or the thoracic surgeon (Crabbe, 2003). If feeding by nasogastric tube produces no symptoms, yet the oral feed is associated with choking, cyanosis, or aspiration, the H-type tracheoesophageal fistula is strongly suspected (Mattei, 2012).

Misdiagnosis of esophageal fistula, especially the H type, results in frequent respiratory infections. Radiographic findings with such infants may reveal patchy infiltrates of the lungs from aspiration pneumonia and air in the bowel (Anuntaseree et al., 2002; Celayir & Erdogan, 2003).

Collaborative Management

If a nurse suspects that a newborn has a tracheoesophageal fistula, he or she allows nothing by mouth (NPO) and notifies the pediatrician immediately. An additional priority is to position the infant prone with the head on a plane elevated to at least 30 degrees to prevent gastric reflux into the lungs. The nurse may pass a nasogastric tube if a test gavage feeding is prescribed and assist with supervised administration of the trial gavage. Suction equipment and an oxygen source must be available immediately in the event of respiratory distress secondary to aspiration. When the newborn is preterm and lacking necessary surfactant, respiratory distress syndrome may complicate treatment. PPV is usually contraindicated with tracheoesophageal fistula because of the danger of abdominal distention.

While the newborn is NPO, the nurse provides opportunities for non-nutritive sucking to promote comfort and security, as well as to help develop the oropharyngeal musculature. Hydration is maintained by IV fluids administered through the umbilical vein. Before corrective surgery, a gastrostomy tube may be inserted for decompression and to minimize gastric dilation and reflux (Wilson et al., 2011). The nurse monitors and maintains patency of the gastrostomy tube to gravity drainage. Underwater seal drainage may be used to prevent air from being sucked into the stomach with

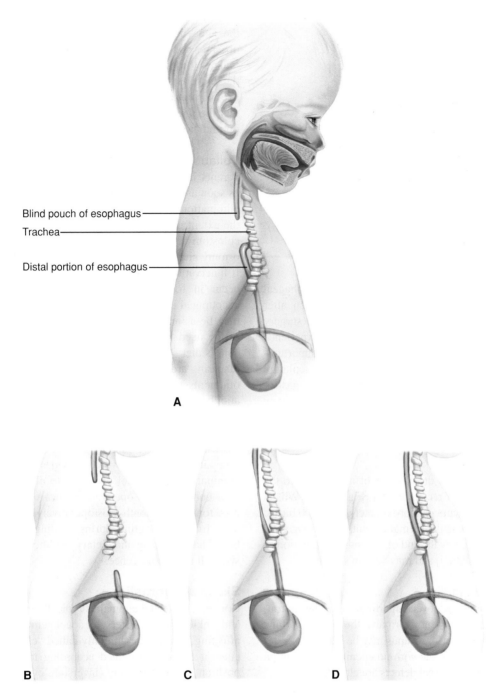

Blind pouch of esophagus

Trachea

Distal portion of esophagus

A

B   C   D

FIGURE 22.14   A: Esophageal atresia, with the distal end of the esophagus attached to the trunk of the trachea and the proximal end of the esophagus forming a blind pouch. **B:** Esophageal atresia without a corresponding fistula. **C:** The rare "H-type" tracheoesophageal fistula. **D:** Tracheoesophageal fistula with a connecting tracheal passageway to both the proximal and distal ends of the esophagus.

respirations, while allowing gas and gastric fluid to escape. With esophageal atresia, the blind pouch must be suctioned frequently, using low, intermittent pressure to prevent overflow of mucus and aspiration. Pneumonia is a frequent postoperative complication because of the high risk for aspiration of gastric secretions and mucus into the trachea. Depending on the extent of sur-

gery, the gastrostomy tube may be left in place postoperatively to provide an alternative feeding route while the internal suture lines heal. Oral feedings can resume when the integrity of the repair is intact, as documented with contrast studies.

Postoperatively, when any pneumonia is resolved and oral feeding is established, the nurse monitors the

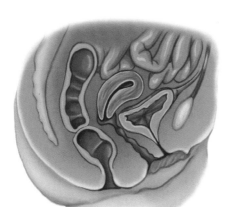

FIGURE 22.15 Imperforate anus.

newborn's eating behaviour. Abnormal esophageal motility may result in residual dysphagia even after surgical correction (Lemoine et al., 2013). If surgery is delayed beyond infancy, the toddler may experience resistance to eating, not having had earlier opportunities to enjoy oral feedings and to develop musculature used for ingestion and swallowing. Incidence of gastroesophageal reflux is also high following repair and may require further interventions for management (Catalano et al., 2011).

Imperforate Anus

Imperforate anus is the absence of an opening to the anus with failure of rectal descent (Fig. 22.15) (Wilson et al., 2011). It occurs in approximately 1 in 5000 births, affecting more male than female infants. This congenital defect can be seen by the end of the embryonic period (7 to 8 weeks' gestation) and may vary in severity.

Assessment Findings

Nurses frequently discover imperforate anus during routine newborn assessment. Normally, the anus is midline and patent. An imperforate anus may be visible with stenosis, totally imperforate with no opening, or absent on the external surface. Anal defects are classified as "low," "intermediate," or "high," depending on where the rectum stops anatomically. Radiographic studies can assist with classification by showing the level at which bowel gas patterns stop in relation to the pubococcygeal line and ischium (Lovvorn et al., 2011).

During newborn assessment, the nurse visualizes the anus and verifies patency by documenting passage of meconium within the first 24 hours of life. With trends toward earlier discharges from the hospital, however, some seemingly normal infants leave the health care facility before 24 hours of life have passed. Thus, nurses advocate for protocols requiring newborns to remain in the facility until they pass meconium.

To test for reflex anal constriction, the nurse strokes the anus lightly with a cotton-tipped applicator and observes for an anal "wink" verifying neurologic normalcy. With high defects, the rectum stops well above the muscle groups that make up the rectal sphincter (Lovvorn et al., 2011). Lack of a wink reflex indicates that the newborn requires stool softeners and fibre for optimal bowel function.

Collaborative Management

Parents need to be informed of the congenital defect as soon as it is diagnosed because of the immediacy of elimination needs. The type of correction depends on the extent of the defect. High defects need immediate colostomy, requiring that parents be taught care of the ostomy site. Low defects are managed with anoplasty. If innervation is damaged or lacking, constipation may occur in formula-fed infants; thus, breastfeeding is encouraged. Even after surgical correction, constipation may be a long-term problem, and parents are advised of the need for stool softeners and added fibre in the child's diet (Wilson et al., 2011). Routine cleaning and diapering are adequate for the young infant. Protective ointments may be used if skin irritation is problematic; however, diapers should be checked regularly and changed promptly to prevent rash.

More complex anorectal anomalies may require extensive corrective surgery done in stages in conjunction with a colostomy, which provides a route for fecal elimination, and bowel diversion to allow for healing after completion of operative repair. A dilator may be used for several months postoperatively to keep the new anus from constricting during healing. The need for bowel habit training and dietary modifications may persist well into adolescence.

Skeletal Anomalies

Congenital skeletal anomalies typically involve the foot and ankle. *Talipes* refers to a congenital foot defect affecting the ankle, commonly called "club foot." Varieties of talipes are named according to the anatomic position of the deformity (inversion, eversion, or flexion). **Talipes equinovarus** is a combination of a downward and inward fixed position of flexion.

Etiology

Incidence of talipes equinovarus is 1 or 2 in 1,000 newborns, affecting boys twice as often as girls (Wilson et al., 2011). Talipes is linked to heredity, and some studies show a relationship between mothers who smoke and idiopathic talipes equinovarus (Parker et al., 2009).

Assessment Findings

Visualization of the lower extremities at birth reveals talipes, which may be unilateral or bilateral. Testing the motion of the affected ankle reveals that the deformity is rigid and resists realignment, which differentiates talipes from the positional deformity seen in LGA newborns (Wilson et al., 2011).

Collaborative Management

Although talipes equinovarus is not life-threatening, it can be upsetting to parents. If untreated, it has the potential to be a major birth defect leading to permanent disability. Referral to a pediatric orthopedic specialist is indicated. Treatment is usually initiated soon after birth, while the foot is malleable. A cast is applied to maintain corrected positioning of the foot (Fig. 22.16). Because of the infant's rapid growth, the foot is recast first every few days, and later, every few weeks. Severe defects or those not responding to manipulation and casting may require surgery.

Once the foot has been correctly aligned, the child will need to perform a series of exercises and wear splints at night to maintain proper positioning. He or she also may require special shoes.

Parents need facts about the nature and treatment of the deformity. Nurses are aware that relatives often experience grief upon seeing the defect. Giving information and listening empathetically are indicated. Treatment usually takes months and requires frequent adjustments and applications of castings, splints, and appliances. Outpatient or clinic nurses usually are involved in assisting with such applications and evaluating the condition of the skin. Such follow-up visits provide opportunities to teach parents and other caregivers how to evaluate the extremity, including checking the toes for warmth and colour and assessing capillary refill, comparing findings bilaterally. Parents also receive instructions in cast care, such as measures to ensure that the cast remains dry and to check for pressure areas, especially around the cast openings.

The nurse verifies parental understanding of the treatment plan and clarifies explanations and instructions given by the orthopedist. Phone contact and follow-up between clinic visits provide encouragement and opportunities for family members to express concerns and ask questions.

Developmental Dysplasia of the Hip

Developmental dysplasia of the hip (DDH) refers to a spectrum of hip abnormalities that involve dysplasia of the acetabulum and results in instability of the hip. The acetabulum does not develop completely and permits the femoral head to be partially or completely moved away from it. It may be present at birth or develop later (Wilson et al., 2011). Acetabular dysplasia (also called preluxation) is deficient development of the acetabulum, which is excessively shallow, and/or the femoral head. Partial displacement of the joint where contact remains between the femoral head and acetabulum is termed subluxation. Dislocation refers to a complete displacement of the joint where there is no contact between the acetabulum and femoral head.

A variety of factors are thought to be implicated in DDH, including family history, intrauterine position and crowding, and breech presentation. It is more common in female infants, thought to be a result of increased susceptibility to maternal secretion of relaxin, which may contribute to laxness of the ligaments (Godley, 2013). Firstborn children are also more susceptible, probably related to an unstretched uterus and tight abdominal muscles that compress the uterine contents (Castañeda, 2009).

Assessment Findings

Following birth, all newborns are routinely assessed for DDH. Visual inspection and a series of manoeuvres pinpoint indicators of the need for further diagnostic testing and referrals.

With the newborn lying on a firm surface and as relaxed as possible, the nurse grasps both ankles and manually extends both legs. This manoeuvre may reveal that one leg appears slightly shorter than the other. With the infant prone, the nurse visually compares the skin

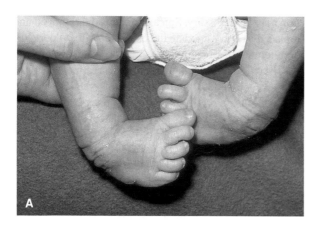

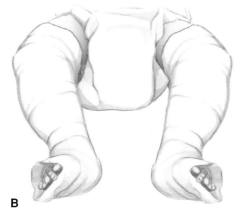

FIGURE 22.16 **A:** Initial appearance of talipes equinovarus (clubfoot). **B:** Application of the casts for treatment.

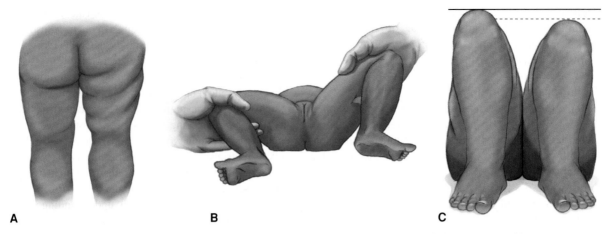

A   **B**   **C**

FIGURE 22.17 Developmental dysplasia of the hip is characterized by (**A**) asymmetric skin folds on the thighs or buttocks; (**B**) limited abduction of the hip; and (**C**) one leg appearing shorter than the other.

folds from gluteal crease to knee, again comparing bilaterally.

With the baby supine, the nurse elicits the Galeazzi sign by flexing the infant's hips and knees to 90 degrees (Das & Paul, 2013). The Galeazzi sign is positive if the nurse detects asymmetry upon visual comparison of the height of the knees. (Fig. 22.17) The Ortolani and Barlow manoeuvres are other methods for detecting DDHs. The sensation of the dislocated hip reducing is felt with the Ortolani manoeuvre, while the Barlow test detects the unstable hip dislocating from the acetabulum. See Nursing Procedure 22.3. The infant is in the supine position with the hips flexed to 90 degrees to perform the Barlow test. "The adducted hip is gently pushed downwards and laterally to see whether it is dislocatable" (Sinha et al., 2012, p. 60). It is considered a positive test when a "chunk" or sensation of posterior movement is felt. Ultrasound will rule out false-positive assessments and confirm the diagnosis of DDH.

Nurses having contact with newborns and young infants are alert for indicators of hip joint laxity that may not have been apparent at birth. Assessments continue throughout health visits until the child is walking with an obviously normal gait.

Collaborative Management

Treatment begins with diagnosis of the condition. The earlier treatment is initiated, the fewer complications the baby experiences, and the more favourable is the prognosis (Wilson et al., 2011). The proximal femoral head is centred in the acetabulum and then splinted with a device to keep the head of the femur in the reduced position. To maintain flexion of the knees and hips and abduction, the Pavlik harness is commonly used for infants up to 6 months of age (Fig. 22.18). When worn continuously until clinical and radiographic examinations are normal, the Pavlik harness maintains reduc-

tion of the femoral head in the acetabulum, allowing muscle and cartilage development for a stable hip. The time required to attain normal examinations varies from 6 weeks to as much as 3 to 5 months (Wilson et al., 2011).

If treatment is delayed and the infant develops adduction contractures, he or she will need more intensive therapy. Traction to slowly and gently stretch the hip to full abduction and hip spica casting to maintain reduction may be necessary. Spica casts must be removed and replaced to accommodate the child's growth. Older children require open reduction.

Because of the lengthy nature of treatment, parents will need to understand the necessity and long-term implications of compliance with prescribed continuous splinting, as well as the importance of maintaining hip flexion and abduction. For example, they will need

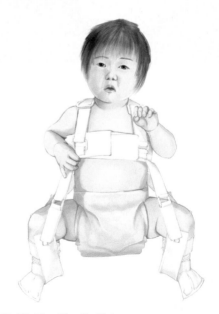

FIGURE 22.18 The Pavlik harness.

NURSING PROCEDURE 22.3

Performing Ortolani and Barlow Manoeuvres

PURPOSE

To evaluate the newborn for evidence of developmental dysplasia of the hip (DDH)

ASSESSMENT AND PLANNING

- Review the newborn's medical record for factors that may predispose him or her to DDH.
- Ask the parents about any past history of congenital problems, including those involving the leg.
- Assess parental knowledge of and previous exposure to the manoeuvres.
- Inspect the newborn while he or she is supine for evidence of apparent limb shortening on one side, and while he or she is prone for asymmetric gluteal and thigh folds.
- Flex both lower extremities at the knee and hip toward the abdomen; observe for differences in the height of the knees.
- Gather equipment
- Flat, clean, warm surface

IMPLEMENTATION

1. Explain the manoeuvres and their rationale to the parents *to help allay their anxiety.*
2. Wash hands; place the supine newborn on a firm, clean, warm surface *to facilitate testing and to minimize heat loss.*
3. Place hands on each lower extremity so that the middle finger is over the greater trochanter and the thumb is on the inner aspect of each thigh. Flex the knees and hips at a 90-degree angle toward the abdomen.
4. Abduct each hip while holding the opposite hip in maximum abduction (*to lock the pelvis*) and applying upward pressure *to determine whether the head of the femur moves into the acetabulum;* listen or feel for a clicking or clucking sound, *which indicates a positive Ortolani sign suggesting hip dislocation.*

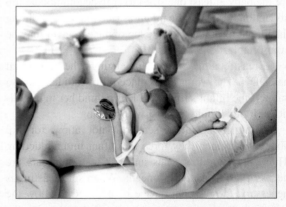

Step 4. Manoeuvre for Ortolani sign.

5. With the infant again in the supine position, apply downward pressure while adducting the hip and maintaining knee flexion at 90 degrees. Note any feeling of the femoral head slipping out of the acetabulum, *which indicates a positive Barlow sign suggesting dislocation.*
6. Return the newborn to a position of comfort.
7. Wash hands; document and report findings.

EVALUATION

- The newborn tolerated the manouvres without difficulty or pain.
- The newborn exhibited no evidence of DDH.

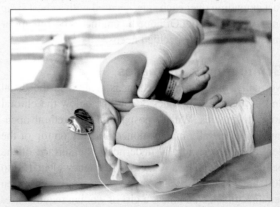

Step 5. Manoeuvre for Barlow sign.

(continued)

NURSING PROCEDURE 22.3 (CONTINUED)
Performing Ortolani and Barlow Manoeuvres

AREAS FOR CONSIDERATION AND ADAPTATION

Life Span Considerations

- Asymmetrical thigh folds may not be reliable indicators of DDH, because an uneven number of folds is a normal finding in some newborns.
- Perform these manoeuvres very gently in the first few days after birth, to prevent persistent dislocation from manoeuvres done too vigorously.
- The earlier the condition is detected, the easier it is to correct; be aware that some newborns exhibit negative signs during initial assessment only to demonstrate evidence of DDH at a later health care visit.
- Inform parents of the need for follow-up testing to confirm the diagnosis.

extra time to bathe and dress the child because they will have to remove and reapply the harness or brace or work around the cast. Parents need a good explanation and demonstration of how to apply the harness; if the infant is left out of the harness for too long a time, success of the intervention may be compromised (Hassan, 2009). Nurses offer praise and encouragement to parents for their efforts. Parents can purchase clothing for the baby at least one size larger to accommodate hip abduction. Carrying the infant astride the hip or holding the infant upright astride the leg of the caregiver may be comfortable.

Breastfeeding can be challenging when an infant has DDH. The woman can place pillows to her side to support the infant's trunk and legs behind her in a traditional football hold to assist with feeding.

Commercial infant seats do not allow for hip abduction; rather, they force the infant into adduction. Thus, special infant seats and car restraint seats are necessary to fit the child's needs. When spica casting is necessary, the restraint device is modified to allow the infant's buttocks to rest on the edge of the seat with the cast extending over each side, secured with a chest strap and a centre buckle. Orthopedic engineers design appliances according to specified needs.

Genitourinary Anomalies

Normally, the urethral opening is centred in the distal end of the penis in males or midline below the clitoral hood in females. With hypospadias, the urethral opening is congenitally malpositioned dorsally on top of the penile shaft or ventrally underneath the surface of the penile shaft. Statistics related to frequency (1 in 150 to 300) are unreliable because hypospadias in females often remains undetected unless a girl or woman requires urethral catheterization, at which point health care providers have difficulty locating the urethral opening.

Hypospadias in males is apparent at birth during inspection of the penile shaft. It is not life-threatening, but male children may be disturbed when the stream of urine sprays sideways. Additionally, a *chordee* (a fibrous band causing downward deflection of the penis) may lead to embarrassment and health-related concerns.

Treatment of hypospadias typically involves corrective surgery. Major associated risks include anaesthesia, bleeding, and infection. Consultation with urology specialists is indicated. Parents need to understand the rationale for *not* circumcising the newborn male with hypospadias, because the foreskin is an ideal tissue for graft that may be needed for the corrective repair. Those families whose religion or culture includes ritual circumcision should investigate the possibility of having the circumcision done immediately before the corrective repair, so that the foreskin can be harvested and used as necessary.

A nurse who notes the obvious defect of hypospadias documents the location of the lesion (dorsal or ventral) and involvement of the glans penis, as well as any chordee. During examination of the newborn, the nurse assesses testicular descent by palpating and rolling the testicles gently between the thumb and forefinger. Such examination is necessary because hypospadias is associated with cryptorchidism. In addition, the nurse evaluates the newborn's urinary stream by applying a pediatric urine collection bag while the newborn remains undiapered.

Most new parents are interested in investigating their newborn to check that everything is "normal"—first counting fingers and toes, and later inspecting the genitals. When a newborn has obvious hypospadias, health care providers inform parents of the genital abnormality as soon as it is identified. The discussion may be distressing for the family, who might fear urologic, sexual, and psychological problems resulting from the defect.

Nurses provide information about the condition and measures to correct it, giving parents photographs of children before and after surgical repair.

SUMMARY

- Many factors can present risks to the fetus and lead to newborn complications. Attempts to identify such risks begin as early as possible with genetic screening, health risk assessments, and early prenatal care and testing. Ongoing nursing assessments and evaluations during the first hours of life also help identify newborns at risk.

- Problems related to newborn size may be categorized as LBW, weight less than 2500 g; VLBW, weight less than 1500 g; and extremely low birth weight, weight of 1000 g or less.

- Newborns also may be classified by their expected size for weeks' gestation as AGA (growth pattern is as expected for gestational age, and weight falls between the 10th and 90th percentiles on an intrauterine growth chart); SGA (weight below the 10th percentile on an intrauterine growth chart for the gestational age); and LGA (weight about the 90th percentile on intrauterine growth charts for gestational age).

- A newborn born any time before 38 weeks' gestation, independent of birth weight, is classified as preterm or premature. A newborn born after 41 weeks' gestation is classified as postterm.

- Key areas to assess for a newborn with complications related to size or gestational age include respiratory status, skin, thermoregulation, glucose levels, feeding, and family coping.

- Nurses establish rapport with parents, caregivers, and other significant family members to develop a trusting relationship. Using goal-directed communication is necessary to elicit information about the family's ability to cope with the complications, family strengths, and resources needed for effective adaptation.

- Oral feedings are preferred if the newborn has adequate sucking and swallowing reflexes, GI functioning, and energy levels. Breast milk is most desirable, especially for preterm newborns. Many premature infants will require more calories, proteins, and minerals than can be supplied by breast milk. For these infants, specially formulated human milk fortifiers may be added to breast milk. If breast milk is not available, specialized formulas containing 80 kcal/100 mL and fortified with calcium, phosphorus, and iron can supply the needed extra calories. Special nipples, called "premie" nipples, are commercially available. They are shorter and softer, making them easier to compress.

- Gavage feedings are indicated for the physiologically stable newborn who cannot ingest sufficient breast milk or formula orally to satisfy nutritive requirements. Trophic feedings (early or minimal enteral feedings) may be used to nourish the gut, promote intestinal maturation, and stimulate motility. Parenteral nutrition may be used for VLBW newborns who are very physiologically immature and cannot ingest or digest breast milk or formula by the enteral route. Any newborn receiving an alternative form of feeding should be provided with non-nutritive sucking.

- Nurses play a key role in promoting family attachment with the newborn experiencing complications. Role modelling of attachment behaviours and allowing time for family members to verbalize feelings are important.

- Hyperbilirubinemia (elevated serum bilirubin level) is manifested by jaundice, a yellow discolouration of the skin and tissues. Mild, self-limiting jaundice (physiologic jaundice) develops on approximately the third day after birth in formula-fed newborns and somewhat later in breast-fed newborns. When hyperbilirubinemia persists or remains untreated, pathologic jaundice occurs. Phototherapy is instituted when TSB levels reach threshold levels determined by the infant's gestational and postnatal ages. Exchange transfusions may be used when jaundice does not respond to intensive phototherapy.

- Congenital heart disease refers to a group of cardiac defects that either change the direction of flow or change the normal structure and function of the heart chambers or great vessels. VSD is the most common of all congenital cardiac anomalies. Other defects include ASD, atrioventricular canal, pulmonary stenosis, patent ductus arteriosus, aortic stenosis, coarctation of the aorta, tetralogy of Fallot, and transposition of the great arteries.

- Congenital diaphragmatic hernia refers to the protrusion of abdominal contents through an abnormality in the diaphragm. As a result, abdominal contents rise up through the defect and occupy space in the thoracic cavity. Surgery is performed as soon after birth as possible.

- Neural tube defects, a group of anomalies involving the brain and spinal cord, include anencephaly, spina bifida, and encephalocele. Spina bifida is the most common neural tube defect and can be manifested in one of three forms: spina bifida occulta, meningocele, or myelomeningocele, the most serious and disabling form. Folic acid supplementation during pregnancy is a major primary prevention strategy.

- Congenital defects of the abdominal wall include omphalocele and gastroschisis. Gentle handling is essential to prevent trauma to the sac or exposed abdominal organs.

- Clefting, which occurs when the embryonic structures of the upper lip, nose, and/or hard and soft palate fail to close and fuse, may be complete or incomplete. The clefting may involve only the lip (unilateral or bilateral), only the palate (hard and/or soft), or a combination of the lip and palate. Surgery is the primary mode of treatment. Parents need much emotional support and teaching.

- Esophageal atresia involves a disruption in the esophageal passageway to the stomach, in which it is closed off and ends in a blind pouch. Without surgical intervention, the newborn has no way to ingest fluid and nutrition. Classic findings include coughing, choking, and cyanosis with feeding, along with excessive salivation and drooling in the side-lying position. Tracheoesophageal fistula involves an abnormal opening between the trachea and esophagus that permits food and fluid to be diverted to the lungs, causing aspiration, and air from the trachea to enter the stomach, causing distention.

- DDH refers to a group of hip abnormalities including a shallow acetabulum, subluxation, or complete dislocation. A positive Galeazzi sign, Ortolani manoeuvre, and Barlow test aid in determining DDH. Diagnostic imaging confirms the diagnosis.

- With hypospadias, the urethral opening is located ventrally (on the underneath surface of the penile shaft) instead of being positioned in the centre in the distal end of the penile shaft.

Questions to Ponder

1. How are the physical characteristics and potential complications of a preterm newborn similar to and yet different from those of a postterm newborn?

2. A Muslim couple requests that their newborn wear a protective amulet during phototherapy for hyperbilirubinemia.
   - Would wearing the amulet pose any health hazard to the newborn?
   - If wearing the amulet is contraindicated, what other options might be available to incorporate cultural and religious practices of the family?

REVIEW QUESTIONS

1. Which of the following should the nurse expect to find when assessing a newborn at 42 weeks' gestation?
   A. Abundant lanugo
   B. Few plantar creases
   C. Dry, scaly skin
   D. Fused eyelids

2. Rupture of a client's membranes revealed thick, green-stained amniotic fluid. Following delivery the neonate has poor tone and is not making respiratory efforts. Which intervention should be the priority immediately following delivery?
   A. Vigourously dry the newborn.
   B. Administer blow-by oxygen.
   C. Assess the apical heart rate.
   D. Intubate the trachea and perform suctioning.

3. When reviewing the medical record of an LGA newborn, which factor in the maternal history should the nurse identify as most likely associated with this condition?
   A. Exposure to rubella in the first trimester
   B. Diabetes
   C. Polyhydramnios
   D. Cervical insufficiency

4. Which of the following risk factors place the neonate at an increased risk of developing significant hyperbilirubinemia?
   A. Female sex
   B. Formula feeding
   C. Postterm delivery
   D. A sibling who had significant jaundice

5. Which of the following assessment findings in a newborn would be suggestive of fetal alcohol spectrum disorder?
   A. Wide, broad upper lip
   B. Short nose
   C. High nasal bridge
   D. Large, protruding eyes

6. When planning the care for a newborn with hyperbilirubinemia who is to receive phototherapy, which intervention should the nurse be most likely to include?
   A. Applying small eye patches to each eye
   B. Keeping the newborn clothed in a T-shirt and diaper
   C. Turning the newborn every 6 to 8 hours
   D. Restricting fluids while the newborn is under the lights

7. Auscultation of a newborn's chest reveals absent breath sounds and audible bowel sounds on the right side. Which of the following conditions would the nurse interpret these findings as suggestive of?
   A. Congenital heart disease
   B. Respiratory distress syndrome
   C. Congenital diaphragmatic hernia
   D. Omphalocele

8. Which of the following expected outcomes would be the highest priority when preparing a newborn with a cleft lip and palate for discharge?
   A. Extended family states that they will help support the new family.
   B. Parents schedule a visit with the plastic surgeon for palate reconstruction.
   C. Parents demonstrate success with appropriate feeding techniques.

D. Siblings exhibit beginning attachment behaviours with the newborn.

9. A nurse suspects that a newborn has a tracheoesophageal fistula. Which intervention would be most appropriate?

A. Encourage the mother to breastfeed on demand.

B. Place the baby prone, elevating the head 30 degrees.

C. Institute positive-pressure ventilation.

D. Prepare for insertion of a gastrostomy tube.

10. A female newborn diagnosed with developmental dysplasia of the hip is to be treated using a Pavlik harness. After teaching the parents about caring for the newborn, which statement by the parents indicates the need for additional teaching?

A. We'll make sure to schedule extra time in the morning to dress her.

B. She seems to like when I carry her astride on my hip.

C. We'll use the harness for 1 month and then she'll be fine.

D. We'll need to check out a special infant car seat for her to use.

REFERENCES

American Academy of Pediatrics Section on Ophthalmology, American Academy of Ophthalmology and Strabismus, and American Association of Certified Orthoptists. (2013) Screening examination of premature infants for retinopathy of prematurity. *Pediatrics, 131*(1), 189–195.

Anuntaseree, W., Patrapinyokul, S., Suntorniohanakul, S., & Thongsuksal, P. (2002). Congenital bronchoesophageal fistula and tracheoesophageal fistula with esophageal atresia. *Pediatric Pulmonology, 33*(2), 162–164.

Arduini, D., & Vendola, M. (2012). The development from fetus to newborn. In G. Buonocore, R. Bracci, & M. Weindling (Eds.), *Neonatology: A practical approach to neonatal diseases* (pp. 7–16). New York: Springer.

Askin, D. F., & Wilson, D. (2011). The high-risk newborn and family. In M. J. Hockenberry & D. Wilson (Eds.), *Wong's nursing care of infants and children* (pp. 314–389). St. Louis, MO: Elsevier.

Aylott, M. (2006). The neonatal energy triangle, Part 2: Thermoregulatory and respiratory adaptation. *Paediatric Nursing, 18*(7), 38–42.

Aziz, K., & Dancey, P.; Canadian Pediatric Society (posted 2004; reaffirmed 2013). Screening guidelines for newborns at risk for low blood glucose. *Paediatric Child Health, 9*(10), 723–729.

Barrington, K. J., & Sankaran, K., (2007, reaffirmed 2011). Guidelines for detection, management and prevention of hyperbilirubinemia in term and late preterm newborn infants. *Paediatric Child Health, 12*(suppl B), 1B–12B. Retrieved from http://www.cps.ca/en/documents/position/hyperbilirubinemia-newborn

Barseghyan, K., Aghajanian, P., & Miller, D. (2012). The prevalence of preterm births in pregnancies complicated with fetal gastroschisis. *Archives of Gynecology and Obstetrics, 286*(4), 889–892.

Bérard, A., Le Tiec, M., & De Vera, M. A. (2012). Study of the costs and morbidities oflate-preterm birth. *Archives of Disease in Childhood: Fetal Neonatal Ed, 97*(5), F329–F334.

Blackburn, S. T. (2013). *Maternal, fetal, & neonatal physiology: A clinical perspective* (4th ed.). St. Louis, MO: Saunders Elsevier.

Boardman, J. P., Wusthoff, C. J., & Cowan, F. M. (2013). Hypoglycaemia and neonatal brain injury. *Archives of Disease in Childhood: Education and Practice Ed, 98*(1), 2–6.

Brown, R. N., & Nicolaides, K. H. (2000). Increased fetal nuchal translucency: Possible association with esophageal atresia. *Ultrasound in Obstetrics and Gynecology, 15*, 631–632.

Brown, V., & Landers, S. (2011). Heat balance. In S. Gardner, B. Carter, M. Enzman-Hines, & J. Hernandez. *Merenstein & Gardner's handbook of neonatal intensive care* (7th ed., pp. 113–133). St. Louis, MO: Mosby.

Bruch, S., Hirschl, R., & Coran, A. (2010). The diagnosis and management of recurrent tracheoesophageal fistulas. *Journal of Pediatric Surgery, 45*(2), 337–340.

Bruzoni, M., & Albanese, C. (2012). Perioperative management of the neonatal patient. In S. Dolgin & C. Hamner (Eds.), *Surgical care of major newborn malformations* (pp. 1–32). Hackensack, NJ: World Scientific.

Buescher, J., & Bland, H. (2011). Care of the newborn. In R. Rakel & D. Rakel (Eds.), *Textbook of family medicine* (8th ed., pp. 402–420). St. Louis, MO: Elsevier.

Cachat, F., Van Melle, G., McGahren, E. D., Reinberg, O., & Norwood, V. (2006). Arterial hypertension after surgical closure of omphalocele and gastroschisis. *Pediatric Nephrology, 21*, 225–229.

Canadian Paediatric Society. (2011). *Addendum to the NRP provider textbook 6th edition: Recommendations for specific modifications in the Canadian context.* Retrieved from http://www.cps.ca/en/nrp-prn/instructor-resources

Caplan, M. (2009). Probiotic and prebiotic supplementation for the prevention of neonatal necrotizing enterocolitis. *Journal of Perinatology, 29*, S2–S6.

Carlo, W., McDonald, S. A., Fanaroff, A. A., Vohr B. R., Stoll, B. J., Ehrenkranz, R. A., et al. (2011). Association of antenatal corticosteroids with mortality and neurodevelopmental outcomes among infants born at 22 to 25 weeks' gestation. *Journal of the American Medical Association, 306*(21), 2348–2358.

Castañeda, P. (2009). Pediatric hip dysplasia and evaluation with ultrasound. *Future Medicine, 3*(5), 465–472.

Catalano, P., Di Pace, M., Caruso, A., Casuccio, A., & De Grazia, E. (2011). Gastroesophageal reflux in young children treated for esophageal atresia: Evaluation with pH-multichannel intraluminal impedance. *Journal of Pediatric Gastroenterology & Nutrition, 52*(6), 686–690.

Celayir, A. C., & Erdogan, E. (2003). Case reports: An infrequent cause of misdiagnosis in esophageal atresia. *Journal of Pediatric Surgery, 38*(9), 1389.

Centers for Disease Control and Prevention. (2013). Facts about cleft lip and cleft palate. Retrieved from http://www.cdc.gov/ncbddd/birthdefects/cleftlip.html

Chitayat, D., Langlois, S., & Wilson, R. D. (2011). Society of Obstetricians and Gynaecologists of Canada (SOGC) Canadian College of Medical Geneticists (CCMG) Clinical Practice Guideline: Prenatal screening for fetal aneuploidy in singleton pregnancies. *Journal of Obstetrics and Gynaecology of Canada, 33*(7), 736–750.

Chua, X., Mohamed, J., & van Bever, HP. (2013). Prevalence of latex allergy in spina bifida patients in Singapore. *Asia Pacific Allergy Journal, 3*(2), 96–99.

Crabbe, D. C. (2003). Isolated tracheo-oesophageal fistula. *Paediatric Respiratory Reviews, 4*, 74–78.

Czerkiewicz, I., Dreux, S., Beckmezian, A., Benachi, A., Salomon, L., Schmitz, T., et al. (2011). Biochemical amniotic fluid pattern for prenatal diagnosis of esophageal atresia. *Pediatric Research, 70*, 199–202.

Das, K., & Paul, B. (2013). Examination of the musculoskeletal system. In K. Das (Ed.), *Clinical medicine* (4th ed., pp. 241–263). London: JP Medical.

Dent, J., & McKenna, K. (2010). Management of haematological disorders. In G. Boxwell (Ed.), *Neonatal intensive care nursing* (2nd ed., pp. 204–229). New York: Routledge.

Dutta, A. K. (2012). Respiratory distress in newborns. In A. K. Sachdeva & M. P. Dutta (Ed.), *Advances in pediatrics* (2nd ed.). New Delhi: Jaypee Brothers Medical Publishers, 83–91.

Evans, N. (2012). Diagnosis of the preterm patent ductus arteriosus: Clinical signs, biomarkers, or ultrasound? *Seminars in Perinatology, 36*(2), 114–122.

Finan, E., Aylward, D., & Aziz, K. (2011). Neonatal resuscitation guidelines update: A case-based review. *Pediatrics & Child Health, 16*(5), 289–291.

Forsythe, E. S., & Allen, P. J. (2013). Health risks associated with late-preterm infants: Implications for newborn primary care. *Pediatric Nursing, 39*(4), 197–201.

Fraser, D. (2012). Complications of positive pressure ventilation. In D. Fraser (Ed.), *Acute respiratory care of the neonate* (pp. 195–238). Petaluma, CA: NICU Ink.

Gardner, S., Enzman-Hines, M., & Dickey, L. (2011). Respiratory diseases. In S. Gardner, B. Carter, M. Enzman-Hines, & J. Hernandez. *Merenstein & Gardner's handbook of neonatal intensive care* (7th ed., pp. 581–677). St. Louis, MO: Mosby.

Gardner, S., & Hernandez, J. (2011). Initial nursery care. In S. Gardner, B. Carter, M. Enzman-Hines, & J. Hernandez. *Merenstein & Gardner's handbook of neonatal intensive care* (7th ed., pp. 78–112). St. Louis, MO: Mosby.

Garofalo, M., & Abenhaim, H. A. (2012). Early versus delayed cord clamping in term and preterm births: A review. *Journal of Obstetrics & Gynaecology Canada, 34*(6), 525–531.

Godley, D. R. (2013). Assessment, diagnosis, and treatment of developmental dysplasia of the hip. *Journal of the American Academy of Physician Assistants, 26*(3), 54–58.

Grant, B., Morgan, G., McCrossan, B., Crealey, G., Sands, A., Craig, B., et al. (2010). Remote diagnosis of congenital heart disease: The impact of telemedicine. *Archives of Disease in Childhood, 95*(4), 276–280.

Greer, M. (2010). Cerebral and spinal malformations. In L. Rowland & T. Pedley (Eds.), *Merritt's neurology* (12th ed., pp. 1035–1059). Philadelphia, PA: Lippincott Williams & Wilkins.

Gyamfi-Bannerman, C. (2012). Late preterm birth: management dilemmas. *Obstetrics & Gynecology Clinics of North America, 39*(1), 35–45.

Hammerman, C., Bin-Nun, A., & Kaplan, M. (2012). Managing the patent ductus arteriosus in the premature neonate: A new look at what we thought we knew. *Seminars in Perinatology, 36*(2), 130–138.

Harijan, P., & Boyle, E. M. (2012). Health outcomes in infancy and childhood of moderate and late preterm infants. *Seminars in Fetal & Neonatal Medicine, 17*(3), 159–162.

Harris, P., Oliver, N., Slater, P., Murdoch, L., & Moss, A. (2010). Safety of neonatal cleft lip repair. *Journal of Plastic Surgery and Hand Surgery, 44*(4–5), 231–236.

Hassan, F. (2009). Compliance of parents with regard to Pavlik harness treatment in developmental dysplasia of the hip. *Journal of Pediatric Orthopaedics, 18*(3), 111–115.

Ives, K., & Austin, T. (2009). Neonatology. In M. Gardiner, S. Eisen, & C. Murphy (Eds.), *Training in pediatrics: The essential curriculum* (pp. 1–28). Oxford: Oxford University Press.

Jones, K., Benirschke, K., & Chambers, C. (2009). Gastroschisis: Etiology and developmental pathways. *Clinical Genetics, 75*(4), 322–325.

Kalyoncu, Ö., Aygün, C., Çetinoğlu, E., & Küçüködük, S. (2010). Neonatal morbidity and mortality of late-preterm infants. *Journal of Maternal-Fetal and Neonatal Medicine, 23*(7), 607–612.

Kaplan, M., Bromiker, R., & Hammerman, C. (2011). Severe neonatal hyperbilirubinemia and kernicterus: Are these still problems in the third millennium? *Neonatology, 100*, 354–362.

Karlsen, K. A. (2013). *The S.T.A.B.L.E. program: Pre-transport/post-resuscitation stabilization care of sick infants guidelines for neonatal healthcare providers* (6th ed.). Salt Lake City: S.T.A.B.L.E. Inc.

Kattwinkel, J. (Ed.). (2011). *Neonatal resuscitation textbook* (6th ed.). Elk Grove Village, IL: American Heart Association, American Academy of Pediatrics.

Kenney, P., Hoover, D., Williams, L., & Iskersky, V. (2011). Cardiovascular diseases and surgical interventions. In S. Gardner, B. Carter, M. Enzman-Hines, & J. Hernandez. *Merenstein & Gardner's handbook of neonatal intensive care* (7th ed., pp. 678–716). St. Louis, MO: Mosby.

Kim, E., Lee, T., & Chae, S. (2009). Effect of unrestricted bottle-feeding on early postoperative course after cleft palate repair. *Journal of Craniofacial Surgery, 20*(8), 1886–1888.

Klauser, C. K., Briery, C. M., Keiser, S. D., Martin, R. W., Kosek, M. A., & Morrison, J. C. (2012). Effect of antenatal tocolysis on neonatal outcomes. *Journal of Maternal & Fetal Neonatal Medicine, 25*(12), 2778–2781.

Klebermass-Schrehof, K., Czaba, C., Olischar, M., Fuiko, R., Waldhoer, T., Rona, Z., et al. (2012). Impact of low-grade intraventricular hemorrhage on long-term neurodevelopmental outcome in preterm infants. *Childs Nervous System, 28*(12), 2085–2092.

Kohr, L. M. (2012). Tetralogy of Fallot and pulmonary atresia with ventricular septal defect. In M. F. Hazinski (Ed.), *Nursing care of the critically ill child* (3rd ed., pp. 348–355). St. Louis, MO: Elsevier.

Kuleva, M., Salomon, L., Benoist, G., Ville, Y., & Dumez, Y. (2012). The value of daily fetal heart rate home monitoring in addition to serial ultrasound examinations in pregnancies complicated by fetal gastroschisis. *Prenatal Diagnosis, 32*(8), 789–796.

Leduc, D., Senikas, V., & Lalonde, A. B. (2009). Active management of the third stage of labour; Prevention and treatment of postpartum hemorrhage. *Journal of Obstetrics & Gynaecology Canada, 31*(10), 980–993.

Lee, J-S. (2010). *Biomedical engineering entrepreneurship.* Hackensack, NJ: World Scientific.

Lemoine, C., Aspirot, A., Le Henaff, G., Piloquet, H., & Levesque, C. (2013). Characterization of esophageal motility following esophageal atresia repair using high-resolution esophageal manometry. *Journal of Pediatric Gastroenterology & Nutrition, 56*(6), 609–614.

Li, D., Rosito, G., & Slagle, T. (2013). Probiotics for the prevention of necrotizing enterocolitis in neonates: An 8-year retrospective cohort study. *Journal of Clinical Pharmacy and Therapeutics, 38*(6), 445–449.

Loder, R. T., & Skopelja, E. N. (2011). The epidemiology and demographics of hip dysplasia. *ISRN Orthopedics, 2011*, 238607.

Lovvorn, H., Glenn, J., Pacetti, A., & Carter, B. (2011). Neonatal surgery. In S. Gardner, B. Carter, M. Enzman-Hines, & J. Hernandez. *Merenstein & Gardner's handbook of neonatal intensive care* (7th ed., pp. 812–847). St. Louis, MO: Mosby.

Magee, L., Sawchuck, D., Synnes, A. & von Dadelszen, P. (2011). Magnesium sulphate for fetal neuroprotection. *Journal of Obstetrics & Gynaecology Canada, 33*(5), 516–529.

Mattei, P. (2012). Double H-type tracheoesophageal fistulas identified and repaired in 1 operation. *Journal of Pediatric Surgery, 47*(11), e11–e13.

McGowan, J., Rozance, P., Price-Douglas, W., & Hay, W. (2011). Glucose homeostasis. In S. Gardner, B. Carter, M. Enzman-Hines, & J. Hernandez. *Merenstein & Gardner's handbook of neonatal intensive care* (7th ed., pp. 353–377). St. Louis, MO: Mosby.

Miltenburg, A. S., van Elburg, R. M., Kostense, P. J., van Geijn, H. P., & Bolte, A. C. (2011). Neonatal morbidity in term neonates is related to gestational age at birth and level of care. *Journal of Perinatal Medicine, 39*, 605–610. doi:10.1515/JPM.2011.070

Morton, N., Fairgrieve, R., Moores, A., & Wallace, E. (2011). Anesthesia for the full-term and ex-premature infant. In G. Gregory & D. Andropoulos (Eds.), *Gregory's pediatric anesthesia* (5th ed., pp. 497–519). New York: Wiley & Sons.

Muglia, L., & Katz, M. (2010). The enigma of spontaneous preterm birth. *New England Journal of Medicine, 362*(6), 529–535.

Nanci, A. (2008). *Ten Cate's oral histology* (7th ed.). St Louis, MO: Elsevier.

Noble, L. M. (2010). Feeding only human milk benefits premies. *AAP Grand Rounds, 24*(1), 3.

Ojha, S., Elvidge, L, Davies, B., & Deorukhkar, A. (2011). Experience of managing oesophageal atresia ± trachea-oesophageal fistula in a tertiary surgical neonatal centre in the UK. *Archives of Diseases of Childhood Fetal & Neonatal Edition, 96*, Fa23–Fa24.

Parker, S., Mai, C., Strickland, M., Olney, R., Rickard, R., Marengo, L., et al. (2009).Multistate study of the epidemiology of clubfoot. *Birth Defects Research, 85*(11), 897–904.

Polito, A., Piga, S., Cogo, P., Corchia, C., Da Fre, M., Di Lallo, D., et al. (2013). Increased morbidity and mortality in very preterm / VLBW infants with congenital heart disease. *Intensive Care Medicine, 39*(6), 1104–1112.

Public Health Agency of Canada. (2012). About FASDFetal Alcohol Spectrum Disorder (FASD). Retrieved from http://www.phac-aspc.gc.ca/fasd-etcaf/about-eng.php

Rahimian, J. (2013). Disproportionate fetal growth. In A. de Cherney, L. Nathan, T. M. Goodwin, & N. Laufer (Ed.), *Current Diagnosis and Treatment Obstetrics and Gynecology* (11th ed.). New York: McGraw-Hill.

Riley, E. P., Infante, M. A., & Warren, K. R.(2011). Fetal alcohol spectrum disorders: an overview. *Neuropsychology Review, 21*(2), 73–80.

Robinson, S. (2012). Neonatal posthemorrhagic hydrocephalus from prematurity: Pathophysiology and current treatment concepts. *Journal Neurosurgery Pediatrics, 9*(3), 242–258.

Sellmer, A., Tauris, L., Johansen, A., & Henriksen, T. (2012). Necrotizing enterocolitis after red blood cell transfusion in preterm infants with patent ductus arteriosus. *Acta Paediatrica, 101*(12), e570–e572.

Sgro, M., Campbell, D., Barozzino, T., & Shah, V. (2011). Acute neurological findings in a national cohort of neonates with severe neonatal hyperbilirubinemia. *Journal of Perinatology, 31,* 392–396.

Shapiro, S. M. (2010). Chronic bilirubin encephalopathy: diagnosis and outcomes. *Seminars in Fetal and Neonatal Medicine, 15*(3), 157–163.

Sharma, R., Hudak, M., Tepas, J., Wludyka, P., Teng, R-J, Hastings, L., et al. (2010). Prenatal or postnatal indomethacin exposure and neonatal gut injury associated with isolated intestinal perforation and necrotizing enterocolitis. *Journal of Perinatology, 30,* 786–793.

Siggers J, Ostergaard, M. V., Siggers, R. H., Skovgaard, K., Mølbak, L., Thymann, T., et al. (2013). Postnatal amniotic fluid intake reduces gut inflammatory responses and necrotizing enterocolitis in preterm neonates. *American Journal Physiology. Gastrointestinal and Liver Physiology, 304*(10), G864–G875.

Simmons, R. (2012). Abnormalities of fetal growth. In C. Gleason & S. Devaskar (Eds.), *Avery's diseases of the newborn* (9th ed., pp. 51–59). Philadelphia, PA: Saunders.

Simpson, K. (2012). Labor and birth. In K. Simpson (Ed.), *Perinatal nursing* (3rd ed., pp. 300–398). Philadelphia, PA: Lippincott Williams & Wilkins.

Singh, A. (2010). Intrauterine growth restriction (IUGR). In S. Trivedi & M. Puri (Eds.), *Management of high-risk pregnancy: A practical approach* (pp. 176–198). London: JP Medical.

Sinha, S., Miall, L., & Jardine, L. (2012). *Essential neonatal medicine* (5th ed.). New York: Wiley & Sons.

Stewart, R., Mavroudis, C., & Backer, C. (2012). Tetralogy of Fallot. In C. Mavroudis & C. Backer (Eds.), *Pediatric cardiac surgery* (4th ed., pp. 410–428). New York: Wiley & Sons.

Stoll, C., Alembik, Y., Dott, B., & Roth, M-P. (2009). Associated malformations in patients with esophageal atresia. *European Journal of Medical Genetics, 52*(5), 287–290.

Tasker, R., McClure, R., & Acerini, C. (2013). *Oxford handbook of paediatrics* (2nd ed). Oxford: Oxford University Press.

Thibodeaux, A., & Mooney-Doyle, K. (2011). Social, cultural, and religious influences on child health promotion. In M. J. Hockenberry & D. Wilson (Eds.), *Wong's nursing care of infants and children* (pp. 20–45). St. Louis, MO: Elsevier.

Van Imhoff, D., Cuperus, F., Dijk, P., Tiribelli, C., & Hulzebos, C. (2012). Physical examination of the newborn. In G. Buonocore, R. Bracci, & M. Weindling (Eds.), *Neonatology: A practical approach to neonatal diseases* (pp. 232–241). New York: Springer.

Wilson, D. (2011). Health problems of the newborn. In M. J. Hockenberry & D. Wilson (Eds.), *Wong's nursing care of infants and children* (pp. 279–313). St. Louis, MO: Elsevier.

Wilson, D., Montagnino, B., & Wilson, K. (2011). Conditions caused by defects in physical development. In M. J. Hockenberry & D. Wilson (Eds.), *Wong's nursing care of infants and children* (pp. 390–463). St. Louis, MO: Elsevier.

Wilson, R. D. (2007). Joint SOGC-Motherrisk clinical practice guideline: Pre-conceptional Vitamin/folic acid supplementation 2007: The use of folic acid in combination with a multivitamin supplement for the prevention of neural tube defects and other congenital anomalies. *Journal Obstetrics and Gynaecology Canada, 29*(12), 1003–1013.

Wolf, A. R., & Jackman, L. (2011). Analgesia and sedation after pediatric cardiac surgery. *Paediatric Anaesthesia, 21*(5), 567–576.

Ziegler, E. E. (2011). Meeting the nutritional needs of the low-birthweight infant. *Annals of Nutrition and Metabolism, 58*(S1), 8–18.

MENOPAUSE AND BEYOND

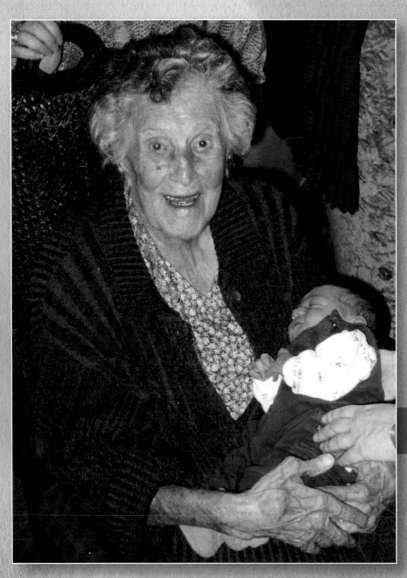

UNIT **6**

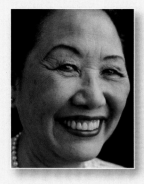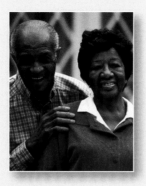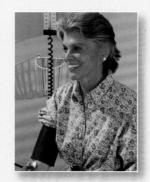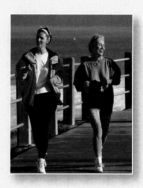

Women whose reproductive years are drawing to a close or have stopped completely make up the fastest-growing segment of the Canadian population. Appropriate holistic care for such clients is a topic of growing importance for nurses and other health care providers, whose encounters with this segment of society are likely to increase significantly with time. In this unit we explore the needs, transitions, concerns, and related care for perimenopausal, menopausal, and older women. We emphasize the health risks and challenges that for some women naturally accompany age-related changes in female physiology, as well as the ways that today's women are diverging from previous generations as a result of social, economic, and political shifts. The inclusion of such content underscores the design and overall philosophy of this text, which is the importance of women's health across the entire lifespan, including, but not limited to, the context of childbearing.

CHAPTER 23

The Menopausal Experience

Carol McDonald and Susan A. Orshan*

 Fran, a 50-year-old married, heterosexual woman, comes to the clinic for a yearly examination. "I notice that I am having more frequent hot flashes," she says. "I wake up at night, drenched. They've really been disrupting my sleep." The client looks pale and tired. Further discussion reveals family transitions. "Both children are now at college, and my husband is working a lot," Fran reports. "It's nice having more time for myself, but sometimes I feel lonely."

 Carol, a 44-year-old married, lesbian woman, experienced menopause 2 years ago. She and her partner have two school-aged, adopted children. Carol has adjusted well to the changes that accompanied her menopause and has tried to optimize her health by making positive lifestyle changes. Her health history includes cigarette smoking since age 18, which she quit 14 months ago. Carol was recently diagnosed with osteopenia. She states, "My mother had osteoporosis and broke her hip. That was a nightmare. I don't want that to happen to me."

You will learn more about Fran's and Carol's stories later. Nurses working with such clients need to understand the material in this chapter to manage care and address issues appropriately. Before beginning, consider the following points related to the above scenarios:

- Based on the information provided, what might be some short-term and long-term priorities for the nurse to establish with each client? Explain your answer.
- What physiologic events form the basis for Fran's symptoms? For Carol's?

*Contributor to first U.S. edition.

- How are the menopausal experiences described similar for each woman? How do they seem different?
- What further details would you expect the nurse to investigate with Fran? With Carol?
- What areas of health promotion, illness prevention, and teaching would the nurse need to address with each client?

LEARNING OBJECTIVES

On completion of this chapter, the reader should be able to:
- Discuss perimenopause and menopause from the viewpoint of health care providers.
- Explain client perspectives on menopause.
- Identify various sociocultural perspectives related to menopause.
- Describe physiologic changes inherent in the menopausal transition and their etiology.
- Identify common psychological adjustments in menopause.
- Summarize the components of assessment focused on menopause-related changes.
- Discuss strategies to enhance the health and comfort of clients experiencing menopausal transition and of their significant others.

KEY TERMS

andropause	osteoporosis
menopause	perimenopause
osteopenia	premature ovarian failure

Almost half of a woman's life is spent after the natural cessation of menstruation known as **menopause**. In Canada, the average age of menopause is 52 years, with most women naturally experiencing this change between 42 and 56 years (Canadian Women's Health Network [CWHN], 2007b). The term menopause is applied retroactively: A woman who has not experienced menstruation for 12 consecutive months is regarded as being in menopause.

Perimenopause is the term given to the period immediately preceding menopause and continuing through the first 12 months of menopause, during which time ovarian hormones fluctuate, resulting in some effects commonly noted with this experience. The duration of perimenopause varies among women and may continue past menopause as estrogen sporadically fluctuates, resulting in postmenopausal vaginal bleeding (Buckler, 2005).

"Menopause is a natural process that occurs in women's lives as part of normal aging" (Edwards & Li, 2013, p. 177). How a woman experiences menopause and the meanings that are given to the experience reflect personal, cultural, and societal perspectives (Deeks, 2004). In some cultures and for some women, menopause represents freedom—freedom from pregnancy, freedom to express wisdom, freedom to redefine themselves and their lives (Hvas, 2006) (Fig. 23.1). Their mothers or other significant older women may have shared their positive views of this change of life; thus, they also look forward to this new life event.

In other cultures and for other women, menopause is perceived as a taboo topic that represents loss—loss of youth, loss of attractiveness, loss of possibilities. These women may be ill-prepared to handle the physiologic and accompanying psychological changes of perimenopause (Deeks & McCabe, 2004). With such a perspective, a woman in her 30s who experiences a hot flash or notices changes in her menstrual cycle may be at a loss to determine what is happening to her body. She may not connect these changes with the beginning

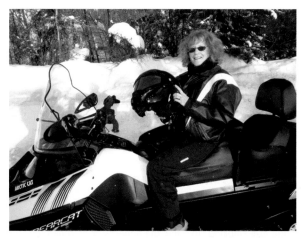

FIGURE 23.1 Many women welcome the menopause transition as providing freedom and opportunities not as available in earlier years.

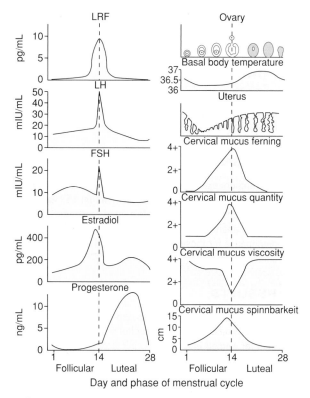

FIGURE 23.2 Hormonal and morphologic changes in the normal menstrual cycle.

of perimenopause and may be embarrassed to ask questions about her experience.

PHYSIOLOGIC BASIS OF NATURALLY OCCURRING PERIMENOPAUSE AND MENOPAUSE

During each normal menstrual cycle, the ovaries produce estrogen and progesterone in varying amounts in a relatively predictable pattern (see Chapter 6). Initially, estrogen is the dominant ovarian hormone, whereas progesterone is dominant in the second half of the cycle preceding menstruation. Fewer ovarian hormones during menstruation stimulate the anterior pituitary to secrete follicle-stimulating hormone (FSH), which in turn stimulates the ovarian follicle to mature and be released midcycle (*ovulation*). FSH decreases before ovulation. In turn, the anterior pituitary gland releases luteinizing hormone (LH) to stimulate the corpus luteum of the ruptured follicle to secrete progesterone and some estrogen (Fig. 23.2).

Follicular atresia, the breakdown of the follicles that would become ova, begins during the fetal period and continues until approximately the time of menopause, when almost all follicles are depleted (Broekmans et al., 2004). As the ovaries age, they secrete less estrogen and progesterone. The anterior pituitary gland responds by increasing secretion of FSH in an attempt to "jump-start" ovarian function, usually at approximately 37.5 years of age (although in women with premature ovarian failure this may occur in their teens or 20s) (Woad et al., 2006). Elevation in FSH increases the rate of follicular atresia, which may result in anovulatory cycles, thus decreasing fertility. This period of decreasing fertility is known

as perimenopause (Society of Obstetricians and Gynaecologists of Canada [SOGC], 2009).

Approximately 6 months to 1 year before the onset of actual menopause, estrogen and progesterone secretion decrease more rapidly. However, sporadic fluctuations in ovarian hormones resulting in postmenopausal bleeding may continue for a few years past the cessation of menstruation (Buckler, 2005; Van Voorhis, 2005).

The age at which menopause occurs naturally is based on several factors. One study showed significant associations between breastfeeding and alcohol consumption with early menopause (Dvornyk et al., 2006). Other factors that influence the time of onset of menopause include family history of early menopause; smoking history; socioeconomic status; and over-all number of lifetime ovulatory cycles, determined by such factors as early onset of menarche, not becoming pregnant, and not using oral contraceptives, which prevent ovulation (Hefler et al., 2006; Kinney et al., 2006). See Research Highlight 23.1.

POTENTIAL CHANGES RELATED TO PERIMENOPAUSE AND MENOPAUSE

The degree to which a woman experiences the physiologic changes of perimenopause and menopause can

● **RESEARCH HIGHLIGHT 23.1**   **Alcohol, Caffeine, and Smoking in Relation to Age at Menopause**

PURPOSE

To identify modifiable factors that might contribute to the onset of menopause, specifically use of alcohol, caffeine intake, and current cigarette smoking.

DESIGN AND PARTICIPANTS

Researchers examined longitudinal data from 494 women between 44 and 60 years of age, of whom 159 experienced menopause. They implemented parametric logistic survival analysis to estimate changes in median age at menopause for those who drank alcohol or caffeine or smoked cigarettes.

RESULTS

Median age at menopause was approximately 2.2 years later for women who drank alcohol 5 to 7 days per week than for women who did not drink alcohol. For those who drank at least 1 day per week, menopause was 1.3 years later. Caffeine intake was not associated with age at menopause. Current smoking of more than 13 cigarettes each day (6%) was linked with menopause approximately 3 years earlier than in women who smoked no or fewer than 13 cigarettes per day.

NURSING IMPLICATIONS

These results reflect a proestrogenic effect of moderate alcohol intake and an antiestrogenic effect of heavy cigarette smoking. To enjoy the benefits of estrogen for longer periods, women may wish to limit smoking and pursue interventions to assist with quitting or modifying this behaviour.

Kinney, A., Kline, J., & Levin, B. (2006). *Maturitas*, *54*(1), 27–38.

---

vary greatly (Fig. 23.3). Although some women experience troubling symptoms during menopause, many women have few, if any, effects of the physiologic changes of menopause. Alexander, a professor at the Yale University School of Nursing and a primary care practitioner, speaks for many women's health advocates as she describes menopause as a normal life transition. This perspective challenges the perception of menopause as a disease requiring biomedical or pharmaceutical intervention (Alexander, 2012).

Common physical changes associated with menopause

Hair

- Thinning of scalp hair
- Darkening or thickening of other body hair, such as facial hair

Skin

- Loss of firmness, tension and fluid
- Decrease in melanocytes, which give skin pigment
- Increased sensitivity to sun exposure

Breasts

- Glandular tissue replaced with fat
- Flattening of form

Urinary system

- Thinning of tissue in bladder and urethra
- Increased risk of urinary tract infections

Bone

- Becomes progressively more porous and brittle
- Increased risk of osteoporosis
- More subject to fractures, especially the shoulder, upper arm and hip

Reproductive system

- Few remaining follicles (egg cells) in ovaries
- Reproductive organs decrease in size
- Vaginal mucosa becomes thinner, less lubricated
- Vaginal pH changes, increasing susceptibility to infection
- Endometriosis disappears

FIGURE 23.3 Common physical changes associated with menopause.

Menstrual Cycle

For most women, the first signs that they are entering perimenopause are changes in the length of their menstrual cycle and amount of flow. Cycle length may shorten 2 to 7 days as a result of a shortened follicular phase from increased FSH. Alternately, cycle length may increase from anovulatory cycles, along with a variation in the amount of flow and periodic midcycle spotting (McVeigh, 2005).

Vasomotor Symptoms

Approximately 65% to 80% of women in North America and Europe experience the "cardinal" vasomotor indicators of menopause (hot flashes), sometimes accompanied by diaphoresis during the day, night, or both (Edwards & Li, 2013; Ratka et al., 2006). Such effects begin during perimenopause and may be related to decreased estrogen levels, although estrogen withdrawal alone does not account for them (Freedman, 2005). For example, some studies have shown a connection between cigarette smoking and increased incidence and intensity of hot flashes, regardless of estrogen levels (Gallicchio et al., 2006; Whiteman et al., 2003). For most women, the hot flash mimics the red flush of embarrassment, appearing on the face, neck, and chest. It may last a few seconds to a few minutes, with an actual increase in skin temperature. For some women, it is accompanied by profuse diaphoresis. Many clients experience hot flashes at night, increasing the likelihood of sleep disturbances (Fig. 23.4).

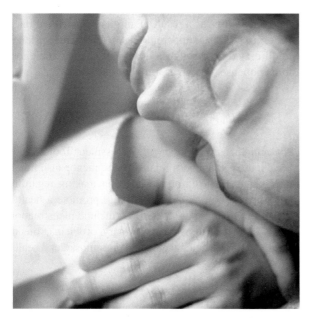

FIGURE 23.4 Vasomotor symptoms occurring during the night, commonly referred to as "night sweats," can contribute to sleep disturbances and subsequent fatigue and depression.

Think back to Fran, the woman at the beginning of the chapter experiencing hot flashes. How would the nurse gather additional information about Fran's symptoms?

Genitourinary Symptoms

The urogenital tract is particularly sensitive to estrogen. During perimenopause and menopause, decreasing estrogen levels lead to thinning, and possible atrophy, of the vaginal mucosa; decreased vaginal lubrication; shortening of the vagina; increased vaginal pH (normal vaginal pH 3.8–4.5); and uterine changes, along with thinning and laxity of the urinary structures, including the urethra and bladder (Ballagh, 2005; Edwards & Li, 2013; Van Voorhis, 2005). These changes increase the client's risk for both urinary tract and vaginal infections.

Fertility

Women's fertility peaks at approximately 24 years and then begins to decrease, with sharp declines between 35 and 40 years (Baird et al., 2005; Burger et al., 2007; Swanton & Child, 2005). Although follicular atresia is responsible for loss of actual oocytes, abnormalities related to meiosis in aging oocytes and decreased hormonal levels are primarily responsible for decreased fertility among women as they age (Burger et al., 2007). Nevertheless, fertility continues to be possible past 40 years. Pregnancy at this stage of life carries higher rates of complications, such as gestational diabetes, preeclampsia, and cesarean birth (see Chapter 12) (Baird et al., 2005; Jacobsson et al., 2004).

Mental Health Changes

For most clients during perimenopause and menopause, more is changing than just their hormones. Many women experience major life events: the stress of family transitions, such as children becoming teenagers or leaving the house for college, divorce, widowhood, or caring for aging family members; career changes, including possible retirement; loss of fertility; and the *perceived* dual loss of youth and attractiveness (Deeks & McCabe, 2004; Gyllstrom et al., 2007). Clients most at risk for depression during this period are those who are sedentary and have been diagnosed previously with depression or who hold negative views of menopause (Dennerstein et al., 2004). Health care providers need to keep in mind that mental health changes in middle age may or may not be related to the hormonal changes of perimenopause and menopause.

Women in midlife may experience hormone-related mood changes, irritability, lethargy, forgetfulness, nervousness, insomnia, and depression (Cohen et al., 2006; Frackiewicz & Cutler, 2000; Woods & Mitchell, 2005). Although these changes may be "labelled" during middle age as premenstrual syndrome, in reality they may be perimenopausal symptoms (Schmidt et al., 2004). It is not certain whether these changes are the result of perimenopause, sleeping difficulties, or the life changes that occur when women reach their 30s or beyond.

Cardiovascular Disease

Coronary artery disease is the number one cause of death for postmenopausal women in western countries (Edwards & Li, 2013). Estrogen is believed to protect women from coronary artery disease and myocardial infarction by increasing the ratio of high-density lipid (HDL) cholesterol to low-density lipid (LDL) cholesterol, increasing vasodilation and improving glucose metabolism. These changes result in a decrease of central abdominal adipose accumulation (Deroo & Korach, 2006). Once the protective mechanisms of estrogen have been diminished, LDL levels that were below those of men before the onset of menopause now exceed those of men, and all the other cardiovascular benefits of estrogen are eliminated as well (Deroo & Korach, 2006). In fact, the rate of death from myocardial infarctions is greater in women than in men (Hoyert et al., 2006). See Chapter 4.

Osteopenia and Osteoporosis

Bone health is an important consideration for women in all stages of life, although in recent years, increasing focus has been placed on bone health for aging women by the media, health care professionals, and the pharmaceutical industry. Although we might note that bone mass peaks between 30 and 35 years of age and decreases after that time, with losses accelerating in conjunction with estrogen deprivation at menopause (Deroo & Korach, 2006; Hobar, 2005), an alternative framing of this concern suggests that bone strength declines as a *natural* part of aging and can result in osteoporosis if precautions are not taken (British Columbia Ministry of Health, 2012). From this perspective **Osteopenia**, meaning a decrease in optimal bone density, can be seen as a part of the aging process that does not necessarily lead to osteoporosis.

Osteoporosis includes both low bone mass density and microarchitectural deterioration of bone tissue, which leads to impaired skeletal integrity and fractures (Andrews et al., 2000). The Osteoporosis Society of Canada states that one in four women and one in eight men over the age of 50 have osteoporosis. Placed in the context of the prevalence with age, osteoporosis "increased with age from approximately 6% at 50 years of age to over 50% above 80 years of age" (Society of Obstetricians and Gynaecologists of Canada [SOGC], 2006, S95). See Chapters 2 and 24.

 Consider Carol, the woman from the beginning of the chapter diagnosed with osteopenia. What is the difference between osteopenia and osteoporosis? Would the nurse consider Carol to be at risk for fractures? What areas would be important for the nurse to assess?

Breast Cancer

Risks for breast cancer are related to many factors, including genetic, environmental, and lifestyle components (see Chapter 4). The amount of exposure to exogenous or endogenous estrogen (or both) increases a person's risk for developing breast cancer. In other words, a woman who experienced early menarche, late menopause, or both; never became pregnant; did not use oral contraceptives; or had some combination of these factors would be exposed to more estrogen through multiple ovulatory cycles than a woman who experienced late menarche, early menopause, or both and had multiple suppressed ovulatory cycles, either through pregnancy or oral contraceptive use. (See Chapter 4 for additional information.)

Other Alterations

Society tends to focus on hormonal changes occurring solely in women of "a certain age." The reality is that some women younger than 40 years, as well as men in midlife, also experience changes related to hormonal alterations. Young women may experience **premature ovarian failure** as a result of surgical or medical interventions, or for no apparent reason (Box 23.1). Men in midlife also go through a hormonal change analogous to menopause, known as **andropause** (Box 23.2).

COLLABORATIVE CARE: MENOPAUSE
Assessment

A comprehensive assessment (Assessment Tool 23.1) of the client's experiences related to the menopause transition can facilitate informed decision making regarding any actions she may wish to take to promote a healthy lifestyle. Important areas of focus include menstruation, vasomotor symptoms, genitourinary problems, mental health, cardiovascular health, and musculoskeletal health.

Menstruation

The nurse obtains the menstrual history, including the onset of menarche and any periods of amenorrhea or episodic cycle changes throughout the years. Providers may wish to encourage clients in perimenopause to

● **BOX 23.1** **Premature Ovarian Failure**

Between 1% and 5% of women younger than 40 years experience premature ovarian failure, also known as premature menopause, decades before their peers become menopausal (Santoro, 2003; Woad et al., 2006). Induced premature ovarian failure occurs in women who undergo an oophorectomy or chemotherapy resulting in an abrupt loss of ovarian function. It may also be related to genetic alterations, such as fragile X or Turner syndrome; enzyme deficiencies, such as galactosemia; autoimmune factors; or unknown causes (Santoro, 2003; Woad et al., 2006).

No characteristic menstrual history exists that would suggest the onset of idiopathic premature ovarian failure (Massin et al., 2006). Although family history appears to exist in some cases, it is by no means universal. In addition, discussions on menstruation may not be considered acceptable in some families, and therefore the histories may not be accurate.

Assessment of women experiencing or suspected of experiencing premature ovarian failure is the same as that of women with perimenopause or menopause. Once the assessment has been completed, serum follicle-stimulating hormone and luteinizing hormone levels will be needed to confirm the suspected medical diagnosis (Popat & Nelson, 2011). Once the diagnosis is confirmed, symptom alleviation is achieved through the same strategies implemented for women with age-appropriate menopause.

Women with premature ovarian failure experience vasomotor instability and genitourinary effects, along with menstrual irregularities that will eventually lead to amenorrhea. In addition, risks for cardiovascular disease and osteoporosis are increased decades earlier than their age-appropriate menopausal peers (Eastell, 2003; Popat & Nelson, 2011).

While women with premature ovarian failure are experiencing menopausal symptoms and decreased fertility, their peer group is focused on pregnancy issues. Although some women with premature ovarian failure are fortunate enough to have a successful pregnancy on their own, most women who wish to become pregnant following a diagnosis achieve pregnancy through medical interventions such as egg donation (Corrigan et al., 2005; Mainini et al., 2003; Pandian et al., 2005; Vandborg & Lauszus, 2006).

Many of these women spend years dealing with lack of support and the absence of a peer group that understands their unique situation—simultaneously experiencing infertility and menopausal symptoms (Groff et al., 2005; Orshan et al., 2001). The International Premature Ovarian Failure Association provides information and support for women with premature ovarian failure. However, this group cannot take away all of the isolation and pain experienced by these women in their interactions with a world that does not understand their situation.

● **BOX 23.2** **Andropause**

Men, as well as women, experience hormonal changes as they enter midlife. Men experience decreased levels of the testicular androgen hormone testosterone, with an ongoing decline of free testosterone levels after 40 years. Although this is a definite decrease, it is very gradual and does not result in a total cessation of exogenous hormones, as found with the loss of ovarian function in women (Vermeulen, 2000). Also, as with women, aging men experience overall changes related to both hormonal changes and life cycle events (Mooradian & Korenman, 2006).

Changes that are hormonal in origin include the following:

● Decreased sexual functioning, with decreased libido and erectile dysfunction (although changes may be secondary to medical conditions, such as diabetes mellitus) (Hafez & Hafez, 2004; Mooradian & Korenman, 2006).

● Alterations in adipose tissue distribution, including increased central and upper body fat (Gould et al., 2000).

● Regression of secondary sex characteristics, including decreased body hair (Vermeulen, 2000).

● Decreased bone mass, resulting in osteoporosis, although at a later age than in women (Hafez & Hafez, 2004; Vermeulen, 2000).

● Disturbances in vasomotor functioning, including hot flashes and diaphoresis (Gould et al., 2000; Vermeulen, 2000).

In addition, several psychological changes may be related to hormonal changes or to life cycle changes, including a shift in concern from career and social interests to family; increased need for affirmation and acceptance; increased awareness of mortality and death; and concerns about self-improvement and personal accomplishments (Mooradian & Korenman, 2006).

● **ASSESSMENT TOOL 23.1** **Guidelines for Perimenopause and Menopause**

1. **Onset of Menarche**: "How old were you the first time that you got your period?"
2. **Characteristics of Cycle**
   Primary Inquiry: "Tell me about any changes in your menstrual cycle that you have noticed during the past 6 months."
   Follow-up Questions:
   - "How many times in the past 6 months have you gotten your period?"
   - "How many days were there between the first day of one period (cycle) and the first day of the next period (cycle)?"
   - "How many pads/tampons did you use per day?"
   - "What colour was the blood?"
   - "Were clots present?"
   - "What changes, if any, have there been in your period (cycle) compared with a few years ago?"
3. **Vasomotor Symptoms**
   Primary Inquiry: "Tell me about any hot flashes that you may have experienced in the last 6 months."
   Follow-up Questions:
   - "Where do you first feel them?"
   - "Where do they spread to on your body?"
   - "When in your menstrual cycle are they most likely to occur?"
   - "What time of day/night do they occur most often?"
   - "If night, do they affect your rest?"
   - "Are they accompanied by sweating?"
   - "Are they more likely to occur if you are feeling warm, eat spicy foods, drink alcohol, or are feeling stressed?"
   - "What, if any, strategies have you found that decrease the frequency of hot flashes?"
   - "What, if any, strategies have you found that decrease the intensity of hot flashes?"
4. **Genitourinary Symptoms**
   Primary Inquiry: "Tell me about any changes you may have been experiencing regarding your urination during the past 6 months."
   Follow-up Questions:
   - "Have you experienced any urinary leakage?"
   - "If yes, are any precipitating factors causing the leakage, such as coughing?"
   - "What actions have you taken to try and decrease the leakage?" (eg, Kegel exercises—recommended; decreasing fluid intake—not recommended)
   - "If so, have you found that they decrease the urine leakage?"
   - "Do you experience any pain when you urinate?"
   - "What is the colour of your urine?"

5. **Sexuality Questions**
   Primary Inquiry: "Tell me about any changes you have been experiencing in your sexual activity during the past 6 months."
   Follow-up Questions:
   - "During sexual activity, have you noticed that your vagina is taking longer to lubricate or is not lubricating as much as it did a few years ago?"
   - "Have you experienced pain with sex?"
   - "What action, if any, have you taken to decrease the pain with sexual activity?" (eg, lubrication, hormone replacement therapy, meditation, relaxation techniques)
6. **Fertility**
   Primary Inquiry: "Tell me about your expectations/plans regarding your fertility at this time."
   Follow-up Questions:
   - "Have you ever been pregnant?"
   - "If yes, how many times?"
   - "What were the outcomes?" (birth, spontaneous abortion, induced abortion)
   - "If no, what actions have you taken to prevent pregnancy?" (abstinence, type of family planning/contraception)
   - "Have you ever breastfed?"
   - "If so, how many children and for how long?"
   - "If you wish to become pregnant, have you begun to attempt to become pregnant?"
   - "How long have you been attempting to become pregnant?"
   - "Are you presently taking any medications to improve your fertility?"
   - "If yes, please name the medications."
7. **Mental Health Changes**
   Primary Inquiry: "Tell me about how your mood has been over the past 6 months."
   Follow-*up Questions*:
   - "Have you experienced any recent changes in your mood, ability to feel happiness or joy, ability to remember things, sleep patterns, irritability, nervousness, or anxiety level?"
   - "If yes, in the past, have you ever felt or been diagnosed as depressed?"
   - "Did you ever experience any of these in the past?"
   - "If yes, which of the symptoms have you experienced and what was happening at that time in your life?"
   - "Have you experienced any recent changes in your life?" (family structure or role changes, career changes, change in perceived fertility status)

(continued)

● **ASSESSMENT TOOL 23.1**   **Guidelines for Perimenopause and Menopause** *(Continued)*

- "How do you feel about entering/being in midlife?"
- "Are you presently or have you previously taken any medications to help improve your mood or feelings about yourself?"

8. **Cardiovascular Disease**

*Prima*ry Inquiry: "Tell me about the health of your heart during the past 6 months."

Follow-*up Questions*:
- "Have you ever been diagnosed with any heart problems?"
- "If yes, what is the name of the heart problem?"
- "Do you presently, or have you previously, smoked cigarettes?"
- "If yes, how many per day?"
- "If you have stopped, when did you stop?"
- "How often do you drink alcohol each week?"
- "What is a typical daily diet?"
- "Do you exercise?"
- "If yes, what type and how often?"

9. **Osteoporosis/Osteopenia**

*Prima*ry Inquiry: "Tell me about the health of your bones during the past 6 months."

Follow-*up Questions*:
- "Have you had a bone density scan?"
- "If yes, when was your last scan?"
- "What were the results?"
- "Have you ever had a broken or fractured bone?"
- "If yes, when?"

- "What was the cause?"
- "Do you presently take calcium supplements? If yes, which one?"
- "If yes, when did you first start?"
- "Are you taking any type of prescribed or non-prescribed herb or medication to promote bone strength?"
- "What, if anything, are you doing to promote bone strength?"

Note: The diet and exercise questions above are also directly related to this section.

10. **Breast Cancer**

*Prima*ry Inquiry: "Tell me about the history of your breast health."

Follow-*up Questions*:
- "Have you ever been diagnosed with breast cancer?"
- "If yes, when was the diagnosis?"
- "What treatment was initiated?"
- "What is your present status?"
- "Do you perform breast self-examination?"
- "How often?"
- "What were the findings?"
- "When was the last time your breasts were examined by a health professional?"
- "What were the findings?"
- "When was your last mammogram?"
- "What were the findings?"
- "Are you presently taking any estrogen-containing preparations (eg, oral contraceptives, hormone replacement therapy)?"

keep a journal or diary recording their menstrual cycles, including the day of the month that menstruation begins and the number of days that the client bleeds. Developing such a diary can facilitate women's understanding of changes in the menstrual cycle and help them identify areas in which they may choose to change habits or initiate interventions. For some clients, this experience is empowering because it increases awareness and feelings of self-actualization.

Vasomotor Symptoms

Determining the presence and potential external etiology is the focus of nursing assessment for vasomotor symptoms. In addition to recording menstrual cycles, providers may choose to encourage clients to document any hot flashes they experience in a diary. A client can list the circumstances surrounding the hot flash, including the time, place, duration, activity immediately

preceding, whether it was accompanied by diaphoresis, and what, if anything, alleviated the discomfort. In this way, the nurse can review the recordings with the client to help her identify precipitating factors to the vasomotor instability (Fig. 23.5). Again, although this technique has value in identifying physiologic patterns, it also empowers women to gain knowledge about their bodies, revealing ways in which they can control and improve health.

Some women experience hot flashes immediately before and during the first few days of menstruation. Precipitating factors include hot temperatures, stress, alcohol, hot drinks, cigarette smoking, and spicy foods (Frackiewicz & Cutler, 2000). Review of the diary could help determine whether any of these or other factors are related to the hot flashes. If they do appear to be related, the client can take actions to avoid the precipitating factors or to limit the effects of the hot flash.

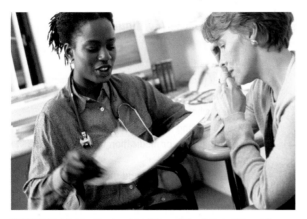

FIGURE 23.5 Reviewing journal findings with a client can help identify patterns in menstrual cycle changes and vasomotor problems. Being able to understand and pinpoint these symptoms can help women feel more in control of anticipating and managing them.

 Remember Fran, the woman from the beginning of the chapter who was complaining of hot flashes? How might a diary help Fran? What causes these vasomotor symptoms?

Genitourinary Problems

Women in perimenopause are often not aware that this is the time they may begin to experience some genitourinary changes. Although the genital and urinary systems are related closely anatomically and physiologically, most women perceive them as two completely different areas. Assessment should reflect their beliefs as much as possible. Sensitivity during questioning is particularly important because many women are embarrassed when discussing issues of elimination and sexuality. Questions regarding the urinary tract may be easier for clients to respond to, so it may be best to begin genitourinary assessment focusing on this area, and then moving to questions related to genital assessment.

The nurse can ask if the woman is experiencing urinary incontinence, urinary tract infections, or both. If responses are positive, the nurse needs to ask additional questions to determine more information about onset and severity.

Assessment of the genital tract focuses on questions about any vaginal infections and dyspareunia (Andrews et al., 2000). If dyspareunia is present, additional sexual information is necessary to determine its effects on the woman's life.

Many women view the reality of decreasing fertility positively because they have either completed their families or decided not to have children. For the growing numbers of women trying to become pregnant during the later years of childbearing, however, issues surrounding fertility may be sensitive. Fertility assessment focuses on fertility history, including the outcome of any previous pregnancies, the client's present desires regarding pregnancy, and, if appropriate, what actions she is taking to achieve her desires—either contraception or fertility enhancement (see Chapters 8 and 10). Assessment of her knowledge regarding fertility choices (eg, birth control side effects, infertility treatments) can be initiated at this time.

Mental Health Status

Assessment of mental health status during perimenopause and menopause focuses on helping the nurse gain insight into the client's past and present health. Together, the nurse and client need to identify personal, familial, and environmental factors that affect mental health and related coping mechanisms. Discussion includes all prescription and over-the-counter medications the client is taking.

Cardiovascular Health

Most women do not consider themselves at risk for cardiovascular disease and may not understand the importance of assessment in this area. Some are frightened to learn that menopausal changes may increase their risk for developing cardiovascular disease. The nurse can provide support and education for clients before initiating cardiovascular assessment and examinations.

Thorough discussion of personal and familial risk factors is needed to assist the client to attain or maintain optimal cardiac health. For all clients, the nurse asks about knowledge concerning present cardiovascular status, along with personal and family history, risk factors, and beneficial activities. In addition, she or he evaluates blood pressure, pulse, and serum total and HDL cholesterol levels to help develop a personalized, realistic plan of care (see Chapter 2).

Bone Health Status

As discussed earlier in this chapter, decreased estrogen levels are partly responsible for the loss of bone density as women age (Andrews et al., 2000; Deroo & Korach, 2006). Risk factors for osteoporosis accumulate across a lifetime and include low body weight, sedentary lifestyle, smoking, excessive alcohol consumption, low sunlight exposure, high-fat diet, inadequate calcium intake or absorption, and excessive caffeine intake, in addition to an early age at menopause, nulliparity, and a family history of osteoporosis (SOGC, 2006; Health Canada, 2008). Some illnesses such as cystic fibrosis, celiac disease, and inflammatory bowel disease, associated with poor calcium absorption, increase risk of low bone density. The use of glucocorticoids is also associated with increased risk for compromised bone health (Health Canada, 2008).

While women of particular ethnic origin appear to be at higher risk for bone fractures, lifestyle factors such as exercise and calcium intake across the lifespan contribute to bone health for all women. There are some differences in bone health among ethnic groups noted in the literature; however, there is a need for further research in this area, particularly regarding the weighting of ethnic differences alongside other risk factors.

It has been reported that differences in bone mineral density (BMD) levels attributed to ethnicity have been reduced or eliminated when height and weight are accounted for in the calculation. This suggests that ethnicity may not be of paramount importance in the assessment process; rather nurses must be aware of the risk factors for osteoporosis discussed above, with particular attention to the discussion of lifestyle risk factors that can be altered or controlled.

The presence of osteopenia and osteoporosis can be determined through ultrasound or, more accurately, through measurements of bone density using dual energy x-ray absorptiometry (DXA) scanning (SOGC, 2006). Measurements that fall below the BMD for young adult women are categorized as osteopenia (1 to 2.5 standard deviations below the young adult mean) or osteoporosis (2.5 standard deviations below the young adult mean). Intervention directed toward a symptomatic woman with a diagnosis of osteopenia should be considered in light of the knowledge that "everyone naturally loses bone density as they age … the standard reference norm on the bone density machines is that of a young woman, making it almost impossible for an older person to have a normal diagnosis" (Sanson, 2005).

 Carol has osteopenia. Based on the information at the beginning of the chapter, what risk factors are found in Carol's health history for osteopenia and potential development of osteoporosis?

Planning/Intervention

Many women view the normal changes in the menstrual cycle as a positive sign that they are moving into the next phase of their life. Other women find the changes of menopause moderately disruptive or uncomfortable but choose to live without intervention in the normal process of menopause. Some of these women find relief of symptoms from the use of alternative therapies. Still other women choose medical or pharmacologic intervention alone, or alongside alternative therapies to alleviate or manage symptoms that disrupt their quality of life. Nursing Care Plan 23.1 highlights the care of a woman experiencing physical and emotional changes related to menopause. For such clients, learning that these changes are a part of normal aging may help alleviate some of their concerns and help them re-evaluate their perception of "normal."

Nurses need to provide anticipatory education to women and their partners so they can correctly and promptly identify any changes that may be related to their changing physiology. Once such changes have been identified, health care providers can work with women to facilitate informed decision making regarding the need for interventions.

Pharmacologic Management

In some cases pharmacologic preparations are prescribed to alleviate symptoms of perimenopause and menopause.

Hormone Replacement Therapy

In the past, women were prescribed hormone replacement therapy (HRT) of estrogen, either with or without progestin, to alleviate the symptoms of menopause. In 2002, the Women's Health Initiative study reported that long-term use of HRT increased risks for breast cancer, cerebrovascular accident, and stroke (Writing Group for the Women's Health Initiative Investigators, 2002). The potential risks posed by HRT has prompted many practitioners to move away from prescribing HRT for all women going through menopausal transitions and to focus more specifically on each client's particular circumstances. As a result of the 2002 study, Health Canada warned that:

> Even short-term use (of Estrogen with or without Progestin) is associated with an increased risk of blood clots, stroke and coronary heart disease. HRT should only be used if your symptoms are severe and if you have been fully informed of the risks (Health Canada, 2004, http://hc-sc.gc.ca/hl-vs/iyh-vsv/med/estrogen-eng.php).

Current practice is for the primary care provider to carefully evaluate the client's health history and work with her to make decisions relative to pharmacologic options. When making management decisions, the client and care provider need to consider the following points:

• The Women's Health Initiative does not recommend using HRT to prevent or to treat heart disease. Clients at risk for cardiovascular problems need a treatment approach focusing on lifestyle modifications, lipid-lowering agents, or both (Writing Group, 2002).

(text continues on page 968)

NURSING CARE PLAN 23.1

•

The Woman Experiencing Menopausal Changes

Fran, described at the start of this chapter, is experiencing hot flashes, sleep problems, and feelings of being alone. Further assessment reveals that her last menstrual period was 1 year ago. Since then, her hot flashes have increased to three to four times per week with diaphoresis. "It's been really upsetting. My children are gone. I'm tired all the time. I'm irritable and moody. I feel so unattractive and unwomanly now!"

NURSING DIAGNOSES

- **Risk for Powerlessness** related to physical and emotional changes associated with menopause.
- **Impaired Adjustment** related to menopausal changes.
- **Sleep Deprivation** related to increased hot flashes and diaphoresis at night.

EXPECTED OUTCOMES

1. The client will identify physiologic and psychological changes accompanying menopause.
2. The client will state ways to increase control over symptoms.
3. The client will identify positive coping strategies.
4. The client will report at least two methods to promote sleep.

INTERVENTIONS	RATIONALES
Assess the client's knowledge about menopause and its accompanying physiologic and psychological changes.	Assessment provides a baseline from which to develop an individualized plan of care.
Review typical menopausal changes; correlate them with the client's current complaints.	Correlation aids in fostering better understanding on the client's part.
Investigate the meaning of menopause to the client and her feelings as a woman, mother, and wife.	Menopause means different things to different women regardless of race or ethnicity. Some view menopause negatively, as a loss of youth and femininity; others may view it positively, as a time for new opportunities.
Remind the client that she is also experiencing other major life changes that reflect growth of her family.	Menopause is also a time of other major life events.
Discuss her concerns, feelings, and perceptions related to menopause and her family and how they are affecting her current situation.	Discussion provides opportunities to emphasize positive aspects; verbalization of concerns establishes sources of stress and problem areas to address.
Explain that many women experience hot flashes of varying intensity and frequency, commonly at night.	This knowledge can help the client feel less alone.

(continued)

NURSING CARE PLAN 23.1 ● The Woman Experiencing Menopausal Changes *(Continued)*

INTERVENTIONS	RATIONALES
Have the client complete a diary detailing her experiences with hot flashes, including time, place, immediately preceding activity, whether it was accompanied by diaphoresis, how long it lasted, and what (if anything) alleviated the discomfort.	The diary can provide clues to possible precipitating factors that the client can then avoid.
Assess the client's usual sleep routine; review measures to promote sleep.	Knowledge of habits aids in formulating appropriate suggestions.
Advise the client to avoid daytime naps and to drink warm milk at bedtime. Encourage a consistent routine before bedtime.	Avoiding daytime naps ensures that the client will be tired at bedtime. Warm milk contains L-tryptophan, a natural sleep aid. Consistency before bed aids in preparing for sleep.
Inquire about past methods used to cope with stressful situations; encourage the client to use methods that were successful; provide additional suggestions for ways to cope with the current situation.	Use of past successful methods enhances the chance of current success. Additional suggestions to deal with the current situation aid in relieving stress associated with outside variables and events and provide the client with various options, thereby promoting a greater feeling of control.
Assist the client to identify her own desires and goals.	Identification of the client's wishes is important in developing strategies appropriate for her.
Provide the client with accurate facts and communicate openly; answer questions.	Open and honest communication promotes trust and helps correct any misconceptions or misinformation.
Review and reinforce the client's positive attributes about herself and her abilities.	Identification of positive attributes provides a foundation for enhancing self-esteem and aids in the realization that the client has an identity, is competent to care for herself, and is worthy of assistance.
Suggest participation in a support group.	Doing so promotes sharing, enhancing the realization that the client is not alone.
Arrange for referral to a mental health specialist if necessary.	A mental health specialist can assist with compromised coping mechanisms, depression, or a previous history of mental health problems.

EVALUATION

1. The client correlates events of menopause with current complaints.
2. The client identifies measures to adapt to changes.
3. The client demonstrates positive coping strategies.
4. The client reports an increase of at least one episode of undisturbed sleep over 1 week.

- Any clients taking HRT require the lowest possible dose. Most clients are advised not to take HRT for more than 5 years.
- Alternatives to HRT include herbal therapies, selective estrogen receptor modulators, and bisphosphonates (see the next discussion). Education related to these products is individualized to the actual agent chosen.

A Cochrane Collaboration review (Marjoribanks et al., 2012) of long term hormone therapy for premenopausal and menopausal women reinforced the concerns identified in 2002. The authors note that the use of combined estrogen/progesterone HRT significantly raises the risk for women over age 65 for venous thrombus embolisms, heart attack, stroke, breast cancer, gall bladder disease, and dementia. Long-term use of HRT estrogen alone increases risk for venous thrombus embolism, stroke, and gall bladder disease. While long-term use of HRT can provide a reduction in the risk of bone fracture, this advantage would need to be carefully weighed against the known significant risks for adverse effects (Marjoribanks et al., 2012).

Selective Estrogenic Receptor Modulators (SERMS)

SERMS, known as "designer estrogens," are estrogenic or antiestrogenic synthetic compounds that target specific organs, thereby avoiding some of the negative effects of estrogen (SOGC, 2009). The ideal SERM would have estrogenic-type activity in the brain, bone, cardiovascular system, and genitourinary system, and antiestrogenic activity in the breast and uterus. This SERM would decrease risks for cognitive impairment, Alzheimer disease, osteoporosis, cardiovascular disease, breast cancer, and endometrial cancer.

Raloxifene (Evista) is a SERMS approved in Canada for the treatment of osteoporosis (SOGC, 2006). As raloxifene does not stimulate either the endometrial lining of the uterus or breast tissue, the risk of cancers in these areas is lower than with the use of traditional HRT.

Bisphosphonates

Bisphosphonates, such as alendronate (Fosamax), inhibit bone loss and increase bone mass density, decreasing fractures. Therapeutic treatment courses may be limited to 3 years to avoid osteomalacia (Cutson & Meuleman, 2000). The woman should take alendronate on an empty stomach and take the medication while upright and have nothing but water for the next 30 minutes (Karch, 2013). These measures decrease the risk for esophagitis and the main side effect, heartburn (Cutson & Meuleman, 2000).

Calcitonin

Calcitonin (Miacalcin) is a polypeptide hormone that increases bone mass density and decreases spinal column fractures. Although there is an injectable form of calcitonin, a new intranasal form is being used, often with good results.

Complementary and Alternative Therapies

Many women find that nonpharmacologic strategies are successful in decreasing the vasomotor effects of menopause; these include regular aerobic exercise, biofeedback, dietary changes, and the use of herbal remedies (CWHN, 2007a). Various sources have provided information about such herbal treatments, including Native American medicine, Eastern medicine, and many European cultures. Some herbs have undergone clinical trials. It is advisable to buy herbs that are standardized, meaning that every tablet contains the same amount of active ingredient. Evidence of a number such as the drug information number (DIN) or the general public (GP) number indicates that Health Canada has reviewed and approved labelling and instructions for use (CWHN, 2007a).

Many herbal remedies are available; Complementary/Alternative Medicine Box 23.1 discusses a few of the more popular forms. For additional information, please refer to the References and Web Resources.

Infection Prevention and Sexual Comfort

Clients can avoid many of the potential difficulties related to genitourinary changes by implementing simple self-care actions. All clients can use such strategies to ensure optimal genitourinary health. For example, methods to decrease risk for infection include wearing cotton underwear and pantyhose with a cotton crotch, avoiding damp or tight-fitting clothing, voiding before and after sexual activity, and cleansing the perineum after defecating by wiping from front to back. Kegel exercises, which strengthen the pubococcygeus muscle, may help improve urinary continence (Harvey, 2003; Hay-Smith & Dumoulin, 2006) and vaginal muscle tone. See Teaching Tips 23.1.

During this life stage, many women find that vaginal lubrication is decreased. Encouraging clients and their partners to increase time spent in foreplay during sexual activities may help promote vaginal lubrication. In addition, the client may wish to apply a water-based vaginal lubricant immediately before sexual activity. Doing so can help minimize problems with dyspareunia resulting from lack of vaginal lubrication. Of course, the nurse will be careful to follow up on whether these measures solve the problem because ongoing pain or discomfort during sex may indicate a need for further physiologic or psychological intervention.

Fertility Control

Many women welcome menopause because of its accompanying effects of eliminating the chance of

● COMPLEMENTARY/ALTERNATIVE MEDICINE 23.1

Herbs for Menopausal Symptom Alleviation

- **Isoflavones**: Also called *phytoestrogens*, these include dietary soy products and black cohosh (*Cimicifuga racemosa*). They are used to alleviate problems related to estrogen loss, such as vasomotor instability and vaginal dryness. For many women, they are viable alternatives to prescription estrogen therapy, although their ability to decrease risks for osteoporosis and cardiovascular disease has not been established (Carroll, 2006; Frackiewicz & Cutler, 2000).
- **Soy products** contain a natural form of dietary estrogen. Their isoflavones are much weaker than those of endogenous estrogen; however, studies have shown fewer vasomotor symptoms, decreased vaginal dryness and bone loss, and lower low-density lipoprotein and total cholesterol levels among people who ingest soy products as part of their regular diet or as a dietary supplement (Cutson & Meuleman, 2000). Research findings on soy protein neither refute nor substantiate claims made by soy proponents (Andrews et al., 2000; Carroll, 2006). Recommended daily intake of soy is 45 g (Frackiewicz & Cutler, 2000). Sources include tofu, soy nuts, and soy milk. A new category of soy-fortified products is aimed at perimenopausal and menopausal women; it includes hot and cold cereals as well as over-the-counter nutritional supplements.
- In North America the herb Black Cohosh has been used to reduce menopausal symptoms, including vasomotor disturbances. Although the Cochrane Collaboration review suggests that studies of the efficacy of the herb have been inconclusive (Leach & Moore, 2012), practitioners report a "history of successful use in practice" (Abascal & Yarnell, 2013). In Canada Black Cohosh is sold under the name Remifemin, and is promoted as a nonprescription alternative to hormone therapy.
- **Dong Quai**: Dong Quai (*Angelica sinensis*), a coumarin, is a traditional Chinese herb with a reputation in the West as the "menopause herb." Although Western medicine uses Dong Quai as both a singular and compound element in herbal preparations, Chinese medicine limits its use to multiple-herb compounds. Research focused on Dong Quai has not validated its use for menopausal symptoms (MedlinePlus, 2013). Dong Quai might interfere with blood clotting, and should not be used in combination with other preparations that also slow blood clotting (MedlinePlus, 2013).

undesired or unintended pregnancy. Because the duration of perimenopause varies and pregnancy remains a possibility for many women well into their 40s, the client and her partner need to make reproductive-control decisions to ensure support for their fertility choices. If a client desires to avoid pregnancy, the nurse can provide her with education regarding options for fertility control (see Chapter 8). Assuming that the client is in good health, these options are much the same as for younger women. Oral contraceptives may be prescribed as a low-dose form of HRT with the added benefit of pregnancy prevention.

Clients who desire pregnancy during this time of their lives need to be aware that chances of conception without intervention are not high. If such intervention is unsuccessful in helping a client achieve pregnancy with

● TEACHING TIPS 23.1   Kegel (Pelvic Floor) Exercises

The pubococcygeus muscle helps support the bladder and uterus in their proper position in the pelvis. Kegel exercises help to strengthen this important muscle of the pelvic floor. The technique is very simple:

- Kegel exercises can be done sitting, standing, or lying down. Only the person who is performing the exercise need know that it is being done. If the woman has trouble identifying the muscle, share with her that it is the muscle used to stop urinating.
- It is helpful for some clients to think of the pubococcygeus muscle as an elevator. In the relaxed position, the muscle is imagined as being at ground floor. The woman slowly and consciously tightens the muscle past the first floor, second floor, third floor, and finally the penthouse.
- The muscle stays at the penthouse for about 10 seconds, and then slowly descend down again to the ground floor.
- This exercise should be repeated about 5 to 10 times, 3 or more times a day.

her own ova, oocyte donation may be a viable option. This and other measures to facilitate pregnancy are discussed in Chapter 10.

Stress Management and Coping

Reinforcing healthy coping strategies, and, if needed, helping clients develop additional strategies to deal with real and potential stresses related to perimenopause and menopause are of primary importance during this life phase. Clients with compromised coping strategies or a history of mental health alterations may benefit from a referral to a mental health specialist. Because previous episodes of depression appear to increase the likelihood of recurrence during this time, nurses need to be aware of symptoms so that they can take appropriate actions immediately to alleviate or prevent depression in their clients (Dennerstein et al., 2004) (see Chapter 5).

Women experiencing insomnia may be exhibiting alterations in mental health that increased sleep will alleviate. For some women, avoiding daytime naps, drinking warm milk at bedtime (contains L-tryptophan), or taking a warm bath may promote relaxation and sleep. Stress management techniques, meditation, and regular exercise also may help. Support groups and psychological counselling may be appropriate for clients experiencing family or career challenges, self-esteem issues, or both.

St. John's wort (*Hypericum perforatum*) has been viewed as a "natural" method of treating depression and anxiety, but there are conflicting views on its efficacy. St. John's wort has multiple known interactions with prescribed medications, including protease inhibitors used for HIV, cyclosporines, digoxins, β-blockers, antidepressants, monoamine oxidase inhibitors, ephedra, and oral contraceptives (Karch, 2013; Williamson, 2005).

Cardiovascular Health

Education regarding the effects of perimenopause and menopause on cardiovascular health is important in helping women understand the increased risks that accompany estrogen depletion. A healthy lifestyle is essential for maintaining or improving cardiovascular health.

Smoking is the most prevalent cause of mortality, followed by inactivity. Women who smoke heavily tend to experience menopause 2 to 3 years earlier than moderate smokers or nonsmokers, and therefore experience estrogen deprivation, along with the negative effects related to lack of estrogen, for a longer time than nonsmokers (Kinney et al., 2006). Clients can be counselled to stop smoking and, if needed, referred to community support groups, over-the-counter medications, or a nurse practitioner or physician for appropriate medication to assist with smoking cessation.

Activity levels need to be evaluated and a safe, effective program of exercise initiated. A referral to an exercise therapist may be appropriate. A combination of aerobic and weight-bearing exercises helps decrease the risk for coronary artery disease, control postmenopausal lipoprotein levels, increase bone and muscle mass, aid sleep, and control weight. It also may decrease depression. Before assisting midlife and older adults in exercises, it is important to remind them of the precautions outlined in Teaching Tips 23.2.

Dietary intake is one of the most important influences over cardiovascular health. A well-balanced, low-fat diet is important in controlling cholesterol. After menopause, women are more likely to gain weight, creating additional strain on the heart (Gavaler & Rosenblum, 2003). To help prevent weight gain, clients need information about changing caloric needs (see Chapter 3). Antioxidants, including vitamins C and E, may help prevent or

---

● **TEACHING TIPS 23.2** Exercise

- **Exercise should be pain free**. Remember, pain can emerge a few days after the exercise, so caution the exerciser to learn to listen to her body.
- **Keep breathing**. This can be crucial in an exerciser who has heart disease or hypertension.
- **Watch out for shoulder and neck tension**. Encourage the exerciser to inhale and, when exhaling, to exhale the stress from shoulders and neck.
- **Maintain good neck alignment**. Demonstrate how a small pillow or rolled-up towel can be placed behind the neck when in a supine position.
- **Hold weights with a neutral wrist**. Demonstrate the technique of holding a weight without bending the wrist backward.

- **Maintain normal spinal curves**. Demonstrate engaging abdominal muscles to protect the spine, rather than weaken the spine by altering its configuration.
- **Evaluate the exerciser's handgrip**. If the exerciser has a tendency to drop objects, encourage the use of a weight that can be strapped onto the exerciser's hand or wrist.
- **Avoid forward bending**. Share with the exerciser that bending increases the risk for spinal fracture.

Adapted from Daniels, D. (2000). *Exercises for osteoporosis*. New York: Hatherleigh Press.

reduce arterial LDL (Andrews et al., 2000). If the client has obesity, diabetes, hypertension, established cardiac problems, or a combination of these conditions, a referral to a nutritionist may be appropriate, because these medical conditions place her at even greater risk for cardiovascular problems.

Osteoporosis Prevention

Preventive care for osteopenia and osteoporosis is a lifestyle choice that optimally begins before perimenopause. A dietary intake high in calcium and regular participation in aerobic and weight-bearing exercise are important to preventing or limiting skeletal deterioration. Health Canada notes it is "often possible to prevent or delay bone loss through healthy living" (2008). An optimum goal is for 30 minutes of weight-bearing exercise each day (CWHN, 2012).

Following menopause, women can be advised to ingest 1,500 mg of calcium per day, along with 400 to 800 IU of vitamin D (Gold, 2005). Vitamin D is required for the absorption of calcium. For Canadian women, sunlight intensity between November and March is not sufficient to support the manufacture of adequate Vitamin D (British Columbia Ministry of Health, 2012). Prescribed medications that can reverse or inhibit further bone loss include specific SERMS, such as raloxifene; bisphosphonates, including alendronate (Fosamax); and HRT. See Nursing Care Plan 23.2.

NURSING CARE PLAN 23.2

●

The Menopausal Woman at Risk for Osteoporosis

 Carol is 44 years old and has been diagnosed with osteopenia, as described at the beginning of the chapter. Further assessment reveals that she exercises occasionally, going for short walks with friends two to three times per month. She says, "Since I stopped smoking, I've cut down my coffee intake to about 2 cups per day. I do use milk as my creamer in the coffee, though, and I try to eat a container of yogurt at least once a week." She denies any use of calcium supplements or herbal remedies. "I know I need to drink more milk, but I'm not a big fan. What else could I do?"

NURSING DIAGNOSES

- **Health-seeking Behaviours** related to risk reduction and alteration in bone integrity.
- **Risk for Injury** related to osteopenia and continued loss of bone mass.

EXPECTED OUTCOMES

1. The client will identify measures to prevent or limit changes in bone integrity.
2. The client will verbalize ways to maintain safety to reduce the risk for fractures.

INTERVENTIONS	RATIONALES
Assess the client's knowledge of osteopenia and osteoporosis.	Assessment provides a baseline from which to develop an individualized plan.
Review the client's history for possible risk factors.	Risk factor identification is the first step in identifying areas that need intervention.
Question the client about food likes and dislikes; review high-calcium foods, encouraging her to eat those she prefers. Discuss foods high in vitamin D. Suggest the use of calcium-fortified foods.	Encouraging the client to select high-calcium foods that she prefers increases the chances for adherence. Vitamin D promotes calcium absorption and prevents further bone loss.

(continued)

NURSING CARE PLAN 23.2 ● The Menopausal Woman at Risk for Osteoporosis (Continued)

INTERVENTIONS	RATIONALES
Encourage the client to reduce her intake of caffeinated beverages; suggest caffeine-free drinks and decaffeinated coffee.	Caffeine interferes with calcium absorption.
Offer positive reinforcement for smoking cessation.	Smoking increases risk for osteoporosis. Positive reinforcement fosters a sense of achievement, helping reduce the chance for relapse.
Review the client's daily routine.	Knowledge of her habits and routine aids in developing appropriate individualized suggestions that match the client's lifestyle.
Encourage the client to increase her activity level; suggest a goal of aerobic weight-bearing exercise for 30 minutes daily; assist her to develop a workable plan based on her daily routine. If possible, encourage the client to exercise outdoors or to otherwise get 30 minutes of sunlight per day.	Aerobic weight-bearing exercise helps slow down bone loss. Weight-bearing exercise helps stimulate new bone formation. Sunlight provides vitamin D, which helps with absorption of calcium.
Question the client about family, friends, or others who might join her in her activities.	Participation of others promotes sharing and provides encouragement for those involved.
Recommend that the client wear well-fitting supportive shoes when exercising; emphasize the need to warm up and cool down.	Proper footwear and warm-up and cool-down exercises are important to reduce the risk for injury.
Provide suggestions for safety measures in the home, such as avoiding throw rugs and loose extension cords that cross the room, having well-lit halls and stairs, using banisters or railings for support, and wearing shoes with nonskid soles.	Environmental safety measures reduce the risk for falls.
Advise the client to use an over-the-counter calcium supplement (1,500 mg/day) with 400–800 IU of vitamin D if necessary.	Calcium supplementation is necessary to replace lost calcium and reduce bone loss.
Arrange for the client to have a follow-up DEXA scan 12–18 months from her first one.	Follow-up scanning is needed to evaluate bone mineral density and any progression of osteopenia to osteoporosis.

EVALUATION

1. The client demonstrates appropriate measures to reduce risk and minimize loss of bone mass.
2. The client remains injury free.

Evaluation

Evaluation varies according to the individualized plan and specific interventions. For all clients, increased understanding of potential changes is paramount. Once interventions have been initiated, they are deemed successful if the client experiences increased comfort and acceptance of the normal age-related changes. If the client and her health care provider choose an intervention or medication regimen, knowledge of expected outcomes, along with side effects and any danger signs, is imperative.

The client needs to understand the possibility of becoming pregnant with a healthy fetus at this time and interventions that may be needed to facilitate or prevent conception. See Chapters 8 and 10 for the evaluation of interventions that may be initiated to control fertility.

Because of societal attitudes toward mental distress, evaluating mental health status and intervention success may be difficult. Determining the client's understanding of the etiology of mental health changes during this period is crucial, as is identifying her awareness of potential interventions. Any changes in mental health status need to be monitored continually, with further actions initiated as needed.

Evaluation of the woman's diet, exercise regimen, and coping skills is necessary to assist her to achieve the most optimal cardiovascular health possible. Awareness of her knowledge level concerning the effects of osteopenia and osteoporosis is also of primary importance. Once such knowledge has been validated, the outcomes of actions or nonactions that she chooses to take can be determined.

SUMMARY

- With aging, the ovaries secrete less estrogen and progesterone, resulting in increased secretion of FSH from the anterior pituitary, which increases the rate of follicular atresia. These developments lead to infertile anovulatory cycles and eventual depletion of ovarian follicles at approximately the time of menopause.
- Physiologic and psychological changes related to perimenopause and menopause are a combination of hormonal influences and lifestyle changes during midlife.
- The earliest signs of perimenopause include changes in menstruation cycle length and flow rate. Health care providers may encourage clients to keep a calendar that records the menstrual cycle and to use the findings to form a plan of care to manage changes.
- Vasomotor instability, including hot flashes and diaphoresis, most likely results from decreased endogenous estrogen.

- Genitourinary changes in menopause include atrophy of the vaginal lining; decreased vaginal lubrication; decreased libido; increased vaginal infections; and increased urinary urge, incontinence, and urinary tract infections.
- Fertility decreases rapidly throughout midlife; however, pregnancy continues to remain a possibility for many women well into their 40s.
- Mental health changes, including depression, irritability, lethargy, and forgetfulness, may be related to hormonal alterations of perimenopause and menopause or may be manifestations of life cycle events.
- Cardiovascular changes, particularly increased risks for cardiovascular disease and myocardial infarction, are related to the lipid and vascular alterations of estrogen depletion.
- Decreased estrogen, along with familial and lifestyle factors, influence the risk for osteoporosis.
- Prescribed pharmacologic measures, particularly HRT, must be carefully considered given the high risk of serious adverse effects of these medications.
- Exercise, dietary intake, biofeedback, and prescribed HRT may be useful in improving vasomotor stability. Complementary treatments to alleviate the symptoms of perimenopause and menopause include isoflavones.
- Anticipatory education to limit or prevent genitourinary problems includes teaching Kegel exercises, explaining the benefits of increasing sexual foreplay, and advising the client to use a vaginal lubricant before sexual activity.
- To prevent or facilitate pregnancy in women during this stage, providers must work with the client to identify her fertility choices and assist with providing contraception or, if needed, referrals for fertility promotion.
- Collaborative care related to mental health includes identification of potential issues, including insomnia and stress, and devising strategies to assist women to achieve mental health, based on the etiology of the changes.
- Beneficial lifestyle choices for cardiovascular health during this stage may include smoking cessation, exercise, and dietary changes. A well-balanced diet contains calcium-rich foods and soy products. Relaxation and stress management are also vital.
- Assisting the client to prevent or control osteopenia and osteoporosis focuses on decreasing controllable risk factors (eg, smoking) and emphasizing the need for appropriate calcium and vitamin D supplementation.
- Premature ovarian failure occurs in women younger than 40 years of age who experience menopausal symptoms from either induced or naturally occurring ovarian failure. In addition, these women are simultaneously experiencing infertility at a time

when many of their peers are experiencing parenthood, leading to potential psychosocial difficulties.

● Andropause is the term used to define the physiologic and psychological changes men begin to experience in midlife. As with women, completely differentiating life cycle changes from decreased hormone levels is difficult. Typical andropause changes include decreased bone mass, vasomotor disturbances, cognitive alterations, and decreased libido.

Questions to Ponder

1. Fran, the 50-year-old woman who has been experiencing menopausal symptoms, has read on the internet that there are natural remedies for her menopausal symptoms, including eating tofu. She thinks she will try some of these remedies and asks what you know about them. What is your response?

2. Carol, the 44-year-old woman with osteopenia, has a limited amount of regular physical activity. What kinds of activities would help build up her bone mass density and prevent bone fractures?

3. During an appointment with an infertility specialist, a 44-year-old woman with no viable ovarian follicles has been advised that if she and her husband wish to become pregnant, one of the most viable options is ova donation. During a counselling session with the nurse, the woman shares that her husband is very excited about the prospect, but that she is ambivalent because the child will not share her genetic traits, but those of her husband and a donor.

    • What are your personal feelings about helping a menopausal woman become pregnant?

    • What additional information might be helpful for the nurse to have before responding?

    • What type of response may provide the woman with some comfort and support regarding her decision?

REVIEW QUESTIONS

1. A 40-year-old client asks the nurse, "When do you think I will go through menopause?" After completing an assessment, the nurse identifies which of the following factors as potentially increasing the woman's risk for early menopause?
    A. Menarche at age 14 years
    B. History of three previous pregnancies
    C. Use of oral contraceptives
    D. Breastfeeding her children

2. A 48-year-old woman comes to her gynecologist's office for a routine checkup. During the visit, she complains of hot flashes accompanied sporadically by excessive diaphoresis. The woman states that her menstrual cycle has remained static for the past 5 years, although before that time, the cycle was longer. She denies experiencing dyspareunia, altered libido, or urinary tract infections. To help determine an appropriate plan for this woman, which question should the nurse ask next?
    A. "How many days is your menstrual cycle now?"
    B. "Can you tell me a bit more about your hot flashes?"
    C. "Are you using a vaginal lubricant during sexual activity?"
    D. "Do you ever eat any soy products?"

3. Which of the following factors increases the likelihood of developing osteoporosis?
    A. Intake of calcium through diet and supplementation
    B. Family history of osteoporosis
    C. Increasing age
    D. Regular weight-bearing activity

4. Which suggestion if made by the nurse would be most appropriate for a menopausal client complaining of dyspareunia?
    A. Perform Kegel exercises three times per day
    B. Apply a water-soluble lubricant before sexual activity
    C. Take a bisphosphonate such as alendronate (Fosamax)
    D. Wear cotton underwear and pantyhose with cotton crotch

5. When assessing a woman who is considering the use of estrogen replacement therapy, a history of which of the following would be of least concern?
    A. Hysterectomy
    B. Chronic severe liver disease
    C. Recent thromboembolism
    D. Breast cancer

6. The nurse is preparing a teaching plan for a local women's community group about menopause. Which of the following would the nurse be least likely to include in the teaching plan?
    A. The average age of menopause is about 51 to 52 years of age
    B. Men experience a change in hormonal levels with aging
    C. Levels of LDL drop with the onset of menopause
    D. Osteoporosis is a major cause of fractures after menopause

7. Which of the following assessment findings might lead the nurse to suspect that a client is experiencing a common adverse effect associated with her prescribed therapy with alendronate (Fosamax)?
    A. Fluid retention
    B. Heartburn
    C. Breast tenderness
    D. Mood alterations

8. A client states that she is taking a medication in the form of a nasal spray to reduce her risk for back fractures. Which medication is she most likely using?
   A. Calcitonin (Miacalcin)
   B. Raloxifene (Evista)
   C. Tamoxifen
   D. Atorvastatin (Lipitor)

9. Which of the following suggestions would the nurse include in a plan of care to promote the cardiovascular health of a menopausal woman?
   A. Limit the intake of vitamin C–containing foods
   B. Perform isometric exercises at least twice weekly
   C. Restrict intake to 1,000 calories per day
   D. Eat foods high in polyunsaturated and monounsaturated fats

10. Nursing assessment of a healthy 27-year-old woman who is attending a gynecologic clinic reveals that, since the woman's healthy pregnancy 2 years earlier, she has had an irregular menstrual cycle, is experiencing periodic hot flashes particularly at night, and complains of dyspareunia. Based on this information, the nurse should anticipate the need to
    A. Provide sexual counselling to the woman.
    B. Suggest a referral to a mental health counsellor.
    C. Assess the woman's level of ovarian hormones.
    D. Determine whether the woman is presently breastfeeding her child.

REFERENCES

Abascal, K., & Yarnell, E. (2013). Night sweats in perimenopause and beyond. *Alternative and Complementary Therapies, 19*(1), 28–32.

Alexander, I. (2012). The history of hormone therapy use and recent controversy related to heart disease and breast cancer arising from prevention trail outcomes. *Journal of Midwifery and Women's Health, 57*(6), 547–557.

Andrews, W. C., Weisman, C. S., Holleran, M. K., Johnson, C., Mort, E. A., O'Kane, M., et al. (2000). Guidelines for counseling women on the management of menopause. Retrieved from http://www.jiwh.org/Resources/Guidelines%20for%20menopause.pdf

Baird, D. T., Collins, J., Egozcue, J., Evers, L. H., Gianaroli, L., Leridon, H., et al. (2005). Fertility and ageing. *Human Reproduction Update, 11*(3), 261–276.

Ballagh, S. A. (2005). Vaginal hormone therapy for urogenital and menopausal symptoms. *Seminars in Reproductive Medicine, 23*(2), 126–140.

British Columbia Ministry of Health. (2012). Health link BC: Osteoporosis. Retrieved from http://www.healthlinkbc.ca/kb/content/major/hw131419.html

Broekmans, F. J., Faddy, M. J., Scheffer, G., & te Velde, E. R. (2004). Antral follicle counts are related to age at natural fertility loss and age at menopause. *Menopause, 11*(6 Pt 1), 607–614.

Society of Obstetricians and Gynaecologists of Canada. (SOGC). (2006). Canadian Consensus Conference on osteoporosis. *Journal of Obstetrics and Gynaecology Canada, 28*, S95–S112.

Buckler, H. (2005). The menopause transition: Endocrine changes and clinical symptoms. *Journal of the British Menopause Society, 11*(2), 61–65.

Burger, H., Hale, G., Robertson, D., & Dennerstein, L. (2007). A review of hormonal changes during the menopausal transition: Focus on findings from the Melbourne Women's Midlife Health Project. *Human Reproduction Update, 13*(6), 559–565.

Canadian Women's Health Network. (2007a). *Alternatives to hormone therapy*. Retrieved from http://www.cwhn.ca/node/40774

Canadian Women's Health Network. (2007b). *What is menopause?* Retrieved from http://www.cwhn.ca/en/node/40801

Canadian Women's Health Network. (2012). *Why not take that bone density test?* Retrieved from http://www.cwhn.ca/en/node/45481

Carroll, D. G. (2006). Nonhormonal therapies for hot flashes in menopause. *American Family Physician, 73*(3), 457–464.

Cohen, L. S., Soares, C. N., Vitonis, A. F., Otto, M. W., & Harlow, B. L. (2006). Risk for new onset of depression during the menopausal transition: The Harvard study of moods and cycles. *Archives of General Psychiatry, 63*(4), 385–390.

Corrigan, E. C., Raygada, M. J., Vanderhoof, V. H., & Nelson, L. M. (2005). A woman with spontaneous premature ovarian failure gives birth to a child with fragile X syndrome. *Fertility and Sterility, 84*(5), 1508.

Cutson, T. M., & Meuleman, E. (2000). Managing menopause. *American Family Physician, 61*(5), 1391–1400.

Deeks, A. A. (2004). Is this menopause? Women in midlife—psychosocial issues. *Australian Family Physician, 33*(11), 889–893.

Deeks, A. A., & McCabe, M. P. (2004). Well-being and menopause: An investigation of purpose in life, self-acceptance and social role in premenopausal, perimenopausal and postmenopausal women. *Quality of Life Research, 13*(2), 389–398.

Dennerstein, L., Guthrie, J. R., Clark, M., Lehert, P., & Henderson, V. W. (2004). A population-based study of depressed mood in middle-aged, Australian-born women. *Menopause, 11*(5), 563–568.

Deroo, B. J., & Korach, K. S. (2006). Estrogen receptors and human disease. *Journal of Clinical Investigation, 116*(3), 561–570.

Dvornyk, V., Long, J. R., Liu, P. Y., Zhao, L. J., Shen, H., Recker, R. R. et al. (2006). Predictive factors for age at menopause in Caucasian females. *Maturitas, 54*(1), 19–26.

Eastell, R. (2003). Management of osteoporosis due to ovarian failure. *Medical and Pediatric Oncology, 41*(3), 222–227.

Edwards, B., & Li, J. (2013). Endocrinology of menopause. *Periodontology 2000, 61*, 177–194.

Frackiewicz, E. J., & Cutler, N. R. (2000). Women's health care during the perimenopause. *Journal of the American Pharmaceutical Association, 40*(6), 800–811.

Freedman, R. R. (2005). Hot flashes: Behavioral treatments, mechanisms, and relation to sleep. *American Journal of Medicine, 118*(12 Suppl. 2), 124–130.

Gallicchio, L., Miller, S. R., Visvanathan, K., Lewis, L. M., Babus, J., Zacur, H. et al. (2006). Cigarette smoking, estrogen levels, and hot flashes in midlife women. *Maturitas, 53*(2), 133–143.

Gavaler, J. S., & Rosenblum, E. (2003). Predictors of postmenopausal body mass index and waist hip ratio in the Oklahoma postmenopausal health disparities study. *Journal of the American College of Nutrition, 22*(4), 269–276.

Gold, D. T. (2005). Elevated calcium requirements for women and unique approaches to improving calcium adherence. *Journal of Reproductive Medicine, 50*(11 Suppl.), 891–895.

Gould, D. C., Petty, R., & Jacobs, H. S. (2000). The male menopause—does it exist? *British Medical Journal, 320*(35), 858–860.

Groff, A. A., Covington, S. N., Halverson, L. R., Fitzgerald, O. R., Vanderhoof, V., Calis, K. et al. (2005). Assessing the emotional needs of women with spontaneous premature ovarian failure. *Fertility and Sterility, 83*(6), 1734–1741.

Gyllstrom, M., Schreiner, P., & Harlow, B. (2007). Perimenopause and depression: Strength of association, causal mechanisms and treatment recommendations. *Best Practice & Research. Clinical Obstetrics & Gynaecology, 21*(2), 275–292.

Hafez, B., & Hafez, E. S. (2004). Andropause: Endocrinology, erectile dysfunction, and prostate pathophysiology. *Archives of Andrology, 50*(2), 45–68.

Harvey, M. A. (2003). Pelvic floor exercises during and after pregnancy: A systematic review of their role in preventing pelvic floor dysfunction. *Journal of Obstetrics and Gynaecology Canada, 25*(6), 451–453.

Hay-Smith, E. J., & Dumoulin, C. (2006). Pelvic floor muscle training versus no treatment, or inactive control treatments, for urinary incontinence in women. *Cochrane Database of Systematic Reviews, 25*(1), CD005654.

Health Canada. (2004). *Benefits and risks of hormone replacement therapy (Estrogen with or without Progestin).* Retrieved from http://www.hc-sc.gc.ca/hl-vs/iyh-vsv/med/estrogen-eng.php

Health Canada. (2008). *Seniors and aging – Osteoporosis.* Retrieved from www.hc-sc.gc.ca/hl-vs/iyh-vsv/diseases-maladies/seniors-aines-ost-eng.php

Hefler, L. A., Grimm, C., Bentz, E. K., Reinthaller, A., Heinze, G., & Tempfer, C. B. (2006). A model for predicting age at menopause in white women. *Fertility and Sterility, 85*(2), 451–454.

Hobar, C. (2005). *Osteoporosis. [E-Medicine].* Retrieved from http://ωωω.emedicine.com/med/topic1693.htm

Hoyert, D. L., Heron, M. P., Murphy, S. L., & Kung, H. (2006). Deaths: Final data for 2003. *National Vital Statistics Reports, 54*(13), 1–120.

Hvas, L. (2006). Menopausal women's positive experience of growing older. *Maturitas, 54*(3), 245–251.

Jacobsson, B., Ladfors, L., & Milsom, I. (2004). Advanced maternal age and adverse perinatal outcome. *Obstetrics and Gynecology, 104*(4), 727–733.

Karch, A. M. (2013). *2013 Lippincott's nursing drug guide.* Philadelphia, PA: Lippincott Williams & Wilkins.

Kinney, A., Kline, J., & Levin, B. (2006). Alcohol, caffeine and smoking in relation to age at menopause. *Maturitas, 54*(1), 27–38.

Leach, M., & Moore, V. (2012). Black Cohosh for menopausal symptoms. The Cochrane Library Collection. Published online September 12, 2012, doi: 10.1002/14651858.CD007244.pub2. Retrieved April 28, 2013.

Learn, C. D., & Higgins, P. G. (1999). Harmonizing herbs. Managing menopause with help from Mother Earth. *AWHONN Lifelines, 3*(5), 39–43.

Mainini, G., Festa, B., Messalli, E. M., Torella, M., & Ragucci, A. (2003). Premature ovarian failure. Clinical evaluation of 32 cases. *Minerva Ginecologica, 55*(6), 525–529.

Marjoribanks, J., Farquhar, C., Roberts, H., & Lethaby, A. (2012). Long term hormone therapy for perimenopausal and postmenopausal women. Cochrane Database Systematic Review, July 11(7). doi: 10.1002/14651858.CD004143.pub4

Massin, N., Czernichow, C., Thibaud, E., Kuttenn, F., Polak, M., & Touraine, P. (2006). Idiopathic premature ovarian failure in 63 young women. *Hormone Research, 65*(2), 89–95.

McVeigh, C. (2005). Perimenopause: More than hot flushes and night sweats for some Australian women. *Journal of Obstetric, Gynecologic, and Neonatal Nursing, 34*(1), 21–27.

MedlinePlus. (2013). *Dong quai.* Retrieved from http://www.nlm.nih.gov/medlineplus/druginfo/natural/936.html

Mooradian, A. D., & Korenman, S. G. (2006). Management of the cardinal features of andropause. *American Journal of Therapeutics, 13*(2), 145–160.

Orshan, S. A., Furniss, K., Forst, C., & Santoro, N. (2001). The lived experience of premature ovarian failure. *Journal of Obstetric, Gynecologic, and Neonatal Nursing, 30*(2), 202–208.

Pandian, Z., Bhattacharya, S., Vale, L., & Tempelton, A. (2005). In vitro fertilization for unexplained subfertility. *Cochrane Database of Systematic Reviews, 18*(2), CD003357.

Popat, V., & Nelson, L. (2011). *Ovarian insufficiency. eMedicine.* Retrieved from http://emedicine.medscape.com/article/271046-overview

Ratka, A., Miller, V., Brown, K., Raut, A., Cipher, D., Meczekalski, B. et al. (2006). Menopausal Vasomotor Symptoms (MVS) Survey for assessment of hot flashes. *Journal of Women's Health, 15*(1), 77–89.

Sanson, G. (2005). The myth of osteoporosis. *Canadian Women's Health Network Magazine, 7*(4). Retrieved from http://www.cwhn.ca/en/node/23265

Santoro, N. (2003). Mechanisms of premature ovarian failure. *Annals of Endocrinology, 64*(2), 87–92.

Schmidt, P. J., Haq, N., & Rubinow, D. R. (2004). A longitudinal evaluation of the relationship between reproductive status and mood in perimenopausal women. *American Journal of Psychiatry, 161*(12), 2238–2244.

Society of Obstetricians and Gynaecologists of Canada. (2009). *Menopause and osteoporosis update.* Guideline No. 222. Retrieved from http://sogc.org/wp-content/uploads/2013/01/Menopause_JOGC-Jan_09.pdf

Swanton, A., & Child, T. (2005). Reproduction and ovarian ageing. *Journal of the British Menopause Society, 11*(4), 126–131.

Vandborg, M., & Lauszus, F. F. (2006). Premature ovarian failure and pregnancy. *Archives of Gynecology and Obstetrics, 273*(6), 387–388.

Van Voorhis, B. J. (2005). Genitourinary symptoms in the menopausal transition. *American Journal of Medicine, 118*(12 Suppl. 2), 47–53.

Vermeulen, A. (2000). Andropause. *Maturitas, 34*, 5–15.

Whiteman, M. K., Staropoli, C. A., Langenberg, P. W., McCarter, R. J., Kjerulff, K. H., & Flaws, J. A. (2003). Smoking, body mass, and hot flashes in midlife women. *Obstetrics and Gynecology, 101*(2), 264–272.

Williamson, E. M. (2005). Interactions between herbal and conventional medicines. *Expert Opinion on Drug Safety, 4*(2), 355–378.

Woad, K. J., Watkins, W. J., Prendergast, D., & Shelling, A. N. (2006). The genetic basis of premature ovarian failure. *Australia and New Zealand Journal of Obstetrics and Gynaecology, 46*(3), 242–244.

Woods, N., & Mitchell, E. (2005). Symptoms during the perimenopause: Prevalence, severity, trajectory, and significance in women's lives. *The American Journal of Medicine, 118*(12 Suppl. 2), 14–24.

Writing Group for the Women's Health Initiative Investigators. (2002). Risks and benefits of estrogen plus progestin in healthy postmenopausal women: Principal results from the Women's Health Initiative randomized controlled trial. *Journal of the American Medical Association, 288*(3), 321–333.

WEB RESOURCES

Canadian Women's Health Network
http://www.cwhn.ca/
Canadian Research Institute for the Advancement of Women
http://www.criaw-icref.ca/
Health Canada
http://www.hc-sc.gc.ca/index-eng.php
Association of Women's Health, Obstetric, and Neonatal Nursing
http://www.awhonn.org/awhonn/
The North American Menopause Society
www.menopause.org
International Premature Ovarian Failure Support Group
http://www.ipofa.org/
Society of Obstetricians and Gynaecologists of Canada
http://www.menopauseandu.ca/index_e.aspx

CHAPTER 24

The Older Postmenopausal Woman

Yvonne M.R. Brown, Janice Kinch, Susan Scanland*, and Christine Bradway*

Ann, an independent and healthy 67-year-old, lives with her husband, daughter, and two grandchildren. She works part-time at the local library and is active in volunteer work. She enjoys gardening and tennis. During a routine checkup, Ann says to the nurse, "I need to discuss something. Lately, I've been having bladder problems. Sometimes when I sneeze or laugh, I leak. Once in a while, when I'm walking home from the library I have to rush inside to make it to the bathroom. I've been waking up at night needing to urinate. I've read a bit about this on the internet, and I'm wondering if I have urinary incontinence."

A home care nurse is working with Lena and Hannah, life partners of 25 years. Hannah, 71 years old, has dementia of the Alzheimer type, late onset. Although Lena, 65 years old, can still care for Hannah at home, she has noticed that Hannah is becoming increasingly disengaged and forgetful. Lena is finding that most of her time is spent caring for Hannah and the house. At one point when they are alone, Lena says to the nurse, "I'd do anything for Hannah, but sometimes I feel so frustrated. The other day she tripped and fell and didn't seem to recognize me when I went to help her. I'm afraid she's going to wander from the house at night. I never thought this would happen to us."

You will learn more about these stories later in this chapter. Before beginning this chapter, consider the following points related to the above scenarios:

*Contributor to first U.S. edition.

- What association might there be with these clients' problems and negative societal feelings and beliefs associated with aging? How might nurses help people understand the differences between normal aging and medical problems more common in older adults?
- Despite some clear differences, what might the women in these scenarios have in common? What problems or circumstances are similar?
- Describe some specific strategies that the nurse might use to show sensitivity and compassion when working with these women.
- How might the nurse promote adaptation and adjustment for these clients?

LEARNING OBJECTIVES

On completion of this chapter, the reader will be able to:
- Facilitate effective communication with an older woman and her family or significant others.
- Elicit an informative health history from an older woman.
- Conduct a comprehensive assessment of an older woman, including lifestyle, medication, nutrition, function, social status, sexuality, safety and the environment, prevention and screening, sleep, and long-term health care wishes.
- Describe age-associated physiologic changes in each major body system, as well as in functional performance.
- Develop the ability to prevent, identify, and intervene in cases of inappropriate medication use and adverse drug reactions in older women.
- Identify women at high risk for common health conditions, such as urinary incontinence, osteoporosis, falls, fractures, and immobility.
- Differentiate typical aging from cognitive and mental disorders such as depression, delirium, and dementia.
- Become familiar with nursing roles in home care, long-term care, and assisted living, with awareness of professional opportunities for registered and advanced practice nurses who specialize in care of older adults.

KEY TERMS

actinic keratoses	hyperthermia
activities of daily living (ADLs)	hypothermia
adverse drug reaction	isolated systolic hypertension
ageism	myocardial ischemia
agnosia	orthostatic (postural) hypotension
anterior vaginal wall prolapse	osteopenia
aphasia	osteoporosis
apraxia	pharmacodynamics
confabulation	pharmacokinetics
cystocele	polypharmacy
delirium	posterior vaginal wall prolapse
dyspareunia	presbycardia
dysphagia	primary caregiver
dysthymia	primary health care provider
elder abuse	sleep phase advancement
elderspeak	syncope
fear of falling	xerostomia
health care advance directives	

omen are living longer than ever before. In 1960 the life expectancy at birth was 74 years for women, and by 2009, women's life expectancy had increased to 83 years (Statistics Canada, 2012a). Demographics in the 21st century will contribute to significant societal changes, with the aging population sector in Canada expected to double by 2031. In 2010 women comprised 56% of the 4.8 million seniors over the age of 65 (Milan & Vézina, 2012). Projections show that, by 2031, of the 9.6 million people 65 years and over, 5.1 million will be women (Milan & Vézina, 2012). The most rapid population growth is occurring in people older than 80 years. Having grown steadily, the population aged 80 and over was estimated at 1.4 million in 2012, 4.1% of the Canadian population. Demographic projections indicate that in 2036, 7.6% of Canadians could be 80 years of age or older (Statistics Canada, 2012b). Increasing numbers of older adults are living beyond 100 years, a group with health, emotional, and social needs previously unconsidered (Fig. 24.1).

An important aspect of the changing Canadian demography is that Canada has one of the most diverse populations in the world. The challenge ahead will be to continue to explore and implement health and social care policies and practices that meet the needs of all Canadian residents and citizens, including the older generations of immigrants and Aboriginal citizens. By the year 2017, Canada's mosaic will have altered dramatically. The projected growth of the Aboriginal population sends a message to health care planners, policy makers, and health care and social welfare profes-

sionals. First Nations people living off reserve, Métis, and Inuit have a higher rate of obesity, diabetes, other chronic illnesses, smoking, and food insecurity than non-Aboriginal people (Statistics Canada, 2013). All Canadian citizens must be treated equally within the social, political, and cultural frameworks of the country. Nurses must be positioned to make this equity occur as they are the health care professionals who come in contact with all population sectors.

Growth in the fields of gerontology and geriatrics has exploded, with fascinating clinical and research knowledge further promoting longevity and quality of life for older adults. Over the past 20 years, experts have defined age by numbers. For the future, experts predict that the focus will shift from describing aging in terms of predefined stages to focusing more on functional capacity and quality of life. The focus will shift as well from making assumptions that all people read and understand the official languages of Canada as they enter the health care system. Older women from other ethnic origins and cultures have needs that must be recognized and respected. The practices of inclusion and respect are key to maintaining Canada's reputation as a model for other countries in health care provision.

In this chapter, we explore the unique needs of older postmenopausal women as they journey through the second half or last third of their lives. We focus on functional status and its relationships to illness and common health conditions seen in older women. We describe assessment of various aspects of the older woman's lifestyle, circumstances, and environment for safety, appropriateness, and satisfaction and analyze

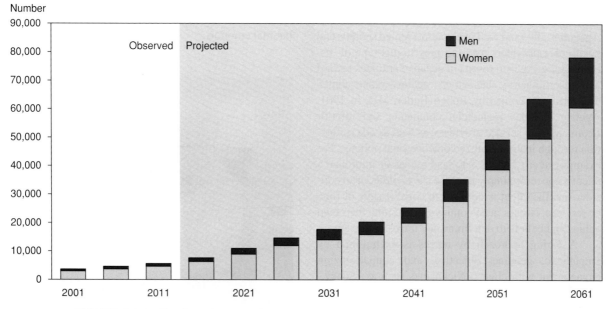

FIGURE 24.1 Number of centenarians in the Canadian population, 2001–2061. (Adapted from Statistics Canada, Census in Brief. Catalogue no. 98–311-X-2011003. Figure 1: Number of Centenarians by Sex, Canada, 2001 to 2061. Released 2012–05–29. This does not constitute an endorsement by Statistics Canada of this product.)

common health conditions and medication use, interweaving their effects and uses in older women. Finally, we provide material that addresses the nursing care of women across levels of function and setting, emphasizing "best practices" of nursing care for older women.

One further issue must be raised. Since mandatory retirement has been abolished in public service and increasingly in private sector organizations, many women over the age of 65 years are choosing to continue to participate in the economic workforce. We must not make any assumptions about the employment status of older women in our care. Regardless of whether a woman has retired or continues to work for salary or as a volunteer, she is still contributing to our society. Respect and recognition of her continuing contributions must be accorded.

COMMUNICATING WITH THE OLDER WOMAN

Effective communication is essential to successful nursing care. Strong communication skills are especially important when dealing with older clients because of the multitude of factors that often affect communication adversely. Language and culture present challenges to teaching, learning, and understanding for nurses who are caring for clients from other countries and cultures. In addition, sensory impairments, effects of acute or chronic illness, medication effects, ageist attitudes on the part of the nurse, sociocultural factors, and a noisy or chaotic environment are all potential barriers to effective communication.

Using Interviewing Skills

Ageism is alive and well in a youth-oriented society, and health care providers may fall prey to this type of discrimination. Ageism results in negative attitudes toward and discriminatory behaviours against older adults. The term was coined by Robert Butler, MD, in 1961. Ageism includes prejudicial comments and inferior treatment from service providers, as well as discrimination through institutionalized practices and policies. For example, ageist beliefs may lead nurses to minimize a client's concerns simply because she is older, or to consider that the client is not "worth" investments of time or services. Nurses must continue to examine their own values and beliefs to determine any traces of ageism.

A caring approach by nurses is exemplified by empathetic, genuine, objective, and nonpatronizing engagement with clients. Nicknames such as "honey," "doll," "sweetie," and "dear" are condescending for older people who have lived full lives, and are to be avoided. See video *Elderspeak* (Yorkcollegepa, 2011). Use of demeaning nicknames and a patronizing tone for older adults is called **elderspeak** and may be as high as 20% in long-term care settings (Jerrard, 2006). An observational study showed that the likelihood of resistance to care behaviour in clients with dementia was significantly greater following use of elderspeak communication rather than normal talk or silence (Williams et al., 2009). Listening is an extremely important skill, as is giving the older person enough time to speak and express her concerns. Keeping interviews on track, however, prevents the client from going off on tangents.

Standing taller than the interviewee may induce feelings of powerlessness and inferiority in her. For this reason, a position that allows for eye-level contact with clients is more appropriate. If an older woman is in a wheelchair, the interviewer sits, facilitating direct eye contact (Fig. 24.2). Because hearing impairment is common in older adults, nurses speak slowly in a normal tone of voice (Miller, 2011). Yelling or speaking loudly often irritates clients with hearing impairment, because they are usually sensitive to loud noises. Inexpensive amplifying devices are available to facilitate communication.

It is important not to interrupt or finish the client's response or sentences, even if she rambles. It is better to let the interviewee complete the thought. If the content is veering off course, the nurse might acknowledge those remarks and return the interviewee to the main topic. It is effective at the interview's onset to let the client know exactly how much time is available and the specific goals of the interview. The nurse can then refer back to this information if the interview drifts off track. Using direct open-ended questions rather than inquiries that result in closed "yes" or "no" responses is important. An example of an open-ended question is, "Tell me about the pain in your hip." It is imperative that nurses assess nonverbal behaviours, which provide clues to internal emotions.

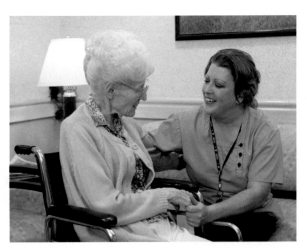

FIGURE 24.2 During discussions, it is imperative to try to maintain eye-level contact with clients, particularly those who require wheelchair assistance.

A quiet background facilitates communication. Examples of methods to enhance a quiet background include closing the door to the room, asking other people who are conversing to leave the room where the interview is being held, and shutting off the television or radio. Nurses also can augment understanding by using gestures, nonverbal language, and alternative communication techniques (eg, word or communication board).

 Consider Ann, the 67-year-old woman from the beginning of the chapter who reported having difficulty controlling her bladder. Describe how the nurse could facilitate an effective interview with Ann.

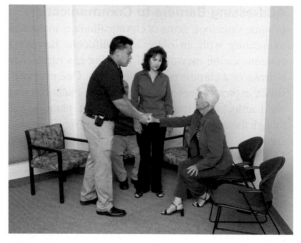

FIGURE 24.3 To convey respect and to establish a trusting and comfortable relationship, the nurse introduces himself or herself to the client first and then acknowledge the presence of significant others who are with her.

Obtaining a Health History

Obtaining a health history from an older person can be a challenging process. Many factors can affect the nurse's ability to obtain information. Older people frequently have atypical presentations of illness, meaning that an illness presents without symptoms or with symptoms different from those that would occur in a young or middle-aged adult. An example is a "silent" myocardial infarction (MI), which may occur without symptoms, or present as confusion or dizziness in the older person, rather than with the classic chest pain found in a middle-aged person (Rosen et al., 2010).

Older adults usually have at least one or more chronic, coexisting illnesses (Rosen et al., 2010). Sometimes it is difficult to sift through multiple symptoms when obtaining a history and determine what is clinically significant. The tendency in older clients is to underreport symptoms, contradicting conventional wisdom that older people overreport symptoms or suffer from excessive anxiety related to symptoms. For example, older women may "normalize" symptoms by attributing them to old age, underestimating their significance, and in turn, reducing the nurse's ability to identify and address important health issues. Some have suggested this behaviour may result from denial regarding symptoms or not wanting to "bother" the health care provider.

Obtaining a history from an older person is more time consuming than with younger clients. The older adult has many years of past medical history to review. Many providers request that older clients complete an informal health status questionnaire before the office visit. Review of previous medical records is essential. It is time-saving to review previous charts before interviewing a client.

Upon meeting an older client, the nurse introduces himself or herself to the client first, and then acknowledge significant others present in the room (Fig. 24.3). She or he asks the client her title (eg, Mrs., Miss, Ms., Dr.), then continue to address the client accordingly unless she requests to be called by her first name. It is more respectful and appropriate for the nurse to direct the conversation to the client rather than to family members. He or she should ask the client's permission to have other family members present during the interview. It is essential to avoid side conversations with the family in the client's presence. Interview time alone with the client is important to explore confidential issues like sexuality, **elder abuse** (neglect, exploitation), or emotional concerns that the client may not want to share with the family. The nurse asks the client her main concern, or why she is visiting today. In addition, he or she evaluates the family's main concern, relating it to the client's chief complaint.

The nurse can track the history of symptoms, including onset as well as changes over time. Discussing previous treatment successes and failures is important. The nurse can use questions like, "What do you mean when you say that you are…?" Quantifying fluctuating symptoms like pain, using a scale studied in older people, is important, as is separating active and past problems and prioritizing the urgency of each current concern.

The nurse inquires about symptoms related to common illnesses that affect elders. These conditions include arthritis, hearing impairment, visual problems, and congestive heart failure (CHF). Usually, clients do not have just one concern but several simultaneous matters. Many complaints are the result of chronic illness, but the nurse must discern whether any complaints are caused by active or acute exacerbation of such chronic illness.

Addressing Barriers to Communication

In some situations, acute or chronic illnesses make communicating with an older adult difficult. Barriers to communication may occur if a person has experienced a stroke or a chronic neurologic illness. One example is Broca expressive aphasia, in which the client has awkward articulation when forming simple phrases, even though the auditory system is preserved. Wernicke aphasia results in fluent speech that is lacking in content. Speech apraxia can develop after a stroke or can result directly from a dementing process in the brain. Dysarthria results from inadequate control of speech caused by muscle weakness. It can develop with neuromuscular diseases or a stroke. It can also occur from muscle paralysis and lack of muscle coordination. Other speech barriers may be seen with Parkinson disease, in which destruction of the basal ganglia affects speech, sometimes rendering speech completely incomprehensible. Neuronal degeneration of the frontal lobes also may affect speech quality. As dementia progresses, the ability to understand abstractions becomes more impaired; it is more difficult for a client to express herself through words. The person's vocabulary narrows, and she has difficulty choosing words. Other barriers to communication include laryngectomy and endotracheal intubation.

The nurse can address communication barriers by being sensitive to them and by addressing them with individualized interventions. Selected examples of nursing interventions to enhance communication are included in Box 24.1.

COMPREHENSIVE ASSESSMENT OF THE OLDER WOMAN

In this section, we address a comprehensive assessment of the older woman in several domains. Areas covered include lifestyle and habits, nutrition, medications, function, social issues, sexuality, safety and the environment, prevention and screening, sleep, and long-term health care wishes.

Lifestyle

When considering the older woman's lifestyle, the nurse assesses health habits, particularly in the areas of smoking, alcohol use, and exercise.

Smoking and Tobacco Use

To conduct assessment of smoking and tobacco use, the nurse asks the client the following questions:

- Do you smoke cigarettes or cigars or use other tobacco products?
- How many years have you smoked?
- What is the number of packs you have smoked over these years (to give a "pack/year" ratio)?

● **BOX 24.1 Interventions to Enhance Communication With Older Adults**

- Take the time to introduce yourself to the client.
- Verbally exchange names and ask the woman what name she prefers to be called (eg, Ms., Dr., Mrs.). Use proper names, unless directed otherwise.
- Use a handshake or touch when introduced. Be sensitive to cultural or gender differences that may indicate discomfort with the use of touch.
- Listen to what the older adult says.
- If at all possible, talk to the woman in a face-to-face position because this enhances verbal and nonverbal communication.
- As much as possible, remove physical barriers (eg, walker, bedside table) that compromise field of vision.
- Modify the environment to facilitate communication:
  - Provide a quiet setting
  - Eliminate competing noises (eg, turn off TV, radio)
  - Assure privacy
  - Optimize lighting by minimizing glare
- Introduce formal screening (eg, depression or cognitive testing) in a matter-of-fact manner. Explain the purpose and ask the client's permission to proceed.

From Miller, C. A. (2011). *Nursing for wellness in older adults. Theory and practice* (6th ed.). Philadelphia, PA: Lippincott Williams & Wilkins.

- Have you ever attempted to stop smoking?
- Have you used any nicotine products or prescription drugs to stop smoking?
- Have you ever quit suddenly ("cold turkey")?
- How long were you successful in nicotine abstinence?
- What psychosocial, behavioural, or physical factors caused you to start smoking again?
- What is your rationale for continuing to smoke?
- Are there other smokers in the household?
- Do your friends smoke?
- Do you spend time in places where there are several smokers?

Alcohol Use

Alcoholism is often a silent syndrome in older women. Typically, clients underestimate or give false low reports of alcohol intake. Older individuals may experience some health benefits from moderate alcohol consumption, but the changes that occur with aging increase the likelihood that alcohol will be harmful (International Center for Alcohol Policies, 1995–2013). Asking about alcohol intake is important: the amount and type of

● **ASSESSMENT TOOL 24.1** **Michigan Alcohol Screening Test-Geriatric Version (MAST-G)**

Please check "yes" or "no" for each question.

QUESTION	YES	NO
1. After drinking have you ever noticed an increase in your heart rate or beating in your chest?		
2. When talking with others, do you ever underestimate how much you actually drink?		
3. Does alcohol make you sleepy so that you often fall asleep in your chair?		
4. After a few drinks, have you sometimes not eaten or been able to skip a meal because you didn't feel hungry?		
5. Does having a few drinks help decrease your shakiness or tremors?		
6. Does alcohol sometimes make it hard for you to remember parts of the day or night?		
7. Do you have rules for yourself that you won't drink before a certain time of the day?		
8. Have you lost interest in hobbies or activities you used to enjoy?		
9. When you wake up in the morning, do you ever have trouble remembering part of the night before?		
10. Does having a drink help you sleep?		
11. Do you hide your alcohol bottles from family members?		
12. After a social gathering, have you ever felt embarrassed because you drank too much?		
13. Have you ever been concerned that drinking might be harmful to your health?		
14. Do you like to end an evening with a nightcap?		
15. Did you find your drinking increased after someone close to you died?		
16. In general, would you prefer to have a few drinks at home rather than go out to social events?		
17. Are you drinking more now than in the past?		
18. Do you usually take a drink to relax or calm your nerves?		
19. Do you drink to take your mind off your problems?		
20. Have you ever increased your drinking after experiencing a loss in your life?		
21. Do you sometimes drive when you have had too much to drink?		
22. Has a doctor or nurse ever said they were worried or concerned about your drinking?		
23. Have you ever made rules to manage your drinking?		
24. When you feel lonely does having a drink help?		

SCORING

Five or more "yes" responses are indicative of an alcohol problem.

---

alcohol consumed daily, weekly, or monthly. Women over the age of 60 are advised not to consume more than seven standard drinks per week or one per day (Substance Abuse and Mental Health Administration and Administration on Aging, 2012). Use of a screening instrument, such as Ewing's (1984) CAGE mnemonic (see Chapter 2), can be helpful as a first step in identifying and documenting alcohol use and dependence in older adults. The Michigan Alcoholism Screening Test-Geriatric Version (MAST-G) is an assessment tool that has been found appropriate for use with elderly people (Assessment Tool 24.1). In addition, questions about falls, dizziness, weight gain, and motor vehicle crashes can provide clues to alcohol use. Guidelines for working with older adults with alcohol disorders are available from a number of sources, including the Canadian Healthy Aging Project (2006).

Exercise

It is important to find out what factors contribute to adherence to or decreased participation in exercise for older women (Fig. 24.4). Questions to ask include the following:

- What do you do to stay physically active?
- Have you had any falls, accidents, or fractures related to physical activity?
- Do you limit your activities because of a fear of falling?
- Do you have any symptoms that interfere with activities (eg, shortness of breath on exertion, leg cramps after walking a certain distance)?

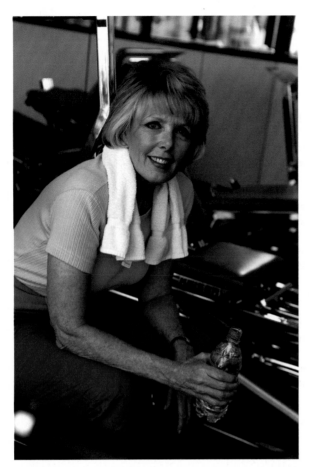

FIGURE 24.4 Exercise in older women can help maintain functional status, as well as contribute to overall health and well-being.

Nutrition

Assessment of the older woman's nutrition is vital. One third of Canada's seniors living at home are at risk for not getting adequate nutrition. Factors such as living alone, depression, multiple medications, and/or impaired ability to shop for or prepare meals contribute to the risk for poor nutrition (Ramage-Morin & Garriguet, 2013). The nurse can take a nutritional history by using the 24-hour food recall, asking the client, "What did you eat in the past 24 hours?" (see Chapter 3).

In addition to asking about a 24-hour food recall, the nurse may also check any available laboratory results to identify the older woman's serum albumin level. A low serum albumin level indicates protein malnutrition, which has been shown to be associated with diminished immune response and impaired muscle and respiratory function. Hospitalized elders have been found to have delayed wound healing, overall increased complications, longer rehabilitation, greater length of hospital stay, and increased mortality (Milne et al., 2009).

The prevention of **osteoporosis** begins in a woman's younger years because bone mineral density (BMD), which accounts for 70% of bone strength, begins to decline in midlife (Masoro, 2010) (see Chapter 2). The nurse can encourage women to eat foods high in calcium, including milk, cheese, yogurt, broccoli and other dark-green vegetables, canned salmon or sardines, ice cream, and custard. Women who are lactose intolerant or who cannot meet daily requirements for dietary calcium can be encouraged to shop for calcium-fortified foods (eg, orange juice, cereal, breads, and waffles).

There is controversy about the use of calcium and vitamin D supplementation for reducing fractures caused by osteoporosis. A 2013 report from the U.S. Preventive Services Task Force concluded that there is no evidence to support such supplementation (Moyer, 2013). However, Osteoporosis Canada states that anyone over the age of 50 is advised to take 1,200 mg of calcium daily, preferably from dietary sources, and from 800 to 2,000 International Unit of vitamin D supplement daily, depending on the risk for vitamin D deficiency (Osteoporosis Canada, 2013).

Because many older adults are more sedentary and drink less fluid than when they were younger, the probability of constipation is increased. As well, some medications have side effects that cause constipation. Many older people drink inadequate amounts of fluid because of declining age-related thirst mechanism; women with urinary incontinence may limit their fluid intake in an effort to control "accidents." Immobility, with decreased ability to reach water sources, is often a cause of dehydration and constipation in older adults. The nurse assesses the intake of high-fibre foods, such as cereals, whole grain breads, and fresh fruits and vegetables, and asks about the client's daily fluid intake. An adequate intake of fluid from any source for women over the age of 50 is 2.7 L per day (Institute of Medicine, 2004). Approximately 80% of fluid intake comes from water and other beverages, with 20% from food (Zelman, 2010). Thus, for women, the recommended daily amount of water and other beverages is about 2.1 L, that is, eight to nine (8-oz) glasses.

Other dietary areas the nurse can evaluate are caffeine intake and weight patterns, paying special attention to increases or decreases of more than 4.5 kg in the past 5 years. Sudden unintentional weight loss could signal the possibility of poverty, functional impairment, social isolation, poor nutritional knowledge, elder abuse, depression, or medical reasons such as poor dentition, dementia, malignancy, or endocrine abnormalities (Rosen et al., 2010). What was the older woman's maximal height as an adult? Older women may decrease several centimetres in height because of osteoporotic vertebral compression fractures. Does the person eat alone? Who prepares her meals? Who shops for groceries and how often? Can the older woman afford nutritious food? All these factors are an important part of the nutritional assessment.

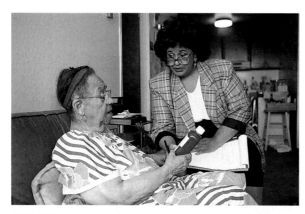

FIGURE 24.5 Adherence to medication regimens depends on several factors, including the client's cognitive capacity and family dynamics. (Photo © Kathy Sloane.)

Medications

Performing a thorough medication history when interviewing an older client is essential. People of all ages may not adhere to medication regimens for a wide variety of reasons (Fig. 24.5). A good way to elicit information about medication use is to ask questions nonjudgementally and to give the older woman ample opportunity to discuss her understanding of over-the-counter and prescription medications. For example, the nurse could ask questions such as, What medications are you currently taking? How many times/days in the last week did you take (or forget to take) your pills? How do you think your medications are working for you? Do you use any herbal, over-the-counter, or recreational drugs on a regular or occasional basis?

The nurse documents the location and telephone number of the client's pharmacy and asks whether the pharmacy makes deliveries. Does the client use any other pharmacies? Does she have adequate or supplemental coverage for medications that are not included for seniors in the provincial formulary? Does the woman order by mail or through the internet any medications from other countries? Would any visual problems interfere with reading medication labels? Will she have problems opening the caps or packaging of the medication containers due to arthritis or weakness?

The nurse should review the client's history for any past experiences with, or current symptoms of, clinical depression. Depression may minimize the motivation necessary to follow a medication regimen. In addition, the nurse should consider whether any confusion is present, because dementia is a common cause of errors in self-administration of medication. The nurse should ask the older woman if she saves and reuses old prescriptions. Does she share medications with friends? How does she store and administer medications? Does she use a special medication container with the times of the day and days of the week? Does she have any history of allergic reactions to drugs (eg, documented rash, hives, anaphylaxis)?

In an older woman, asking about the history of **adverse drug reactions** is equally important. These events are not allergic reactions; rather, they are defined as "harmful, unintended reactions to medicines that occur at doses normally used for treatment" (World Health Organization, 2008, p.1). For example, an older woman may experience muscle degeneration as a result of a statin prescribed for controlling cholesterol (WHO, 2008). Although adverse drug reactions are not unique to older adults, risk increases with age, primarily as a result of polypharmacy. In 2010 and 2011, more than 27,000 seniors 66 years and over (1 in 200) were admitted to hospital for an adverse drug reaction. The rate for people under the age of 65 was 1 in 1,000. Although seniors represented only 14.2% of the Canadian population, they accounted for 57.6% of the hospitalizations related to adverse drug reactions. Drug most commonly involved included anticoagulants, antineoplastics, opioids and related analgesics, glucocorticoids, and nonsteroidal anti-inflammatory drugs (Canadian Institute for Health Information, 2013).

Ideally, the nurse will take the client's medication history through the "brown-bag" approach. In an office visit setting, the receptionist, upon booking the appointment, asks the client to bring to the visit all her medications, including over-the-counter drugs, ointments, eye drops, herbs, and vitamins. In the home setting, the nurse can duplicate the brown-bag approach by assessing the client's medication cabinet, with her permission. The nurse also inquires what medications other providers have prescribed. Is the **primary health care provider** coordinating medications prescribed by other specialists? The nurse should ask the older woman about her use of eye drops, ointments, creams, herbal drinks, foods, vitamins, and other supplements. Herbal preparations may interact with the multiple medications that many older adults take. It is important to ask about laxatives because some older clients forget to include them as medications. Another influence on a woman's well-being may be whether or not she is taking hormone replacement therapy (HRT).

The nurse also evaluates storage issues. Keeping medications safe from young children and others during child care or elder care responsibilities is essential to prevent accidental poisoning or overdose. The older woman may benefit from using pillbox organizers to assist her in taking the right medication in the right quantity at the right time. If she is unable to sort her medications into the organizer, a caregiver can help with this task.

Function

Functional assessment is an essential piece of a comprehensive geriatric assessment. In the hospitalized elderly,

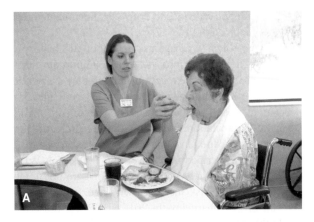

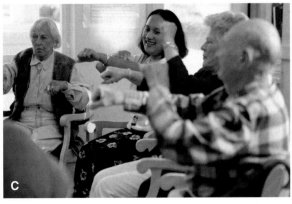

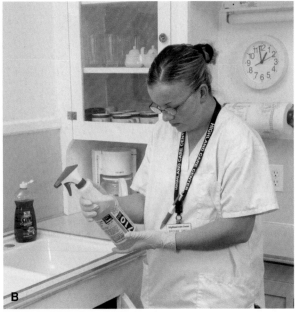

FIGURE 24.6 **A:** Nurses may assist clients with basic ADLs such as feeding. **B:** An example of assisting with instrumental ADLs may involve doing housework. **C:** Nurses may help clients with advanced ADLs through facilitating attendance at recreational or occupational tasks.

functional status is a strong predictor of functional decline, rehospitalization, and death after discharge (Volpato et al., 2010). The ability of an older woman to function may affect her living arrangements, relationship with others, quality of life, and overall health. It is important for the nurse to assess and document baseline functional level when the older woman is well. Health care professionals can then use these findings for comparison if illnesses, adverse drug reactions, delirium, dementia, or depression change the client's level of function. They can also use the information gathered to communicate with one another about what constitutes a baseline for the client on a daily basis. The main reason to assess function is to determine whether the older woman's living arrangements and social support match her functional needs. Knowing the woman's activity level has major implications for both her safety and quality of life.

Activities of Daily Living

Activities of daily living (ADLs) are those functions necessary for independent living. *Basic* ADLs include self-care tasks such as bathing, dressing, toileting, maintaining continence, feeding, and transferring. *Instrumental* ADLs are those activities that further enhance the client's ability to live independently. Examples include shopping for groceries; driving or using public transportation; using the telephone; preparing meals; doing housework, repair work, and laundry; taking medications; and handling finances. *Advanced* ADLs refer to the client's ability to fulfill societal, community, and family roles as well as participate in recreational or occupational tasks (Ward & Reuben, 2012) (Fig. 24.6).

When reviewing ADLs, the may ask, How do you...? for each component. Older adults needing assistance with basic ADLs usually require live-in assistance from family members or health care personnel or placement in long-term care facilities such as nursing homes. Elders with deficits in instrumental ADLs may live at home by themselves but are dependent on others to assist in completion of these tasks. Assisted living and personal care facilities are rapidly growing in number to meet instrumental ADL and ADL needs of elders who do not require skilled or total nursing care. A woman's ability to complete advanced ADLs depends on her ability to complete instrumental ADLs.

 Recall Lena and Hannah, who were described at the beginning of the chapter. How might the nurse expect Lena's ability to complete ADLs to compare with that of Hannah?

Mobility

Performance-based testing of functional status focuses primarily on transfers, gait, and balance. The nurse asks the client to stand from the seated position in a hard-backed chair while keeping her arms folded. Inability to complete this task suggests weakness of the lower extremities or quadriceps, and is highly predictive of future disability. Once the client is standing, the nurse can observe her walking back and forth over a short distance, ideally with any usual walking aid. Abnormalities of gait include path deviation; diminished step height, length, or both; trips, slips, or near falls; and difficulty turning. The tasks of rising from the chair, walking 3 m, turning around and returning to the chair, turning, and then sitting back down in the chair (without using arms) make up the "Timed Up and Go" test (Mathias et al., 1986; Podsiadlo & Richardson, 1991). Most people take 10 seconds or less to complete this task. People who take 14 seconds or more are at increased risk for falls (Saskatoon Health Region, 2002–2013). Assessment Tool 24.2 contains an algorithm to predict a client's risk for falls.

● **ASSESSMENT TOOL 24.2**   **Algorithm for Fall Prevention in Older Adults**

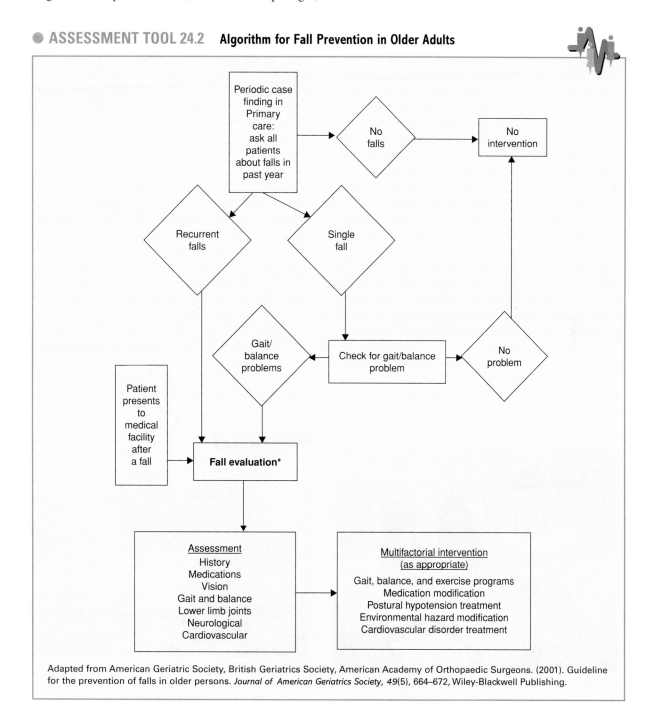

Adapted from American Geriatric Society, British Geriatrics Society, American Academy of Orthopaedic Surgeons. (2001). Guideline for the prevention of falls in older persons. *Journal of American Geriatrics Society, 49*(5), 664–672, Wiley-Blackwell Publishing.

Social Aspects

Exploring the woman's relationships is an integral part of social assessment. How are her relationships with loved ones, children, grandchildren, friends, and coworkers? Does she prefer activities alone, like reading, or group activities offered in many senior citizens' centres? Is she employed? What is or was her main occupation? What are/were her activities and hobbies? Does the client volunteer in the community or serve on boards? Does she have child care responsibilities for grandchildren or caregiving responsibilities for other adults or elders? (Fig. 24.7).

Another component of social assessment is what the woman does on a 24-hour basis. Does she travel? If so, what distance does she travel? Is this a change from previous social or travel patterns? How does she get around? Can she make and reach appointments? What does she do for recreation and socialization? Changes in usual social activity patterns can indicate a subtle or acute change in physical or mental health. The social assessment includes asking the older person whom she can depend on if she needs assistance or in an emergency. Women with functional impairment need regular, dependable assistance with instrumental ADLs and advanced ADLs.

Many older women belong to community seniors' clubs and organizations. They watch out for each other and provide support and friendship as they age together. They are interested in sharing information and learning new things. They want to be knowledgeable about current health information and to be included in the decision making and planning around their own health care (Kinch & Jacubec, 2004). An increasing number of seniors use computers and social media sites to communicate with others and to search for information. In the United States, 30% to 40% of seniors use social media sites and social networking sites. Seniors use e-mail, search engines, and other online information sources at rates similar to younger people (Perceptions of Libraries, 2010).

Some researchers have shown a relationship between spiritual faith and health. Lawler-Row and Elliott (2009) found that spiritual well-being contributed to the prediction of psychological and subjective well-being, physical symptoms, and depression. Understanding individual spiritual perspectives is important, but there are barriers to assessing spirituality, including health professionals' discomfort in addressing spirituality, and lack of training and time for assessment (Lavretsky, 2010). There are no widely accepted measures of spirituality in clinical practice, but some of the measuring tools include items such as beliefs, attitudes, religious orientation, faith development, fundamentalism, attitudes toward death, church involvement, character traits such as optimism, forgiveness, and the ability to find meaning and purpose in life, or feelings of peacefulness, gratitude, harmony, and general well-being (Lavretsky, 2010).

Sexuality

This vital component of the client's history is often avoided. Comfort with discussing sexuality is learned through experience, increased knowledge, and openness to other sexual orientations. When assessing the sexuality and sexual needs of the older woman, the nurse may begin by asking the client if she has questions or concerns in this area that she would like to discuss. The nurse may ask whether the woman is currently in an intimate relationship (Fig. 24.8).

Is there difficulty with sexual intimacy as a result of any physical disability? Does the couple have a close relationship without sexual intercourse? This is an appropriate time to provide information about sexual health. For example, the concept of self-pleasure or masturbation as

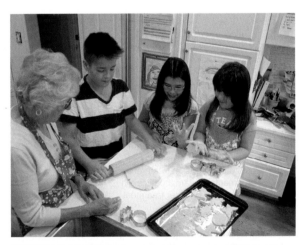

FIGURE 24.7 Many grandmothers are providing primary and part-time care for their grandchildren.

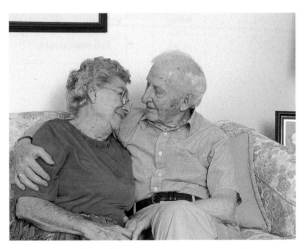

FIGURE 24.8 Sexual and romantic relationships continue into older adulthood; nurses need to assess the older woman's satisfaction with the quality of her sexual life.

a normal and satisfying practice could be introduced. If cognitive impairment or depression exists in a life partner, how has the relationship changed? Do they need any special counselling to minimize or remove health care barriers interfering with sexual activity?

Has the client or her partner had any difficulty or problems achieving orgasm? Is orgasm an important aspect of their lovemaking? Has the use of medications affected orgasmic ability or capacity? For example, selective serotonin reuptake inhibitors (SSRIs), commonly used to treat depression, may cause alterations in sexual function. Is the client undergoing any major financial, physical, or emotional stressors? Is there a history of violence in the relationship? If a person is not in a monogamous relationship for a long period, does she ever have unprotected sexual intercourse? Does she engage in high-risk behaviours or have multiple partners? Is there a history of blood transfusion in the 1980s? Is there a history of sexually transmitted infections (STIs)? Has the woman ever been diagnosed with hepatitis, which may increase the risk for other STIs? If she is in a heterosexual relationship, have there been any problems with her male partner having erectile dysfunction? If so, has he used any erectile aids, medications, or other treatments? What has worked?

Health care professionals tend to make heteronormative assumptions about sexual orientation, relationships, and activities of older clients, closing the door to learning important information about their lesbian, gay, bisexual, and other differently oriented clients (Brotman et al., 2007; Röndahl et al., 2006). In a study of lesbian women's health care experiences, three important aspects of health care professionals' abilities were identified. First, awareness: Can the health care professional facilitate disclosure of a lesbian orientation? Second, does the professional acknowledge and respect the lesbian orientation? And third, does the professional have adequate medical knowledge to know about specific health concerns of lesbian women (Bjorkman & Malterud, 2009)? If the woman is a lesbian, does she currently have a partner? Has she had any problems in her relationship with her partner? Does her sexual orientation influence any health problems, relationship changes, or barriers to obtaining health care services or benefits?

Contrary to popular myth, sexual activity forms only a part of the lives of lesbian women, so it is important for the nurse to understand additional factors that may create stress in a relationship. Significant changes and stress may occur if either or both women also have primary caregiving responsibilities for aging parents, family members, or siblings. According to a 2004 study, 46% of lesbian, gay, bisexual, and transgender adults older than 50 years were currently providing or had provided caregiving for family members in the past 5 years, with 84% of the care recipients being parents (Cantor et al., 2004). In a Canadian study of gay and lesbian seniors and their caregivers, Brotman et al. (2007) identified a number of themes, including discrimination, the process of "coming out," caregiver roles, and support.

Prevention and Screening

The nurse needs to help the postmenopausal woman take an active role in preventing future illness, functional decline, and disability. Fragility fractures, a consequence of osteoporosis, are a major cause of functional decline and lead to excess mortality, morbidity, chronic pain, admission to institutions, and economic costs (Papaioannou et al., 2010). Fragility fractures comprise 80% of all fractures in postmenopausal women over the age of 50. The focus on prevention and treatment of osteoporosis and fractures has shifted from treatment of low BMD to an integrated approach for prevention of fragility fractures. Canadian guidelines focus on assessment and management of women and men over the age of 50 who are at high risk for fractures (Papaioannou et al., 2010).

A detailed history and a focused physical examination will identify risk factors for low BMD, falls, and fractures. A woman's height can be measured annually to identify the possibility of vertebral fractures. If she has fallen in the past year, additional assessments may be carried out, including her ability to get out of a chair without using her arms (Papaioannou et al., 2010). Indications for a DEXA or DXA (dual-energy x-ray absorptiometry) scan to determine low BMD include age 65 years and over, a previous fragility fracture, prolonged use of corticosteroids, current smoking, high alcohol intake, a vertebral fracture identified by x-ray, low body weight or major weight loss, rheumatoid arthritis, or having had a parent with a hip fracture. **Osteoporosis** is defined as BMD of 2.5 or more standard deviations below the peak bone mass for young adults, that is, a T-score at or below −2.5. The 10-year risk of a major fracture, that is, hip, vertebra, or proximal humerus, can be estimated by using the BMD T-score of the neck of the femur (Papaioannou et al., 2010). **Osteopenia** refers to bone density below normal, but above the level defined as osteoporosis (Fig. 24.9).

A woman with osteoporosis or at risk for osteoporosis can improve her physical function, decrease pain, improve muscle strength and balance, and possibly reduce the risk for hip fracture by doing resistance-training and/or weight-bearing exercises. She can improve her balance through exercises such as tai chi. Home safety assessment should be carried out for women with visual impairment and others at high risk for falls (Papaioannou et al., 2010).

Is the client up-to-date on her adult immunizations? These include influenza vaccine annually for all women

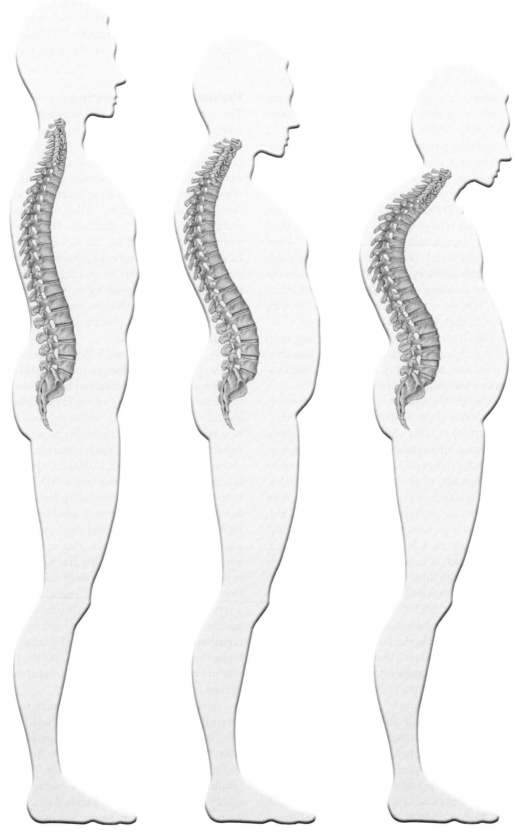

FIGURE 24.9 Osteoporosis in an older woman.

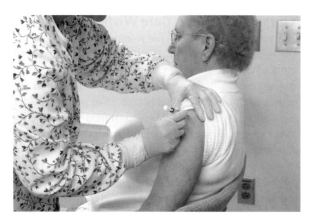

FIGURE 24.10 Regular immunizations for older clients are an essential health maintenance practice.

65 years of age and over, and pneumococcal vaccine to prevent pneumococcal pneumonia (Fig. 24.10). The pneumococcal vaccine is administered once for those 65 years of age or older, or for younger women with chronic illness (Public Health Agency of Canada, 2012d). Public Health Agency of Canada (PHAC) also recommends that older adults receive a diphtheria–tetanus booster every 10 years. Women who travel out of country can consult their public health travel clinic for advice regarding immunizations relevant to their travel area. It is important to continue all immunizations as long as the person has some functional ability, or if she would likely be treated for the illness that the immunization would prevent. One illness that can be prevented is herpes zoster (shingles), a reactivation of the varicella (chicken pox) virus. Shingles can be very painful and may lead to long-term postherpetic neuralgia. The vaccine is recommended for persons 60 and over, without contraindications, who have had previous varicella infection (Public Health Agency of Canada, 2012a).

The nurse can determine whether the client is up-to-date with cancer screening tests appropriate for age, functional status, and life expectancy. A meta-analysis of screening for breast cancer using mammography showed a reduction in breast cancer mortality in women between the ages of 40 and 69, but no significant effect in women 70 and older (Fitzpatrick-Lewis et al., 2011). The Canadian Cancer Society (2011) recommends that women between the ages of 50 and 69 have a mammogram every 2 years, unless they have factors that put them at increased risk for breast cancer. They also suggest that after the age of 70, women should talk to their doctor about the need for screening.

The risk for cervical cancer decreases as women age. The Canadian Task Force on Preventive Health Care (2013) published cervical screening recommendations for women who are asymptomatic and who are or have been sexually active. These recommendations do not apply to women with symptoms of cervical cancer, previous abnormal screening results, those who do not have a cervix, or who are immunosuppressed. According to these recommendations, women aged 30 to 69 are advised to have routine screening every 3 years. Women 70 and over who have had three successive negative Pap tests in the last 10 years do not need further screening. Women 70 or over who have not been screened adequately should continue to be screened until they have three negative tests.

According to the Canadian Cancer Society (2012) the death rate from colorectal cancer could be reduced significantly if screening was to take place widely among the Canadian population. They recommend that men and women of age 50 and over have a stool test (fecal occult blood test or fecal immunochemical test) at least every 2 years, with a positive test followed up by a colonoscopy or double-contrast barium enema and flexible sigmoidoscopy.

There are exceptions to age-based routine screening, including older women with a short life expectancy or whose multiple health problems or dementia would cause them to find screening burdensome. Screening needs to be individualized for each older woman, rather than being simply age based.

Sleep

Sleep disorders are common in older women; thus, an accurate sleep history is vital. Does the client have difficulty falling or staying asleep? Symptoms to assess for include nocturia, pain, and shortness of breath. Does the client's partner or significant other report any loud snoring, as with sleep apnea? Persons experiencing sleep apnea have a heightened risk of suffering adverse cardiovascular events, such as cardiac or respiratory failure (Sigurdson & Ayas, 2007). Does the partner observe any periods when it seems that the client stops breathing or has coarse inspiratory noises? Does the client have early morning awakening and difficulty falling back to sleep? Clinical depression often presents with early morning awakening several hours before usual waking time. Anxiety may make it difficult to fall asleep, because the person may ruminate over worries rather than relaxing. Dementia may cause reversal of the sleep/wake cycle. **Sleep phase advancement** occurs frequently in older adults, meaning that they go to bed and rise earlier than when they were younger.

Is the client spending more time than usual awake in bed? This is a common consequence of age-associated sleep changes. Does she take any medication to induce sleep? If so, is the medication a benzodiazepine or a nonbenzodiazepine sleep agent? How long has she been taking the drug? What is the dosage? How often does she use this? Has she noticed any daytime drowsiness that interferes with driving or operating other machinery? Has daytime fatigue contributed to any accidents or falls?

The nurse should inquire about sleep patterns. Does the client go to sleep and awaken the same time each day? Does she avoid activities such as television before going to bed? Does she avoid drinking large amounts of fluid, having caffeine, or exercising close to bedtime? How many episodes of nocturia does the person have each night? Can she return to sleep after voiding? Does she suffer from panic attacks during the night? Are any nightmares related to a traumatic event, such as sudden death of a spouse or child? Upon wakening during the night, does the client remain in bed or get out of bed for a diversional relaxing activity? Does she get any exercise during the day and sunlight exposure to improve the quality of her sleep? The Pittsburgh Sleep Quality Index is a useful instrument by which nurses can assess sleep disorders in their clients (Smyth, 2012). See Research Highlight 24.1.

Long-Term Health Care Wishes

The nurse needs to assess the woman's long-term wishes for health care. Has the client determined her **health care advanced directives** that define her wishes regarding aggressive life extension measures? Who holds the power of attorney for health care? The power of attorney for health care should be determined when a person is competent. It is much more difficult for the family if this decision is not made. Is there a will for the woman's estate? Does she have an attorney? Is the woman knowledgeable about estate planning? A referral to a social worker might help decision making in this area.

AGE-ASSOCIATED PHYSIOLOGIC CHANGES IN OLDER WOMEN

Physical aging is a universal phenomenon among living beings. Every person has unique physiologic changes and a general health status based on multiple variables

---

● RESEARCH HIGHLIGHT 24.1 Examining the Feasibility of Implementing Specific Nursing Interventions to Promote Sleep in Hospitalized Elderly Patients

BACKGROUND

Sleep problems in the elderly have been well documented in the literature. Sleep deprivation can have adverse effects on the body and places older adults at increased risk for anxiety, depression, and delirium. Sleep problems may be related to normal age changes or to medical diagnoses. Evidence-based nursing strategies to promote sleep quality are limited.

PURPOSE

The purpose of this experimental pilot study was to examine the feasibility of implementing specific nursing interventions to promote sleep in hospitalized older adults.

DESIGN

Eight medical patients in a teaching hospital were enrolled in the study each week over a 16-week period. Four were randomly assigned to the control group and four to the experimental group. The final sample consisted of 59 patients, aged 65 to 94, approximately half of whom were female. The experimental group received a sleep protocol intervention while the control group received the usual nighttime care.

RESULTS

This study implemented a sleep protocol for hospitalized older adults to promote sleep, increase ease in falling asleep, improve sleep quality, and increase the ability to remain asleep. Although this hypothesis was only partially supported, patients in the experimental group showed a significant improvement in sleep quality and ability to remain asleep. It was also hypothesized that the patients who received the sleep intervention would use fewer sleep medications than those in the control group. This hypothesis was supported. Experimental group patients identified sleep protocol preferences such as personal hygiene, awareness of normal bedtime, receiving a back rub, straightening bed linens, and receiving a bedtime snack.

NURSING IMPLICATIONS

Although a number of challenges were identified in implementation of the protocol, the study provides initial evidence that it is feasible to implement a sleep protocol in an acute care setting. Additional research is necessary to examine the effectiveness of a nursing sleep protocol in hospitalized older adults.

From Lareau, R., Benson, L., Watcharotone, K., & Manguba, G. (2008). Examining the feasibility of implementing specific nursing interventions to promote sleep in hospitalized elderly patients. *Geriatric Nursing, 29*(3), 197–206.

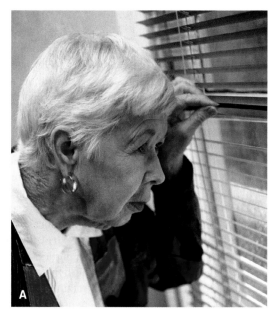
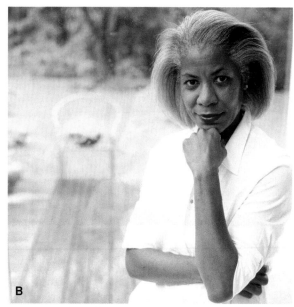

FIGURE 24.11   Both these women are 73 years old. The effects of aging vary based on many parameters, including genetics, ethnicity, general health, nutrition, stress, and other circumstances.

(Fig. 24.11). Such factors include genetics, family history, and lifestyle behaviours affecting health. Emotional, functional, and financial variables interplay in health outcomes, morbidity, and mortality. Patterns of physiologic changes in elders have been described over the past 20 years; however, it is important for the nurse to consider these changes in the context of the individual client. Aging does affect all body systems.

General Appearance

The recent popularity of cosmetic surgery, injections, and procedures has made age estimation more difficult, especially in women. Facial aging consists of decreasing skin turgor, especially around the eyes and below the chin. The depth and number of wrinkles increase with age, as do furrows between the eyebrows. Facial lines are accentuated with increasing years. Facial hair, eyebrows, and hair become more coarse and grey. The skin often has sun-damaged areas of darker pigmentation, and **actinic keratoses** (waxy-appearing lesions of various sizes). Tiny circular cherry angiomas are seen occasionally on the face, chest, and abdomen (Fig. 24.12).

Fair-skinned, blue-eyed individuals are at highest risk for basal cell carcinoma; however, older women of all backgrounds are susceptible because this is the most common type of skin cancer. Basal cell carcinoma commonly presents on sun-exposed areas such as the face, ears, neck, and dorsal aspects of the hands and knees. Basal cell carcinoma is circular, beginning as a small nodule with a central indentation. It gradually increases in size, with the circular (donut-shaped) border becom-

ing more raised, having a translucent appearance. Squamous cell carcinoma and malignant melanoma also may occur in older adults (Fig. 24.13).

Gait Changes

General movement slows with advancing years, although there is considerable variance among older adults, depending on health status, level of activity, and amount of exercise. Gait speed declines. The centre of gravity often changes from straight vertical to more anterior from the base of support at the hips and below. Arm swing decreases slightly with age, as does the height of the gait swing. The foot does not clear the floor at a height that it does in younger people. Range of motion of the hips and knees frequently is limited because of osteoarthritis. Pain and foot deformities as a result of arthritic conditions and hallux valgus (bunion) can alter the biomechanics of walking (Fig. 24.14).

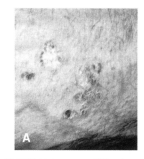
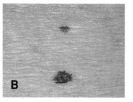

FIGURE 24.12   Skin changes in aging include (**A**) actinic keratoses and (**B**) cherry angiomas.

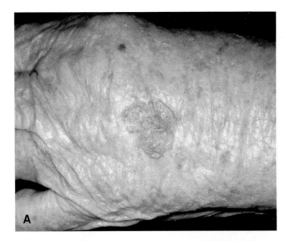

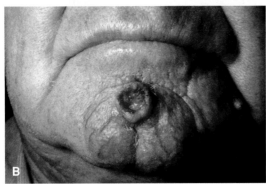

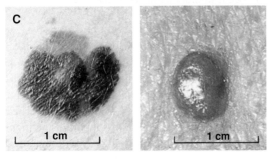

FIGURE 24.13 The incidence of skin cancer rises sharply for older adults. **A:** Basal cell carcinoma. **B:** Squamous cell carcinoma. **C:** Malignant melanoma.

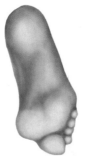

FIGURE 24.14 Bunions can cause gait abnormalities and other problems.

Vital Signs

Alterations in vital signs require special attention. Infections in older adults often present without fever (Rosen et al., 2010), so the nurse pays sharp attention to respiratory and pulse rates, as well as subtle cognitive changes. Use of a thermometer that records low temperatures is important, because older adults are at increased risk for hypothermia as a result of age-associated thermoregulatory changes.

Proper measurement techniques are especially important. The nurse should measure blood pressure in both arms during initial examination and periodically thereafter. Occlusive atherosclerotic disease of the subclavian or brachial artery often reduces systolic pressure in one arm. **Orthostatic (postural) hypotension** is common among older adults, particularly after meals (Higginson, 2012). Orthostatic hypotension is a risk factor for syncope, falls, and fracture (Higginson, 2012). To assess for orthostatic hypotension, blood pressure and heart rate are measured after 5 minutes supine and at 1 and 3 minutes after standing. The definition is a drop of greater than 20 mm Hg systolic and/or 10 mm Hg diastolic (Higginson, 2012). Symptoms such as light-headedness, dizziness, or tachycardia may also accompany orthostatic hypotension.

Cardiovascular System

Cardiovascular disease (CVD) is a leading killer of Canadian women and an important public health concern (Heart and Stroke Foundation, 2013). Historically, the rate of diagnostic accuracy in women with CVD has been lower than in men. Studies have enrolled significantly fewer women than men, and results have not traditionally been reported by gender. Both women and men may experience typical or nontypical symptoms such as nausea, sweating, or pain in the arm, throat, or jaw. Nevertheless, the most common symptom of myocardial ischemia (decreased coronary blood flow) or acute MI (an infarct in the myocardium) in women and men is still chest pressure, squeezing, fullness, burning, heaviness, or pain (Heart and Stroke Foundation, 2013). Women may also experience neck, shoulder, or upper back pain; abdominal discomfort; or unusual fatigue (Mayo Clinic, 2014). The term "silent ischemia" or "silent MI" is used to describe ischemia or infarction without symptoms in older adults. Atypical presentations of ischemia or MI may include the sudden onset of confusion, syncope, or a fall, and may occur without the classic symptoms of chest pain, dyspnea, and nausea common in younger and middle-aged people. Some people later recall that their silent heart attack was mistaken for indigestion, nausea, muscle pain, or a bad case of the flu (Grogan, 2011).

Another change in the cardiovascular system is an increased incidence of **isolated systolic hypertension (ISH)**, defined as systolic BP greater than 140 mm Hg, accompanied by a diastolic BP less than 90 mm Hg. ISH increases the risk of heart attack and stroke (Musini et al., 2009). Both cardiac output and peripheral vascular resistance affect blood pressure. With aging, changes occur in the cardiovascular system. The large arteries thicken and stiffen as the result of collagen and calcium deposits and loss of elastic fibres in the medial layer. These changes cause the systolic blood pressure to increase, whereas the diastolic pressure may decline. The wall of the left ventricle thickens but the cavity size does not change, resulting in decreased early filling and increased filling pressure, with symptoms of dyspnea. The left atrium enlarges, increasing the risk for atrial fibrillation. Cardiovascular reserve diminishes, leading to a lowering of the threshold for heart failure. Deficits in beta-adrenergic activity contribute to reduced cardiovascular performance during exercise (Fleg & Strait, 2012).

It is important to know the benefits and harms of antihypertensive treatment in older people. Drug treatment trials show that there is benefit in treating the elderly and very elderly patients with systolic hypertension. However, there is uncertainty as to the optimal target for systolic blood pressure. Allen et al., (2013) found that drug treatment trials have not provided evidence to support lowering systolic blood pressure in elderly patients to less than 140; they suggest that a systolic blood pressure between 140 and 160 mm Hg is acceptable in individuals at low risk. Padwal et al. (2013) further commented that there is no arbitrarily defined point at which blood pressure reduction reduces vascular events, and below which it does not. "Thus, choosing a single, specific systolic threshold that applies equally to every patient and every age group is difficult" (Padwal et al., 2013, paragraph 3). The Canadian Hypertension Education Program (CHEP) recommends an arbitrary target of less than 140 for individuals at low risk and under 130 for people with risk factors such as diabetes and emphasizes the importance of both lifestyle modification and medication for treatment (Padwal et al., 2013).

Respiratory System

Age-associated anatomic and physiologic changes in the respiratory system affect an older woman's breathing ability. Skeletal deformities, the most notable being kyphosis, may accompany aging, and are more accentuated with osteoporosis. The resulting increase in the chest's anterior–posterior diameter affects lung expansion. Decreased lung tissue elasticity affects the efficiency of air exchange. Calcification of the thoracic wall leads to increased susceptibility to infection and atelectasis. There may be increased risk of aspiration as a result of atrophy of the cilia. Decreased respiratory muscle strength causes a decreased response to

hypoxia and hypercapnia, and decreased PaO_2 causes increased sensitivity to the effects of narcotics (Kane et al., 2009).

Dyspnea is a common, complex, and often debilitating symptom frequently reported by older people. It has been defined as "a subjective experience of breathing discomfort that consists of qualitatively distinct sensations that vary in intensity" (Parshall et al., 2012, page 435). Dyspnea can accompany a variety of clinical conditions, such as asthma and chronic obstructive pulmonary disease (COPD), CHF, pulmonary hypertension, renal disease, anxiety disorders, or panic attacks. The person may describe a sensation of work or effort in breathing, tightness in the chest, and air hunger/unsatisfied inspiration. The health care professional may observe signs such as tachypnea, use of accessory muscles, and intercostal retractions. Dyspneic symptoms should be investigated and treated according to the underlying cause (Parshall et al., 2012).

Mortality from pneumonia is the fifth leading cause of death among elderly people (Rosen et al., 2010.) The nurse should assess the client's risk factors for pneumonia, which include comorbidities such as COPD, asthma, diabetes, CHF, and any other condition that lowers resistance to infection (Centers for Disease Control, 2013). To prevent pneumonia, it is important that women older than 65 years receive the pneumococcal vaccine (Public Health Agency of Canada, 2012b).

Smoking increases the risk for the development of COPD, an umbrella term for a number of diseases including chronic bronchitis and emphysema (Public Health Agency of Canada, 2013). The main symptoms of COPD are a long-lasting cough, sputum production, wheezing, dyspnea, and weight loss (Canadian Lung Association, 2013). The nurse should encourage smoking cessation in older adults and assist them to set goals for quitting and for enrolling in a smoking cessation program.

Asthma, an episodic reversible airway disease, causes inflammation and edema of the respiratory mucosa with excessive sputum production and bronchial spasm. Symptoms include wheezing, dyspnea, increased use of accessory muscles, intercostal muscle retractions, nasal flaring, diaphoresis, cyanosis, and tachypnea.

Gastrointestinal System

The normal gastrointestinal tract has the capacity for unimpaired absorption, digestion, and defecation. Anorexia usually has a defined etiology in older clients. The most frequent presentations are with clinical depression, side effects from medications, thyroid disorders, constipation, and cancer. Weight loss usually correlates with anorexia, which can decrease strength, functional status, and immunity.

Xerostomia

Xerostomia or dry mouth from decreased salivary secretions, is common in older adults and most often occurs as a result of medication side effects (Turner & Ship, 2007). In addition to xerostomia, older adults commonly suffer from several other oral health problems. Missing teeth, periodontal infections, or loose dentures will affect the ability to chew a solid diet. Oral health is important in older adults: the nurse should inquire about oral health and instruct women in measures to minimize or treat common oral health problems. Nursing measures include encouraging regular professional dental care, regular brushing and flossing, adequate fluid intake to prevent dehydration, regular medication review to identify drugs potentially causing or exacerbating xerostomia (eg, anticholinergic medications), and use of artificial saliva products as necessary to treat xerostomia.

Dysphagia

Dysphagia (difficulty swallowing) can result from motility disorders, medications, vascular changes, strokes, and other neuromuscular disorders. Clients with impaired swallowing are at risk for aspiration pneumonia. The nurse should assess the client's history for dysphagia for solids, liquids, or both; he or she should observe for any dysphagia during meals.

Gastroesophageal reflux disease (GERD) affects millions of people, and the potential for developing this disease increases with age. The older woman may describe her symptoms as "heartburn," or as hoarseness, dry cough, a feeling like there is something stuck in the throat, dysphagia, or chronic sore throat. Acid reflux may result from a number of underlying conditions such as use of certain medications and decreased saliva production (Gillson, 2012).

Diverticular disease occurs in about half of all people over the age of 60. Diverticula are small outpouchings in the lining of the colon, most commonly in the sigmoid colon. Most people do not have any discomfort or symptoms. However, sometimes the diverticula become inflamed and the person experiences abdominal pain that may come on either suddenly or over a period of days. This complication, diverticulitis, can lead to bleeding, infections, perforations in the colon, or blockages. Diverticular disease is thought to be caused by low-fibre diets and constipation and is commonly treated with a high-fibre diet (National Digestive Diseases Information Clearing House, 2012) (Fig. 24.15).

Genitourinary System

Women may encounter changes in their sexual activities during the postmenopausal phase of their lives. **Dyspareunia** (pain with sexual intercourse) may occur with vaginal atrophy. This is the result of decreased vaginal

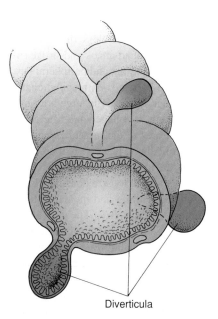

Diverticula

FIGURE 24.15 The formation of diverticula places older women at risk for constipation, bloating, distention, and discomfort. Acute inflammation causes diverticulitis, in which the diverticula may rupture and bleed.

lubrication related to estrogen reduction. Libido in older women may be more related to testosterone rather than to estrogen. Physical conditions such as arthritis, urinary or bowel difficulties, pelvic surgery, fatigue, or headaches may decrease libido, as well as some medications. Anxiety or depression as well as long-term stress can diminish sexual responsiveness (Mayo Clinic, 2012). Clients with arthritic functional disabilities may benefit from use of the left lateral position for pelvic examinations. This position is assumed with the woman's knees flexed with greater flexion in the right hip.

Ovarian size decreases with aging. Palpable ovaries are abnormal in older women. This finding or increased uterine size needs evaluation for cancer. Women with uterine prolapse may have low back pain, fecal or urinary incontinence, or a palpable mass. On pelvic examination an **anterior vaginal wall prolapse** (cystocele) or **posterior vaginal wall prolapse** (enterocele or rectocele) can be identified (see Chapters 4 and 19). Postmenopausal vaginal bleeding has many causes; this finding requires evaluation for endometrial carcinoma or other malignancies (Breijer et al., 2010).

Peripheral Vascular System

Clients with coronary or cerebrovascular atherosclerotic disease frequently have peripheral vascular disease (Table 24.1). Intermittent claudication causes pain, burning, or discomfort in the muscles of the legs during exercise. It disappears when resting. It may be missed in older women who are not ambulatory. It is important to assess for jugular venous pulsation or distention with the client in the sitting position, especially for

● TABLE 24.1 **Arterial Versus Venous Insufficiency**

Characteristic	Chronic Arterial Insufficiency	Chronic Venous Insufficiency
Pain	Intermittent, especially at rest	None to aching on dependency
Pulses	Decreased or absent	Normal, although difficult to feel
Colour	Pale or dusky red	Normal or cyanotic on dependency
Temperature	Cool	Normal
Edema	Absent or mild	Present, often marked
Skin changes	Thin, shiny, atrophic, with hair loss over feet and thick toenails	Brown discolouration around the ankles; possible skin thickening and scarring
Ulceration	Toes or trauma points on feet	Possibly at sides of ankle
Gangrene	May develop	Does not develop

those with heart failure. Peripheral edema is common in venous insufficiency and heart failure.

The nurse should examine the peripheral arteries carefully and perform carotid palpation gently and unilaterally. The nurse should check capillary filling time in the client's toes by applying firm pressure to them. Full colour should return in 3 to 5 seconds. Arterial insufficiency often appears as lower extremity pallor. Arterial occlusion may exhibit with severe pain, pallor, or erythema. Lower extremity assessment includes assessing venous return because decreased competence is common in older women. Mild or severe varicosities may be visible in the older woman's lower extremities. Erythema may result from cellulitis, dermatitis, or phlebitis. Decreased hair distribution in the lower extremities is frequent in arterial insufficiency (Kane et al., 2009).

The nurse should assess for any lower extremity ulcers. Venous insufficiency ulcers typically are large, medial, and irregular and often extend to the subcutaneous level. They frequently have "leaky" drainage. Arterial insufficiency ulcers tend to present laterally on the lower extremities.

Any client with diabetes needs regular foot examinations by a nurse and a podiatrist, with evaluation for areas of pressure, breakdown, or necrosis to prevent amputation of a lower extremity (Fig. 24.16). Osteomyelitis of the bone is a frequent complication of diabetic foot ulcers and requires intensive intravenous therapy and infectious disease consultation as well as vascular studies to prevent loss of the foot or lower leg.

Neurologic System

With aging comes a gradual decrease in brain weight and change in appearance. Brain shrinkage is due to both a decrease in size of the large neurons and due to fewer neurons. Cell losses in the limbic system have a significant effect on memory. Within the cells there are alterations in synaptic activity, biochemical changes, mitochondrial DNA mutations, accumulation of iron

and other pigments, and a decline in concentrations of neurotransmitters. Although amyloid and neurofibrillary plaques develop in the brains of mentally sound older individuals, there are larger numbers of them in individuals with dementia. There is a decline in cerebral blood flow and cerebral metabolic rate, related to cerebral atherosclerosis. Postmortem examination has shown that approximately 25% of individuals older than 70 have one or more cerebral infarcts. In addition to the changes in the brain there are losses of nerve cells and myelinated fibres in the spinal cord (Ropper & Samuels, 2009).

Reaction time slows. Decreased baroreceptor function or cerebral blood flow can cause **syncope**, a loss of consciousness with decreased postural tone. Reflexes decrease, especially in the lower extremities. Obtaining ankle reflexes in older adults is particularly difficult. Joints become more flexed with decreased muscle

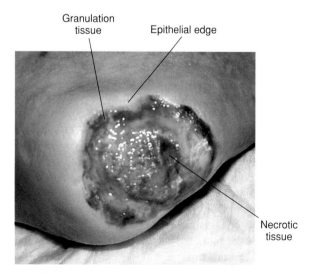

Granulation tissue

Epithelial edge

Necrotic tissue

FIGURE 24.16 Older clients with immobility, diabetes, and other problems need regular skin assessments to prevent bedsores and related complications.

strength. Age-associated intention tremors increase with movement and are absent at rest.

Extremes in environmental temperatures pose risks for older women. **Hypothermia** occurs when the rectal temperature is 35°C or below. The body's ability to regulate temperatures and sense cold may lessen with age. As well, some older adults may not be able to communicate that they are cold or cannot get to a warm location because of immobility (Mayo Clinic, 2011). Hypothermia deaths in the elderly rise during episodes of very cold weather when older people may not be able to afford to pay their heating bills (The Telegraph, 2012).

Conversely, women may experience **hyperthermia**. Heat stroke, which causes death in many older adults, results from excessive heat storage with a decreased ability to rid the body of heat through evaporation, radiation, and conduction. Signs of heat exhaustion include dizziness, weakness, anorexia, nausea, vomiting, body warmth, headache, or dyspnea. If the body temperature continues to be elevated above 40.6 degrees, symptoms escalate to psychosis, delirium, or coma. Mortality is as high as 80% from heat stroke (Kane et al., 2009).

Musculoskeletal System

Difficulty with mobility and performance of ADLs is commonly related to the decreased muscle and bone mass and deterioration and drying of joint cartilage that accompanies aging physiology and chronic illness (Kane et al., 2009). In a longitudinal study, researchers investigated modifiable factors underlying onset of ADL disability. Three physical performance-based measurements—functional reach, climbing steps, and comfortable walking speed—were measured for predictability of ADL disability. The participants were 113 nondisabled community-dwelling women with a mean age of 79.5 years at baseline. After 9 years, one quarter of the women had disabilities in ADLs. All three performance measurements were predictive of the onset of ADL disability, with walking speed having the strongest predictive value (Idland et al., 2013). In another study, researchers examined the effects of combined resistance and aerobic training sessions in a group of 72 women from 60 to 74 years old. All women had increased strength and aerobic fitness and decreased fat mass (Hunter et al., 2013).

The nurse should assess the mobility status of the older woman. Nursing assessment includes gait evaluation, unilateral favouring of an extremity, joint swelling, muscle atrophy, paralysis, or muscle weakness. Observation of the older woman performing ADLs provides an ideal and practical musculoskeletal assessment. The nurse can do so in the office setting by observing the client ambulating, transferring into a chair or examination table, or rising from a wheelchair. It is important for the acute care and long-term care nurse to advance mobility as medically indicated. Significant bone loss can occur during periods of immobility.

Osteoarthritis is extremely common in older women and is a result of degeneration of the cartilage in the joints, causing bones to rub together, with accompanying pain, swelling, and stiffness. It occurs particularly in the knees, hips, feet, spine, and hands. The nurses should assess for osteoarthritis by checking the client for decreased range of motion, joint swelling, tenderness when pressure is put on the joint, and crepitus, a grating sound, when joints are moved. Bony enlargements may be present in the joints of the hands (WebMed, 2013a).

Rheumatoid arthritis, an autoimmune disorder, is characterized by bilateral symmetric inflammation of affected joints, and usually affects the hands, wrists, knees, and feet. The joint becomes swollen, very painful, and warm to the touch, and rheumatoid nodules may appear under the skin (WebMed, 2013b). It often involves the metacarpal and proximal interphalangeal joints (Fig. 24.17).

Pharmacology of Aging

Drug expenditures comprise the most rapidly growing health care cost in Canada. Whereas drug benefit programs help cover the costs of prescription medications for seniors, all governments are examining strategies to ensure costs to seniors are kept down, while continuing and promoting optimal use of required medications. Public drug spending on seniors increased from $603.5 million in 2002 to $1 billion in 2008. A large percentage of the drugs prescribed are for cardiovascular conditions, including cholesterol-lowering statins. The majority of seniors are using multiple drugs; 62% of seniors on public drug programs are using five or more drug classes and the number of drug classes increases with age (Canadian Institute for Health Information, 2010).

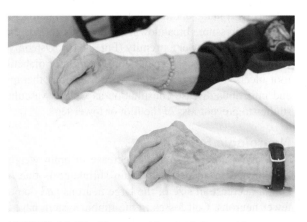

FIGURE 24.17 Rheumatoid arthritis in an older woman.

According to a Canadian survey reported by Ramage-Morin (2009), 97% of all residents of health care institutions and 76% of seniors living in private households had taken some form of medication in the previous 2 days. Women were more likely than men to have taken medications, and seniors aged 75 to 84 were more likely to have done so than those aged 65 to 74. Concurrent use of five or more medications was reported by 53% of seniors in institutions and 13% of those in private households. This amounts to over a half million seniors taking multiple medications: approximately 94,000 in institutions and 445,000 in households. Almost 78% took medications that act on the nervous system, such as analgesics, antipsychotics, anxiolytics, hypnotics, and sedatives. Laxatives, antacids, drugs to control diabetes, and drugs to treat peptic ulcers and flatulence were taken by 71% of the seniors. Cardiovascular medications, including diuretics and antihypertensives, were taken by close to half of all seniors (Ramage-Morin, 2009).

Multiple medication use of prescription and over-the-counter remedies (**polypharmacy**) by seniors is dangerous and expensive and can lead to adverse drug reactions because of comorbidity and physiologic changes that come with aging. Mortality increases for individuals who take six or more medications, with the highest risk for those taking 10 or more (Little & Morley, 2013). Reasons for people taking multiple medications include comorbidity, multiple prescribing physicians, inappropriate prescribing, and access to different pharmacies, as well as self-medication with over-the-counter and alternative products (Ramage-Morin, 2009). It must be remembered, however, that in certain chronic illnesses, multiple medications are necessary, for example, in hypertension, heart failure, and diabetes. It is important for the nurse and other health care professionals to conduct regular reviews of the drugs that older clients are taking.

The field of **pharmacokinetics** in aging examines how the older adult's body handles drugs. The field of **pharmacodynamics** examines the effect of drugs on the older person's body. Many factors influence how the older body uses drugs. *Absorption* appears to be the least affected parameter. However, drug *distribution* differences can occur. A decline in serum albumin, for example, in poor nutrition, can increase the amount of drug available for action, particularly in protein-bound drugs. Because of the decline in total body water and lean body mass, drugs that distribute in body compartments, such as antimicrobials, digoxin, lithium, and alcohol may result in higher concentrations than expected from a usual dosage in a younger adult. Drugs that distribute in body fat, such as psychotropic agents, may have a longer half-life and prolongation of effect in an older person. *Metabolism* of drugs in an older person is complex and difficult to predict. It depends on metabolic pathways in the liver and other factors such as gender and smoking. The effect of aging on the *excretion* of drugs, on the other hand, is more predictable, linked to renal function, decline in muscle mass, state of hydration, cardiac output, and renal disease. *Tissue responsiveness* to drugs, that is, pharmacodynamic changes, may cause an older person to be more sensitive to some drugs, for example, benzodiazepines, and less sensitive to others (Kane et al., 2009).

COMMON CONDITIONS FOUND IN OLDER WOMEN

Urinary Incontinence

Incontinence is defined as any involuntary leakage of urine (Canadian Continence Foundation, 2009). Conservative estimates of the prevalence are that "7% of Canadian women experience some form of moderate to severe incontinence on a daily basis" (Canadian Continence Foundation, 2009, page 4). The actual incidence is difficult to ascertain because of the stigma and embarrassment associated with incontinence.

Incontinence can cause cellulitis, pressure ulcers, and urinary tract infections. It increases the risk for falls, institutionalization, and mortality. It can lead to stress, isolation, depression, and limitation of activities and can affect interpersonal relationships and sexual function. It has a negative impact on concentration and self-confidence. Estimates are that incontinence costs Canadians over $7.5 billion annually, including direct costs to individuals ($1,500 annually), employers (9 million days of lost work), and $1.95 billion in health care costs (Canadian Continence Foundation, 2009).

Types

- *Stress incontinence:* leaking of urine associated with coughing, sneezing, straining, exercise, or any other type of exertion. Fifty percent of individuals with incontinence have stress incontinence.
- *Urge incontinence:* urine leaks when there is a sudden uncontrollable urge to empty the bladder. It is a key symptom of the overactive bladder syndrome.
- *Overflow incontinence:* constant leaking or dribbling from a full bladder.
- *Mixed incontinence:* a combination of stress and urge incontinence.
- *Functional incontinence:* stems from external factors like the client's inability to reach the toilet in time to void. It accompanies cognitive problems like dementia or delirium, and can also be caused by a lack of personnel to assist clients in toileting. Another possible cause is any medications, such as hypnotics or

tranquilizers, that slow psychomotor functioning, delaying time to get to the bathroom.

 Remember Ann, the 67-year-old from the beginning of the chapter who is having bladder problems? Based on Ann's statements, which type of incontinence would the nurse suspect?

Etiology and Pathophysiology

Aging alone does not cause incontinence, but several age-related changes contribute to its development. With age, bladder capacity decreases, residual urine increases, and involuntary bladder contractions become more common. Diminished estrogen and laxity of pelvic floor muscles associated with prior childbirths or surgeries predispose to stress incontinence. Decreased estrogen can cause atrophic vaginitis and urethritis, with symptoms of dysuria and urgency (Kane et al., 2009). An acronym for potentially reversible conditions that can lead to incontinence is **DRIP: D**elirium, **R**estricted mobility, **R**etention, **I**nfection, **I**nflammation, **I**mpaction, **P**olyuria, **P**harmaceuticals (Kane et al., 2009, page 223).

Assessment Findings

The assessment of urinary incontinence begins with direct observation, a brief history, and a physical examination (Kane et al., 2009). Bladder diaries kept for 2 to 3 days are helpful in determining a diagnosis. Examples of diaries are available online (American Urological Association Foundation, 2011; National Kidney and Urologic Diseases Information Clearinghouse, 2010). The nurse should choose the type that best fits the setting and the individual client. For example, complex diaries provide a large amount of information but are not likely to be useful for women with moderate to severe cognitive impairment. The nurse should review the bladder diary and use the information as a starting point for further investigation and treatment. Typical areas covered in the bladder diary include the following:

* Did the client urinate in the toilet?
* When did episodes of incontinence occur?
* What was the associated activity at the time of leakage?
* Was an urge present?
* What was the type and amount of fluid intake?

Further investigation may include urinalysis, which can identify bacteria, glucose, protein, or blood in the urine. A postvoid residual volume measures the urine in the bladder after a completed void. This can be done by two methods. The easiest method involves use of a portable ultrasound device. The second method is urinary catheterization after voiding to measure the quantity of retained urine, with removal of the catheter after specimen collection. Postvoid residual readings above 200 mL should be further investigated (Kane et al., 2009).

A pelvic examination can assess for atrophic vaginitis, masses, prolapse, cystocele, rectocele, or enterocele. A rectal examination is needed to evaluate for fecal impaction or rectal masses. Women with palpable pelvic or bladder prolapse require referral to a provider specializing in incontinence, such as an advanced practice continence nurse, urologist, or gynecologist. A neurologic consult may be in order if a neurologic condition is the cause of the incontinence.

Other tests may be done by specialists and include urinometry, which measures urine flow with a disposable urine flow meter. Cystometrography produces pressure measurements within the bladder if the bladder is filled and also records intra-abdominal pressure with a rectal probe. Cystometrics are helpful to diagnose detrusor overactivity and sphincter dysfunction.

Collaborative Management

Numerous treatment modalities are available for incontinence, depending on the type. Various surgical procedures and several medications may be useful in the management; however, if possible, noninvasive, nonmedical therapies should be used as first-line treatment strategies.

Nonmedical therapies for incontinence include elimination of bladder irritants such as alcohol, aspartame, and carbonated beverages, especially for women suffering from urge incontinence or symptoms of an overactive bladder. Limiting fluid intake after 9 PM may reduce nighttime incontinence. Voiding pattern corrections may also assist in alleviating symptoms.

The nurse should encourage the client to empty her bladder completely with each void. Telling the client to pause when voiding is complete and to wait another minute to retry voiding again may help. Scheduled voiding regimens are helpful for women with stress, urge, overflow, or functional incontinence. The nurse should evaluate the client's voiding schedule and inquire about episodes of incontinence. Using this information, he or she can suggest an individualized voiding schedule as a way to minimize or alleviate incontinence. For example, a woman with urge incontinence approximately every 3 hours may benefit from reorganizing her daily routine to include bathroom breaks every 2 to 2½ hours. Nursing Care Plan 24.1 provides information related to the care of a woman with urinary incontinence.

Prompted voiding is another nursing strategy whereby prescribed voiding schedules are adjusted to the client's voiding pattern. It is used for stress, urge,

NURSING CARE PLAN 24.1

●

The Older Client Experiencing Urinary Incontinence

 Remember Ann, the older woman struggling with bladder problems, described at the beginning of this chapter? Upon examination, the nurse finds that Ann's perineal area is slightly reddened and irritated. She states, "Sometimes I don't always make it to the bathroom. I've started to wear thin panty liners just in case."

NURSING DIAGNOSES

- **Stress Incontinence** related to age-associated changes in pelvic muscles and support structures and increased abdominal pressure
- **Deficient Knowledge** related to urinary incontinence
- **Urge Incontinence** related to bladder contractions

EXPECTED OUTCOMES

1. The client will identify situations that affect urinary elimination.
2. The client will define urinary incontinence and possible contributing factors.
3. The client will report fewer episodes of stress and urge incontinence.

INTERVENTIONS	RATIONALES
Assess the client's knowledge base and current understanding about urinary incontinence	Assessment provides a baseline from which to develop an individualized teaching plan
Assess for possible contributing factors to urinary incontinence; review with the client possible factors that may lead to urinary incontinence	Atrophic vaginitis, medications, and acute or chronic conditions can lead to transient urinary incontinence
Question the client about any additional complaints related to urinary elimination, such as pain or burning. Obtain a urine dipstick and culture and sensitivity as ordered	Hyperglycemia of diabetes or urinary tract infection can be a cause of urinary incontinence
Assist with obtaining a postvoid residual urine volume	Elevated postvoid residual volumes require further evaluation
Complete or assist with a pelvic examination	Pelvic examination reveals clues to possible genitourinary conditions such as atrophic vaginitis, masses, uterine prolapse, cystocele, or rectocele that may lead to urinary incontinence
Instruct the client in how to keep a bladder diary for 2 to 3 days; review diary with the client	Diary provides additional information from which to determine a diagnosis and plan of care
Prepare the client for testing, such as pad test or urodynamic tests	Testing provides clues to the underlying cause of the client's urinary incontinence
Instruct the client to eliminate alcohol, aspartame, carbonated beverages, and smoking	These substances are bladder irritants
Suggest that the client limit her intake of fluids after dinner in the evening	Limiting fluids after this time may help to reduce nighttime urinary incontinence

(continued)

NURSING CARE PLAN 24.1 ● The Older Client Experiencing Urinary Incontinence (Continued)

INTERVENTIONS	RATIONALES
Encourage the client to empty her bladder completely with each voiding; assist her to set up a voiding schedule based on her lifestyle and activity level	Complete bladder emptying reduces the risk for residual urine remaining in the bladder. Voiding schedules aid in minimizing and reducing episodes of urinary incontinence
Instruct the client in pelvic muscle exercises, including assistance with finding the correct muscles, optimal technique, and suggested number of times to perform the exercise (see Chapter 23)	Pelvic muscle exercises help to strengthen and tone these supportive muscles

EVALUATION

1. The client identifies realistic measures to manage urinary elimination.
2. The client describes the underlying processes and factors involved in urinary incontinence.
3. The client demonstrates an increase in control over urinary elimination.

NURSING DIAGNOSIS

Risk for Impaired Skin Integrity related to urinary leakage and incontinence

EXPECTED OUTCOMES

1. The client identifies measures to reduce risk for perineal irritation.
2. The client exhibits a reduction in perineal redness and irritation.

INTERVENTIONS	RATIONALES
Assess the client's current measures for perineal hygiene	Assessment provides a baseline from which to develop an individualized plan of care
Instruct the client to wash and dry the perineal area with mild soap and warm water after each voiding and bowel movement	Cleansing after elimination reduces the risk for further irritation and possible infection
Encourage the client to avoid perfumed soaps, lotions, or scented items, such as panty liners	Perfumes and scented items can further irritate the area
Instruct the client to use cotton underwear	Cotton allows air to circulate, decreasing the risk for perineal irritation
Advise the client to keep the area as dry as possible; encourage her to change panty liners frequently	Increased moisture in the area can lead to further irritation and excoriation

EVALUATION

1. The client exhibits a perineal area that is clean, dry, and intact without evidence of redness, irritation, or excoriation.
2. The client demonstrates measures to promote perineal hygiene.

and functional incontinence, but not for overflow incontinence. Caregivers monitor the client's toileting and prompt her to void on a 2- to 3-hour schedule, as well as offering positive reinforcement for maintaining continence and attempting to void. This is helpful for cognitively or physically impaired clients; however, it requires significant commitment and effort on the part of the caregiver.

Pelvic floor muscle exercises (Kegel) are used to treat stress, urge, and mixed incontinence (Spencer, 2012). The nurse should instruct women by explaining the purpose of the exercises, helping clients find the correct muscles to exercise, and instructing clients on the optimal technique. See Chapter 23 for more information on these exercises. Resources that can be used for and by women with urinary incontinence have been developed and are available on the internet (Continence Conversation, 2013; Registered Nurses Association of Ontario, 2012).

Falls and Fractures

Control of posture by the central nervous system is determined by proprioception, sensory input, and vestibular input. Older adults have a righting reflex in which vestibular receptors detect any loss of stability. Muscles will oppose a postural sway. Younger adults correct weight shift at the hip, whereas older people use the feet instead of the hip to correct any shift in body posture. Older adults take a rapid step forward or backward to prevent being thrown off balance. They use protective reflexes by extending the arms to restore balance or to secure a surface.

Falls are the most frequent cause of injuries in people aged 65 years and over, accounting for 90% of hip and wrist fractures and 60% of head injuries (Robinovitch et al., 2013). Incidence of falls increases with age and varies according to where a person lives, that is, in the community, in a long-term care setting, or during an acute hospitalization. More than one third of community-dwelling people over the age of 65 fall each year, and more than half of them have recurrent falls (Rosen et al., 2010). About 30% of elderly people living independently and 50% of those in long-term care fall at least once each year (Robinovitch et al., 2013).

Etiology and Pathophysiology

Falls may result from internal (intrinsic) or environmental (extrinsic) factors. Intrinsic causes include syncope, sudden leg weaknesses, dizziness, orthostatic hypotension, side effects of medications, acute illnesses, heart disease, transient ischemic attacks, stroke, and Parkinson disease (Kane et al., 2009). One study identified the most common intrinsic cause of falling as incorrect weight shifting when performing daily activities such as walking, turning, reaching, or standing up from sitting (Robinovitch et al., 2013; Ubelacker, 2012) (Research Highlight 24.2).

Extrinsic factors include environmental hazards such as excessive bed height, inadequate lighting or assistive devices, loose carpets, inappropriate use of side rails, an unfamiliar environment, slippery or uneven surfaces, or poor building design. Risk-taking behaviours such as climbing ladders, using unsafe furniture for reaching items, and poor choice of footwear contribute to falls.

Complications

The most common injuries after a fall are fractures of the hip, femur, humerus, wrist, and ribs, and painful soft tissue injuries. These injuries usually result in hospitalization, with subsequent risks of immobilization and iatrogenic illnesses (Kane et al., 2009).

Østbye et al. (2004), using data from the longitudinal Canadian Study of Health and Aging, concluded that pain and mobility problems were common sequelae of fractures in elderly people. After any lower-body fracture, walkers or wheelchairs were needed by more than 30% of the people, and more than 50% reported moderate or severe pain. The researchers also concluded that older women are at most risk. Whether a fall becomes a fracture depends on various factors, including BMD, fall risk factors, the older adult's biomechanical protective responses, and the amount of local shock when hitting the surface.

Vertebral fractures in women may cause a gradual loss of height affecting stature. It is estimated that between 6% and 21% of postmenopausal women have at least one vertebral deformity. Functional limitations for these women include respiratory compromise, risk for further vertebral and other fractures, reduced quality of life, and increased mortality (Clark et al., 2012). Paraspinal muscles shorten, and pain from muscle fatigue relating to postural maintenance occurs. Pain may become chronic, even after the vertebral fracture heals. Dowager hump or postmenopausal cervical kyphosis in the upper back may occur and further complicate gait, balance, and functional capacity, decreasing the woman's quality of life.

Another fall complication is **fear of falling** in which an older person becomes afraid to resume a previous level of ambulation. This fear can cause anxiety or panic. The nurse should watch to see whether the client clutches others while ambulating or transferring, maintains contact with environmental objects, or uses the wall to steady during ambulation. The nurse then should intervene through consultation with physical therapy for physical strengthening, as well as instituting measures to decrease anxiety, such as offering psychological support (Fig. 24.18). Some researchers found that a group-based balance training program had

● **RESEARCH HIGHLIGHT 24.2** Video Capture of the Circumstances of Falls in Elderly People Residing in Long-Term Care: An Observational Study

BACKGROUND

Falls are the most frequent cause of injuries in people 65 years and over, accounting for 90% of hip and wrist fractures and 60% of head injuries. About 30% of elderly people living independently and 50% of those in long-term care fall at least once each year. Many studies have used interviews or incident reports to study falls in the elderly.

PURPOSE

This study may add to the limited amount of objective evidence about how and why falls occur.

DESIGN

Videotaping was used to conduct an observational study in two long-term care facilities in British Columbia, over a period of 3 years. The researchers captured 227 falls by 130 individuals. A team of at least three experts analyzed each fall, using a consensus approach and selecting the best available answers from a structured questionnaire.

RESULTS

The researchers found that the major cause of falls was incorrect weight shifting, that is, leaning too far past the body's centre of gravity when performing daily activities such as walking, turning, reaching, or standing up from sitting. Other causes were tripping or stumbling, hitting or bumping into an object, loss of support and collapse. Slipping accounted for only six of the falls.

IMPLICATIONS

Each of these activities needs to be targeted in risk assessment and prevention strategies for falls. Several clinical instruments, such as the "Timed Up and Go" test, incorporate a multitask approach, but many residents of long-term care units cannot perform the tests due to mobility or cognitive impairments. There is a need to develop instruments that assess mobility and balance applicable to those residents. This study has implications for modifications of the environment and furniture design, as 25% of the trips happened when a foot was caught on a chair or table leg. Transferring was responsible for 21% of the falls, suggesting the need for exercises to improve muscle strength and consistent use of improved assistive devices when moving to and from chairs. Because this research identified the activities leading to the imbalance and falls, caregivers can be made aware of which activities are most likely to result in a fall.

LIMITATIONS

The study only included falls in common areas of long-term care facilities, not bedrooms or bathrooms, and not in community home-based settings.

Robinovitch, S., Feldman, F., Yang, Y., Schonnop, R., Leung, P., Sarraf, T. et al. (2013). Video capture of the circumstances of falls in elderly people residing in long-term care: An observational study. *Lancet, 381*, 47–54.

---

a beneficial effect on gait, balance, and fear of falling (Halvarsson et al., 2013).

Assessment Findings

According to the American Geriatrics Society (2013), a fall evaluation is an assessment that includes the following:

- Examination of vision, gait and balance, and lower extremity joint function
- Examination of basic neurologic function, including mental status, muscle strength, lower extremity peripheral nerves, proprioception, reflexes, tests of cortical, extrapyramidal, and cerebellar function
- Assessment of basic cardiovascular status, including heart rate and rhythm, postural pulse, and blood pressure
- Examination of feet and footwear

The "Timed Up and Go" test (Mathias et al., 1986; Podsiadlo & Richardson, 1991) is a good assessment of functional ability, useful as well for assessment of gait, balance, and postural control. Another excellent assessment of posture and stability is the chair stand test. The client rises from the chair with hands crossed over the chest, which should take less than 30 seconds to complete.

Collaborative Management

After extensive analysis of research and practice, the Registered Nurses Association of Ontario (2005, 2011) developed a Best Nursing Practice Guideline, with a 2011 supplement to reflect new evidence, related to falls in the elderly. The guidelines recommend a number of fall prevention strategies, including assessment of risk on admission to hospital or care home, as well as after a fall

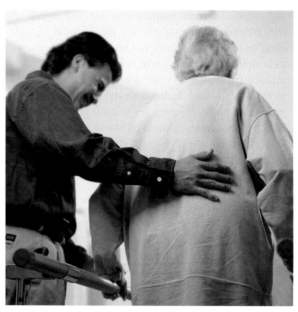

FIGURE 24.18 A physical therapist can assist clients having problems related to mobility.

has occurred. The guidelines include an examination of strategies such as strength and balance training exercises, dietary intake of vitamin D to improve muscle strength, calcium for osteoporosis prevention, environmental modifications, periodic medication reviews among the elderly in health care settings, and tai chi (RNAO, 2005, 2011).

Postfall investigation incident reporting forms (Registered Nurses' Association of Ontario, n.d.) include questions such as:

* Was the fall observed? If so, by whom?
* Was the person previously identified as being at high risk for a fall?
* Does she have a history of falls?
* What footwear was she wearing?
* What was she doing at the time of the fall?
* Where did the fall occur?
* Was a restraint in place at the time of the fall?
* What mechanical and/or assistive devices were in use?
* What was her mental and physical status at the time?
* What was the environmental status at the time of the fall?
* What medications has she taken in the past 48 hours?
* Was she transferred to hospital?
* Were the family and physician notified?

Tsung-Jung et al. (2012) found that long-term tai chi exercise is a good choice in an exercise program to improve balance and reduce the risk of falling in the elderly. Another important factor in decreasing the risk for falls is assessment of visual acuity. It is also important that any adaptive device that an older woman uses (eg, cane and walker) has been professionally fitted. Thin-soled, well-fitting flat shoes will maximize propriocep-

tion and decrease the likelihood of tripping. High heels in older women cause more instability, because they decrease plantar flexion and effective gait. They may also catch on rugs, steps, or wooden decks. A podiatry consult is essential in older women with foot deformities because bunions or painful heels or toes can affect both ambulation and balance. Orthotics worn inside the shoe can be customized to minimize the person's biomechanical abnormalities of gait and to prevent pressure areas in the feet. Foot hygiene, with proper podiatric nail care, will help prevent gait abnormalities and falls.

The nurse can encourage clients to keep a fall diary. The client can do so for 1 to 2 weeks to find the precipitating factors before and during each fall episode. The client should note the date, time, and location of the fall, as well as her activity at the time of the fall, along with related symptoms. Women at high risk for falling may wish to consider hip protectors as one component of a multimodal approach to fall prevention.

Delirium, Dementia, and Depression

Although the incidence of delirium, dementia, and depression rises with advanced age, these mental health conditions are neither synonymous with aging nor are they inevitable. Because assessment and caregiving strategies are complex and require specialized knowledge, an interdisciplinary approach and partnership with family members are needed.

Delirium

Delirium is an acute or subacute alteration in mental status especially common in older people. It is a potentially fatal condition that may go unrecognized in hospitalized older adults. It is classified as a neurocognitive disorder in the Diagnostic and Statistical Manual of Mental Disorders (DSM-5) (American Psychiatric Publishing Association, 2013). It has been estimated that 25% to 50% of older patients admitted to hospital are delirious on admission or develop delirium during their hospital stay (Kane et al., 2009). Signs and symptoms may include illusions, restlessness, picking at bedclothes, attempting to get out of bed, drowsiness, anxiety, fear, irritability, anger, or apathy (Kane et al., 2009).

Although the exact pathophysiologic mechanisms for delirium are unknown, common contributing factors include infection, pain, cardiac or cerebrovascular events, adverse drug reactions, and metabolic abnormalities. Other causes include any acute event such as dehydration or exacerbation of a chronic health problem, which can upset the older person's frail homeostatic balance. Even fecal impaction and urinary retention can cause delirium, as can transfer to unfamiliar surroundings if sensory input is limited (Kane et al., 2009).

The Confusion Assessment Method (CAM) is a valid and reliable assessment for delirium (Inouye,

1998; Inouye et al., 1990; Thomas et al., 2012). It is frequently used in hospitals, but it can be applied across clinical settings. See Assessment Tool 24.3.

Another way to assess delirium is to perform digit span testing. The examiner recites one, two, or three numbers to the client at a rate of one digit per second. The client then repeats the numbers. The tester increases the numbers by one each time. People without cognitive impairment can usually remember seven digits forward and four digits backward. If a client has difficulty with this or with spelling the word "world" backward, the likelihood of delirium is high.

The first and most important step in managing delirium is to identify the delirium and then to treat the causative factors. The nurse should work collaboratively with other members of the health care team to reach these goals. For example, the nurse should assess the client's current medications for any agents that may be causing or exacerbating the delirium (eg, sedatives, hypnotics, analgesics). Other nursing measures to treat delirium include early correction of dehydration, urinary tract infection, or pneumonia in a medically induced delirium. Environmental measures such as minimization of unnecessary stimuli and noise, use of hearing aids and eyeglasses, removal of indwelling urinary catheters and physical restraints, and early mobilization activities will assist hospitalized or bed-bound older adults with delirium (Fong et al., 2009).

Dementia

Dementia is "a clinical syndrome involving a sustained loss of intellectual functions and memory of sufficient severity to cause dysfunction in daily living" (Kane et al., 2009, page 154). Dementia has numerous causes,

---

● **ASSESSMENT TOOL 24.3**   **Confusion Assessment Method Shortened Version Worksheet**

EVALUATOR: _____   DATE: _____

I. ACUTE ONSET AND FLUCTUATING COURSE   **BOX 1**

   a. Is there evidence of an acute change in mental status from the   No _____   Yes _____
      patient's baseline?

   b. Did the (abnormal) behaviour fluctuate during the day, that is,   No _____   Yes _____
      tend to come and go or increase and decrease in severity?

II. INATTENTION

   Did the patient have difficulty focusing attention, for example,   No _____   Yes _____
   being easily distractible or having difficulty keeping track of what
   was being said?

III. DISORGANIZED THINKING   **BOX 2**

   Was the patient's thinking disorganized or incoherent, such as
   rambling or irrelevant conversation, unclear or illogical flow of   No _____   Yes _____
   ideas, or unpredictable switching from subject to subject?

IV. ALTERED LEVEL OF CONSCIOUSNESS
   Overall, how would you rate the patient's level of consciousness?

   _____ Alert (normal)

   | _____ Vigilant (hyperalert)   No _____   Yes _____
   | _____ Lethargic (drowsy, easily aroused)
   | _____ Stupor (difficult to arouse)
   | _____ Coma (unarousable)

Do any checks appear in this box?

If all items in Box 1 are checked and at least one item in Box 2 is checked, a diagnosis of delirium is suggested.

Adapted from Inouye, S.K., van Dyck, C.H., Alessi, C.A., Balkin. S., Siegal, A.P., & Horwitz, R.I. (1990). Clarifying confusion: The confusion assessment method. A new method for detection of delirium. *Annals of Internal Medicine, 113*, 941–948.

including Alzheimer disease, vascular dementia, and other degenerative disorders. In 2011 there were 747,000 people living with dementia in Canada, that is, 14.9% of all Canadians over the age of 65 (Alzheimer Society Canada, 2013). Alzheimer disease is a fatal, progressive, and degenerative disease that destroys brain cells. This progressive dementia is characterized by loss of memory, difficulty with day-to-day tasks, and changes in mood and behaviour (Alzheimer Society Canada, 2012). It is *not* part of normal aging, but rather a form of neuropathology accompanied by neurotransmitter changes.

Assessment Findings. Onset of symptoms in Alzheimer disease is gradual, with manifestations of cognitive and functional decline occurring over months to years. Symptoms may include **aphasia,** a disturbance in language not related to mechanical aspects of speech. Individuals substitute words or forget simple words (Fig. 24.19). **Apraxia** is the inability to carry out motor tasks despite intact motor and sensory function. People may have difficulty performing familiar tasks such as preparing a meal or using a vacuum cleaner. **Agnosia** refers to failure to recognize or identify objects despite intact basic sensory function (Kane et al., 2009). They may become lost on their own street, not knowing how they got there or how to get home. Their judgement may be impaired and they have problems with abstract thinking. They may misplace things—an iron in the freezer or a watch in the sugar bowl (Alzheimer Society Canada, 2012).

Progression of the disease causes additive neuronal destruction (Fig. 24.20). Behavioural symptoms

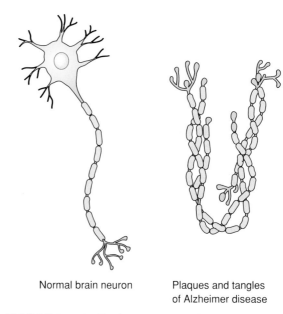

Normal brain neuron   Plaques and tangles of Alzheimer disease

FIGURE 24.20 The brain neurons of clients with Alzheimer disease are marked by tangles and plaques not found in the healthy brain.

such as agitation, insomnia, delusions, hallucinations, and wandering may occur. Paranoia and suspiciousness are common. Sleep cycle disruptions often develop with Alzheimer disease. Other behaviours include apathy, combativeness, hoarding behaviours, and physical or verbal aggression.

Many older clients suffering from Alzheimer disease and other chronic cognitive impairments try to conceal their symptoms. **Confabulation** (telling imaginary stories to fill gaps in the memory of an event) is a common defense mechanism that many use when they realize they are dealing with early cognitive loss.

Safety assessment in women in the early stages of cognitive impairment includes potential household dangers and a driving history. Have there been any motor vehicle crashes or close calls? Does the spouse, partner, or others worry about the client's driving pattern? Was the woman ever lost for a significant time when driving the car? Have passengers compensated for any driving deficit (eg, telling the driver when to stop, when to turn)? Impaired cognition can also affect a woman's ability to take medication as prescribed, putting her at risk for underdosing and overdosing.

Diagnosis is based on a multifactorial process that includes laboratory and diagnostic workups to rule out other causes of cognitive impairment (eg, delirium, depression, or neurologic disorders). The most important diagnostic clue is the history of cognitive loss, which the nurse gathers from the client, family members, or significant others. Other essential components of the dementia workup include a health history and physical examination.

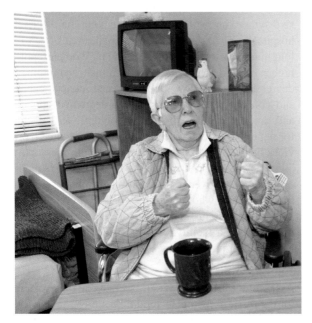

FIGURE 24.19 The communication problems associated with Alzheimer disease can be particularly frustrating for clients.

If the health history reveals forgetfulness, changes in instrumental ADLs, personality, or mood, the nurse should identify when symptoms began, subsequent functional losses, the effects of these cognitive and functional changes, and alterations in social functioning. The nurse should ask about a family history of Alzheimer disease as one way to identify familial onset. The nurse should use a delicate and calm approach when questioning the client about memory changes and cognitive loss. The client's statements may differ significantly from those of the family members. The client must undergo a complete physical examination, with special attention given to the neurologic component to rule out focal deficits and other disorders presenting as dementia.

Collaborative Management. There is currently no cure for Alzheimer disease, but medications may help with some of the symptoms such as decline in memory, language, thinking abilities, and motor skills. Not everyone will respond to the medications, but those who do will have improved quality of life that may last for several years. For mild to moderate Alzheimer disease, three cholinesterase inhibitors are approved for use in Canada: Aricept, Exelon, and Reminyl. For moderate to advanced Alzheimer disease, Aricept can be used, and Ebixa, one of a group of NMDA receptor antagonists, has been conditionally approved. Medications are also available to help manage symptoms such as sleep disruption (Alzheimer Society Canada, 2013).

Think back to Lena and her partner, Hannah, described at the beginning of the chapter. Would cholinesterase inhibitors be appropriate for use with Hannah?

Researchers have explored the relationship between statin therapy and a lower incidence of Alzheimer disease. A comprehensive report published in the Cochrane Reviews did not support the efficacy of statins in the prevention of Alzheimer disease (Kelly, 2009). Other drugs, including estrogen, vitamin E, *Ginkgo biloba,* and nonsteroidal anti-inflammatory agents, have been tried for dementia, but have not been shown to be effective in either prevention or treatment. There is no evidence to support the use of vitamin B supplementation to improve cognition (Kane et al., 2009).

Some practitioners prescribe psychotropic drugs for management of behavioural and emotional symptoms. Although there is very little research into a polypharmacy approach to the treatment of Alzheimer disease, some studies are looking at the concurrent use of psychoactive medications, such as antidepressants and/or hypnotics along with cholinesterase inhibitors, or the addition of an emergency medication such as one of the benzodiazepines (Wood & Weiner, 2013).

Nursing Care Plan 24.2 highlights the management of a client with Alzheimer disease and her caregiver.

Lena is providing care to her partner, Hannah, who has Alzheimer disease. Suppose Lena asks, "I've heard that *G. biloba* helps to improve memory. Would this help Hannah?" How should the nurse respond?

Access to support for caregivers throughout the stages of progression of Alzheimer disease is important. Recently, the Alzheimer Society of Ontario partnered with MedicAlert in a program called *Finding Your Way,* a nationwide program to help identify the person who has wandered and assist her in a safe return home (Alzheimer Society Ontario, 2013). The Alzheimer Society of Canada has extensive information for caregivers as well as local chapters in each province that provide support and education for caregivers. These chapters can be located through the Society website (www.alzheimer.ca).

Depression

Depression is the most common mental health problem in the elderly and affects individuals, families, and communities. It is estimated that 14% to 20% of the elderly who live in the community experience depressive symptoms, with higher rates among the elderly in hospital (12% to 45%), and even higher rates (40%) in long-term care facilities (Wiese, 2011). Women report a higher incidence of depression than men. Symptoms of depression include low mood; reduced interest, energy, and concentration; poor sleep and decreased appetite; and preoccupation with health problems. Risk factors for depression include being widowed or divorced, previous depression, brain changes, disabling illness, polypharmacy, excessive alcohol use, low social support, or being a caregiver for a person with a major disease. Elderly people who are depressed often have a decline in functional status and may require increased care or placement in a facility, causing family stress, a higher likelihood of physical illnesses, and poor recovery from illness (Wiese, 2011).

Assessment Findings. When assessing an older woman for depression, the nurse should be alert to factors that can precipitate a depressive episode, such as recent bereavement, moving from home to another place such as a nursing home, financial crisis, decline in health,

NURSING CARE PLAN 24.2

●

Clients Dealing With Dementia

Think back to Lena, the woman caring for Hannah, her partner of 25 years who has Alzheimer disease. Lena tells the home care nurse, "I feel so frustrated sometimes, and tired. I think I'm just going to fall apart. But I can't leave Hannah."

NURSING DIAGNOSES

- **Caregiver Role Strain** related to being overwhelmed by responsibilities, fatigue, and depression
- **Risk for Injury** related to fatigue and partner's cognitive changes secondary to dementia
- **Ineffective Coping** related to demands of caring for ill partner
- **Deficient Knowledge** related to the care of a person experiencing cognitive decline

EXPECTED OUTCOMES

1. The client will experience fewer feelings of being overwhelmed.
2. The client will verbalize measures to aid in dealing with responsibilities.
3. The client will identify appropriate plans for needed relief.
4. The client and her partner will remain free of injury.
5. The client will identify appropriate methods for coping with and caring for the partner's decreasing health status.

INTERVENTIONS	RATIONALES
Assess the client's daily routine, including caregiving tasks necessary and the partner's ability to participate in care activities	Assessment provides a baseline from which to develop an appropriate individualized plan of care. Information about the client's routine and partner's ability to participate provides clues to areas in which the family may need assistance
Assess the client's strengths, limitations, and ability to manage caretaking activities	Sleep deprivation, physical injury, and social isolation may occur if the client does not have the adequate resources and abilities
Work with the client to develop a schedule of care that includes help from family and friends on a regular rotating basis	Dividing caretaking responsibilities promotes physical endurance and emotional stability
Develop a list of emergency contacts and their phone numbers	An emergency contact list is important to allow for quick access to assistance in a crisis, thereby minimizing feelings of being overwhelmed
In early stages recommend that the client and family attend to legal matters such as creating wills and preparing an *advance directive*. Suggest establishing *power of attorney* for health care, designating who may make decisions if the client becomes incompetent	Dealing with legal matters before the client experiences severe cognitive changes is essential to ensure that the appropriate person has access to unencumbered funds and follows the partner's wishes regarding health care decisions

(continued)

NURSING CARE PLAN 24.2 ● Clients Dealing With Dementia *(Continued)*

INTERVENTIONS	RATIONALES
Teach the client about measures to maintain partner's safety including: • Maintaining consistency in routine • Removing hazards, such as footstools and small tables, from areas where the client walks, and keeping the areas well lit • Ensuring that partner wears some type of medical alert identification • Keeping a current photograph of the partner in the medical record	Consistency reduces confusion. Removing obstacles and slippery surfaces promotes safer ambulation. Adequate lighting reduces the risk for injury secondary to environmental hazards. Clients with Alzheimer disease are known to wander and not recall their current residence. Having the means to identify the client aids in search-and-rescue efforts
Instruct the client in measures to promote partner's self-care including: • Opening food containers and cutting food into bite-sized pieces in later stages • Offering the partner fluids and snacks at 2-hour intervals while awake • Ensuring scheduled toileting • Providing partner with self-care devices such as comb and toothbrush and reviewing its use • Modifying clothing with hook and loop fasteners or suspenders	Self-care promotes independence and self-esteem for the partner while alleviating some of the client's stress associated with caregiving. Minimal assistance facilitates self-care. Adequate fluid and food intake promotes adequate hydration and nutrition. Regular toileting reduces the potential for incontinence. Clients with Alzheimer disease commonly experience forgetfulness related to the names of items, their purpose, and their use. Clothing modifications promote independence in dressing
Instruct the client in measures to promote communication with partner, such as using short, simple explanations and directions, allowing time for the partner to answer, reducing environmental stimuli and noise, and keeping partner focused on one task at a time	Clients with Alzheimer disease commonly experience problems in communication secondary to the decline in cognitive function
Provide information about agencies that offer supportive services; initiate referral to agencies if appropriate. If necessary, arrange for additional help from a home care agency	Additional support from outside agencies provides the client with assistance to deal with her and her partner's needs
Assess for caregiver stress and depression	Caregivers often have difficulty balancing their personal and professional needs with caregiving demands, which can contribute to depression

EVALUATION

1. The client seeks relief from caregiving responsibilities at least 1 or 2 days a week.
2. The client implements measures to deal with responsibilities.
3. The client and partner use appropriate measures to maintain safety.
4. The client uses appropriate strategies and techniques to deal with partner's declining health status.

family or marital problems, social isolation, and persistent sleep difficulties (Wiese, 2011).

A common assessment tool to evaluate depression in the elderly is the Geriatric Depression Scale (GDS) Short Form, which is a 15-item questionnaire evaluating life satisfaction, helplessness, hopelessness, and energy (Assessment Tool 24.4). A longer version is a 30-item scale, also called the GDS (Yesavage, 1988).

Some elderly people consume large amounts of prescription medications. Many pharmacologic agents can cause depression in elders (Kane et al., 2009). The nurse should complete a thorough medication review to determine whether any new symptoms of depression are associated with new or discontinued medications. Hoarding

of medications may be indicative of intent to attempt suicide; therefore, it is critical to assess for adherence to medication regimes as well as for polypharmacy.

Suicide rates are high in the elderly, with an average of 1.3 suicides daily in Canadian seniors (Wiese, 2011), and more men than women committing suicide (Statistics Canada, 2012c). In 2009, of the 90 women aged 65 years and older who committed suicide, most were between 65 and 69 (Statistics Canada, 2012c). These numbers may continue to grow as a result of the aging population. Although both men and women attempt suicide, women are less likely to use methods that are not as lethal and they are more likely to survive than men (Wikipedia, 2013). Between 2000 and

● ASSESSMENT TOOL 24.4 Short Form: Geriatric Depression Scale

NAME _____ AGE _____ SEX _____ DATE _____

WING _____ ROOM _____ PHYSICIAN _____ ASSESSOR _____

SCORING SYSTEM

Answers indicating depression are highlighted. Each **bold faced** answer counts one (1) point.

1. Are you basically satisfied with your life?	YES/**NO**
2. Have you dropped any of your activities and interests?	**YES**/NO
3. Do you feel that your life is empty?	**YES**/NO
4. Do you often get bored?	**YES**/NO
5. Are you in good spirits most of the time?	YES/**NO**
6. Are you afraid that something bad is going to happen to you?	**YES**/NO
7. Do you feel happy most of the time?	YES/**NO**
8. Do you often feel helpless?	**YES**/NO
9. Do you prefer to stay in your room/facility, rather than going out and doing new things?	**YES**/NO
10. Do you feel you have more problems with memory than most?	**YES**/NO
11. Do you think it is wonderful to be alive?	YES/**NO**
12. Do you feel worthless the way you are now?	**YES**/NO
13. Do you feel full of energy?	YES/**NO**
14. Do you feel that your situation is hopeless?	**YES**/NO
15. Do you think that most people are better off than you?	**YES**/NO

Score greater than 5 = Probable Depression   SCORE _____

Notes/Current Medications: _____

_____

_____

INSTRUCTIONS FOR USE

1. Choose a quiet place, preferably the same location each time the test is administered.
2. The administration of this test should not be immediately after some mental trauma or unsteady period.
3. Speak in a soft pleasant tone.
4. Answer all questions by circling the answer (yes or no) to the question.
5. Add the total number of **BOLD FACED** answers circled and record that number in the "SCORE" box.
6. Scores totalling five (5) points or more indicate probable depression.

A 30-item version of the GDS is also available. Address inquiries regarding this scale to: Jerome A. Yesavage, M.D. http://www.stanford.edu/~yesavage/

2009 the most commonly used method of suicide in older adults was hanging, followed by firearms and poisoning. The methods used by women of all ages were largely hanging and poisoning (Navaneelan, 2012).

Suicide prevention includes being aware of the warning signs. These signs may include thinking and talking of death; substance abuse; feelings of hopelessness, helplessness, or purposelessness; feelings of being trapped; withdrawal from social contacts; anxiety; agitation; anger; or mood changes. Immediate warning signs often include threatening to hurt or kill oneself; looking for ways to kill oneself; and talking or writing about death, dying, or suicide, if these actions are out of the ordinary. Good health practices, strong social networks, support of family and friends, and active interests are factors that protect against suicide (Centre for Suicide Prevention, 2012).

Collaborative Management. Treatment of depression includes management to reverse the current episode and ongoing assessment and treatment to prevent a recurrence. Several classifications of medications are used to treat depression; given the incidence of comorbidities in older adults, caution is required to avoid exacerbating the medical condition or causing adverse events. For example, dementia, cardiovascular problems, diabetes, and Parkinson disease can worsen with anticholinergic drugs (Wiese, 2011). It is also important to minimize drug–drug interactions because of the many drugs that elderly people may be taking.

Tricyclic antidepressants were used for many years; however, these drugs are lethal in overdose and are avoided for this reason. The SSRIs have lower anticholinergic effects than older antidepressants. Despite a low side effect profile, a small percentage of elders may develop hyponatremia, especially with high doses of SSRIs. Other side effects include nausea, dry mouth, insomnia, somnolence, agitation, diarrhea, excessive sweating, and, less commonly, sexual dysfunction. Some SSRIs have a better safety profile than others and a lower potential for drug–drug interactions. Some of the newer antidepressants are relatively safe in the elderly. The nurse should become familiar with any antidepressants her client may be taking, and in particular, interactions between drugs and effect of drugs on any comorbid diseases (Wiese, 2011).

Electroconvulsive therapy (ECT) has re-emerged as a first-line treatment for depression in the elderly. The recovery is faster compared with medication and is considered to be an alternative treatment for severe depression, particularly when an individual has not responded to antidepressants, is acutely suicidal, or is unable to take medications because of other medical problems (Wiese, 2011).

Pain

Pain is a frequent symptom among older women with chronic health conditions. It is often underdiagnosed and undertreated, especially in long-term care residents who have dementia and cannot verbalize their pain. Thorough interdisciplinary assessment and evaluation are necessary and may reveal underlying causes of the pain, pointing to interventions that can relieve pain at its source (American Geriatrics Society, 2009). Many older people underreport pain, and even pain that is causing severe impairment may not be reported for a variety of personal, cultural, or psychological reasons (AGS, 2009). The *Numeric Rating Scale* (NRS) is the pain intensity scale most widely used with older adults. In this scale, the individual is asked to rate her pain on a scale of 0 to 10, with 0 being no pain and 10 being the worst pain imaginable. Studies have shown that the NRS, *Faces Pain Scale,* and *Verbal Descriptor Scale* can be used effectively with adults who have cognitive impairment (Flaherty, 2012).

When taking the client's history for pain, the nurse should evaluate characteristics like intensity, frequency, character, location, duration, and precipitating, aggravating, and alleviating factors. The nurse should assess the level of pain within the context of the woman's functional status and document the effect of pain on appetite, sleep, energy, mood, exercise, cognition, and sexual, social, and personal issues (Fig. 24.21). The nurse should evaluate the client's history of use of analgesics, previous and current medications, over-the-counter drugs, complementary/alternative therapies, and alcohol. He or she needs to note the effectiveness of previously tried treatments, including the client's satisfaction with current pain treatment. Clients with intact cognition can use a pain log or diary to assess intensity, use of medications, and response to treatments.

The physical examination for pain includes its location and any sites of pain radiation. The musculoskeletal and neurologic physical examinations must be thorough.

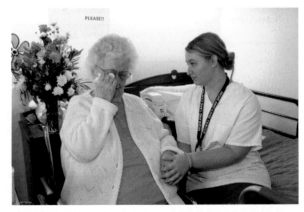

FIGURE 24.21 Discussing and documenting a client's pain and its effects are essential nursing interventions.

● **BOX 24.2** Common Pain Behaviours in Cognitively Impaired Elderly People

Facial Expressions

- Slight frown; sad, frightened face
- Grimacing, wrinkled forehead, closed or tightened eyes
- Any distorted expression
- Rapid blinking

Verbalizations, Vocalizations

- Sighing, moaning, groaning
- Grunting, chanting, calling out
- Noisy breathing
- Asking for help
- Verbal abuse

Body Movements

- Rigid, tense body posture, guarding
- Fidgeting
- Increased pacing, rocking
- Restricted movement
- Gait or mobility changes

Changes in Interpersonal Interactions

- Aggressive, combative, resisting care
- Decreased social interactions
- Socially inappropriate, disruptive
- Withdrawn

Changes in Activity Patterns or Routines

- Refusing food, appetite change
- Increase in rest periods
- Sleep, rest pattern changes
- Sudden cessation of common routines
- Increased wandering

Mental Status Changes

- Crying or tears
- Increased confusion
- Irritability or distress

Note: Some patients demonstrate little or no specific behaviour associated with severe pain.

From American Geriatrics Society. (2002). Guidelines on the management of persistent pain in older persons. *Journal of the American Geriatrics Society, 50*(6), S205–S224.

Psychosocial evaluation includes the effects of pain on social, recreational, and occupational functioning. In clients with cognitive impairment, the nurse should assess for any new onset or exacerbation of delirium, dementia, or depression. The nurse should look for nonverbal clues to pain and observe cognitively impaired clients during ambulation and transferring (Box 24.2).

Initiation of nonpharmacologic pain management can be an essential part of care. For example, referral to physical therapy and occupational therapy may help prevent pain that arises from muscular atrophy, immobility, or compromised muscle strength.

The American Geriatrics Society (2009) has guidelines for pharmacologic pain management in older adults. For episodic pain, medications can be prescribed as needed, as long as the client is able to request pain medication. In cognitively impaired individuals, pain medications should be given before pain is anticipated. For continuous pain, medications should be provided around the clock to maintain optimal analgesic blood concentration. These individuals should also have short-acting analgesics prescribed for breakthrough pain (AGS, 2009).

Key recommendations include starting with acetaminophen for mild to moderate pain, because of low cost, high efficacy, and low toxicity. Guidelines also recommend opioid analgesics for severe pain or pain not controlled by NSAIDs (AGS, 2009).

When managing pain in older adults, prevention of related constipation is an important nursing intervention. Constipation is a common side effect of opioids. A stool softener may be prescribed when initiating narcotic therapy. Another important measure is ensuring the client's safety in the environment. Sedative effects of pain medication may increase the risk for falls and confusion. In addition, the nurse should evaluate the client for any problems with enuresis because pain medications may cause older adults to sleep through nocturnal urges to void.

The nurse serves as a client advocate, helping to prevent suffering from undiagnosed and undertreated pain. The nurse should ensure that ongoing pain assessment, medication management, and nonpharmacologic pain management continue on a predetermined schedule, with appropriate documentation and reporting to the primary health care provider.

NURSING CARE OF THE HOMEBOUND OR COMMUNITY-RESIDING WOMAN

Government-supported home care and private nursing agencies are the main sources of skilled nursing care for older adults who continue to live in their own homes or elsewhere in the community. The role of the home care nurse working with older women is complex, independent, and potentially rewarding. The nurse is in the unique position of assisting the woman to maximize function and maintain independence in the most desired setting: her own home. The role of the home health nurse has increased significantly in the past 20 years. Whereas services and service providers vary across the country, intravenous infusions, wound therapy, catheter care, and special nutritional supplementation devices are now routine home nursing interventions. The home care evaluation is vital because the nurse reports findings to the primary health care provider.

Observation of family dynamics and communication is integral to home assessment. The **primary caregiver** is usually a family member, significant other, or friend who assists the client to meet her functional needs. The primary caregiver may be living with the client or may reside in his or her own home. In today's mobile society, the nurse often communicates from a distance with the primary caregiver or the person with medical decision-making abilities for the client if the client becomes mentally incapacitated.

The nurse should determine whether the client can accomplish ADLs with assistance from the primary caregiver. The caregiver may provide assistance with instrumental ADLs such as shopping, cooking, cleaning, laundry, and transportation for laboratory testing and physician visits. The primary caregiver often organizes medications for the client, picks up prescriptions, pays bills, and handles other money management activities. The nurse needs to determine whether the primary caregiver's availability to assist with these activities meets the client's functional needs.

Older women with more significant functional impairments need assistance with basic ADLs. Often in such cases, the primary caregiver assists with bathing, ambulating, transferring from various positions, and getting to the toilet. If the primary caregiver cannot meet these needs and the client experiences problems with personal hygiene or falls during transfers or trips to the bathroom, the client requires a higher level of care (Fig. 24.22).

The nurse should connect clients lacking needed primary caregiver assistance with outside community agencies. To do so, the nurse needs to be aware of the woman's financial status, approximate income, and other financial resources (eg, investments, assets, retirement benefits, savings accounts, government pensions, and subsidies). Some community services are based on income eligibility and sliding scale status (fees charged based on the person's ability to pay). The visiting nurse needs to know whether her client has supplemental insurance or other types of health care funding to assist with community services.

Home care nurses, or home health nurses as they are sometimes called, work with interprofessional teams of

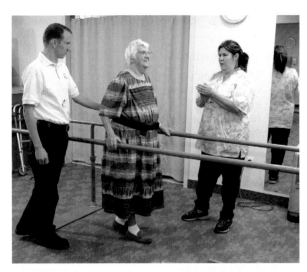

FIGURE 24.22 Clients who need assistance with ambulation, feeding, and other basic ADLs and who do not have adequate support from primary caregivers require a higher level of nursing intervention.

community caregivers, such as program case managers, social workers, occupational therapists, physiotherapists, or speech and language therapists. They assess clients who may need personal care homes or assisted living facilities, as well as determine long-term care home eligibility for clients who need a higher level of care.

Other sources of community support include pharmacies and grocery stores that make home deliveries, "Meals on Wheels" or church-related food programs, and special transportation offered by community services (eg, wheelchair van, low-cost bus transportation to and from health care appointments). Ideally, the nurse is aware of any local optometrists, dentists, or podiatrists who make home visits. The nurse can recommend these providers to the primary health care provider or directly to families. Many insurance programs such as Blue Cross offer special visual and auditory support to subsidize adaptive devices to clients with sensory impairments. Some organizations such as the Canadian National Institute for the Blind (CNIB) have related support and counselling for older adults suffering from sensory deficits.

Senior citizens' centres offer historical, educational, and recreational trips, as well as specialized classes in such areas as painting, tai chi, and computer use. The greatest advantage of these centres is that they provide an age-appropriate outlet for older people to form new relationships and networks (Fig. 24.23).

Local libraries may have bookmobiles. For clients with visual impairments, they supply books on audiocassette or compact disk for auditory reading enjoyment. Caregiver support groups have increased in availability and number and are often advertised on television bulletin boards and in local newspapers. Support groups can be general, for example, for chronic illness, or specific,

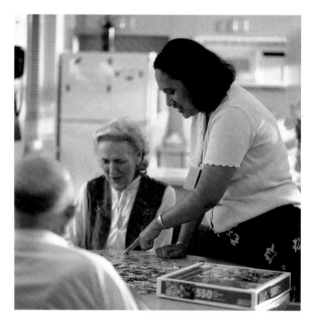

FIGURE 24.23 Senior citizens' centres provide a strong social and recreational outlet for older women and men.

such as the Alzheimer Society of Canada, which has local chapters in each province (www.alzheimer.ca). These support groups offer a network of informal support from other clients and primary caregivers.

The nurse should be aware of professional, scientifically based internet sites related to specific disorders. Busy family members appreciate knowing where to access authentic and research-based information on clinical illnesses or syndromes. The nurse should also be familiar with local and regional health care providers who may have a special interest in Alzheimer disease, geriatric depression, and urinary incontinence or other conditions seen in older adults. He or she needs to know of any gerontology programs with nurses, nurse practitioners, social workers, or psychologists specializing in care of older adults in the local area. The nurse can suggest consultation with such specialists to the primary health care provider, or directly to the family members for discussion with the primary health care provider.

The home health nurse is knowledgeable regarding reputable home health product suppliers. These agencies may come to the client's home and measure for proper use of adaptive devices such as canes, walkers, or wheelchairs. There are emergency call systems available to elderly people living alone at home. These electronic services respond to a call from the client through an electronic device worn around the client's neck or wrist, or placed on an accessible table. The client presses the call button at specific times each day or if in distress. A call is immediately put through to the client and if there is no response, the service agent will notify the predetermined next of kin or significant other. Programs offering

telephone reminders for the client to take medications on time are available in some communities.

The home health nurse has a "golden" opportunity to observe family dynamics. It is important for the nurse to assess how family members are coping and assisting with loss of ADLs in an older person. If involved with live-in or part-time caretaking, how are the primary caregivers coping? How has this task changed their family and work lives? Do the caregiver's siblings share responsibilities? Does the primary caregiver have the physical and emotional ability, motivation, intelligence, time, and financial resources to implement and monitor the plan of care? Caregiving can be expensive and may be a financial stressor. How is assisting the client affecting the primary caregiver's health and financial status? It is important for the nurse to assess this because he or she may be the connecting agent for financial and social assistance.

The nurse visiting the home should assess for signs of potential caregiver burden or burnout. Brunshaw (2012) listed 10 signs of caregiver burnout.

- Feeling unusually tense, irritable, or agitated with others
- Being irritable and angry toward the ill/disabled individual
- Feeling sad, tearful, or dissatisfied with life in general
- Feeling exhausted and overwhelmed
- Withdrawal from friends and enjoyable activities due to loss of desire and/or energy
- Lowered immunity: getting sick more often and taking an unusually long time to recover
- Increased need for medications and/or use of drugs or alcohol
- Feeling out of control in attempts to manage usual daily routine, with no sense of how to regain that control any time soon
- Trouble sleeping and/or disturbing dreams
- Change in appetite

ELDER ABUSE

One in five Canadians believes they know of an elderly person who might be experiencing abuse. "Elder abuse is any action by someone in a relationship of trust that results in harm or distress to an older person" (Public Health Agency of Canada, 2012c. page 1). The abuse may be physical, psychological, and/or financial, with financial being the most commonly reported type. The abuser might be a family member, a friend, someone who provides assistance with basic needs, or a health care provider. Although elder abuse and neglect can be difficult to detect, the nurse should assess the older woman for signs of fear, anxiety, depression, or passivity in relation to a family member, friend, or care provider; unexplained physical injuries; dehydration, poor nutrition, or poor hygiene; improper use of medication; confusion about new legal documents such as a new will or a new mortgage; sudden drop in cash flow or financial holdings; and reluctance to speak about the situation (Public Health Agency of Canada, 2012c).

If elder abuse or neglect is suspected, it is important for the nurse to talk to her client and ask questions about her experience, while respecting her values and right to make decisions. The nurse should seek consent or permission before taking any action and should respect confidentiality and privacy rights. The nurse can assist her client in accessing help or support (Canadian Centre for Elder Law, 2011).

There is no national reporting system for elder abuse in Canada, but there are response teams available in most areas, usually through the city or regional police services. There are differences in standards and reporting across the country because of the structure of federal and provincial systems. Criminal, family violence, adult protection, and adult guardianship laws apply across Canada and can help protect seniors from abuse and neglect. Forms of abuse such as fraud, assault, uttering verbal threats, and criminal harassment are considered crimes under the Criminal Code of Canada. Civil laws vary by province and territory. Abuse of power of attorney is an offence within provincial/territorial jurisdiction. Many provinces and territories have laws that provide additional protection for older adult victims of abuse and a range of social service interventions to protect those with physical or mental deterioration. Some jurisdictions have legislation regarding abuse of people in the care of an institution, and most jurisdictions provide protection to victims of family violence (Public Health Agency of Canada, 2012e).

The nurse's legal obligation to report abuse, neglect, or risk depends on several factors: What province or territory does the older woman live in? What agency is responsible for her care? Does she live in the community or in a care facility? Does she need support or assistance or is she unable to care for herself? Is there risk for abuse or has abuse already happened? Has a criminal act occurred? "A Practical Guide to Elder Abuse and Neglect Law in Canada" (Canadian Centre for Elder Law, 2011) contains reporting information that is province- and territory-specific.

NURSING CARE OF THE OLDER WOMAN IN OTHER ENVIRONMENTS

Assisted living facilities or personal care facilities offer nursing care to older adults who need assistance with ADLs or who are unsafe or uncomfortable living inde-

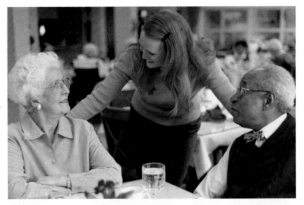

FIGURE 24.24 Shared social experiences, such as dining and recreation, are one of the strongest benefits of assisted living facilities for older clients.

pendently. These housing arrangements often allow for aging in place, that is, the woman would not have to move to other facilities if her status changes. Progression of care needs determines the need for minimal assistance or more complex care within a long-term care facility.

Assisted living facilities offer meals in a shared dining room (Fig. 24.24). Some facilities also provide small kitchens in each resident's room or apartment. Transportation, cosmetology, laundry, and social and recreational activities are available in some facilities. Physicians with an interest in caring for older adults are usually attached to these facilities for residents who have no family physician. Geriatricians and home health nurses can be consulted to provide primary health care assessment and specialty services (eg, incontinence evaluation and management, psychogeriatric evaluations).

Long-term care facilities provide higher levels of complex care to the residents. There is usually a mix of staff, from personal care assistants, or aides, Licensed Practical Nurses, Registered Practical Nurses (Ontario), Registered Psychiatric Nurses (Manitoba and west), to Registered Nurses. Many provinces or health care regions have variations of care provision, but generally the Registered Nurses or Registered Psychiatric Nurses provide ongoing assessment and decision making for everyday direct care given by personal care assistants or aides. Nurses assess residents and plan their care, implement and evaluate care plans, and administer direct care, medications, and treatments.

There is movement toward employing nurse practitioners in long-term care facilities to work along with advanced practice nurses. Wound care and ostomy nurses, continence nurse specialists, and advanced practice nurses with various specialty skills often provide consultation in the long-term care setting. Psychogeriatric or psychiatric clinical nurse specialists and geriatric or psychiatric nurse practitioners may be consulted in long-term care settings for management of depression and behavioural problems.

Care given in long-term care settings requires interdisciplinary collaboration. Nurses meet regularly with other team members and the client's family to evaluate and discuss the needed changes to the client's plan of care. Other team members include dietitians; physiotherapists, occupational and speech therapists; psychologists; medical directors; or attending physicians. The consulting pharmacist is a valuable team member whom nurses can consult regarding medication use and drug interactions. He or she can help identify clients at high risk for adverse drug reactions. The recreational therapist is responsible for implementing socialization and structured activity programs during waking hours.

Standards of excellence in care and clinical and operational performance in long-term care facilities are promoted through accreditation. Many institutions across the country participate voluntarily in the rigorous program of assessment, evaluation, and guidance from Accreditation Canada. System-wide areas assessed include governance, leadership and management, infection prevention and control, and medication management, whereas population-specific and service excellence standards address specific sectors, services, conditions, and populations (Accreditation Canada, 2013).

The Canadian Gerontological Nursing Association (http://www.cgna.net/) provides specific education and support through research, conferences, workshops, and special programs to nurses who focus on caring for the older adult. Certification in gerontologic nursing is an asset to nurses working with aging people. The Canadian Nurses Association Certification Program encourages nurses to achieve recognition for attaining the standard of professional competencies in their chosen area of nursing practice (http://www.cna-aiic.ca/en/).

SUMMARY

- Nurses in the 21st century will care for an expanding aging population that is expected to double by 2031 to 9.6 million. The most rapid population growth is occurring in people older than 80 years. An unprecedented number of women older than 85 years and a rapidly growing number of female centenarians mean women are living longer with one or more chronic illnesses.
- Data gathering and communicating with the postmenopausal woman require self-evaluation for ageist attitudes, allowing extra time for history taking, and excellent communication techniques to compensate for the deficiencies in vision, hearing, and cognition that some women experience in later years.
- Comprehensive assessment of the postmenopausal woman includes evaluation of lifestyle activities within the context of personal and family medical history. A detailed medication history is necessary

because many older women experience adverse drug events that mimic common geriatric syndromes. Physiologic and physical examination findings are different from those in younger adults; all organ and body systems are affected by the aging process. The greatest indicator of the postmenopausal woman's health is her functional status, which tells the nurse of the woman's basic, instrumental, and advanced activities of daily living. The social history is important. As age or chronic illnesses increase, a woman may need to expand utilization of her social support system. The nurse must realize sexual needs exist in women during the later phases of life and should assess and address them with respect and concern for the individual.

- Screening for osteoporosis is essential near the time of menopause because failure to identify and treat women with osteoporosis has a major impact on the quality of life during the later years. Sleep assessment and client education regarding proper sleep hygiene is important. Postmenopausal women may be affected by hormonal changes, sleep phase advancement, depression, anxiety, or cognitive changes, all of which may alter sleep patterns and affect the woman's energy level and overall health.
- Geriatric syndromes affect many women and have a major impact on quality of life. Unfortunately, these syndromes are not always assessed and treated. The nurse needs to understand the various types of urinary incontinence. Falls should be evaluated with a specific falls history and physical evaluation. The nurse needs to use the assessment tools available for detection of delirium, depression, and dementia, as well as contributing causes. Persistent pain is often underdiagnosed and undertreated. The nurse can assess pain using standard pain tools and will document response to treatment.
- The nurse working with elderly women must understand the levels of care that women may move through in the later phase of their lives. Independent living with outpatient or ambulatory care, home care, assisted living, and long-term care offer various opportunities for nurses to work with older women. The nurse needs to assist the woman in planning health care and advanced directives for her later years. It is essential for the nurse to support the caregiver/care recipient dyad.

Questions to Ponder

1. Recalling Ann, the 67-year-old woman with bladder incontinence, what dietary and lifestyle modifications might the nurse suggest to help reduce the incidence of bladder leakage? What exercises will help strengthen the muscles that support her bladder?

2. Remember Lena and Hannah from the earlier part of the chapter. What safety precautions will Lena need to take to keep Hannah safe as her dementia progresses?

3. How would you counsel a 55-year-old woman regarding ways to preserve her level of health?

4. Name several reasons why the rates of diagnosis for and treatment of dementia, depression, and delirium remain below an acceptable level of care.

5. Your grandmother is 85 years old and has lived at home, in assisted living, and in a long-term nursing home setting. Describe the roles of nurses who have cared for her in each setting.

REVIEW QUESTIONS

1. When obtaining the health history from an older adult woman, which question would be most appropriate for the nurse to use?
   A. "Do you live with your son and daughter-in-law?"
   B. "How are you feeling today, sweetie?"
   C. "What can you tell me about your shoulder pain?"
   D. "Are you having any pain right now?"

2. The nurse is assessing a 74-year-old client's instrumental activities of daily living. Which area should the nurse include in this assessment?
   A. Ability to dress self
   B. Meal preparation
   C. Senior-centre activities
   D. Volunteer work

3. The nurse is preparing a presentation on osteoporosis for a local community women's group comprising women ranging in age from 50 to 75 years. As part of the presentation, the nurse should stress that older women should
   A. Increase their calcium intake by taking calcium supplements
   B. Eat foods high in calcium
   C. Take vitamin D supplements
   D. Have a bone scan

4. When assessing an older client, which of the following findings should the nurse consider most significant?
   A. Crackles on lung auscultation
   B. Decreased arm swing with walking
   C. Systolic blood pressure drop of 10 mm Hg on standing
   D. Decrease in forced vital capacity

5. Which of the following should the nurse keep in mind when administering medications to an older woman?
   A. A decrease in adipose tissue allows for an increase in the drug's duration of effect.
   B. Drug absorption is incomplete in the older adult woman, leading to erratic responses.
   C. The half-lives of drugs are shortened as a result of the decrease in renal function with age.
   D. The risk for adverse drug reactions is increased because of decreased serum albumin levels.

6. The home health care nurse arrives at the home of a 78-year-old client who has had a surgical repair of her fractured hip. The nurse is developing a plan to reduce the client's risk for falling that focuses on extrinsic factors. Which areas should the nurse address? Select all that apply.
   A. Throw rugs in the kitchen
   B. Absence of grab bars in the shower
   C. Client's recent surgery on her hip
   D. Complaints of forgetfulness
   E. Electrical cord running across the living room

7. The physician prescribes a cholinesterase inhibitor for a woman with Alzheimer disease. Which drug should the nurse expect to administer?
   A. Memantine (Ebixa)
   B. Vitamin E
   C. Donepezil (Aricept)
   D. Diazepam

8. An older client is diagnosed with depression and is to receive Zoloft, a drug in the SSRI class. The nurse teaches her about possible side effects. Which of the following should the nurse include as most common?
   A. Sexual dysfunction
   B. Orthostasis
   C. Sedation
   D. Constipation

9. The nurse is discussing the side effects of the opioid medication that has been prescribed for her client's persistent pain. Which of the following side effects should she include?
   A. Constipation
   B. Change in body weight
   C. Confusion
   D. Enuresis

10. An 88-year-old client is being cared for by her daughter in her daughter's home. The client has moderate dementia and needs assistance with bathing, dressing, and toileting. The daughter, a 65-year-old retired school teacher, lives with her 72-year-old husband. The husband, who had a stroke approximately 3 years ago, has some left-sided weakness and moderate osteoarthritis. The nurse making a home visit would most likely identify which nursing diagnosis as the priority?
    A. Self-care deficit: bathing
    B. Risk for caregiver role strain
    C. Risk for injury
    D. Impaired urinary elimination

REFERENCES

Accreditation Canada. (2013). *Access to standards.* Retrieved from http://www.accreditation.ca/about-us

Allen, M., Kelly, K., & Fleming, I. (2013). Hypertension in elderly patients: Recommended systolic targets are not evidence based. *Canadian Family Physician, 59*(1), 19–21. Retrieved from http://www.cfp.ca/content/59/1/19.full

Alzheimer Society Canada. (2012). *Alzheimer's disease.* Retrieved from http://www.alzheimer.ca/en/About-dementia/Dementias/Alzheimer-s-disease

Alzheimer Society Canada. (2013). *Drugs approved for Alzheimer's disease.* Retrieved from http://www.alzheimer.ca/en/Living-with-dementia/Treatment-options/Drugs-approved-for-Alzheimers disease

Alzheimer Society Ontario. (2013). *Finding your way.* Retrieved from http://www.alzheimer.ca/en/on/Finding-Your-Way/Tools-and-resources

American Geriatrics Society. (2009). Pharmacological management of persistent pain in older persons. New York: American Geriatrics Society, *57*(8). doi:10.1111/j.1532-5415.2009.02376.x. Retrieved from http://www.americangeriatrics.org/files/documents/2009_Guideline.pdf

American Geriatrics Society. (2013). Prevention of falls in older persons. *AGS/BGS clinical practice guideline.* Retrieved from http://www.americangeriatrics.org/health_care_professionals/clinical_practice/clinical_guidelines_recommendations/prevention_of_falls_summary_of_recommendations/

American Psychiatric Association. (2013). *Diagnostic and statistical manual of mental disorders* (5th ed., pp. 596–602). Washington, DC: American Psychiatric Publishing.

American Urological Association Foundation. (2011). *Bladder diary instructions.* Retrieved from http://www.urologyhealth.org/SUI/_documents/_pdf/AUAF_SUI_Bladder_Diary.pdf

Bjorkman, M., & Malterud, K. (2009). Lesbian women's experiences with health care: A qualitative study. *Scandinavian Journal of Primary Health Care, 27*(4), 238–243. Retrieved from http://www.ncbi.nlm.nih.gov/pmc/articles/PMC3413916/

Breijer, M., Timmermans, A., van Doom, H., Mol, B., & Opmeer, B. (2010). Diagnostic strategies for postmenopausal bleeding. *Obstetrics and Gynecology International, 2010,* 850812. doi:10.1155/2010/850812. Retrieved from http://www.ncbi.nlm.nih.gov/pmc/articles/PMC2821624/

Brotman, S., Ryan, B., Collins, S., Chamberland, L., Cormier, R., Julien, D. et al. (2007). Coming out to care: Caregivers of gay and lesbian seniors in Canada. *Gerontologist, 47*(4), 490–503. Retrieved from http://search.proquest.com.cyber.usask.ca/docview/211027564?accountid=14739

Brunshaw, J. (2012, June 12). *Compassion fatigue and caregiver burnout.* Health Council of Canada blog. Retrieved from http://healthcouncilcanada.blogspot.ca/2012/06/compassion-fatigue-and-caregiver.html

Canadian Cancer Society. (2011). *Breast cancer screening guidelines.* Retrieved from http://www.cancer.ca/Canada-wide/Prevention/Getting%20checked/Breast%20cancer%20NEW.aspx?sc_lang=en

Canadian Cancer Society. (2012). *Colorectal cancer.* Retrieved from http://www.cancer.ca/Canada-wide/Prevention/Getting%20checked/Colorectal%20cancer%20screening.aspx?sc_lang=en

Canadian Centre for Elder Law. (2011). A practical guide to elder abuse and neglect law in Canada. *British Columbia Law Institute.* Retrieved from http://yourlegalrights.on.ca/sites/all/files/Practical_Guide_English_Rev_JULY_2011.pdf

Canadian Continence Foundation. (2009). *Impacts of incontinence in Canada.* Retrieved from http://www.canadiancontinence.ca/pdf/impacts-of-incontinence.pdf

Canadian Healthy Aging Project. (2006). *Responding to older adults with substance abuse, mental health and gambling challenges.* Toronto, ON, Canada: Centre for Addiction and Mental Health. Retrieved from http://www.sheridancollege.ca/About%20Sheridan/Sheridan%20Research/Centres/SERC/Your%20Health%20Marketplace/Mental%20Health/~/media/WF_03_Research_010/responding_older_adults.ashx

Canadian Institute for Health Information. (2010). Seniors and prescription drug use. *Series on seniors.* Retrieved from http://www.cihi.ca/CIHI-ext-portal/pdf/internet/SENIORS_DRUG_INFO_EN

Canadian Institute for Health Information. (2013). Adverse drug reaction-related hospitalizations among seniors 2006–2011. Analysis in Brief. March. Retrieved from https://secure.cihi.ca/free_products/Hospitalizations%20for%20ADR-ENweb.pdf

Canadian Lung Association. (2013). *Lung diseases, COPD.* Retrieved from http://www.lung.ca/diseases-maladies/copd-mpoc/signs-signes/index_e.php

Canadian Task Force on Preventive Health Care. (2013). *Screening for cervical cancer.* Retrieved from http://canadiantaskforce.ca/guidelines/screening-for-cervical-cancer/

Cantor, M. H., Brennan, M., & Shippy, R. A. (2004). *Caregiving among older lesbian, gay, trans-sexual and transgender New Yorkers.* New York, NY: National Gay and Lesbian Task Force Policy Institute. Retrieved from http://www.thetaskforce.org/downloads/reports/reports/CaregivingAmongOlderLGBT.pdf

Centers for Disease Control. (2013). *Vaccines and preventable diseases: Pneumococcal disease in-short.* Retrieved from http://www.cdc.gov/vaccines/vpd-vac/pneumo/in-short-both.htm

Centre for Suicide Prevention. (2012). Plus 65 at the end of the day. *Suicide Prevention Toolkit.* Retrieved from http://suicideinfo.ca/LinkClick.aspx?fileticket=cmFwRL4DMJw%3D&tabid=563

Clark, E., Gould, V., Morrison, L., Ades, A., Dieppe, P., & Tobias, J. H. (2012). Randomized controlled trial of a primary care–based screening program to identify older women with prevalent osteoporotic vertebral fractures: Cohort for skeletal health in Bristol and Avon (COSHIBA). *Journal of Bone and Mineral Research, 27,* 664–671. doi:10.1002/jbmr.1478. Retrieved from http://onlinelibrary.wiley.com/doi/10.1002/jbmr.1478/full

Continence Conversation. (2013). *Continence toolkit.* Retrieved from http://continenceconversation.com/community-toolkit/

Fitzpatrick-Lewis, D., Hodgson N., Ciliska, D., Peirson, L., Gauld, M., & Liu, Y. (2011). *Breast cancer screening.* Hamilton, ON: Mc Master University. Retrieved from http://site.ebrary.com.cyber.usask.ca/lib/usask/docDetail.action?docID=10516309

Flaherty, E. (2012). Pain assessment for older adults. *Try this: Best practices in nursing care to older adults: General assessment series, 7.* Retrieved from http://consultgerirn.org/uploads/File/trythis/try_this_7.pdf

Fleg, J., & Strait, J. (2012). Age associated changes in cardiovascular structure and function: A fertile milieu for future disease. *Heart Failure Reviews, 17*(4–5), 545–554. doi:10.1007/s10741–011–9270–2. Springer Science + Business Media, LLC, Retrieved from http://link.springer.com/article/10.1007/s10741–011–9270–2?LI=true#page-2

Fong, T., Tulebaev, S., & Inouye, S. (2009). Delirium in elderly adults: Diagnosis, prevention and treatment. *Nature Reviews Neurology, 5*(4), 210–220. Retrieved from http://www.ncbi.nlm.nih.gov/pmc/articles/PMC3065676/

Gillson, S. (2012). GERD in the elderly. *Heartburn. About. com.* Retrieved from http://heartburn.about.com/od/gerdacidrefluxdisease/a/Gerd-In-The-Elderly.htm

Grogan, M. (2011). What is a silent heart attack? *Mayo Clinic Health Information.* Retrieved from http://www.mayoclinic.com/health/silent-heart-attack/AN02146

Halvarsson, A., Franzén, E., Farén, E., Olsson, E., Oddsson, L., & Stahle, A. (2013). Long-term effects of new progressive group balance training for elderly people with increased risk of falling—a randomized control trial. *Clinical Rehabilitation, 27*(5), 450–458. doi:10.1177/0269215512462908. Abstract retrieved from http://cre.sagepub.com/content/early/2012/10/31/0269215512462908.abstract

Heart and Stroke Foundation. (2013). Women and heart disease and stroke. *Heart Disease.* Retrieved from http://www.heartandstroke.com/site/c.ikIQLcMWJtE/b.3484041/k.D80A/Heart_disease__Women_and_heart_disease_and_stroke.htm

Higginson, L. (2012). Orthostatic hypotension. *Merck manual for health care professionals. Cardiovascular disorders.* Retrieved from http://www.merckmanuals.com/professional/cardiovascular_disorders/symptoms_of_cardiovascular_disorders/orthostatic_hypotension.html?qt=postural%20hypotension%20elderly&alt=sh

Hunter, G., Bickel, C., Fisher, G., Neumeier, W., & McCarthy, J. (2013). Training and energy expenditure in older women. *Medicine and Science in Sports and Exercise*, Europe PubMed Central. Abstract retrieved from http://europepmc.org/abstract/MED/23377831

Idland, G., Petterson, R., Avlund, K, & Bergland, A. (2013). Physical performance as long-term predictor of onset of activities of daily living (ADL) disability: A 9-year longitudinal study among community-dwelling older women. *Archives of Gerontology and Geriatrics, 56*(3), 501–506. http://dx.doi.org/10.1016/j.archger.2012.12.005, Abstract retrieved from http://www.sciencedirect.com/science/article/pii/S0167494312002440

Inouye, S.K. (1998). Delirium in hospitalized older patients: Recognition and risk factors. *Journal of Geriatric Psychiatry and Neurology, 11*, 118–125.

Inouye, S.K., Van Dyck, C.H., Alessi, C.A., Balkin, S., Siegal, A.P., & Horwitz, R.I. (1990). Clarifying confusion: The confusion assessment method. A new method for detection of delirium. *Annals of Internal Medicine, 113*, 941–948.

Institute of Medicine. (2004). Dietary reference intakes: Water, potassium, sodium, chloride, and sulfate. *Consensus Report*. Retrieved from http://www.iom.edu/reports/2004/dietary-reference-intakes-water-potassium-sodium-chloride-and-sulfate.aspx

International Center for Alcohol Policies. (1995–2013). Alcohol and the elderly. *ICAP blue book*, (Module 23.1–23.8). Retrieved from http://www.icap.org/LinkClick.aspx?fileticket=JrDTh3DzjMw%3d&tabid=181

Jerrard, J. (2006). Eliminate elderspeak and restore dignity. *Caring for the Ages, January*. American Medical Directors Association, Inc. Retrieved from http://cfa.gcnpublishing.com/fileadmin/content_pdf/cfa/archive_pdf/vol7iss1/60009_main.pdf

Kane, R.L., Ouslander, J.G., Abrass, I.B., & Resnick, B. (2009). *Essentials of clinical geriatrics* (6th ed.). New York, NY: McGraw-Hill.

Kelly, J. (2009, April 16). Statins fail to prevent dementia, Alzheimer's disease. *Medscape Medical News*. Retrieved from http://www.medscape.com/viewarticle/591119

Kinch, J., & Jacubec, S. (2004). Out of the multiple margins: Older Canadian women managing their health care. *Canadian Journal of Nursing Research, 36*(4), 90–108.

Lavretsky, H. (2010). Spirituality and aging. *Aging Health, 6*(6), 749–769. Retrieved from http://www.medscape.com/viewarticle/740654

Lawler-Row, K., & Elliott, J. (2009). The role of religious activity and spirituality in the health and well-being of older adults. *Journal of Health Psychology, 14*(1),43–52. Abstract retrieved from http://www.unboundmedicine.com/medline/citation/19129336/The_role_of_religious_activity_and_spirituality_in_the_health_and_well_being_of_older_adults_

Little, M., & Morley, A. (2013). Reducing polypharmacy: Evidence from a simple quality improvement initiative. *Journal of the American Medical Directors Association, 14*(3), 152–256. Abstract retrieved from http://www.jamda.com/article/S1525-8610(12)00420-3/abstract

Masoro, E. (2010). Physiology of aging. In H. Fillit, K. Rockwood, & K. Woodhouse (Eds.), *Brockelhurst's textbook of geriatric medicine and gerontology* (7th ed., Chapter 9). Philadelphia, PA: Saunders Elsevier.

Mathias, S., Nayak, U. S. L., & Isaacs, B. (1986). Balance in elderly patients: The "get up and go" test. *Archives of Physical Medicine Rehabilitation, 67*, 387–389.

Mayo Clinic Staff. (2011). Hypothermia. *Patient Care and Health Information, Diseases and Conditions*. Mayo Foundation for Medical Education and Research. Retrieved from http://www.mayoclinic.org/diseases-conditions/hypothermia/basics/definition/con-20020453

Mayo Clinic Staff. (2012). Female sexual dysfunction. *Patient Care and Health Information, Diseases and Conditions*. Mayo Foundation for Medical Education and Research. Retrieved from http://www.mayoclinic.org/diseases-conditions/female-sexual-dysfunction/basics/definition/con-20027721

Mayo Clinic Staff. (2014). Heart disease in women: Understand symptoms and risk factors. *Patient Care and Health Information, Diseases and Conditions*. Mayo Foundation for Medical Education and Research. Retrieved from http://www.mayoclinic.org/diseases-conditions/heart-disease/in-depth/heart-disease/art-20046167

Milan, A., & Vézina, M. (2012). Senior Women. *Women in Canada: A Gender-based Statistical Report*. Statistics Canada, Catalogue no. 890503-X. Retrieved from http://www.statcan.gc.ca/pub/89-503-x/2010001/article/11441-eng.htm

Miller, C.A. (2011). *Nursing for wellness in older adults.* (6th ed.). Philadelphia, PA: Wolters Kluwer Health/Lippincott Williams & Wilkins.

Milne A., Potter, J, Vivanti, A. & Avenell, A. (2009). Protein and energy supplementation in elderly people at risk from malnutrition. *Cochrane Database of Systematic Reviews, 2*. Art. No.: CD003288. doi:10.1002/14651858.CD003288.pub3. Abstract retrieved from http://summaries.cochrane.org/CD003288/protein-and-energy-supplementation-in-elderly-people-at-risk-from-malnutrition

Moyer, V. (2013). Vitamin D and calcium supplementation to prevent fractures in adults: U. S. Preventive Services Task Force recommendation statement. *Annals of Internal Medicine, 158*(9), 691–696, Clinical Guideline, February. Retrieved from http://annals.org/article.aspx?articleid=1655858

Musini, V., Tejani, A., Bassett, K., & Wright, J. (2009). Pharmacotherapy for hypertension in the elderly. *The Cochrane Database of Systematic Reviews*. John Wiley & Sons, Ltd. doi:10.1002/14651858.CD000028.pub2

National Digestive Diseases Information Clearing House. (2012). *Diverticulosis and diverticulitis*. Retrieved from http://www.digestive.niddk.nih.gov/ddiseases/pubs/diverticulosis/index.aspx

National Kidney and Urologic Diseases Information Clearinghouse. (2010). *Daily bladder diary*. Retrieved from http://kidney.niddk.nih.gov/kudiseases/pubs/diary/index.aspx

Navaneelan, T. (2012). Suicide rates: An overview. *Health at a glance*. Statistics Canada, catalogue no. 82–624-X, charts 2 and 3. Retrieved from http://www.statcan.gc.ca/pub/82–624-x/2012001/article/11696-eng.htm

Østbye, T., Walton, R., Steenhuis, R., & Hodsman, A. (2004). Predictors and sequelae of fractures in the elderly: The Canadian Study of Health and Aging (CSHA). *Canadian Journal on Aging, 23*(3), 245–251.

Osteoporosis Canada. (2013, February 28). *Position statement on calcium and vitamin D for overall bone health*. Retrieved from http://www.osteoporosis.ca/despite-recent-studies-calcium-and-vitamin-d-remain-important-nutrients-for-overall-bone-health/

Padwal, R., Kaczorowski, J., Herman, R., Khan, N., Quinn, R., Tobe, S. et al. (2013). Systolic blood pressure targets: Additional considerations beyond age. Response to Allen et al., Hypertension in elderly patients: Recommended systolic targets are not evidence based, published on-line, *Canadian Family Physician*. Retrieved from http://www.cfp.ca/content/59/1/19.full/reply#cfp_el_12303

Papaioannou, A., Morin, S., Cheung, A., Atkinson, S., Brown, J., Feldman, S. et al. (2010). 2010 clinical practice guidelines for the diagnosis and management of osteoporosis in Canada: Summary. *Canadian Medical Association Journal, 182*(17), 1864–1873. doi:10.1503/cmaj.100771. Retrieved from http://www.cmaj.ca/content/182/17/1864.full

Parshall, M., Schwartzstein, R., Adams, L., Banzett, R., Manning, H., Bourbeau, J. et al. (2012). An official American Thoracic Society statement: Update on the mechanisms, assessment, and management of dyspnea. *American Journal of Respiratory and Critical Care Medicine, 185*(4), 425–452. Retrieved from http://www.thoracic.org/statements/resources/respiratory-disease-adults/update-on-mamd.pdf

Perceptions of Libraries. (2010). *Seniors' use of social sites soars*. Retrieved from http://www.oclc.org/content/dam/oclc/reports/2010perceptions/seniors.pdf

Podsiadlo, D., & Richardson, S. (1991). The timed "Up and Go": A test of basic functional mobility for frail elderly persons. *Journal of the American Geriatrics Society, 38*, 142–148.

Public Health Agency of Canada. (2012a). Active vaccines, herpes zoster. *Canadian immunization guide, Part 4*. Retrieved from http://www.phac-aspc.gc.ca/publicat/cig-gci/

Public Health Agency of Canada. (2012b). Active vaccines, pneumococcal vaccine. *Canadian immunization guide, Part 4*. Retrieved from http://www.phac-aspc.gc.ca/publicat/cig-gci/

Public Health Agency of Canada. (2012c). Elder abuse: It's time to face the reality. *Health promotion, national clearinghouse on family violence*. Retrieved from http://www.phac-aspc.gc.ca/ncfv-cnivf/sources/age/age-abuse-broch/index-eng.php

Public Health Agency of Canada. (2012d). Immunization of adults. *Canadian immunization guide, Part 3*. Retrieved from http://www.phac-aspc.gc.ca/publicat/cig-gci/

Public Health Agency of Canada. (2012e). Preventing abuse and neglect of seniors. *The Chief Public Health Officer's Report on the State of Public Health in Canada 2010*. Chapter 4: Setting conditions for healthy aging. Retrieved from http://www.phacaspc.gc.ca/cphorsphc-respcacsp/2010/fr-rc/cphorsphc-respcacsp-07-eng.php

Public Health Agency of Canada. (2013). *Chronic Obstructive Pulmonary Disease (COPD)*. Retrieved from http://www.phac-aspc.gc.ca/cd-mc/crd-mrc/copd-mpoc-eng.php

Ramage-Morin, P. (2009). Medication use among senior Canadians. *Health Reports, 20*(1), 37–44. Statistics Canada, catalogue no. 82–003-XPE. Retrieved from http://www.statcan.gc.ca/pub/82–003-x/2009001/article/10801-eng.htm

Ramage-Morin, P., & Garriguet, D. (2013). Nutritional risk among older Canadians. *Health Reports, 24*(3), 3–13. Statistics Canada, catalogue No. 82–003-x. Retrieved from http://www.statcan.gc.ca/pub/82–003-x/82–003-x2013003-eng.htm

Registered Nurses' Association of Ontario. (n.d.). Post fall investigation. Falls: Assessment tools. *Best practices toolkit*. Retrieved from http://ltctoolkit.rnao.ca/resources/falls#Risk-Assessment-Tools

Registered Nurses Association of Ontario. (2005, 2011). *Best nursing practice guideline: Prevention of falls and fall injuries in the older client*. Retrieved from http://rnao.ca/sites/rnao-ca/files/Prevention_of_Falls_and_Fall_Injuries_in_the_Older_Adult.pdf

Registered Nurses Association of Ontario. (2012). *Talking with Your Health care provider: What can I do about urinary incontinence?* Retrieved from http://uida.rnao.ca/sites/uida.rnao.ca/files/documents/Uninary-Incontinence-Decision-Aid_0.pdf

Robinovitch, S., Feldman, F., Yang, Y., Schonnop, R., Leung, P., Sarraf, T. et al. (2013). Video capture of the circumstances of falls in elderly people residing in long-term care: An observational study. *Lancet, 381*, 47–54. Published Online October 17, 2012 http://dx.doi.org/10.1016/ S0140–6736(12)61263-X. Retrieved from http://www.sciencedirect.com.cyber.usask.ca/science/article/pii/S014067361261263X

Röndahl, G., Innala, S., & Carlsson, M. (2006). Heterosexual assumptions in verbal and non-verbal communication in nursing. *Journal of Advanced Nursing, 56*(4), 373–381. Retrieved from http://onlinelibrary.wiley.com/doi/10.1111/j.1365–2648.2006.04018.x/abstract

Ropper, A. & Samuels, M. A. (2009). The neurology of aging: Morphologic and physiologic changes in the aging nervous system. *Victor's Principles of Neurology* (9th ed.). Chapter 29. New York: McGraw-Hill.

Rosen, S., Koretz, B., & Reuben, D. (2010). Presentation of disease in old age. In H. Fillit, K. Rockwood, & K. Woodhouse (Eds.), *Brockelhurst's textbook of geriatric medicine and gerontology* (7th ed., Chapter 34). Philadelphia, PA: Saunders Elsevier.

Saskatoon Health Region. (2002–2013). Timed up and go test. *Falls prevention screening and referral tools. Programs and services*. Retrieved from http://www.saskatoonhealthregion.ca/your_health/ps_ip_falls_screening_tools_related_documents.htm

Sigurdson, K., & Ayas, N.T. (2007). The public health and safety consequences of sleep disorders. *Canadian Journal of Physiological Pharmacology, 85*, 179–183.

Smyth, C. (2012). *The Pittsburgh Sleep Quality Index (PSQI). Try this: Best practices nursing care to older adults, 6.1*. New York: New York University: Hartford Institute for Geriatric Nursing.

Spencer, J. (2012). Continence promotion. *Nursing for Women's Health, 16*(4), 337–340. Retrieved from http://onlinelibrary.wiley.com.cyber.usask.ca/doi/10.1111/j.1751–486X.2012.01753.x/full

Statistics Canada. (2012a). Life expectancy at birth. *CANSIM Table 102–0512*, Catalogue no. 84–537-XIE. Retrieved from http://www.statcan.gc.ca/tables-tableaux/sum-som/l01/cst01/health26-eng.htm

Statistics Canada. (2012b). Population by age and sex. *Annual demographic estimates: Canada, provinces and territories*. Catalogue no. 91–215-X. Retrieved from http://www.statcan.gc.ca/pub/91–215-x/2012000/part-partie2-eng.htm

Statistics Canada. (2012c). Suicides and suicide rate, by sex and by age group. *CANSIM Table 102–0551*. Retrieved from http://www.statcan.gc.ca/tables-tableaux/sum-som/l01/cst01/hlth66b-eng.htm

Statistics Canada. (2013). Study: Select health indicators of First Nations people living off reserve, Métis and Inuit, 2007–2010. *The Daily*, January 29. Retrieved from http://www.statcan.gc.ca/daily-quotidien/130129/dq130129b-eng.pdf

Substance Abuse and Mental Health Administration & Administration on Aging. (2012). Alcohol misuse and abuse prevention. *Older Americans behavioral health. Issue Brief 2*. Retrieved from http://www.aoa.gov/AoARoot/AoA_Programs/HPW/Behavioral/docs/Older_Americans_Issue%20Brief%202_Alc%20Misuse_508_12JUN06_dr.pdf

The Telegraph. (2012, February 13). Hypothermia deaths double over five years. *Health News*. Retrieved from http://www.telegraph.co.uk/health/healthnews/9078273/Hypothermia-deaths-double-over-five-years.html

Thomas, C., Kreisel, S., Oster, P., Driessen, M., Arolt, V., & Inouye, S. (2012). Diagnosing delirium in older hospitalized adults with dementia: Adapting the Confusion Assessment Method to International Classification of Diseases, Tenth Revision, Diagnostic Criteria. *Journal of the American Geriatrics Society, 60*(8), 1471–1477. doi:10.1111.1532–5415.04066.x. Retrieved from http://onlinelibrary.wiley.com.cyber.usask.ca/doi/10.1111/j.1532–5415.2012.04066.x/full

Tsung-Jung, H., Sheng-Chang, C., Tung-Wu, L., & Jaung-Geng, L. (2012). Influence of long-term Tai-Chi Chuan training on standing balance in the elderly. *Biomedical Engineering; Applications, Basis and Communications, 24*, 1. Abstract retrieved from http://www.worldscientific.com/doi/abs/10.4015/S1016237212002913

Turner, M., & Ship, J. (2007). Dry mouth and its effects on the oral health of elderly people. *Journal of the American Dental Association, 139*(3), 252–253.

Ubelacker, S. (2012, October 17). Videotaping shows most falls among elderly due to incorrect weight-shifting: Study. *The Canadian Press*. Retrieved from http://www.canada.com/health/Videotaping+shows+most+falls+among+elderly+incorrect+weightshifting/7399779/story.html

University of Michigan. (1991). Michigan alcohol screening test-geriatric version (MAST-G). Ann Arbor, Michigan: National Serious Mental Illness Treatment Resource and Evaluation Center and University of Michigan Medical School.

Volpato, S., Cavalier, M., Sioulis, F., Guerra, G., Maraldi, C., Zuliani, G. et al. (2010). Predictive value of the Short Physical Performance Battery following hospitalization in older patients. *The Journals of Gerontology, 66A*(1), 89–96. Abstract retrieved from http://biomedgerontology.oxfordjournals.org/content/66A/1/89.short

Ward, K., & Reuben, D. (2013). Comprehensive geriatric assessment. *UpToDate*. Retrieved from http://www.uptodate.com/contents/comprehensive-geriatric-assessment

WebMed. (2013a). *Osteoarthritis Health Center*. Retrieved from http://www.webmd.com/osteoarthritis/default.htm

WebMed. (2013b). *Rheumatoid Arthritis Health Center*. Retrieved from http://www.webmd.com/rheumatoid-arthritis/guide/rheumatoid-arthritis-basics

Wiese, B. (2011). Geriatric depression: The use of antidepressants in the elderly. *BC Medical Journal, 53*(7), 341–347. Retrieved from http://web.ebscohost.com.cyber.usask.ca/ehost/pdfviewer/pdfviewer?sid=e3d0ae1e-c9ab-45d8-acfe-4b3fa18fb2ae%40sessionmgr12&vid=2&hid=24

Wikipedia. (2013). *Sex differences in suicide*. Retrieved from http://en.wikipedia.org/wiki/Sex_differences_in_suicide

Williams, K., Herman, R., Gajewski, B., & Wilson, K. (2009). Elderspeak communiction: Impact on dementia care. *American Journal of Alzheimer's Disease and Other Dementias, 24*(1): 11–20. Retrieved from http://www.ncbi.nlm.nih.gov/pmc/articles/PMC2823803/

Wood, J. & Weiner, M. (2013). Pharmacological treatment of behavioral and emotional symptoms of Alzheimer's disease; a case for polypharmacy. *Neurodegenerative Disease Management, 3*(1), 35–42. Retrieved from http://search.proquest.com.cyber.usask.ca/docview/1283305883/fulltextPDF?accountid=14739

World Health Organization. (2008). Medicines: Safety of medicines-adverse drug reactions. *Media Centre, Fact Sheet No 293.* Retrieved from http://www.who.int/mediacentre/factsheets/fs293/en/index.html

Yesavage, J. A. (1988). Geriatric depression scale. *Psychopharmacology Bulletin, 24,* 709.

Yorkcollegepa. (2011, August 11). ElderSpeak. *YouTube video.* Retrieved from http://www.youtube.com/watch?v=cRs1iOI_Q-Q

Zelman, K. (2010). The wonders of water. *WebMD information and resources.* Retrieved from http://www.webmd.com/a-to-z-guides/features/wonders-of-water

Answers to Case-Based Questions

1. The nurse can investigate options such as having her husband or the children assume some responsibility for planning and cooking healthy meals. If Elaine's youngest is in junior high school, these children are old enough to provide such assistance. Elaine also might consider making and freezing extra nutritious meals on the weekends and simply reheating them (or having her family do so) on the nights she works. The nurse can encourage the client to discuss with her husband the need for him to help with house duties, now that she is working outside the home.

2. Taohua's family support systems seem challenging. She cannot rely on her parents and seems dependent on her aunt, who may have limited resources for appropriate nutrition and health care.

3. The nurse could schedule Elaine's appointment at a time that is convenient and does not compromise work attendance for the client. Also, the nurse can emphasize that monitoring and checking health now may wind up being a long-term financial saving if doing so helps prevent chronic and expensive problems such as hypertension or depression.

4. The nurse needs to respect Taohua's wish for confidentiality, while emphasizing the importance of going to regular prenatal appointments, eating and resting adequately, and taking prenatal vitamins if the client is considering maintaining the pregnancy. The nurse can refer her to community resources that might be able to help provide some assistance.

5. The nurse may be concerned about the family's reaction to the pregnancy. The relatives may be resistant to supporting another person in their household and may try to influence the client's decisions relative to the pregnancy. Taohua's options include continuing with the pregnancy and keeping the baby, continuing with the pregnancy and giving the baby up for adoption, or terminating the pregnancy. She needs to consider each of these options within the context of her relationship with Robert, her current and future living arrangements, the culture of her family in China, and her plans for her education. It would be helpful for you to know more about Taohua's own cultural beliefs related to pregnancy, since these may differ from those of her family.

6. The nurse can examine the parameters of the study with Elaine to see if she qualifies for participation, and then explore with her whether the additional money that might come from the study is worth the risk in postponing medication. The nurse also needs to consider whether the study really might positively influence the client's problem for which medication was prescribed and whether Elaine's participation could be a potentially effective intervention.

1. Renee has voiced concern about being at a healthy weight. The nurse needs to explore whether Renee's beliefs about what actually is a healthy weight are accurate. In addition, the nurse should evaluate the client's commitment to making and adhering to a plan, especially in light of her statement about being so busy.

2. The nurse needs to ask Renee what she knows about this diet she found on the internet and if she knows who has endorsed it. In addition the nurse should discuss with Renee why is considering this particular diet.

3. Jill's BMI is about 22.

4. Renee may prefer exercises that can include her son. For example, she might take brisk walks while

pushing her son in a stroller. She could join a community facility that offers baby-sitting while clients exercise. Alternatively, Renee could arrange for someone to watch her son at night while she attends a local gym.

5. Linda is experiencing menopause. Most bone loss occurs within the first 5 to 7 years after cessation of menstruation. Linda works 50 hours a week and spends most of that time sitting at a computer. Inactivity thus may be a risk factor. She also reports that she does not like milk, so low calcium intake may be a risk factor.

6. Linda can eat low-fat yogurt or cheese. She also can consume soy-based beverages with added calcium, calcium-fortified breakfast cereals and fruit juices, and dark green leafy vegetables. If necessary, she also can take calcium supplements.

7. In addition to the information normally gathered during a health assessment, the nurse needs to obtain a thorough reproductive history because this is Jill's first reproductive health visit. Critical information includes age at menarche, menstrual history (cycle frequency, duration, and typical flow), and any signs and symptoms of premenstrual syndrome. Also, the nurse should evaluate Jill's sexual activity, use of safer-sex practices, and method of contraception (as well as her awareness of various types). Another important measure would be to evaluate Jill's knowledge about fertility and sexually transmitted infections.

8. Being sensitive to the fact that this is Jill's first time and that she may have experienced some form of sexual abuse in the past the nurse would provide her an opportunity to discuss any underlying sexual or trauma related issues. The nurse would have this discussion while Jill is still fully dressed. It would be important to explain the procedure fully to Jill, answer any questions and if necessary rebook an appointment for a later date. The nurse might need to see Jill again before she feels comfortable enough to have the examination.

9. Linda might apply a water-soluble lubricant (eg, K-Y jelly) before or during sexual intercourse. She and her partner also might extend foreplay to enhance lubrication.

10. Linda should undergo a yearly mammogram. She should undergo a Pap smear and pelvic examination annually with the option of every 1 to 3 years after three consecutive normal results, as long as she has minimal or no risk factors for cervical cancer. The nurse also should encourage her to perform monthly breast self-examinations.

CHAPTER 3

1. Sheila might be at risk for inadequate protein, vitamin B_{12}, iron, and zinc.

2. Betsy's BMI is 18.

3. With a prepregnancy BMI of 27, Sheila was overweight prior to her pregnancy and should gain approximately 0.3 kg per week during pregnancy. She is in her third trimester, so her weight should be between 73 and 77 kg.

4. Appropriate suggestions include other dairy products such as yogurt, cheese, and ice cream. Nondairy products that are high in calcium include green leafy vegetables (eg, kale, broccoli), sesame seeds, tofu, and calcium-fortified juices and breads.

5. Betsy's statement reflects self-focus, a key aspect of adolescent development. The nurse should determine the exact meaning of the statement and work to correct any misinformation.

6. The nurse should begin by exploring what foods Betsy dislikes and her concerns about becoming "fat." Lack of knowledge about sound nutritional intake may promote the ingestion of empty calories and unhealthy foods, such as those high in saturated fat or low in vitamins and minerals. Next, the nurse should address Betsy's typical dietary intake, possibly using a 24-hour recall, to gather data about the types and amounts of food that the client eats. Results can help the nurse target areas for additional instruction. A third key area is to assess Betsy's food preferences, which will help nurse and client develop an individualized nutritional plan that promotes Betsy's sense of autonomy and contributes to her participation.

CHAPTER 4

1. Vaginal discharge with itching and irritation might indicate an STI. The nurse should further investigate whether Lela has dysuria, pelvic pain, intermenstrual bleeding, or other general symptoms of STIs. He or she also should ask about the amount and characteristics of the discharge and obtain cultures for diagnostic evaluation of the exact cause.

2. The nurse needs to find out the colour of the vaginal discharge, which is grey/white or watery with bacterial vaginosis. The nurse also should ask about any odour of the discharge which, with bacterial vaginosis, is fishy and especially noticeable after intercourse. To confirm a diagnosis of bacterial vaginosis, a specimen of vaginal fluid needs to be obtained and examined for a pH greater than 4.5 with evidence of bacterial vaginosis organisms.

3. Jade has a family history of breast cancer; no information is given about other genetic risks. Her reproductive history reveals pregnancy at 19 years and menarche at 11 years. Studies show that women who experience their first full-term pregnancy before 22 years are at decreased risk, whereas women who experience menarche before 12 years appear to be at increased risk. Jade's inconsistent physical activity may be a risk, because increased exercise has been associated with a decreased risk for breast cancer.

4. Jade's statements imply lack of understanding of the causes of and risks associated with breast cancer. A priority nursing diagnosis for her is "Lack of Knowledge."

CHAPTER 5

1. Dina would be at Erikson's stage of "intimacy vs. isolation," and thus would be concerned with developing mature attachments and making commitments. Her decisions during this stage can have far-reaching consequences into midlife.

2. Dina's statements reflect hopelessness and desperation. Factors placing her at risk for self-harm include the many demands on her time and attention, isolation associated with a language barrier, low self-esteem, and sense of shame about her Arabic background. The nurse should complete a suicide assessment and refer Dina for mental health services.

3. Gladys is easily distracted and seems to be responding to something or someone other than the nurse. Her behaviour may suggest a response to auditory hallucinations. Also, Gladys says that voices may be coming from the fetus. Although she says it would be unusual, she thinks that it could happen. Thus, she is manifesting false beliefs. The nurse needs to realize that experiencing hallucinations can be frightening to Gladys. It is important to create a calm environment, reassure Gladys that you want to help her, and help her to focus on reality rather than the hallucination.

4. Dina thinks she is responsible for the abuse and is making excuses for her husband's behaviour. Her statements indicate that she is in the enduring phase.

5. The nurse should investigate Gladys's comment closely. Alcohol use/abuse during pregnancy poses numerous fetal risks and may be contributing to the client's auditory hallucinations. Further investigation (eg, with the CAGE questionnaire) would help iden-

tify Gladys's patterns of alcohol use. Once the nurse has more information, interventions can be initiated, such as teaching about the fetal effects of maternal alcohol use and making referrals for support in assisting Gladys to stop drinking.

6. Akathisia refers to continuous observable restlessness. Gladys may exhibit such behaviours as fidgety movements, arm or leg swinging, pacing, inability to stand or sit still for more than a few minutes, and foot-to-foot rocking when standing.

CHAPTER 6

1. Gender identity is reflected in a person's sense of maleness or femaleness, as well as in his or her acceptance and internalization of the roles of that gender. Kendra's appearance and dress suggest acceptance of her "femaleness." The initial information indicates that she is comfortable with her gender role.

2. Rochelle's concerns are common for many parents of teens. The nurse should respond calmly, paying particular attention to the meaning behind Rochelle's statements. First, the nurse should determine any specific concerns or fears. For example, is Rochelle afraid that Kendra may become pregnant or develop an STI? Once Rochelle has pinpointed her worries, the nurse can then address them. He or she can explain that many teens are preoccupied with sexual issues and developments related to changes in hormones, appearance, and body functions. The nurse could mention that dating prepares adolescents for mature relationships and helps them improve their social skills. Throughout the discussion, the nurse can reinforce that teens are striving for identity, self-confidence, self-esteem, and trust in preparation for future mature relationships.

3. The nurse should review whether the client has indeed experienced menopause and when this happened. He or she should ask Patti whether sexual problems coincided with changes in menstrual function and if the couple took any measures at the time to address the difficulties.

4. The nurse would shift the focus of assessment from exploration of the client's age and physiology to a discussion of how long she has been attracted to other women and how she feels about her sexual orientation. The nurse could then refer the client to appropriate resources for assistance in working through her feelings, accepting her identity, and figuring out her future relative to her marriage and sexual orientation.

CHAPTER 7

1. The couple is preparing for a new role as parents. Pregnancy affects each partner, as well as the overall family unit. Olivia expresses anxiety by stating that she is "overwhelmed." Possibly she is concerned about being a good mother; maybe she worries about how the baby will change her lifestyle. She also notes changes in Tyler's behaviour. He also may be anxious about potential changes in responsibilities, or he may be struggling to cope with his wife's feelings. Many changes are occurring even before the baby is born.

2. The birth mother is grieving and needs the opportunity to hold and spend time with the baby, acquainting herself with the newborn before beginning to accept her loss. Although she has initially relinquished the newborn to Jacob and Rachel, the birth mother can still change her mind. Therefore, during this interaction, the nurse should be alert for statements or behaviours that might indicate that the birth mother is unsure of or felt pressured into making the decision.

CHAPTER 8

1. Determine exactly what Veena means. If Veena says that she wants to be responsible for what is used and how, then a diaphragm may be appropriate. How comfortable is Veena with touching herself? Does she have the manual dexterity to apply spermicide to the diaphragm, as well as to insert and remove it?

2. Explore options with the client that provide hormonal contraception but do not need as much maintenance as daily-dose methods require. Examples may include the contraceptive patch or Depo-Provera.

3. Explore Kenya's reasons for choosing natural family planning. She may have misconceptions that need to be corrected. In addition, the nurse should assess Kenya's knowledge about her menstrual cycle and period of fertility. A major area of focus is the client's menstrual history, including information about menarche, cycle length, and regularity. Because some methods of natural family planning involve checking cervical mucus, the nurse needs to know how comfortable Kenya is with touching her genitals to do so. The nurse also can discuss the possibility of including Darrell in future sessions to ensure that both partners understand that success with natural family planning requires the couple to abstain from intercourse during fertile days.

4. Perform a thorough health history that reviews full medical, sexual, family, and social details. Information about lifestyle, financial status, plans for future pregnancy, and involvement of a partner is crucial to helping Veena make an informed decision. In addition, the nurse should gather information about any cultural, religious, or personal beliefs that may influence Veena's options. Determine exactly what the client knows about the various types of contraception, being alert to any misconceptions. Doing so helps to form the basis for an appropriate contraceptive education plan.

CHAPTER 9

1. Multiple factors were probably involved. The fetus had severe physical and congenital abnormalities that likely would have required advanced care throughout the child's life. Providing such care may have caused physical, emotional, and financial stressors that were too numerous for Gina to have felt she could handle.

2. The gestation would be in the first trimester. Thus, the abortion method may be vacuum aspiration or methotrexate and misoprostol.

3. The gestation would be in the second trimester. Thus, the abortion method may be dilatation and evacuation or induction of labour with misoprostol and oxytocin.

CHAPTER 10

1. Stacy is verbalizing a common myth related to infertility. The nurse should clearly and tactfully explain that infertility is a medical condition with a wide range of causes, and should further investigate whether cultural or religious beliefs are influencing the client.

2. In some cases, a definitive cause of infertility cannot be determined. The best response is to address Ted's concerns honestly and openly, making sure to approach the topic empathetically. In addition, the nurse should explore what coping methods the couple has used, reinforce positive strategies, and provide ongoing support. They may benefit from participation in support groups or from community resources and counselling.

3. The nurse should clarify what Stacy means by "the doctors couldn't find anything wrong." Did both Stacy and her ex-husband undergo fertility testing? If so, what types of testing were performed? If fertility testing was not completed, then the nurse should ask how the couple and doctors concluded that nothing was wrong.

4. Through laparoscopy, examiners can explore the internal organs to identify problems such as adhesions, structural abnormalities, and endometrial implants that may be the cause of infertility. In addition, dye instilled through laparoscopy can reveal tubal patency, the shape of the uterine cavity, and any defects that could interfere with embryonic implantation or development.

5. The most appropriate recommendation is gamete intrafallopian transfer (GIFT), in which eggs are retrieved, but then eggs and sperm are deposited directly into the fallopian tubes. Thus, fertilization occurs within the woman, not in a laboratory. All eggs are deposited, with none left to be available for cryopreservation or destruction.

CHAPTER 11

1. Based on Table 11.4, a fetus between 13 to 16 weeks can weigh 60 to 200 g.

2. Using the typical obstetrical standard of 40 weeks, the pregnancy embryologically would be at 10 weeks' gestation. This would be the fetal period of development.

3. Down syndrome is a *trisomy,* a common form of aneuploidy, which is characterized by the addition or deletion of one or more (but fewer than 23) chromosomes. Down syndrome involves trisomy of chromosome 21.

4. A genogram would provide additional information about the family members with the chronic conditions of concern. The health care provider could then better understand how close these relatives are to the client to better evaluate the risks. The client also mentions a distant cousin with a problem, which may need more investigation.

CHAPTER 12

1. Pregnant teens face numerous challenges. Nurses working with them need to assess physical and psychosocial status. Adolescents need adequate nutrition, sleep, and rest to promote growth and development. Needs for nutrition, sleep, and rest also increase during pregnancy. Thus, dietary intake and activity/rest patterns would be key areas of concern. In addition, adolescents are striving for identity and a sense of independence. Pregnancy, however, causes changes in identity and compounds a client's need for outside support. The nurse should examine the teen's current living situation and the physical, psychological, and social support available from family, the father of the child and possibly his family, friends, and the community.

2. Striae gravidarum indicate small ruptures in the skin's connective layer. These marks appear with each pregnancy; although they may fade, they never disappear completely. Because Millie has been pregnant twice before, she most likely would have stretch marks. As her current pregnancy progresses, she probably will develop more striae gravidarum.

3. By 12 weeks' gestation, the client most likely would have a softened cervix (Goodell sign); a dark violet colouration of her cervix, vagina, and vulva (Chadwick sign); and a softened lower part of the uterus (Hegar sign). In addition, uterine enlargement will probably be noticeable, because Millie is a multigravida. The fundus should be palpable just above the symphysis pubis. Lastly, her serum hCG level should be elevated.

4. According to the information originally presented, this is Millie's third pregnancy and both of her children were born at term. Therefore, her history of past pregnancies would be 3–2–0–0–2. According to the changed history, she had a spontaneous abortion and a living child born prematurely. Therefore, this past pregnancy history would be documented as 4–1–1–1–2.

CHAPTER 13

1. Because Lindsey has an active 2-year-old, child care could be a source of stress. If Lindsey works outside the home, the family's financial situation could be compromised. Lindsey, too, may experience increased anxiety over the fetus. She may feel isolated or that she is missing out on normal activities. All these elements can alter family dynamics and relationships.

2. Keyla has a family history of diabetes, most likely type 2. She also belongs to an ethnic group that is considered at high risk for the disease. It is recommended that she would have been screened during the first trimester of her pregnancy.

3. The nurse needs to explain the differences between gestational and type 2 diabetes and how treatment plans are individualized for each client. He or she should review the effects of pregnancy on glucose control and the need to closely monitor glucose levels to ensure healthy maternal and fetal outcomes.

4. Lindsey has two main risk factors: multiparity and hypertension in previous pregnancies.

5. Risks include abruptio placentae, acute renal failure, pulmonary edema, cerebral hemorrhage, preeclampsia, eclampsia, and intrauterine growth restriction.

CHAPTER 14

1. Monique needs information about the labour process and measures used to control labour pain. She and her husband need to understand the different approaches to labour and birth that are available, so that they can make an informed decision that best meets their preferences.

2. Shelley and Joel might want to consider a number of questions when evaluating information found on the web for reliability and credibility including: is the author of the material qualified to provide the information; what is the purpose of the document/information; how current is the information/is the information updated regularly; is the information factual or opinion/biased; and are references and other sources that have been used cited?

3. The nurse should first explore with Monique the stories that she has been hearing about labour and her understanding of them. This will provide the nurse with baseline information and will provide the opportunity to correct any misconceptions or provide additional information. In addition, the nurse would provide information about both non-pharmacologic and pharmacologic pain relief measures, including information about risks and benefits to assist Monique and Joel with decision making. The nurse would provide support for any decisions made, even if they might not be consistent with decisions he/she might make for themselves.

4. Monique's consideration of epidural analgesia reflects the current trend to medicated birth and the increased use of epidural anaesthesia to cope with labour pain.

CHAPTER 15

1. Tyrese reports increased urination and decreased abdominal tightness, both of which suggest that lightening has occurred. She mentions a backache, which may be from mild and early uterine contractions, pressure on the sacroiliac joint from the effects of relaxin, or both. The nurse needs to further assess these symptoms. First, he or she should explore if Tyrese has any burning or pain with the urinary frequency to rule out a possible urinary tract infection. Also, the nurse should measure fundal height to determine if lightening has indeed occurred. He or she should inspect Tyrese's abdomen for any change in shape, which would indicate that the uterus has moved forward. The nurse should ask for details about the backache, including frequency, duration, intensity, and accompanying symptoms. A backache that fluctuates regularly, increases in intensity, or is accompanied by pelvic pressure or cramping is sug-

gestive of labour. Other assessments would include evaluation for cervical dilatation and effacement.

2. Cervical dilatation = 1; cervical effacement = 1; station = 1; cervical consistency = 2; cervical position = 1. The total score would be 6.

3. Labour tends to be prolonged when the fetus is in the occiput posterior position. The mother usually has increased back pain, primarily because the fetal head is usually not well flexed. The nurse would need to assess for back pain and have the client rate her pain, using this information to institute measures of comfort.

4. Increased stress could affect the progress of labour. Worry can increase anxiety, possibly compounding pain perception and leading to a need for additional relief measures.

5. The FHR pattern described is suggestive of variable decelerations, which usually are associated with compression of the umbilical cord. The nurse should immediately change Yolanda's position and then reassess the FHR to determine if the position change corrected the problem. The nurse may need to change the client's position again and reassess to ensure that the pattern has returned to baseline.

6. Because Yolanda reports moderate contractions with a frequency of every 7 to 8 minutes and a duration of approximately 45 to 60 seconds, she is most likely in the active phase of the first stage of labour.

7. The nurse should expect the contractions to increase in intensity, frequency, and duration. The client most likely will begin to indicate she is experiencing rectal pressure and the need to push or bear down once cervical dilation is completed.

CHAPTER 16

1. This is Carlotta's first pregnancy, so she may be anxious, uncertain, or fearful about the unknown. In addition, she expresses that she is tired and has concerns about pain and hoping that she will not need an epidural. Her postterm status may be another source of stress. Her boyfriend's presence can be helpful. Depending on how labour progresses, both of them may need additional support.

2. Frequent maternal position changes (eg, getting on the hands and knees, side-lying, sitting, walking, using a birthing ball) may help open the pelvis further to promote fetal turning. Throughout, team members must provide pain-relief measures and support so that Beverly changes positions safely and without discomfort.

3. Carlotta is postterm, with subsequent increased risks for fetal morbidity and mortality. Examples include

inadequate fetal nutrition and oxygenation secondary to decreased placental function and increased risk for meconium staining (and aspiration).

4. This Bishop's score is 9, which indicates a cervix favourable and suitable for induction. A score of 8 or more indicates an increased likelihood that labour will begin soon on its own.

5. Carlotta is to receive 2 mU/ minute; in 1 hour (60 minutes) she would receive 120 mU. There are 10 mU in 1 mL, so 120 mU would be present in 12 mL.

CHAPTER 17

1. Marnie's contractions reflect the latent phase of the first stage of labour. Her cervix most likely is beginning to dilate, and effacement is starting. As she moves to the active phase of the first stage, contraction frequency and intensity will increase significantly. Marnie probably will experience more pain from these contractions. At the transition phase, contractions will peak in intensity, occur frequently, and last longer. The intensity of the pain associated with contractions may lead to increased anxiety, irritability, and feelings of loss of control, possibly compounding her pain level.

2. Contributing factors would include the extent of pain with each previous labour, the duration of these prior experiences, the speed and effectiveness of actions to control past pain, measures used for relief, support from others (eg, staff, husband, family), coping methods used and their effectiveness, cultural background and beliefs about labour pain, and any concomitant stressors.

3. Promethazine causes drowsiness and sedation for 2 to 8 hours; it has been 3 hours since it was administered. Thus, ambulation might place Felicia at risk for injury. The nurse should ask whether Felicia is experiencing any drowsiness or sedation. In addition, he or she should check Felicia's vital signs. If Felicia's condition is stable, the nurse might place the head of the bed upright to see how the client tolerates the position change. Next, the nurse might have Felicia dangle her legs at the side of the bed. If Felicia remains stable, then the nurse might try ambulating with her to the bathroom, staying with her at all times to prevent injury.

4. The nurse should explain that it may take 2 to 3 days for Marnie to excrete 95% of the meperidine. Breastfeeding women may have residual amounts of this drug in their breast milk up to 56 hours after administration of a 50-mg dose. The meperidine in the woman's system can be transferred to the newborn through the breast milk. Because the newborn liver is immature and cannot readily metabolize the medication, the baby who has received meperidine in this manner tends to exhibit problems with latching on and sleepiness.

5. The FACES pain rating scale probably would be best. Marnie could easily point to the face depicting her pain level, thus avoiding any miscommunication because of a language barrier.

6. Key measures to treat postdural headache involve hydration. The nurse should encourage Felicia to increase intake of water and caffeinated beverages. An IV infusion of lactated Ringer solution at 150 cc/ hour may help replace the lost cerebrospinal fluid. The nurse should encourage consumption of caffeine, because it causes cerebral vasoconstriction. The client should be placed on bed rest. Analgesics may be beneficial, but this measure is not always effective. If none of these measures are effective, an epidural blood patch may be necessary.

CHAPTER 18

1. Nadia's estrogen and progesterone levels should decrease dramatically. Subsequently, her prolactin level should be greatly increased, which would allow her to produce milk for nursing.

2. Jody is being seen on her sixth postpartum day. Using the rule that uterine involution progresses 1 cm each day, the nurse would expect to palpate the fundus approximately 6 cm below the umbilicus. In addition, Jody should have lochia serosa (pale pink colour).

3. The nurse should teach Chelsea about Nadia's physiologic and psychological changes at this time. He or she should explain what to expect for her partner, the baby, and herself. The nurse should emphasize how Chelsea can best promote Nadia's and her own adaptation to the parental role. Suggestions may focus on aiding Nadia to obtain adequate rest and sleep and ways that support people can assist both women during this transition.

4. The nurse should begin by explaining how hormonal changes help prepare the breasts for nursing. Next, he or she should reassure Jody that while her breasts have filled with milk, lack of newborn stimulation eventually will cause milk production to stop, easing discomfort. Until then, Jody can take measures to ease pain, such as wearing a supportive bra and applying cool compresses to the breasts. The nurse should remind Jody to avoid nipple and breast stimulation.

5. The most common cause of a fundus displaced from midline and above its expected position is a distended bladder. First, the nurse should palpate the

bladder for distention. Then, he or she should check whether Nadia has voided; if not, the nurse should encourage her to do so. If Nadia cannot void, she may require catheterization. If a distended bladder is not the cause, the nurse should anticipate the need for uterine massage.

CHAPTER 19

1. Factors placing Rosanna at increased risk for post-partum hemorrhage include multiparity, prolonged labour, and labour augmentation with oxytocin. In addition, she may have a distended bladder because she has not yet voided, which interferes with uterine contraction and further compounds her risk for hemorrhage.

2. This finding is highly suggestive of a distended bladder, which interferes with uterine involution. The nurse should assess the bladder for distention and initiate measures to promote voiding. If possible, he or she can help Rosanna to the bathroom to void on the toilet. Promoting the normal sitting position for urination may be all that is necessary. In addition, the nurse can employ other techniques to stimulate voiding, such as turning on the faucet so that the client hears the sound of running water, placing Rosanna's hand in a basin of warm water, and running warm water over her perineum. Also, the nurse should anticipate the need for catheterization to relieve the urinary distention.

3. The nurse needs to ask Leslie about the pattern of her fever, including times of day when it is highest. Fever associated with endometritis typically peaks in the evening and has irregular spikes. In addition, the nurse should ask what the client means about her incision being very sore. Is the site itself sore? Is the client having abdominal pain in the area of the incision? Is she experiencing tenderness when she touches the area? Abdominal pain and tenderness on palpation suggest endometritis. The nurse also should ask Leslie about vaginal drainage, including amount, colour, and, most importantly, odour. The drainage of endometritis is usually malodorous.

4. Typical signs and symptoms of an infected incision include redness, swelling, induration, and warmth. In addition, the edges of the wound may be beginning to separate. Serosanguinous or purulent drainage may be oozing from the area. Palpation of the site would reveal tenderness and potentially fluid accumulation that may drain as serosanguinous or purulent.

CHAPTER 20

1. Apgar scores of 5 at 1 minute and 6 at 5 minutes suggest that Thomas may be having some problems with the extrauterine transition. Subsequently, the nurse should continue assigning scores every 5 minutes up to 20 minutes. Depending on the newborn's status, the nurse also should anticipate the need for resuscitative measures.

2. The nurse should teach the mother to use mild non-medicated soaps for bathing the newborn. Perfumed soaps can be absorbed percutaneously; if alkaline, they can alter the pH of the newborn's skin and thus compromise its protective function.

3. William should have received both vitamin K IM and erythromycin ointment to the eyes.

4. Thomas is most likely losing heat through convection. Although he is clothed, he is lying uncovered on a bed, probably near a doorway. If the bed is near a window on the exterior wall, he might lose heat via radiation.

5. Because William's serum bilirubin level was only mildly elevated and he did not require phototherapy, he probably has physiologic jaundice and is not at risk for bilirubin-related brain damage. After discharge, his parents should watch for any increased sleepiness, decreased feeding, or decreased wet or dirty diapers which may indicate that his bilirubin levels are increasing. If his parents notice any of these symptoms, they should take him to their health care provider for further assessment

6. The nurse would approach Thomas calmly and use the bulb syringe to suction his mouth and nose to prevent aspiration. While clearing his airways, the nurse should explain to his mother what is happening and the rationale for the actions used, while at the same time reassuring her that such choking can happen normally in newborns. The nurse also needs to teach the mother how to use the bulb syringe and to help her gain confidence in her ability to care for her son. Follow-up guidance, reassurance, and support are also important.

CHAPTER 21

1. It is important to explore with Lindsay her expectations and her feelings and experiences so far with breastfeeding. In addition, the effects of the cesarean surgery and the increased demands of caring for a newborn may have left Lindsay overly tired. The nurse should investigate the support available

to Lindsay, such as from a partner or other family members. Lack of support would further compound her difficulties.

2. Breastfeeding would not be advised if Joelle had a herpes simplex virus lesion on her breast. In this case, the nurse should instruct Joelle to temporarily pump and discard breast milk until the lesion healed. Once healed, she could then resume breastfeeding.

3. At 6 weeks postpartum, Lindsay is producing mature human milk.

4. Lindsay's incision site may be contributing to discomfort with specific feeding positions. Women who have had cesarean births may find the football hold and side-lying position comfortable for nursing. The side-lying position also would allow Lindsay to rest during feedings. An alternative would be the over-the-shoulder position with the mother lying down.

5. A breastfed infant typically eats 8 to 12 times over 24 hours. The nurse should instruct Joelle to look for satiety cues, such as the infant falling off the breast, pushing the nipple from the mouth, or stopping sucking. Other indicators of successful breastfeeding include 6 to 8 wet diapers over 24 hours (by days 4 to 7 of life) and 3 to 4 stools per day (by day 3 of life).

CHAPTER 22

1. Mitchell, born at 30 weeks' gestation, would be classified as preterm. His birth weight was 1590 g; therefore, he would be classified as low birth weight (LBW). If he had been born at this weight at term, Mitchell would have been classified as small for gestational age (SGA)

2. Mitchell is LBW and thus would most likely need an endotracheal tube of 3.5 to 4 mm.

3. Because Mitchell is intubated and on a ventilator, he most likely would require enteral or parenteral nutrition. He also needs measures to assist him with nonnutritive sucking.

4. The nurse should allow Danita to express her feelings while demonstrating ongoing respect for all family members. Open and empathetic communication is essential. The nurse can point out the baby's family-related characteristics, such as Madeline having Danita's nose or eyes. In addition, the nurse should emphasize normal newborn characteristics (eg, alertness, strong grasp). In addition, the nurse should encourage Danita to touch, stroke, and hold Madeline

to facilitate closeness. Throughout interactions, the nurse plays a key role in teaching Danita and Louie about the high success rate in repair of the cleft.

5. Breastfeeding is possible when a newborn has a cleft lip because breast tissue can close off the cleft effectively. In cases of cleft palate, the ability to conduct breastfeeding depends on the degree of separation of the palate. If the palate is widely separated, breastfeeding would be difficult. In this case, the nurse would encourage Danita to pump her breasts for milk and then to feed it to Madeline through special nipples or appliances, as appropriate.

CHAPTER 23

1. The nurse could ask open-ended questions to elicit more information about the hot flashes. Asking Fran to describe her symptoms would be an appropriate way to start. Because the client states that she is experiencing hot flashes more often, the nurse needs to determine what she means specifically. For example, the nurse should ask about the frequency of episodes each week and if they occur during the day, at night, or both. Where does she first sense the hot flashes? Are there any factors that seem to precipitate them (eg, stress, alcohol consumption, spicy food intake)? What, if anything, relieves them?

2. Osteopenia refers to a decrease in optimal bone density, a part of the aging process that does not necessarily lead to osteoporosis. Osteoporosis includes both low bone mass density and deterioration of bone tissue. Carol may be at risk for fractures. The nurse can review three major areas: nutritional information for calcium intake; medication history for use of calcium supplements, prescribed or nonprescribed herbs or medications, or both, to promote bone strength; and activity and exercise patterns.

3. A diary might help Fran to identify the pattern of and precipitating factors for hot flashes. In addition, writing in a journal might increase her sense of control over the situation. If precipitating factors are obvious, then the client and nurse could develop a plan to help minimize occurrences. Diary keeping also provides an opportunity for Fran to learn about the changes in her body. Moreover, the diary can act as a means to evaluate how successful the plan is. Vasomotor symptoms are thought to be caused by decreased estrogen levels, although estrogen withdrawal alone does not entirely account for them.

4. Carol's risk factors for osteopenia and osteoporosis include Caucasian race, early age at menopause, family history of osteoporosis, and a history of smoking.

CHAPTER 24

1. The nurse should be empathetic, genuine, objective, and nonpatronizing. The client's chief concern is the elimination problem, which is a sensitive and private topic. Thus, the nurse should close the examining room door or curtain during history taking. The nurse also should not attribute the problem to the client's age without further inquiry and should use open-ended questions to gather specifics. Observing nonverbal behaviours as the client describes the problem can provide clues about her emotional status.

2. Lena, the primary caregiver, should be able to complete basic ADLs. She might need assistance in completing instrumental ADLs (eg, grocery shopping, doing household repairs), because of the time she spends caring for Hannah. Lena's ability to complete advanced ADLs probably is severely constrained, based on her statements about the time spent assisting Hannah and managing the home. Hannah needs assistance with basic ADLs, and her ability to perform instrumental ADLs and advanced ADLs would be curtailed severely because of her cognitive changes and the need for Lena to provide for her care.

3. Ann reports urine leakage when she coughs or sneezes, which suggests stress incontinence. She also reports needing to rush to the bathroom, suggesting urge incontinence. Therefore, the nurse should suspect mixed incontinence.

4. Cholinesterase inhibitors are appropriate for clients with moderate to severe Alzheimer disease, such as Hannah. In addition, the nurse should determine the onset of Hannah's Alzheimer disease, because these drugs are most effective when started early.

5. Studies have not shown use of *Ginkgo biloba* as effective for mild to moderate Alzheimer disease. Therefore, the nurse would caution Lena against its use for Hannah.

Answers and Rationales for End-of-Chapter Review Questions

CHAPTER 1

No review questions

CHAPTER 2

1. **B.** Studies show that women are more likely to exercise consistently if they do so with a companion. Clients can become discouraged with exercise if they focus on long-term goals, because results can be slow. Ideally, people should vary aerobic, flexibility, and weight-bearing exercises.

2. **D.** Clients are most likely to continue exercises that reflect their preferences. Metabolic rate and nutrient intake would not form the basis for a program. The client may not want to change her appearance.

3. **A.** Regular alcohol consumption can decrease bone density, which may lead to osteoporosis. Protein is not a prevention or management strategy for osteoporosis, nor is how the client divides exercise. Weight-bearing exercise helps prevent osteoporosis.

4. **D.** Of the items presented, fresh orange juice has the most calcium.

5. **C.** Menopause decreases risk for iron-deficiency anemia, which is a natural potential complication of the monthly blood loss of menstruation. The other clients are still menstruating.

6. **C.** Diabetes can alter normal vaginal pH and flora, creating an environment favourable to yeast overgrowth. Osteoporosis, lactation, and postpartum status are not common risk factors for yeast infection.

7. **C.** Ideally, the first Pap smear is performed before a woman is sexually active. Regularly participating in low-impact aerobic exercise, consuming calcium daily, and consistently performing monthly breast self-examinations are correct health-promotion strategies.

8. **D.** HPV is the most frequent virus linked to cervical cancer.

9. **A.** Research has shown no link between oral contraceptives and cervical cancer. Identified risk factors for cervical cancer include early sexual intercourse, multiple partners, and smoking.

CHAPTER 3

1. **D.** Women of normal prepregnancy weight should gain 11.5 to 16 kg over three trimesters. Gaining 7.3 kg per trimester is more than recommended, while 6.8 to 9 kg in total is insufficient. The client should consume foods she enjoys as part of a healthy, balanced pregnancy diet.

2. **A.** Folic acid supplementation can help prevent neural tube defects if maternal stores are adequate before the client conceives. Supplementation needs

to be ongoing. Adequacy of stores of folic acid is not related to the menstrual cycle. Waiting until the client has missed a period or pregnancy has been confirmed is too late to initiate preventive supplementation.

3. **B.** *Eating Well with Canada's Food Guide* is a source for suggesting selections from various food groups to help design a balanced diet. It is not a retrospective tool for analysis of actual food consumption.

4. **A.** Frequent nursing can stimulate the milk supply. Supplemental feedings may confuse the baby, disrupting breastfeeding. Switching to formula feeding should not be the first strategy if the woman wants to continue nursing. Caffeinated beverages can interfere with milk production.

5. **B & C.** Potatoes and watermelon are high-glycemic-index foods. Seven-grain bread and lentils are high in fibre, thus have a low glycemic index.

6. **C.** Clients trying to control total cholesterol level should consume no more than 30% of total daily calories from fat.

7. **A**

8. **D.** This client is postmenopausal and no longer losing iron during monthly menstruation.

9. **A.** Vegan diets may be low in nutrients found in meat: B_{12}, iron, and zinc.

10. A. The recommended adequate intake of calcium during pregnancy is 1,000 mg/day.

11. D. Vitamin C is lacking in people who smoke.

CHAPTER 4

1. **D.** Although joint pain is common with systemic lupus erythematosus, inflammation and swelling of multiple joints are more common with rheumatoid arthritis. With systemic lupus erythematosus, a butterfly-shaped facial rash is common. Diagnostic tests may show an abnormal C-reactive protein level, an elevated erythrocyte sedimentation rate, and a positive antinuclear antibody titer.

2. **C.** Chlamydia can reside in the cervix for many years, damaging the fallopian tubes. Resulting pelvic inflammatory disease may cause fertility problems. Although early mild symptoms may include purulent vaginal discharge with urination, the infection often is asymptomatic. Painless ulcer formation suggests syphilis. Chlamydia is not treated with penicillin.

3. **D.** A T-4 cell count at or below 200/mm^3 indicates AIDS.

4. **D.** Genital herpes is caused by a virus; thus, an antiviral agent such as acyclovir (Zovirax) would be the most likely treatment. Azithromycin, ofloxacin, and metronidazole are commonly used medications for bacterial STIs.

5. **B.** Knowing one's breasts is important to identify any early changes that might occur. Most women diagnosed with breast cancer first identify a change in their breast on their own. More women die from lung cancer than breast cancer each year. Many who develop breast cancer have no risk factors other than aging. Risks are increased for women older than 60 years.

6. **A.** Numbness or tingling on the chest wall and inner arm is normal for up to 1 year after surgery; it does not need to be reported. Clients should not carry or lift anything more than 7.5 kg. Blood pressure measurements, infusions, and injections are contraindicated in the involved arm. Sleeping on or wearing tight garments around the affected arm could impair circulation.

7. **B.** The client is seeking information; therefore, explaining the underlying hormonal contribution is most appropriate. Telling her that she probably has an infection is incorrect and nontherapeutic. Advising her that menstrual cramps are normal and asking if she needs a prescription are inappropriate, because these responses ignore the client's need for information.

8. **D.** Abnormal vaginal bleeding and frequent vaginal bleeding are common symptoms of leiomyomas. High fever and pain on cervical movement suggest pelvic inflammatory disease. Dysmenorrhea and irregular vaginal bleeding are common with endometriosis. Abnormal bleeding in menopause with pelvic pain suggests endometrial cancer.

9. **A.** Routine Pap testing is the best method for detecting cervical dysplasia and preventing cancer. CA-125 testing is used to screen for ovarian cancer. Condoms are preventive against STIs. Perineal hygiene is important for health, but does not prevent against cervical dysplasia.

10. **C.** Antibiotics are prescribed for 7 to 10 days to treat cystitis. The client should complete the entire prescription to fully eradicate the bacteria. Urinating after intercourse helps reduce the risk of infection. Recurrences need prompt and thorough treatment to prevent upper UTIs. Cranberry juice has been found to decrease recurrent UTIs, especially in older women.

CHAPTER 5

1. **C.** While exercise can help with stress management, the duration the client suggests may be ineffective. The other measures may assist with stress management.

2. **B.** The first step is to make sure that the client recognizes she is being abused. Only after the client has expressed awareness of the abuse can the nurse assist her with escape, new housing, and documentation of injuries for future litigation.

3. **C.** The client needs to admit her problem and develop a realistic body image. Until then, other interventions will be largely ineffective.

4. **A.** Psychoactive drugs treat mental illness, but may have teratogenic effects, depending on their levels of risk. They act not only on target sites, but on other parts of the body. While these drugs are effective, many are considered unsafe or potentially unsafe in pregnancy.

5. **C.** The client's stoic behaviours reflect an effort to regain control. Her response may be normal for her and not necessarily indicative of another problem. Whether she is handling the situation well and whether she is concerned about her physical injuries are subjective issues.

6. **B.** The nurse should ensure that he or she understands the client's specific issue by restating it in similar words. The client is not focusing on health insurance or other life changes. Giving opinions about how the client has managed money is a value judgement, which is not therapeutic.

7. **C.** Any suggestive statements need further exploration about potential for suicide so that the nurse can take action to protect the client's safety. The family's feelings are secondary, as is the client's career. How long the client has felt this way is less important than protecting safety.

8. **C.** Ongoing fatigue is a primary symptom of postpartum depression.

9. **C.** Neglect of hygiene is an indicator of depression. Cleanliness and attention to dress may indicate that the client's mood is improving. While a strong social support network is helpful, it will not directly reflect effectiveness of interventions unless there is evidence that the client is interacting with members of this group regularly. Healthy eating and regularly exercising are good health promotion activities, but usually are not direct indicators of a client's mood.

10. **A.** The most important aspect of care for the client with schizophrenia is ensuring that she takes her medications and receives ongoing treatment to monitor for relapses. Relying on the client's reports about voices and powers may be problematic if the client is neglecting her treatment plan. Many clients with schizophrenia have difficulty functioning adequately for long enough to sustain employment or to participate in the community.

CHAPTER 6

1. **D.** Many parents confuse sexual orientation with gender identity. They may question whether small children who adopt behaviours associated with the opposite sex are homosexual.

2. **B.** Children of preschool age commonly adopt behaviours of the opposite sex without the activity being related to sexual orientation or preferences.

3. **A**

4. **C.** Menopause is the absence of menstrual cycles for 12 months or more. Nevertheless, Mary may still become pregnant if she has continued to ovulate.

5. **C.** Short stature is commonly associated with premature testosterone production and secretion.

6. **A.** Several medications can lead to problems with erectile function. While understanding the partner's view of the problem may be necessary, the first step should be pinpointing the cause of the problem. Exercise and sexual practices should not have an influence on erectility.

7. **B.** Teens need to know how to protect themselves against STIs. Providing birth control to a teen who does not want to engage in sexual activity might lead to confusion. Many homosexuals are aware of their orientation before adolescence. Forcing children to discuss sexual issues can lead to communication problems.

CHAPTER 7

1. **B**

2. **C**

3. **A.** Family processes focus on roles and decision making. Illnesses, discipline, and recreation are tied to family functions.

4. **B.** Open discussion of problems reflects healthy family communication. Third-party interpretations, refusing to share internal views, and discrepancies

between words and feelings are signs of dysfunctional communication.

5. **D.** Closed adoption means that no contact occurs between birth and adoptive parents. Rights and circumstances in open adoptions vary. Children in closed adoptions sometimes learn about their biologic parents later in life. Parental satisfaction with adoption is not solely tied to type.

6. **D**

CHAPTER 8

1. **B.** Combined oral contraceptives affect the clotting mechanism, thereby increasing the risk of thromboembolic events. Fibrocystic breast changes and irritable bowel syndrome are not contraindications. Smokers older than 35 years should not use combined oral contraceptives because of their increased risk of myocardial infarction.

2. **D**

3. **D**

4. **B.** A reservoir should remain at the tip of the condom to collect ejaculate. The man should put on the condom as soon as the penis is erect, because some fluid may leak before ejaculation. He should remove the condom carefully while the penis remains erect to avoid spilling the contents. A new condom for each sexual act prevents breakage/leakage.

5. **A.** Studies have found that repeated and high doses of the spermicide nonoxynol-9 have been associated with increased risk of vaginal lesions, which may increase the risk of acquiring HIV infection an increased risk of HIV transmission.

6. **C.** Combined oral contraceptives will not prevent STIs.

7. **A**

8. **A.** Methods that contain estrogen, such as combined oral contraceptives, the vaginal contraceptive ring, and the contraceptive patch, are not suggested for breastfeeding women.

9. **B.** Use of a diaphragm during menstruation may increase risk of toxic shock syndrome. The woman should leave the diaphragm in place for 6 to 8 hours after intercourse. With repeated acts of intercourse, the client should leave the diaphragm in place and insert more spermicide into the vagina. The woman should replace her diaphragm every 2 years or if the device is leaking.

10. **B**

CHAPTER 9

1. **C.** Nurses should not share personal beliefs with clients, even when asked, because doing so may influence a client's independent decision making. Many nurses who believe abortion is unacceptable work successfully in women's health.

2. **C**

3. **A.** The nurse should first identify his or her own beliefs and biases about abortion. Nurses are obligated to discuss with clients the full range of options available to them with respectful attitudes for all possibilities. Nurses should never imply or make it evident that they find one option more acceptable than another. In addition, the nurse must ensure that the client has the necessary information to make an independent decision.

4. **C.** Vacuum aspiration involves administration of a local anaesthetic followed by insertion into the cervix of a thin plastic catheter attached to a suction or syringe for evacuation of the contents.

5. **C.** Discharge teaching should include information about notifying the health care provider if elevated temperature, excessive cramping or tenderness, or excessive bleeding develops. Other teaching should cover avoiding the use of tampons and sexual activity while she is actively bleeding, expecting bleeding similar to that of a heavy menstrual period, and expecting menses to resume 4 to 6 weeks after the procedure. Strong narcotic analgesics should not be necessary.

6. **D.** The client should receive anti-D immune globulin to prevent Rh isoimmunization.

CHAPTER 10

1. **D.** Infertility evaluations begin with a normal health assessment and progress in invasiveness, as necessary. The other methods come after a health history and physical examination.

2. **D.** Some cases of infertility cannot be explained through testing. While testing can be stressful, it is more important for the nurse to ensure that clients understand they may not receive answers. Encouraging clients to continue with testing is inappropriate. While review of each test is helpful, this is not the best response.

3. **B.** Ferning is the only response that indicates ovulation.

4. **B.** Men should deliver the ejaculate to the laboratory within a specified time. The container does not

need to be sterile. It should be kept at body temperature. The client does not need to avoid ejaculating for 3 days prior to providing a specimen.

5. **B.** Clients who are trying to conceive should expect ovulation once their basal body temperature begins to rise after being at its lowest point within that cycle.

6. **B.** Studies have not shown a link between previous induced abortions and infertility. The client does not mention a history of spontaneous abortion. No evidence supports the idea of infertility being linked to guilt or remorse about past events.

7. **C.** Cigarette smoking has been liked with impaired fertility.

8. **A.** Impaired fecundity is the term used when a woman can become pregnant but cannot continue the gestation to a point of viability.

9. **A.** Of the options listed, obesity is a potential risk factor for infertility.

10. **B.** Infertility medications are taken by women, not men.

CHAPTER 11

1. **D.** Through physical examination, the health care provider would be able to identify the client's exhibited characteristics. Genogram, chromosome analysis, and DNA analysis all would focus on "hidden" genetic or molecular components of the person's makeup.

2. **C**

3. **B**

4. **C**

5. **A.** Finding out if chromosomal abnormalities contributed to previous pregnancy losses is the first step in determining the client's risk for recurrent miscarriage.

6. **A.** False-positive quad screening results are most commonly related to misdated pregnancies.

7. **C.** Caucasians are at increased risk for cystic fibrosis. A client without a family history of this problem could still be a carrier. Preventive care would involve screening for carrier status.

8. **C**

9. **C.** There is a small risk of pregnancy loss associated with amniocentesis. There may be some discomfort associated with the amniocentesis. Women

need to have an empty bladder during the test to decrease the risk of accidental injury to the bladder. The amniocentesis is conducted concurrently with ultrasound which is used to guide insertion of the needle and decrease contact with fetal parts, umbilical cord, and placenta.

10. **B.** Of these options, reviewing the screening tests performed is the most important.

CHAPTER 12

1. **B.** Women older than 35 years tend to be aware of their increased risk for miscarriage and often express related concerns. Nothing in the information presented suggests that the client fears the unknown, may not want to be pregnant, or is experiencing changes in her mental health.

2. **B.** The nurse should review with each client aspects of culture and religion of importance to the client. Some people do not follow all the traditions of their culture or faith. An interpreter would be needed only if the client does not understand English. Although the client is Muslim, she may not observe Friday as a religious day. Nothing indicates that additional time is needed.

3. **B.** Urinary frequency usually occurs in the first and third trimesters, when the uterus and fetal head (once lightening occurs) put pressure on the bladder. Urinary frequency at other times may indicate infection, which may predispose the client to pyelonephritis and preterm labour. Nasal stuffiness is a normal finding, resulting from elevated estrogen levels. Tingling in the breasts is normal as they enlarge and vascularity increases. Darkened spots on the nose and cheeks result from increased circulating hormones. Such spots usually fade after childbirth.

4. **D.** Ultrasound can detect movement of the fetal heart as early as the seventh week. This positive sign of pregnancy has no other possible cause. The woman will not be able to feel the fetus move until 18 to 20 weeks' gestation, which will delay the reassurance she seems to need now. Until a positive sign is confirmed, no evidence proves definitely that she is pregnant. A positive result on a pregnancy test may be caused by reasons other than pregnancy.

5. **C.** G is the client's total pregnancies, including the current one; (4) T is the number of term births at 37 or more weeks' gestation; (1) P is the number of preterm births after 20 weeks', but before 37 weeks' gestation; (1) A is the number of pregnancies that ended in spontaneous or therapeutic abortion; (1) L is the number of children currently alive (3).

6. C. Naegele's rule begins with the first day of the last normal period, subtracts 3 months (September 2), and adds 7 days (September 9). The EDD is September 9.

7. A. Low heels will assist with varicose veins. The client should not massage the area. Pregnant women should not indiscriminately increase exercise. Varicose veins may not disappear after birth.

8. A. While these symptoms are normal for the stage of pregnancy, the nurse should investigate each to ensure that they are not the result of other, more serious, causes.

9. B. Emptying a cat's litter box predisposes a pregnant woman to toxoplasmosis, which can lead to spontaneous abortion if contracted in the first trimester or to congenital infection in the newborn if contracted in the last trimester. There is no problem with close contact with dogs or cats; the only precaution is avoidance of changing the cat's litter box.

10. A. These findings would result in a score of 10 on the biophysical profile, indicating a healthy fetus. The fetus has demonstrated activity by stretching, flexing arms and legs, and moving. Nothing indicates sleep, need for immediate birth, or fetal compromise.

CHAPTER 13

1. C. The risk of asthma exacerbation during pregnancy is related directly to asthma severity. The most common exacerbation period in pregnancy is from gestational weeks 24 to 36.

2. A. Women with chronic hemolytic anemia may appear jaundiced from hemolysis of RBCs. They may suffer from gallstones (cholelithiasis) and splenomegaly. Severe bone pain is associated with acute sickle cell crisis.

3. D. During labour, the pregnant woman with HIV may receive antibiotic therapy at least 4 hours before birth to protect the fetus/newborn. Intravenous retroviral therapy also may be used. Procedures such as rupturing the membranes and using internal electronic fetal monitoring are avoided to reduce the risk of vertical transmission. Cesarean birth is under investigation as a way to decrease perinatal HIV transmission.

4. B. Hypotonia is associated with congenital rubella syndrome. Fetal effects of parvovirus include anemia, fetal non-immune hydrops, and fetal death in the second or third trimester.

5. A. The woman is describing common findings associated with pyelonephritis. The temperature typically spikes and then returns to normal or even progresses to hypothermia. Acute renal failure is manifested by signs and symptoms such as fluid imbalances, changes in vital signs, malaise, irritation, and disorientation. Gestational hypertension is indicated by blood pressure greater than or equal to 140/90 mm Hg or diastolic pressure greater than or equal to 90 mm Hg with or without proteinuria. Hypoglycemia would be indicated by decreased blood glucose levels, hunger, weakness, dizziness, confusion, headache, diaphoresis, and irritability.

6. C. Self-monitoring of blood glucose typically involves testing a blood sample, obtained by fingerstick, with a glucose meter. Usually, the pregnant client needs to monitor her blood glucose level four times a day (prandial and preprandial) and record the results on a written log to allow for easy tracking of patterns. Testing is not limited to one sample a day before breakfast. Eating a light snack or administering insulin before testing would interfere with test accuracy.

7. C. Although the nurse might refer the client to a local shelter or give her information about such resources, this action is the least important.

8. D. Oral fluid intake would not be allowed until the client has not vomited for 48 hours.

9. B. Often the first indication of magnesium toxicity is absence of deep tendon reflexes, such as the knee-jerk reflex. Muscle weakness is a possible side effect of magnesium therapy, whereas flaccid paralysis occurs with toxicity. Seizures suggest eclampsia. A respiratory rate of 18 bpm is within normal parameters.

10. D. A complete molar pregnancy is a form of gestational trophoblastic disease, in which trophoblastic villi abnormally proliferate and degenerate. Although gestational tissue is found, the pregnancy is not viable. The statement about an umbilical cord indicates that the client needs more teaching about gestational trophoblastic disease. Complete molar pregnancy increases the risk for choriocarcinoma, a dangerous and rapidly spreading malignancy. After dilatation and curettage for gestational trophoblastic disease, the client must undergo follow-up testing of her hCG levels for 1 year to evaluate for malignancy. Because of the cancer risk, the client must be careful to avoid pregnancy for 1 year after gestational trophoblastic disease.

CHAPTER 14

1. **A.** Respect in birth is a major benchmark for the mother's satisfaction and ability to move past the experience and provide for her newborn. Use of nonpharmacologic pain-relief methods, extent of childbirth education, and past experiences with pain all influence who controls the decision about how a woman gives birth.

2. **D.** Information on the prevention of birth defects would not be included in a class that focused on preparation for birth, labour and birth. It would be appropriate to include stages of labour, breathing exercises, and pain control techniques.

3. **C.** The self help movement arose from second wave feminism. Women learned about childbirth by careful observation and attending births until physicians assumed significant control over information as births moved into hospitals. Lactation consultants are a more recent phenomenon.

4. **B.** Psychoprophylaxis emphasizes strategies such as controlled breathing, abdominal stroking, and pressure application to prevent pain rather than the use of chemicals to remove it. The Dick-Read method focuses on breaking the fear–tension–pain cycle by creating healthy bodies and attitudes able to deal with the strong physical sensations of labour and birth.

5. **D.** Reassuring her that she does not need the information does not address her needs. It is important to take advantage of any opportunity to provide informal education. Information can be provided over the telephone or during prenatal visits with the health care provider.

6. **C.** Mindfulness approaches to childbirth preparation incorporate ways of being present during birth. Whether walking, swaying, chanting, or rubbing their bellies, women have sought and often found ways of being present or mindful of their experience of labour and what they need for comfort.

7. **B.** A doula provides continuous support to the woman before, during, and after childbirth.

8. **D.** Nurses assist childbearing women today by recommending reliable sources of information.

9. **D.** To promote health literacy for childbearing is the best description of the purpose of perinatal education today.

10. **C.** Health literacy does not include the ability to navigate the health care system.

CHAPTER 15

1. **B.** The pelvis or buttocks of the fetus lying over the pelvic inlet indicates this as the presenting part and would be documented as a breech presentation. With a cephalic presentation, the head is the presenting part; a shoulder presentation indicates that the shoulder is the presenting part. Transverse refers to fetal lie.

2. **A.** A presenting part that has descended to a level at or past the pelvic inlet is said to be engaged. Floating indicates that the presenting part has not yet entered the true pelvis. A −1 station indicates that the presenting part is 1 cm above the ischial spines. Crowning refers to the appearance of the fetal head at the perineum.

3. **D.** The most effective way to assess the intensity of contractions is to palpate the uterine fundus for tightening. Auscultating with a Doppler ultrasound would provide information about fetal heart rate. Although observing the client's facial expression and asking her to rate intensity would help determine her pain, this information would not be as effective as actual palpation.

4. **B.** Duration is the time from the beginning to the end of a single contraction. Frequency is the time from the beginning of one contraction to the beginning of the next contraction. Acme refers to the peak of a contraction. Intensity refers to the strength of the contraction.

5. **D.** After spontaneous rupture of membranes, umbilical cord prolapse is possible, so the nurse should first assess FHR for any changes that may indicate fetal distress because of a cord prolapse. If FHR remains stable, then the nurse should test the fluid with Nitrazine paper to assess if the leakage was indeed amniotic fluid. The nurse should then assist with cleaning the perineum and notify the primary care provider.

6. **B.** Before auscultating FHR, the nurse first determines the location of the fetal back, where the strongest heart sounds are transmitted. Because the fetal back is toward the mother's left side and the fetus is vertex, auscultation should begin in the left lower quadrant.

7. **A.** An FHR that slows during the peak of a contraction and then returns to baseline indicates an early deceleration. It is considered a normal physiologic response. Uteroplacental insufficiency and uterine hyperstimulation would lead to late decelerations, in which the FHR would decrease after the peak of a contraction and end after the contraction. Umbilical cord compression would be demonstrated by variable decelerations.

8. B. A doula is a professionally trained supportive companion who focuses on supporting the labouring woman through each contraction. The doula's focus is the client, not the primary care provider or partner. The doula may provide information to assist the woman in making decisions or support the woman's choices, but does not make decisions for her.

9. A. The characteristics presented are found with the latent phase of the first stage of labour. During the transition phase, cervical dilatation and effacement are complete, with relatively strong contractions and beginning urges to bear down. The second stage is characterized by the strong urge to push as the fetus moves through the birth canal, perineal bulging, and ultimately birth. The third stage involves separation and expulsion of the placenta.

10. C. An episiotomy is a surgical incision of the perineum to enlarge the outlet. An amniotomy is artificial rupturing of the membranes. Labour augmentation involves the use of medication to enhance contractions. Effacement refers to the thinning of the cervical tissue.

CHAPTER 16

1. D. Oxytocin would likely be contraindicated because it could further exacerbate hypertonic uterine contractions, interfering with fetal oxygenation. Intravenous fluid therapy is appropriate to maintain hydration and electrolyte balance. Intramuscular morphine may be used to inhibit the uncoordinated contraction pattern. A short-acting barbiturate may be ordered to promote rest.

2. C. Both before and after ECV, the client should undergo a nonstress test to evaluate fetal well-being. An ultrasound may be used before ECV to determine adequate amniotic fluid volume, which would increase the chances of success with ECV. An emergency cesarean birth may be done instead of or in addition to ECV, if fetal or maternal distress or complications occur during the procedure. The McRobert maneuver is used for shoulder dystocia.

3. A. The woman whose fetus is in the OP position typically has back pain with contractions. She may describe her labour primarily as back pain. Fetal heart sounds may be auscultated at the umbilicus or laterally, rather than in the lower abdominal quadrants. Palpating the fetal back may be difficult with OP positioning. In a breech presentation, the buttocks are the presenting part.

4. B. Tocolytic therapy is generally used when preterm labour has been definitively diagnosed, gestational age is greater than 20 weeks but less than 36 weeks, fetal weight is estimated as less than 2,500 g, and the fetal lung profile shows signs of immaturity. Preterm labour is diagnosed with regular uterine contractions and rupture of membranes.

5. D. The Bishop scoring method assigns a score of 0 to 2 for each of five factors: cervical dilation, cervical length, station, consistency, and position. A total of 8 or more indicates a cervix suitable for induction, which increases the likelihood of a successful vaginal birth.

6. A. A battledore placenta is not considered clinically significant. In velamentous placenta, the umbilical vessels course unprotected for long distances through the membranes to insert into the placental margin. If they pass over the internal cervical os, they are at risk for compression by the presenting fetal part. This type also is at risk for tearing when the membranes rupture. In circumvallate placenta, the membranes fold back on the fetal surface of the placenta, exposing part of the umbilical cord. Such exposure increases the risk of hemorrhage both before and after birth. In succenturiate placenta, one or more small accessory lobes develop in the membranes at a distance from the main placenta. Connecting vessels may tear during birth or with rupture of the membranes. After placental expulsion, retention of one or more lobes in the uterus can cause maternal postpartum hemorrhage.

7. C. With umbilical cord prolapse, interventions focus on relieving pressure of the fetal presenting part on the cord. The knee-chest, Trendelenburg, or Sims lateral position is effective in achieving this.

8. B. When oxytocin is being administered, the goal is for contractions to occur every 2 to 3 minutes, lasting 45 to 60 seconds. Resting tone should not exceed 20 mm Hg; contraction intensity should not be above 60 mm Hg.

9. A. A transverse incision is made in the thinnest and least active portion of the uterus, thus minimizing blood loss. The area is easiest to repair, decreasing the chances of uterine rupture with subsequent pregnancies. Suturing occurs in two layers, which seals off the incision and helps to prevent lochia from entering the peritoneal cavity. A classic or vertical incision allows rapid access to the fetus if complications develop. It also allows for the birth of a fetus in breech presentation younger than 34 weeks. Closure requires three layers of absorbable sutures. Unfortunately, a classic incision requires cutting into the full thickness of the uterine corpus.

CHAPTER 17

1. **B.** Malignant hyperthermia is a hypermetabolic response to common inhalation anaesthetics (eg, halothane) and depolarizing muscle relaxants (eg, anectine) used with general anaesthesia.

2. **D.** Clients can receive inadvertent spinal anaesthesia during epidural insertion if the needle pierces the spinal column. The hole created by the needle allows spinal fluid leakage. Severe headaches can occur with initial ambulation because of the sudden shift in spinal fluid volume.

3. **C.** While all the interventions help with relaxation and pain management, giving nalbuphine and promethazine would produce the most optimal pain relief at this time. Secobarbital is usually given early in labour; however, this drug provides rest and sedation only. Nonpharmacologic methods may be inadequate to relieve pain. It is too early to administer epidural anaesthesia.

4. **A.** Somatic pain is a deeper pain associated with the later phases of the first stage and with the second stage of labour.

5. **C**

6. **C.** The client will be able to assess her own pain using a 0–10 point numeric rating scale. Unless there is a communication barrier, the Wong-Baker FACES pain scale would not be an appropriate scale.

7. **D.** The area of injection described is the epidural space outside the spinal column.

8. **B.** It can take 2 to 3 days for the body to excrete 95% of meperidine. Meperidine that remains during this time is excreted in breast milk, causing the breastfed newborn to be sleepy and have problems with latching.

9. **C.** The client is experiencing hypotension from the epidural. The most immediate response is to increase IV fluids and to give oxygen by face mask. The nurse should try to rectify the problem with increased IV fluids and oxygen therapy before calling the anaesthesiologist. Ephedrine is the last action if the others fail to rectify the problem.

CHAPTER 18

1. **A.** Although urinary overflow can be seen as frequency, the amounts voided are lesser than the 500 mL this client is voiding. Diuresis in the first week postpartum is normal. Although frequency is a symptom of a urinary tract infection, no other assessment data suggest this problem. Trauma to the pelvic muscles usually manifests as urinary retention, not frequency.

2. **D.** The fundus should be at or 2 to 3 fingerbreadths below the umbilicus during the fourth stage of labour. A fundus above the umbilicus may be the result of uterine blood clots, retained placental fragments, or a full bladder. Each condition predisposes the woman to postpartum hemorrhage. Moderate rubra at this time is normal, as is a decreased pulse rate. Abdominal pains are commonly related to breastfeeding.

3. **C.** Normal hemoglobin is 120 to 160 g/L. For several days after birth, this value fluctuates near pregnancy level and then rises. The WBC normally is elevated (25,000 to 30,000 × 10⁹/L) during the postpartum period. Normal hematocrit values are 0.37 to 0.47. Normal serum iron is 7 to 32 mmol/L.

4. **B.** Although lochia will increase if the uterus is atonic, these developments may not occur simultaneously. If the nurse cannot feel the fundus in the abdomen, it is atonic and requires massage for contraction. Oxytocin may be ordered, but administration should be a secondary action on the second day and implemented only if fundal massage does not result in uterine contraction. The second day postpartum is too early for the fundus to be so low in the abdomen.

5. **D.** Menstruation may return normally in women who are breastfeeding any time from 8 weeks to 18 months. Menstruation may return in women who do not breastfeed as early as 6 weeks. Although women who breastfeed may have menstruation return as early as 6 to 8 weeks, stating that it can be expected may cause increased anxiety if it occurs later.

6. **B.** Warm compresses facilitate vasodilation, provide comfort, and assist with the movement of blood and milk. Lanolin ointment is appropriate for painful nipples. Cool compresses facilitate vasoconstriction, which decreases milk production. Expression of milk may contribute to engorgement because the breasts produce milk in relation to demand.

7. **C.** Postpartum depression has no absolute set of symptoms; each case is unique. Bipolar disorder is more common with postpartum psychosis than with postpartum depression. Shortness of breath and sensations of smothering are associated with anxiety disorders. It is important for the safety of both mother and baby that the nurse asks questions that may be considered sensitive (eg, if she has had any thoughts of harming herself or her baby).

8. **B.** How the client became pregnant is irrelevant. Her partner is part of her family, and the nurse should include her in all aspects of care. Acting as though nothing is different about the client may lead the woman to feel that her sexual orientation is being minimized or negated. The nurse may choose to ask the woman if she wishes the nurse to tell anyone else about her sexual orientation; however, the nurse should not do so without the client's consent.

9. **C.** Implementing teaching every time the nurse is with the client is overwhelming. Postpartum women often have difficulty taking in a lot of new material. It is better to determine and to focus on essential information.

10. **B.** Women may experience difficulty voiding up to 14 hours postpartum. A full bladder can displace the fundus upward and contribute to uterine atony, which may be the cause of the increased flow. If assessment of the bladder reveals that it is not distended, then the nurse should massage the boggy uterus. The nurse can take these actions without notifying a physician. No evidence suggests clots. The nurse may administer oxytocin to stimulate uterine contraction; however, he or she should implement the other steps first.

CHAPTER 19

1. **C.** Urinary catheterization would increase risk for urinary tract infection, not endometritis. Premature rupture of membranes, prolonged labour, cesarean birth, multiple vaginal examinations, placement of intrauterine catheters or fetal scalp electrodes, and manual removal of the placenta are known risk factors that may introduce bacterial organisms into the uterine cavity.

2. **B.** Bleeding from a genital laceration typically is bright red and appears to spurt. Dark red, steady bleeding and a boggy uterus suggest uterine atony. Purulent lochia suggests uterine infection.

3. **C.** Rosanna has a full bladder that is preventing the uterus from contracting.

4. **C.** A vulvar hematoma presents as a tense fluctuant mass with ecchymosis on the vulvar area. Signs of uterine prolapse are dysmenorrhea, irregular periods, low back pain, infertility, recurrent vaginal infections, urinary incontinence, dyspareunia, varicose veins, and aching legs. Parametritis is the extension of a uterine infection into the broad ligament, manifested by prolonged fever, lateral extension of abdominal pain, rebound tenderness, and a firm tender mass in one or both adnexa. Uterine

inversion refers to dropping of the fundus into the endometrial cavity, possibly extending beyond the cervical os. Findings include a nonpalpable fundus, profuse bleeding, and obvious alterations during abdominal examination.

5. **B.** The priority is to restore circulating volume through intravenous fluid therapy, thereby helping to restore and maintain hemodynamic stability. Although late postpartum hemorrhage and intrauterine infection are highly correlated, this is not the priority. Surgical curettage is performed only when nonsurgical interventions are ineffective. Applying ice to the perineum may promote vasoconstriction to that area, but it is used only in the first 24 hours after birth.

6. **C.** The nurse can check on the progress of wound healing when she/he changes the dressing.

7. **B.** Limiting the frequency of urination can lead to urinary stasis and UTIs. Instead, the woman should empty her bladder frequently. Other behaviours to prevent UTIs include a high fluid intake to flush the bladder, good perineal hygiene, and a front-to-back wiping motion before and after voiding or bowel movements.

8. **C.** The nurse should encourage breastfeeding to ensure emptying, thereby preventing milk stasis.

9. **D.** Deep vein thrombosis is characterized by unilateral leg pain, swelling, warmth, calf tenderness on ambulation, inequality in size of the lower extremities, and enlargement and warmth of the vein over the site of the thrombus. Dyspnea, sudden chest pain, and hemoptysis are indicative of a pulmonary embolism.

10. **A.** The main medical therapy for a client with peripartum cardiomyopathy is angiotensin-converting enzyme (ACE) inhibitors. Although anticoagulant therapy may be ordered to reduce the risk of thrombotic and embolic complications, it is not the main treatment. NSAIDs are used to treat mild to moderate pain and superficial thrombophlebitis. Cephalosporin antibiotics are often used to treat mastitis.

11. **C.** This finding is most likely with postpartum depression. Hallucinations, delusions, and confusion are associated with postpartum psychosis.

CHAPTER 20

1. **C.** Blood vessels in the fetal lungs are tightly constricted; blood pressure is high (high pulmonary vascular resistance). The systemic blood pressure in the fetus is low (low systemic vascular resistance).

2. A. Gestational age, sex, muscle tone, weight, length, and head circumference are important to note, but not as essential as colour, respirations, and heart rate. Temperature is not measured in the first minute of life.

3. C. Central cyanosis denotes lack of oxygen to the tissues and necessitates supplemental oxygen. Acrocyanosis and circumoral cyanosis usually are normal in the first 24 hours of life. Jaundice is a yellowish colour to the skin or sclera, indicating excess bilirubin in the blood.

4. B. Apgar scores reflect the newborn's response to the extrauterine environment and resuscitative efforts, which are not delayed until Apgar scores are determined. Apgar scores are assigned at 1 and 5 minutes of age; if the 5-minute score is not at least 7, additional scores are assigned every 5 minutes thereafter up to 20 minutes of age. The Apgar score, particularly at 1 minute, is not sufficient evidence on which to base neurologic outcome.

5. A. These are some symptoms of hypoglycemia, although it is important to remember that some infants with hypoglycemia are asymptomatic.

6. B. Duskiness (central cyanosis) indicates lack of oxygen to the tissues. Because the baby is pink when crying (and breathing through the mouth), the nurse should suspect nasal or upper airway obstruction (the airway may be blocked when the baby quiets and closes the mouth).

7. A. These are the normal expected parameters for a newborn's initial voiding and passing of meconium.

8. A. This is the only correct answer. None of the other statements is accurate.

9. B. Infants should be placed supine for sleeping to reduce risk for SIDS.

10. A. Although signs of newborn illness can be vague, major indicators of sepsis are respiratory distress and temperature instability. Newborns manifest temperature instability more often than fever as a sign of illness; soft, frequent stools (not diarrhea) do not indicate illness in a newborn. Newborns have a reduced capacity to sweat and do not shiver, except as a late response to hypothermia. Periodic breathing is normal in the newborn. Nevus simplex is a "stork bite mark," a commonly found vascular birthmark.

CHAPTER 21

1. A. Crying is a late sign of hunger. Early cues include licking or smacking lips and sucking on fingers.

2. C. Weight loss is not obligatory for breastfeeding mothers. Breastfed babies usually gain weight at a slower rate than do bottle-fed babies. Maternal–child bonding can (and should) occur regardless of chosen feeding type.

3. B. The mother is forcing the infant to finish each bottle, which is probably causing emesis from too great a volume of feeding.

4. D. Information about what the baby eats can help the nurse to assess the adequacy of the fluid intake.

5. A. Heating a feeding under warm, running water allows for quick, even heating without the risk of hot spots that can occur with use of the microwave, or the risk of bacterial contamination by leaving the bottle out to warm at room temperature.

6. D. A woman should pump every 3 hours and once during the night. It is recommended to pump between 12 to 15 minutes each time.

7. A. A breastfed baby needs to eat 8 to 12 times in a 24-hour period.

8. B. A palpable breast lump in a lactating woman with warmth at the site likely indicates a plugged milk duct.

CHAPTER 22

1. C. A postterm newborn most likely would exhibit dry, scaly skin. Lanugo is absent; plantar creases are deep and numerous. Abundant lanugo and few plantar creases are typical findings in preterm newborns. If the newborn is very preterm, the eyelids may be fused.

2. D. Green, thick, stained amniotic fluid suggests meconium, which places the newborn at risk for meconium aspiration syndrome. Deep tracheal suctioning is indicated when the infant is not making any respiratory effort and has poor tone. It should be done before the newborn takes the first breath. All stimulation of the newborn, including drying the skin, must be delayed until the vocal cords have been visualized and deep endotracheal suctioning has been done. Other interventions, such as drying the baby, administering blow-by oxygen and assessing apical heart rate, would be accomplished later, once the airway is cleared of meconium.

3. B. Risk factors associated with LGA newborns include maternal history of diabetes, excessive pregnancy weight gain, high maternal birthweight, previous LGA infant, maternal pregravid obesity, multiparity, and fetal exposure to high estrogen levels. Exposure to rubella in the first trimester is associated with congenital heart disease. Polyhydramnios and incompetent cervix are associated with preterm birth.

4. D. Factors contributing to risk for developing hyperbilirubinemia include a previous family history, ethnic background, birth trauma, and illness.

5. B. Characteristics of fetal alcohol spectrum disorder include a short nose; a flat, thin upper lip; small eyes with short slits for openings; a flattened midface and profile; and a low nasal bridge.

6. A. Small patches on both eyes protect them from the phototherapy lights. During phototherapy, the newborn should be unclothed to expose the maximum surface area of skin. The nurse needs to turn the newborn frequently, not just every 6 to 8 hours, to maximize exposure. Dehydration is possible with phototherapy because of increased insensible fluid loss. Additional fluids most likely will be necessary.

7. C. Congenital diaphragmatic hernia refers to an abnormality that allows the abdominal contents to rise up and protrude through the defect and occupy space in the thoracic cavity. Auscultation reveals absent or decreased breath sounds and audible bowel sounds on the side with the herniation. Common manifestations of congenital heart disease include tachycardia, tachypnea, poor or prolonged feeding, pallor, cold extremities, murmurs, and irritability. Manifestations of respiratory distress syndrome include rapid, irregular respirations, tachycardia, and central cyanosis. An omphalocele is a sac containing abdominal contents that protrudes through the external abdominal surface at the base of the umbilical cord.

8. C. The highest priority is for the newborn to receive adequate nutrition, which requires adaptive techniques because of the craniofacial defect. An outcome in which parents demonstrate success with feeding is most important. Support from extended family members, a scheduled visit to the surgeon, and sibling attachment are important, but are not as high priorities.

9. B. The nurse should position the newborn prone and elevate the head at least 30 degrees to prevent gastric reflux into the lung. In addition, the nurse should give the newborn nothing by mouth and notify the paediatrician immediately. The nurse may pass a nasogastric tube if a test gavage feeding is prescribed. A gastrostomy tube would not be used.

10. C. Treatment for developmental dysplasia of the hip is typically lengthy. The parent's statement about

using the harness for 1 month indicates a need for more instruction. Parents often need extra time to remove and reapply the harness during bathing and dressing the newborn. Carrying the newborn astride the hip or holding her upright on the leg can be helpful for her caregivers. Commercial infant seats do not allow for hip abduction; therefore, special infant seats and car restraints are necessary.

CHAPTER 23

1. D. Although age of menopause varies among women, factors correlated with it include breastfeeding, alcohol consumption, family history of early menopause, smoking history, early onset of menarche, never becoming pregnant, and never using oral contraceptives.

2. B. The nurse needs to gather more information about the client's symptoms (hot flashes). The nurse can best obtain answers by using open-ended questions. Asking about the client's menstrual cycle is not directly related to her symptoms. Inquiring about the use of a vaginal lubricant presumes that the client is experiencing vaginal dryness or dyspareunia, which she has not described. Although soy products have been associated with decreased vasomotor symptoms, this question would be more appropriate once the nurse has gathered additional information.

3. B, C. Adequate calcium intake and regular weight-bearing activity may help prevent osteoporosis. A family history of osteoporosis and the decreased estrogen that accompanies the aging process are some of the factors that increase the likelihood of developing osteoporosis.

4. B. Dyspareunia is related to a decrease in or lack of vaginal lubrication. Using a water-based lubricant immediately before sexual activity and increasing sexual foreplay may help promote vaginal lubrication. Kegel exercises would help manage urinary incontinence. A bisphosphonate would be useful in preventing osteoporosis. Wearing cotton underwear and panty hose with a cotton crotch helps to reduce the risk of infection.

5. A. Estrogen replacement therapy is appropriate for women who have undergone a hysterectomy. HRT is absolutely contraindicated in women who have active or chronic severe hepatic disease, active or recent thromboembolic disease, and undiagnosed abnormal vaginal bleeding. HRT is potentially contraindicated in women with breast cancer, active or recent (within 5 years) endometrial cancer, history of thromboembolic disease, history of gallbladder disease, seizure disorders, and migraine headaches.

6. **C.** With menopause, loss of estrogen protection leads to increased LDL levels, exceeding those of men. In addition, women lose other cardiovascular benefits of estrogen. The average age of menopause is 51.4 years. Men, like women, experience hormonal changes with aging. Osteoporosis is a leading cause of impaired skeletal integrity and fractures after menopause.

7. **B.** A common adverse effect of alendronate (Fosamax) is heartburn. Fluid retention, breast tenderness, and mood alterations are common adverse effects associated with HRT.

8. **A.** Calcitonin (Miacalcin), available in injectable and intranasal forms, increases bone mass density and decreases backbone fractures. Raloxifene (Evista) is an oral selective estrogenic receptor modulator approved for prophylactic treatment of osteoporosis. Tamoxifen may be prescribed to prevent breast cancer recurrence. Atorvastatin is an antihyperlipemic agent.

9. **D.** The nurse should encourage clients to eat foods high in polyunsaturated and monounsaturated fats, while reducing intake of foods with saturated and trans fats. Antioxidants, such as vitamins C and E, may help prevent or reduce arterial LDLs. Aerobic exercise is important for cardiovascular health. Restricting intake to 1,000 cal/day is not appropriate. Although the client may need to decrease her caloric intake, it still needs to be balanced and individualized according to her specific needs and circumstances.

10. **C.** Assessing ovarian hormone levels is key to determining if the client is experiencing premature ovarian failure. Once the nurse has obtained these levels, he or she can plan further interventions. Referrals for counselling depend on the situation. Breastfeeding is not relevant.

CHAPTER 24

1. **C.** When communicating with older adults, nurses should use direct, open-ended questions to elicit information. Asking about shoulder pain allows the client to describe her feelings in her own words. Asking the client about her living situation and if she is having pain right now are direct questions that could be important; however, they would elicit only "yes" or "no" answers, limiting the client's responses. Although asking a general lead-in question about how the client is feeling would be appropriate, calling her "sweetie" would be patronizing and incorrect.

2. **B.** Instrumental ADLs further enhance the client's ability to live independently. They include such things as preparing meals, shopping for groceries, driving, doing housework, and handling finances. Ability to dress oneself is an example of a basic ADL. Participation in senior centre activities and volunteer work are examples of advanced ADL.

3. **(all of the above).** Eating foods high in calcium helps prevent decrease in bone mineral density and should begin in a woman's younger years. Although dietary supplementation with calcium and Vitamin D is controversial, Osteoporosis Canada states that anyone over the age of 50 is advised to take 1,200 mg of calcium daily, preferably from dietary sources, and from 800 to 2,000 IU of vitamin D supplement daily, depending on the risk for vitamin D deficiency. Indications for a Bone (DEXA) scan to determine low BMD include: age 65 years and over, a previous fragility fracture, prolonged use of corticosteroids, current smoking, high alcohol intake, low body weight or major weight loss, rheumatoid arthritis, or having had a parent with a hip fracture.

4. **A.** Crackles, the most common physical finding in older adults, are always abnormal because they indicate inadequate air exchange, which is a potential source of infection. Decreased arm swing with walking is a normal age-associated change. A decrease in systolic blood pressure of 20 mm Hg or more or in diastolic blood pressure of 10 mm Hg or more indicates orthostasis. Decreases in forced vital capacity of 25 to 30 mL per year are age-associated respiratory system changes resulting from atrophy of the intercostal muscles and decreased diaphragmatic strength.

5. **D.** Decreased serum albumin levels can lead to an increased amount of free active drug, which subsequently leads to more adverse drug reactions and toxic effects. Adipose tissue increases, not decreases; as a result, fat/lipid-soluble drugs have increased tissue and decreased plasma concentrations. The result is a longer duration of effect by the drug on the body. Drug absorption in the older adult is complete, but at a slower rate. Renal function decreases in older adults. Drugs excreted by the kidneys take longer to clear the body; thus, their half-lives are prolonged.

6. **A, B, and E.** Extrinsic factors are environmental hazards. Examples may include throw rugs; clutter; missing grab bars or rails in the bathroom, tub, or shower; exposed wires or cords; carpet holes or folds; poorly placed light switches; lack

of a raised toilet seat; and no use of slip-resistant materials or surfaces on a floor, tub, or shower. The client's recent hip surgery and complaints of forgetfulness would be considered intrinsic (internal) factors.

7. C. Donepezil (Aricept), rivastigmine (Exelon), and galantamine (Reminyl) are examples of cholinesterase inhibitors used to treat AD. Memantine (Ebixa) works on the glutamate neurotransmitter system. Vitamin E is used with cholinesterase inhibitors and memantine to help delay the progression of moderately severe cases of AD. Divalproex (Depakote), an anticonvulsant, has been shown to reduce impulsivity and agitation in clients with AD.

8. A. The most common side effect associated with sertraline (Zoloft), a selective serotonin reuptake inhibitor (SSRI), is sexual dysfunction.

9. A, C, D. Constipation is a common side effect of opioid analgesics. A stool softener may be prescribed when initiating narcotic therapy. Sedative effects of pain medication may increase the risk for falls and confusion. Pain medications may cause older adults to sleep through nocturnal urges to void. Change in body weight is not a common side effect.

10. B. Based on the scenario, the client's daughter is most likely taking care of both her husband and her mother. The mother requires assistance with basic ADLs. The husband probably needs help because of his history of cerebrovascular accident, weakness, and osteoarthritis. Thus, the daughter would be at risk for caregiver role strain.

Breathing Instructions for Labour and Childbirth

Cleansing Breathing. This breathing is like the "bread of a sandwich," done at the beginning and end of each contraction. The breathing "filler" varies with the strength of the contraction. At the beginning and end of each contraction, take in a long breath through the nose; exhale out the mouth. Inhalation should be as long as exhalation.

Slow-paced Breathing. This is exactly as the name describes—breathing done when the client is not having a contraction and is relaxed and calm. Slow-paced breathing helps relax the muscles, thus increasing uterine contraction and moving oxygen-rich blood to the uterus and fetus. After a cleansing breath, continue to breathe very slowly and deeply, directly into the uterus. The pace should be half as fast as normal breathing. Once the contraction ends, repeat the cleansing breath and visualize something relaxing.

Modified-paced Breathing. When slow-paced breathing no longer effectively allows the client to stay "on top" of the contraction, **modified-paced breathing** should begin. The pace is about twice as fast as normal breathing. It is similar to running a race. You start slow; as you gain momentum, you pick up speed. As speed increases, breathing rate increases and becomes shallower. After a cleansing breath, breathe with the contraction, increasing the rate with the contraction intensity. Breathing is focused mainly on the lungs, not the uterus, because you need to increase your breathing rate. To do so, you need to make the breaths shallower. Focus your breathing on expanding the lungs and therefore increasing the oxygen available to the fetus. Finish with a cleansing breath.

Some people find difficulty with modified-paced breathing because they breathe so quickly (hyperventilate) that they become dizzy and may feel faint. If this happens, place your hand (or a bag) over your nose and mouth. Breathing will automatically slow because you will be inhaling carbon dioxide that you just exhaled. Another way to stop hyperventilating is to focus on your coach's face and to breathe in time with him or her.

Patterned-paced Breathing. This pattern requires more concentration than the previous "fillers." It is more effective against hyperventilation and will help decrease the chance of inadvertently pushing before your body is ready. Naturally, start with a cleansing breath; then follow this pattern: inhale, exhale, inhale, blow. Force the blow from pursed lips. Repeat until the contraction ends, and then complete with a cleansing breath. If you feel the urge to push, which may happen at the height of the contraction and indicates that the fetus has moved down in your pelvis, repeat the blowing without inhaling or exhaling. Once the urge to push has passed, restart the original pattern: inhale, exhale, inhale, blow. Complete with a cleansing breath.

Remember that just because the fetus is low in the pelvis, it does not mean that the cervix is open enough to facilitate birth. Do not to push until it has been determined via manual vaginal examination that the cervix is dilated enough to allow the fetus to pass through.

Page numbers in italics denote figures; page numbers followed by *t* indicate tables.